D1278500

The Cytokine Handbook
Second Edition

For Robyn, Andrew, Natalie and Emma

The Cytokine Handbook
Second Edition

edited by
Angus W. Thomson

Departments of Surgery and
Molecular Genetics and Biochemistry,
School of Medicine,
University of Pittsburgh,
USA

Academic Press
Harcourt Brace & Company, Publishers
London   San Diego   New York
Boston   Sydney   Tokyo   Toronto

ACADEMIC PRESS LIMITED
24–28 Oval Road
LONDON NW1 7DX

U.S. Edition Published by
ACADEMIC PRESS INC.
San Diego, CA 92101

This book is printed on acid free paper

A catalogue record for this book is available from the British Library

ISBN 0-12-689661-5

Typeset by Paston Press Ltd, Loddon, Norfolk, England
Printed in Great Britain by St Edmundsbury Press Ltd, Bury St Edmunds, Suffolk

Contents

Preface to the First Edition xiii
Preface to the Second Edition xv

Foreword xvii
Joost J. Oppenheim

CHAPTER 1 **Immunology of Cytokines: 1
An Introduction**
Jan Vilček and Junming Le

CHAPTER 2 **Molecular Genetics of 21
Cytokines**
Gordon W. Duff

CHAPTER 3 **Interleukin-1 31**
Charles A. Dinarello

CHAPTER 4 **Interleukin-2 and the 57
Interleukin-2 receptor**
Mark A. Goldsmith and Warner C. Greene

CHAPTER 5 **Interleukin-3 81**
John W. Schrader

CHAPTER 6 **Interleukin-4 99**
Jacques Banchereau and Mary Ellen Rybak

CHAPTER 7 **Interleukin-5 127**
Colin J. Sanderson

CHAPTER 8 **Interleukin-6 145**
Toshio Hirano

CHAPTER 9 **Interleukin-7 169**
Howard Edington and
Michael T. Lotze

CHAPTER 10 **Interleukin-8 and Related 186
Chemotactic Cytokines**
Jo Van Damme

CHAPTER 11 **Interleukin-9 209**
Jean-Christophe Renauld and
Jacques Van Snick

CHAPTER 12   **Interleukin-10 223**
                              Tim R. Mosmann

CHAPTER 13   **Interleukin-12 239**
                   Herbert H. Zeh III, Hideaki Tahara and
                                Michael T. Lotze

CHAPTER 14   **Interleukins 13, 14 and 15 257**
                   Angus W. Thomson and Michael T. Lotze

CHAPTER 15   **Interferons 265**
                             Edward De Maeyer and
                        Jacqueline De Maeyer-Guignard

CHAPTER 16   **Tumour Necrosis Factor-Alpha 289**
                                Kevin J. Tracey

CHAPTER 17   **Tumour Necrosis Factor-Beta 305**
                           Lymphotoxin-Alpha
                               Nancy H. Ruddle

CHAPTER 18   **Transforming Growth Factor-Beta 319**
                                Rik Derynck

CHAPTER 19   **Granulocyte-Macrophage Colony 343**
                          Stimulating Factor
                             John E.J. Rasko and
                             Nicholas M. Gough

CHAPTER 20   **Granulocyte Colony Stimulating 371**
                         Factor and its Receptor
                             Shigekazu Nagata

CHAPTER 21   **Colony Stimulating Factor 1 387**
                 (Macrophage Colony Stimulating Factor)
                             E. Richard Stanley

CHAPTER 22   **The Chemokines 419**
                               Thomas J. Schall

CHAPTER 23   **Prospects for Cytokines 461**
                       in Human Immunotherapy
                   Catherine Haworth, Ravindir Nath Maini and
                                Marc Feldmann

CHAPTER 24   **Future Prospects of Therapy with** **489**
                      Haemopoietic Growth Factors
                      Peter G. Bardy, Angel F. Lopez
                      M. Frances Shannon and Mathew A. Vadas

CHAPTER 25   **Biological and Immunological** **507**
                      Assays for Cytokines
                      Andrew J.H. Gearing, Judith E. Cartwright and
                      Meenu Wadhwa

CHAPTER 26   **Cytokines and their Receptors** **525**
                      as Potential Therapeutic Targets
                      R. Geoffrey P. Pugh-Humphreys and
                      Angus W. Thomson

CHAPTER 27   **The Phylogeny of Cytokines** **567**
                      Christopher J. Secombes

CHAPTER 28   **Future Cytokines: Interleukin 2001** **595**
                      Scott K. Durum

                      Index   603

Contributors

Jacques Banchereau Schering-Plough, Laboratory for Immunological Research, 69571 Dardilly cedex, France

Peter G. Bardy Vancouver General Hospital, Division of Hematology & Leukemia, 910 West 10th Av, Vancouver BC, Canada V5Z 4E3

Judith E. Cartwright British Biotechnology Ltd, Clinical Research & Development, 4–10 The Quadrant, Barton Lane, Abingdon, Oxon OX14 3YS, UK

Jo Van Damme Universiteit Leuven, Rega Institute, Minderbroedersstraat 10, B-3000 Leuven, Belgium

Rik Derynck UC San Francisco, Department of Growth & Development, San Francisco, CA 94143-0640, USA

Charles A. Dinarello Tufts University School of Medicine, New England Medical Center Hospitals Department of Medicine, 750 Washington Street, Box 68, Boston, MA 02111, USA

Gordon W. Duff University of Sheffield, Department of Medicine & Pharmacology, Section of Molecular Medicine, M Floor, Royal Hallamshire Hospital, Sheffield S10 2JF, UK

Scott K. Durum Laboratory of Molecular Immunoregulation, National Cancer Institute, Building 560, Room 31-45, Frederick, MD 21702-1201, USA

Howard Edington University of Pittsburgh School of Medicine, Department of Molecular Genetics & Biochemistry, 497 Scaife Hall, Pittsburgh, PA 15261, USA

Marc Feldmann The Charing Cross Sunley Research Centre, 1 Lurgan Avenue, Hammersmith, London W6 8LW, UK

Andrew J.H. Gearing British Biotechnology Ltd, Clinical Research & Development, 4–10 The Quadrant, Barton Lane, Abingdon, Oxon OX14 3YS, UK

Mark A. Goldsmith Gladstone Institute of Virology and Immunology, San Francisco General Hospital, PO 419100, San Francisco, CA 94141-9100, USA

Nick Gough The Walter & Eliza Hall Institute of Medical Research, PO Royal Melbourne Hospital, Parkwill, Victoria 3050, Australia

Warner C. Greene Departments of Medicine and Microbiology and Immunology, University of California, San Francisco, California 94141-900, USA

Catherine Haworth Leicester Royal Infirmary Child Health Unit, Leicester LE1 5WW, UK

Toshio Hirano Biomedical Research Center, Osaka University Medical School, Division of Molecular Oncology, 2-2 Yamada-oka, Suita, Osaka 565, Japan

Junming Le NYU Medical Center, Department of Miocrobiology, 550 First Avenue, New York, NY 10016, USA

Angel F. Lopez The Hanson Centre for Cancer Research, Institute of Medical & Veterinary Science, Box 14 Rundle Mall PO, Adelaide, SA 5000, Australia

Michael T. Lotze University of Pittsburgh School of Medicine, Department of Molecular Genetics & Biochemistry, 497 Scaife Hall, Pittsburgh, PA 15261, USA

Edward De Maeyer URA 1343 du CNRS, Institut Curie, Section de Biologie, Centre Universitaire, 91405 Orsay cedex, France

Jacqueline De Maeyer-Guignard URA 1343 du CNRS, Institut Curie, Section de Biologie, Centre Universitaire, 91405 Orsay cedex, France

Ravindir Nath Maini The Charing Cross Sunley Research Centre, 1 Lurgan Avenue, Hammersmith, London W6 8LW, UK

Tim R. Mosmann University of Alberta, Department of Immunology, Medical Sciences Bldg, Room 865, Edmonton, Alberta T6G 2H7, Canada

Shigekazu Nagata Osaka Bioscience Institute, Department of Molecular Biology, 6-2-4 Furuedai, Suita-shi, Osaka 565, Japan

Joost J. Oppenheim National Cancer Institute, Building 560, Room 21-89A, Frederick, MD 21702-1201, USA

R. Geoffrey P. Pugh-Humphreys University of Aberdeen, Department of Zoology, Tillydrone Avenue, Aberdeen AB9 2TN, UK

John E. Rasko The Walter & Eliza Hall Institute of Medical Research, PO Royal Melbourne Hospital, Parkwill, Victoria 3050, Australia

Jean-Christophe Renauld Ludwig Institute for Cancer Research, Avenue Hippocrate 74, UCL 7459, B-1200 Brussels, Belgium

Nancy H. Ruddle Yale University School of Medicine, Department of Epidemiology & Public Health, 60 College Street, PO Box 3333, New Haven, CT 06510, USA

Mary Ellen Rybak Schering-Plough Research Institute, Kenilworth, USA

Colin J. Sanderson Institute for Child Health Research, Perth, Australia

Thomas Schall Genentech Inc, Department of Immunology, 460 Point San Bruno Blvd, South San Francisco, CA 94080, USA

John W. Schrader University of British Columbia Department of Medicine, UBC Biomedical Research Center, 2222 Health Sciences Mall, Vancouver BC, Canada V6T 1Z4

Christopher J. Secombes University of Aberdeen, Department of Zoology, Tillydrone Avenue, Aberdeen AB9 2TN, UK

M. Frances Shannon The Hanson Institute for Cancer Research, Institute of Medical & Veterinary Science, Box 14 Rundle Mall PO, Adelaide, SA 5000, Australia

Jacques Van Snick Ludwig Institute for Cancer Research, Avenue Hippocrate 74, UCL 7459, B-1200 Brussels, Belgium

E. Richard Stanley Albert Einstein College of Medicine, Department of Developmental Biology & Cancer, Jack & Pearl Resnick Campus, 1300 Morris Park Avenue, Bronx, NY 10461, USA

Hideakei Tahara University of Pittsburgh School of Medicine, Department of Molecular Genetics & Biochemistry, 497 Scaife Hall, Pittsburgh, PA 15261, USA

Angus W. Thomson Departments of Surgery and Molecular Genetics & Biochemistry, University of Pittsburgh, Pittsburgh, PA, USA

Kevin J. Tracey North Shore University Hospital, Cornell University Medical College, Department of Surgery/Division of Neurosurgery, 300 Community Drive, Manhasset, NY 11030, USA

Mathew A. Vadas The Hanson Institute for Cancer Research, Institute of Medical & Veterinary Science, Box 14 Rundle Mall PO, Adelaide, SA 5000, Australia

Jan Vilček NYU Medical Center, Department of Miocrobiology, 550 First Avenue, New York, NY 10016, USA

Meenu Wadhwa NIBSC, Blanche Lane, South Mimms, Hertfordshire, UK

Herbert H. Zeh III University of Pittsburgh School of Medicine, Department of Molecular Genetics & Biochemistry, 497 Scaife Hall, Pittsburgh, PA 15261, USA

Preface to the First Edition

Cytokines feature at the forefront of biomedical research. An understanding of their properties is now essential for the immunology student, researcher and teacher and for today's medical practitioner who needs to understand immunologic disease and immunological approaches to therapy. The pace with which this ever-expanding field has developed has been rapid enough to exceed the most optimistic expectations and to bewilder the most assiduous student. Cytokine research is expected to provide the key to pharmacological manipulation of the immune response and commands the attention of a massive and highly focussed biotechnology industry. The chapters in this book are a good representation of the areas to which molecular biology has been most successfully applied. Biotechnology companies provide most of the pure, well characterized cell growth regulatory and effector molecules used in academic and industrial laboratories or in clinical medicine as diagnostic tools or therapeutic agents.

Cytokines represent a sought-after symposium theme in immunology, molecular biology and molecular genetics. The cytokine literature ranges from the most basic to the applied. Unfortunately, technical advances, rapid expansion and diversification have prompted narrower specialization and reduced the ease of communication. The aim of this book is to inform and to provide detailed information and reference material on the many aspects of pure and applied cytokine science. These include the molecular characteristics of cytokines, their genes and receptors, the cellular sources and targets of cytokines, their biological activities and as best can presently be defined, their mechanisms of action. Confronted with such a vast amount of new information, up-to-date coverage is an almost unattainable goal. The scope of cytokine research could only be effectively covered in a multi-authored volume and it is indeed fortunate that each chapter is written by a leading authority(ies). Although many chapters focus on individual cytokines, it is also apparent that aspects such as cell sources, molecular structure, purification and bioassay have many features in common. A certain amount of duplication is therefore, inevitable. The cytokine network, cytokine interactions, the roles of cytokines in disease pathogenesis and the therapeutic applications of cytokine research are dealt with in detail. In attempting to provide comprehensive coverage, a chapter on phylogeny has been included. The last chapter was commissioned to provide both perspective and a somewhat sobering view of the future.

I am indebted to the many authors around the world who have so generously devoted their knowledge, energy and time to the creation of this book. I also wish to acknowledge the support of Dr Susan King, and her staff at Academic Press in London, whose skill and energy were essential in the genesis of *The Cytokine Handbook*.

Angus W. Thomson,
University of Pittsburgh

Preface to the Second Edition

In the Preface to the First Edition, it was stated that to produce a book that provided up-to-date coverage of all aspects of the cytokine field was an 'almost unattainable goal'. Since the First Edition went to press in the spring of 1991, advancement both in our knowledge and understanding of the cytokine network has been predictably rapid, fully justifying the publishers' faith in a Second Edition of the Cytokine Handbook within 3 years. The original chapters have been revised and updated, and, with few exceptions, this has been undertaken by the original authors. Synthesis of information in the context of the cytokine network has again been a key objective. Every effort has been made to maintain currency and it is in promptly fulfilling this goal that the contributing authors deserve great credit. 'New' cytokines have, of course, emerged and continue to 'appear'. Thus, this new edition features individual chapters on IL-9, IL-10 and IL-12, with a 'stop-press' overview of IL-13 and even newer molecules that are candidates for designation as interleukins IL-14 and IL-15.

What constitutes a new interleukin? The assignation of a new designation depends on several clearly defined criteria, recently established by a sub-committee of the nomenclature committee of the International Union of Immunological Societies (Paul *et al.*, 1992). The criteria laid down include molecular cloning and expression, a unique nucleotide and inferred amino acid sequence, and the availability of a neutralizing monoclonal antibody. Furthermore, the granting of a new interleukin designation requires that the candidate molecule be a natural product of cells of the immune system (defined loosely as lymphocytes, monocytes and other leukocytes). The new interleukin must also mediate a potentially important function in immune responses and exhibit an additional function(s) so that a simple, functional name might not be adequate. Finally, these characteristic features should have been described in a peer-reviewed publication.

This new edition incorporates separate chapters on G-CSF, M-CSF and GM-CSF, whereas in the first edition, only one chapter – on 'colony stimulating factors' – covered the properties of these molecules. A chapter is also now afforded to TGF-β, which exhibits both inhibitory and stimulatory effects on a variety of cell types and is a potent immunosuppressant. Another significant and substantial new chapter concerns 'chemokines'. IL-8 (the 'highest' interleukin designation afforded a separate chapter in the first edition) was the first member of the chemokine family to be identified. More recently, other low molecular weight chemotactic polypeptides have been discovered that play a key role in cell activation and chemotaxis during the inflammatory response. These include RANTES (*R*egulated upon *A*ctivation, *N*ormal *T* *E*xpressed and *S*ecreted!), macrophage chemotactic and activating factor (MCAF), macrophage inflammatory protein (MIP) -1α and MIP-1β. All share a conserved, four cysteine motif and can be further subclassified on the spacing of the conserved cysteine residues.

Evaluation of the clinical potential of cytokines is one of the most exciting challenges of contemporary medicine. In addition, and in contradistinction to cytokine or cytokine gene therapy, the emergence of a new class of therapeutic agents, comprising soluble cytokine receptors (e.g. soluble (s) IL-1R, sTNFR, sIFN-γR), receptor antagonists (e.g. IL-1ra) and counter-regulatory cytokines, represents one of the most important developments in the cytokine field in recent years. Successes in the sequencing, cloning and expression of cytokine receptors has facilitated production and evaluation of their therapeutic utility in several acute and chronic cytokine-mediated diseases. This exciting and challenging development is one of the themes covered under the several chapters devoted to therapeutic aspects of cytokine biology.

The last few years have seen the advent of new approaches to interrogating the roles of cytokines *in vivo*. Thus cytokine gene 'knockout' mice and mice transgenic for cytokine gene reporter constructs are likely to provide new knowledge about the *in vivo* role(s) of cytokines, especially in experimental autoimmune disorders, cancer or infectious diseases that may be difficult to mimic satisfactorily *in vivo*. The molecular genetics of cytokines (reviewed in chapter 2) is yet another new and exciting aspect of this key field of contemporary molecular biology and medicine that has provided the impetus for the second edition of *The Cytokine Handbook*. Those who acquire knowledge by reading this book, or who are stimulated by the implications of the recent developments described herein, owe thanks to the many experts around the world who have so generously given of their valuable time, energy and expertise. The cordial and enthusiastic support of these scientists and clinicians has been an impelling influence that would be difficult to overrate. I am indebted to my colleague Dr Mike Lotze for constructive suggestions, Ms Shelly Conkin for valuable secretarial help and to Dr. Tessa Picknett and her colleagues at Academic Press in London for their resolute support and guidance in ensuring that the notion of a second edition became a tangible reality.

Angus W. Thomson

REFERENCE

Paul, W.E., Kishimoto, T., Melchers, F., Metcalf, D,, Mosmann, T., Oppenheim, J., Ruddle, N. and Van Snick, J. (1992). *Clin. Exp. Immunol.* **88**, 367.

Foreword

Joost. J. Oppenheim

Laboratory of Molecular Immunoregulation
National Cancer Institute
Frederick, Maryland 21702-1201, USA

What Are Cytokines?

As so aptly discussed by Vilček and Le in the introductory chapter of *The Cytokine Handbook*, cytokines are regulatory peptides that can be produced by virtually every nucleated cell type in the body and they have pleiotropic regulatory effects on haematopoietic and many other cell types that participate in host defence and repair processes. Cytokines therefore include lymphocyte-derived factors known as 'lympho-kines', monocyte-derived factors called 'monokines', haematopoietic 'colony stimu-lating factors' and connective tissue 'growth factors'.

How Did Lymphokines Come to be Discovered?

The possibility that cell-derived factors mediate biological activities was first suggested by experiments of Rich and Lewis (1932). They observed that migration of neutrophils and macrophages was inhibited in cultures of tuberculin-sensitized tissues and that macrophages were sometimes killed if incubated with antigens. Waksman and Matoltsy (1958) observed that macrophages in monolayer cultures were actually stimulated rather than damaged by exposure to tuberculin antigens. George and Vaughan (1962) improved the technique of evaluating migration of mononuclear cells using capillary tubes. This approach was then used concurrently by David *et al.* (1964) and Bloom and Bennet (1965) to show that antigens could stimulate sensitized lymphocytes to produce macrophage migration inhibitory factors (MIF). At about the same time, supernatants of mixed leukocyte cultures were found by Kasakura and Lowenstein (1965) to be 'blastogenic' for lymphocytes in leukocyte cultures. This 'blastogenic factor' (BF) was subsequently called 'lymphocyte mitogenic factor' (LMF). This was followed by the discovery by Ruddle and Waksman (1968) of a cytotoxic lymphocyte-derived mediator called 'lymphotoxin'. Consequently, the various biological activities secreted by cul-tured antigen-stimulated lymphocytes provided *in vitro* models for the pathogenesis of *in vivo* delayed hypersensitivity reactions. For example, the recruitment of the mononuclear cell infiltrates to inflammatory sites were attributable to the activities of a lymphocyte-derived chemotactic factor (LCF) (Ward *et al.*, 1969). MIF and the macrophage aggregation factor (MAgF) (Lolekha *et al.*, 1970) presumably served to retain cells at inflammatory sites. The necrotic centres of some granulomas could be attributed to the cytodestructive activity of lymphotoxin (LT) (Kolb and Granger, 1968; Ruddle and Waksman, 1968), and the presence of lymphoblasts and frequent mitotic figures to lymphocyte-derived mitogenic factors (LMF) (Kasakura and Lowen-stein, 1965). Identification of macrophage activating factor (MAF) (Nathan *et al.*, 1971) and lymphocyte-derived immune interferon (IFN-γ) (Green *et al.*, 1969) served to explain the basis for acquired resistance to infectious organisms. These biochemically undefined, lymphocyte-derived activities were termed 'lymphokines' in 1969 by Dumonde *et al*. Discovery of the lymphokines revolutionized the conceptual basis of cell-mediated immunity and these biological activities were considered '*in vitro corre-lates*' of cell-mediated immunity.

What Led to the Recognition that Lymphokines were Cytokines?
Gery and coworkers in 1971–4 showed that the lymphocyte activating factor (LAF) was produced by adherent monocytes and macrophages (Gershon and Kondo, 1971; Gery *et al.*, 1971; Gershon *et al.*, 1974). This was the first demonstration of the existence of non-lymphocyte-derived 'monokines'. Based on this information and his own obser-vations that some replicating non-lymphoid cell lines, as well as virally infected non-lymphoid cells, could also produce lymphokine-like MIF and chemotactic factors, Stanley Cohen, in 1974, proposed that all these mediators including lymphokines should therefore be called 'cytokines' (Cohen *et al.*, 1974). This resulted in the conceptual transformation of lymphokines from subjects of interest to a minor subset of immunologists to cytokines that function as bidirectional intercellular signals between somatic and myeloid as well as lymphoid cells, with potential impact on a broad range of biological processes.

What Was the Origin of the Interleukin Terminology?
By 1978, the confusing plethora of eponyms in existence for monocyte- and lymphocyte-derived activities motivated investigators at the Second International Lymphokine Workshop held near Interlaken, Switzerland to propose more inclusive 'neutral' terms for these biological activities. The researchers recognized that the numerous monokine and lymphokine activities they were detecting with a variety of bioassays actually had numerous properties in common. This gave the erroneous impression that these cytokine activities, each with their own name, could all be attributable to one or two molecular entities. Dr Werner Paetkau proposed that LAF/BAF/MCF be renamed interleukin-1 (IL-1), while LMF/BF/TCGF should be called IL-2 (Mizel and Farrar, 1979). The interleukin terminology symbolized the broader roles of these cytokines, and with the progressive increase in the number of inter-leukins, now 15, has led to an explosive increase in the interest of investigators from a variety of disciplines in these molecules.

What Developments have Galvanized the Study of Cytokines?
The development of tissue culture techniques enabled immunologists in the 1960s to detect the presence of factors in tissue culture supernatants with effects on the mobility, proliferation, differentiation and functional capabilities of lymphocytes and other leukocytes. Cytokines are very potent and active at pg to ng concentrations. Thus, they are present at only trace levels. This makes it particularly difficult to biochemically isolate and identify these peptides. These factors, which were originally disparagingly termed 'lymphodrek', could be purified only with the development of improved chromatography and microsequencing techniques in the late 1970s. The fortuitous development of molecular biology and monoclonal antibody technologies accelerated the identification of cytokines in the 1980s and have made abundant quantities available

in recombinant form during the past decade. This has resulted in an information explosion that is reflected by *The Cytokine Handbook*.

Why do Cytokines Exist?

The evolutionary development of large multicellular organisms presumably required the development of intercellular messengers such as hormones and cytokines to permit marshalling of co-ordinated cellular responses. According to Dr Gerald Edelman the structural homology between adhesion proteins that mediate cell-contact-dependent interactions and cytokine ligands suggests that the soluble cytokines evolved from cell-associated signals (Grumet *et al.*, 1991).

How are Cytokines Different from Hormones?

Endocrine hormones, which are generally produced by specialized glands, are present in the circulation and serve to maintain homeostasis. In contrast, cytokines usually act over short distances as autocrine or paracrine intercellular signals in local tissues and (with the exception of macrophage-colony stimulating factor (M-CSF), stem cell factor, erythropoietin and transforming growth factor β (TGFβ), only occasionally spill over into the circulation and initiate systemic reactions. Except for the aforementioned four examples, cytokines are generally not produced constitutively, but are generated in emergencies to contend with challenges to the integrity of the host. Cytokines, like hormones, achieve these ends by mobilizing and activating a wide variety of target cells to grow and perform their functions. However, the functions of cytokines are distinct from those of hormones, since they serve to maintain the integrity of the host by mediating the differentiation between self- and non-self, through damage control and by promotion of reparative processes.

Why Should we be Interested in Cytokines?

Recombinant cytokines provide useful laboratory probes for studying the cell biology of immunity and inflammation. Cytokines are the major orchestrators of our host defence processes and, as such, are involved in response to exogenous and endogenous insults, repair and restoration of homeostasis. In addition, cytokines appear to play a major role in development and some of them may account for as yet unidentified embryonic inductive factors. The study of cytokines is also elucidating the mechanisms underlying pathophysiological processes. Cytokines mediate not only host responses to invading organisms, tumours, and trauma, but also maintain our capacity for daily survival in our germ-laden environment. Detection of cytokines in disease states may provide useful diagnostic tools. The therapeutic utility of administration of pharmacological doses of cytokines is being explored in a wide variety of infectious diseases and in immunocompromised patients with AIDS, autoimmune diseases and neoplasias.

Why a Cytokine Handbook?

Studies of cytokines has drawn scientists from a multiplicity of fields including immunologists, hematologists, molecular biologists, neurobiologists, cell biologists, biochemists, physiologists, and others. Consequently, the burgeoning field of cytokine research is unique and interdisciplinary. The chapters in this handbook cover the structure and functions of cytokines, their genes, receptors, mechanisms of signal transduction and clinical applications. This second edition of the *Cytokine Handbook* is necessary, at this relatively early date, to keep up with rapid developments in this dynamic discipline. All the chapters, and even this foreword, have been updated and a number of new chapters by internationally renowned experts have been added to cover Interleukins 9, 10, 12, 13–15, TGF-β, the haematopoietic colony stimulating factors for granulocytes and macrophages (GM-CSF, G-CSF and M-CSF) and the chemotactic cytokines or 'chemokines'. This Handbook provides us with the opportunity to keep up with the rapidly evolving studies of cytokines.

REFERENCES

Bloom, B.R. and Bennet, B. (1966). *Science* **153**, 80–82.

Cohen, S., Bigazzi, P.E. and Yoshida, T. (1974). *Cell. Immunol.* **12**, 150–159.

David, J.R., Al-Askari, S., Lawrence, H.S. and Thomas, L. (1964). *J. Immunol.* **93**, 264–273.

Dumonde, D.C., Wolstencroft, R.A., Panayi, G.S., Matthew, M., Morley, J. and Howson, W.T. (1969). *Nature* **224**, 38–42.

George, M. and Vaughan, J.H. (1962). *Proc. Soc. Exp. Biol. Med.* **111**, 514–521.

Gershon, R.K. and Kondo, K. (1971). *Immunology* **21**, 903–914.

Gershon, R.K., Gery, I. and Waksman, B.H. (1974). *J. Immunol.* **112**, 215–221.

Gery, I., Gershon, R.K. and Waksman, B.H. (1971). *J. Immunol.* **107**, 1778–1780.

Green, J.A., Cooperland, S.R. and Kibnick, S. (1969). *Science* **164**, 1415–1417.

Grumet, M., Mauro, V., Burgoon, M.P., Edelman G.M. and Cunningham, B.A. (1991). *J. Cell. Biol.* **113**, 1399–1412.

Kasakura, S. and Lowenstein, L. (1965) *Nature* **205**, 794–798.

Kolb, W.P. and Granger, G.A. (1968). *Proc. Natl. Acad. Sci. USA* **61**, 1250–1255.

Lolekha, S., Dray, S. and Gotoff, S.P. (1970). *J. Immunol.* **104**, 296–304.

Mizel, S.B. and Farrar, J.F. (1979). *Cel. Immunol.* **48**, 433–436.

Nathan, C.F., Karnovsky, M.L. and David, J.R. (1971). *J. Exp. Med.* **133**, 1356–1376.

Rich, A.R. and Lewis, M.R. (1932). *Bull. Johns Hopkins Hosp.* **50**, 115–131.

Ruddle, N.H. and Waksman, B.H. (1968). *J. Exp. Med.* **128**, 1267–1279.

Waksman, B.H. and Matoltsy, M. (1958). *J. Immunol.* **81**, 220–234.

Ward, P.A., Remold, H.G. and David, J.R. (1969). *Science* **163**, 1079–1081.

Chapter 1

Immunology of Cytokines: An Introduction

Jan Vilček and Junming Le

Department of Microbiology, New York University Medical Center, New York,
NY 10016, USA

GENERAL FEATURES OF CYTOKINES

Origins of Cytokine Research

The field of cytokine research as it exists today has evolved from four originally independent sources. The first and probably most significant source is immunology and, more specifically, the field of lymphokine research. The origins of lymphokine research can be traced to the mid-1960s when it was demonstrated that lymphocyte-derived secreted protein mediators regulate the growth and function of a variety of leukocytes. It soon became apparent that monocytes too are the source of important proteins (monokines) that can modulate leukocyte function.

The second source of cytokine research springs from the study of the interferons. Originally described in the 1950s as selective antiviral agents, interferons gradually became recognized as proteins exerting a broad range of actions on cell growth and differentiation, both within and without the immune system. As a result, the dividing line between lymphokines/monokines and the interferons began to dwindle and today it is clear that interferons are cytokines.

The third source of cytokine research is the field of haematopoietic growth factors, i.e. colony stimulating factors (CSFs). In addition to promoting the growth and differentiation of haematopoietic stem cells, colony stimulating factors have been shown to regulate some functions of fully differentiated haematopoietic cells, thus blurring the dividing line between these agents and lymphokines/monokines.

The fourth source of cytokine research springs from the study of growth factors acting on non-haematopoietic cells. One might be reluctant to count 'classical' growth factors, such as PDGF, EGF, FGF or NGF, among the cytokines. Nevertheless, it is clear that, in addition to promoting cell growth, many of these agents exert other effects, which might be referred to as 'cytokine-like' actions. Moreover, at least one of the offsprings of growth factor research, i.e. transforming growth factor-β (TGF-β), is now considered a true cytokine.

The Cytokine Handbook, 2nd ed.
ISBN 0–12–689661–5

A Brief Outline of the History of Cytokine Research

The beginnings of lymphokine research are usually traced to the demonstration that migration of normal macrophages is inhibited by material released from sensitized lymphocytes upon exposure to antigen (Bloom and Bennett, 1966; David, 1966). The putative factor responsible for this action was termed macrophage migration inhibitory factor (MIF). The description of MIF activity was followed by the discovery of lymphotoxin activity in supernatants of activated lymphocyte cultures (Ruddle and Waksman, 1968; Williams and Granger, 1968). Dumonde *et al.* (1969) coined the term 'lymphokine' to designate 'cell-free soluble factors (responsible for cell-mediated immunological reactions), which are generated during interaction of sensitized lymphocytes with specific antigen'.

Among the lymphokines a central role in the regulation of T-cell growth and function is played by interleukin-2 (IL-2). It has been known since the early 1970s that lymphocytes can produce one or more factor(s) mitogenic for other lymphocytes (reviewed by Oppenheim *et al.*, 1970). Morgan *et al.* (1976) reported that supernatants of mitogen-activated human mononuclear cells could support the continuous growth of human bone-marrow-derived T-cells. The responsible mitogenic factor is IL-2, then designated T-cell growth factor (TCGF) and also known under a variety of other names that are, by now, largely forgotten (Aarden *et al.*, 1979).

The first monocyte/macrophage-derived cytokine described was tumour necrosis factor (TNF), which was originally identified as a cytotoxic protein present in the serum of animals sensitized with Bacillus Calmette–Guerin and challenged with LPS (Carswell *et al.*, 1975). In addition to its direct cytotoxicity for some tumour cells *in vitro*, TNF was identified as the mediator of LPS-induced haemorrhagic necrosis of Meth A sarcoma in mice.

Among the first monocyte-derived cytokines described is also lymphocyte activation factor (LAF), now known as interleukin-1 (IL-1). LAF activity, defined as a mitogenic signal for thymocytes, was originally detected in supernatants of adherent cells isolated from human peripheral blood (Gery *et al.*, 1971). Other investigators described activities that are now known to be mediated by IL-1 under a variety of other names, e.g. mitogenic protein, leukocytic pyrogen, endogenous pyrogen, B-cell-activating factor, leukocyte endogenous mediator, etc. (reviewed by Oppenheim *et al.*, 1979; Aarden *et al.*, 1970).

While the early studies of lymphokines and monokines were largely the domain of immunologists who sought a better understanding of delayed-type hypersensitivity and other cell-mediated immune reactions, interferons were the brainchildren of virologists. Interferon was first described by Isaacs and Lindenmann (1957) as a factor produced by a variety of virus-infected cells capable of inducing cellular resistance to infection with homologous or heterologous viruses. That interferons would affect immune reactions was initially not even suspected. However, several years later, Wheelock (1965) described a functionally related virus-inhibitory protein (today known as IFN-γ) produced by mitogen-activated T lymphocytes. It is now known that T-cell- and NK-cell-derived IFN-γ is structurally completely distinct from the large family of IFN-α/β proteins, which are produced by a variety of cell types, including monocytes, NK cells and B cells in addition to sundry nonhaematopoietic cells (reviewed by De Maeyer and De Maeyer-Guignard, 1988; Vilček, 1990).

CSFs are proteins whose major function is to support the proliferation and differentiation of haematopoietic cells. Their name reflects the early observation that CSFs promote the formation of granulocyte or monocyte colonies in semisolid medium (Pluznik and Sachs, 1965; Bradley and Metcalf, 1966). Years of effort by many groups of investigators have led to the isolation and characterization of several distinct proteins, to be described in greater detail elsewhere in this volume (see chapters 19–21).

Many proteins that can stimulate the growth of nonhaematopoietic cells have been identified; best known among these are epidermal growth factor (EGF), platelet-derived growth factor (PDGF), fibroblast growth factors (FGF), to name just a few. Although these and other growth factors are generally not included among the cytokines, some cytokine-like actions of classical growth factors on immunocytes and other cells have been described. DeLarco and Todaro (1978) described a growth factor, originally termed sarcoma growth factor, whose most interesting property was that it promoted the growth of normal rat fibroblasts in soft agar. Since then, two families of 'transforming growth factors' have been identified—TGF-α and TGF-β; these are distinct peptides with very different spectrums of biological activity. TGF-α is closely related to EGF whereas the TGF-β protein family appears to play important roles not only in cell growth control and neoplasia but also in inflammation and immunoregulation. Among the important actions of TGF-β proteins are the recruitment and activation of mononuclear cells, promotion of wound healing, fibrosis and angiogenesis, and a potent immunosuppressive action on numerous functions of T lymphocytes (Roberts and Sporn, 1990). Based on what is known about the actions of TGF-β proteins today, these polypeptides undoubtedly qualify for inclusion among the cytokines.

Cytokine Nomenclature

Inasmuch as the cytokine field evolved from several separate sources, a unifying concept of what cytokines are has been slow to emerge. The term 'lymphokine', which originally denoted the product of sensitized lymphocytes exposed to specific antigen (Dumonde et al., 1969), has been often used less discriminately for secreted proteins from a variety of cell sources, affecting the growth or functions of many types of cells. To dispel the incorrect notion that such proteins could be produced by lymphocytes alone, Cohen et al. (1974) proposed the term 'cytokines'. After a long-standing reluctance, 'cytokine' is becoming the preferred designation for these proteins. A group of participants at the Second International Lymphokine Workshop held in 1979 proposed the term 'interleukin' in order to develop 'a system of nomenclature . . . based on (the proteins') ability to act as communication signals between different populations of leukocytes' (Aarden et al., 1979). As a first step, the group introduced the names 'IL-1' and 'IL-2' for two important cytokines, which until then had been described under a variety of different names. As of this writing, the interleukin series has reached 13 (Minty et al., 1993). Although the name 'interleukin' implies that these agents function as communication signals among leukocytes, Aarden et al. (1979) suggested that the term should not be reserved for factors that can act only on leukocytes. Indeed, a number of the proteins that have been labelled as interleukins not only are produced by a variety of nonhaematopoietic cells but also affect the functions of many diverse somatic cells (e.g. IL-1 or IL-6). Whereas many cytokines are now termed interleukins, others remain to be known by their older names (e.g. IFN-α/β, IFN-γ, TNF, lymphotoxin, TGF-β, leukocyte inhibitory factor (LIF), most CSFs and many others). Although these older names are easier to remember, they suggest only one (i.e. the earliest recognized) function of these pleiotropic agents.

In summary, the state of cytokine nomenclature is less than ideal. A look at the history helps to understand how the present situation has arisen, but this does not make it any easier, especially for outsiders, to remember the features and designations of individual cytokines. With new cytokines being rapidly characterized (and named), no relief is in sight.

Cytokines, Hormones and Growth Factors

Having outlined their history and nomenclature, it is appropriate to try to define what cytokines are. We propose the following general definition: 'Cytokines are regulatory proteins secreted by white blood cells and a variety of other cells in the body; the pleiotropic actions of cytokines include numerous effects on cells of the immune system and modulation of inflammatory responses'. Since no short definition can encompass all essential properties, cytokines are best defined by a set of characteristic features, as listed in Table 1.

In reviewing the characteristic features of cytokines outlined in Table 1, it is evident that many of these properties are shared by two other groups of protein mediators, namely growth factors and hormones. The relationship between cytokines and growth factors was mentioned earlier in this chapter. Although the division is rather tenuous, one difference is that the production of growth factors (e.g. PDGF, EGF or TGF-α) tends to be constitutive and not as tightly regulated as that of cytokines. Another difference is that, unlike cytokine actions, the major actions of growth factors are targeted at nonhaematopoietic cells.

It is also not easy to distinguish clearly between cytokines and classical polypeptide hormones (Table 2). One of the major distinguishing features is that classical hormones are produced by specialized cells, e.g. insulin is produced by β cells of the pancreas,

Table 1.   Characteristic features of cytokines.

Cytokines are simple polypeptides or glycoproteins with a molecular weight $\leq$30 kDa (some cytokines form higher molecular mass oligomers). Only one known cytokine, IL-12, is a heterodimer.

Constitutive production of cytokines is usually low or absent; production is regulated by various inducing stimuli at the level of transcription or translation.

Cytokine production is transient and the action radius is usually short (typical action is autocrine or paracrine, not endocrine).

Cytokines produce their actions by binding to specific high affinity cell surface receptors (K_d in the range of 10^{-9}–10^{-12} M).

Most cytokine actions can be attributed to an altered pattern of gene expression in the target cells. Phenotypically, cytokine actions lead to an increase (or decrease) in the rate of cell proliferation, change in cell differentiation state and/or a change in the expression of some differentiated functions.

Although the range of actions displayed by individual cytokines can be broad and diverse, at least some action(s) of each cytokine is (are) targeted at haematopoietic cells.

Table 2. Distinguishing features between polypeptide hormones and cytokines.

Hormones		Cytokines	
Characteristic Features	Exceptions	Characteristic Features	Exceptions
Secreted by one type of specialized cells		Made by more than one type of cells	IL-2, IL-3, IL-4, IL-5, IFN-γ, LT are made only by lymphoid cells
Each hormone is unique in its action		Structually dissimilar cytokines have an overlapping spectrum of actions ('redundancy')	
Restricted target cell specificity and a limited spectrum of actions	Insulin	Multiple target cells and multiple actions ('ambiguity')	
Act at a distant site (endocrine mode of action)		Usually have short action radius (autocrine or paracrine mode of action)	Many (e.g., TNF, IL-1 or IL-6 in septic shock)

growth hormone by the anterior pituitary and parathormone by the parathyroid. In contrast, cytokines tend to be produced by less specialized cells, and more often than not, several unrelated cell types can produce the same cytokine (e.g. IL-1 is produced by monocytes/macrophages, mesangial cells, NK cells, B cells, T cells, neutrophils, endothelial cells, smooth muscle cells, fibroblasts, astrocytes and microglial cells). However, there are exceptions (e.g. IL-2, IL-3, IL-4, IL-5, lymphotoxin and IFN-γ are produced only by lymphoid cells, especially T cells). Perhaps the most characteristic features of cytokines, those that distinguish them from hormones, are the redundancy and ambiguity of cytokine actions, i.e. the fact that structurally dissimilar cytokines (e.g. TNF-α/β and IL-1α/β) show remarkable similarities in their actions (Le and Vilček, 1987), and that individual cytokines tend to exert a multitude of actions on different cells and tissues.

Despite some differences, it is apparent that cytokines, growth factors and polypeptide hormones together form a large family of extracellular signalling molecules featuring fundamentally similar mechanisms of action. This conclusion is supported by the recent finding that receptors for several cytokines and hormones (i.e. IL-2, IL-3, IL-4, IL-5, IL-6, IL-7, GM-CSF, G-CSF, erythropoietin, prolactin and growth hormone) show several common structural features (Bazan, 1989; D'Andrea et al., 1989; Gearing et al., 1989; Taga and Kishimoto, 1992). A structural similarity has been described between the receptors for PDGF and macrophage CSF (M-CSF) (Roberts et al., 1988). In addition, similar molecular pathways transmit signals from the growth factor, polypeptide hormone or cytokine receptors to the nucleus. A common feature is that ligand binding to the respective receptors leads to the sequential activation of sets of cellular kinases and subsequent activation of nuclear transcription factors. Several components in the signal transduction pathways are shared by cytokines, growth factors and polypeptide hormones. Rapid progress is being made in the elucidation of signal transduction pathways responsible for cytokine actions (Taga and Kishimoto, 1992).

CYTOKINE NETWORKS

Synergistic and Antagonistic Interactions

Most of the recent studies of cytokine actions have been carried out with homogeneous cytokine preparations produced by recombinant DNA techniques. These studies have led to the assembly of an enormous body of information on the spectrum of actions displayed by individual cytokines. A very informative catalogue of the repertoire of actions exerted by the major cytokines was recently compiled by Burke *et al.* (1993); most of this information was derived from the analysis of recombinant cytokine actions in various *in vitro* systems.

Although this recently accumulated information is very useful, it may not provide a realistic picture of the functions of these cytokines in the intact organism. One reason is the previously mentioned ambiguity and redundancy in cytokine actions. Another reason is that actions of cytokines can be profoundly influenced by the milieu in which they act and especially by the presence or absence of other biologically active agents, such as other cytokines, as well as hormones, growth factors, prostaglandins, etc. Cytokine action is contextual (Sporn and Roberts, 1988). Under natural conditions a cell rarely, if ever, encounters only one cytokine at a time. Rather, a cell is likely to be exposed to a cocktail of several cytokines and other biologically active agents, with the resulting biological action reflecting various synergistic and antagonistic interactions of the agents present. A certain pattern of characteristic features of cytokine actions has emerged that might be referred to as 'molecular philosophy of cytokine actions' (Table 3).

To achieve a better understanding of the actions of cytokines under natural conditions, investigators have begun to analyse mixtures of two or more cytokines. Many examples of synergistic actions have been documented. While it is impossible to include in this chapter a comprehensive survey of the myriad of synergistic or antagonistic interactions that have been reported, some typical examples will be mentioned.

Synergistic interactions are more likely to occur between cytokines that exert related but not identical actions than between cytokines that are functionally closely related. This conclusion is supported by a comparison of the interactions of TNF-α/TNF-β with IL-1α/IL-1β and IFN-γ. As will be explained in other chapters in this volume, TNF-α and TNF-β (the latter is also known as lymphotoxin, LT) bind to the same receptors; IL-1α and IL-1β also share common receptors that are distinct from the TNF receptors. A third distinct receptor exists for IFN-γ (the IFN-γ receptor is distinct from the IFN-α/β receptor). Despite the fact that TNF and IL-1 bind to different receptors, they exert many similar actions both *in vitro* and in the intact organism (Le and Vilček, 1987; Neta *et al.*, 1992). However, relatively few examples of a synergistic action between TNF and IL-1 have been described (Neta *et al.*, 1992; Lee *et al.*, 1993). The reason for this infrequent synergy is likely to be that TNF and IL-1 often may act through similar intracellular signalling pathways. For example, both TNF and IL-1 are potent activators in the transcription factor NF-κB (Lowenthal *et al.*, 1989; Osborn *et al.*, 1989; Shirakawa *et al.*, 1989) and this action is responsible for the activation of expression of several genes by TNF or IL-1.

In contrast, a large number of publications describe synergistic actions of TNF and IFN-γ. For example, IFN-γ was found to potentiate the cytotoxic action of TNF on

Table 3. Molecular philosophy of cytokine actions.

Ambiguity	A cytokine tends to have multiple target cells and multiple actions
Redundancy	Different cytokines may have similar actions
Synergism/Antagonism	Exposure of cells to two or more cytokines at a time may lead to qualitatively different responses
Cytokine cascade	A cytokine may increase (or decrease) the production of another cytokine
Receptor transmodulation	A cytokine my increase (or decrease) the expression of receptors for another cytokine

tumour cells (Lee *et al.*, 1984; Fransen *et al.*, 1986). Other examples of synergistic actions of TNF and IFN-γ include enhancement of CSF-1 and granulocyte (G)-CSF production by monocytes or lymphocytes (Lu *et al.*, 1988), induction of differentiation of human myeloid cell lines (Trinchieri *et al.*, 1986), antiviral activity (Wong and Goeddel, 1986), and the induction of nitric oxide production in murine macrophages (Ding *et al.*, 1988). It is significant that while TNF and IFN-γ act on similar target cells, and they tend to partly overlap in their ability to activate genes in the target cells (Beresini *et al.*, 1988; Lee *et al.*, 1990), they are likely to exert their actions through intracellular pathways that are quite distinct. However, some intracellular signalling pathways appear to be shared by TNF and IFN-γ, such as their ability to induce transcription factor IRF-1, which is thought to be involved in the regulation of expression of IFN-β and of some IFN-induced genes (Fujita *et al.*, 1989; Reis *et al.*, 1992).

Not only can a mixture of two cytokines produce an action that represents more than the sum of the separate actions of the individual cytokines (classical definition of a synergistic effect), but a cytokine mixture can result in actions that are qualitatively different from those seen with the individual cytokines. For example, in the HT29 colon carcinoma cell line, TNF-α alone or IFN-γ alone, even at high concentrations, do not exert marked effects on cell viability. However, when the two cytokines are applied together a rapid and marked cytotoxic action ensues (Feinman *et al.*, 1987).

Although not as frequently documented, there are also many examples of antagonistic interactions among cytokines. Since, in many types of cells, IFNs tend to inhibit growth whereas some other cytokines stimulate growth, the presence of IFN (either IFN-α/β or IFN-γ) together with a growth-stimulating cytokine (or growth factor) will result in a mutually antagonistic relationship (De Maeyer and De Maeyer-Guignard, 1988). Other examples of an antagonistic interaction include the actions of IL-4 and IFN-γ on the synthesis of immunoglobulin subclasses in B cells (Snapper *et al.*, 1988), or the inhibitory action of IFN-α/β on IFN-γ-induced enhancement of class II HLA antigen expression (Ling *et al.*, 1985; Kamijo *et al.*, 1993b). Analysis of the synergistic or antagonistic interactions involving pairs of cytokines help us to appreciate the complexities of cytokine actions in the intact organism. Nevertheless, it seems that the experimental systems employed still greatly underestimate the variables influencing the actions of cytokines *in vivo*.

Stimulatory and Inhibitory Actions of Cytokines on Cytokine Production

Another characteristic feature of cytokines is their ability to stimulate or inhibit the production of other cytokines. As a result, many cytokine actions are indirect, i.e. they may cause an increase or decrease in the level of production of other cytokines, which then results in an altered biological response. Among the earliest discovered examples of such an indirect action was the demonstration that the mitogenic action of IL-1 in murine thymocytes involves the stimulation of IL-2 production, and that IL-2 is the actual effector molecule responsible for the stimulation of thymocyte proliferation (Smith *et al.*, 1980).

The stimulatory effect of IL-1 on IL-2 production and the role of this interaction in T-cell proliferation has become a paradigm for the actions of many other cytokines. In addition to IL-2, IL-1 was found to stimulate the production of IL-6 (Content *et al.*, 1985), GM-CSF (Zucali *et al.*, 1986), IL-8 (Matsushima *et al.*, 1988) and monocyte chemotactic and activating factor, MCAF (Larsen *et al.*, 1989) in various types of cells. All of these cytokines are also induced by TNF, in accord with the many other similarities seen between the actions of IL-1 and TNF (Le and Vilček, 1987; Neta *et al.*, 1992). In monocytes both TNF and IL-1 are also autostimulatory and, in addition, they stimulate each other's production (Neta *et al.*, 1992). Other known examples of stimulatory interactions involve the ability of IL-2 and IFN-γ to augment IL-1, TNF-α, IL-6 and TNF-β production (Svedersky *et al.*, 1985; Collart *et al.*, 1986; Kamijo *et al.*, 1993a), and the stimulation of IFN-γ production by IL-2 (Torres *et al.*, 1982). IL-12 (natural killer-cell stimulatory factor) induces IFN-γ production in T and NK cells and appears to be a major regulator of IFN-γ production in the intact organism (Trinchieri *et al.*, 1993).

Although not as numerous as the reports of stimulatory interactions, there is increasing evidence of inhibitory actions of cytokines on cytokine production. One example is the inhibitory action of IL-4 (Hart *et al.*, 1989) or IL-6 (Aderka *et al.*, 1989) on the production of TNF or IL-1 by monocytic cells. IL-10 is a cytokine whose major biological function appears to be inhibition of cytokine production by Th1 cells and by monocytes/macrophages (Fiorentino *et al.*, 1991). Many of the immunosuppressive and anti-inflammatory actions of TGF-β also appear to result from its ability to suppress cytokine production in T cells and mononuclear phagocytes (Roberts and Sporn, 1990). Finally, the recently identified cytokine IL-13 showed a strong inhibitory activity on inflammatory cytokine production (IL-6, IL-1β, TNF-α, IL-8) in LPS-stimulated monocytes (Minty *et al.*, 1993).

Analysis of the mechanisms of these stimulatory and inhibitory interactions is still in its infancy, but the preliminary impression is that both transcriptional and post-transcriptional events are involved. A case in point is the action of TGF-β on TNF and IL-1 production in monocytes (Chantry *et al.*, 1989a). TGF-β was found to increase transcription of IL-1α, IL-1β and TNF-α mRNAs. However, the actual release of the corresponding proteins tended to be inhibited, apparently owing to an inhibition of translation. IFN-β was found to inhibit TNF-stimulated IL-8 synthesis in some cells at the transcriptional level, but an inhibition of IL-8 production by IFN at the post-transcriptional level was also reported (Oliveira *et al.*, 1992; Aman *et al.*, 1993).

Transmodulation of Cytokine Receptors

Another mechanism important in the network of cytokine actions is the modulation of the level of cytokine receptor expression. One of the most thoroughly studied models involves induction of the high-affinity IL-2 receptor on T cells by IL-1 (Kaye *et al.*, 1984; Lowenthal *et al.*, 1986). Appearance of high-affinity receptors is the consequence of the induced expression of the IL-2 receptor complex, mainly due to the regulation of its p55 or α chain (Smith, 1988; Hatakeyama *et al.*, 1989). Other cytokines, including TNF and IL-6 (Noma *et al.*, 1987; Lowenthal *et al.*, 1989), can also affect IL-2 receptor expression, though perhaps not as efficiently as IL-1.

Other examples of the modulation of cytokine receptors include the stimulatory action of the interferons, especially IFN-γ, on the expression of TNF receptors on many different cell lines (Aggarwal *et al.*, 1985). This action might contribute to the widely documented synergism between IFN-γ and TNF. Conversely, TNF was also shown to upregulate IFN-γ binding (Raitano and Korc, 1990). TNF, in turn, was shown to increase the expression of EGF receptors in human fibroblasts (Palombella *et al.*, 1987); this latter action correlates with the mitogenic effect of TNF in this type of cell. However, in some other cells TNF was found to produce a transient downregulation of EGF receptors (Bird and Saklatvala, 1989).

In some instances receptor transmodulation by cytokines results in a reduced level of receptor expression. One example is the downregulation of TNF receptors by IL-1, probably mediated by the activation of protein kinase C (Holtman and Wallach, 1987).

How Essential are Cytokines?

The important roles of cytokines in the regulation of immune and inflammatory responses are now clearly recognized. Availability of purified, potent cytokine preparations and the use of transgenic mouse models has helped to define the major actions of cytokines and their *in vivo* functions. However, the extensive redundancy and ambiguity in cytokine actions makes it difficult to predict how unique and essential individual cytokine actions are in the intact organism. The quest to learn how cytokines function in their natural environment of the intact host has been greatly aided by the development of the technique of targeted gene disruption, which utilizes the introduction of suitable constructs into the genome of murine embryonic stem cells. Genetically altered embryonic stem cells are then introduced into the blastocyst *in utero*, leading eventually to the transmission of the disrupted gene through the germ line.

Gene targeting has been used for the disruption of several cytokine and cytokine-receptor genes in the mouse (Table 4). With the exception of LIF, the gene 'knockout' did not interfere with embryo development, indicating that these cytokines or cytokine receptors alone were not essential during embryogenesis. With the exception of the TGF-β1 and IL-10 knockout, the mice also developed normally after birth and they showed no overt abnormalities for several weeks or longer, following birth. Experimental analysis of the mice with deletions of the IL-2, IL-4, IFN-γ or IFN-γ receptor genes showed various types of changes in their immune responses (Table 4). In general, these alterations were relatively subtle and they became apparent only under specific

Table 4. Analysis of cytokine and cytokine receptor functions by gene-knockout studies in mice.

Targeted Gene	Major Changes in Phenotype	References
IL-2	Reduced polyclonal T cell responses; altered Ig subsets; increased mortality; ulcerative colitis	Schorle *et al.* (1991) Sadlack *et al.* (1993)
IL-4	Reduced T$_{H2}$ cytokine production; reduced helminth-induced eosinophilia and IgE production; reduced IgG1 levels	Kühn *et al.* (1991) Kopf *el al.* (1993)
IL-10	Retardation of growth; anaemia; enterocolitis	Kühn *et al.* (1993)
TGF-β1	Death at 3–4 weeks of age owing to massive inflammatory response	Shull *et al.* (1992) Kulkarni *et al.* (1993)
LIF	Failure of blastocyst implantation in the uterus	Stewart *et al.* (1992)
CNTF	Atrophy and loss of motor neurons	Masu *et al.* (1993)
IFN-γ	Increased sensitivity to mycobacterial infection; increased T-cell proliferation *in vitro*	Dalton *el al.* (1993)
IFN-γ receptor	Increased sensitivity to infection with Listeria, vaccinia virus, Leishmania and mycobacteria; decreased production of TFN, IL-1 and IL-6; decreased sensitivity to LPS toxicity	Huang *et al.* (1993) Kamijo *et al.* (1993a)
IFN-α/β receptor	Increased sensitivity to virus infections	M. Aguet, personal communication
p55 TNF receptor	Increased sensitivity to infection with Listeria; decreased sensitivity to LPS toxicity	Pfeffer *et al.* (1993) Rothe *et al.* (1993)
p75 TNF receptor	Decreased sensitivity to LPS toxicity	D.V. Goeddel, personal communication

experimental conditions. Disruption of the genes for IFN-γ, the IFN-γ receptor or the p55 TNF receptor resulted in a loss of the ability of these mice to survive experimental infections with some normally nonlethal intracellular infectious agents, including *Listeria monocytogenes*, *Mycobacterium bovis* or vaccinia virus. The most dramatic changes were seen in the TGF-β1 knockout mice which developed massive inflammatory lesions in multiple organs and died 3–4 weeks after birth. The latter result clearly establishes that the anti-inflammatory action of endogenous TGF-β1 (likely due to the ability of TGF-β1 to suppress inflammatory cytokine production) is essential for animal survival. Many more cytokine- and cytokine-receptor-gene knockout studies are now in progress, and their results are likely to be reported in the near future. The breeding of mice with deletions of multiple cytokine or cytokine receptor genes is also being attempted.

Are gene knockout studies providing realistic information about cytokine functions in the intact organism? There is no doubt that the technique represents a very powerful tool for functional analysis and a wealth of information about the roles of cytokines will emerge from these studies. However, complete deletion of gene function may promote the development of compensatory mechanisms that are not normally operative if the deleted gene is functional. Hence, it is possible that gene knockout studies may underestimate the value of specific cytokines or cytokine receptors in a fully functional organism.

SOME MAJOR IMMUNOREGULATORY ACTIONS OF CYTOKINES

Regulation of T-Cell Growth and Differentiation

Although numerous cytokines have been described to function as T-cell growth factors, IL-2 is widely considered to play a pivotal role under most circumstances in T-cell proliferation. The IL-2 receptor exists in low-, intermediate-, and high-affinity forms, comprising various combinations of at least three distinct subunits: the α (p55), β (p75) and γ (p64) chains (Sharon et al., 1986; Bich-Thuy et al., 1987; Waldmann, 1989; Takeshita et al., 1992; Voss et al., 1993). While all three subunits directly interact with IL-2, the p75 β and p64 γ chains may be required for IL-2 internalization and signal transduction (Asao et al., 1990, 1993; Arima et al., 1992).

Both IL-2 and IL-4 were found to trigger human intrathymic pre-T cells ($CD7^+2^+1^-3^-4^-8^-$) to proliferate in the absence of mitogen. The IL-4-induced proliferation is independent of the IL-2 pathway, as it cannot be inhibited by anti-IL-2R antibody (Barcena et al., 1990). Similarly, IL-7 stimulates the proliferation of $CD4^-8^-$ thymocytes in the absence of mitogen, and this activity is not affacted by antibodies to IL-2 or IL-4 (Henney, 1989). These results thus indicate that both IL-4 and IL-7 can act as authentic T-cell growth factors independent of IL-2. In contrast to IL-2, IL-4 and IL-7, the cytokines IL-1, IL-6 or TNF alone fail to induce resting thymocytes to proliferate (Le et al., 1988; Ranges et al., 1988). However, IL-1, IL-6 and TNF all enhance IL-2-induced thymocyte proliferation, whereas only IL-6 augments IL-4-induced proliferation (Suda et al., 1990).

More potent growth stimulation by these cytokines has been observed in preactivated T cells. Thus, IL-4 stimulates the proliferation of preactivated thymocytes and T cells of both the $CD4^+$ and $CD8^+$ phenotypes in the presence of antibodies to IL-2 or to the IL-2R (Spits et al., 1987; Brown et al., 1988). Moreover, IL-2 and IL-4 are produced by different subsets of murine $CD4^+$ cells (T_{H1} and T_{H2}, respectively). The proliferation of T-cell clones producing IL-4, but not IL-2, can be totally dependent on the synthesis of autocrine IL-4 (Cherwinski et al., 1987). Highly purified mature T cells were shown to proliferate in response to IL-7 in the presence or absence of mitogens, and the target cells include both the $CD4^+$ and $CD8^+$ subpopulations of T cells (Welch et al., 1989; Armitage et al., 1990; Londei et al., 1990). In mitogen-activated purified murine T cells, significant proliferation of $CD4^+$ cells was obtained when both IL-6 and IL-1 were present, while IL-6 alone induced $CD8^+$ cell proliferation (Le et al., 1989; Vink et al., 1990). IL-12 also shows a direct mitogenic effect on T cells and NK cells preactivated by various stimuli (Perussia et al., 1992).

Involvement of complex mechanisms in cytokine-mediated stimulation of activated T-cell proliferation has been proposed. Thus, IL-1, IL-4, IL-6, IL-7 and TNF can induce an enhanced expression of the IL-2R on T cells (Schwab et al., 1985; Scheurich et al., 1987; Le et al., 1988; Mitchell et al., 1989; Armitage et al., 1990), which may partly account for the synergism of these cytokines with IL-2 in T-cell proliferation. Both IL-6 and IL-7 stimulate the clonal expansion of activated T cells via IL-2-dependent and IL-2-independent pathways (Le et al., 1988; Lotz et al., 1988; Chazen et al., 1989; Morrissey et al., 1989), yet anti-IL-6 antibody shows no effect on IL-7-induced T-cell activation (Morrissey et al., 1989). Conversely, although IL-1-induced thymocyte proliferation appears to be related to the production of endogenous IL-6 and IL-7 (a potent inducer of IL-6) (Helle *et al.*, 1989; Herbelin *et al.*, 1992), other mechanisms are likely to operate (Suda *et al.*, 1990). IL-9 enhances the proliferation of T cells following prolonged activation (Houssiau *et al.*, 1993). In contrast, TGF-β appears to serve as a major negative regulator of T-cell growth. TGF-β was shown to inhibit IL-2-dependent T-cell proliferation, most likely owing to a suppression of the IL-2-induced enhanced expression of the IL-2R and transferrin receptors (Kehrl *et al.*, 1986). IL-1- and IL-7-stimulated thymocyte proliferation is also inhibited by TGF-β (Chantry *et al.*, 1989b). By an indirect action on accessory cells, IL-10 shows inhibitory effects both on cytokine production and antigen-specific proliferation of T_{H1} cells (Fiorentino *et al.*, 1989; de Waal Malefyt *et al.*, 1991).

Cytokines also play important roles in T-cell differentiation. Both IL-2 and IL-4 can promote differentiation of pre-T cells into phenotypically mature T cells. It was found that the majority of T cells induced to mature by IL-4 preferentially express the TCR-γ/δ, whereas T cells generated in response to IL-2 mostly express the TCR-α/β (Barcena *et al.*, 1990). Generation of cytolytic T lymphocytes (CTLs) from precursor cells requires both antigen and cytokine signals. IL-6 was shown to induce differentiation of $CD8^+$ CTL from murine thymocytes in the presence of IL-2, and their cytotoxicity can be enhanced by IFN-γ (Takai *et al.*, 1988). Limiting dilution analysis showed that in mixed lymphocyte cultures, IL-2, IL-4 and IL-7 induce CTL generation with essentially identical frequencies, although IL-2-induced CTL clones showed greater average lytic activity than either IL-4 or IL-7. Approximately half of the CTL precursors that responded to IL-7 proliferated and differentiated in an IL-2-independent manner, and the other half did so via an IL-2-dependent pathway (Alderson *et al.*, 1990). TGF-β was found to inhibit CTL generation in a dose-dependent fashion. TNF plays a role in CTL differentiation, as addition of antibodies to TNF significantly inhibited CTL generation, and addition of TNF can also reverse TGF-β-induced inhibition (Ranges *et al.*, 1987). Cytokines may also play important roles in the differentiation of T helper cells. Recent evidence has shown that IL-12 can preferentially induce antigen-stimulated differentiation of T_{H1} cells, while neutralization of endogenous IL-12 promotes T_{H2} cell differentiation (Manetti *et al.*, 1993). Because the production of IL-12 is enhanced by IFN-γ (a T_{H1} cell product) and inhibited by IL-10 and IL-4 (T_{H2} cell products), relative expression levels of these cytokines may critically influence the direction of T_{H1}-type versus T_{H2}-type immune responses (Trinchieri *et al.*, 1993).

Regulation of B-Cell Growth and Differentiation

The earliest identified cells committed to the B-cell lineage are pro-B cells, which differentiate into pre-B cells with rearranged μ-chain genes. After rearrangement of light-chain genes, pre-B cells differentiate into mature B cells expressing surface Ig. IL-7 stimulates the proliferation of both pro-B and pre-B cells, and shows no ability to induce differentiation of these cell compartments (Namen *et al.*, 1988; Takeda *et al.*, 1989). Mature B cells fail to respond to IL-7 even in the presence of anti-Ig (Henney, 1989). In contrast, a wide range of cytokines, including IL-1, IL-2, IL-4, IL-5, IL-10, IL-13, IFN-α, IFN-β, IFN-γ and LT, have been described to stimulate the growth of mature B cells activated by *Staphylococcus aureus*, anti-Ig, or other stimuli (Howard *et al.*, 1982; Lantz *et al.*, 1985; Kehrl *et al.*, 1987; Morikawa *et al.*, 1987; Freedman *et al.*, 1988; Takatsu *et al.*, 1988; Rousset *et al.*, 1992; Minty *et al.*, 1993).

Table 5. Regulation of Ig isotype expression by cytokines in LPS-stimulated murine B cells.[a]

	IL-4	IFN-γ	IL-5	TGF-β
IgG1	↑	↓	↑	↓
IgG2a	↓	↑		
IgG2b	↓	↓		↑
IgG3	↓	↓		
IgM			↑	↓
IgA			↑	↑
IgE	↑	↓		

[a] ↑, Stimulation; ↓, inhibition; blank space indicates either no effect or lack of information.

IL-4 plays important roles in B-cell activation and proliferation. It induces striking increases in the expression of MHC class II antigens and CD23 molecules (IgE receptor) of resting B cells (Noelle *et al.*, 1984; Defrance *et al.*, 1987), and prepares these cells to enter the S phase in response to anti-IgM or other B-cell mitogens (Rabin *et al.*, 1985). Interactions of IL-4 with other cytokines in B-cell activation have been recognized. Thus, IFN-γ was shown to inhibit the growth-stimulating and class II antigen-enhancing effects of IL-4 on resting B cells (Mond *et al.*, 1986; Rabin *et al.*, 1986). IL-1 appears to synergize with IL-4 in B-cell clonal expansion, suggesting a growth-promoting effect of IL-1 on activated B cells (Peschel *et al.*, 1987). In contrast, IL-4 antagonizes the B-cell growth-promoting effect of IL-2 (Defrance *et al.*, 1988).

During B-cell differentiation, Ig isotype production is regulated by various cytokines (Table 5). LPS-stimulated mouse spleen B cells synthesize predominantly IgM, IgG2b, and IgG3. Addition of IL-4 enhances IgG1 and IgE secretion, and reduces IgG2b and IgG3 synthesis (Vitetta *et al.*, 1985; Coffman *et al.*, 1986). IL-5 stimulates mainly IgM and IgA synthesis (Takatsu *et al.*, 1988). IFN-γ preferentially enhances IgG2a production (Snapper and Paul, 1987a), whereas TGF-β selectively augments IgA and IgG2b synthesis (Lebman *et al.*, 1990; McIntyre *et al.*, 1993). In human B cells, IL-13 induces IgG4 and IgE synthesis independent of IL-4, although IL-13 and IL-4 may share common signalling pathways (Punnonen *et al.*, 1993). It was found that IL-5 synergizes with IL-4 to promote IgE secretion (Coffman *et al.*, 1987), IL-2 or IL-5 enhances TGF-β-induced IgA production by LPS-stimulated B cells (Sonoda *et al.*, 1989; Lebman *et al.*, 1990), and IL-10 cooperates with TGF-β in inducing IgA secretion by anti-CD40-activated B cells (Defrance *et al.*, 1992). Interestingly, IL-4-induced enhanced IgG1 and IgE synthesis is inhibited by IFN-γ, whereas IL-4 suppresses the stimulation of IgG2a expression by IFN-γ (Snapper and Paul, 1987a).

The selected Ig isotype production could result from either cytokine-directed Ig heavy-chain switching, or a selection of precommitted B cells. The effect of IL-4 appears to involve Ig class switching, as IL-4 enhances IgG1 secretion in surface IgG$^-$/IgM$^+$ B cells (Snapper and Paul, 1987b). Similar observations suggest that IFN-γ and TGF-β also act as isotype-specific switch factors for IgG2a and IgA, respectively (Snapper and Paul, 1987a; Sonoda *et al.*, 1989). In contrast, available evidence suggests that IL-5 functions by inducing differentiation of precommitted B cells, as IL-5 fails to induce IgA synthesis in surface IgA$^-$/IgM$^+$ B cells (Harriman *et al.*, 1988).

Somewhat differently, isotype (IgE and IgA) regulation by IL-4 and IL-5 in human B cells generally requires the presence of specific B-cell activating agents, such as T cells or PMA (Callard and Turner, 1990). Different activation signals may largely determine the outcome of isotype switching. For example, IL-4 induced IgE secretion in enriched B-cell preparations containing T cells. In purified B cells preactivated with *S. aureus*, however, IL-4 failed to stimulate IgE secretion, but induced IgM and IgG production (Yokota *et al.*, 1988).

Another cytokine important in the differentiation of activated B cells into Ig-secreting cells is IL-6, which shows minimal effects on B-cell proliferation (Le and Vilček, 1989). IL-6 induces enhanced Ig secretion by EBV-transformed B cells and PWN-stimulated B cells, and it appears to act at the late-stage of B-cell maturation (Muraguchi *et al.*, 1988). Using purified human B cells, it was shown that IL-6 lacks the ability to induce Ig secretion by *S. aureus*-stimulated B cells, but markedly enhances the induction of all isotypes of Ig by *S. aureus* and IL-2, suggesting that IL-2 may function as a costimulator in IL-6-induced B-cell differentiation (Splawski *et al.*, 1990).

Macrophage Activation

Macrophages can be produced from bone marrow precursor cells by stimulation with M-CSF, GM-CSF, G-CSF or IL-3, among which M-CSF is the only CSF specific for macrophages. In murine systems, M-CSF is a potent growth factor; bone marrow precursor cells and tissue macrophages strongly proliferate in response to M-CSF, and form colonies in growth medium (Meltzer *et al.*, 1990). For human monocyte cultures, M-CSF functions as a survival and differentiation factor, instead of a growth factor (Becker *et al.*, 1987).

Macrophages are able to display tumoricidal and antimicrobial activities mediated, at least partly, by TNF and/or reactive nitrogen intermediates. While IFN-γ is the best characterized, and probably the most potent monocyte/macrophage-activating cytokine (Le *et al.*, 1983; Nathan *et al.*, 1983), other cytokines are able to exhibit stimulation of macrophage cytotoxicity or microbicidal activity. Thus, IL-4 can activate murine peritoneal macrophages to show increased tumoricidal activity (Crawford *et al.*, 1987). In some situations IL-7 and GM-CSF activate monocytes to kill tumour target cells in the apparent absence of LPS (Grabstein *et al.*, 1986; Alderson *et al.*, 1991). GM-CSF also stimulates macrophages to inhibit *Trypanosoma cruzi* and release hydrogen peroxide (Reed *et al.*, 1987). Other cytokines that have been reported to induce enhanced tumoricidal activity of monocytes/macrophages include IL-1, IL-2, IFN-α and TNF (Philip and Epstein, 1986; Philip, 1988). Pretreatment of monocytes with M-CSF significantly increases IFN-γ-induced tumoricidal activity, due apparently to the increased TNF production stimulated by M-CSF (Sampson-Johannes and Carlino, 1988).

The expression of class II histocompatibility antigens on antigen-presenting macrophages is crucial in the initiation of an immune response. Many cytokines are known to regulate class II antigen expression. IFN-γ was the first cytokine described to increase the expression of class II antigens (Sztein *et al.*, 1984). In contrast to IFN-α and IFN-β that stimulate mainly the expression of class I antigens, IFN-γ induces enhanced expression of both class I and class II antigens in macrophages and other types of cells (Kelley *et al.*, 1984). As a result of increased class II antigen expression, the antigen-presenting ability of IFN-γ-treated cells is augmented (Zlotnik *et al.*, 1983). Similarly, IL-4 is capable of inducing both class I and class II antigens in certain subsets of macrophages (Crawford *et al.*, 1987; Stuart *et al.*, 1988), and of enhancing their antigen-presenting ability (Zlotnik *et al.*, 1987). In murine bone marrow-derived macrophages, GM-CSF induces high levels of Ia expression, similar to the levels induced by IFN-γ. IL-3 also induces class II antigens in murine peritoneal macrophages, and the kinetics of IL-3-induced Ia expression is distinct from that induced by IFN-γ, IL-4 or GM-CSF (Frendl and Beller, 1990). In contrast, M-CSF not only suppresses the basal levels of Ia, but also inhibits GM-CSF- or IFN-γ-induced Ia expression (Willman *et al.*, 1989). IL-10 was shown to inhibit strongly the constitutive and inducible expression of class II molecules on monocytes and macrophages, thereby suppressing antigen-specific T-cell proliferation (de Waal Malefyt *et al.*, 1991). In human monocytes IFN-γ can increase the expression of HLA-DR, -DP and -DQ antigens, whereas IL-4 and GM-CSF selectively enhance HLA-DR and -DP antigen expression (Gerrard *et al.*, 1990). Recently, IL-13 was found to induce human monocyte differentiation and enhance the expression of class II antigens (McKenzie *et al.*, 1993). Therefore, the type of cytokines produced by activated T cells in the process of antigen presentation may determine the specific pattern of macrophage functions.

REFERENCES

Aarden, L.A. *et al.* (1979). *J. Immunol.* **123**, 2928–2929.
Aderka, D., Le, J. and Vilček, J. (1989). *J. Immunol.* **143**, 3517–3523.
Aggarwal, B.B., Eessalu, T.E. and Hass, P.E. (1985). *Nature* **318**, 665–666.
Alderson, M.R., Sassenfeld, H.M. and Widmer, M.B. (1990). *J. Exp. Med.* **172**, 577–587.
Alderson, M.R., Tough, T.W., Ziegler, S.F. and Grabstein, K.H. (1991). *J. Exp. Med.* **173**, 923–930.
Aman, M.J., Rudolf, G., Goldschmitt, J., Aulitzky, W.E., Lam, C., Huber, C. and Peschel, C. (1993). *Blood* **82**, 2371–2378.
Arima, N., Kamio, M., Imada, K., Hori, T., Hattori, T., Tsudo, M., Okuma, M. and Uchiyama, T. (1992). *J. Exp. Med.* **176**, 1265–1272.
Armitage, R.J., Namen, A.E., Sassenfeld, H.M. and Grabstein, K.H. (1990). *J. Immunol.* **144**, 938–941.
Asao, H., Takeshita, T., Nakamura, M., Nagata, K. and Sugamura, K. (1990). *J. Exp. Med.* **171**, 637–644.
Asao, H., Takeshita, T., Ishii, N., Kumaki, S., Nakamura, M. and Sugamura, K. (1993). *Proc. Natl Acad. Sci. USA* **90**, 4127–4131.
Barcena, A., Toribio, M.L., Pezzi, L. and Martinez-A, C. (1990). *J. Exp. Med.* **172**, 439–446.
Bazan, J.F. (1989). *Biochem. Biophys. Res. Commun.* **164**, 788–895.
Becker, S., Warren, M.K. and Haskill, S. (1987). *J. Immunol.* **139**, 3703–3709.
Beresini, M.H., Lempert, M.J. and Epstein, L.B. (1988). *J. Immunol.* **140**, 485–493.
Bich-Thuy, L.T., Dukovich, M., Peffer, N.J., Fauci, A.S., Kehrl, J.H. and Greene, W.C. (1987). *J. Immunol.* **139**, 1550–1556.
Bird, T.A. and Saklatvala, J. (1989). *J. Immunol.* **142**, 126.
Bloom, B.R. and Bennett, B. (1966). *Sicience* **153**, 80–82.
Bradley, T.R. and Metcalf, D. (1966). *Aust. J. Exptl Biol. Med. Sci.* **44**, 287–300.
Brown, M., Hu-Li, J. and Paul, W.E. (1988). *J. Immunol.* **141**, 504–511.
Burke, F., Naylor, M.S., Davies, B. and Balkwill, F. (1993). *Immunol. Today* **14**, 165–170.
Callard, R.E. and Turner, M.W. (1990). *Immunol. Today* **11**, 200–203.
Carswell, E.A., Old, L.J., Kassel, R.L., Green, S., Fiore, N. and Williamson, B. (1975). *Proc. Natl Acad. Sci. USA* **72**, 3666–3670.
Chantry, D., Turner, M., Abney, E. and Feldmann, M. (1989a). *J. Immunol.* **142**, 4295–4300.
Chantry, D., Turner, M. and Feldmann, M. (1989b). *Eur. J. Immunol.* **19**, 783–786.
Chazen, G.D., Pereira, G.M.B., LeGros, G., Gillis, S. and Shevach, E.M. (1989). *Proc. Natl Acad. Sci. USA* **86**, 5923–5927.
Cherwinski, H.M., Schumacher, J.H., Brown, K.D. and Mosmann, T.R. (1987). *J. Exp. Med.* **166**, 1229–1244.
Coffman, R.L., Ohara, J., Bond, M.W., Carty, J., Zlotnik, A. and Paul, W.E. (1986). *J. Immunol.* **136**, 4538–4541.

Coffman, R.L., Shrader, B., Carty, J., Mosmann, T.R. and Bond, M.W. (1987). *J. Immunol.* **139**, 3685–3690.

Cohen, S., Bigazzi, P.E. and Yoshida, T. (1974). *Cell Immunol.* **12**, 150–159.

Collart, M.A., Belin, D., Vassalli, J.-D., De Kossodo, S. and Vassalli, P. (1986). *J. Exp. Med.* **164**, 2113–2118.

Content, J., De Wit, L., Poupart, P., Opdenakker, G., Van Damme, J. and Billiau, A. (1985). *Eur. J. Biochem.* **152**, 253–257.

Crawford, R.M., Finbloom, D.S., Ohara, J., Paul, W.E. and Meltzer, M.S. (1987). *J. Immunol.* **139**, 135–141.

Dalton, D.K., Pitts-Meek, S., Keshav, S., Figari, I.S., Bradley, A. and Stewart, T.A. (1993). *Science* **259**, 1739–1742.

D'Andrea, A.D., Fasman, G.D. and Lodish, H.F. (1989). *Cell* **58**, 1023–1024.

David, J.R. (1966). *Proc. Natl Acad. Sci. USA* **56**, 73–77.

Defrance, T., Aubry, J.P., Rousset, F., Vanbervliet, B., Bonnefoy, J.Y., Arai, N., Takebe, Y., Yokota, T., Lee, F., Arai, K., DeVries, J. and Banchereau, J. (1987). *J. Exp. Med.* **165**, 1459–1467.

Defrance, T., Vanbervliet, B., Aubry, J.P. and Banchereau, J. (1988). *J. Exp. Med.* **168**, 1321–1337.

Defrance, T., Vanbervliet, B., Brière, F., Durand, I., Rousset, F. and Banchereau, J. (1992). *J. Exp. Med.* **175**, 671–682.

DeLarco, J.E. and Todaro, G.J. (1978). *Proc. Natl Acad. Sci. USA* **75**, 4001–4005.

De Maeyer, E. and De Maeyer-Guignard, J. (1988). *Interferons and Other Regulatory Cytokines*, John Wiley and Sons, New York.

de Waal Malefyt, R., Haanen, J., Spits, H., Roncarolo, M., te Velde, A., Figdor, C., Johnson, K., Kastelein, R., Yssel, H. and DeVries, J.E. (1991). *J. Exp. Med.* **174**, 915–924.

Ding, A.H., Nathan, C.F. and Stuehr, D.J. (1988). *J. Immunol.* **141**, 2407–2412.

Dumonde, D.C., Wolstencroft, R.A., Panayi, G.S., Matthew, M., Morley, J. and Howson, W.T. (1969). *Nature* **224**, 38–42.

Feinman, R., Henriksen-DeStefano, D., Tsujimoto, M. and Vilček, J. (1987). *J. Immunol.* **138**, 635–640.

Fiorentino, D.F., Bond, M.W. and Mosmann, T.R. (1989). *J. Exp. Med.* **170**, 2081–2095.

Fiorentino, D.F., Zlotnik, A., Vieira, P., Mosmann, T.R., Howard, M., Moore, K.W. and O'Garra, A. (1991). *J. Immunol.* **146**, 3444–3451.

Fransen, L., Van Der Heyden, J., Ruysschaert, R. and Fiers, W. (1986). *Eur. J. Cancer Clin. Oncol.* **22**, 419–426.

Freedman, A.S., Freeman, G., Whitman, J., Segil, J., Daley, J. and Nadler, L.M. (1988). *J. Immunol.* **141**, 3398–3404.

Frendl, G. and Beller, D.I. (1990). *J. Immunol.* **144**, 3392–3399.

Fujita, T., Reis, L.F.L., Watanabe, N., Kimura, Y., Taniguchi, T. and Vilček, J. (1989). *Proc. Natl Acad. Sci. USA* **86**, 9936–9940.

Gearing, D.P., King, J.A., Gough, N.M. and Nicola, N.A. (1989). *EMBO J.* **8**, 3667–3676.

Gerrard, T.L. Dyer, D.R. and Mostowski, H.S. (1990). *J. Immunol.* **144**, 4670–4674.

Gery, I., Gershon, R.R. and Waksman, B.M. (1971). *J. Immunol.* **107**, 1778–1780.

Grabstein, K.H., Urdal, D.L., Tushinski, R.J., Mochizuki, D.Y., Price, V.L., Cantrell, M.A., Gillis, S. and Conlon, P.J. (1986). *Science* **232**, 506–508.

Harriman, G.R., Kunimoto, D.Y., Elliott, J.F., Paetkau, V. and Strober, W. (1988). *J. Immunol.* **140**, 3033–3039.

Hart, P.H., Vitti, G.F., Burgess, D.R., Whitty, G.A., Piccoli, D.S. and Hamilton, J.A. (1989). *Proc. Natl Acad. Sci. USA* **86**, 3803–3807.

Hatakeyama, M., Tsudo, M., Minamoto, S., Kono, T., Doi, T., Miyata, T., Miyasaka, M. and Taniguchi, T. (1989). *Science* **244**, 551–556.

Helle, M., Boeije, L. and Aarden, L.A. (1989). *J. Immunol.* **142**, 4335–4338.

Henney, C.S. (1989). *Immunol. Today* **10**, 170–173.

Herbelin, A., Machavoine, F., Schneider, E., Papiernik, M. and Dy, M. (1992). *J. Immunol.* **148**, 99–105.

Houssiau, F.A., Renauld, J.-C., Stevens, M., Lehmann, F., Lethe, B., Coulie, P.G. and Van Snick, J. (1993). *J. Immunol.* **150**, 2634–2640.

Howard, M., Farrar, J., Hilfiker, M., Johnson, B., Takatsu, K., Hamaoka, T. and Paul, W.E. (1982). *J. Exp. Med.* **155**, 914–923.

Huang, S., Hendriks, W., Althage, A., Hemmi, S., Blüethmann, H., Kamijo, R., Vilček, J., Zinkernagel, R.M. and Aguet, M. (1993). *Science* **259**, 1742–1745.

Isaacs, A. and Lindenmann, J. (1957). *Proc. Roy. Soc. (London) Series B* **147**, 258–267.

Kamijo, R., Le, J., Shapiro, D., Havell, E.A., Huang, S., Aguet, M., Bosland, M. and Vilček, J. (1993a). *J. Exp. Med.* **178**, 1435–1440.

Kamijo, R., Shapiro, D., Le, J., Huang, S., Aguet, M. and Vilček, J. (1993b). *Proc. Natl Acad. Sci. USA* **90**, 6626–6631.

Kaye, J., Gillis, S., Mizel, S.B., Shevach, E.M., Malek, T.R., Dinarello, C.A., Lachman, L.B. and Janeway, C.A. (1984). *J. Immunol.* **133**, 1339–1345.

Kehrl, J.H., Wakefield, L.M., Roberts, A.B., Jakowlew, S., Alvarez-Mon, M., Derynck, R., Sporn, M.B. and Fauci, A.S. (1986). *J. Exp. Med.* **163**, 1037–1050.

Kehrl, J.H., Alvarez-Mon, M., Delsing, G.A. and Fauci, A.S. (1987). *Science* **238**, 1144–1146.

Kelley, V.E., Fiers, W. and Strom, T.B. (1984). *J. Immunol.* **132**, 240–245.

Kopf, M., Le Gros, G., Bachmann, M., Lamers, M.C., Blüethmann, H. and Köhler, G. (1993). *Nature* **362**, 245–248.

Kühn, R., Rajewsky, K. and Müller, W. (1991). *Science* **254**, 707–710.

Kühn, R., Löhler, J., Rennick, D., Rajewsky, K. and Müller, W. (1993). *Cell* **75**, 263–274.

Kulkarni, A.B., Huh, C.-G., Becker, D., Geiser, A., Lyght, M., Flanders, K.C., Roberts, A.B., Sporn, M.B., Ward, J.M. and Karlsson, S. (1993). *Proc. Natl Acad. Sci. USA* **90**, 770–774.

Lantz, O., Grillot-Courvalin, C., Schmitt, C., Fermand, J.-P. and Brouet, J.C. (1985). *J. Exp. Med.* **161**, 1225–1230.

Larsen, C.G., Zachariae, C.O.C., Oppenheim, J.J. and Matsushima, K. (1989). *Biochem. Biophys. Res. Comm.* **160**, 1403–1408.

Le, J. and Vilček, J. (1987). *Lab. Invest.* **56**, 234–248.

Le, J. and Vilček, J. (1989). *Lab. Invest.* **61**, 588–602.

Le, J., Prensky, W., Yip, Y.K., Chang, Z., Hoffman, T., Stevenson, H.C., Balazs, I., Sadlik, J.R. and Vilček, J. (1983). *J. Immunol.* **131**, 2821–2826.

Le, J., Fredrickson, G., Reis, L.F.L., Diamantstein, T., Hirano, T., Kishimoto, T. and Vilček, J. (1988). *Proc. Natl Acad. Sci. USA* **85**, 8643–8647.

Le, J., Fredrickson, G., Pollack, M. and Vilček, J. (1989). *Ann. N.Y. Acad. Sci.* **557**, 444–453.

Lebman, D.A., Lee, F.D. and Coffman, R.L. (1990). *J. Immunol.* **144**, 952–959.

Lee, S.H., Aggarwal, B.B., Rinderknecht, E., Assisi, F. and Chiu, H. (1984). *J. Immunol.* **133**, 1083–1086.

Lee, T.H., Klampfer, L., Shows, T.B. and Vilček, J. (1993). *J. Biol. Chem.* **268**, 6154–6160.

Lee, T.H., Lee, G.W., Ziff, E.B. and Vilček, J. (1990). *Mol. Cell. Biol.* **10**, 1982–1988.

Ling, P.D., Warren, M.K. and Vogel, S.N. (1985). *J. Immunol.* **135**, 1857–1863.

Londei, M., Verhoef, A., Hawrylowicz, C., Groves, J., DeBerardinis, P. and Feldmann, M. (1990). *Eur. J. Immunol.* **20**, 425–428.

Lotz, M., Jirik, F., Kabouridis, P., Tsoukas, C., Hirano, T., Kishimoto, T. and Carson, D.A. (1988). *J. Exp. Med.* **167**, 1253–1258.

Lowenthal, J.W., Cerottini, J.-C. and MacDonald, H.R. (1986). *J. Immunol.* **137**, 1226–1231.

Lowenthal, J.W., Ballard, D.W., Bogerd, H., Bohnlein, E. and Greene, W.C. (1989). *J. Immunol.* **142**, 3121–3128.

Lu, L., Walker, D., Graham, C.D., Waheed, A., Shadduck, R.K. and Broxmeyer, H.E. (1988). *Blood* **72**, 34–42.

McIntyre, T.M., Klinman, D.R., Rothman, P., Lugo, M., Dasch, J.R., Mond, J.J. and Snapper, C.M. (1993). *J. Exp. Med.* **177**, 1031–1037.

McKenzie, A.N.J., Culpepper, J.A., de Waal Malefyt, R., Briere, F., Punnonen, J., Aversa, G., Sato, A., Dang, W., Cocks, B.G., Menon, S., DeVries, J.E., Banchereau, J. and Zurawski, G. (1993). *Proc. Natl Acad. Sci. USA* **90**, 3735–3739.

Manetti, R., Parronchi, P., Giudizi, M.G., Piccinni, M.-P., Maggi, E., Trinchieri, G. and Romagnani, S. (1993). *J. Exp. Med.* **177**, 1199–1204.

Masu, Y., Wolf, E., Holtman, B., Sendtner, M., Brem, G. and Thoenen, H. (1993). *Nature* **365**, 27–32.

Matsushima, K., Morishita, K., Yoshimura, T., Lavu, S., Kobayashi, Y., Lew, W., Appella, E., Kung, H.F., Leonard, E.J. and Oppenheim, J.J. (1988). *J. Exp. Med.* **167**, 1883–1893.

Meltzer, M.S., Skillman, D.R., Hoover, D.L., Hanson, B.D., Turpin, J.A., Kalter, D.C. and Gendelman, H.E. (1990). *Immunol. Today* **11**, 217–223.

Minty, A., Chalon, P., Derocq, J.-M., Dumont, X., Guillemot, J.-C., Kaghad, M., Labit, C., Leplatois, P., Liauzun, P., Miloux, B., Minty, C., Casellas, P., Loison, G., Lupker, J., Shire, D., Ferrara, P. and Caput, D. (1993). *Nature* **362**, 248–250.

Mitchell, L.C., Davis, L.S. and Lipsky, P.E. (1989). *J. Immunol.* **142**, 1548–1557.
Mond. J.J., Carman, J., Sarma, C., Ohara, J. and Finkelman, F.D. (1986). *J. Immunol.* **137**, 3534–3537.
Morgan, D.A., Ruscetti, F.W. and Gallo, R. (1976). *Science* **193**, 1007–1010.
Morikawa, K., Kubagawa, H., Suzuki, T. and Cooper, M.D. (1987). *J. Immunol.* **139**, 761–766.
Morrissey, P.J., Goodwin, R.G., Nordan, R.P., Anderson, D., Grabstein, K.H., Cosman, D., Sims, J., Lupton, S., Acres, B., Reed, S.G., Mochizuki, D., Eisenman, J., Conlon, P.J. and Namen, A.E. (1989). *J. Exp. Med.* **169**, 707–716.
Muraguchi, A., Hirano, T., Tang, B., Matsuda, T., Horii, Y., Nakajima, K. and Kishimoto, T. (1988). *J. Exp. Med.* **167**, 332–344.
Namen, A.E., Lupton, S., Hjerrild, K., Wignall, J., Mochizuki, D.Y., Schmierer, A., Mosley, B., March, C.J., Urdal, D., Gillis, S., Cosman, D. and Goodwin, R.G. (1988). *Nature* **333**, 571–573.
Nathan, C.F., Murray, H.W., Wiebe, M.E. and Rubin, B.Y. (1983). *J. Exp. Med.* **158**, 670–689.
Neta, R., Sayers, T. and Oppenheim, J.J. (1992). In *Tumor Necrosis Factor: Structure, Function and Mechanism of Action* (eds B.B. Aggarwal and J. Vilček), Marcel Dekker, Inc., New York, pp. 499–566.
Noelle, R., Krammer, P.H., Ohara, J., Uhr, J.W. and Vitetta, E.S. (1984). *Proc. Natl Acad. Sci. USA* **81**, 6149–6153.
Noma, T., Mizuta, T., Rosen, A., Hirano, T., Kishimoto, T. and Honjo, T. (1987). *Immunol. Lett.* **15**, 249–253.
Oliveira, I.C., Sciavolino, P.J., Lee, T.H. and Vilček, J. (1992). *Proc. Natl Acad. Sci. USA* **89**, 9049–9053.
Oppenheim, J.J., Mizel, S.B. and Meltzer, M.S. (1979). In *Biology of the Lymphokines* (eds S. Cohen, E. Pick and J.J. Openheim), Academic Press, New York, pp. 291–323.
Osborn, L., Kunkel, S. and Nabel, G.J. (1989). *Proc. Natl Acad. Sci. USA* **86**, 2336–2340.
Palombella, V.J., Yamashiro, D.J., Maxfield, F.R., Decker, S.J. and Vilček, J. (1987). *J. Biol. Chem.* **262**, 1950–1954.
Perussia, B., Chan, S., D'Andrea, A., Tsuji, K., Santoli, D., Pospisil, M., Young, D., Wolf, S. and Trinchieri, G. (1992). *J. Immunol.* **149**, 3495–3502.
Peschel, C., Green, I., Ohara, J. and Paul, W.E. (1987). *J. Immunol.* **139**, 3338–3347.
Pfeffer, K., Matsuyama, T., Kündig, T.M., Wakeham, A., Kishihara, K., Shahinian, A., Wiegmann, K., Ohashi, P.S., Krönke, M. and Mak, T.W. (1993). *Cell* **73**, 457–467.
Philip, R. and Epstein, L.B. (1986). *Nature* **323**, 86–89.
Philip, R. (1988). *J. Immunol.* **140**, 1345–1349.
Pluznik, D.H. and Sachs, L. (1965). *J. Cell. Comp. Physiol.* **66**, 319–324.
Punnonen, J., Aversa, G., Cocks, B.G., McKenzie, A.N.J., Menon, S., Zurawski, G., de Waal Malefyt, R. and DeVries, J.E. (1993). *Proc. Natl Acad. Sci. USA* **90**, 3730–3734.
Rabin, E.M., Ohara, J. and Paul, W.E. (1985). *Proc. Natl Acad. Sci. USA* **82**, 2935–2939.
Rabin, E.M., Mond, J.J., Ohara, J. and Paul, W.E. (1986). *J. Immunol.* **137**, 1573–1576.
Raitano, A.B. and Korc. M. (1990). *J. Biol. Chem.* **265**, 10466–10472.
Ranges, G.E., Figari, I.S., Espevik, T. and Palladino, M.A. (1987). *J. Exp. Med.* **166**, 991–998.
Ranges, G.E., Zlotnik, A., Espevik, T., Dinarello, C.A., Cerami, A. and Palladino, M.A. (1988). *J. Exp. Med.* **167**, 1472–1478.
Reed, S.G., Nathan, C.F., Pihl, D.L., Rodricks, P., Shanebeck, K., Conlon, P.J. and Grabstein, K.H. (1987). *J. Exp. Med.* **166**, 1734–1746.
Reis, L.F.L., Harada, H., Wolchok, J.D., Taniguchi, T. and Vilček, J. (1992). *EMBO J.* **11**, 185–193.
Roberts, A.B. and Sporn, M.B. (1990). In *Peptide Growth Factors and Their Receptors I, Handbook of Experimental Pharmacology 95/II.* (eds M.B. Sporn and A.B. Roberts), Springer-Verlag, Berlin, pp. 419–472.
Roberts, W.M., Look, T., Roussel, M.F. and Scherr, C.J. (1988). *Cell* **55**, 655–661.
Rothe, J., Lesslauer, W., Lötscher, H., Lang, Y., Koebel, P., Köntgen, F., Athage, A., Zinkernagel, R., Steinmetz, M. and Blüethman, H. (1993). *Nature* **364**, 798–802.
Rousset, F., Garcia, E., Defrance, T., Péronne, C., Vezzio, N., Hsu, D., Kastelein, R., Moore, K.W. and Banchereau, J. (1992). *Proc. Natl Acad. Sci, USA* **89**, 1890–1893.
Ruddle, N.H. and Waksman, B.H. (1968). *J. Exp. Med.* **128**, 1267–1280.
Sadlack, B., Merz, H., Schorle, H., Schimpl, A., Feller, A.C. and Horak, I. (1993). *Cell* **75**, 253–261.
Sampson-Johannes, A. and Carlino, J.A. (1988). *J. Immunol.* **141**, 3680–3686.
Scheurich, P., Thoma, B., Ucer, U. and Pfizenmaier, K. (1987). *J. Immunol.* **138**, 1786–1790.
Schorle, H., Holtschke, T., Hünig, T., Schimpl, A. and Horak, I. (1991). *Nature* **352**, 621–624.
Schwab, R., Crow, M.K., Russo, C. and Weksler, M.E. (1985). *J. Immunol.* **135**, 1714–1718.

Sharon, M., Klausner, R.D., Cullen, B.R., Chizzonite, R. and Leonard, W.J. (1986). *Science* **234**, 859–863.

Shirakawa, F., Chedid, M., Suttles, J., Pollok, B.A. and Mizel, S.B. (1989). *Mol. Cell. Biol.* **9**, 959–964.

Shull, M.M., Ormsby, I., Kier, A.B., Pawlowski, S., Diebold, R.J., Yin, M., Allen, R., Sidman, C., Proetzel, G., Calvin, D., Annunziata, N. and Doetschman, T. (1992). *Nature* **359**, 693–699.

Smith, K.A., Lachman, L.B., Oppenheim, J.J. and Favata, M.F. (1980). *J. Exp. Med.* **151**, 1551–1556.

Smith, K.A. (1988). *Science* **240**, 1169–1176.

Snapper, C.M. and Paul, W.E. (1987a). *Science* **236**, 944–947.

Snapper, C.M. and Paul, W.E. (1987b). *J. Immunol.* **139**, 10–17.

Snapper, C.M., Finkelman, F.D. and Paul, W.E. (1988). *Immunol. Rev.* **102**, 51–76.

Sonoda, E., Matsumoto, R., Hitoshi, Y., Ishii, T., Sugimoto, M., Araki, S., Tominaga, A., Yamaguchi, N. and Takatsu, K. (1989). *J. Exp. Med.* **170**, 1415–1420.

Spits, H., Yssel, H., Takebe, Y., Arai, N., Yokota, T., Lee, F., Arai, K., Banchereau, J. and DeVries, J.E. (1987). *J. Immunol.* **139**, 1142–1147.

Splawski, J.B., McAnally, L.M. and Lipsky, P.E. (1990). *J. Immunol.* **144**, 562–569.

Sporn, M.B. and Roberts, A.B. (1988). *Nature* **332**, 217–220.

Stewart, C.L., Kaspar, P., Brunet, L.J., Bhatt, H., Gadi, I., Köntgen, F. and Abbondanzo, S.J. (1992). *Nature* **359**, 76–79.

Stuart, P.M., Zlotnik, A. and Woodward, J.G. (1988). *J. Immunol.* **140**, 1542–1547.

Suda, T., Murray, R., Guidos, C. and Zlotnik, A. (1990). *J. Immunol.* **144**, 3039–3045.

Svedersky, L.P., Nedwin, G.E., Goeddel, D.V. and Palladino, M.A. Jr. (1985). *J. Immunol.* **134**, 1604–1608.

Sztein, M.B., Steeg, P.S., Johnson, H.M. and Oppenheim, J.J. (1984). *J. Clin. Invest.* **73**, 556–565.

Taga, T. and Kishimoto, T. (1992). *FASEB J.* **6**, 3387–3396.

Takai, Y., Wong, G.G., Clark, S.C., Burakoff, S.J. and Herrmann, S.H. (1988). *J. Immunol.* **140**, 508–512.

Takatsu, K., Tominaga, A., Harada, N., Mita, S., Matsumoto, M., Takahashi, T., Kikuchi, Y. and Yamaguchi, N. (1988). *Immunol. Rev.* **102**, 107–135.

Takeda, S., Gillis, S. and Palacios, R. (1989). *Proc. Natl Acad. Sci. USA* **86**, 1634–1638.

Takeshita, T., Asao, H., Ohtani, K., Ishii, N., Kumaki, S., Tanaka, N., Munakata, H., Nakamura, M. and Sugamura, K. (1992). *Science* **257**, 379–382.

Torres, B.A., Farrar, W.L. and Johnson, H.M. (1982). *J. Immunol.* **128**, 2217–2219.

Trinchieri, G., Kobayashi, M., Rosen, M., Loudon, R., Murphy, M. and Perussia, B. (1986). *J. Exp. Med.* **164**, 1206–1225.

Trinchieri, G., Wysocka, M., D'Andrea, A., Rengaraju, M., Aste, M., Kubin, M., Valiante, N.M. and Chehimi, J. (1993). In *Progress in Growth Factor Research*, Vol. 4 (ed. J.K. Heath), Pergamon Press, pp. 355–368.

Vilček, J. (1990). In *Peptide Growth Factors and Their Receptors II, Handbook of Experimental Pharmacology 95/II* (eds M.B. Sporn and A.B. Roberts), Springer-Verlag, Berlin, pp. 3–38.

Vink, A., Uyttenhove, C., Wauters, P. and Van Snick, J. (1990). *Eur. J. Immunol.* **20**, 1–6.

Vitetta, E.S., Ohara, J., Myers, C., Layton, J., Krammer, P.H. and Paul, W.E. (1985). *J. Exp. Med.* **162**, 1726–1731.

Voss, S.D., Leary, T.P., Sondel, P.M. and Robb, R.J. (1993). *Proc. Natl Acad. Sci. USA* **90**, 2428–2432.

Waldmann, T.R. (1989). *Annu. Rev. Biochem.* **58**, 875–911.

Welch, P.A., Namen, A.E., Goodwin, R.G., Armitage, R. and Cooper, M.D. (1989). *J. Immunol.* **143**, 3562–3567.

Wheelock, E.F. (1965). *Science* **149**, 310–311.

Williams, T.W. and Granger, G.A. (1968). *Nature* **219**, 1076–1077.

Willman, C.L., Stewart, C.C., Miller, V., Yi, T. and Tomasi, T.B. (1989). *J. Exp. Med.* **170**, 1559–1567.

Wong, G.H.W. and Goeddel, D.V. (1986). *Nature* **323**, 819–822.

Yokota, T., Arai, N., DeVries, J., Spits, H., Banchereau, J., Zlotnik, A., Rennick, D., Howard, M., Takebe, Y., Miyatake, S., Lee F. and Arai, K. (1988). *Immunol. Rev.* **102**, 137–187.

Zlotnik, A., Shimonkevitz, R.P., Gefter, M.L., Kappler, J. and Marrack, P. (1983). *J. Immunol.* **131**, 2814–2820.

Zlotnik, A., Fischer, M., Roehm, N. and Zipori, D. (1987). *J. Immunol.* **138**, 4275–4279.

Zucali, J.R., Dinarello, C.A., Oblon, D.J., Gross, M.A., Anderson, L. and Weiner, R.S. (1986). *J. Clin. Invest.* **77**, 1857–1863.

Chapter 2

Molecular Genetics of Cytokines

Gordon W. Duff

Section of Molecular Medicine, University of Sheffield, Sheffield, UK

CYTOKINES IN CHRONIC INFLAMMATORY DISEASE

As extracellular signalling molecules that coordinate the inflammatory and immune responses, cytokines have many roles in the normal processes of host defence against infection and injury. They also appear to be involved, at many stages, in the mechanisms of autoimmunity and the pathogenesis of chronic inflammatory diseases (CID). Diseases that fall into this category include rheumatoid arthritis and other chronic inflammatory arthritides, diabetes and its complications, connective tissue diseases such as systemic lupus erythematosus (SLE) and scleroderma, inflammatory bowel diseases, inflammatory skin diseases, and possibly even arteriosclerosis could be classified in this way. Common pathological features of these cytokine-related conditions include inflammatory cell infiltration of target organs, loss of normal cellular components and tissue damage. Such diseases also have in common their chronicity, being more or less life-long once established, and a tendency to occur in families.

The genetic basis for the familial tendencies of common CIDs has not been defined fully in any particular case. However, it seems likely, on epidemiological grounds and studies of monozygotic and dizygotic twins that genetic factors contribute to disease susceptibility and severity, though environmental factors are also important or even critical for the development of clinical disease. Thus, common familial diseases appear to be multifactorial with the involvement of an unknown number of genes and unknown environmental factors (Table 1).

In many cases, associations between CIDs and alleles or haplotypes of the major histocompatibility complex (MHC) have been established. These associations have

Table 1. A list of some major multifactorial diseases that show familial clustering.

Inflammatory joint disease
Diabetes
Arteriosclerosis
Inflammatory skin diseases
Inflammatory bowel diseases
Connective tissue diseases

The Cytokine Handbook, 2nd ed.
ISBN 0–12–689661–5

mostly been interpreted as 'immune response' gene effects and more recently in terms of the genetically defined ability of MHC molecules to accommodate a particular linear peptide and interact with a T-cell antigen receptor. This mechanism could explain the immunopathogenic component of familial CIDs.

Within the MHC, diseases are often associated with quite extensive haplotypes, making it difficult to distinguish which particular allele(s) may contribute to pathogenesis and which may be associated with disease through physical linkage to the true disease-related alleles. Not only can it be difficult, for practical reasons, to assess the contribution of an individual allele within an MHC haplotype, but it seems certain that susceptibility to or severity of many CIDs is determined also by other unknown genes that are located outside of the MHC. Progress in defining these non-MHC genes has been, until recently, somewhat slow.

CYTOKINES AS CANDIDATE GENES

There are several approaches to the identification of disease-associated genes. When the mechanisms of disease are not known, linkage analysis of the disease phenotype within families may identify first the chromosome and then the chromosomal region where the gene is located. In the human genome, there are now so many well-spaced polymorphic markers for each chromosome that linkage analysis in families can relatively easily locate disease genes in monogenic diseases with quite a high degree of resolution. Clearly, linkage analysis becomes more difficult in multigenic and multi-factorial diseases unless major single-gene effects are present.

Another approach is to propose putative genes that may be important. This is often possible when there is some understanding of the disease process. Thus, a 'candidate' gene in this sense is a hypothesis to be tested. The macrophage-derived cytokines that control the inflammatory response would seem to be reasonable 'candidate genes' in CIDs. Not only are they active in the pathogenesis of many CIDs (Duff, 1989) but they also show stable inter-individual differences in rates of production (Molvig et al., 1988).

In order to test the hypothesis that cytokine genes may contribute to CIDs it is necessary to seek polymorphic markers within these genes and then to ascertain whether there are differences in allelic frequencies between populations of unrelated individuals with a CID and a relevant 'healthy' population. If a disease-associated allele emerges from such a population analysis another question is raised: does the identified gene, itself, contribute to the disease process or is it a chromosomal 'marker' for a more important contributory gene with which it is physically linked? Clearly, if a candidate gene has been proposed on the basis of a biological role in the disease process and is then found to possess a disease-associated allele its likelihood of being a contributory gene may be greater. This would be particularly true if the polymorphism resulted in an altered protein or in altered regulation of the gene. The latter might result in a quantitative difference in gene regulation (e.g. increased rate of gene transcription) or a qualitative difference in gene regulation (e.g. a change in gene transcription in response to a specific signalling pathway or in a particular cell type). Thus, the DNA that comprises eukaryotic genes is divided into stretches that contain information for coding RNA (exons) broken up by intervening, non-coding sequences (introns). The DNA 'upstream' of the first exon (5' flanking region)

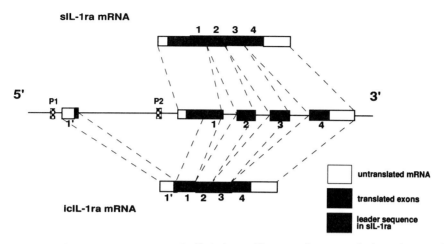

Fig. 1. Structure of the IL-1 receptor antagonist (IL-1ra) gene. The genomic structure is shown between the two alternative mRNA sequences. The genomic sequence is divided into exons (numbered boxes) and introns (intervening sequences between exons). Upstream of exons 1' and 1, the alternative promoters are indicated by P1 and P2. Cells, such as macrophages, use the downstream promoter (P2) and make an mRNA that encodes a leader sequence. This is translated into a secreted form of the IL-1 receptor antagonist (sIL-1ra). Other cell types, such as skin keratinocytes, use the upstream promoter (P1) and generate an alternative mRNA that lacks the coding region for a leader sequence. This is translated as an intracellular form of the IL-1 receptor antagonist (icIL-1ra).

contains short nucleotide sequences that bind transcription factors and thereby controls the process of gene transcription (the promoter region (Fig. 1). Not all of the RNA is translated into protein. Whether it is translated or not, it can affect the production of protein, e.g. untranslated sequences at the 3' end influence the stability of the mRNA of many cytokine genes. Short DNA sequences in the 5' or 3' flanking regions or within the gene itself can act to increase gene transcription (enhancer sequences) or to reduce it (repressor sequences).

TUMOUR NECROSIS FACTOR AND THE MHC

The search for disease-related polymorphisms in cytokine genes is relatively recent since specific probes for their identification have been available for less than a decade. Because of its biological properties and its location within the MHC, there was early interest in potential disease-related alleles of the tumour necrosis factor (TNF) locus and the first such observation was made in mice (Jacob and McDevitt, 1988). A restriction fragment length polymorphism within the TNF-α gene of lupus-prone (NZB × NZW) F$_1$ mice correlated with reduced production of TNF-α and was thought to be related to the development of the lupus-like nephritis in these mice (Jacob and McDevitt, 1988).

In humans early attempts to find TNF polymorphisms that might be associated with MHC haplotypes met with mixed success (Choo et al., 1988; Partanen and Koskimies, 1988; Fugger et al., 1989b). It was possible to relate an NcoI restriction fragment length polymorphism (RFLP) at the TNF locus to HLA-B and a DR haplotype (Choo et al., 1988). This RFLP polymorphism was also related to modest changes in TNF production

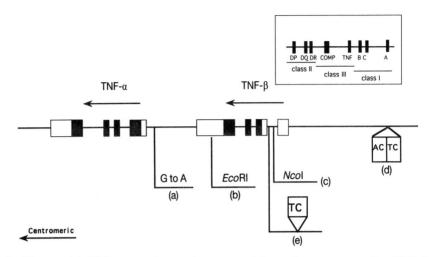

Fig. 2. Diagram of the TNF genes on human chromosome 6 (insert shows structure of the MHC). The TNF-α and TNF-β genes are in tandem (both containing four exons). The position of the known polymorphic markers are indicated: a, Wilson *et al.* (1993); b, Webb and Chaplin (1990); c, Nedospasov *et al.* (1991); d, e, Messer *et al.* (1991). The positions of the microsatellites (TC and AC repeats) are indicated. The distance between TNF-α and TNF-β is 1100 bp.

rates *in vitro* (Fugger *et al.*, 1989a). Associations between HLA types and TNF-α production rate *in vitro* have also been noted (Bendtzen *et al.*, 1988; Jacob *et al.*, 1991b). Despite these promising associations no relationship was found between the TNF RFLP and HLA-associated diseases such as multiple sclerosis and optic neuritis (Fugger *et al.*, 1990). In fact, the *Nco*I RFLP at the TNF locus was, when it was characterized, found to be located within the first intron of the TNF-β gene (Webb and Chaplin, 1990; Messer *et al.*, 1991a). This polymorphism was shown also to be correlated with an amino acid variation at position 26 of TNF-β (lymphotoxin) and also with a reduced rate of TNF-β production (Messer *et al.*, 1991a).

The search for further and possibly more informative polymorphisms at the TNF locus continued with the identification of four dinucleotide repeats of variable length (microsatellites). Of these, two were 3.5 kb upstream of the TNF-β gene, one was some 10 kb downstream of the TNF-α gene and one TC repeat was located within the first intron of the TNF-β gene (Nedospasov *et al.*, 1991) (Fig. 2). While the previously discussed polymorphisms are within the TNF-β gene, or at some distance from the tandem TNF genes, polymorphisms have also been described in the promoter region of the murine TNF-α gene (Jongeneel *et al.*, 1990) and at position −308 within the promoter region of the human TNF-α gene (Wilson *et al.*, 1992) (Fig. 3).

TNF POLYMORPHISM AND DISEASES

Several studies have tested whether there may be disease-associated or functionally different alleles of the TNF locus. No association was found between TNF-β polymorphism and the low TNF-β production rates seen in patients with primary biliary cirrhosis (Messer *et al.*, 1991b) and, likewise, there was no relation between

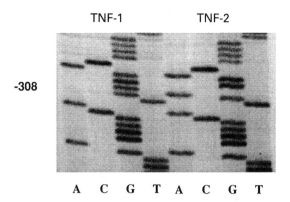

TNF-1   TNF-2

-308

A   C   G   T   A   C   G   T

Fig. 3. Sequencing gel from two individuals shows single-base transition in the TNF-α gene sequence at position −308 from the transcription start site. An individual who is homozygous for the common allele (TNF-1) has G at position −308, while an individual who is homozygous for the rarer allele (TNF-2) shows an A at this position.

TNF-β polymorphism and ankylosing spondylitis (Verjans *et al.*, 1991). Associations were found between TNF microsatellites and other loci within the MHC including Class I, II and III alleles (Jongeneel *et al.*, 1991). More recently, the single-base transition polymorphism within the human TNF-α promoter has been highly associated with the 'autoimmune haplotype' HLA-A1, B8, DR3 (Wilson *et al.*, 1993). The TNF-β gene *Nco*I RFLP also correlates with MHC ancestral haplotypes including HLA-A1, B8, DR3 (Dawkins *et al.*, 1989; Abraham *et al.*, 1993) This HLA haplotype has also been associated with increased TNF-α production by lymphoid cell lines *in vitro* (Jacob *et al.*, 1990; Abraham *et al.*, 1993). In the light of these associations it is not surprising that TNF alleles have been found at raised frequencies in diseases associated with the HLA-A1, B8, DR3 haplotype. For example the TNF-β RFLP has been associated with Graves' disease of the thyroid (Badenhoop *et al.*, 1992) and also with SLE (Bettinotti *et al.*, 1993). An association has also been found between SLE and the TNF-α base-transition polymorphism in the 5′ region (Wilson *et al.*, 1994). With this polymorphism, the association was even stronger between the TNF-α rare allele and the presence of anti-Ro and anti-La autoantibodies (Wilson *et al.*, 1994).

In all of these studies, however, the association between disease and DR3 has been stronger than that between disease and TNF, suggesting that the TNF association results from linkage dysequilibrium between the TNF locus and the DR3 locus. It is only in the lupus-prone mouse strains where disease susceptibility, TNF-α production rate and TNF-α genotype have been associated in a way that suggests a direct involvement of the TNF gene product in disease pathogenesis (Jacob *et al.*, 1991a). These mice have a promoter region polymorphism within the TNF-α gene and it remains to be seen whether the promoter region polymorphism in the human TNF-α gene is also associated with the production-rate phenotype. Although these issues remain outstanding, it is now clear that polymorphisms at the TNF locus form part of extended MHC haplotypes such as the A1, B8, DR3 ancestral haplotype that has been associated with a range of autoimmune human diseases.

Table 2.   Chromosomal locations on the long arm of human chromosone 2 of the IL-1 gene cluster and related genes.

IL-1α	2q 13
IL-1β	2q 13–21
IL-1ra	2q 13–14.1
IL-1 receptor type I	2q 12
IL-1 receptor type II	2q 12–22

THE INTERLEUKIN 1 GENE CLUSTER

The interleukin-1 gene cluster comprising IL-1α, IL-1β and IL-1 receptor antagonist is located on the long arm of human chromosome 2. The IL-1 receptor type I (and possibly IL-1 receptor type II) are also located on 2q (Table 2). Recently, three IL-1 ligand genes have all been mapped to a 430 Kb stretch of DNA (Nicklin *et al.*, 1994). The gene products of these loci have been implicated extensively in CIDs of all types and in chronic inflammatory arthritis such as rheumatoid arthritis in particular (Eastgate *et al.*, 1988).

Several different polymorphisms have been found and characterized within the IL-1 gene cluster. They include single base changes in 5′ flanking DNA of IL-1 β (di Giovine *et al.*, 1992) and IL-1α (McDowell *et al.*, 1994) as well as polymorphic variable number tandem repeats (VNTR polymorphism) in IL-1α and IL-1 receptor antagonist. In IL-1α, the VNTR is made up of a 46-bp stretch of DNA that is repeated from five to 19 times within intron 6. There are six alleles, of which the most frequent has 9 repeats (62%) and the second most frequent (23%) has 18 repeats (Bailly *et al.*, 1993). Each repeat stretch contains sites of potential significance in gene regulation, in particular a glucocorticoid response element and a potential binding site for the transcription factor SP-1. There is also an uncharacterized *Taq* I restriction fragment length polymorphism in the IL-1 gene cluster that is detected with IL-1β probes (Pociot *et al.*, 1992).

The IL-1 receptor antagonist is a very powerful anti-inflammatory agent *in vivo*. Within the IL-1 receptor antagonist (IL-1ra) gene there is a VNTR polymorphism in intron 2. This comprises an 86-bp tandem repeat and there are five alleles with four repeats being the common allele (74%) and two repeats the next most frequent allele (22%) (Tarlow *et al.*, 1993) (Fig. 4). These repeat stretches, like those in IL-1 α, also

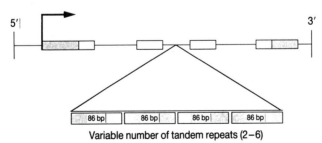

Variable number of tandem repeats (2–6)

Fig. 4.   Diagram to show the nature of the VNTR polymorphism in intron 2 of the human IL-1ra gene. An 86 bp stretch is tandemly repeated up to six times. Four repeats is the commonest allele (74%) while two repeats is the next commonest allele (22%).

Table 3. Some associations between polymorphisms of the IL-1 gene cluster and chronic inflammatory diseases (CID).

CID	Comment	Reference
Systemic lupus erythematosus (SLE)	Especially discoid rash and photosensitivity (IL-1ra)	Blakemore *et al.* (1994)
Juvenile chronic arthritis	Especially with iridocyclitis (IL-1α)	McDowell *et al.* (1994)
Ulcerative colitis	Especially total colonic involvement (IL-1ra)	Mansfield *et al.* (1994)
Psoriasis	Especially hospital populations (IL-1ra)	Cork *et al.* (1993)
Diabetes	Diabetic complications (IL-1ra)	Gonzalez *et al.* (1994)
Diabetes	Type 1	Pociot *et al.* (1992)
Alopecia Areata	Especially Alopecia Universalis	Tarlow *et al.* (1994)
Lichen sclerosus	Especially with extra-genital involvement	Clay *et al.* (1994)

contain potential binding sites for transcription factors but no function has yet been demonstrated for any of these IL-1 gene cluster polymorphisms.

DISEASE ASSOCIATION WITH POLYMORPHISMS IN THE IL-1 GENE CLUSTER

Several associations have been found between the polymorphic markers of the IL-1 gene cluster region and a range of CIDs (Blakemore *et al.*, 1994; Cork *et al.*, 1993; McDowell *et al.*, 1994; Gonzalez *et al.*, 1994; Mansfield *et al.*, 1994) (Table 3). These associations represent statistically significant differences in allele frequencies between disease populations and matched control populations. What the significance may be in terms of disease pathogenesis is not yet known, but studies to relate cytokine production rates to the genetic markers of the IL-1 gene cluster and direct testing *in vitro* of the functional significance of these polymorphisms in gene regulation is currently being investigated. There has been one report associating an IL-1β RFLP with IL-1β secretion *in vitro* (Pociot *et al.*, 1992). It is notable that in the clinical diseases that show associations with the IL-1 gene cluster there have been many reports implicating the products of these loci in their pathogenesis (Dinarello and Wolff, 1993).

MARKERS OF SUSCEPTIBILITY OR SEVERITY?

The disease associations that have been established with IL-1 gene cluster polymorphisms have been detected by comparing allele frequencies in disease and in normal populations. In this way it is possible to generate hypotheses about susceptibility genes which, of course, may be quite normal 'alleles of the locus'. This is in contrast to a mutation in a single gene leading to a disease. For example, mutations in the gene that encodes IL-2 receptor γ chain 'cause' X-linked severe combined immunodeficiency disease (SCID) (Noguchi *et al.*, 1993). Whether genetic linkage analysis will show that other diseases can be mapped to single genes encoding cytokines or their receptors remains to be seen.

The data collected to date seem to indicate that IL-1 gene polymorphisms represent markers of disease severity. For example, in ulcerative colitis the carriage rate of IL-1ra

28 G.W. Duff

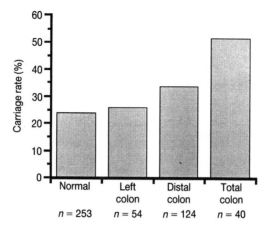

Fig. 5. Allele carriage rate of IL-1ra allele 2 in patients with ulcerative colitis. The carriage rate in a normal population is shown. The carriage rate in patient groups increases with increasing colonic involvement. Number of patients in each group are shown beneath columns.

allele 2 increases in populations with increasing extent of colonic involvement (Mansfield *et al.*, 1994) (Fig. 5).

CONCLUSION

The discovery in recent years of polymorphisms in cytokine and related genes has made it possible to test allelic associations with chronic inflammatory diseases. In the case of the pro-inflammatory cytokine TNF-α, the picture is complicated because of haplotypic association with other loci of the MHC. An allele of TNF-α is associated with the MHC haplotype A1, B8, DR3 which is itself associated with several autoimmune diseases such as SLE, Type I diabetes and Graves' disease. TNF-α, therefore, is also associated genetically with these diseases but it might be difficult to isolate the effect of the single gene from that of the extended haplotype.

The IL-1 gene cluster on chromosome 2 also has several polymorphic markers and it has been possible to find disease-associated alleles in CIDs such as SLE, ulcerative colitis, psoriasis and juvenile chronic arthritis. IL-1α, IL-1β and IL-1 receptor antagonist have all been implicated in the pathogenesis of these disorders but it is still possible that the polymorphisms in this gene cluster are merely markers for stronger disease-related genes elsewhere on chromosome 2. Studies are in progress to resolve this and also to test directly the effect of these polymorphisms on gene function and the production rate of the cytokine.

For many years, the genes of the MHC were the focus of attention for investigators interested in the genetic basis of common inflammatory diseases. It would now appear that genetic analysis of the cytokine system will also contribute to the understanding of the multifactorial nature of these conditions.

Since the days of Garrod, clinical genetics has regarded "genetic diseases" as those where a recent mutation in a critical gene leads directly to the production of disease. With the progress in molecular genetics in the last decade, we can now extend the idea of "genetic diseases" to those common conditions where DNA variation in the normal human population contributes to susceptibility or to the severity of disease and its clinical outcome. This chapter has focused on sterile inflammatory conditions but we can be confident that similar insights will be forthcoming in the lethal infections (such as malaria, septic shock, meningococcal and HIV disease) and also in cancers. The clinical potential for selection of specific therapeutic approaches seems clear.

REFERENCES

Abraham, L.J., French, M.A.H. and Dawkins, R.L. (1993). *Clin. Exp. Immunol.* **92**, 14–18.

Badenhoop, K., Schwarz, G., Schleusener, J. *et al.* (1992). *J. Clin. Endocr. & Metab.* **74**, 287–291.

Bailly, S., di Giovine, F.S. and Duff, G.W. (1993). *Human Genetics* **91**, 85–86.

Bendtzen, K., Morling, N., Fomsgaard, A. *et al.* (1988). *Scand. J. Immunol.* **28**, 599.

Bettinotti, M.P., Hartung, K., Deicher, H. *et al.* (1993). *Immunogenetics* **37**, 449–454.

Blakemore, A.I.F., Tarlow, J.K., Gordon, C., Emery, P. and Duff, G.W. (1994). *Arthritis & Rheumatism*, in press.

Choo, S.Y., Spies, T., Strominger, J.L. and Hansen, J. (1988). *Hum. Immunol.* **23**, 86.

Clay, F.E., Tarlow, J.K., Blakemore, A.I., Harrington, C.I., Lewis, F., Cork, M.J. and Duff, G.W. (1994). *Human Genetics*, in press.

Cork, M.J., Tarlow, J.K., Blakemore, A.I.F., McDonagh, A.J.G., Messenger, A.G., Bleehan, S.S. and Duff, G.W. (1993). *J. Invest. Dermatol.* **100**(4), 736.

Dawkins, R.L., Leaver, A., Cameron, P.U. *et al.* (1989). *Hum. Immunol.* **26**, 91–97.

di Giovine, F.S., Takhsh, E., Blakemore, A.I.F. and Duff, G.W. (1992). *Human Mol. Genetics.* **1**, 353.

Dinarella, C.A. and Wolff, S.M. (1993). *New Eng. J. Med.* **328**, 106–113.

Duff, G.W. (1989). *Lancet* **i**, 1432–1435.

Eastgate, J.A., Symonds, J.A., Wood, N.C., Grinlington, F.M., di Giovine, F.S. and Duff, G.W. (1988). *Lancet* **ii**, 706–709.

Fugger, L., Bendtzen, K., Morling, N. *et al.* (1989a). *Eur. J. Haematol.* **43**, 255–256.

Fugger, L., Morling, N., Ryder, L.P. *et al.* (1989b). *Scand. J. Immunol.* **30**, 185–189.

Fugger, L., Morling, N., Sandberg-Wollheim, M. *et al.* (1990). *J. Neuroimmunol.* **27**, 85–88.

Gonzalez, A.-M., Blakemore, A.I.F., Tarlow, J.K., Cox, A., Wilson, R.M., Ward, J.D. and Duff, G.W. (1994). *Diab. Med.*, in press.

Jacob, C.O. and McDevitt, H.O. (1988). *Nature* **331**, 356–358.

Jacob, C.O., Hwang, F., Lewis, G.D. and Stall, A.M. (1991a). *Cytokine* **3**, 551–561.

Jacob, C.O., Lewis, G.D. and McDevitt, H.O. (1991b). *Immunol. Res.* **10**, 156.

Jacob, C.P., Fronek, Z., Lewis, G.D., Koo, M., Hansen, J.A. and McDevitt, H.O. (1990). *Proc. Natl Acad. Sci. USA* **87**, 1233–1237.

Jongeneel, C.V., Acha-Orbea, H. and Blankenstein, T. (1990). *J. Exp. Med.* **171**, 2141–2146.

Jongeneel, C.V., Briant, L., Udalova, I.A. *et al.* (1991). *Proc. Natl Acad. Sci. USA* **88**, 9717–9721.

McDowell, T.L., Symons, J.A., Ploski, R., Førre, Ø. and Duff, G.W. (1993). *B. J. Rheum.* **32**(Suppl. 1): 162.

McDowell, T., Symons, J.A., Ploski, R., Førre, Ø. and Duff, G.W. (1994). (submitted).

Mansfield, J.C., Holden, H., Tarlow, J.K., di Giovine, F.S., McDowell, T.L., Wilson, A.G., Holdsworth, C.D. and Duff, G.W. (1994). *Gastroenterol* **106**, 637–642.

Messer, G., Spengler, U., Jung, M.C. *et al.* (1991a). *J. Exp. Med.* **173**, 209–219.

Messer, G., Spengler, U. and Jung, M.C. *et al.* (1991b). *Scan. J. Immunol.* **34**, 735–740.

Molvig, J., Back, L., Cristensen, P. *et al.* (1988). *Scand. J. Immunol.* **27**, 705.

Nedospasov, S.A., Udalova, I.A., Kuprash, D.V. and Turetskaya, R.L. (1991). *J. Immunol.* **147**, 1053–1059.

Nicklin, M.J., Weith, A. and Duff, G.W. (1994). *Genomics* **19**, 382–384.

Noguchi, M., Yi, H. and Rosenblatt, H.M. (1993). *Cell* **73**, 147–157.

Partanen, J. and Koskimies, S. (1988). *Scand. J. Immunol.* **28**, 313–316.

Pociot, F., Mølvig, J., Wogensen, L. *et al.* (1992). *Euro. J. Clin. Invest.* **22**, 396–402.

Tarlow, J.K., Blakemore, A.I.F., Lennard, A., Solari, R., Hughes, H., Steinkasserer, A. and Duff, G.W. (1993). *Human Genetics* **91**, 403–404.

Tarlow, J.K., Clay, F.E., Cork, M.J., Blakemore, A.I., McDonagh, A.J., Messinger, A.G. and Duff, G.W. (1994). *J. Inv. Dermatol.*, in press.

Verjans, G.M.G.M., van der Linden, S.M., van Eys, G.J.J.M. *et al.* (1991). *Arthritis & Rheumatism* **34**, 486–489.

Webb, G.C. and Chaplin, D.D. (1990). *J. Immunol.* **145**, 1278–1285.

Wilson, A.G., di Giovine, F.S., Blakemore, A.I.F. and Duff, G.W. (1992). *Human Mol. Genetics* **1**, 353.

Wilson, A.G., de Vries, N., Pociot, F., di Giovine, F.S., van der Putte, L.B. and Duff, G.W. (1993). *J. Exp. Med.* **177**, 557–560.

Wilson, A.G., Gordon, C., di Giovine, F.S., de Bries, N., van de Putte, L.B.A., Emery, P. and Duff, G.W. (1994). (submitted)

Interleukin-1

Charles A. Dinarello

Department of Medicine, Tufts University School of Medicine and the New England Medical
Center, Boston, Massachussetts 02111, USA

INTRODUCTION

Interleukin-1 (IL-1) is primarily an inflammatory cytokine, whereas IL-2 and other cytokines are primarily growth factors for lymphocytes. IL-1 is more closely related to tumour necrosis factor (TNF) than any other cytokine, although the structure and receptors for IL-1 and TNF are clearly distinct. IL-1 is biologically active in the low pM or even fM range. In contrast, clotting factors, complement components and IL-8 are active in the nM range. There is little evidence that cytokines such as IL-1 play a role in normal homeostasis such as hormonal regulation, metabolism or in physiological regulation through, for example, temperature or blood pressure. On the other hand, since IL-1 is related to some growth factor cytokines, for example, fibroblast growth factor, it may be involved in repair of tissues and may play a role in the daily wear and tear of tissue breakdown and cell growth. In addition, following damage, growth factor polypeptides are produced in large amounts and may play a fundamental role in fibrosis. However, it is unclear, in the absence of injury, whether IL-1 is needed. The skin and epithelial cells, being exposed to the external environment, may require IL-1. There is abundant IL-1 in the skin, some epithelial lining cells and in the brain. Repair of nerve injury appears to require IL-1 (Guenard *et al.*, 1991).

During inflammation, injury, immunological challenge or infection, IL-1 is produced and because of its multiple biological properties, this cytokine appears to affect the pathogenesis of disease. Most studies on IL-1 are derived from experiments in which bacterial products such as lipopolysaccharide (LPS) endotoxins from Gram-negative bacteria or exotoxins from Gram-positive organisms are used to stimulate macrophage cells. In general, the production of several cytokines are induced by microbes or their products. Although cytokines are thought to play a role in the outcome of disease, only a few have been directly implicated as mediators of the pathogenic mechanisms by which illness causes death of the host. Recent studies using specific cytokine antagonism have shed considerable light on which cytokines appear to be playing a critical role. This review will focus on interleukin-1 (IL-1) as a cytokine of primary and strategic importance to the outcome of disease, particularly inflammatory and infectious diseases.

The Cytokine Handbook, 2nd ed.
ISBN 0–12–689661–5

A distinction is made between the local effects of IL-1 and the consequences of systemic blood levels. The ultimate function of the host defence system is the elimination of the invading organism whether by phagocytosis and antibody formation, as is the case in most bacterial infections, or the induction of cytotoxic T-cells for elimination of virus-infected cells. Inflammation is the price the host pays for an efficient and effective defence system. In the case of IL-1, high systemic blood levels have not been a characteristic of patients with sepsis compared with other cytokines, for example TNF or IL-6. Nevertheless, IL-1 is a potent inducer of hypotension and shock and, together with TNF, can be lethal in experimental animals. Humans are particularly sensitive to the pyrogenic and hypotensive properties of IL-1: a single intravenous injection of IL-1 of 10 ng/kg induces fever (39°C), and hypotension is consistently observed at 100 ng/kg; 300 ng/kg is the maximal dose tolerated because of the resulting severe fall in blood pressure (Smith *et al.*, 1992).

The local effects of IL-1 appear to induce neutrophil and macrophage emigration, lower pain thresholds and to release secondary lipid-derived mediators. For example, the family of neutrophil and monocyte chemotactic cytokines are important in local inflammation and likely mediate some of the effects of IL-1. The best-characterized member of this cytokine family is IL-8 (also called neutrophil activating protein-1); for the purposes of this overview, the entire family of chemotactic peptides will be considered as represented by IL-8. IL-1 is a potent inducer of IL-8 synthesis from monocytes, fibroblasts and endothelial cells. Concentrations of IL-1 of 1 pg/ml will induce IL-8 production in fibroblast cultures. In monocytes stimulated with bacterial endotoxin, 50% of the IL-8 produced is *via* an intermediate action of IL-1 (Porat *et al.*, 1992) and IL-8 produced from endothelial cells stimulated with activated platelets is by an IL-1-dependent pathway (Kaplanski *et al.*, 1993). Therefore, because of the potency of IL-1, local inflammation can be IL-1 mediated, in part, through the induction of IL-8.

The last 10 years of IL-1 research has focused on the structure and biological properties of this cytokine; these have recently been reviewed in detail (Dinarello, 1991). IL-1 research has now shifted to the study of receptors and anti-IL-1 strategies. These later studies have gained increasing importance in combating inflammatory and life-threatening aspects of this molecule. They include methods for limiting IL-1 synthesis, secretion, processing or interaction with its cell-bound receptors. The concept presented in this overview is that blocking systemic levels of IL-1 can be a life-saving clinical strategy in certain clinical situations but total IL-1 blockade may leave the host with less than optimal defence and repair mechanisms.

STRUCTURE, RECEPTORS AND SIGNAL TRANSDUCTION

IL-1 Structure

There are two distinct genes for IL-1: these have been named IL-1α and IL-1β. Each gene is located on chromosome 2 and codes for the IL-1α and β proteins, respectively. Both forms of IL-1 are first synthesized as larger, precursor molecules. The precursors for IL-1α and β have molecular masses of 31 000 Da, but unlike most proteins, both forms lack the series of amino acids, sometimes called 'leader sequences', that enable a

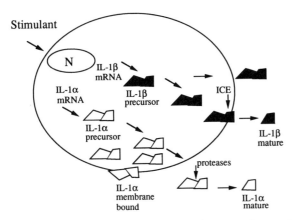

Fig. 1. Production and secretion of interleukin-1 (IL-1). A stimulant such as endotoxin activates a monocyte to transcribe the genes for IL-1α and IL-1β. Both forms of IL-1 are first synthesized as larger precursors. Most of the IL-1α remains intracellular or is expressed on the surface of the membrane. Proteases cleave IL-1α precursor into a mature form. The IL-1β precursor is cut by a specific interleukin-1β converting enzyme (ICE) to its mature form. Secretion of IL-1β takes place after the action of ICE; however, the IL-1β precursor is also found outside cells where it may be cleaved by other proteases.

precursor protein to be inserted into the Golgi, cleaved to a smaller or so-called 'mature' size and transported out of the cell.

For both forms of IL-1, the mature size is mostly 17 000 Da. Mature IL-1α and IL-1β have different amino acid sequences, sharing only 26% similarity; however, structurally the two isoforms of IL-1 are related at the three-dimensional level. Both IL-1α and IL-1β have been crystallized (Preistle *et al.*, 1988, 1989) and the amino acids critical for receptor binding and the stability of their structures have been identified. The third member of the IL-1 gene family is the IL-1 receptor antagonist (IL-1Ra). The three members of the IL-1 family recognize and bind to the same cell surface receptors. IL-1α and IL-1β binding to the IL-1 receptors transmits a signal whereas IL-1Ra does not.

IL-1 is rapidly synthesized by mononuclear cells, primarily monocytic phagocytes, when stimulated by microbial products or inflammatory agents. Because of the lack of a leader peptide, most IL-1α remains in the cytosol of cells. There is some evidence that IL-1α may function as an autocrine messenger in the skin. There is also evidence that the precursor of IL-1α is transported to the surface of the cell where it has been identified as 'membrane' IL-1 (Brody and Durum, 1989). Surface-bound IL-1α precursor is biologically active.

In human monocytes, between 40–60% of IL-1β is transported out of the cell but in contrast to IL-1α, IL-1β enters the circulation. Various mechanisms for transport include exocytosis from vesicles, active transport via multiple-drug-resistance carrier proteins, 'leakiness' or following cell death. Unlike the IL-1α precursor, the IL-1β precursor requires cleavage for optimal biological activity. Several common enzymes will cut the IL-1β precursor into smaller and more active forms. However, one particular protease appears highly specific for cleaving the IL-1β precursor from 31 000 to 17 500, its most active form (Cerretti *et al.*, 1992; Thornberry *et al.*, 1992) (Fig. 1). This enzyme is known as the IL-1β converting enzyme (ICE). ICE is a member of the cysteine protease family. ICE does not cleave the IL-1α precursor.

Other enzymes have been found which cleave the IL-1α precursor but these seem less specific than ICE.

Although both IL-1β and IL-1α have glycosylation sites, the majority of biological studies have concentrated on recombinant forms of IL-1 expressed in *Escherichia coli*, which lacks the ability to glycosylate. Glycosylation by expression in yeast has not increased specific activity over that of the nonglycosylated form (Casagli *et al.*, 1989). However, naturally produced membrane IL-1α may be a glycosylated form of IL-1. Mannose residues may be responsible for the binding of membrane IL-1α to the surface of macrophage via cell-surface lectin recognition of mannose sites (Brody and Durum, 1989).

Subpeptides of IL-1β have varying degrees of biological activity, although compared with mature IL-1β, their specific activities are low. A nonapeptide consisting of residues 163–171 activated T cells, stimulates glycosaminoglycan synthesis, is an adjuvant and recruits anti-tumour reactivity *in vivo*, but lacks pro-inflammatory and pyrogenic properties (Antoni *et al.*, 1989; Boraschi *et al.*, 1990). Interestingly, the amino acids which comprise the nonapeptide are missing in the IL-1Ra. A single point substitution in the human IL-1β of arginine 127 to glycine results in a 100-fold loss in biological activity on T cells without diminishing receptor–ligand binding (Gehrke *et al.*, 1990). However, this amino acid change results in a misfolding of IL-1 rather than the arginine being directly involved with signal transduction. Changing the aspartic acid at position 151 to tyrosine in the mature IL-1α results in loss of PGE$_2$ induction and fibroblast growth but retention of T-cell responses (Yamayoshi *et al.*, 1990). This mutein also antagonizes IL-1α and IL-1β induction of PGE$_2$ and functions like a receptor antagonist.

IL-1 Receptors

At present, there are two primary distinct gene products for IL-1 receptors (IL-1R); both are members of the immunoglobulin superfamily. The cDNAs for these receptors have been cloned (Sims *et al.*, 1988; McMahon *et al.*, 1991). The type I receptor (IL-1RI) is an 80 kDa glycoprotein prominently found on endothelial cells, hepatocytes, fibroblasts, keratinocytes and T lymphocytes whereas the type II receptor (IL-1RII) is a 68 kDa glycoprotein prominently found on B lymphocytes, monocytes and neutrophils. The type I receptor preferentially binds IL-1α and the type II receptor preferentially binds IL-1β. However, each member of the IL-1 family can bind to either receptor. The extracellular regions of the type I and II receptors share 28% amino acid homology; both have a single transmembrane segment but the IL-1RII has only a short cytosolic segment (Fig. 2). The IL-1RI is the primary signal transducing receptor and is found on nearly all cells. The longer cytoplasmic domain of the type I receptor has no intrinsic tyrosine kinase activity. The IL-1RII appears not to be capable of forming a complex with the type I receptor and is not involved in transducing a signal. Binding of IL-1 to the chimaeric receptor comprised of the extracellular portion of the type II receptor fused to the cytoplasmic domain of the type I receptor results in a biological signal (Heguy *et al.*, 1993). Glycosylation of IL-1RI appears to be important for the affinity of the ligand (Mancilla *et al.*, 1992).

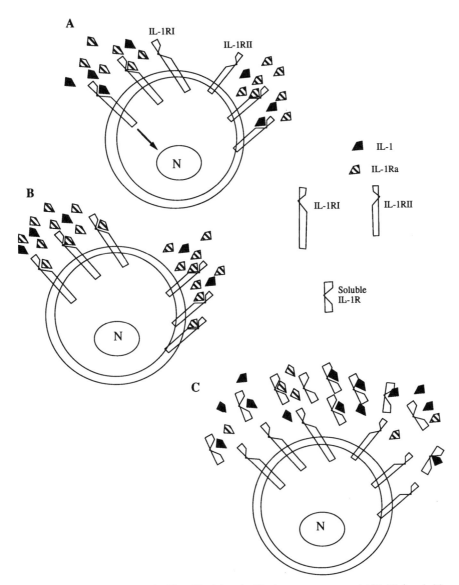

Fig. 2. Interactions between interleukin-1 (IL-1), interleukin-1 receptor antagonist (IL-1Ra) and either cell-bound or soluble IL-1 receptors (IL-1RI, IL-1RII). (A). Cell with the two types of IL-1 receptors. IL-1 shown can be either ·IL-1α or IL-1β. The IL-1RI and IL-1RII have similar extracellular structures and both bind IL-1α or IL-1β or IL-1Ra. There is partial occupancy of either type of IL-1 receptors by IL-1 and partial occupancy by IL-1Ra. In this cell, IL-1 is still able to trigger a biological response as indicated by the arrow towards the nucleus (N) from the type I receptor. (B). The cell is exposed to excess of IL-1Ra compared with IL-1 so that all IL-1 receptors are occupied by IL-1Ra. Under these conditions, no cellular activation occurs as IL-1 cannot bind to IL-1RI. (C). Cells exposed to soluble (extracellular domain) of IL-1R (either type I or type II). Either type of soluble IL-1R binds to IL-1 so that IL-1 cannot bind to and activate its cell surface receptors. If enough soluble IL-1R are present, all IL-1 is bound and no cell activation takes place.

Regulation of IL-1 Receptors

Studies have shown that various agents and cytokines increase the number of surface receptors on a variety of cells. IL-1 itself, however, downregulates IL-1 surface receptors on T cells and this takes place via a mechanism of IL-1 suppression of steady-state mRNA coding for the type I receptor (Ye *et al.*, 1992). IL-1RI gene expression is upregulated by corticosteroids, epidermal growth factor, IL-4 and IL-2. Despite evidence that the type I receptor is regulated, recent genomic cloning of the human type I IL-1R has revealed a lack of a TATA and CAAT box (Ye *et al.*, 1993). The promoter region for the human IL-1RI shares striking similarity to those of house-keeping genes rather than highly regulated genes. There are three distinct promoter regions of the human IL-1R gene, each RNA species containing considerable secondary structures.

Signal Transduction

One of the important characteristics of IL-1 signal transduction is that as few as 2% of IL-1 receptors need be occupied for a biological response to occur. To date, there is no single mechanism of signal transduction which accounts for the biological effects of IL-1 following its engagement of the type I receptor. These have included G-protein coupling (O'Neill *et al.*, 1990), activation of cAMP (Mizel, 1990), hydrolysis of phospholipids (Rosoff *et al.*, 1988) and activation of sphingomyelinase (Mathias *et al.*, 1993). Early events following IL-1 binding to the type I receptor are associated with the formation of intracellular kinases that phosphorylate various proteins, receptors and transcription factors (nuclear binding proteins): heat-shock protein (p27) is one example of cytosolic proteins (Guesdon and Saklatvala, 1991), epidermal growth factor receptor is an example of one of the receptors that are phosphorylated (Bird and Saklatvala, 1990) and NFκB is an example of one of the nuclear factors that are activated by IL-1 (Stylianou *et al.*, 1992). The most frequently reported phosphorylations associated with IL-1 activation of cells are on serine and threonine residues.

Recent studies have identified the activation of nuclear binding proteins within 15 min of IL-1 binding. Late events are most often linked to new gene transcription and the synthesis of new proteins. There is an increasing list of new genes and proteins synthesized by cells following exposure to IL-1. There are also some genes whose expression is reduced by IL-1, for example albumin and lipoprotein lipase, but these are few compared with the number of genes whose expression is either initiated or upregulated by IL-1. Some of these have been reviewed (Dinarello, 1991).

There can be confusion about the early and late effects of IL-1. For example, within 6–8 min following the intravenous injection of IL-1, elevated body temperature (fever) is initiated and this event is clearly mediated by PGE_2 synthesis. In the case of fever, the increase in hypothalamic PGE_2 is caused by IL-1-mediated release of arachidonic acid from phospholipids of cell membranes. Once released, arachidonic acid is rapidly converted to prostaglandins and/or leukotrienes by their respective 'household' enzymes. This rapid release and oxygenation of arachidonic acid accounts for the short time-frame of an IL-1 effect such as fever. This action of IL-1 should not be confused with the ability of IL-1 to induce gene expression for cyclooxygenases. For example, cells exposed to IL-1 *in vitro* will synthesize large amounts of PGE_2 but this is through

IL-1-induced cyclooxygenase gene expression (Raz *et al.*, 1988) and the PGE_2 levels that result can be elevated for several days.

The early and late events of IL-1 are likely due to the same signalling mechanism. The early event associated with fever requires the rapid release of arachidonic acid and IL-1 induces the hydrolysis of phospholipids from cell membranes within 3–5 min (Rosoff *et al.*, 1988). This action of IL-1 would account for such a rapid event. Several groups have reported that IL-1 causes a rapid but transient increase in diacyl glycerol release from either phosphatidylcholine or phosphatidylethanoloamine (Rosoff, 1989). TNF has also been reported to release arachidonic acid from phosphatidylcholine. The hydrolysis of phospholipids by specific phospholipase C generates diacyl glycerol. Resident diacyl glycerol lipase cleaves arachidonic acid from the number two position and the release of arachidonic acid is the rate-limiting step in the formation of prostaglandins and leukotrienes.

The hydrolysis of phosphatidylcholine requires phosphatidylcholine-specific phospholipase C; however, the activation of phosphatidylcholine-specific phospholipase C takes place without an increase in cytosolic calcium. With few exceptions, studies fail to observe a change in cytosolic calcium associated with IL-1 (Rosoff, 1989).

New gene expression and protein synthesis induced in cells stimulated by IL-1 are linked to phosphorylations of various nuclear binding proteins which then, in turn, activate new gene expression. In T cells stimulated with agonists for the T-cell receptor, the addition of IL-1 increases the amount of c-jun and c-fos, the two components of the AP-1 factor (Muegge *et al.*, 1989). AP-1 sites are present in the promoter region of many genes whose expression is increased following incubation with IL-1, including the promoter regions for IL-1 itself and IL-1Ra. Recent studies have examined more carefully the role of c-jun and c-fos transcription in activating AP-1 motifs following addition of IL-1.

IL-1 AS A MEDIATOR OF DISEASE

Microorganisms produce lethal toxins which, upon entrance into the circulation cause hypotension, decreased perfusion of vital organs, acidosis and death. It makes no difference whether these are endotoxins from Gram-negative bacteria or exotoxins from Gram-positive organisms (Ikejima *et al.*, 1988). A significant breakthrough came when blocking TNF reduced death in mice from a lethal endotoxin challenge (Beutler *et al.*, 1985) or in baboons given a lethal injection of *E. coli* bacteria (Tracey *et al.*, 1987). Similar studies showed that blocking IL-1 using the IL-1 receptor antagonist (IL-1Ra) also prevents lethal shock in mice, rabbits and baboons (Ohlsson *et al.*, 1990; Alexander *et al.*, 1991; Fischer *et al.*, 1992a; Wakabayashi *et al.*, 1991a). Together, these experiments clearly established that blocking a cytokine would prevent a host-mediated, self-destructive process. In Phase III clinical trials, either anti-TNF monoclonal antibodies or IL-1Ra have been effective in reducing deaths in some humans with septic shock syndrome. These anti-cytokine agents are also effective in reducing acute, noninfectious disease which is characterized by generalized cytokine-activated endothelium. Therefore, the septic shock syndrome falls into a category which is now termed the Systemic Inflammatory Response Syndrome, SIRS (Bone, 1993). Although the septic shock syndrome accounts for most cases of SIRS, other diseases such as acute pancreatitis, organ rejection and disseminated intravascular coagulation fulfill the criteria for SIRS. Cytokines, particularly IL-1 and TNF, play a critical role in mediating SIRS.

Production of IL-1 During Models of Disease in Animals

Specific cDNAs of rabbit IL-1α and IL-1β (Cannon *et al.*, 1989) have been used to study gene expression for IL-1 *in vivo*. New transcription was observed in various tissues as early as 15 min after an intravenous injection of a nonlethel dose of endotoxin. Rabbit IL-1 was measured in the circulation and tissues at 30 min with peak levels from 2–4 h after the endotoxin injection (Clark *et al.*, 1991). Nearly every tissue examined produced IL-1, although the highest levels were found in the liver, spleen, and lung (Clark *et al.*, 1991). During bacteraemia in rabbits injected with *E. coli* organisms, plasma levels of IL-1β are elevated to over 2000 pg/ml (Wakabayashi *et al.*, 1991a,b). IL-1β reached peak levels 180 min after the infusion of organisms and IL-1β levels correlated with the degree of hypotension ($r = 0.87$, $P < 0.01$) (Wakabayashi *et al.*, 1991b). Although IL-1α levels in human plasma are rarely elevated, in the rabbit model of severe sepsis, IL-1α levels correlated with IL-1β levels but were fivefold lower (Wakabayashi *et al.*, 1991b). Cell death and release of intracellular contents may account for the presence of IL-1α in the plasma of these rabbits. One does not need bacterial lipopolysaccharide to induce shock or IL-1. Using heat-killed *Staphylococcus epidermidis*, we observed a degree of hypotension that was comparable to that produced by *E. coli*, and which correlated with IL-1β levels (Wakabayashi *et al.*, 1991b). In those studies using *Staphylococcus epidermidis*, there was no detectable endotoxin in the circulation.

Circulating IL-1 in Humans

Experimental endotoxaemia in humans is a useful tool with which to study the production of cytokines. A single intravenous injection into healthy human subjects of *E. coli* endotoxin at 3–4 ng/kg induces fever, cytokinaemia and several haematological and endocrinological changes characteristic of infection and inflammation (Dinarello *et al.*, 1981; Watters *et al.*, 1985, 1986; Revhaug *et al.*, 1988; Cannon *et al.*, 1990). Using this model, elevated levels of TNF-α and IL-1β have been measured (Michie *et al.*, 1988; Cannon *et al.*, 1990) which reach peak plasma levels at 90 and 180 min, respectively, as has been observed in animals (Wakabayashi *et al.*, 1991a,b). Unless the plasma is extracted in chloroform (Cannon *et al.*, 1988), IL-1β is not detectable following this dose of LPS. Elevated levels of IL-1β are also found in patients with infections (Cannon *et al.*, 1990, 1992). IL-1β and TNF-α levels correlate in some patients directly with the APACHE II (Acute Physiology And Chronic Health Evaluation) score, which is an index of disease severity. In other studies, a single determination of circulating levels of these cytokines does not correlate with the severity of disease (Cannon *et al.*, 1992). This may be related to the episodic nature of cytokine release.

Production of IL-1 from Cells

A large number of studies have used the production of cytokines from peripheral blood mononuclear cells (PBMC) *in vitro* as an indicator of disease activity. Other cells have included pulmonary alveolar macrophages and peritoneal macrophages. In general, IL-1 is not present in these cells when taken from healthy subjects; however, PBMC cultured *in vitro* from patients with a variety of diseases such as rheumatoid arthritis, osteomalacia, sepsis and vasculitis produced elevated amounts of IL-1. This subject has been reviewed previously (Dinarello, 1991).

THE BIOLOGICAL EFFECTS OF IL-1

Expression of Various Genes in Cells Exposed to IL-1

A fundamental property of IL-1's role in mediating disease includes its ability to induce a wide variety of genes. In some cases, IL-1 induces new transcripts such as serum amyloid A protein (Ramadori *et al.*, 1985) or IL-1 itself (Dinarello *et al.*, 1987), whereas for other genes, the effect of IL-1 represents stabilization and prolonging of mRNA half-life. This has been observed for GM-CSF (Demetri *et al.*, 1989; Ernst *et al.*, 1989; Griffin *et al.*, 1990). In general, IL-1 stimulates new transcripts for several protoonco-genes (Bottazzi *et al.*, 1990). Recent studies by Rangnekar and coworkers have described five 'early' genes induced by IL-1 in melanoma cells which appear to suppress the growth of these cells (Rangnekar *et al.*, 1992). However, it is important to note that IL-1 suppresses the expression of other genes, for example albumin, cytochrome P450, and aromatase by reducing new transcription.

IL-1 Infusion Mimics Shock

Many of the biological effects of IL-1 are similar to those observed during a toxic event; however, recent studies in humans have confirmed data from animal experiments. IL-1α or IL-1β have been administered to humans in Phase I trials. Systemic adminis-tration of intravenous IL-1 from 1–10 ng/kg has produced fever, sleepiness, anorexia, generalized myalgias, arthralgias, and headache. However, the most dramatic biologi-cal response to IL-1 was observed at doses of 100 ng/kg or higher. In those patients a rapid fall in blood pressure takes place (Smith *et al.*, 1992). Because of these results, the dose-limiting toxicity for IL-1 of hypotension has been set at 300 ng/kg. In some patients receiving 1 μg/kg, stage IV hypotension was reported (Smith *et al.*, 1992). The subcutaneous route is associated with fewer side effects. Laboratory data confirm the neutrophilia-inducing property of IL-1, but increased circulating platelets have also been observed (Tewari *et al.*, 1990). In general, the experience of IL-1 in humans is consistent with observations in the rabbit and other animals.

   In the rabbit, a single intravenous injection of 10 μg/kg of recombinant human IL-1β resulted in a shock-like state with hypotension, neutropenia and thrombocytopenia (Okusawa *et al.*, 1988). This has been confirmed in studies using IL-1α in baboons (Fischer *et al.*, 1991). The mechanism for the hypotensive effect of IL-1 appears to be the generation of at least three small-molecular-weight mediators: cyclooxygenase products (Okusawa *et al.*, 1988), platelet activating factor and nitric oxide (Beasley *et al.*, 1991). The fall in circulating leukocytes and platelets is thought to be caused by the stimulation of endothelial adhesion molecules, a particularly important property of IL-1. The effects of IL-1 in inducing a shock-like state are potentiated by coinfusion of

TNF. The potentiation of IL-1 and TNF has been observed in anaesthetized (Okusawa *et al.*, 1988) as well as in the conscious rabbit (Tredget *et al.*, 1988). In the conscious rabbit, injection of IL-1 and TNF together induced a fall in mean arterial pressure, onset of lactic acidosis and glucose intolerance. Many effects of IL-1 and TNF are synergistic in a variety of models *in vitro* and *in vivo*.

IL-1 Effects on the Central Nervous System

IL-1 is a potent pyrogen. Even at the lowest doses of IL-1 admistered to humans (1 ng/kg), some patients developed fever (Tewari *et al.*, 1990). In experimental animals, IL-1 induces slow-wave sleep and decreases rapid eye movement sleep. Compared with molecules of similar size, however, IL-1 does not cross the blood–brain barrier and does not enter the substance of the central nervous system (Coceani *et al.*, 1988). However, the rapid (5 min) induction of fever, sleep and the release of a variety of neuropeptides suggest that IL-1 readily affects structures in the central nervous system. It is likely that IL-1 acts on the special endothelial cells of the periventricular organs where the blood–brain barrier is interrupted; furthermore, arachidonic acid metabolites are released from these cells. IL-1Rs are found distributed throughout the brain. Glial and possibly neuronal cells synthesize IL-1.

Changes in Hepatocytes Caused by IL-1

IL-1 induces increases in normal hepatic proteins two- to three-fold, but the synthesis of pathological proteins can increase 100-fold to 1000-fold. One such protein, serum amyloid A protein, contributes to the development of secondary amyloidosis. Both *in vitro* and *in vivo*, IL-1 induces hepatocytes to synthesize fibrinogen, complement components, factor B, metallothioneins, and various clotting factors. Some of these effects are via the intermediate production of IL-6, leukemia inhibitory factor and/or ciliary neurotropic factor. In isolated hepatocytes, IL-1 decreases the transcription of RNA coding for albumin, transferrin, lipoprotein lipase and cytochromes. Recent studies have focused on the role of IL-1 in the hyperlipidaemia associated with infections. IL-1 reduces gene expression for lipoprotein lipase but, in addition, also stimulates fatty acid synthesis by increasing hepatic citrate levels (Grunfeld *et al.*, 1990). There is also a role for IL-1 in the hypertriglyceridaemia of infection.

Catabolic Effects of IL-1

Although early studies suggested that IL-1 played a role in the negative nitrogen balance often associated with chronic disease by inducing muscle proteolysis, subsequent studies have not confirmed that isolated muscle tissues incubated with IL-1 *in vitro* release amino acids (Moldawer *et al.*, 1988). However, IL-1 likely contributes to the development of negative nitrogen balance because IL-1 administration in combination with TNF increases loss of mean body mass (Flores *et al.*, 1989). In addition, IL-1 reduces food intake in experimental animals. It should be pointed out that animals given daily injections of IL-1 exhibit tachyphylaxis to the anorectic property of IL-1 (Hellerstein *et al.*, 1989; Mrosovsky *et al.*, 1989). IL-1 also induces hypoglycaemia and this effect may be due to the ability of IL-1 to increase insulin (Wogensen *et al.*, 1988) or the synthesis of glucose transporters, thus increasing intracellular glucose levels (Bird *et al.*, 1990). The mechanism of IL-1-induced anorexia is thought to be due to a direct effect on the liver which subsequently affects the hypothalamic appetite centre (Hellerstein *et al.*, 1989). This concept is supported by a study in which systemically administered antibodies to the IL-1RI blocks the weight loss associated with inflammation (Gershenwald *et al.*, 1990).

Vascular Wall Effects of IL-1

Arterial perfusion with IL-1 increases prostanoid synthesis, which lowers the pain threshold to bradykinin (Schweizer *et al.*, 1988). TNF potentiates these effects of IL-1 whereas pretreatment with cyclooxygenase inhibitors blocks the response. IL-1 also inhibits vascular smooth muscle contraction (Beasley *et al.*, 1989) independent of prostaglandin synthesis. The inhibition of smooth muscle contraction by IL-1 appears to be due to an L-arginine-dependent increase in nitric oxide production, leading to increased guanylate cyclase activity (Beasley *et al.*, 1991).

Cultured endothelial cells exposed to IL-1 express adhesion molecules, which leads to the adherence of leukocytes to endothelial surfaces. These IL-1-treated endothelial cells also increase procoagulant activity, tissue factor, PGE_2, PGI_2, platelet activating factor, and plasmingen activator inhibitor production (Rossi *et al.*, 1985; Dejana *et al.*, 1987). The pro-inflammatory effect of IL-1 on endothelial cells likely plays a role in vasculitis (Movat *et al.*, 1987).

Endocrinologic Effects of IL-1

Within 10 min of an intravenous injection of IL-1, several neuropeptides are released into the systemic circulation; increased corticotropin releasing factor (ACTH), endorphins, vasopressin and somatostatin are induced by IL-1 whereas IL-1 inhibits thyroid releasing hormone-induced prolactin release. The effect of IL-1 on ACTH release is via a cyclooxygenase metabolite pathway. It has been proposed that IL-1-induced corticosteroids (via direct and indirect ACTH action) represents a biological negative-feedback loop since corticosteroids inhibit cytokine gene expression (Del Rey *et al.*, 1987). The IL-1-induced corticosteroids serve some protective effect since adrenalectomized mice are markedly sensitive to the IL-1-induced lethality (Bertini *et al.*, 1988).

Haematopoietic Effects of IL-1

There are various levels at which IL-1 affects haematopoiesis. IL-1 induces the production of GM-CSF, G-CSF, M-CSF, IL-3 (Bagby *et al.*, 1986; Zucali *et al.*, 1986; Zsebo *et al.*, 1988) and acts synergistically with CSFs and IL-6 on a haematopoiesis, particularly at the stem cell level. The increased production of these factors can be through new mRNA transcription or as in the case of GM-CSF, through stabilization of mRNA (Bagby, 1989; Griffin *et al.*, 1990). IL-1, by itself, has no effect on stem cell proliferation or differentiation but requires CSFs such as IL-3 or IL-6. Stem cell factor is a unique cytokine which synergizes with CSFs (McNiece *et al.*, 1990); it is possible that IL-1's activity on stem cells is a result of induction of stem cell factor or synergy with this cytokine.

The necessary cofactor for colony formation after bone marrow treatment with cytotoxic drugs was originally described as haemopoietin-1; during molecular cloning, haemopoietin-1 was identified as IL-1α; IL-1β also possesses haemopoietin-1 activity. A single injection of IL-1 stimulates circulating CSFs, protects stem cells, and accelerates the return of granulocytes following cytotoxic drugs or irradiation (Schwartz *et al.*, 1987; Neta *et al.*, 1988; Fibbe *et al.*, 1989; Oppenheim *et al.*, 1989). IL-1 suppresses erythroid precursors.

COMPARISON OF IL-1 WITH TNF AND IL-6

IL-1 and TNF

The biological properties of TNF share remarkable similarities to those of IL-1. When the two cytokines are used together in experimental studies, the net effect often exceeds the additive effect of each cytokine. Potentiation or synergism between these two molecules has been demonstrated in the induction of a shock-like state (Okusawa *et al.*, 1988), on fibroblast production of PGE$_2$, on the cytotoxic effects on insulin-producing β cells of the islets of Langerhans (Mandrup-Poulsen *et al.*, 1987) and muscle proteolysis in rats (Flores *et al.*, 1989). The synergism between these two cytokines seems to be due to second message molecules rather than upregulation of cell receptors; in fact, IL-1 reduces TNF receptors (Holtmann and Wallach, 1989; Wallach *et al.*, 1989).

IL-1 and IL-6

In some models, the production of IL-6 appears to be under the control of IL-1; for example, mice subjected to an inflammatory event induced by intramuscular injection of turpentine fail to produce IL-6 when pretreated with anti-IL-1 receptor antibodies (Gershenwald *et al.*, 1990). In baboons injected with *E. coli*, anti-TNF antibodies prevent the appearance of IL-6 in the circulation (Fong *et al.*, 1989). IL-IRa reduces the amount of endotoxin-stimulated IL-6 produced by human monocytes *in vitro* (Granowitz *et al.*, 1992a,d) and *in vivo* (Henricson *et al.*, 1991). Levels of IL-6 often correlate with the amount of fever and severity of disease in patients with infections. The best correlations of the severity of disease with any plasma cytokine are clearly those with IL-6, not IL-1 or TNF. However, it is important to note that unlike IL-1 and TNF, there is no evidence that IL-6 is a lethal cytokine.

IL-6 does not cause shock in mice or primates regardless of the amount given, either alone or with TNF. In humans, intravenous administration of IL-6 at 30 μg/kg has not produced hypotension, whereas at 100 ng/kg IL-1 induces a fall in blood pressure in nearly all patients (Smith *et al.*, 1992). IL-6 suppresses LPS- and TNF-induced IL-1 production (Schindler *et al.*, 1990e). In general, IL-6 appears to be an anti-inflammatory cytokine. The spectrum of acute-phase proteins induced by IL-6 includes many anti-proteases and one interpretation of the biological significance of IL-6 is the anti-inflammatory property of these anti-proteases.

PREVENTING IL-1 EFFECTS

What Controls IL-1 Gene Expression and Synthesis?

Gene Expression and Translational Control

The two forms of IL-1 appear to be under separate transcriptional control (Turner *et al.*, 1989; Yamato *et al.*, 1989). Critical to understanding IL-1 gene expression is the exquisite sensitivity to LPS. In human blood monocytes, 10–20 pg/ml of LPS which is found in routine tissue culture media induce IL-1 production. When subjected to ultrafiltration to remove IL-1-inducing substances (Schindler and Dinarello, 1990), there is no IL-1β or IL-1α gene expression in circulating monocytes of healthy subjects by Northern hybridization, *in situ* hybridization or polymerase chain reaction. However, adherence of monocytes to glass or polystyrene triggers IL-1β gene expression (Schindler *et al.*, 1990a). Transcription of IL-1β mRNA is rapid; in macrophage cell lines, endothelial, smooth muscle, and blood monocytes, LPS-stimulated IL-1β RNA transcription is observed within 15 min (Libby *et al.*, 1986a,b; Fenton *et al.*, 1987, 1988; Schindler *et al.*, 1990a). Peak accumulation of mRNA occurs after 3–4 h, is sustained for 6–8 h and then decreases rapidly. There is synthesis of a transcriptional repressor as well as an increase in the half-life of the mRNA (Fenton *et al.*, 1987, 1988). Conversely, using IL-1 as a stimulus of its own gene expression, steady-state levels are slower to rise and are sustained for 30 h (Schindler *et al.*, 1990c).

Transcription and translation of IL-1 are distinct and dissociated processes. Transcription without translation can be observed following adherence of blood monocytes to surfaces, or exposure to recombinant C5a, β-glucan polymers, or calcium ionophore (Yamoto *et al.*, 1989; Schindler *et al.*, 1990a,b,d); in each case, steady-state mRNA levels for IL-1β are comparable with those using 1 ng/ml of LPS but unlike LPS, there is no translation of the IL-1 mRNA into protein. The half-life of mRNA is unchanged in using these stimuli suggesting that accelerated destruction of mRNA is not the explanation for the failure of translation (Schindler *et al.*, 1990b). Cells containing untranslated IL-1 mRNA are 'primed' and small amounts of other stimuli (LPS or IL-1 itself) rapidly trigger translation and this results in more IL-1 synthesis than non-primed cells. Another stimulus, heat-killed *S. epidermidis*, primarily delivers a translational signal (Schindler *et al.*, 1990a).

IL-1 stimulates its own gene expression and synthesis in blood monocytes, fibroblasts, endothelial and smooth muscle cells (Dinarello *et al.*, 1987; Warner *et al.*, 1987a,b). TNF (Dinarello *et al.*, 1986), GM-CSF (Sisson and Dinarello, 1988) and M-CSF also stimulate IL-1 production. In the strict absence of endotoxins, interferon-γ (IFN-γ) does not stimulate IL-1 transcription or synthesis but rather suppresses IL-1-induced IL-1 production (Ghezzi and Dinarello, 1988) at the level of transcriptional activation (Schindler *et al.*, 1990c). Conversely, IFN-γ augments transcription, translation and secretion of LPS-induced IL-1 (Schindler *et al.*, 1990c; Ucla *et al.*, 1990). Although IFN-γ augments LPS-induced IL-1 production, LPS-induced IL-1 transcription is suppressed by IL-4 (Hart *et al.*, 1989; Vannier *et al.*, 1992), IL-6 (Schindler *et al.*, 1990d), transforming growth factor β (TGF-β) (Chantry *et al.*, 1989), IL-10 and IL-13.

Corticosteroids suppress IL-1 transcription and synthesis when added before initiation of transcription (Knudsen *et al.*, 1987); they are less effective when added after transcription. IL-1 transcription is unaffected by specific inhibitors of the

5-lipoxygenase pathway (Sirko *et al.*, 1991). The 13-lipoxygenase pathway products may be involved in the early events of transcription (Schade *et al.*, 1987). The importance of lipoxygenase products in the production of IL-1 has been demonstrated in blood monocytes taken from human volunteers consuming eicosapentaenoic (N-3) fatty acid dietary supplements or a diet rich in these fatty acids (Endres *et al.*, 1989b; Meydani *et al.*, 1990, 1993); a 50–70% reduction in *ex vivo* IL-1β total synthesis has been consistently observed.

Role of cAMP in IL-1 Production

LPS, prostaglandins and prostacyclin have almost no effect on transcription but reduce translation of IL-1 (Knudsen *et al.*, 1986a). Blocking cyclooxygenase increases production of IL-1. Prostaglandin-induced suppression of IL-1 translation appears to be via the induction of cAMP. The addition of PGE or dibutyryl cAMP suppresses LPS-induced IL-1 synthesis (Knudsen *et al.*, 1986a; Hurme, 1990).

The effects of cAMP on IL-1 synthesis and gene expression depend on the type of stimulant used for IL-1 production. For example, histamine, which reduces LPS-induced IL-1 synthesis via a cAMP pathway, enhances IL-1-induced IL-1 synthesis and gene expression (Vannier and Dinarello, 1993). Similarly, PGE$_2$ enhances IL-1-induced IL-1, and this is reduced by cyclooxygenase inhibitors (Vannier and Dinarello, 1993).

Strategies for Blocking Secretion and Processing

Secretion of IL-1

IL-1α and IL-1β lack classic signal peptides; hence, a considerable amount of IL-1 remains in the precursor form and cell-associated. Precursor IL-1α is thought to be biologically active and capable of binding to cell surface receptors. This would suggest that there are intracellular receptors for IL-1α, and one possible site is the nucleus. Anti-sense IL-1α prevents cultured endothelial cells from their programmed cell apoptosis (Maier *et al.*, 1990). In addition, an intracellular form of the IL-1Ra may block IL-1α in keratinocytes from these same functions (Haskill *et al.*, 1991).

Despite the lack of a signal peptide, IL-1β does get out of the cell. The amount of IL-1 which is 'secreted' depends upon the cell type and the conditions of stimulation. For example, the blood monocyte appears to be highly efficient in secreting IL-1β compared with endothelial cells, smooth muscle cells or fibroblasts. Nearly all IL-1α remains cell-associated (Endres *et al.*, 1989a; Lonnemann *et al.*, 1989). There are three populations of human monocytes: one population produces both IL-1α and IL-1β and the other two populations produce either IL-1α or IL-1β (Barkley *et al.*, 1989; Andersson *et al.*, 1992). With heat-killed *S. epidermidis* as a stimulus, nearly all IL-1β is secreted from monocytes. In cells stimulated with IL-1α or IL-2, nearly all IL-1β remains cell-associated (Dinarello *et al.*, 1987; Numerof *et al.*, 1988, 1990).

It is still unclear how IL-1 is transported from the cytosol to the extracellular compartment, but evidence suggests that a multiple-drug-resistance glycoprotein may be involved in this event (Young and Krasney, 1991). Secretion and processing to the mature peptide appear to be linked events, although some studies demonstrate that pro-IL-1β can be secreted intact (Auron *et al.*, 1987) and then later cleaved by serine proteases present in inflamed tissue. IFN-γ enhances the amount of IL-1β which is secreted from monocytes stimulated with endotoxin (Schindler *et al.*, 1990b) and this may be via IFN's ability to suppress PGE$_2$ synthesis. Inhibiting prostaglandins by indomethacin also increases the secretion of IL-1β.

IL-1 Converting Enzyme

Mature IL-1β has an *N*-terminus at the alanine position 117 (Van Damme *et al.*, 1985) but other naturally occurring *N*-termini have been reported (Knudsen *et al.*, 1986b; Mizutani *et al.*, 1991). A 22 kDa intermediate peptide is found in the supernatants of monocytes (Auron *et al.*, 1987; Beuscher *et al.*, 1988), suggesting that pro-IL-1β can be secreted prior to generation of the mature peptide. When cell injury occurs, this contributes to the release of pro-IL-1β. However, IL-1β is found outside the cell under conditions in which there is no IL-1α nor lactic acid dehydrogenase.

Elastase, plasmin, cathepsin G, collagenase, and other serine proteases have been implicated in the cleavage of pro-IL-1β into an active 17 kDa carboxyl fragment (reviewed in Dinarello, 1991). ICE is a cytosolic endopeptidase that specifically cleaves IL-1β at the alanine position (Black *et al.*, 1988; Kostura *et al.*, 1989). This protease is not found in fibroblasts but rather in monocytes. The cDNA coding for ICE has been cloned (Cerretti *et al.*, 1992; Thornberry *et al.*, 1992). It appears to be a unique cysteine protease. A dermal mast-cell chymase also accomplishes cleavage (Mizutani *et al.*, 1991). Blockade of ICE has been proposed as a strategy for preventing the effects of IL-1 in disease. Some viruses contain genes coding for a protein specifically inhibiting an ICE-like enzyme (Ray *et al.*, 1992).

IL-1Ra

Specific Receptor Blockade by IL-1Ra

Naturally occurring substances that specifically inhibit IL-1 activity have been detected in the serum of human volunteers injected with bacterial LPS (Dinarello *et al.*, 1981), supernatants of human monocytes adhering to IgG-coated surfaces (Arend *et al.*, 1985) and urine of patients with monocytic leukaemia (Seckinger and Dayer, 1987). A glucocorticoid-induced substance from keratinocytes also specifically blocks IL-1 (Stosic-Grujicic and Lukic, 1992). The 'IL-1 inhibitor' (Arend *et al.*, 1985, 1989; Seckinger *et al.*, 1987; Seckinger and Dayer, 1987) is a 23–25 kDa protein. It has been purified from the urine of patients with monocytic leukaemia (Seckinger *et al.*, 1987; Seckinger and Dayer, 1987; Mazzei *et al.*, 1990) and IgG-stimulated monocytes (Hannum *et al.*, 1990). This naturally occurring IL-1 inhibitor blocked the ability of IL-1 to stimulate synovial cell PGE$_2$ production, thymocyte proliferation, and decreased insulin release from isolated pancreatic islet cells (Balavoine *et al.*, 1986; Seckinger *et al.*, 1987; Seckinger and Dayer, 1987; Dayer-Metroz *et al.*, 1989).

The IL-1 urinary inhibitor blocked the binding of IL-1 to cells and did not possess agonist activity (Seckinger *et al.*, 1987). After purification from human monocytes (Hannum *et al.*, 1990) and urine (Mazzei *et al.*, 1990) and the confirmation of its mode of activity (Hannum *et al.*, 1990), the IL-1 inhibitor was re-named IL-1Ra. Antibodies produced to the recombinant human IL-1Ra recognize the purified urinary IL-1 inhibitor of Seckinger and Dayer, establishing that the IL-1 inhibitor and IL-1Ra are the same molecule (Seckinger *et al.*, 1990). An IL-1 inhibitor for the M20 myelomono-cytic cell line (Barak *et al.*, 1986) does not share identity with the IL-1Ra (Barak *et al.*, 1991).

IL-1Ra binds to the IL-1RI with near equal affinity as IL-1α or IL-1β (Eisenberg *et al.*, 1990) but does not transmit a signal on a variety of cells *in vitro* (Dripps *et al.*, 1991). IL-1Ra also recognizes the type II receptor (Granowitz *et al.*, 1991). In humans receiving large amounts of IL-1Ra intravenously, likewise, there have been no agonist-like activities (see below). The most likely explanation for the lack of biological activity of IL-1Ra is that the receptor binding sites for IL-1α, IL-1β and IL-1Ra are nearly the same but that IL-1Ra lacks a critical component of the three-dimensional structure which is responsible for triggering the receptor (Fig. 2). This structure appears to be the amino acids forming the loop of the nonopeptide (see above). Thus, a model for IL-1 binding to its receptor by sites not involved in triggering is proposed.

IL-1Ra Blocks IL-1 Activity In Vitro and In Vivo

Recombinant IL-1Ra blocks the activity of IL-1 administered to various animals. Rabbits (Ohlsson *et al.*, 1990) or baboons (Fischer *et al.*, 1991) injected with IL-1 develop hypotension which is prevented by prior administration of the IL-1Ra. However, what happens when IL-1 receptors are blocked in models of acute or chronic disease where several cytokines are produced? This has been studied in animal models. The results demonstrate that IL-1 receptor blockade significantly reduces the severity of disease, including those associated with infections, inflammation and metabolic disturbances (Arend, 1991; Dinarello and Thompson, 1991). Table 1 lists some of the effects of IL-1Ra administration in animal models of disease. In many of these models,

Table 1. Effects of specific blockade of the action of IL-1[a,b]

Improved survival in endotoxin-injected mice and rabbits and in newborn rats with *Klebsiella pneumoniae*-induced infection.
Diminution of shock in rabbits and baboons from *Escherichia coli* or *Staphylococcus epidermidis* bacteremia
Diminution of *Streptococcus* wall-induced arthritis in rats
Reduction in colonic tissue neutrophil infiltration in rabbits with immune-complex-induced inflammatory bowel disease
Delay in onset of spontaneous diabetes in bio-breeding rats
Decreased hypoglycaemia and production of CSF in mice after administration of endotoxin
Reduced proliferation of human acute myeloblastic and chronic myelogenous leukaemia cells
Decreased neutrophil accumulation in inflammatory peritonitis in mice
Decreased sciatic nerve regeneration in mice
Decreased severity of graft versus host disease in mice
Decreased lung neutrophil accumulation in rats following endotoxin
Improved survival of cardiac allografts in mice
Reduction in severity of experimental autoimmune encephalomyelitis in mice.
Lessening of anorexia and production of interleukin-6 in mice during turpentine-induced myositis

---

[a]Data are compiled, in part, from the following references: Arend (1991), Dinarello (1991) and Dinarello and Thompson (1991).
[b]These studies used IL-1Ra to block IL-1, except those for cardiac allograft rejection and experimental autoimmune encephalomyelitis in which soluble IL-1 receptors were used (Fanslow *et al.*, 1990; Jacobs *et al.*, 1991) and in reducing anorexia associated with inflammation, in which antibodies to the IL-1 type I receptor were used (Gershenwald *et al.*, 1990).

local inflammation plays a key role. The ability of IL-1Ra to block IL-1- and LPS-induced IL-8 production (Porat *et al.*, 1992) may be a major component of the anti-inflammatory properties of IL-1Ra.

In mice and rabbits injected with lethal doses of LPS, prior administration of IL-1Ra reduces the number of deaths (Ohlsson *et al.*, 1990; Alexander *et al.*, 1991). Decreased hypotension was observed in baboons treated with IL-1Ra and then given *E. coli* (Fischer *et al.*, 1991). We have studied the effects of IL-1Ra in two models of septic shock in the rabbits: Gram-negative sepsis caused by *E. coli* and Gram-positive infections by *S. epidermidis*. In the first model, we observed no deaths in rabbits receiving IL-1Ra when challenged with *E. coli* whereas control rabbits receiving saline had a 50% mortality when challenged with the bacteria (Wakabayashi *et al.*, 1991a). Following the injection of *E. coli*, mean blood pressure fell in both groups and this fall coincided with the appearance of TNF in the circulation. After the early episode of hypotension, blood pressure returned to pre-*E. coli* challenge levels in rabbits treated with IL-1Ra. We concluded that IL-1Ra was blocking the IL-1 effects which take place at 180 min and are associated with the IL-1 plasma peak. We also examined the effect of IL-1Ra in the model of Gram-positive sepsis and observed an almost complete block of hypotension, including the early fall in blood pressure associated with the TNF levels (Aiura *et al.*, 1993). In newborn rats, a lethal *Klebsiella* infection is blocked by a single injection of IL-1Ra (Mancilla *et al.*, 1993).

IL-1Ra in Human Subjects

Humans have been injected with IL-1Ra. In a Phase I trial, healthy volunteers were given a 3-h intravenous infusion of IL-1Ra from 1 to 10 mg/kg (Granowitz *et al.*, 1992c). Mean blood levels for volunteers receiving the 10 mg/kg dose were $29 \pm 2 \mu g/ml$. Post-infusion plasma levels fell rapidly and the initial half-life was 21 ± 3 min with a terminal half-life of 108 ± 18 min. Plasma clearance was 2.0 ± 0.3 ml/min.kg and less than 3.5% of the administered dose was recovered in the urine using an immunoreactive detection assay. The clearance of IL-1Ra from the plasma did not correlate with creatinine clearance.

In that study, there were no indications of agonist activity (clinical signs or symptoms) at any dose level (Granowitz *et al.*, 1992c). No changes were observed in hormonal or biochemical parameters. Haematological profiles were also unchanged. Considering the plasma levels of IL-1Ra were 100 000 times higher than those of IL-1β detected in the circulation of patients with severe sepsis (Cannon *et al.*, 1992), we conclude that IL-1Ra possesses no agonist activity and that short-term blockage of IL-1 receptors does not affect homeostatis (Granowitz *et al.*, 1992c).

Healthy humans have also been injected intravenously with a bolus of *E. coli* bacterial endotoxin (3 ng/kg) and at the same time received a 3-h infusion of IL-1Ra (Granowitz *et al.*, 1992a). Control subjects injected with endotoxin received a 3-h infusion of saline. IL-1Ra did not significantly reduce the fever or constitutional symptoms induced by endotoxin IL-1Ra (Granowitz *et al.*, 1992b). However, there was a statistically significant reduction in the endotoxin-induced neutrophilia (47%) and a complete reversal of the transient suppression of mitogen-induced mononuclear cell proliferation associated with endotoxaemia (Granowitz *et al.*, 1992b).

There have been two clinical trials testing the efficacy of IL-1Ra in patients with the sepsis syndrome (also called SIRS). The first trial compared four groups of 25 patients each; one group received placebo and the three other groups received increasing doses of IL-1Ra infused intravenously over 72 h. The two highest doses of 1 or 2 mg/kg.h (5 g or 10 g) revealed a significant reduction in 28-day mortality compared with placebo. The mortality rate in the placebo group was 44% and the reduction in mortality of the two groups of patients treated with IL-1Ra was 40% and 63%, respectively ($P = 0.015$).

The study was expanded to 893 patients in 63 hospitals in eight countries. This Phase III double-blind, placebo-controlled trial tested two doses of IL-1Ra (1 and 2 mg/kg.h for 72 h). Mortality in the placebo group was 34%, 31% in patients receiving 1 mg/kg.h and 29% in patients treated with 2 mg/kg.h ($P = 0.22$). However, a subgroup of 595 patients at high risk of death were analysed according to the severity of their disease as assessed by APACHE II scores. In this high-risk subgroup, mortality in patients receiving placebo was 45%, 37% in the group treated with 1 mg/kg.h and 35% in patients receiving 2 mg/kg.h (a 22% reduction in mortality, $P = 0.032$, Wilcoxon) (Fisher *et al.*, 1993).

These clinical data support laboratory and animal studies demonstrating that blockade of IL-1 is effective as the severity of disease increases. In less-severe models, blocking IL-1 receptors has little or no effect (Fischer *et al.*, 1992a; Aiura *et al.*, 1993). The studies in patients also confirm previous conclusions from animal experiments that high circulating levels of IL-1Ra ($>30 \mu g/ml$) are required for IL-1 receptor blockade *in vivo* (Ohlsson *et al.*, 1990).

The Production of IL-1 and IL-1Ra

Endotoxin is a stimulator of both IL-1 and IL-1Ra in human monocytes and each protein is produced by the same cell (Andersson *et al.*, 1992). The differential production of IL-1 compared with IL-1Ra can be observed in human blood monocytes under several conditions; for example, IL-1β is transcribed and synthesized in cells before IL-1Ra (Arend *et al.*, 1991). Immune complexes or IgG do not stimulate IL-1 synthesis or IL-1 mRNA, whereas in the same cell culture, large amounts of IL-1Ra are synthesized (Arend *et al.*, 1990; Poutsiaka *et al.*, 1991). However, preventing cell–cell contact prevents IL-1Ra synthesis but increases IL-1β production (Poutsiaka *et al.*, 1991).

Cytokines themselves exhibit differential regulation of production of IL-1Ra and IL-1. TGF-β, IL-4 (Vannier *et al.*, 1992), IFN-α (Tilg *et al.*, 1993) and GM-CSF are examples of cytokines that primarily increase IL-1Ra production with no significant increase in IL-1 synthesis. In the case of GM-CSF, 1–2 ng/10^6 monocytes of IL-1β or IL-1α are synthesized (Sisson and Dinarello, 1988) whereas these same cells produce 15–20 ng of IL-1Ra (Poutsiaka *et al.*, 1991). Although IFNs can potentiate the production of IL-1 in the presence of endotoxin (Schindler *et al.*, 1990b), they are themselves not inducers of IL-1. However, IFN in the absence of other stimuli triggers IL-1Ra production both *in vitro* and *in vivo* in human subjects (Tilg *et al.*, 1993). A special case exists for TGF-β and IL-4. These cytokines suppress the transcription of IL-1 in cells stimulated with LPS or IL-1 itself; however, in these same cells, IL-1Ra gene expression is upregulated by IL-4 (Vannier *et al.*, 1992).

The Balance of IL-1 and IL-1Ra

It remains unclear whether the relative concentration of IL-1 versus IL-1Ra has an impact on the outcome of disease. At present, only plasma levels are available for comparison. One important consideration is that monocyte/macrophage IL-1Ra contains a leader sequence, is found in the Golgi apparatus (Andersson *et al.*, 1992) and is transported out of cells, as are most secretory proteins. Conversely, IL-1β lacks a leader sequence and various amounts remain in the cytosol of the cell. Nevertheless, several studies have compared the plasma levels of IL-1Ra and IL-1β in various human disease states. In health, circulating levels of IL-1Ra are consistently in the 200–300 pg/ml range and stressful conditions such as a 3-h intravenous infusion of saline or a subcutaneous injection of saline do not result in elevation of these basal levels (Granowitz *et al.*, 1991; Fischer *et al.*, 1992b; Tilg *et al.*, 1993). In contrast, plasma IL-1Ra levels rise dramatically during experimental endotoxaemia in humans to 6–8000 pg/ml (Granowitz *et al.*, 1991; Fischer *et al.*, 1992b). IL-1Ra is found elevated in the circulation of septic humans with a variety of infectious or inflammatory diseases (Fischer *et al.*, 1992b). There is a positive correlation of serum creatinine and plasma IL-1Ra levels in patients with renal failure (Pereira *et al.*, 1992).

The dysregulation in production of the agonist and antagonist in human disease has been studied by Rambaldi and Cozzolino. Cells from each of 11 patients studied spontaneously expressed the gene for IL-1β, whereas leukaemic cells from only one of 11 patients expressed IL-1Ra following stimulation (Rambaldi *et al.*, 1991).

During experimental endotoxaemia in humans (Granowitz *et al.*, 1991), in sepsis (Fischer *et al.*, 1992b) or in systemic juvenile rheumatoid arthritis (Prieur *et al.*, 1987), large amounts of circulating IL-1Ra have been measured. In contrast, circulating IL-1β during infection in humans rarely exceeds 1 ng/ml (Cannon *et al.*, 1990, 1992). During experimental endotoxaemia in humans, levels of IL-1β reach a maximal concentration of 150–200 pg/ml after 3–4 h, and then fall rapidly; in these same individuals, the peak levels of IL-1Ra occur after 4 h, exceed the molar concentration of IL-1β by 100-fold and are sustained for 12 h (Granowitz *et al.*, 1991). During *E. coli* sepsis in baboons, peak IL-1Ra levels are also at 100-fold molar excess to those of IL-1β and levels are elevated 8–10 h later (Fischer *et al.*, 1992b).

Thus, production of a small amount of IL-1 but a large amount of the IL-1Ra appears to be a natural response in infectious diseases of bacterial origin. However, in terms of systemic treatment in humans and animals, a 100 000-fold plasma excess of IL-1Ra to IL-1 is needed to reduce mortality compared with a 100-fold excess which occurs naturally. Endogenously produced systemic levels of IL-1Ra may be inadequate in overwhelming infection or acute inflammation. Providing exogenous IL-1Ra in pharmacologic levels appears to have beneficial effects, as observed in animal models. However, tissue levels of endogenously produced IL-1Ra may contribute to limiting the severity of disease (Miller *et al.*, 1993).

Antibodies to IL-1 Receptors

Antibodies have been produced to the IL-1RI on murine cells (Chizzonite *et al.*, 1989; Lewis *et al.*, 1990). These have been used to block IL-1 effects *in vitro* and *in vivo*. For example, in animal models of infection and inflammation, anti-IL-1RI antibodies have reduced disease severity and the administration of these antibodies reveals that systemic responses of animals to IL-1 is via IL-1RI. For example, mice given intraperitoneal injections of IL-1 develop peritonitis with large numbers of neutrophils; however, prior treatment with anti-IL-1RI prevents the influx of neutrophils, synthesis of serum amyloid A protein and circulating IL-6 levels (Chizzonite *et al.*, 1989). Anti-IL-1RI also blocks the neutrophil influx in response to endotoxin by 50%. Mice given an intramuscular injection of turpentine manifest several acute-phase changes typical of inflammation such as decreased food intake, weight loss (lean and fat loss), IL-6 production, hepatic synthesis of amyloid P component, and elevated corticosterone levels. When anti-IL-1RI was given prior to the inflammatory event, 80–90% of the intensity of these responses was reduced, with the exception of elevated corticosterone levels (Gershenwald *et al.*, 1990). The protective effect of IL-1 on lethal radiation appears to be due to the type I receptor since anti-type I receptor antibodies block this IL-1 response and also the protective response induced by LPS (Neta *et al.*, 1990). This demonstrates that other cytokines such as IL-6 induced by the turpentine inflammation or LPS are secondary to the production and activity of IL-1.

The advantage of the anti-IL-1RI antibodies is that they block IL-1 effects for several hours to days whereas IL-1Ra blood levels need to be sustained at sufficiently high levels to block IL-1 effects. In animals and humans, this is in the range 20–30 μg/ml. Using either method, however, blocking of nearly all the IL-1R appears to be necessary because occupancy of as few as 5% of the IL-1R is sufficient to trigger an IL-1 response. At present, the number of available IL-1R on the surface of the endothelium in a rabbit is unknown but an intravenous bolus injection of 100 ng/kg of IL-1 to rabbits produces fever. The calculated peak blood levels in these animals is less than 100 pg/ml; a sustained level of 5 μg/ml of IL-1Ra is required to block this IL-1-induced fever (Dinarello *et al.*, 1992).

In vitro, a concentration of IL-1 of 10 pg/ml is a potent stimulus for IL-8 synthesis from blood monocytes. However, the calculated number of IL-1R occupied at 10 pg/ml is approximately 5%. This represents the 'spare receptor' hypothesis of IL-1 in which most of the receptors are not needed for a biological response (Ye *et al.*, 1992). Figure 2 illustrates the effects of partial or full IL-1R blockade. Another explanation for high levels of IL-1Ra may be the rapid excretion of IL-1Ra into the urine, whereas anti-IL-1R antibodies remain in the circulation for longer periods of time. In addition, during sepsis the numbers of IL-1R on circulating neutrophils increase dramatically and this increase may require more IL-1Ra.

Soluble IL-1 Receptors

The extracellular domain of the IL-1RI has been expressed and shown to bind both forms of IL-1 (see Fig. 2). When the recombinant soluble IL-1RI was given to mice undergoing heart transplantation, survival of the heterotopic allografts was increased. Lymph nodes directly injected with allogeneic cells have reduced hyperplasia with the use of the soluble IL-1RI (Fanslow *et al.*, 1990). Administration of soluble IL-1R to rats with autoimmune encephalomyelitis reduced the severity of the paralysis and delayed the onset of neurologic disease (Jacobs *et al.*, 1991). However, it is unclear from these experiments how much of the effects of the soluble type I receptor are due to decreased inflammation rather than decreased immuno-responsiveness.

Conditioned media from the IL-1RII-bearing Raji cells contain the soluble form (35–45 kDa) of the IL-1RII (Giri *et al.*, 1990). An IL-1-binding protein (soluble form of an IL-1R) was found circulating in humans with inflammatory disease and appears to be related to the type II receptor (Symons *et al.*, 1991). The type II receptor binds IL-1β

preferentially over that of IL-1α and may serve as a natural, circulating inhibitor of IL-1β in the blood. Some viruses produce proteins that have a high homology to the extracellular domain of the type II receptor and this appears to serve a protective role preventing IL-1-mediated activation of host defence systems.

DOES IL-1 BLOCKADE IMPAIR HOST DEFENCE?

Effect of IL-1 on Host Defence Mechanisms

Administration of a single, low dose of IL-1 protects animals against a variety of lethal and noxious events. In general, the protective effect of IL-1 is most effective when the cytokine is administered 24 h prior to the challenge (van der Meer *et al.*, 1988). For example, pretreatment with IL-1 reduces lethal hyperoxia in rats, bacterial cell wall arthritis in rats, antigen-induced histamine release in guinea pigs, immune-complex-mediated colitis in rabbits, endotoxin-induced liver damage and lethal radiation in mice. Pretreatment with IL-1 has also been used in a variety of bacterial infections such as cerebral malaria, and fungal and bacterial infections in normal and granulocytopenic mice. Although in models of infection in granulocytopenic mice there is the possibility of IL-1 accelerating bone marrow recovery, this is not the mechanism of protection and neither is protection related to a cyclooxygenase product (van der Meer *et al.*, 1988). However, protection against colitis and hyperoxia are mediated, in part, by IL-1-stimulated prostaglandins (Cominelli *et al.*, 1990; White and Ghezzi, 1989). Explanations for how a single, low dose of IL-1 can be so effective in affording protection include the ability of IL-1 to downregulate the TNF and IL-1 receptors (Wallach *et al.*, 1988; Ye *et al.*, 1992), induce oxygen scavenger molecules, or the release of corticosteroids.

Effects of IL-1Ra on Host Defence

From both animal and *in vitro* cell cultures, short-term blocking of IL-1 receptors does not appear to be immunosuppressive. In short-term animal models, twice daily administration of IL-1Ra has not affected cytotoxic T-cell responses nor impaired antibody formation (Faherty *et al.*, 1992). *In vitro*, IL-1Ra has not affected natural killer cell function nor the mixed leukocyte reaction (Nicod *et al.*, 1992). Because IL-1 induces PGE_2, and PGE_2 is a potent immunosuppressive agent for lymphocyte function, blocking IL-1 with IL-1Ra may result in some augmentation of lymphocyte function, particularly when monocytes are present in the cultures. In humans given daily injections of IL-1Ra for rheumatoid arthritis, lymphocyte function and lymphocyte phenotypes have not been affected after several weeks. Blood levels of IL-1Ra of 25 μg/ml in healthy humans did not affect *ex vivo* lymphocyte proliferation (Granowitz *et al.*, 1992c).

We have studied the effect of increasing doses of IL-1Ra administered to newborn rats infected with *Klebsiella pneumoniae*. A single dose of IL-1Ra of 5 mg/kg just prior to infection reduced mortality from 80% to 40% ($P < 0.05$). Administration of 5 mg/kg on two consecutive days did not improve survival nor did increasing IL-1Ra from 10 to 20 mg/kg. In contrast, administering 30 or 40 mg/kg of IL-1Ra resulted in a significant increase in mortality when compared with vehicle-injected controls ($P < 0.001$) (Mancilla *et al.*, 1993). These results suggest that blocking IL-1 receptors reduces IL-1-mediated death but that near-complete blockade of IL-1R can also be detrimental. Apparently, in this model, blockade of most IL-1R is beneficial and consistent with other data on IL-1R blockade in models of infection. We assume that at the higher doses of IL-1Ra, small amounts of IL-1, essential for the ability of these newborn rats to survive their infection, are being blocked. This interpretation would also be consistent with the observation that low doses of IL-1 are protective.

ACKNOWLEDGEMENTS

The studies mentioned in this chapter are supported by NIH Grant AI 15614. The author thanks K. Aiura, B.D. Clark, J.G. Cannon, J.A. Gelfand, E.V. Granowitz, G. Kaplanski, J. Kennedy, G. Lonnemann, J. Mancilla, L.C. Miller, S.F. Orencole, R. Porat, L. Shapiro, E. Vannier, T. Wilckens, Sheldon M. Wolff and K. Ye. Parts of this chapter have been adapted from previously published reviews on interleukin-1 (Dinarello, 1991; Dinarello and Wolff, 1993).

REFERENCES

Aiura, K., Gelfand, J.A., Wakabayashi, G., Burke, J.F., Thompson, R.C. and Dinarello, C.A. (1993) *Infect Immun.* **61**, 3342–3350.

Alexander, H.R., Doherty, G.M., Buresh, C.M., Venzon, D.J. and Norton, J.A. (1991). *J. Exp. Med.* **173**, 1029–1032.

Andersson, J., Björk, L., Dinarello, C.A., Towbin, H. and Andersson, U. (1992). *Eur. J. Immunol.* **22**, 2617–2623.

Antoni, G., Presentini, R., Perin, F., Nencioni, L., Villa, L. and Censini, S. (1989). *Adv. Exp. Med. Biol.* **251**, 153–160.

Arend, W.P. (1991). *J. Clin. Invest.* **88**, 1445–1451.

Arend, W.P., Joslin, F.G. and Massoni, R.J. (1985) *J. Immunol.* **134**, 3868–3875.

Arend, W.P., Joslin, F.G., Thompson, R.C. and Hannum, C.H. (1989). *J. Immunol.* **143**, 1851–1858.

Arend, W.P., Welgus, H.G., Thompson, R.C. and Eisenberg, S.P. (1990). *J. Clin. Invest.* **85**, 1694–1697.

Arend, W.P., Smith, M.F., Jr, Janson, R.W. and Joslin, F.G. (1991). *J. Immunol.* **147**, 1530–1536.

Auron, P.E., Warner, S.J., Webb, A.C. *et al.* (1987). *J. Immunol.* **138**, 1447–1456.

Bagby, G.C., Jr. (1989). *Blood Rev.* **3**, 152–161.

Bagby, G.C.J., Dinarello, C.A., Wallace, P., Wagner, C., Hefeneider, S. and McCall, E. (1986). *J. Clin. Invest.* **78**, 1316–1323.

Balavoine, J.F., de Rochemonteix, B., Williamson, K., Seckinger, P., Cruchaud, A. and Dayer, J.M. (1986). *J. Clin. Invest.* **78**, 1120–1124.

Barak, V., Treves, A.J., Yanai, P., Halperin, M., Wasserman, D., Biran, S. and Braun, S. (1986). *Eur. J. Immunol.* **16**, 1449–1452.

Barak, V., Peritt, D., Flechner, I. *et al.* (1991). *Lymphokine Cytokine Res.* **10**, 437–442.

Barkley, D., Feldmann, M. and Maini, R.N. (1989). *J. Immunol. Methods* **120**, 277–283.

Beasley, D.S., Cohen, R.A. and Levinsky, N.G. (1989). *J. Clin. Invest.* **83**, 331–335.

Beasley, D., Schwartz, J.H. and Brenner, B.M. (1991). *J. Clin. Invest.* **87**, 602–608.

Bertini, R., Bianchi, M. and Ghezzi, P. (1989). *J. Exp. Med.* **167**, 1708–1712.

Beuscher, H.U., Nickells, M.W. and Colten, H.R. (1988). *J. Biol. Chem.* **263**, 4023–4028.

Beutler, B., Milsark, I.W. and Cerami, A. (1985). *Science* **229**, 869–871.

Bird, T.A. and Saklatvala, J. (1990). *J. Biol. Chem.* **265**, 235–240.

Bird, T.A., Davies, T., Baldwin, S.A. and Saklatvala, J. (1990). *J. Biol. Chem.* **265**, 13578–13583.

Black, R.A., Kronheim, S.R., Cantrell, M., Deeley, M.C., March, C.J. and Prickett, K.S. (1988). *J. Biol. Chem.* **263**, 9437–9442.

Bone, R.C. (1993). *JAMA* **268**, 3452–3455.

Boraschi, D., Antoni, G., Perni, F., Villa, L., Nencioni, L., Ghiara, P., Presentini, R. and Tagliabue, A. (1990). *Eur. Cytokine* **1**, 21–26.
Bottazzi, B., Nobili, N. and Mantovani, A. (1990). *J. Immunol.* **144**, 4878–4882.
Brody, D.T. and Durum, S.K. (1989). *J. Immunol.* **143**, 1183.
Cannon, J.F., van der Meer, J.W., Kwiatkowski, D., Endres, S., Lonneman, G., Burke, J.F. and Dinarello, C.A. (1988). *Lymphokine Res.* **7**, 457–467.
Cannon, J.G., Clark, B.D., Wingfield, P. *et al.* (1989). *J. Immunol.* **142**, 2299–2306.
Cannon, J.G., Friedberg, J.S., Gelfand, J.A., Tompkins, R.G. Burke, J.F. and Dinarello, C.A. (1992). *Crit. Care Med.* **20**, 1414–1419.
Cannon, J.G., Tompkins, R.G., Gelfand, J.A., Michie, H.R., Stanford, G.G., van der Meer, J.W.M., Endres, S., Lonneman, G., Corsetti, J., Chernow, B., Wilmore, D.W., Wolf, S.M. and Dinarello, C.A. (1990). *J. Inf. Dis.* **161**, 79–84.
Casagli, M.C., Borri, M.G., Bigio. M. *et al.* (1989). *Biochem. Biophys. Res. Commun.* **162**, 357–363.
Cerretti, D.P., Kozlosky, C.J., Mosley, B. *et al.* (1992). *Science* **256**, 97–100.
Chantry, D., Turner, M., Abney, E. and Feldmann, M. (1989). *J. Immunol.* **142**, 4295–4300.
Chizzonite, R., Truitt, T., Kilian, O.L. *et al.* (1989). *Proc. Natl Acad. Sci. USA* **86**, 8029–8033.
Clark, B.D., Bedrosian, I., Schindler, R. *et al.* (1991). *J. Appl. Physiol.* **71**, 2412–2418.
Coceani, F., Lees, J. and Dinarello, C.A. (1988). *Brain Res.* **446**, 245–250.
Cominelli, F., Nast, C.C., Llerena, R., Dinarello, C.A. and Zipser, R.D. (1990). *J. Clin. Invest.* **85**, 582–586.
Dayer-Metroz, M.D., Wollheim, C.B., Seckinger, P. and Dayer, J.M. (1989). *J. Autoimmun.* **2**, 163–171.
Dejana, E., Breviario, F., Erroi, A. *et al.* (1989). *Blood* **69**, 695–699.
Del Rey, A., Besedovsky, H., Sorkin, E. and Dinarello, C.A. (1987). *Ann. N.Y. Acad. Sci.* **496**, 85–90.
Demetri, G.D., Zenzie, B.W., Rheinwald, J.G. and Griffin, J.D. (1989). *Blood* **74**, 940–946.
Dinarello, C.A. (1991). *Blood* **77**, 1627–1652.
Dinarello, C.A. and Thompson, R.C. (1991). *Immunol. Today* **12**, 404–410.
Dinarello, C.A. and Wolff, S.M. (1993). *N. Engl. J. Med.* **328**, 106–113.
Dinarello, C.A., Rosenwasser, L.J. and Wolff, S.M. (1981). *J. Immunol.* **127**., 2517–2519.
Dinarello, C.A., Cannon, J.G., Wolff, S.M. *et al.* (1986). *J. Exp. Med.* **163**, 1433–1450.
Dinarello, C.A., Ikejima, T. and Warner, S.J. (1987). *J. Immunol.* **139**, 1902–1910.
Dinarello, C.A., Zhang, X.X., Wen, H.D., Wolf, S.M. and Ikejima, T. (1992). In *The Effect of Interleukin-1 Receptor Antagonist on IL-1, LPS,* Staphylococcus epidermidis *and Tumor Necrosis Factor Fever* (eds T. Bartfai and D. Ottoson), Pergamon Press, Oxford, 11–18.
Dripps, D.J., Brandhuber, B.J., Thompson, R.C. and Eisenberg, S.P. (1991). *J. Biol. Chem.* **266**, 10331–10336.
Eisenberg, S.P., Evans, R.J., Arend, W.P. *et al.* (1990). *Nature* **343**, 341–346.
Endres, S., Cannon, J.G., Ghorbani, R. *et al.* (1989a). *Eur. J. Immunol.* **19**, 2327–2333.
Endres, S., Ghorbani, R., Kelley, V.E. *et al.* (1989b). *N. Engl. J. Med.* **320**, 265–271.
Ernst, T.J., Ritchie, A.R., Demetri, G.D. and Griffin, J.D. (1989). *J. Biol. Chem.* **264**, 5700–5703.
Faherty, D.A., Claudy, V., Plocinski, J.M. *et al.* (1992). *J. Immunol.* **148**, 766–771.
Fanslow, W.C., Simms, J.E., Sassenfeld, H. *et al.* (1990). *Science* **248**, 739–742.
Fenton, M.J., Vermeulen, M.W., Clark, B.D., Webb, A.C. and Auron, P.E. (1988). *J. Immunol.* **140**, 2267–2273.
Fenton, M.J., Clark, B.D., Collins, K.L., Webb, A.C., Rich, A. and Auron, P.E. (1987). *J. Immunol.* **138**, 3972–3979.
Fibbe, W.E., van der Meer, J.W.M., Falkenburg, J.H.F., Hamilton, M.S., Kluin, P.M. and Dinarello, C.A. (1989). *Exp. Hematol.* **17**, 805–808.
Fischer, E., Marano, M.A., Barber, A.E. *et al.* (1991). *Am. J. Physiol.* **261**, R442–R449.
Fischer, E., Marano, M.A., van Zee, K.J. *et al.* (1992a). *J. Clinc. Invest.* **89**, 1551–1557.
Fischer, E., Van Zee, K.J., Marano, M.A. *et al.* (1992b). *Blood* **79**, 2196–2200.
Fisher, C.J., Dhainaut, J.F., Pribble, J. and Knaus, W. Group, I.—1.P.I.S. (1993). *13th Int. Sym. Intensive Care Emerg. Med. Brussels* (Abst.).
Flores, E.A., Bistrian, B.R., Pomposelli, J.J., Dinarello, C.A., Blackburn, G.L. and Istfan, N.W. (1989). *J. Clin. Invest.* **83**, 1614–1622.
Fong, Y., Tracey, K.J., Moldawer, L.L. *et al.* (1989). *J. Exp. Med.* **170**, 1627–1633.
Gehrke, L., Jobling, S.A., Paik, L.S., McDonald, B., Rosenwasser, L.J. and Auron, P.E. (1990). *J. Biol. Chem.* **265**, 5922–5925.

Gershenwald, J.E., Fong, Y.M., Fahey, T.J. *et al.* (1990). *Proc. Natl Acad. Sci. USA* **87**, 4966–4970.
Ghezzi, P. and Dinarello, C.A. (1988). *J. Immunol* **140**, 4238–4244.
Giri, J., Newton, R.C. and Horuk, R. (1990). *J. Biol. Chem.* **265**, 17416–17419.
Granowitz, E.V., Mancilla, J., Clark, B.D. and Dinarello, C.A. (1991a). *J. Biol. Chem.* **266**, 14147–14150.
Granowitz, E.V., Santos, A., Poutsiaka, D.D. *et al.* (1991b). *Lancet* **338**, 1423–1424.
Granowitz, E.V., Clark, B.D., Vannier, E., Callahan, M.V. and Dinarello, C.A. (1992a). *Blood* **79**, 2356–2363.
Granowitz, E.V., Porat, R., Mier, J.W. *et al.* (1992b). *Clin. Res.* **40**, 651A (abst.).
Granowitz, E.V., Porat, R., Mier, J.W. *et al.* (1992c). *Cytokine* **4**, 353–360.
Granowitz, E.V., Vannier, E., Poutsiaka, D.D. and Dinarello, C.A. (1992d). *Blood* **79**, 2364–2369.
Griffin, J.D., Cannistra, S.A., Sullivan, R., Demetri, G.D., Ernst, T.J. and Kanakura, Y. (1990). *Int. J. Cell Cloning* **1**, 35–44.
Grunfeld, C., Soued, M., Adi, S., Moser, A.H., Dinarello, C.A. and Feingold, K.R. (1990). *Endocrinology* **127**, 46–52.
Guenard, V., Dinarello, C.A., Weston, P.J. and Aebischer, P. (1991). *J. Neurosci. Res.* **29**, 396–400.
Guesdon, F. and Saklatvala, J. (1991). *J. Immunol.* **147**, 3402–3407.
Hannum, C.H., Wilcox, C.J., Arend, W.P. *et al.* (1990). *Nature* **343**, 336–340.
Hart, P.H., Vitti, G.F., Burgess, D.R., Whitty, G.A., Piccoli, D.S. and Hamilton, J.A. (1989). *Proc. Natl Acad. Sci. USA* **86**, 3803–3807.
Haskill, S., Martin, M., VanLe, L. *et al.* (1991). *Proc. Natl Acad. Sci. USA* **88**, 3681–3685.
Heguy, A., Baldari, C.T., Censini, S., Ghiara, P. and Telford, J.L. (1993). *J. Biol. Chem.* **268**, 10490–10494.
Hellerstein, M.K., Meydani, S.N., Meydani, M., Wu, K. and Dinarello, C.A. (1989). *J. Clin. Invest.* **84**, 228–235.
Henricson, B.E., Neta, R. and Vogel, S.N. (1991). *Infect. Immun.* **59**, 1188–1192.
Holtmann, H. and Wallach, D. (1987). *J. Immunol.* **139**, 1161–1167.
Hurme, M. (1990). *FEBS Lett.* **263**, 35–37.
Ikejima, T., Okusawa, S., van der Meer, J.W. and Dinarello, C.A. (1988). *J. Inf. Dis.* **158**, 1017–1025.
Jacobs, C.A., Baker, P.E., Roux, E.R. *et al.* (1991). *J. Immunol.* **146**, 2983–2989.
Kaplanski, G., Porat, R., Aiura, K., Erban, J.K., Gelfand, J.A. and Dinarello, C.A. (1993). *Blood* **81**, 2492–2495.
Knudsen, P.J., Dinarello, C.A. and Strom, T.B. (1986a). *J. Immunol.* **137**, 3189–3194.
Knudsen, P.J., Dinarello, C.A. and Strom, T.B. (1986b). *J. Immunol.* **136**, 3311–3316.
Knudsen, P.J., Dinarello, C.A. and Strom, T.B. (1987). *J. Immunol.* **139**, 4129–4134.
Kostura, M.J. Tocci, M.J., Limjuco, G. *et al.* (1989). *Proc. Natl Acad. Sci. USA* **86**, 5227–5231.
Lewis, C., Mazzei, G. and Shaw, A. (1990). *Eur. J. Immunol.* **20**, 207–213.
Libby, P., Ordovas, J.M., Auger, K.R., Robbins, A.H., Birinyi, L.K. and Dinarello, C.A. (1986a). *Am. J. Pathol.* **124**, 179–185.
Libby, P., Ordovas, J.M., Birinyi, L.K., Auger, K.R. and Dinarello, C.A. (1986b). *J. Clin. Invest.* **78**, 1432–1438.
Lonnemann, G., Endres, S., van der Meer, J.W., Cannon, J.G., Kock, K.M. and Dinarello, C.A. (1989). *Eur. J. Immunol.* **19**, 1531–1536.
McMahon, C.J., Slack, J.L., Mosley, B. *et al.* (1991). *EMBO J.* **10**, 2821–2832.
McNiece, I., Langely, K. and Zsebo, K. (1990). *Blood* **76**(Suppl.), 154a.
Maier, J.A.M., Voulalas, P., Roeder, D. and Maciag, T. (1990). *Science* **249**, 1570–1574.
Mancilla, J., Ikejima, I. and Dinarello, C.A. (1992). *Lymphokine and Cytokine Research* **11**, 197–205.
Mancilla, J., Garcia, P. and Dinarello, C.A. (1993). *Infect. Immunol.* **61**, 926–932.
Mandrup-Poulsen, T., Bendtzen, K., Dinarello, C.A. and Nerup, J. (1987). *J. Immunol.* **139**, 4077–4082.
Mathias, S., Younes, A., Kan, C.-C., Orlow, I., Joseph, C. and Kolesnick, R.N. (1993). *Science* **259**, 519–522.
Mazzei, G.J., Seckinger, P.L., Dayer, J.M. and Shaw, A.R. (1990). *Eur. J. Immunol.* **20**, 683–689.
Meydani, S.N., Endres, S., Woods, M.M. *et al.* (1990). *J. Nutr.*
Meydani, S.N., Lichtenstein, A.H. and Cornwall, S. (1993). *J. Clin. Invest.*
Michie, H.R., Manogue, K.R., Spriggs, D.R. *et al.* (1988). *N. Engl. J. Med.* **318**, 1481–1486.
Miller, L.C., Lynch, E.A., Isa, S., Logan, J.W., Dinarello, C.A. and Steere, A.C. (1993). *Lancet* **341**, 146–148.
Mizel, S.B. (1990). *Immunol. Today* **11**, 390–391.
Mizutani, H., Schecter, N., Zazarus, G., Black, R.A. and Kupper, T.S. (1991). *J. Exp. Med.* **174**, 821–825.
Moldawer, L.L., Andersen, C., Gelin, J. and Lundholm, K.G. (1988). *Am. J. Physiol.* **254**, G450–G456.
Movat, H.Z., Burrowes, C.E., Cybulsky, M.I. and Dinarello, C.A. (1987). *Am. J. Pathol.* **129**, 463–476.

Mrosovsky, N., Molony, L.A., Conn, C.A. and Kluger, M.J. (1989). *Am. J. Physiol.* **257**, R1315–R1321.

Muegge, K., Williams, T.M., Kant, J. *et al.* (1989). *Science* **246**, 249–251.

Neta, R., Oppenheim, J.J. and Douches, S.D. (1988). *J. Immunol.* **140**, 108–111.

Neta, R., Plocinski, J.M. *et al.* (1990). *Blood* **76**, 57–62.

Nicod, L.P., el Haber, F. and Dayer, J.-M. (1992). *Cytokine* **4**, 29–35.

Numerof, R.P., Aronson, F.R. and Mier, J.W. (1988). *J. Immunol.* **141**, 4250–4257.

Numerof, R.P., Kotick, A.N., Dinarello, C.A. and Mier, J.W. (1990). *Cell Immunol.* **130**, 118–128.

O'Neill, L.A.J., Bird, T.A. and Saklatvala, J. (1990). *Immunol Today* **11**, 392–394.

Ohlsson, K., Bjork, P., Bergenfeldt, M., Hageman, R. and Thompson, R.C. (1990). *Nature* **348**, 550–552.

Okusawa, S., Gelfand, J.A., Ikejima, T., Connolly, R.J. and Dinarello, C.A. (1988). *J. Clin. Invest.* **81**, 1162–1172.

Oppenheim, J.J., Neta, R., Tiberghien, P., Gress, R., Kenny, J.J. and Longo, D.L. (1989). *Blood* **74**, 2257–2263.

Pereira, B.J.G., Poutsiaka, D.D., King, A.J. *et al.* (1992). *Kidney Int.* **42**, 1419–1424.

Porat, R., Poutsiaka, D.D., Miller, L.C., Granowitz, E.V. and Dinarello, C.A. (1992). *FASEB J.* **6**, 2482–2486.

Poutsiaka, D.D., Clark, B.D., Vannier, E. and Dinarello, C.A. (1991). *Blood* **78**, 1275–1281.

Priestle, J.P., Schar, H.P. and Grutter, M.G. (1988). *EMBO J.* **7**, 339–343.

Preistle, J.P., Schar, H.P. and Grutter, M.G. (1989). *Proc. Natl Acad. Sci. USA* **86**, 9667–9671.

Prieur, A.M., Kaufmann, M.T., Griscelli, C. and Dayer, J.M. (1987). *Lancet* **ii**, 1240–1242.

Ramadori, G., Sipe, J.D., Dinarello, C.A., Mizel, S.B. and Colten, H.R. (1985). *J. Exp. Med.* **162**, 930–942.

Rambaldi, A., Torcia, M., Bettoni, S. *et al.* (1991). *Blood* **78**, 3248–3253.

Rangnekar, V.V., Waheed, S. and Rangnekar, V.M. (1992). *J. Biol. Chem.* **267**, 6240–6248.

Ray, C.A., Black, R.A., Kronheim, S.R. *et al.* (1992). *Cell* **69**, 597–604.

Raz, A., Wyche, A., Siegel, N. and Needleman, P. (1988). *J. Biol. Chem.* **263**, 3022–3028.

Revhaug, A., Michie, H.R., Manson, J.M. *et al.* (1988). *Arch. Surg.* **123**, 162–170.

Rosoff, P.M. (1989). *Lymphokine Res.* **8**, 407–413.

Rosoff, P.M., Savage, N. and Dinarello, C.A. (1988). *Cell* **54**, 73–81.

Rossi, V., Breviario, F., Ghezzi, P., Dejana, E. and Mantovani, A. (1985). *Science* **229**, 174–176.

Schade, U.F., Burmeister, I. and Engel, R. (1987). *Biochem. Biophys. Res. Comm.* **147**, 695–700.

Schindler, R. and Dinarello, C.A. (1990). *Bio. Techniques* **8**, 408–413.

Schindler, R., Clark, B.D. and Dinarello, C.A. (1990a). *J. Biol. Chem.* **265**, 10232–10237.

Schindler, R., Gelfand, J.A. and Dinarello, C.A. (1990b). *Blood* **76**, 1631–1638.

Schindler, R., Ghezzi, P. and Dinarello, C.A. (1990c). *J. Immunol.* **144**, 2216–2222.

Schindler, R., Lonnemann, G., Shaldon, S., Koch, K.M. and Dinarello, C.A. (1990d). *Kidney Int.* **37**, 85–93.

Schindler, R., Mancilla, J., Endres, S., Ghorbani, R., Clark, S.C. and Dinarello, C.A. (1990e). *Blood* 40–47.

Schwartz, G.N., MacVittie, T.J., Vigneulle, R.M. *et al.* (1987). *Immunopharmacol. Immunotoxicol.* **9**, 371–389.

Schweizer, A., Feige, U., Fontana, A., Muller, K. and Dinarello, C.A. (1988). *Agents Actions* **25**, 246–251.

Seckinger, P. and Dayer, J.M. (1987). *Ann. Inst. Pasteur/Immunol.* **138**, 461–516.

Seckinger, P., Lowenthal, J.W., Williamson, K., Dayer, J.M. and MacDonald, H.R. (1987). *J. Immunol.* **139**, 1546–1549.

Seckinger, P., Klein-Nulend, J., Alander, C., Thompson, R.C., Dayer, J.M. and Raisz, L.G. (1990). *J. Immunol.* **145**, 4181–4184.

Sims, J.E., March, C.J., Cosman, D. *et al.* (1988). *Science* **241**, 585–589.

Sirko, S., Schindler, R., Doyle, M.J., Weisman, S.M. and Dinarello, C.A. (1991). *Eur. J. Immunol.* **21**, 242–250.

Sisson, S.D. and Dinarello, C.A. (1988). *Blood* **72**, 1368–1374.

Smith, J.W., Urba, W.J., Curti, B.D. *et al.* (1992). *J. Clin. Oncol.* **10**, 1141–1152.

Stosic-Grujicic, T. and Lukic, M.L. (1992). *Immunol.* **75**,

Stylianou, E., O'Neill, L.A.J., Rawlinson, L., Edbrooke, M.R., Woo, P. and Saklatvala, J. (1992). *J. Biol. Chem.* **267**, 15836–15841.

Symons, J.A., Eastgate, J.A. and Duff, G.W. (1991). *J. Exp. Med.* **174**, 1251–1254.

Tewari, A., Buhles, W.C., Jr. and Starnes, H.F. Jr. (1990). *Lancet* **336**, 712–714.

Thornberry, N.A., Bull, H.G., Calaycay, J.R. *et al.* (1992). *Nature* **356**, 768–774.

Tilg, H., Mier, J.W., Vogel, W. *et al.* (1993). *J. Immunol.* **150**, 4687–4692.

Tracey, K., Fong, Y., Hesse, D.G. *et al.* (1987). *Nature* **330**, 662–664.

Tredget, E.E., Yu, Y.M., Zhong, S. *et al.* (1988). *Am. J. Physiol.*

Turner, M., Chantry, D.G.B., Barrett, K. and Feldmann, M. (1989). *J. Immunol.* **143**, 3556–3561.

Ucla, C., Roux-Lombard, P., Fey, S., Dayer, J.-M. and Mach, B. (1990). *J. Clin. Invest.* **85**, 185–191.

Van Damme, J., De Ley, M., Opdenakker, G., Billiau, A. and De Somer, P. (1985). *Nature* **314**, 266–268.

van der Meer, J.W.M., Barza, M., Wolf, S.M. and Dinarello, C.A. (1988). *Proc. Natl Acad. Sci. USA* **85**, 1620–1623.

Vannier, E. and Dinarello, C.A. (1993). *J. Clin. Invest.* **92**.

Vannier, E., Miller, L.C. and Dinarello, C.A. (1992). *Proc. Natl Acad. Sci. USA* **89**, 4076–4080.

Wakabayashi, G., Gelfand, J.A., Burke, J.F., Thompson, R.C. and Dinarello, C.A. (1991a). *FASEB J.* **5**, 338–343.

Wakabayashi, G., Gelfand, J.A., Jung, W.K., Connolly, R.J., Burke, J.F. and Dinarello, C.A. (1991b). *J. Clin. Invest.* **87**, 1925–1935.

Wallach, D., Holtmann, H., Aderka, D. *et al.* (1989). *Lymphokine Res.* **8**, 359–363.

Wallach, D., Holtmann, H., Engelmann, H. and Nophar, Y. (1988). *J. Immunol.* **140**, 2994–2999.

Warner, S.J.C., Auger, K.R. and Libby, P. (1987a). *J. Exp. Med.* **165**, 1316–1331.

Warner, S.J.C., Auger, K.R. and Libby, P. (1987b). *J. Immunol.* **139**, 1911–1917.

Watters, J.M., Bessey, P.Q., Dinarello, C.A., Wolff, S.M. and Wilmore, D.W. (1985). *Surgery* **98**, 298–306.

Watters, J.M., Bessey, P.Q., Dinarello, C.A., Wolff, S.M. and Wilmore, D.W. (1986). *Arch. Surg.* **121**, 179–190.

White, C.W. and Ghezzi, P. (1989). *Biother.* **1**, 361–367.

Wogensen, L.D., Mandrup, P.T., Markholst, H. *et al.* (1988). *Acta Endocrinol. (Copenhagen).* **117**, 302–306.

Yamayoshi, M., Ohue, M., Kawashima, H. *et al.* (1990). *Lymph. Res.* **9**, 405–413.

Yamoto, K., el-Hajjaoui, Z. and Koeffler, H.P. (1989). *J. Cell Physiol.* **139**, 610–616.

Ye, K., Dinarello, C.A. and Clark, B.D. (1993). *Proc. Natl Acad. Sci. USA* **90**, 2295–2299.

Ye, K., Koch, K.-C., Clark, B.D. and Dinarello, C.A. (1992). *Immunol.* **75**, 427–434.

Young, P.R. and Krasney, P.A. (1991). *Cytokine* **3**, 472 (abs).

Zsebo, K.M., Yuschenkoff, V.N., Schiffer, S. *et al.* (1988). *Blood* **71**, 99–103.

Zucali, J.R., Dinarello, C.A., Oblon, D.J., Gross, M.A., Anderson, L. and Weiner, R.S. (1986). *J. Clin. Invest.* **77**, 1857–1863.

Chapter 4

Interleukin-2 and the Interleukin-2 Receptor

Mark A. Goldsmith[1] and Warner C. Greene[2,3]

[1]Gladstone Institute of Virology and Immunology and Departments of Medicine[2] and Microbiology and Immunology[3], University of California, San Francisco, California 94141-900, USA

INTRODUCTION

Interleukin-2 (IL-2) was first identified in 1975 as a growth-promoting activity for bone-marrow-derived T lymphocytes (Morgan *et al.*, 1976). Since then, the spectrum of its recognized biological activity has expanded significantly to include direct effects on the growth and differentiation not only of T cells but also of B lymphocytes, natural killer (NK) cells, lymphokine-activated killer (LAK) cells, monocytes, macrophages and oligodendrocytes. The biological effects of IL-2 are mediated through the binding of this growth factor to specific receptors present on these various cellular targets. The functional, high-affinity IL-2 receptor (IL-2R) is composed of three distinct, membrane-associated subunits: a 55 kDa α chain (IL-2Rα, Tac, p55), a 70–75 kDa β chain (IL-2Rβ, p70/75) and a 64 kDa γ chain (IL-2Rγ, p64). While these individual subunits alone bind IL-2 with very low affinity, heterodimerization and heterotrimerization of the subunits permit binding with intermediate and high affinity, respectively. Although substantial progress has been made in defining the biochemical and molecular properties of IL-2 and of its cellular receptor, the precise mechanism by which this ligand–receptor complex transduces growth-promoting intercellular signals remains unclear. However, several studies suggest that activation of a receptor-associated tyrosine kinase(s) may be involved. The general structural and functional properties of the IL-2/IL-2R system are discussed in the following sections.

STRUCTURE AND MOLECULAR BIOLOGY OF IL-2

IL-2 is a 15.5 kDa glycoprotein produced by activated T cells. Some studies suggest that activated B cells may also share the ability to produce IL-2 (Taira *et al.*, 1987; Walker *et al.*, 1988). The complete primary structure of IL-2 in seven mammalian species has been deduced by the cloning of human (Devos *et al.*, 1983; Taniguchi *et al.*, 1983), gibbon ape (Chen *et al.*, 1985), murine (Kashima *et al.*, 1985; Yokota *et al.*, 1985), bovine (Cerretti *et al.*, 1986; Reeves *et al.*, 1986), rat (McKnight *et al.*, 1989), sheep (Seow *et al.*, 1990), and porcine (Goodall *et al.*, 1991) IL-2 cDNAs. Substantial similarity is seen across

```
Human        APTSSST---  ----------  -KKTQLQLEH  LLLDLQMILN  GINNYKNPKL   36
Gibbon ape   APTSSST---  ----------  -KKTQLQLEH  LLLDLQMILN  GINNYKNPKL   36
Cow          APTSSST---  ----------  -GNTMKEVKS  LLLDLQLILE  KVKNPENLKL   36
Sheep        APTSSST---  ----------  -GNTMKEVKS  LLLDLQLILE  KVKNPENLKL   36
Pig          APTSSST---  ----------  -KNTKKQLEP  LLLDLQLILK  EVKNYENADL   36
Mouse        APTSSSTSSS  TAEAQQQQQQ  QQQQQQHLEQ  LLMDLQELLS  RMENYRNLKL   50
Rat          APTSSPA---  ----------  -KETQQHLEQ  LLLDLQVLLR  GIDNYKNLKL   36


Human        TRMLTFKFYM  PK-KATELKH  LQCLEEEELKP  LEEVLNLAQS  KNFHLR-PRD   84
Gibbon ape   TRMLTFKFYM  PK-KATELKH  LQCLEEEELKP  LEEVLNLAQS  KNFHLR-PRD   84
Cow          SRMHTFDFYV  PKVNATELKH  LKCLLEELKL  LEEVLDLAPS  KNLNPREIKD   86
Sheep        SRMHTFNFYM  PKVNATELKH  LKCLLEELKL  LEEVLDLAPS  KNLNTREIKD   86
Pig          SRMLTFKFYM  PK-QATELKH  LQCLVEELKA  LEGVLNLGQS  KNSDSANIKE   85
Mouse        PRMLTFKFYL  PK-QATELKD  LQCLEDELGP  LRHVLDLTQS  KSFQLEDAEN   99
Rat          PMMLTFKFYL  PK-QATELKH  LQCLFNELGA  LQRVLDLTQS  KSFHLEDAGN   85


Human        LISNINVIVL  ELKGSETTFM  CEYADETATI  VEFLNRWITF  CQSIISTLT-   133
Gibbon ape   LISNINVIVL  ELKGSETTFM  CEYADETATI  VEFLNRWITF  CQSIISTLT-   133
Cow          SMDNIKRIVL  ELQGSETRFT  CEYDDATVNA  VEFLNKWITF  CQSIMSTMT-   135
Sheep        SMDNIKRIVL  ELQGSETRFT  CEYDDATVKA  VEFLNKWITF  CQSIMSTMT-   135
Pig          SMNNINVIVL  ELKGSETSFK  CEYDDETVTA  VEFLNKWITF  CQSIMSTLT-   134
Mouse        FISNIRVTVV  KLKGSDNTFE  CQFDDESATV  VDFLRRWIAF  CQSIISTSPQ   149
Rat          FISNIRVTVV  KLKGSENKFE  CQFDDEPATV  VEFLRRWIAI  CQSIISTMTQ   135
```

Fig. 1. Deduced primary sequences of mature IL-2 molecules from several mammalian species. Sequences are aligned to maximize display of homologies, and are shown using the one-letter amino-acid designation. Extensive similarities are evident across these species, including many perfectly conserved (boxed) and partially conserved residues. The mouse IL-2 molecule has an unusual insertion of 12 Gln residues at the N-terminus. Sequences were deduced from the cDNA sequences contained in the GenBank. See text for references.

these species (Fig. 1), including strict conservation of all three cysteine residues. The 153-aminoacid human IL-2 primary translation product undergoes several post-translational processing events, including cleavage of a 20-residue signal peptide, addition of carbohydrate to the threonine residue at position 3, and formation of a disulphide bond between the cysteines located at positions 58 and 105. This latter modification is essential for bioactivity, whereas the addition of carbohydrate appears to be dispensable (Robb et al., 1983).

The human IL-2 gene has been mapped to chromosome 4q bands 26–28 (Siegel et al., 1984). The inducible expression of this gene is controlled primarily at a transcriptional level via a 5′ enhancer element (Fujita et al., 1983; Holbrook et al., 1984; Siebenlist et al., 1986). Several functional cis-acting regulatory sequences have been identified within the IL-2 enhancer, including binding sites for NFAT-1, NF-𝜘B, AP-1 and octamer proteins (Durand et al., 1988; Shaw et al., 1988; Hoyos et al., 1989; Muegge et al., 1989; Serfling et al., 1989). In addition, IL-2 gene expression is also controlled at a post-transcriptional level involving instability of IL-2 mRNA, apparently mediated through AU-rich sequence motifs present in the 3′-untranslated region of the IL-2 mRNA (Shaw and Kamen, 1986). For a more complete discussion of these aspects of IL-2 gene regulation, recent reviews are suggested (Crabtree, 1989; Muegge and Durum, 1989; Ullman et al., 1990).

The three-dimensional structure of the human IL-2 protein remains the subject of some controversy. A proposed X-ray crystal structure at 3 Å resolution (Fig. 2A) contains six helical domains involving 89 amino acids or 67% of the molecule

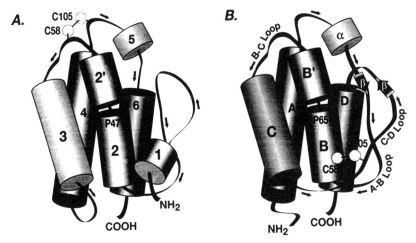

Fig. 2. Models of three-dimensional structure of human IL-2. (A) Model of structure derived from X-ray crystallographic analysis. (B) Model derived from secondary structure predictions and correlations with other members of cytokine family. See Bazan (1992) for detailed discussion. Figure modified from Bazan, 1992 with permission of the author and the publisher.

(Brandhuber *et al.*, 1987). An alternative structure was subsequently proposed (Fig. 2B) based upon secondary structure predictions derived from a comparison of the primary sequence of IL-2 with those of several related cytokines (Bazan, 1992). This alternative model, which contains four core α-helices and two crossover loops containing β strands, appears to accommodate the X-ray scaffold data while incorporating the results of mapping studies of receptor-binding epitopes by mutagenesis (see 'Structural Considerations in Subunit Cooperation and Ligand Binding'). Higher resolution crystallographic analysis should provide a more definitive structure.

IL-2 RECEPTOR COMPOSITION

The IL-2Rα Subunit

Progress in the characterization of the human high-affinity IL-2 receptor complex was facilitated by the development both of a sensitive IL-2 bioassay (Gillis *et al.*, 1978) and of a receptor-binding assay (Robb *et al.*, 1981). Purified, radiolabelled IL-2 for these receptor-binding assays was either isolated from IL-2-secreting cell lines (Gillis and Watson, 1980) or produced by recombinant DNA methodology (Taniguchi *et al.*, 1983). Another major advance in the analysis of the IL-2 receptor was the generation of anti-receptor monoclonal antibodies. The first such anti-IL-2 receptor antibody was prepared using tumour cells from a patient with adult T-cell leukaemia as the immunogen (Uchiyama *et al.*, 1981). This antibody did not bind to normal resting T cells but did react strongly with mitogen-activated T cells, hence the name anti-Tac (T activated). This monoclonal antibody blocks the binding of IL-2 to the high-affinity IL-2 receptor and also inhibits IL-2-induced proliferation (Leonard *et al.*, 1982; Miyawaki *et al.*, 1982; Robb and Greene, 1983). In immunoprecipitation assays, anti-Tac reacted

```
 -21  MDSYLLMWGLLTFIMVPGCQAELCDDDPPEIPHATFKAMAYKEGTMLNCE
                        ▲                                ▲

  30  CKRGFRRIKSGSLYMLCTGNSSHSSWDNQCQCTSSATRNTTKQVTPQPEE
      ▲                   ▲           ▲ ▲

  80  QKERKTTEMQSPMQPVDQASLPGHCREPPPWENEATERIYHFVVGQMVYY
                               ▲

 130  QCVQGYRALHRGPAESVCKMTHGKTRWTQPQLICTGEMETSQFPGEEKPQ
      ▲                ▲                ▲

 180  ASPEGRPESETSCLVTTTDFQIQTEMAATMETSIFTTEYQVAVAGCVFLL
                  △                            △

 230  ISVLLLSGLTWQRRQRKSRRTI    251
```

Fig. 3. Predicted primary sequence and features of human IL-2Rα. Underline, signal peptide; bold underline, transmembrane domain; double underline, N-linked glycosylation sites; closed triangles, Cys residues thought to participate in intramolecular disulphide bonds; open triangle, additional Cys residues. Sequence deduced from cDNA sequence contained in the GenBank. See text for references.

with the same 55 kDa glycoprotein recognized by IL-2 (Leonard *et al.*, 1982; Robb and Green, 1983). N-terminal amino acid sequencing of the Tac antigen permitted the isolation of full-length human IL-2Rα cDNA clones (Cosman *et al.*, 1984; Leonard *et al.*, 1984; Nikaido *et al.*, 1984). In addition, murine IL-2Rα cDNAs were isolated by low-stringency hybridization with the human IL-2Rα cDNA probe (Miller *et al.*, 1985).

The human IL-2Rα gene was cloned (Nikaido *et al.*, 1984; Leonard *et al.*, 1985a) and localized to chromosome 10p band 14–15 (Leonard *et al.*, 1985b). The highly inducible nature of the IL-2Rα gene promoter has been studied in considerable detail. As in the case of the IL-2 gene, transcriptional activation of the IL-2Rα gene is mediated through an enhancer element containing multiple regulatory sites, including the NF-×B, CArG and SpI binding sites (for a review, see Greene *et al.*, 1989; Muegge and Durum, 1989).

The primary translation product from the IL-2Rα gene contains 272 amino acids (Fig. 3). After cleavage of the 21-amino-acid signal peptide, the mature 251-residue IL-2Rα polypeptide exhibits a molecular mass of 33 kDa. Post-translational processing involving N- and O-linked glycosylation, sulphation and serine/threonine phosphorylation culminates in surface display of the 55 kDa IL-2Rα subunit (Leonard *et al.*, 1983, 1985c). The majority of the IL-2Rα chain (219 amino acids) is positioned outside the cell. There are 11 cysteine residues in this extracellular region, some of which are involved in intrachain disulphide bridges: Cys-3 is linked to Cys-147; Cys-131 is linked to Cys-163; Cys-28, 30 is linked to Cys-59, 61; and Cys-46 may be linked to Cys-104 (Rusk *et al.*, 1988). Disruption of any of these disulphide bonds by site-directed mutagenesis greatly reduces the ability of the corresponding protein to bind IL-2 or anti-Tac (Rusk *et al.*, 1988). There are two sites for N-linked sugar attachment, both of which are utilized. However, glycosylation at these sites is required neither for intracellular transport of the receptor nor for IL-2 binding (Cullen *et al.*, 1988). Many sites are present for the addition of O-linked sugar, which occurs in the Golgi and appears to be needed for normal transport of the receptor to the cell membrane.

The single transmembrane region of the IL-2Rα protein is 19 amino acids long, while the cytoplasmic tail consists of only 13 amino acids. This intracellular region contains six basic residues which presumably constitute a stop-transfer sequence that aids in anchoring the receptor protein within the plasma membrane. This region is unlikely to exhibit an intrinsic catalytic function involved in signal transduction, and its small size led to the prediction that the formation of functional IL-2R might involve additional unidentified receptor subunits. This notion found support in transfection assays, where IL-R2α expression in nonlymphoid cells resulted in only low-affinity binding sites (Sabe *et al.*, 1984; Greene *et al.*,1985) but both high- and low-affinity binding sites in lymphoid cells (Hatakeyama *et al.*, 1985; Wano *et al.*, 1987a). These findings suggested that lymphoid cells provide one or more proteins that participate in the formation of the high-affinity IL-2R.

The IL-2Rβ Subunit

Several groups observed that certain lymphoid cells respond to IL-2 in the apparent absence of IL-2Rα. Specifically, NK cells and SKW6.4 B cells were found to respond to high doses of IL-2 even in the presence of anti-Tac (Ortaldo *et al.*, 1984; Ralph *et al.*, 1984; Trinchieri *et al.*, 1984). In addition, gibbon ape MLA 144 T cells and the NK-like human YT leukaemic cells were observed to bind IL-2 with a unique intermediate affinity, and to lack reactivity with anti-Tac. Binding of ^{125}I-IL-2 to these or related cells followed by chemical cross-linking and immunoprecipitation with anti-IL-2 antibodies revealed a novel IL-2-binding protein of approximately 70–75 kDa (Sharon *et al.*, 1986; Tsudo *et al.*, 1986; Dukovich *et al.*, 1987; Robb *et al.*, 1987; Techigawara *et al.*, 1987). Using YT cells or other p70–75-bearing cells as immunogens, several monoclonal antibodies were prepared against the p70–75 IL-2-binding protein (Nakamura *et al.*, 1989; Takeshita *et al.*, 1989; Tsudo *et al.*, 1989a). One of these antibodies, Mikβ1 (Tsudo *et al.*, 1989a), was successfully employed in expression screening of a YT cDNA library, resulting in the isolation of p70 cDNA clones and the identification of p70 as the IL-2Rβ subunit (Hatakeyama *et al.*, 1989a). Mouse IL-2Rβ cDNAs were subsequently isolated by cross-hybridization using the human IL-2Rβ cDNA (Kono *et al.*, 1990). In addition, the human IL-2Rβ gene has recently been mapped to chromosome 22 (Gnarra *et al.*, 1990).

Sequencing of the full-length IL-2Rβ cDNA yielded a predicted primary translation product of 551 amino acids (Fig. 4). The receptor contains a putative signal peptide 26 amino acids in length, and the mature IL-2Rβ protein is composed of 525 amino acids with a calculated molecular mass of 58 kDa. The extracellular portion of IL-2Rβ has 214 amino acids with four potential sites for *N*-linked glycosylation and eight cysteine residues. Among these cysteines are two canonical pairs with characteristic spacing, as found in other members of the cytokine receptor superfamily (Bazan, 1990). A hydrophobic stretch of 25 amino acids (residues 215–239) forms the single membrane-spanning region, followed by a 286-amino-acid cytoplasmic domain. This region is particularly rich in proline and serine residues (42 and 30 residues, respectively) and also contains a preponderance of negatively charged amino acids. A consensus sequence found in the tyrosine kinases, Gly–X–Gly–X–X–Gly (Hanks *et al.*, 1988) is not present, although there are six tyrosine residues in the cytoplasmic domain that form potential sites for phosphorylation.

Little is yet known about the regulation of expression of the IL-2Rβ gene. Some normal cell populations, including NK cells, monocytes and at least a subset of resting T cells, constitutively express IL-2Rβ at the cell surface in the absence of IL-2Rα (Dukovich *et al.*, 1987; Nishi *et al.*, 1988; Ben Aribia *et al.*, 1989; Ohashi *et al.*, 1989;

```
 -26  MAAPALSWRLPLLILLLPLATSWASAAVNGTSQFTCFYNSRANISCVWSQ
                                       ==      ▲     == ▲
  25  DGALQDTSCQVHAWPDRRRWNQTCELLPVSQASWACNLILGAPDSQKLTT
             ∧              == ▲            ▲
  75  VDIVTLRVLCREGVRWRVMAIQDFKPFENLRLMAPISLQVVHVETHRCNI
              ∆                                       ∧ ==
 125  SWEISQASHYFERHLEFEARTLSPGHTWEEAPLLTLKQKQEWICLETLTP
      ==                                          ∧
 175  DTQYEFQVRVKPLQGEFTTWSPWSQPLAFRTKPAALGKDTIPWLGHLLVG
                        •••••
 225  LSGAFGFIILVYLLINCRNTGPWLKKVLKCNTPDPSKFFSQLSSEHGGDV
      ━━━━━━━━━━━━━━━━━
 275  QKWLSSPFPSSSFSPGGLAPEISPLEVLERDKVTQLLLQQDKVPEPASLS

 325  SNHSLTSCFTNQGYFFFHLPDALEIEACQVYFTYDPYSEEDPDEGVAGAP
                         )              )  )  )
 375  TGSSPQPLQPLSGEDDAYCTFPSRDDLLLFSPSLLGGPSPPSTAPGGSGA
                       )
 425  GEERMPPSLQERVPRDWDPQPLGPPTPGVPDLVDFQPPPELVLREAGEEV

 475  PDAGPREGVSFPWSRPPGQGEFRALNARLPLNTDAYLSLQELQGQDPTHL
                                           )
 525  V
```

Fig. 4. Predicted primary sequence and features of human IL-2Rβ. Underline, signal peptide; bold underline, transmembrane domain; double underline, potential N-linked glycosylation sites; closed triangles, Cys residues that are characteristic of members of cytokine receptor superfamily; open triangle, additional Cys residues; closed circles, WSXWS sequence; open circles, cytoplasmic Tyr residues. Sequence deduced from cDNA sequence contained in the GenBank. See text for references.

Tsudo *et al.*, 1989a; Yagita *et al.*, 1989). In unstimulated peripheral-blood T cells, IL-2Rβ may be constitutively expressed in CD8$^+$ mature T cells but is inducible in CD4$^+$ T cells (Ohashi *et al.*, 1989; Tsudo *et al.*, 1989a). IL-2Rβ expression in B cells may be upregulated by IL-2 in some circumstances (Nakanishi *et al.*, 1992).

The IL-2Rγ Subunit

Cloning of cDNAs encoding the IL-2Rα and IL-2Rβ chains failed to solve all of the mysteries surrounding the multiple affinity forms of the IL-2R. For example, the observation that transfection of the IL-2Rβ cDNA into nonlymphoid cells failed to generate an IL-2 binding site while transfection into lymphoid cells generated the expected binding sites (Hatakeyama *et al.*, 1989a) suggested the possibility of an additional lymphoid-specific receptor component. Indeed, cross-linking studies using ^{125}I-labelled IL-2 in conjunction with the cell lines YT and MLA-144 had previously revealed several unidentified proteins with molecular masses of 83–92 kDa expressed on the surface of these cells that appeared to be involved in IL-2 binding (Dukovich *et al.*, 1987; Robb *et al.*, 1987). After a variety of candidate molecules were proposed, a technical advance was made when coimmunoprecipitation studies were performed in the presence of IL-2. Such studies identified a 64 kDa protein that was associated with IL-2Rβ, but which exhibited a unique peptide map (Takeshita *et al.*, 1990). Related studies demonstrated a quantitative relationship between the levels of this protein

-22 <u>MLKPSLPFTSLLFLQLPLLGVGLN<u>TT</u>I</u>LTPNGNEDTTADFFLTTMPTDSL

 29 SVSTLPLPEVQCFVFNVEYM<u>NCT</u>W<u>NSS</u>SEPQPT<u>NLT</u>LHYWYKNSDNDKVQ
                 ▲   ▲▲

 79 KCSHYLFSEEITSGCQLQKKEIHLYQTFVVQLQDPREPRRQATQMLKLQN
   ▲   ▲

129 LVIPWAPE<u>NLT</u>LHKLSESQLELNWNNRFLNHCLEHLVQYRTDWDHSWTEQ
                               △

179 SVDYRHKFSLPSVDGQKRYTFRVRSRFNPLCGSAQHW<u>SEW</u>SHPIHWG<u>SNT</u>
                           △   ●●●●●

229 <u>SKENPFLFALEAVVISVGSMGLIISLLCVYFWLE</u>RTMPRIPTLKNLEDLV

279 TEYHGNFSAWSGVSKGLAESLQPDYSERLCLVSEIPPKGGALGEGPGASP
    ()   ()

329 CNQHSPYWAPPCYTLKPET   347
    ()   ()

Fig. 5. Predicted primary sequence and features of human IL-2Rγ. Underline, signal peptide; bold underline, transmembrane domain; double underline, potential N-linked glycosylation sites; closed triangles, Cys residues that are characteristic of members of cytokine receptor superfamily; open triangle, additional Cys residues; closed circles, WSXWS sequence; open circles, cytoplasmic Tyr residues. Sequence deduced from cDNA sequence contained in the GenBank. See text for references.

associated with IL-2Rβ and the number of intermediate affinity binding sites in a particular cell line (Takeshita *et al.*, 1992b; Voss *et al.*, 1992).

Recently, a cDNA clone encoding this putative receptor component (termed the γ chain) was obtained by sequencing this protein to deduce nucleotide sequences for cloning by reverse transcriptase polymerase chain reaction (RT-PCR) using polyadenylated RNA from a lymphoid cell line (Takeshita *et al.*, 1992a). The amplified product was used to screen a cDNA library from this cell line, resulting in the isolation of a clone that contained an open reading frame for a 369-residue polypeptide. This protein (Fig. 5) contains a putative 22-amino-acid signal peptide at the N-terminus, a 255-amino-acid extracellular domain, a 29-amino-acid hydrophobic transmembrane domain, and an 86-amino-acid C-terminal cytoplasmic domain. The predicted extracellular domain contains several features that are characteristic of cytokine receptors, including six potential N-linked glycosylation sites, four conserved cysteines, and the canonical WSXWS (Trp–Ser–X–Trp–Ser) motif. It is notable that consensus sequence analysis also suggested the presence of an SH2 subdomain in the cytoplasmic tail, although the absence of several critical features of functional SH2 domains in the molecule raises doubt about its biologic significance. In addition, four leucine residues with heptameric spacing located in a predicted α-helical region of the extracellular domain raise the possibility of a leucine zipper motif that may be involved in protein–protein interaction.

Reconstitution studies with this cDNA clone in fibroblastoid cells demonstrated that the IL-2Rβ and IL-2Rγ subunits could cooperate to generate an intermediate-affinity receptor, while coexpression of all three subunits, (α, β, and γ) resulted in high-affinity binding (Takeshita *et al.*, 1992a). Somewhat surprisingly, the putative intermediate affinity βγ heterodimer exhibited a higher K_d (4.6 nM) than the intermediate affinity receptor that had been previously described (K_d in the 0.5–1.0 nM range). Whether this lower affinity is simply the result of technical variation among various reported studies or reveals previously unrecognized additional complexity in the receptor system is currently unknown.

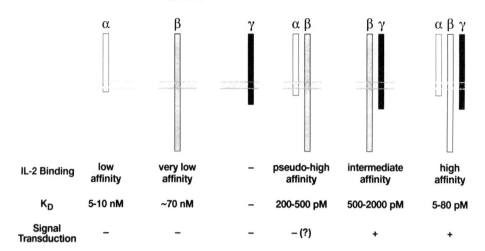

	α	β	γ	α β	β γ	α β γ
IL-2 Binding	low affinity	very low affinity	–	pseudo-high affinity	intermediate affinity	high affinity
K_D	5-10 nM	~70 nM	–	200-500 pM	500-2000 pM	5-80 pM
Signal Transduction	–	–	–	– (?)	+	+

Fig. 6. Multiple forms of IL-2R. Shown are the ligand binding and signal transduction properties of monomeric, heterodimeric, and heterotrimeric forms of the receptor as explained in the text.

THE MULTIMOLECULAR IL-2R COMPLEX

Cooperation by IL-2R Subunits Generates Multiple Binding Affinities for IL-2

The identification and subsequent cloning of the IL-2Rγ chain has helped to clarify the molecular basis of multiple binding sites with distinct binding affinities for IL-2 (Fig. 6). The IL-2Rα chain alone is the low-affinity receptor form (K_d 10–20 nM). In contrast, no binding to the IL-2Rγ chain alone has been reported to date. The IL-2Rβ chain, which alone binds IL-2 with extremely low affinity (K_d 70–100 nM), can cooperate with IL-2Rα to generate a 'pseudo-high affinity' binding site (K_d 100–500 pM) or with IL-2Rγ to generate an 'intermediate-affinity' binding site (K_d 500 pM–2 nM) when expressed on lymphoid cells or multiply transfected nonlymphoid cells. The tri-molecular $\alpha\beta\gamma$ complex, present on activated T cells or multiply transfected non-lymphoid cells, represents the 'high affinity' IL-2R (K_d 10–80 pM). Such bimolecular and trimolecular partnerships among these subunits therefore serve to expand dramatically the dynamic range of IL-2 binding. Thus, historical paradoxes regarding the differential binding properties of these subunits expressed on lymphoid or nonlymphoid hosts have been largely resolved with the recent recognition that many, if not all, lymphoid cells express IL-2Rγ endogenously (Takeshita *et al.*, 1992a).

The distinct binding affinities of the three forms of the receptor derive from the unique binding kinetics inherent to each of the subunits. Specifically, IL-2 binding to IL-2Rα is characterized by rapid rates of both association and dissociation ($t_{1/2}$ is 4 s and 6 s, respectively), and these kinetics determine its low affinity binding property (Lowenthal and Greene, 1987; Wang and Smith, 1987). Binding to IL-2Rβ alone (expressed on a nonlymphoid cell) is characterized by a relatively slower dissociation rate ($t_{1/2}$ 1.6 min) and, by inference from its K_d, a much slower association rate (Ringheim *et al.*, 1991). Intriguingly, the higher affinity of IL-2 binding to the IL-2R$\alpha\beta$ heterodimer results primarily from the rapid association kinetics contributed by α, with a small contribution by the somewhat slower dissociation kinetics of β (net $\alpha\beta$

association $t_{1/2}$ 30 s and net dissociation $t_{1/2}$ 18.5 min) (Ringheim *et al.*, 1991). Although IL-2Rγ alone has not been demonstrated to bind IL-2, participation of γ in a $\beta\gamma$ heterodimeric complex confers dramatically slower dissociation kinetics on the receptor ($t_{1/2}$ 255 min) (Ringheim *et al.*, 1991). Recent studies provide evidence that γ contributes directly to the IL-2 binding site in heterodimeric complexes (Voss *et al.*, 1993), a finding that is consistent with its influence on ligand-binding kinetics.

Thus, it appears that the resultant multimolecular IL-2 receptor complexes exhibit the most 'favourable' properties of each of the component subunits. Accordingly, complexes containing IL-2Rα exhibit rapid association kinetics while those containing IL-2Rγ exhibit slow dissociation kinetics. $\alpha\beta$ and $\beta\gamma$ heterodimers therefore display intermediate binding properties, while the $\alpha\beta\gamma$ complex exhibits rapid association kinetics ($t_{1/2}$ 37 s) and slow dissociation kinetics ($t_{1/2}$ 285 min) with a resulting net binding affinity that is higher than those of the heterodimeric complexes (Lowenthal and Greene, 1987; Ringheim *et al.*, 1991). Although there is no evidence that receptor complexes lack γ function *in vivo*, these subunit pairing studies have been crucial in defining the contributions of each subunit to the functional IL-2-binding sites.

Structural Considerations in Subunit Cooperation and Ligand Binding

Features of the Receptor

These important collaborations among receptor components imply critical intramolecular interactions within the IL-2R complex. Evidence now strongly suggests that α and β directly interact with one another, since they are cointernalized by IL-2 (Fung *et al.*, 1988; Kuziel *et al.*, 1993) and since preformed heterodimers can be detected in some systems (Saragovi and Malek, 1988). Although comparable evidence regarding γ has not been reported, the observation that γ confers more efficient ligand internalization properties on $\alpha\beta$ receptors implies formation of complete heterotrimers (Takeshita *et al.*, 1992a). Likewise, direct contact between IL-2 and IL-2Rγ in the presence of IL-2Rβ implies such subunit interactions (Voss *et al.*, 1993).

Evidence has recently been reported that suggests functional subunit interactions extending beyond mere passive association. Specifically, an analogue of IL-2 containing a Phe substitution for Ala-42 demonstrates no detectable binding to IL-2Rα alone yet retains intermediate binding affinity for $\beta\gamma$ (K_d of 2.1 nM) and higher-affinity binding for $\alpha\beta\gamma$ (K_d of 160 pM) complexes (Grant *et al.*, 1992). Thus, participation of α in the receptor complex confers enhanced binding properties on other constituents of the complex, independently of its own direct contact with IL-2. The simplest model to account for this enhancement holds that physical interaction between IL-2Rα and β produces a conformational change in one or both subunits that alters the structure of the ligand-binding site. Similar conformational effects might also be exerted by the γ subunit, although no studies in this regard have been reported.

An important step in defining the structural basis of subunit cooperation was taken recently when the three-dimensional X-ray crystal structure of the extracellular domain of the growth hormone receptor containing growth hormone ligand was solved (Devos *et al.*, 1992). Consistent with prior biophysical studies (Cunningham *et al.*, 1991) was the finding that the growth hormone receptor is homodimeric. The structure further revealed that the N-terminal half of each subunit contributed to a ligand-binding crevice, and that the membrane-proximal half of each contained residues that were closely approximated to residues of the partner subunit. The theoretical secondary structure analysis has suggested that the IL-2Rβ and IL-2Rγ chains may assume similar three-dimensional conformations since they are part of a structurally related cytokine receptor superfamily, of which the growth hormone receptor is the prototype (Bazan, 1990; Bazan, J.F., personal communication). Further studies will be needed to determine how these principles apply to assembly and function of the heterotrimeric IL-2R.

Finally, although little is known about IL-2Rγ, some details have emerged about the ligand contact residues and subunit assembly domains within the α and β subunits. In IL-2Rα, both internal deletion and truncation studies have demonstrated that the N-terminal 163 amino acid residues (derived from exons 1–4) contain all the information necessary for binding to IL-2 (Cullen *et al.*, 1988; Robb *et al.*, 1988; Rusk *et al.*, 1988). Furthermore, residues 1–6 and 35–43 (derived from exon 2) appear to be essential both for IL-2 binding as well as for recognition by several anti-receptor antibodies; His-120 (from exon 4) also appears to be critical (Robb *et al.*, 1988). In addition, antibodies that selectively block high-affinity binding sites without impairing low-affinity binding by IL-2Rα depend upon α residues 158–160 (derived from exon 4), suggesting that this domain may be involved in subunit interactions that are necessary for assembly of a high-affinity binding site rather than in direct contact with IL-2 (Robb *et al.*, 1988). Finally, the cytoplasmic domain of IL-2Rα does not appear to play a critical role in assembly of the high-affinity trimolecular receptor complex (Kondo *et al.*, 1987).

In IL-2Rβ, the N-terminal 212 residues of the extracellular domain appear to be sufficient for ligand binding at very low affinity (Tsudo *et al.*, 1990). Specific segments that appear to be critical determinants of ligand binding include residues 194–197 (Miyazaki *et al.*, 1991) and residues 132–134 (Imler *et al.*, 1992). It is noteworthy that residues 194–198 constitute the extracellular, membrane-proximal WSXWS (Trp–Ser–X–Trp–Ser) motif that is common to many members of the cytokine receptor family. It is not known whether these two domains actually participate directly in ligand binding or instead contribute to receptor conformation or subunit interactions; some evidence suggests that residues 132–134 may contribute directly to the binding site (Imler *et al.*, 1992). Further structure–function correlations are needed to complete the emerging picture of the ligand binding function of the IL-2R.

Features of IL-2
An outline of the structural requirements for IL-2 itself has begun to emerge from the X-ray crystallographic analyses described previously along with site-directed mutagenesis studies. Deletion experiments indicated clearly that the N-terminal 20 amino-acid residues of IL-2 are critical to its interaction with the receptor (Ju *et al.*, 1987). Likewise, antibodies directed against residues 8–27 block binding of IL-2 to high-affinity receptors (Kuo and Robb, 1986). Moreover, Asp-20 is conserved across seven species reported to date, and substitution of Lys at this position in human IL-2 results in loss of bioactivity and of binding to receptor complexes containing IL-2Rβ (Collins *et al.*, 1988; Zurawski and Zurawski, 1989). These results suggest that residue(s) in the N-terminal α-helical segment of IL-2 may interact directly with the ligand-binding domain of IL-2Rβ or IL-2Rγ. Conversely, replacement of Phe-42 with Ala or of Arg-38 with

Glu or Ala results in markedly diminished binding to IL-2Rα and to high-affinity receptors, while permitting substantial residual bioactivity (Weigel *et al.*, 1989; Sauve *et al.*, 1991; Grant *et al.*, 1992); the A–B interloop (Fig. 2B) encompassing these residues may therefore contain the contact residues for IL-2Rα, allowing mutations within this region to abrogate selectively its α interaction without interfering with its binding to βγ. A reciprocal selective impairment of binding to βγ without precluding binding to αβ results from mutation of Gln-141 in the murine IL-2 molecule (Zurawski *et al.*, 1990), suggesting that the *C*-terminal D α-helix (Fig. 2B) containing this residue is the site of contact with IL-2Rγ. Thus, although a higher resolution molecular dissection is needed, a simple structural model of the quaternary complex would place the β and γ chains contacting opposite faces of the bound IL-2, with the α chain supporting the ligand via binding at one end (Bazan, J.F., personal communication). It is possible that the precise stereochemistry of this multimolecular receptor–ligand complex is a crucial determinant of receptor activation.

FUNCTION OF THE IL-2/IL-2R SYSTEM

Biology of IL-2 and IL-2R

The *de novo* synthesis and secretion of IL-2 and the expression of high-affinity IL-2R represent early consequences of antigen- or mitogen-induced activation of mature resting T cells. The subsequent interaction of IL-2 with the high-affinity receptors promotes the rapid clonal expansion of the effector T-cell population originally activated by antigen (reviewed by Smith, 1980; Robb *et al.*, 1984). The subsequent decline in both IL-2 synthesis and high-affinity receptor display probably contributes to the normal termination of the T-cell immune response. In addition to its growth-promoting function, IL-2 stimulates T cells to produce other lymphokines, including interferon-γ (IFN-γ) (Farrer *et al.*, 1982) and IL-4 (Howard *et al.*, 1983), revealing its capacity to act as a differentiation signal.

While the role of IL-2 in the growth of T cells activated via the T-cell receptor (TCR) by antigen is well established, evidence has emerged that suggests that the IL-2/IL-2R system might also function in the thymus during the early stages of T-cell development prior to the acquisition by thymocytes of a cell-surface CD3–TCR complex. The identification of T-cell progenitors within the human thymus that constitutively express the IL-2Rβ chain and secrete low levels of IL-2 has led to the suggestion that an autocrine pathway might promote the growth of these immature thymocytes (De la Hera *et al.*, 1986, 1987; Toribio *et al.*, 1989). Furthermore, it is conceivable that IL-2 might even be involved in signalling for the rearrangement and expression of TCR genes (Toribio *et al.*, 1988). The nature of the activation signals for IL-2 and IL-2Rβ gene expression in these progenitors remains unknown, although an interaction with thymic stromal elements and induction by other cytokines represent attractive mechanisms.

In the murine thymus, high levels of IL-2Rα have been detected on fetal and adult immature thymocytes (Ceredig *et al.*, 1985; Habu *et al.*, 1985; Hardt *et al.*, 1985; Raulet, 1985; Von Boehmer *et al.*, 1985) and IL-2 binding studies on fetal thymocytes revealed both high- and low-affinity IL-2 receptors (Zuniga-Pflucker *et al.*, 1990). As in the case of human thymocytes, mouse fetal T-cell precursors also express IL-2 mRNA, as revealed by *in situ* hybridization (Carding *et al.*, 1989). In contrast to human thymocytes, when mouse precursor T cells are isolated from the fetal or adult thymus and cultured either with or without exogenous IL-2, their proliferative response is minimal (Ceredig *et al.*, 1985; Raulet, 1985; Von Boehmer *et al.*, 1985; Bluestone *et al.*, 1987; Garni-Wagner *et al.*, 1990). However, when intact murine fetal thymic lobes, but not cell suspensions, are cultured in high-affinity levels of IL-2 (20 pM), there is a significant *in vitro* proliferative response (Zuniga-Pflucker *et al.*, 1990). Some experiments suggest that expression of the IL-2Rα chain also may be essential for the normal emergence of mature T cells in the mouse, as the development of these T cells is inhibited in thymic organ culture in the presence of anti-IL-2Rα monoclonal antibodies (Jenkinson *et al.*, 1987) and in newborn mice whose mothers have been treated with the anti-IL-2Rα antibodies (Tentori *et al.*, 1988). However, the importance of IL-2/IL-2R interactions during thymocyte maturation remains uncertain since mice lacking IL-2 synthesis retain normal thymocyte and peripheral T-cell development (Schorle *et al.*, 1991). Further studies are needed to clarify these apparent contradictions.

Although antigen activation of resting T cells is normally followed by induction of the IL-2 gene, cell surface display of high-affinity IL-2R and clonal expansion of the activated cells, engagement of the TCR on self-antigen-specific mature thymocytes and peripheral T cells has been shown to induce a state of clonal anergy, apparently as a result of selective inhibition of IL-2 gene expression (Rammensee *et al.*, 1989; Bonneville *et al.*, 1990). The failure of self-reactive T cells to produce IL-2 may contribute to the establishment of tolerance to self-determinants (reviewed by Ramsdell and Fowlkes, 1990; Schwartz, 1990).

Other lymphoid cell populations also express IL-2R and respond to IL-2. For example, B cells activated by antigen or mitogen bear high-affinity IL-2R, although at five- to tenfold lower levels than do activated T cells (Waldmann *et al.*, 1984). A recent study demonstrates that although resting B cells constitutively express both IL-2Rα and β, expression of β is preferentially upregulated by either IL-2R or IL-4, while expression of α is preferentially induced by B-cell mitogens (Nakanishi *et al.*, 1992). Furthermore, IL-2 can support the growth of B cells (Jelinek and Lipsky, 1987; Nakanishi *et al.*, 1992), the induction of Ig secretion by B cells (Jelinek and Lipsky, 1987) and the induction of J-chain synthesis leading to assembly and secretion of IgM (Tigges *et al.*, 1989).

NK cells also constitutively express IL-2Rβ. These cells not only proliferate in response to high doses of IL-2 but also produce IFN-γ and exhibit enhanced cytolytic activity (Ortaldo *et al.*, 1984; Trinchieri *et al.*, 1984). Similarly, incubation of normal resting T lymphocytes in high concentrations of IL-2 results in the expansion of a population of lymphoid cells that has potent cytolytic activity against fresh tumour target cells (reviewed in Rosenberg and Lotze, 1986). These LAK cells and their precursors have been characterized extensively. The generation of these cells *in vitro* and *in vivo* for use in adoptive immunotherapy protocols represents an area of active investigation (Rosenberg and Lotze, 1986). Unfortunately, the clinical utility of IL-2 may be limited by its toxicity at high doses, one manifestation of which is a profound capillary-leak syndrome (for review, see Chang and Rosenberg, 1989).

IL-2 function is not limited to cells of the lymphoid lineage. Myeloid cell populations such as bone-marrow-derived macrophage precursors (Baccarini *et al.*, 1989) and primary peripheral blood monocytes (Ohashi *et al.*, 1989) express cell surface IL-2Rβ but not IL-2Rα. Both blood monocytes and alveolar macrophages can be induced to express IL-2Rα by treatment with IFN-γ and/or LPS (Herrmann *et al.*, 1985; Holter *et al.*, 1986, 1987; Hancock *et al.*, 1987), and the stimulated cells bear both high- and low-affinity IL-2 binding sites (Holter *et al.*, 1987). IL-2Rα has also been detected on alveolar macrophages obtained from patients with active pulmonary sarcoidosis (Hancock *et al.*, 1987). Prolonged exposure to high doses of IL-2 results in proliferation and differentiation of macrophage precursors (Baccarini *et al.*, 1989), enhancement of the cytolytic activity of peripheral blood monocytes *in vitro* (Malkovsky *et al.*, 1987) and enhancement of macrophage antibody-dependent tumoricidal activity (Ralph *et al.*, 1988).

Cells outside the immune system may also be directly sensitive to the biological effects of IL-2. For example, isolated oligodendrocytes are reactive with an anti-IL-2Rα monoclonal antibody (Saneto *et al.*, 1986) and IL-2 has been reported to mediate both growth stimulation (Benveniste and Merrill, 1986) and growth inhibition (Saneto *et al.*, 1986).

Signal Transduction by the IL-2R

The minimal IL-2R complex competent to transduce signals appears to be the $\beta\gamma$ heterodimer. For example, lymphoid cells expressing only $\beta\gamma$ rapidly internalize surface-bound IL-2 (Robb and Greene, 1987). In addition, this heterodimer mediates induction by IL-2 of cytolytic activity and of proliferation in NK cells (Siegel *et al.*, 1987; Tsudo *et al.*, 1987; Kehrl *et al.*, 1988) and monocytes (Malkovsky *et al.*, 1987; Baccarini *et al.*, 1989) as well as secretion of Ig by certain B cells (Ralph *et al.*, 1984). Furthermore, in certain established T-cell lines IL-2R$\beta\gamma$ mediates a signal by IL-2 for growth arrest (Hatakeyama *et al.*, 1989a; Tsudo *et al.*, 1989b). Despite these findings, the relative contribution of each of the three recognized subunits to the complete receptor signalling programme has not been elucidated. In addition, the biochemical pathways comprising these signal transduction events remain largely undefined. Evidence has accumulated against important roles for many of the traditional second messengers, including hydrolysis of phosphatidylinositols and mobilization of intracellular free calcium, activation of protein kinase C, and induction of guanylate or adenylate cyclase (Mills *et al.*, 1986; Valge *et al.*, 1988; Tigges *et al.*, 1989).

Phosphorylation in Signalling

Like many other receptors the IL-2R undergoes phosphorylation of cytoplasmic residues during receptor-mediated signalling, suggesting a possible contribution by cellular kinases in the signalling process. The first recognized IL-2-receptor phosphorylation event was serine- and threonine-phosphorylation of the cytoplasmic domain of IL-2Rα upon exposure to PMA (Shackelford and Trowbridge, 1991), but this event was later demonstrated by site-directed mutagenesis studies to be nonessential for either receptor downregulation or transmission of proliferative signals (Hatakeyama *et al.*, 1986). Subsequently, inducible phosphorylation on tyrosine residues of IL-2Rβ

(Sharon et al., 1989; Asao et al., 1990; Mills et al., 1990) and of other cellular proteins (Morla et al., 1988; Saltzman et al., 1988; Merida and Gaulton, 1990) was observed, suggesting activation of a receptor-associated tyrosine kinase. Similarly, IL-2-induced phosphorylation of cytoplasmic tyrosine residues of IL-2Rγ was also reported (Sugamura et al., 1990). While the role of these phosphorylation events in receptor function or regulation remains unknown, these observations imply the activation of a tyrosine kinase functionally linked to the IL-2R.

The absence in IL-2R subunits of the cardinal ATP-binding site of protein kinases (Gly–X–Gly–X–X–Gly; Hanks et al., 1988) strongly argues against an intrinsic kinase function in the receptor itself. However, recent in vitro kinase studies demonstrated the association of both a tyrosine kinase and a serine/threonine kinase activity with the IL-2R complex (Fung et al., 1991; Michiel et al., 1991). Further characterization has suggested that a receptor-associated 97 kDa protein contains intrinsic tyrosine kinase activity (Garcia et al., 1992). However, direct proof of a functional role for these kinases in receptor-mediated signalling has not yet been reported.

Several members of the src family of nonreceptor tyrosine kinases have been postulated to play central roles in IL-2R function. The first observation that prompted this hypothesis was the induction by IL-2, in certain cell lines, of serine/threonine-phosphorylation of the lymphoid-specific kinase p56^{lck}, accompanied by an increase in its specific activity (Horak et al., 1991). Subsequent cotransfection experiments demonstrated a physical association between IL-2Rβ and p56^{lck} that is mediated by the C-terminal catalytic domain of p56^{lck} rather than by its SH2 domain (Hatakeyama et al., 1991). Similarly, a physical association between p59^{fyn} and IL-2Rβ was demonstrated in lymphoid cells lacking p56^{lck} (Minami et al., 1993). Surprisingly, although receptor-mediated induction of p56^{lck} activity and phosphorylation were observed in certain situations (Hatakeyama et al., 1991; Horak et al., 1991; Minami et al., 1993), several studies have revealed IL-2 receptor competence in cells lacking p56^{lck} and/or p59^{fyn} (Mills et al., 1992; Otani et al., 1992), implying either kinase redundancy and promiscuity or a nonessential contribution by these kinases to receptor signalling function.

Other kinases have also been postulated to contribute to IL-2R function. Activation of phosphatidylinositol-3-kinase (P13K) by IL-2 has been reported, an event that appears to depend upon an unidentified upstream tyrosine kinase (Augustine et al., 1991; Merida et al., 1991, 1993). In addition, activation of ribosomal p70 S6 kinase by IL-2 has been observed (Calvo et al., 1992; Kou et al., 1992; Terada et al., 1992); the significance of these observations was bolstered by the concomitant finding that this induction of kinase activity is prevented by the macrolide rapamycin, a recognized inhibitor of IL-2-mediated progression through cell cycle. Finally, both the expression and catalytic activity of the nonreceptor tyrosine kinase Raf-1 is regulated by IL-2 (Turner et al., 1991; Zmuidzinas et al., 1991), and this induction could be the proximal event leading to enhancement of S6 kinase activity and consequent progression through cell cycle. It may be noteworthy also that the GTP-bound (active) form of p21^{ras} is promoted by IL-2 (Graves et al., 1992), and that this induction is blocked by the protein tyrosine kinase inhibitor herbimycin (Izquierdo et al., 1992; Izquierdo and Cantrell, 1993). Therefore, although the data reported to date are largely circumstantial, it is tempting to speculate that a receptor-regulated tyrosine kinase(s) mediates activation of p21^{ras}, leading to activation of Raf-1 and S6 kinase with resultant progression through cell cycle.

Regulation of Gene Transcription

Among the many events observed following triggering of the IL-2R is selective activation of transcription. One of the earliest reported targets is the gene encoding IL-2Rα, the induction of which is an important step in the generation of high-affinity IL-2 receptors (Depper *et al.*, 1985; Smith and Cantrell 1985; Le Gros *et al.*, 1987; Kehrl *et al.*, 1988). A wide range of stimuli can induce the IL-2Rα promoter, including antigen, IL-1 and TNFα, PHA and PMA, and HTLV-1 Tax (Depper *et al.*, 1984; Andrew *et al.*, 1985; Lowenthal *et al.*, 1985, 1989; Inoue *et al.*, 1986; Bich-Thuy *et al.*, 1987; Cross *et al.*, 1987; Lee *et al.*, 1987; Maruyama *et al.*, 1987; Siegel *et al.*, 1987; Siekevitz *et al.*, 1987; Wano *et al.*, 1987b). Induction of IL-2Rα expression by IL-2 may be mediated, at least in part, by the transcription factor NF-κB, since IL-2 can induce NF-κB activation (Arima *et al.*, 1992). The biological significance of IL-2-mediated induction of IL-2Rα is not certain, but it is a central element in the paracrine model of clonal expansion.

An array of proto-oncogenes associated with cell cycle regulation is also activated upon ligation of the IL-2R. Despite some variability displayed in different cell-culture model systems, induction of transcripts for *c-myc, c-myb,* and the AP-1 factors *c-fos/c-jun* have been observed upon exposure to IL-2 (Granelli-Piperno *et al.*, 1986; Stern and Smith, 1986; Reed *et al.*, 1987; Shibuya *et al.*, 1992). Similarly, transcripts for the cyclin family and *cdc2* family of cell cycle regulators are induced by IL-2 (Shibuya *et al.*, 1992). Such associations perhaps are not surprising since these factors are intimately linked with progression through cell cycle and consequent proliferation. The precise contribution of each to the integrated biologic response remains to be determined.

Structural Features of IL-2R Influencing Signalling Function

Structure–function correlations for cytokine and other cellular receptors are beginning to emerge, primarily derived from mutagenesis studies of the cytoplasmic domains of receptor chains. To date, an essential role for the IL-2Rα chain beyond enhancing ligand binding has not been revealed. Indeed, in an early study deletion of the 10 C-terminal cytoplasmic amino acids of this subunit did not seem to impair delivery of proliferation signals by the IL-2R$\alpha\beta\gamma$ heterotrimer (Kondo *et al.*, 1987). More extensive analysis will be needed to determine conclusively whether or not this chain makes a functional contribution to receptor signalling.

In contrast, several deletions and substitutions of the cytoplasmic domain of the IL-2Rβ subunit have yielded provocative results. For example, deletion of a serine-rich stretch of residues (IL-2Rβ amino acids 267–322) completely abrogated transduction of a proliferative signal by IL-2 through the $\alpha\beta\gamma$ heterotrimer, while leaving intact the ligand-binding and internalization properties of the receptor (Hatakeyama *et al.*, 1989a, b). Deletion of this domain (termed S domain) also abrogated induction of expression of the proto-oncogenes *c-fos* (Hatakeyama *et al.*, 1990) and *c-myc* (Satoh *et al.*, 1992; Merida *et al.*, 1993), coimmunoprecipitation of tyrosine kinase activity with the receptor (Fung *et al.*, 1991), induction of intracellular protein tyrosine kinase activity (Merida *et al.*, 1993), and activation of p21^{ras} (Satoh *et al.*, 1992). The S domain is also essential for the induction of NF-κB by IL-2 (Arima *et al.*, 1992). Moreover, although the S deletion did not prevent physical association of p56^{lck} with IL-2Rβ, induction of its tyrosine kinase activity by IL-2 was abrogated (Minami *et al.*, 1993).

Intriguingly, this deletion spans a 15-amino-acid region with notable homology to a similarly located segment in many other members of the cytokine receptor superfamily, including IL-2Rγ. This domain, termed 'Box 2', has been shown to contain critical amino acid residues in the signalling competence of other cytokine receptors (Murakami et al., 1991). That at least part of the essential function of the S region lies in Box 2 was proven by the finding that substitution of Pro for Leu-299 of IL-2Rβ abrogated delivery of growth signals by the $\alpha\beta\gamma$ receptor (Mori et al., 1991) as well as induction of p56^{lck} tyrosine kinase activity (Minami et al., 1993). Further molecular analysis is needed to define precisely the role of this region as well as of another conserved region ('Box 1') lying N-terminal to the SD and Box 2 regions.

A second segment of β that appears to have an important functional role is a 46-amino-acid region that is rich in acidic residues (Hatakeyama et al., 1989a). While deletion of this region (residues 313–382, termed 'A') did not prevent proliferation driven by IL-2 (Hatakeyama et al., 1989b), it did eliminate physical association with p56^{lck} (Hatakeyama et al., 1991), induction of c-fos transcription (Hatakeyama et al., 1992), as well as activation of p21^{ras} (Satoh et al., 1992). Thus, this deletion appears to define a domain lying C-terminal to Box 1 and Box 2 that functions selectively in certain signal transduction functions of the IL-2R.

Potentially noteworthy is the finding that replacement of the conserved Ser residues in the extracellular IL-2Rβ WSXWS motif resulted in slightly diminished, but still evident, growth signal transduction by IL-2 (Miyazaki et al., 1991). This finding raises the possibility that this extracellular domain contributes to association with other molecules involved in signal transmission. Although structure–function studies with the associated IL-2Rγ have not yet been reported, the presence of cytoplasmic Box 1 and Box 2 domains as well as Tyr residues that undergo phosphorylation suggest that this chain will be found to play a significant role in signal transduction.

A highly schematic and speculative cartoon of the current body of knowledge is depicted in Fig. 7. Further information will be needed to assemble a high-resolution picture of receptor subunit stoichiometry, conformational features, and dynamic molecular associations that comprise signal transduction competence. The observation that induction of homodimerization by introduction of an inter-chain disulphide bond in the erythropoietin receptor leads to constitutive receptor activation may have important implications for the IL-2R (Yoshimura et al., 1990; Watowich et al., 1992). The extension of such principles from the prototypical homodimeric receptors for growth hormone and for erythropoietin to the heterotrimeric IL-2R awaits additional molecular investigation.

PATHOLOGY AND CLINICAL IMPLICATIONS

The biological significance of cytokine/cytokine receptor systems is emphasized by several clinical syndromes and animal models in which such regulatory molecules may play a pathogenetic role. For example, leukaemic T-cell lines derived from patients with the adult T-cell leukaemia/lymphoma syndrome often display extremely high levels of IL-2Rα (for a review, see Yodoi and Uchiyama, 1992). Although it has been hypothesized that this receptor expression is elicited by the Tax product derived from the aetiologic human retrovirus HTLV-I, the genesis of receptor expression may be more complex than this simple model. Nevertheless, it remains an attractive possibility

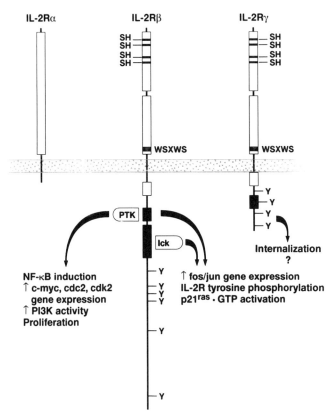

Fig. 7. Speculative schematic of signal transduction by the IL-2R. Characteristic Cys residues in extracellular domains of IL-2Rβ and γ are indicated (-SH), as are the WSXWS motifs. Cytoplasmic Tyr residues are indicated (-Y). the proximal 'Box 1' and distal 'Box 2' domains are shown as shaded boxes below the transmembrane regions. The more distal boxed region in β represents a part of the 'acidic' or 'A' domain. In β, both Box 2 and the A domain are required for activation of p56[lck] (lck) and for induction of several signal transduction responses, as indicated. Coimmunoprecipitation with β of an as yet unidentified protein tyrosine kinase (PTK) activity depends on the 'serine-rich' or 'S' domain that contains Box 2. To date, the only specific biologic response attributable to γ is ligand-induced internalization (Takeshita *et al.*, 1992a), although other functions are likely to be found.

that aberrant receptor expression may play a contributing role at some stage in the development of this disease by eliciting inappropriate proliferative signals. Intriguingly, mice deficient in IL-2 production (generated by homologous recombination) demonstrate normal thymocyte and peripheral T-cell development but subsequently become severely immunocompromised during further maturation (Schorle *et al.*, 1991; Sadlack *et al.*, 1993). A striking demonstration of the critical role of the IL-2 receptor in human immune function was revealed by recent studies of X-linked severe combined immunodeficiency (X-SCID), in which three X-SCID patients were shown to have genetic defects that map to the IL-2Rγ gene locus (Noguchi *et al.*, 1993). These patients carried point mutations that resulted in premature termination of translation of the IL-2Rγ chain. Although not yet proven in reconstitution studies, it appears that these genetic defects are the likely cause of this disease, which is characterized by severely impaired cell-mediated and humoral immunity. These studies thus imply a critical role for IL-2Rγ in normal immune function. Since two of the mutations resulted in truncation of the cytoplasmic domain of this receptor (deletion of 62 and 81 amino acids, respectively), such natural variants provide an initial 'roadmap' for defining critical domains within this receptor subunit. It has not been determined whether or not other subunits of the IL-2 receptor or of other cytokine receptors might be similarly affected in other forms of congenital immunodeficiency. It is also tempting to speculate that the profound clinical effects of these mutations may indicate a broader role of the IL-2Rγ protein in immune processes. For example, sharing of common receptor subunits by different cytokine receptors has been demonstrated in other receptor systems (for a review, see Miyajima *et al.*, 1992), and further studies will be needed to determine whether or not IL-2Rγ is itself a common subunit to a family of cytokine receptors. Finally, several poxviruses have been found to contain transduced homologues of mammalian cytokine receptors (Smith *et al.*, 1990; Upton *et al.*, 1991, 1992; Alcami and Smith, 1992; Spriggs *et al.*, 1992). Such 'viroceptors' appear to constitute virulence factors for the viruses, in which a receptor homologue is used to antagonize the normal cytokine system. Although no such IL-2 viroceptor has been reported to date, further studies will be needed to define the complete viroceptor family.

CONCLUSIONS AND FUTURE DIRECTIONS

The IL-2R is now recognized as a heteromultimeric receptor complex that is responsible for mediating a variety of critical cellular responses to extracellular IL-2 in several cell types. Cellular, biochemical, genetic and structural studies have begun to provide a framework for understanding the molecular basis of ligand binding, subunit assembly and interaction, and signal transduction. IL-2 likely lies in a binding crevice generated by the *N*-terminal regions of IL-2Rα, β and γ, with more distal domains of these subunits interacting in some manner to facilitate assembly of the complex into a high-affinity receptor configuration. This configuration, which is at least partly dependent upon the binding of IL-2, permits the discharge of signals into the cell that lead to biological responses such as progression through cell cycle and induction of effector or differentiation genes. The contributions of conformational shifts and intramolecular interactions in the transition to an active signal transduction state remain undefined. Within the IL-2Rβ cytoplasmic region certain domains have been identified that are essential for competence to transmit specific signals. A complete map of such domains within β and other subunits awaits further analysis, as does an elucidation of the molecular principles underlying a domain design. Many constituents of the entire signal transduction apparatus also remain unidentified, although a cadre of tyrosine kinases and other enzymes that may participate in the signal transduction process is beginning to emerge. The specific role(s) of such catalytic components in effecting or regulating signal transmission are under intense scrutiny through molecular and biochemical strategies. Finally, the pathogenetic roles that the IL-2R may play in human lymphoid malignancies and immunodeficiency syndromes has been the subject of extensive investigation and of recent discovery. A thorough understanding of the molecular basis of IL-2/IL-2R function is an essential element to defining the aetiology of such disease states and to identifying potential therapeutic strategies for the future.

ACKNOWLEDGEMENTS

The authors acknowledge the excellent secretarial assistance of Ms Diane Gearhart in the preparation of this manuscript. M.A.G. was a Fellow in the UCSF AIDS Program sponsored by the National Institutes of Health, and both M.A.G. and W.C.G. are supported by the J. David Gladstone Institutes.

REFERENCES

Alcami, A. and Smith, G.L. (1992). *Cell* **71**, 153–167.
Andrew, M.E., Churilla, A.M., Malek, T.R., Braciale, V.L. and Braciale, T.J. (1985). *J. Immunol.* **134**, 920–925.
Arima, N., Kuziel, W.A., Grdina, T.A. and Greene, W.C. (1992). *J. Immunol.* **149**, 83–91.
Asao, H., Takeshita, T., Nakamura, M., Nagata, K. and Sugamura, K. (1990). *J. Exp. Med.* **171**, 637–644.
Augustine, J.A., Sutor, S.L. and Abraham, R.T. (1991). *Mol. Cell. Biol.* **11**, 4431–4440.
Baccarini, M., Schwinzer, R. and Lohmann, M.M. (1989). *J. Immunol.* **142**, 118–125.
Bazan, J.F. (1990). *Proc. Natl Acad. Sci. USA* **87**, 6934–6938.
Bazan, J.F. (1992). *Science* **257**, 410–413.
Ben Aribia, M., Moire, N., Metivier, D., Vaquero, C., Lantz, O., Olive, D., Charpentier, B. and Senik, A. (1989). *J. Immunol.* **142**, 490–499.
Benveniste, E.N. and Merrill, J.E. (1986). *Nature* **321**, 610–613.
Bich-Thuy, L., Dukovich, M., Peffer, N.J., Fauci, A.S., Kehrl, J.H. and Greene, W.C. (1987). *J. Immunol.* **139**, 1550–1556.
Bluestone, J.A., Pardoll, D., Sharrow, S.O. and Fowlkes, B.J. (1987). *Nature* **326**, 82–84.
Bonneville, M., Ishida, I., Itohara, S., Verbeek, S., Berns, A., Kanagawa, O., Haas, W. and Tonegawa, S. (1990). *Nature* **344**, 163–165.
Brandhuber, B.J., Boone, T., Kenney, W.C. and McKay, D.B. (1987). *Science* **238**, 1707–1709.
Calvo, V., Crews, C.M., Vik, T.A. and Bierer, B.E. (1992). *Proc. Natl Acad. Sci. USA* **89**, 7571–7575.
Carding, S.R., Jenkinson, E.J., Kingston, R., Hayday, A.C., Bottomly, K. and Owen, J.J. (1989). *Proc. Natl Acad. Sci. USA* **86**, 3342–3345.
Ceredig, R., Lowenthal, J.W., Nabholz, M. and MacDonald, H.R. (1985). *Nature* **314**, 98–100.
Cerretti, D.P., McKereghan, K., Larsen, A., Cantrell, M.A., Anderson, D., Gillis, S., Cosman, D. and Baker, P.E. (1986). *Proc. Natl Acad. Sci. USA* **83**, 3223–3227.
Chang, A.E. and Rosenberg, S.A. (1989). *Semin. Surg. Oncol.* **5**, 385–390.
Chen, S.J., Holbrook, N.J., Mitchell, K.F., Vallone, C.A., Greengard, J.S., Crabtree, G.R. and Lin, Y. (1985). *Proc. Natl Acad. Sci. USA* **82**, 7284–7288.
Collins, L., Tsien, W.H., Seals, C., Hakimi, J., Weber, D., Bailon, P., Hoskings, J., Greene, W.C., Toome, V. and Ju, G. (1988). *Proc. Natl Acad. Sci. USA* **85**, 7709–7713.
Cosman, D., Cerretti, D.P., Larsen, A., Park, L., March, C., Dower, S., Gillis, S. and Urdal, D. (1984). *Nature* **312**, 768–771.
Crabtree, G.R. (1989). *Science* **243**, 355–361.
Cross, S.L., Feinberg, M.B., Wolf, J.B., Holbrook, N.J., Wong, S.F. and Leonard, W.J. (1987). *Cell* **49**, 47–56.
Cullen, B.R., Podlaski, F.J., Peffer, N.J., Hosking, J.B. and Greene, W.C. (1988). *J. Biol. Chem.* **263**, 4900–4906.
Cunningham, B.C., Ultsch, M., De, V.A., Mulkerrin, M.G., Clauser, K.R. and Wells, J.A. (1991). *Science* **254**, 821–825.
De la Hera, A., Toribio, M.L., Marquez, C., Marcos, M.A., Cabrero, E. and Martinez, A.C. (1986). *Eur. J. Immunol.* **16**, 653–658.
De la Hera, A., Toribio, M.L., Marcos, M.A., Marquez, C. and Martinez, C. (1987). Eur. J. Immunol. **17**, 683–687.
Depper, J.M., Leonard, W.J., Kronke, M., Noguchi, P.D., Cunningham, R.E., Waldmann, T.A. and Greene, W.C. (1984). *J. Immunol.* **133**, 3054–3061.
Depper, J.M., Leonard, W.J., Drogula, C., Kronke, M., Waldmann, T.A. and Greene, W.C. (1985). *Proc. Natl Acad. Sci. USA* **82**, 4230–4234.

Devos, R., Plaetinck, G., Cheroutre, H., Simons, G., Degrave, W., Tavernier, J., Remaut, E. and Fiers, W. (1983). *Nucl. Acids Res*. **11**, 4307–4323.

Devos, A., Ultsch, M. and Kossiakoff, A.A. (1992). *Science* **255**, 306–312.

Dukovich, M., Wano, Y., Le, thi, Bich-Thuy, L., Katz, P., Cullen, B.R., Kehrl, J.H. and Greene, W.C. (1987). *Nature* **327**, 518–522.

Durand, D.B., Shaw, J. P., Bush, M. R., Replogle, R.E., Belagaje, R. and Crabtree, G.R. (1988). *Mol. Cell. Biol*. **8**, 1715–1724.

Farrar, J.J., Benjamin, W.R., Hilfiker, M.L., Howard, M., Farrar, W.L. and Fuller, F.J. (1982). *Immunol. Rev*. **63**, 129–166.

Fujita, T., Takaoka, C., Matsui, H. and Taniguchi, T. (1983). *Proc. Natl Acad. Sci. USA* **80**, 7437–7441.

Fung, M.R., Ju, G. and Greene, W.C. (1988). *J. Exp. Med*. **168**, 1923–1928.

Fung, M. R., Scearce, R.M., Hoffman, J. A., Peffer, N.J., Hammes, S.R., Hosking, J.B., Schmandt, R., Kuziel, W.A., Haynes, B.F. and Mills, G.B. (1991). *J. Immunol*. **147**, 1253–1260.

Garcia, G.G., Evans, G.A., Michiel, D.F. and Farrar, W.L. (1992). *Biochem. J*. **285**, 851–856.

Garni-Wagner, B., Witte, P.L., Tutt, M.M., Kuziel, W.A., Tucker, P.W., Bennett, M. and Kumar, V. (1990). *J. Immunol*. **144**, 796–803.

Gillis, S. and Watson, J. (1980). *J. Exp. Med*. **152**, 1709–1719.

Gillis, S., Ferm, M.M., Ou, W. and Smith, K.A. (1978). *J. Immunol*. **120**, 2027–2032.

Gnarra, J.R., Otani, H., Wang, M.G., McBride, O.W., Sharon, M. and Leonard, W.J. (1990). *Proc. Natl Acad. Sci. USA* **87**, 3440–3444.

Goodall, J.C., Emery, D.C., Bailey, M., English, L.S. and Hall, L. (1991). *Biochim. Biophys. Acta* **1089**, 257–258.

Granelli-Piperno, A., Andrus, L. and Steinman, R.M. (1986). *J. Exp. Med*. **163**, 922–937.

Grant, A.J., Roessler, E., Ju, G,. Tsudo, M., Sugamura, K. and Waldmann, T.A. (1992). *Proc. Natl Acad. Sci. USA* **89**, 2165–2169.

Graves, J.D., Downward, J., Izquierdo, P.M., Rayter, S., Warne, P.H. and Cantrell, D.A. (1992). *J. Immunol*. **148**, 2417–2422.

Greene, W.C., Robb, R.J., Svetlik, P.B., Rusk, C.M., Depper, J.M. and Leonard, W.J. (1985). *J. Exp. Med*. **162**, 363–368.

Greene, W.C., Bohnlein, E. and Ballard, D.W. (1989). *Immunol. Today* **10**, 272–278.

Habu, S., Okumura, K., Diamantstein, T. and Shevach, E.M. (1985). *Eur. J. Immol*. **15**, 456–460.

Hancock, W.W., Muller, W.A. and Cotran, R.S. (1987). *J. Immunol*. **138**, 185–191.

Hanks, S.K., Quinn, A.M. and Hunter, T. (1988). *Science* **241**, 42–52.

Hardt, C., Diamantstein, T. and Wagner, H. (1985). *J. Immunol*. **134**, 3891–3894.

Hatakeyama, M., Kawahara, A., Mori, H., Shibuya, H. and Taniguchi, T. (1992). *Proc. Natl Acad. Sci., USA* **89**, 2022–2026.

Hatakeyama, M., Minamoto, S., Uchiyama, T., Hardy, R.R., Yamada, G. and Taniguchi, T. (1985). *Nature* **318**, 467–470.

Hatakeyama, M., Minamoto, S. and Taniguchi, T. (1986). *Proc. Natl Acad. Sci. USA* **83**, 9650–9654.

Hatakeyama, M., Tsudo, M., Minamoto, S., Kono, T., Doi, T., Miyata, T., Miyasaka, M. and Taniguchi, T. (1989a). *Science* **244**, 551–556.

Hatakeyama, M., Mori, H., Doi, T. and Taniguchi, T. (1989b). *Cell* **59**, 837–845.

Hatakeyama, M., Kono, T., Kobayashi, N., Kawahara, A., Levin, S.D., Perlmutter, R.M. and Taniguchi, T. (1991). *Science* **252**, 1523–1528.

Hatakeyama, M., Kawahara, A., Mori, H., Shibuya, H. and Taniguchi, T. (1992). *Proc. Natl Acad. Sci. USA* **89**, 2022–2026.

Herrmann, F., Cannistra, S.A., Levine, H. and Griffin, J.D. (1985). *J. Exp. Med*. **162**, 1111–1116.

Holbrook, N.J., Lieber, M. and Crabtree, G.R. (1984). *Nucl. Acids Res*. **12**, 5005–5013.

Holter, W., Grunow, R., Stockinger, H. and Knapp, W. (1986). *J. Immunol*. **136**, 2171–2175.

Holter, W., Goldman, C.K., Casabo, L., Nelson, D.L., Greene, W.C. and Waldmann, T.A. (1987). *J. Immunol*. **138**, 2917–2922.

Horak, I.D., Gress, R.E., Lucas, P.J., Horak, E.M., Waldmann, T.A. and Bolen, J.B. (1991). *Proc. Natl Acad. Sci. USA* **88**, 1996–2000.

Howard, M., Matis, L., Malek, T.R., Shevach, E., Kell, W., Cohen, D., Nakanishi, K. and Paul, W.E. (1983). *J. Exp. Med*. **158**, 2024–2039.

Hoyos, B., Ballard, D.W., Bohnlein, E., Siekevitz, M. and Greene, W.C. (1989). *Science* **244**, 457–460.

Imler, J.L., Miyajima, A. and Zurawski, G. (1992). *EMBO J.* **11**, 2047–2053.

Inoue, J., Seiki, M., Taniguchi, T., Tsuru, S. and Yoshida, M. (1986). *EMBO J.* **5**, 2883–2888.

Izquierdo, M. and Cantrell, D.A. (1993). *Eur. J. Immunol.* **23**, 131–135.

Izquierdo, M., Downward, J., Graves, J.D. and Cantrell, D.A. (1992). *Mol. Cell. Biol.* **12**, 3305–3312.

Jelinek, D.F. and Lipsky, P.E. (1987). *Adv. Immunol.* **40**, 1–59.

Jenkinson, E.J., Kingston, R. and Owen, J.J. (1987). *Nature* **329**, 160–162.

Ju, G., Collins, I, Kaffka, K.L., Tsien, W.H., Chizzonite, R., Crowl, R., Bhatt, R. and Kilian, P.L. (1987). *J. Biol. Chem.* **262**, 5723–5731.

Kashima, N., Nishi, T.C., Fujita, T., Taki, S., Yamada, G., Hamuro, J. and Taniguchi, T. (1985). *Nature* **313**, 402–404.

Kehrl, J.H., Dukovich, M., Whalen, G., Katz, P., Fauci, A.S. and Greene, W.C. (1988). *J. Clin. Invest.* **81**, 200–205.

Kondo, S., Kinoshita, M., Shimizu, A., Saito, Y., Konishi, M., Sabe, H. and Honjo, T. (1987). *Nature* **327**, 64–67.

Kono, T., Doi, T., Yamada, G., Hatakeyama, M., Minamoto, S., Tsudo, M., Miyasaka, M., Miyata, T. and Taniguchi, T. (1990). *Proc. Natl Acad. Sci. USA* **87**, 1806–1810.

Kuo, C.J., Chung, J., Fiorentino, D.F., Flanagan, W.M., Blenis, J. and Crabtree, G.R. (1992). *Nature* **358**, 70–73.

Kuo, L.M. and Robb, R.J. (1986). *J. Immunol.* **137**, 1538–1543.

Kuziel, W.A., Ju, G., Grdina, T.A. and Greene, W.C. (1993). *J. Immunol.* **150**, 3357–3365.

Le Gros, G., Shackell, P.S., Le, G.J. and Watson, J.D. (1987). *J. Immunol.* **138**, 478–483.

Lee, J.C., Truneh, A., Smith, M.J. and Tsang, K.Y. (1987). *J. Immunol.* **139**, 1935–1938.

Leonard, W.J., Depper, J.M., Uchiyama, T., Smith, K.A., Waldmann, T.A. and Greene, W.C. (1982). *Nature* **300**, 267–269.

Leonard, W.J., Depper, J.M., Robb, R.J., Waldmann, T.A. and Greene, W.C. (1983). *Proc. Natl Acad. Sci. USA* **80**, 6957–6961.

Leonard, W.J., Depper, J.M., Crabtree, G.R., Rudikoff, S., Pumphrey, J., Robb, R.J., Kronke, M., Svetlik, P.B., Peffer, N.J. and Waldmann, T.A. (1984). *Nature* **311**, 626–631.

Leonard, W.J., Depper, J.M., Kanehisa, M., Kronke, M., Peffer, N.J., Svetlik, P.B., Sullivan, M. and Greene, W.C. (1985a). *Science* **230**, 633–639.

Leonard, W.J., Donlon, T.A., Lebo, R.V. and Greene, W.C. (1985b). *Science* **228**, 1547–1549.

Leonard, W.J., Depper, J.M., Kronke, M., Robb, R.J., Waldmann, T.A. and Greene, W.C. (1985c). *J. Biol. Chem.* **260**, 1872–1880.

Lowenthal, J.W. and Greene, W.C. (1987). *J. Exp. Med.* **166**, 1156–1161.

Lowenthal, J.W., Tougne, C., MacDonald, H.R., Smith, K.A. and Nabholz, M. (1985). *J. Immunol.* **134**, 931–939.

Lowenthal, J.W., Ballard, D.W., Bogerd, H., Bohnlein, E. and Greene, W.C. (1989). *J. Immunol.* **142**, 3121–3128.

McKnight, A.J., Mason, D.W. and Barclay, A.N. (1989). *Immunogenetics* **30**, 145–147.

Malkovsky, M., Loveland, B., North, M., Asherson, G.L., Gao, L., Ward, P. and Fiers, W. (1987). *Nature* **325**, 262–265.

Maruyama, M., Shibuya, H., Harada, H., Hatakeyama, M., Seiki, M., Fujita, T., Inoue, J., Yoshida, M. and Taniguchi, T. (1987). *Cell* **48**, 343–350.

Merida, I. and Gaulton, G.N. (1990). *J. Biol. Chem.* **265**, 5690–5694.

Merida, I., Diez, E. and Gaulton, G.N. (1991). *J. Immunol.* **147**, 2202–2207.

Merida, I., Williamson, P., Kuziel, W.A., Greene, W.C. and Gaulton, G.N. (1993). *J. Biol. Chem.* **268**, 6765–6770.

Michiel, D.F., Garcia, G.G., Evans, G.A. and Farrar, W.L. (1991). *Cytokine* **3**, 428–438.

Miller, J., Malek, T.R., Leonard, W.J., Greene, W.C., Shevach, E.M. and Germain, R.N. (1985). *J. Immunol.* **134**, 4212–4217.

Mills, G.B., Stewart, D.J., Mellors, A. and Gelfand, E.W. (1986). *J. Immunol.* **136**, 3019–3024.

Mills, G.B., May, C., McGill, M., Fung, M., Baker, M., Sutherland, R. and Greene, W.C. (1990). *J. Biol. Chem.* **265**, 3561–3567.

Mills, G.B., Arima, N., May, C., Hill, M., Schmandt, R., Li, J., Miyamoto, N.G. and Greene, W.C. (1992). *Int. Immunol.* **4**, 1233–1243.

Minami, Y., Kono, T., Yamada, K., Kobayashi, N., Kawahara, A., Perlmutter, R.M. and Taniguchi, T. (1993). *EMBO J.* **12**, 759–768.
Miyajima, A., Hara, T. and Kitamura, T. (1992). *Trends Biochem. Sci.* **17**, 378–382.
Miyawaki, T., Yachie, A., Uwadana, N., Ohzeki, S., Nagaoki, T. and Taniguchi, N. (1982). *J. Immunol.* **129**, 2474–2478.
Miyazaki, T., Maruyama, M., Yamada, G., Hatakeyama, M. and Taniguchi, T. (1991). *EMBO J.* **10**, 3191–3197.
Morgan, D.A., Ruscetti, F.W. and Gallo, R. (1976). *Science* **193**, 1007–1008.
Mori, H., Barsoumian, E.L., Hatakeyama, M. and Taniguchi, T. (1991). *Int. Immunol.* **3**, 149–156.
Morla, A.O., Schreurs, J., Miyajima, A. and Wang, J.Y. (1988). *Mol. Cell. Biol.* **8**, 2214–2218.
Muegge, K. and Durum, S.K. (1989). *New Biol.* **1**, 239–246.
Muegge, K., Williams, T.M., Kant, J., Karin, M., Chiu, R., Schmidt, A., Siebenlist, U., Young, H.A. and Durum, S.K. (1989). *Science*, **246**, 249–251.
Murakami, M., Narazaki, M., Hibi, M., Yawata, H., Yasukawa, K., Hamaguchi, M., Taga, T. and Kishimoto, T. (1991). *Proc. Natl Acad. Sci. USA* **88**, 11349–11353.
Nakamura, Y., Inamoto, T., Sugie, K., Masutani, H., Shindo, T., Tagaya, Y., Yamauchi, A., Ozawa, K. and Yodoi, J. (1989). *Proc. Natl Acad. Sci. USA* **86**, 1318–1322.
Nakanishi, K., Hirose, S., Yoshimoto, T., Ishizashi, H., Hiroishi, K., Tanaka, T., Kono, T., Miyasaka, M., Taniguchi, T. and Higashino, K. (1992). *Proc. Natl Acad. Sci. USA* **89**, 3551–3555.
Nikaido, T., Shimizu, A., Ishida, N., Sabe, H., Teshigawara, K., Maeda, M., Uchiyama, T., Yodoi, J. and Honjo, T. (1984). *Nature* **311**, 631–635.
Nishi, M., Ishida, Y. and Honjo, T. (1988). *Nature* **331**, 267–269.
Noguchi, M., Yi, H., Rosenblatt, H.M., Filipovich, A. H., Adelstein, S., Modi, W. S., McBride, O. W. and Leonard, W. J. (1993). *Cell* **73**, 147–157.
Ohashi, Y., Takeshita, T., Nagata, K., Mori, S. and Sugamura, K. (1989). *J. Immunol.* **143**, 3548–3555.
Ortaldo, J.R., Mason, A.T., Gerard, J.P., Henderson, L.E., Farrar, W., Hopkins, R.F., Herberman, R.B. and Rabin, H. (1984). *J. Immunol.* **133**, 779–783.
Otani, H., Siegel, J.P., Erdos, M., Gnarra, J.R., Toledano, M.B., Sharon, M., Mostowski, H., Feinberg, M.B., Pierce, J.H. and Leonard, W.J. (1992). *Proc. Natl Acad. Sci. USA* **89**, 2789–2793.
Ralph P., Jeong, G., Welte, K., Mertelsmann, R., Rabin, H., Henderson, L.E., Souza, L.M., Boone, T.C. and Robb, R.J. (1984). *J. Immunol.* **133**, 2442–2445.
Ralph, P., Nakoinz, I. and Rennick, D. (1988). *J.Exp. Med.* **167**, 712–717.
Rammensee, H.G., Kroschewski, R. and Frangoulis, B. (1989). *Nature* **339**, 541–544.
Ramsdell, F. and Fowlkes, B.J. (1990). *Science* **248**, 1342–1348.
Raulet, D.H. (1985). *Nature* **314**, 101–103.
Reed, J.C., Alpers, J.D., Scherle, P.A., Hoover, R.G., Nowell, P.C. and Prystowsky, M.B. (1987). *Oncogene* **1**, 223–228.
Reeves, R., Spies, A.G., Nissen, M.S., Buck, C.D., Weinberg, A.D., Barr, P.J., Magnuson, N.S. and Magnuson, J.A. (1986). *Proc. Natl Acad. Sci. USA* **83**, 3228–3232.
Ringheim, G.E., Freimark, B.D. and Robb, R.J. (1991). *Lymphokine Cytokine Res.* **10**, 219–224.
Robb, R.J. and Greene, W.C. (1983). *J. Exp. Med.* **158**, 1332–1337.
Robb, R.J. and Greene, W.C. (1987). *J. Exp. Med.* **165**, 1201–1206.
Robb, R.J., Munck, A. and Smith, K.A. (1981). *J. Exp. Med.* **154**, 1455–1474.
Robb, R.J., Kutny, R.M. and Chowdhry, V. (1983). *Proc. Natl Acad. Sci. USA* **80**, 5990–5994.
Robb, R.J., Greene, W.C. and Rusk, C.M. (1984). *J. Exp. Med.* **160**, 1126–1146.
Robb, R.J., Rusk, C.M., Yodoi, J. and Greene, W.C. (1987). *Proc. Natl Acad. Sci. USA* **84**, 2002–2006.
Robb, R.J., Rusk, C.M. and Neeper, M.P. (1988). *Proc. Natl Acad. Sci. USA* **85**, 5654–5658.
Rosenberg, S.A. and Lotze, M.T. (1986). *Annu. Rev. Immunol.* **4**, 681–709.
Rusk, C.M., Neeper, M.P., Kuo, L.M., Kutny, R.M. and Robb, R.J. (1988). *J. Immunol.* **140**, 2249–2259.
Sabe, H, Kondo, S., Shimizu, A., Tagaya, Y., Yodoi, J., Kobayashi, N., Hatanaka, M., Matsunami, N., Maeda, M. and Noma, T. (1984). *Mol. Biol. Med.* **2**, 379–396.
Sadlack, B., Schorle, H., Schimpl, A., Merz, H., Feller, A.C. and Horak, L. (1993). *J. Cell. Biochem.* **17**, 54.
Saltzman, E.M., Thom, R.R. and Casnellie, J.E. (1988). *J. Biol. Chem.* **263**, 6956–6959.
Saneto, R.P., Altman, A., Knobler, R.L., Johnson, H.M. and De, V.J. (1986). *Proc. Natl Acad. Sci. USA* **83**, 9221–9225.
Saragovi, H. and Malek, T.R. (1988). *J. Immunol.* **141**, 476–482.

Satoh, T., Minami, Y., Kono, T., Yamada, K., Kawahara, A., Taniguchi, T. and Kaziro, Y. (1992). *J. Biol. Chem.* **267**, 25423–25427.

Sauve, K., Nachman, M., Spence, C., Bailon, P., Campbell, E., Tsien, W.H., Kondas, J.A., Hakimi, J. and Ju, G. (1991). *Proc. Natl Acad. Sci. USA* **88**, 4636–4640.

Schorle, H., Holtschke, T., Hunig, T., Schimpl, A. and Horak, I. (1991). *Nature* **352**, 621–624.

Schwartz, R.H. (1990). *Science* **248**, 1349–1356.

Seigel, L.J., Harper, M.E., Wong, S.F., Gallo, R.C., Nash, W.G. and O'Brien, S.J. (1984). *Science* **223**, 175–178.

Seow, H.F., Rothel, J.S., Radford, A.J. and Wood, P.R. (1990). *Nucl. Acids Res.* **18**, 7175.

Serfling, E., Barthelmas, R., Pfeuffer, I., Schenk, B., Zarius, S., Swoboda, R., Mercurio, F. and Karin, M. (1989). *EMBO J.* **8**, 465–473.

Shackelford, D.A. and Trowbridge, I.S. (1991). *Cell Regul.* **2**, 73–85.

Sharon, M., Klausner, R.D., Cullen, B.R., Chizzonite, R. and Leonard, W.J. (1986). *Science* **234**, 859–863.

Sharon, M., Gnarra, J.R. and Leonard, W.J. (1989). *J. Immunol.* **143**, 2530–2533.

Shaw, G. and Kamen, R. (1986). *Cell* **46**, 659–667.

Shaw, J.P., Utz, P.J., Durand, D.B., Toole, J.J., Emmel, E.A. and Crabtree, G.R. (1988). *Science* **241**, 202–205.

Shibuya, H., Yoneyama, M., Ninomiya, T.J., Matsumoto, K. and Taniguchi, T. (1992). *Cell* **70**, 57–67.

Siebenlist, U., Durand, D.B., Bressler, P., Holbrook, N.J., Norris, C.A., Kamoun, M., Kant, J.A. and Crabtree, G.R. (1986). *Mol. Cell. Biol.* **6**, 3042–3049.

Siegel, J.P., Sharon, M., Smith, P.L. and Leonard, W.J. (1987). *Science* **238**, 75–78.

Siekevitz, M., Feinberg, M.B., Holbrook, N., Wong, S.F. and Greene, W.C. (1987). *Proc. Natl Acad. Sci. USA* **84**, 5389–5393.

Smith, C.A., Davis, T., Anderson, D., Solam, L., Beckmann, M.P., Jerzy, R., Dower, S.K., Cosman, D. and Goodwin, R.G. (1990). *Science* **248**, 1019–1023.

Smith, K.A. (1980). *Immunol. Rev.* **51**, 337–357.

Smith, K.A. and Cantrell, D.A. (1985). *Proc. Natl Acad. Sci. USA* **82**, 864–868.

Spriggs, M.K., Hruby, D.E., Maliszewski, C.R., Pickup, D.J., Sims, J.E., Buller, R.M. and VanSlyke, J. (1992). *Cell* **71**, 145–152.

Stern, J.B. and Smith, K. A. (1986). *Science* **233**, 203–206.

Sugamura, K., Takeshita, T., Asao, H., Kumaki, S., Ohbo, K., Ohtani, K. and Nakamura, M. (1990). *Lymphokine Res.* **9**, 539–542.

Taira, S., Matsui, M., Hayakawa, K., Yokoyama, T. and Nariuchi, H. (1987). *J. Immunol.* **139**, 2957–2964.

Takeshita, T., Goto, Y., Tada, K., Nagata, K., Asao, H. and Sugamura, K. (1989). *J. Exp. Med.* **169**, 1323–1332.

Takeshita, T., Asao, H., Suzuki, J. and Sugamura, K. (1990). *Int. Immunol.* **2**, 477–480.

Takeshita, T., Asao, H., Ohtani, K., Ishii, N., Kumaki, S., Tanaka, N., Munakata, H., Nakamura, M. and Sugamura, K. (1992a). *Science* **257**, 379–382.

Takeshita, T., Ohtani, K., Asao, H., Kumaki, S., Nakamura, M. and Sugamura, K. (1992b). *J. Immunol.* **148**, 2154–2158.

Taniguchi, T., Matsui, H., Fujita, T., Takaoka, C,. Kashima, N., Yoshimoto, R. and Hamuro, J. (1983). *Nature* **302**, 305–310.

Tentori, L., Longo, D.L., Zuniga, P.J., Wing, C. and Kruisbeek, A.M. (1988). *J. Exp. Med.* **168**, 1741–1747.

Terada, N., Lucas, J.J., Szepesi, A., Franklin, R.A., Takase, K. and Gelfand, E.W. (1992). *Biochem. Biophys. Res. Commun.* **186**, 1315–1321.

Teshigawara, K., Wang, H.M., Kato, K. and Smith, K.A. (1987). *J. Exp. Med.* **165**, 223–238.

Tigges, M.A., Casey, L.S. and Koshland, M.E. (1989). *Science* **243**, 781–786.

Toribio, M.L., de, la, Hera, A., Borst, J., Marcos, M.A., Marquez, C., Alonso, J.M., Barcena, A. and Martinez, C. (1988). *J. Exp. Med.* **168**, 2231–2249.

Toribio, M.L., Gutierrez, R.J., Pezzi, L., Marcos, M.A. and Martinez, C. (1989). *Nature* **342**, 82–85.

Trinchieri, G., Matsumoto, K.M., Clark, S.C., Seehra, J., London, L. and Perussia, B. (1984). *J. Exp. Med.* **160**, 1147–1169.

Tsudo, M., Kozak, R. W., Goldman, C.K. and Waldmann, T.A. (1986). *Proc. Natl Acad. Sci. USA* **83**, 9694–9698.

Tsudo, M., Goldman, C.K., Bongiovanni, K.F., Chan, W.C., Winton, E.F., Yagita, M., Grimm, E.A. and Waldmann, T.A. (1987). *Proc. Natl Acad. Sci. USA* **84**, 5394–5398.

Tsudo, M., Kitamura, F. and Miyasaka, M. (1989a). *Proc. Natl Acad. Sci. USA* **86**, 1982–1986.
Tsudo, M., Karasuyama, H., Kitamura, F., Nagasaka, Y., Tanaka, T. and Miyasaka, M. (1989b). *J. Immunol.* **143**, 4039–4043.
Tsudo, M., Karasuyama, H., Kitamura, F., Tanaka, T., Kubo, S., Yamamura, Y., Tamatani, T., Hatakeyama, M., Taniguchi, T. and Miyasaka, M. (1990). *J. Immunol.* **145**, 599–606.
Turner, B., Rapp, U., App, H., Greene, M., Dobashi, K. and Reed, J. (1991). *Proc. Natl Acad. Sci. USA* **88**, 1227–1231.
Uchiyama, T., Broder, S. and Waldmann, T.A. (1981). *J. Immunol.* **126**, 1393–1397.
Ullman, K.S., Northrop, J.P., Verweij, C.L. and Crabtree, G.R. (1990). *Annu. Rev. Immunol.* **8**, 421–452.
Upton, C., Macen, J.L., Schreiber, M. and McFadden, G. (1991). *Virology* **184**, 370–382.
Upton, C., Mossman, K. and McFadden, G. (1992). *Science* **258**, 1369–1372.
Valge, V. E., Wong, J. G., Datlof, B. M., Sinskey, A. J. and Rao, A. (1988). *Cell* **55**, 101–112.
Von Boehmer, H., Crisanti, A., Kisielow, P. and Haas, W. (1985). *Nature* **314**, 539–540.
Voss, S.D., Sondel, P.M. and Robb, R.J. (1992). *J. Exp. Med.* **176**, 531–541.
Voss, S.D., Leary, T.P., Sondel, P.M. and Robb, R.J. (1993). *Proc. Natl Acad. Sci. USA* **90**, 2428–2432.
Waldmann, T.A., Goldman, C.K., Robb, R.J., Depper, J.M., Leonard, W.J., Sharrow, S.O., Bongiovanni, K.F., Korsmeyer, S.J. and Greene, W.C. (1984). *J. Exp. Med.* **160**, 1450–1466.
Walker, E., Leemhuis, T. and Roeder, W. (1988). *J. Immunol.* **140**, 859–865.
Wang, H.M. and Smith, K.A. (1987). *J. Exp. Med.* **166**, 1055–1069.
Wano, Y., Cullen, B.R., Svetlik, P.A., Peffer, N.J. and Greene, W.C. (1987a). *Mol. Biol. Med.* **4**, 95–109.
Wano, Y., Feinberg, M., Hosking, J.B., Bogerd, H. and Greene, W.C. (1987b). *Proc. Natl Acad. Sci. USA* **85**, 9733–9737.
Watowich, S.S., Yoshimura, A., Longmore, G.D., Hilton, D.J., Yoshimura, Y. and Lodish, H.F. (1992). *Proc. Natl Acad. Sci. USA* **89**, 2140–2144.
Weigel, U., Meyer, M. and Sebald, W. (1989). *Eur. J. Biochem.* **180**, 295–300.
Yagita, H., Nakata, M., Azuma, A., Nitta, T., Takeshita, T., Sugamura, K. and Okumura, K. (1989). *J. Exp. Med.* **170**, 1445–1450.
Yodoi, J. and Uchiyama, T. (1992). *Immunol. Today* **13**, 405–411.
Yokota, T., Arai, N., Lee, F., Rennick, D., Mosmann, T. and Arai, K. (1985). *Proc. Natl Acad. Sci. USA* **82**, 68–72.
Yoshimura, A., Longmore, G. and Lodish, H.F. (1990). *Nature* **348**, 647–649.
Zmuidzinas, A., Mamon, H.J., Roberts, T.M. and Smith, K.A. (1991). *Mol. Cell. Biol.* **11**, 2794–2803.
Zuniga-Pflucker, J., Smith, K.A., Tentori, L., Pardoll, D.M., Longo, D.L. and Kruisbeek, A.M. (1990). *Dev. Immunol.* **1**, 59–66.
Zurawski, S.M. and Zurawski, G. (1989). *EMBO J.* **8**, 2583–2590.
Zurawski, S.M., Imler, J.L. and Zurawski, G. (1990). *EMBO J.* **9**, 3899–3905.

Chapter 5

Interleukin-3

John W. Schrader

The Biomedical Research Centre, University of British Columbia, Vancouver,
British Columbia, Canada V6T 1Z3

INTRODUCTION

Interleukin 3 (IL-3) acts on numerous target cells within the haemopoietic system, so it is not surprising that it was discovered independently by a number of laboratories studying different biological activities. It went under a variety of names including persisting-cell-stimulating factor, histamine-producing cell-stimulating factor, multi-CSF, multilineage haemopoietic growth factor, Thy-1 inducing factor, CFUs stimulating activity, CSF-2α, CSF-2β, haemopoietic-cell growth factor, mast-cell growth factor, eosinophil-CSF, megakaryocyte-CSF, erythroid-CSF, burst-promoting activity, neutrophil-granulocyte-CSF, haemopoietin-2 and synergistic activity. It was only with the biochemical purification (Ihle *et al.*, 1983; Clark-Lewis *et al.*, 1984), molecular cloning and expression (Fung *et al.*, 1984; Yokota *et al.*, 1984), and chemical synthesis (Clark-Lewis *et al.*, 1986) that it was conclusively established that a single protein mediated all of these bioactivities.

CELLULAR TARGETS OF IL-3

Although there are reports that IL-3 may affect the growth of certain epithelial cells, e.g. in carcinomas of the colon (Berdel *et al.*, 1989), the action of IL-3 on normal cells appears to be restricted to derivatives of the pluripotential haemopoietic stem cell. IL-3, however, has the broadest target specificity of any of the haemopoietic growth factors. The range of target cells can be summarized as including progenitor cells of every lineage derived from the pluripotential haemopoietic stem cells, with the likely exception of cells committed to the T- and B-lymphoid lineages. Thus, IL-3 can stimulate the generation and differentiation of macrophages, neutrophils, eosinophils, basophils, mast cells, megakaryocytes and erythroid cells (summarized in Schrader *et al.*, 1988). Moreover, IL-3 acts on primitive pluripotential stem cells, stimulating the growth *in vitro* of colonies containing mixtures of myeloid and erythroid cells, and stimulates both *in vitro* and *in vivo* the division of cells (CFUs) that form splenic colonies in irradiated mice (Iscove *et al.*, 1989). IL-3 also directly or indirectly promotes the survival *in vitro* of cells able to repopulate mice with T and B lymphocytes (Schrader *et al.*, 1988).

In vitro, haemopoietic progenitor cells rapidly die if cultured in tissue culture medium alone. Like other haemopoietic growth factors, IL-3 prevents death and promotes survival *in vitro*. Populations of mast cells generated by culturing murine bone-marrow cells in IL-3 remain dependent on IL-3, not only for their continual proliferation, but also for their survival. When they are deprived of IL-3 *in vitro* and cultured in medium alone, IL-3-dependent cells undergo apoptosis (Williams, G.T., *et al.*, 1990). This reaction to the withdrawal of IL-3 may be a control mechanism to ensure that the massive proliferation of the haemopoietic system that can be induced by the release of IL-3 (and other haemopoietic growth factors) during emergency situations like infections, is rapidly terminated when the emergency is over and that levels of the growth factors drop. Experiments demonstrating the rapid disappearance of IL-3-dependent cells that have been injected into normal animals lacking detectable IL-3 (Schrader and Crapper, 1983; Crapper *et al.*, 1984a) are consistent with this notion.

In common with other haemopoietic growth factors, IL-3 affects not only immature haemopoietic cells but also the mature members of some lineages. For example, the subset of mast cells associated with mucosal surfaces depend upon IL-3 for survival (Crapper *et al.*, 1984a; Schrader *et al.*, 1988). IL-3 also regulates the levels of major histocompatibility antigens on these mast cells, blocking the increased levels of expression induced by interferon-γ (Wong *et al.*, 1984).

IL-3 induces limited division of well-differentiated murine macrophages and enhances their phagocytosis of yeast (Crapper *et al.*, 1985; Chen *et al.*, 1988). IL-3 stimulation of macrophages results in increased levels of class II major histocompatibility complex antigens and LFA-1 (Frendl and Beller, 1990), and increased levels of mRNA encoding IL-1 (Frendl *et al.*, 1990a), IL-6 and TNF-α (Frendl *et al.*, 1990b).

Murine megakaryocytes differentiate *in vitro* in the presence of IL-3 (Ishibashi and Burstein, 1986). Human basophils are activated by IL-3 (Hirai *et al.*, 1988: Kurimoto *et al.*, 1989) and IL-3 stimulates the survival of human eosinophils (Rothenberg *et al.*, 1988) as well as increasing antibody-dependent cell-mediated cytotoxity, phagocytosis, and superoxide anion production in response to stimulation with f-met-leu-phe (Lopez *et al.*, 1987).

LYMPHOID CELLS

The question of whether IL-3 has a key role in regulating the production of T or B lymphocytes has been controversial. Some of this confusion has stemmed from the fact that unfortunate misconceptions or errors in earlier literature have taken some time to be widely recognized.

The early report that first used the term interleukin-3 (Hapel *et al.*, 1981), erroneously ascribed to IL-3 the property of stimulating the growth of helper T lymphocytes. The cells misidentified as helper T lymphocytes were, in fact, contaminating cells of the myelomonocytic leukaemia WEHI-3B, that had been used as a source for purification of the IL-3.

The confusion in this study may, in part, have been related to the fact that WEHI-3B cells express the Thy-1 antigen. At that time the Thy-1 antigen was thought to be a specific marker for T lymphocytes among lympho-haemopoietic cells in the mouse.

However, IL-3 induces the expression of high levels of the Thy-1 antigen on haemopoietic progenitor cells, including the precursors of macrophages and neutrophils (Schrader et al., 1982).

Another erroneous link between IL-3 and lymphocytic cells was based on the notion that IL-3 played a critical role in T-lymphocyte development. This arose from the observation that IL-3 induced increased levels of the enzyme 20-α-hydroxy-steroid-dehydrogenase in spleen cells from athymic mice and the hypothesis that this enzyme was specific for the T lymphocyte lineage (Ihle et al., 1981). Ihle and colleagues (1983) used the induction of 20-α-hydroxy-steroid-dehydrogenase as the basis of the assay used for the first purification to homogeneity of IL-3. However, the notion that this enzyme was restricted to T lymphocytes was disproved by the demonstration that IL-3 (and GM-CSF) induced this enzyme in cells of a number of myeloid lineages, including mast cells (Hapel and Young, 1988).

T LYMPHOCYTES

As noted above, pluripotential stem cells capable of ultimately giving rise to T and B lymphocytes may be affected directly or indirectly by IL-3 (Schrader et al., 1988). There is evidence that relatively small subsets of mature T cells may respond to IL-3 in the human (Londei et al., 1989). However, at present there is no evidence that thymic development or the function of the common subsets of T lymphocytes are directly influenced by IL-3.

B LYMPHOCYTES

Palacios and colleagues reported that IL-3 responsive clones of pre-B-lymphocytes could be obtained with high frequency from fetal liver (Palacios et al., 1984). However, there are no published accounts of the reproduction or extension of this work from the laboratories of either Palacios or others. Rennick and colleagues (1989) have reported that IL-3 could synergize with a stromal cell factor in stimulating the proliferation of murine pre-B-lymphocytes. There is evidence that IL-3 directly or indirectly affects cells that can give rise to B lymphocytes in irradiated animals (Schrader et al., 1988).

Palacios has reported the generation of a small number of IL-3-dependent cell lines that had the capacity to give rise to B lymphocytes in irradiated animals (Palacios and Steinmetz, 1985). Furthermore there are IL-3-dependent lines that can be induced to undergo B-cell differentiation and immunoglobulin gene rearrangement (Kinashi et al., 1988). However, it is unclear how frequently and how reproducibly such cell lines can be obtained. A proportion of a subset of human acute lymphoblastic leukaemias classified as B-cell precursors have also been shown to respond to IL-3 (Uckun et al., 1989).

Recently, Hirayama and colleagues (1992) reported the in vitro growth of primitive lympho-haemopoietic stem cells that could give rise to both myeloid cells and B lymphocytes. The growth of these stem cells was optimally supported by combinations of Steel or stem-cell factor (SLF) with IL-6, IL-11, or GM-CSF. The generation of B lymphocytes in secondary cultures required the presence of IL-7 and SLF. Interestingly, IL-3 was ineffective, either alone or with SLF, in maintaining the potential to generate B lymphocytes in the primary cultures. This suggests that IL-3 lacked the capacity to maintain or generate cells capable of giving rise to B lymphocytes in response to IL-7 and SLF.

In summary, primitive haemopoietic stem cells that are ultimately capable of giving rise to cells contributing to the B- or T-lymphocyte lineages probably respond to IL-3. Such cells, or their more committed progeny, can give rise to immortal cell-lines or leukaemia cells. However, there is as yet no compelling evidence that IL-3 has a significant, direct influence on B-cell development.

SYNERGIES WITH OTHER CYTOKINES

As is common among cytokines, IL-3 shows strong synergistic activities with other cytokines. For example in man, IL-3 synergizes with CSF-1 in producing macrophages, and with G-CSF in producing neutrophils. Both in humans and in mice, IL-3 synergizes with a number of cytokines such as CSF-1 and IL-1 in maximally stimulating the growth of primitive haemopoietic stem cells. In the mouse, the effect of IL-3 in promoting the growth of mast cells can be enhanced by IL-4, IL-9 and IL-10.

STRUCTURE

IL-3 has broad structural similarities with other interleukins and haemopoietic growth factors. It is a relatively small protein, with a polypeptide chain of 140 amino acids in the mouse (Fung et al., 1984; Yokota et al., 1984) and 133 in the human (Yang et al., 1986), and is heavily glycosylated. There are no marked amino acid sequence homologies with other peptide regulatory factors, although the fact that the genes for GM-CSF and IL-3 are closely linked (Yang et al., 1988) supports a common evolutionary ancestry.

Interestingly, IL-3 and a number of other cytokines including IL-1β, IL-2, GM-CSF and erythropoietin, share a short motif of amino acids at the N-terminus. This is characterized by an N-terminal alanine followed, in most instances, by a proline (Schrader et al., 1986a). The functional significance of this structural feature is obscure; in the case of IL-3 and GM-CSF it can be removed without affecting biological activity in vitro (Clark-Lewis et al., 1986, 1988).

X-ray diffraction studies of three other members of the family of cytokines that bind to members of the haemopoietin receptor superfamily, IL-2, GM-CSF, and IL-4 have demonstrated striking homologies in their three-dimensional structures. The fact that the receptor for IL-3 consists of a common β chain shared with GM-CSF and IL-5 in the human and an α chain that is highly homologous to the α chains bonding IL-5 and GM-CSF, suggests that the three-dimensional structure of IL-3 will closely resemble that of IL-5 and GM-CSF.

Analysis of structural analogues of IL-3 and of the effect on biological activity of antibodies specific for defined parts of the polypeptide chain have yielded information on the structural determinants of IL-3 bioactivity. IL-3 was the first protein of its size to be synthesized successfully by automated chemical methods (Clark-Lewis et al., 1986). This technique, shown by Clark-Lewis to be useful for the synthesis of cytokines in general, including mouse and human IL-3, IL-4, IL-6, GM-CSF and human IL-8, allowed a relatively rapid examination of the effects of deleting parts of the IL-3 molecule on bioactivity. In the case of mouse IL-3, these studies showed that the first 16, and the final 22 amino acids, could be deleted with very little loss of biological activity, suggesting that residues 17–118 could form all the structures essential for interaction with the receptor (Clark-Lewis *et al.*, 1986). Interestingly Clark-Lewis and colleagues showed earlier that the *N*-terminal half of IL-3 alone, i.e. residues 1–79, had detectable biological activity although the specific activity of this analogue was very low (Clark-Lewis *et al.*, 1986).

The notion that the *N*-terminus of IL-3 is not involved in interactions with the receptor, is supported by the fact that polyclonal antibodies specific for a peptide corresponding to residues 1–29 of IL-3 had relatively weak ability to neutralize IL-3 bioactivity (Ziltener *et al.*, 1987). Moreover, antibodies to peptide 1–29 bind to IL-3 molecules that have been allowed first to interact with the IL-3 receptor (Duronio *et al.*, 1991). In contrast, antibodies to peptides corresponding to residues 44–75 (Ziltener, unpublished data) and 91–112 (Ziltener *et al.*, 1987) strongly neutralize bioactivity, suggesting that these residues are part of, or are close to, the site or sites that interact with the IL-3 receptor.

Studies on human IL-3 (Lokker *et al.*, 1990) have identified two regions as targets of neutralizing antibodies. One is a linear epitope around residues 32–35, and the other, defined by conformational epitopes, maps nearer the *C*-terminus.

Because the IL-3 receptor is made up of at least two distinct polypeptide chains, both of which associate closely with IL-3 (Duronio *et al.*, 1991), distinct regions of the IL-3 molecule will be involved in binding to the two chains of the receptor. Based on the analysis of structural requirements of GM-CSF and IL-5 binding by Kastelein and colleagues (Kastelein and Shanafelt, 1993), it appears that residues in the most *N*-terminal α-helix of IL-3 will be critical for interaction with the β chain.

There are other important properties of the IL-3 molecule, apart from its ability to interact with its receptor, that will be regulated by its structure. These include its clearance and half-life in the plasma and its ability to interact with extracellular matrix. Natural IL-3 occurs in a diversity of glycoforms generated by the addition of carbohydrate groups. Whereas the synthesized polypeptide has a M_r of 14K upon sodium dodecyl sulphate (SDS)–polyacrylamide gel electrophoresis, IL-3 released from its natural source, activated T lymphocytes, runs as multiple bands, with major groups of bands with M_r around 22K, 28K and 36K (Ziltener *et al.*, 1988). Different T-cell clones appear to produce different proportions of the differently glycosylated forms (Ziltener, unpublished data). Carbohydrate on IL-3 of T-cell origin is exclusively *N*-linked (Ziltener *et al.*, 1988).

The glycosylation patterns of IL-3 produced by the other physiological source, the activated mast cell, has not been determined. IL-3 produced by recombinant DNA techniques in unnatural sources such as Chinese hamster ovary cells or COS cells, exhibit a broad smear of differently glycosylated species on SDS–gel electrophoresis, that is quite different from the pattern of distinct bands seen with IL-3 from the natural source T lymphocytes (Ziltener *et al.*, 1988).

The function of these extensive carbohydrate modifications of the IL-3 polypeptide is unknown. The clearance rate or stability of IL-3 in the blood, do not appear to be grossly affected by the presence or absence of carbohydrate. Ziltener and colleagues purified heavily, lightly and moderately glycosylated forms of IL-3 from T lymphocytes and demonstrated that, at least *in vitro*, they had the same specific activities and target specificities as deglycosylated material (Ziltener *et al.*, 1988). It is conceivable that the degree or type of glycosylation could regulate interaction with the extracellular matrix and influence diffusion or localization in tissues. One study of *in vitro* interactions of IL-3 with extracellular matrix material found that glycosylated and nonglycosylated IL-3 was bound equally well (Roberts *et al.*, 1988) but this does not exclude the importance of more subtle effects, such as those involving the matrix associated with particular stromal cells *in vivo*.

SOURCES OF IL-3

T Lymphocytes

The major physiological source of IL-3 is the activated T lymphocyte (Schrader and Nossal, 1980; Schrader, 1981; Niemeyer *et al.*, 1989). There is as yet no clear understanding of the mechanisms that regulate the spectrum of cytokines produced in response to a given antigen. It is evident that the type or form of antigen and the presence of adjuvants influence the range and quantity of cytokine produced.

Mast Cells

Recently it has been shown that mast cells can produce IL-3 when IgE Fc receptors are crosslinked (Burd *et al.*, 1989; Wodnar-Filipowicz *et al.*, 1989). The physiological significance of this phenomenon has yet to be established: it may serve to activate or prime other cells in the vicinity of an allergic response. These could include mast cells themselves, macrophages, as well as other haemopoietic cells.

Interaction of mast cells with fibroblasts *in vitro* can also lead to the accumulation of IL-3 mRNA in mast cells (Razin *et al.*, 1990). The physiological significance of this is unclear. It may depend upon the expression of the kit-ligand, SLF, on the surface of the fibroblasts and this may only occur in abnormal situations, for example during inflammation. Mast cells appear to express the kit receptor protein constitutively and the ability of SLF to stimulate mast cell growth, could conceivably involve the autocrine action of IL-3. As discussed below it is possible that interaction of haemopoietic stem and progenitor cells, expressing the c-kit protein, with stromal cells expressing SLF, could result in a similar phenomenon.

IL-3 IN NORMAL AND IMMUNOLOGICALLY STIMULATED ANIMALS

IL-3 is undetectable in the blood of normal animals (Crapper *et al.*, 1984b). In support of the notion that IL-3 is not present in significant quantities in the blood and extracellular fluids of normal mice, IL-3-dependent cell lines die when injected into normal mice, although they survive if the mice are provided with an artificial source of IL-3 (Schrader and Crapper, 1983; Crapper *et al.*, 1984b).

IL-3 can remain undetectable in the serum of animals undergoing immune responses (Crapper *et al.*, 1984a). However, in these instances, evidence for the local production of IL-3 at sites of immunological activation can be found (Crapper *et al.*, 1984a). For example, cells from lymph nodes draining the site of injection of an antigen but not from normal lymph nodes produce IL-3 when incubated overnight in tissue culture medium (Crapper *et al.*, 1984a). The local release of IL-3 at sites where T cells are activated results in a characteristic histological 'foot print', namely the local accumulation of mast cells generated by the action of IL-3 on undifferentiated precursors (Crapper and Schrader, 1983).

In cases where there is massive activation of T lymphoctyes, for example graft-versus-host disease, small amounts of IL-3 can be detected in the serum (Crapper and Schrader, 1986). Another phenomenon that might be accounted for by the release of IL-3 into the serum was the transient appearance of histamine-producing cell stimu-lating factor (HCSF) reported in the serum following the challenge of an immunized animal with a parasite antigen (Abbud-Filho *et al.*, 1983). It is intriguing to speculate that these experiments reflect the rapid release of IL-3, not from the T lymphocytes but from mast cells activated by interaction of specific IgE with the injected antigen.

IL-3 IN THE SERUM

The half-life of intravenously injected IL-3 is short, being in the order of only 40 min (Crapper *et al.*, 1984a). A major part of this IL-3 is destroyed in the kidney. IL-3 does not appear to be bound to larger molecules in the serum (Crapper and Schrader, 1986) and enters the glomerular filtrate. Small amounts are detectable in the urine of animals with high serum levels of IL-3, but most of the filtered IL-3 appears to be resorbed and destroyed in the renal tubules (Crapper *et al.*, 1984b).

The release of IL-3 *in vivo* appears to be associated with stimulation of all of the various types of haemopoietic cells predicted from the *in vitro* activities of IL-3. For example, in certain phases of graft-versus-host disease in mice, increases occur in the number of mast cells and their precursors and of immature myeloid and erythroid cells in the spleen (Crapper and Schrader, 1986). This coincides with the appearance of small amounts of IL-3 in the serum.

Since T-cell activation results in the release of multiple cytokines affecting haemo-poiesis, including IL-4, IL-5, IL-6 and GM-CSF, a clearer picture of the effects of IL-3 release *in vivo* came from experiments in which mice were inoculated with WEHI-3B, a tumour that produces IL-3 constitutively as a result of insertion of a retroviral DNA into one copy of the IL-3 gene (Ymer *et al.*, 1985). Mice with a localized, subcutaneous tumour of WEHI-3B showed dramatic stimulation of haemopoiesis in the spleen, with increased numbers of myeloid cells, mast cells and megakaryocytes (Crapper *et al.*, 1984a). Interestingly, the levels of IL-3 in the serum of these mice were relatively low (less than 2 ED_{50} units/ml) suggesting that the chronic maintenance of low concen-trations of IL-3 in the serum could achieve marked effects on haemopoiesis.

The effects of IL-3 vary in different tissues depending upon the local availability of the different types of target cells. For example, in the gut mucosa, committed mast-cell precursors are relatively frequent, whereas progenitors of other haemopoietic lineages are relatively rare (Crapper and Schrader, 1983). In this tissue the local release of IL-3 induces a mastocytosis. In organs like the murine spleen, where there is a higher frequency of haemopoietic stem and progenitor cells of various lineages, IL-3 stimu-lates increases of myeloid and erythroid cells as well as more modest increases in mast cells and their progenitors (Crapper and Schrader, 1983).

ADMINISTRATION OF IL-3

Administration of IL-3 *in vivo* is complicated by the relatively rapid clearance of IL-3 from the circulation. The subcutaneous administration of 2000 ED_{50} units of chemically synthesized IL-3 three times a day for 3 days resulted in increases in splenic weight and in the number of mast cells and the progenitors of mast cells, neutrophils and macrophages and in CFUs (Schrader *et al.*, 1986b). Similar results were obtained using *Escherichia coli*-derived material (Kindler *et al.*, 1985; Metcalf, 1988).

The administration of human IL-3 to primates and more recently humans indicates broadly similar effects (Donahue *et al.*, 1988; Mayer *et al.*, 1989). IL-3 may have particular utility in stimulating platelet production (Monroy *et al.*, 1990).

ROLE OF IL-3 IN STEADY-STATE HAEMOPOIESIS

There is compelling evidence that IL-3 serves as the link between the immune system (that senses intrusion of foreign substances into the body) and the haemopoietic system that generates the phagocytic and granulocytic cells that mediate defence and repair. There is little evidence, however, that IL-3 is involved in steady-state production of blood cells, despite its potent ability to stimulate almost all phases of haemopoiesis.

The absence of IL-3 in normal serum and the evidence that links its production, whether by T lymphocytes or mast cells to immunological activation, argue against a role for IL-3 in mediating steady-state haemopoiesis in unperturbed animals. Moreover, the production of a range of haemopoietic cells—including progenitor cells and stem cells capable of generating myeloid, erythroid and lymphoid cells—can occur *in vitro* in long-term bone-marrow culture systems in which IL-3 bioactivity is undetectable (Eliason *et al.*, 1988). These cultures can support the survival of IL-3-dependent cells that are unresponsive to other growth factors like GM-CSF, CSF-1 or G-CSF despite the absence of IL-3 (Schrader *et al.*, 1984), suggesting the presence of alternative mechanisms for example involving SLF.

One mechanism that permits the survival and limited growth of IL-3-dependent mast cells has been clarified by characterization of the protein products of the *W* and *Sl* loci as, respectively, a growth-factor receptor and its ligand. Both *W* and *Sl* mutant mice exhibited a macrocytic anaemia and a deficiency of mast cells that were caused in the case of *W* mice by a defect expressed in cells including the haemopoietic stem cells and its derivatives and in the case of the *Sl* mice by a defect in the microenvironment expressed in tissues including the bone marrow, spleen and skin. Fujita and colleagues (1988a,b) showed that IL-3-dependent mast cells from normal mice, but not *W* mutant mice, could survive and proliferate in the absence of IL-3, provided they were allowed to contact fibroblasts from normal mice. Fibroblasts from *Sl* mice could not maintain mast-cell survival. The demonstration that the *W* mutations involved the tyrosine-kinase receptor encoded by the c-kit gene (Chabot *et al.*, 1988; Geissler *et al.*, 1988) and that IL-3-dependent mast cells retained expression of this receptor, made mast cells an obvious substrate for assays designed to detect the ligand for this receptor. The kit-ligand SLF has been shown to be a homodimer encoded, as expected, by the *Sl* locus (Anderson *et al.*, 1990; Copeland *et al.*, 1990; Huang *et al.*, 1990; Williams, D. E., *et al.*, 1990; Zsebo *et al.*, 1990a,b).

INTERACTIONS BETWEEN C-KIT SIGNALLING PATHWAYS AND IL-3

IL-3 produced in response to immunological activation of T lymphocytes or mast cells is unlikely to be involved in steady-state haemopoiesis. Moreover, there is no evidence that IL-3 is constitutively produced by stromal cells in the bone marrow. We have been examining a third possibility, namely that IL-3 may be produced by haemopoietic stem and progenitor cells themselves and play an autocrine role in steady-state haemopoiesis.

One piece of evidence has been our observation that when mast cells interact with fibroblasts they accumulate IL-3 mRNA (Razin *et al.*, 1990). It is conceivable that this accumulation of IL-3 mRNA in the mast cell results from stimulation by SLF. By analogy, the action of SLF on haemopoietic stem and progenitor cells in the bone marrow could also involve the induction of the autogenous production of IL-3 by haemopoietic cells themselves. At present this is only speculative. The question of whether IL-3 (whether produced in small amount by stromal cells or, as hypothesized here, by haemopoietic cells themselves) has a critical role in steady-state haemopoiesis will only be resolved by analysis of 'knock-out' mice in which the IL-3 genes have been artificially inactivated.

LINKS BETWEEN STRESS AND STEADY-STATE HAEMOPOIESIS

Whether or not small amounts of IL-3 play a subtle role in steady-state haemopoiesis, it is clear that IL-3 is an important mediator of the response of the haemopoietic system to stress. The local release of IL-3 from activated T lymphocytes, and in severe immunological stress, its release into the serum, result in accelerated cycling of stem and progenitor cells and large increases in the production of differentiated cells of multiple lineages.

IL-3 and the other cytokines released during stress not only increase blood cell production but also modulate the types of cells produced. The stress response thus involves not only acceleration of the normal mechanisms of haemopoiesis but also overriding of some of the normal processes that regulate the proportions of the different cell-types that are produced. Usually this is thought to result from the positive effects of a lineage-specific factor such as G-CSF or IL-5, that either stimulate committed progenitor cells or, alternatively, direct the differentiation of less-committed progenitors. However, another component of this overriding process could be the disengagement of normal regulatory mechanisms.

There is some evidence that IL-3 may be involved in such a disengagement of steady-state mechanisms. Thus, exposure to high levels of IL-3 leads to the down-regulation of c-kit mRNA and protein in both mast cells and cell-lines corresponding to haemopoietic progenitor cells (Welham and Schrader, 1991). GM-CSF and erythropoietin have similar downregulatory effects on expression of c-kit. The downregulation of c-kit by high levels of IL-3 (as well as GM-CSF and erythropoietin) may be part of a mechanism that overrides steady-state regulatory processes and facilitates control of the rate and cellular composition of blood cell production by cytokines released during stress.

One aspect of this overriding process may be simply the facilitation of the exit of stem and early progenitor cells from the bone marrow. The kit-ligand exists in a cell-bound form as a transmembrane protein (Anderson *et al.*, 1990; Flanagan and Leder, 1990;

Martin *et al.*, 1990) and thus may function as one of the adhesion proteins that retains stem and progenitor cells in the bone-marrow microenvironment. Downregulation of c-kit by IL-3 may therefore facilitate the release of stem cells and early committed progenitors from the bone-marrow microenvironment. The administration of IL-3 has been shown to result in an increase of stem cells in the circulation (Monroy *et al.*, 1990). Seeding of stem and progenitor cells into the blood to sites where cytokine release is occurring would allow the local generation of the appropriate effector cells at sites of inflammation.

RECEPTOR FOR IL-3

Many of the most exciting recent data about cytokines have concerned their receptors. In a relatively short period a picture has emerged of a family of haemopoietin receptors that in contrast with their ligands, share easily recognizable structural features. The family now includes at least one chain of the receptors for IL-3, as well as IL-2, IL-4, IL-5, IL-6, IL-7, IL-9, IL-11, IL-12, GM-CSF, G-CSF, ciliary neutrophilic factor, leukaemia inhibitory factor, oncostatin-M, and erythropoietin (Bazan, 1990). The prolactin and growth hormone receptors are more distantly related. The receptors are homodimers (growth hormone, G-CSF) or are heterodimers containing at least two chains that are members of the superfamily. The IL-2 receptor consists of at least three chains, two of which, the larger β and γ chains, are members of the haemopoietin-receptor superfamily.

In the human, the IL-3 receptor is a heterodimer made up of two members of the haemopoietin receptor superfamily. The α chain binds IL-3 with low affinity and is homologous with two other α chains that bind GM-CSF and IL-5, respectively. The larger β chain is shared by the human IL-3, IL-5, and GM-CSF receptors. While showing no direct affinity for either human IL-3, IL-5 or GM-CSF, the common β chain can interact with any of the three distinct α chains and their ligand to generate three specific high-affinity ligand–receptor complexes (Gearing *et al.*, 1989; Miyajima *et al.*, 1990; Kitamura *et al.*, 1991; Tavernier *et al.*, 1991).

In the mouse, a duplication of the gene encoding the shared β chain has occurred. One gene (*AIC-2B*) encodes a β chain that is functionally equivalent to that in the human, binding neither IL-3, IL-5 nor GM-CSF, but interacting with specific α chains in the presence of the respective ligands to form high-affinity receptors (Kitamura and Miyajima, 1992). The duplicated gene, *AIC-2A*, in contrast, has a low affinity for IL-3 (Itoh *et al.*, 1990) and interacts only with the IL-3-specific α chain. Thus, in the mouse there are two types of IL-3 receptor; the functional significance of this is unknown. The intracellular portions of *AIC-2A* and *AIC-2B* are very similar and no differences in the signals they transmit have been detected. Both chains of the IL-3 receptor interact closely with IL-3 and can be detected by crosslinking studies with radiolabelled IL-3 as a 70 K and 120 K IL-3-binding species (Duronio *et al.*, 1992).

IL-3 MEDIATED SIGNAL TRANSDUCTION

Information on the amino sequence of the α and β chains of the IL-3 receptor has provided few clues to the mechanism by which ligand binding activates intercellular signalling. The cytoplasmic domain of the α chain is short and has no homologies with known enzymes. Although there are experiments with the homologous α chain of the GM-CSF receptor that suggest that the cytoplasmic domain of the α chain is not essential for generation, at least, of a proliferative signal (Sakamaki *et al.*, 1992) this does not appear to be the case for the IL-3 α-chain (Orban and Schrader, unpublished observations).

The β chain of the IL-3 receptor has a large cytoplasmic domain, but like other receptor subunits in the haemopoietic-receptor superfamily, lacks any homologies with enzymes. Analysis of the function of cells transfected with mutant genes encoding β chains, in which elements of the cytoplasm tail have been deleted, have shown that much of the cytoplasmic domain can be deleted without completely abrogating the capacity to transmit a proliferative signal (Sakamaki *et al.*, 1992).

It is unclear how ligand binding activates intracellular events. Association of IL-3 with the α chain is stabilized by interaction of IL-3 and the α chain with the β chain. However, high-affinity binding is not essential for activation of the receptor. Thus, mutants of GM-CSF that only bind with low affinity can stimulate the growth of murine-factor-dependent cells (Shanafelt and Kastelein, 1992). These experiments suggest that the key signalling event is a conformational change that results from interaction of the α and β chains and does not depend directly on high-affinity binding and interaction of the ligand with the β chain. While a conformational change in the β chain induced by association with ligand-bound α chain could be the signal that engages downstream signalling molecules such as a tyrosine kinase, it seems more likely that signalling is initiated by dimerizations of β chains. This might be achieved by αβ dimers associating with a free β chain or another αβ dimer.

In the case of the related IL-2-receptor β chain, there is evidence for a physical association between the active receptor and the tyrosine kinase, Lck (Hatakeyama *et al.*, 1991). However, IL-2 action is not dependent on the presence of Lck, suggesting that other related kinases may substitute. IL-3 results in modest activation of the src-family kinase member lyn (O'Connor *et al.*, 1992; Torigoe *et al.*, 1992) but a dramatic activation of the JAK-2 tyrosine kinase which together with related kinases is also activated by other cytokines. At present, however, the precise roles of these tyrosine kinases in the signalling process is unknown. Nevertheless, it is clear that one of the earliest detectable changes, occurring within seconds of IL-3 binding its receptor, is the phosphorylation of a set of proteins on tyrosine residues (Ferris *et al.*, 1988; Morla *et al.*, 1988). These tyrosine phosphorylation events can be subdivided into two groups: those specifically associated with stimulation by IL-3 (and in most cases GM-CSF and IL-5, since the receptors share one chain) and those that are shared with multiple growth factors, all of which must activate the common paths that regulate general aspects of cell growth.

Comparison of the tyrosine-phosphorylated events stimulated in mast cells by IL-3 with those stimulated by SLF has allowed identification of a set of IL-3-specific tyrosine-phosphorylated events (Welham and Schrader, 1992). One of these is tyrosine phosphorylation of the β chain of the IL-3 receptor (Isfort *et al.*, 1988; Duronio *et al.*, 1992). Over a period of 10 min the β chain of the IL-3 receptor increases in apparent molecular weight, shifting from M_r 125 000, in unstimulated cells to M_r 135–150 000. Much of this increase in apparent molecular weight appears to result from concomitant serine–threonine phosphorylation (Duronio *et al.*, 1992).

Another protein that is phosphorylated on tyrosine specifically in response to IL-3,

IL-5, and GM-CSF but not IL-2 or SLF or CSF-1 is a protein with a M_r of 68K (Duronio *et al.*, 1992; Welham and Schrader, 1992). The function of the protein is unknown but it is the major species associated with PI-3 kinase after IL-3 stimulation (Duronio, Welham and Schrader, unpublished data).

Because IL-3 exerts effects common to most haemopoietic growth factors, such as stimulation of proliferation or enhanced survival, it would be expected that the intracellular signals triggered by IL-3 would include many that are shared by other growth factors. One such event is activation of $p21^{ras}$ (Satoh *et al.*, 1991; Duronio *et al.*, 1992). This is dependent on tyrosine kinase activity (Duronio *et al.*, 1992), the key event probably being tyrosine phosphorylation of a protein termed SHC. We have shown that the prominent 55K protein that is tyrosine-phosphorylated in response to IL-3 (as well as GM-CSF, IL-5, IL-2, SLF and CSF-1) is SHC (Welham, Duronio and Schrader, unpublished data). This protein is known to associate with GRB-2, a small protein that interacts in turn with SOS, a guanine-nucleotide exchange factor that probably is responsible for activating $p21^{ras}$. The link between tyrosine phosphorylation of SHC and activation of $p21^{ras}$ is strengthened by the observation that IL-4, which fails to activate $p21^{ras}$ (Duronio *et al.*, 1992; Satoh *et al.*, 1992), also fails to stimulate tyrosine phosphorylation of SHC (Welham, Duronio and Schrader, unpublished data).

Another event common to all growth factors described with the notable exception of IL-4 (Welham *et al.*, 1994) is activation of erk/MAP-kinases. IL-3, in common with GM-CSF, IL-5, and IL-2, as well as SLF and CSF-1, activates erk/MAP-kinases (Welham *et al.*, 1992). Activation of these enzymes is known to require tyrosine phosphorylation, and the two proteins of M_r 42K and 44K that are phosphorylated on tyrosine in response to the IL-3 have been shown to correspond to erk-2 and erk-1 MAP kinases (Welham *et al.*, 1992).

There is good evidence that IL-3 activates, via a tyrosine-kinase-dependent mechanism, a common path along which lie SHC, GRB-2, SOS, $p21^{ras}$, raf-1 and MAP-kinases. MAP-kinases are known to activate the $p90^{rsk}$ S6 kinase which phosphorylates SRF, a protein that regulates transcription of the *c-fos* gene, and also to phosphorylate important regulatory residues on *c-jun*. Thus, there are emerging details of paths which link the IL-3 receptor with regulation of transcriptional activators like the AP-1 complex made up of *c-fos* and *c-jun* proteins.

IL-3 also resembles other growth factors in that it stimulates increases in levels of *c-myc* RNA (Chang *et al.*, 1991). However, this is likely to occur via a distinct common path from that outlined above. One indication is the fact that IL-4, while failing to activate the SHC, ras, MAP-kinase path, nevertheless stimulates increases in *c-myc* and *c-jun* RNA (Wieler and Schrader, unpublished observations). IL-3-induced increases in *c-jun* mRNA levels have been reported to be independent of tyrosine-kinase activity and to involve protein kinase C, although results of experiments using kinase inhibitors must be interpreted with caution (Mufson *et al.*, 1992). Experiments in which the effect of deletions in the β chain of the IL-3 receptor have been analysed have indicated that deletion of a region necessary for tyrosine phosphorylation of a p85 substrate did not affect the ability of the receptor to stimulate increases in levels of *c-myc* mRNA, and support the notion that there are at least two distinct, common signal transduction paths triggered by this class of receptor (Satoh *et al.*, 1992).

Another common pathway activated by IL-3 and many other growth factors involves activation of the enzyme PI-3' kinase (Gold *et al.*, 1994). The function of this enzyme is unknown. Since it is activated by IL-4 (Wang *et al.*, 1992; Gold *et al.*, 1994) it would appear to lie on a common path, distinct from that including p21^{ras} and MAP-kinases.

There is evidence that IL-3 results in translocation of protein kinase C from the cytoplasm to the cell membrane (Farrar *et al.*, 1985; Whetton *et al.*, 1988b; Pelech *et al.*, 1990). No increased turnover of phosphatidyl inositol has been observed (Whetton *et al.*, 1988a), although there is some evidence of increased turnover of phosphatidyl choline (Duronio *et al.*, 1989) and this may account for generation of diacylglycerol and activation of protein kinase C.

In summary, the binding of IL-3 induces conformational changes in its receptor that result in activation of, as yet, completely characterized tyrosine kinases. Some of the subsequent events, such as activation of p21^{ras}, clearly depend on tyrosine-kinase activity. In other cases, such as activation of protein kinase C or of stimulation of increased levels of *c-myc* RNA, it has not been formally shown that activation of an upstream tyrosine-kinase is involved. Further work on molecular characterization of the cellular response to IL-3/IL-5/GM-CSF should further clarify the mechanisms that activate paths common to the action of most growth factors and identify components specific for the IL-3 response that may be useful as targets for potential antagonists.

CLINICAL SIGNIFICANCE OF IL-3

The ability of IL-3 to stimulate early members of haemopoietic differentiation pathways suggests that it may have specific clinical uses. Promising results in accelerating the recovery of bone marrow following bone-marrow transplantation or damage to the bone marrow by cytotoxic drugs have been obtained with G-CSF and GM-CSF (Morstyn *et al.*, 1990). These factors seem effective in reducing the period of neutropenia. However, there are indications that, unlike G-CSF and GM-CSF, IL-3 may stimulate an increase in platelet levels (Ganser *et al.*, 1990b). Animal experiments suggest that sequential administration of IL-3 and the G-CSF or GM-CSF may provide optimal stimulation of myelopoiesis (Donahue *et al.*, 1988; Mayer *et al.*, 1989). Because of the likelihood that optimal protocols will involve the use of multiple cytokines, it will be some time before the ultimate clinical potential of IL-3 and combinations of other cytokines are clear.

Other potential uses for IL-3 are in the treatment of conditions such as aplastic (Ganser *et al.*, 1990a) or other anaemia (Halperin *et al.*, 1989; Dunbar *et al.*, 1991). In mice it has been shown that the administration of IL-3 (but not erythropoietin) prevents death from acute anaemia (Shibata *et al.*, 1990). IL-3 may be useful in managing certain infections. There is some evidence that IL-3 may have a favourable influence on Herpes simplex infection in mice (Chan *et al.*, 1990).

IL-3 antagonists may become available in the future. These may prove useful in the management of diseases such as bronchial asthma and allergies where mast cells play a central role. Experimental models in which antibodies that neutralize IL-3 have been used as models of IL-3 antagonists have given encouraging results. Anti-IL-3 antibodies in combination with anti-GM-CSF antibodies block the development of cerebral malaria in mice (Grau *et al.*, 1988) and anti-IL-3 antibodies, in combination with anti IL-4 antibodies, block the mastocytosis seen in the parasitized mice (Madden *et al.*, 1991). The administration of IL-3 aggravates leishmaniasis in mice (Feng *et al.*, 1988); *in vitro* anti-IL-3 antibodies have been shown to synergize with anti-IL-4 antibodies in unmasking a macrophage-activating activity present in supernatants of cells from *Leishmania* infected mice (Liew *et al.*, 1989). Analysis of the relative resistance or susceptibility to various diseases of mice in which IL-3 genes have been artificially deleted should yield helpful information on possible therapeutic use of IL-3 agonists and antagonists.

The fact that, in man, the receptors for IL-3, IL-5 and GM-CSF share a common β chain, which plays an important role in signal transduction, raises the possibility of developing antagonists that will specifically block the activity of this trio of cytokines. Because IL-3, IL-5 and GM-CSF promote the production and survival of eosinophils, basophils and mast cells that increase in number at sites of allergic reactions, drugs that block these actions could provide a new approach to the treatment of bronchial asthma or allergic diseases.

In the mouse a number of myeloid leukaemias have been described in which pathological activation of an IL-3 gene was a key oncogenic event. The constitutive production of IL-3 resulted in autostimulation of growth of the myeloid cell (Schrader and Crapper, 1983; Ymer *et al.*, 1985; Leslie and Schrader, 1989). In some instances the growth of such autostimulatory leukaemias may be blocked by anti-IL-3 antibodies (Schrader and Ziltener, unpublished data). Autostimulatory production of IL-3 however does not appear to be an important oncogenic mechanism in human myeloid leukaemia, although the leukaemia cells usually respond to IL-3 (Budel *et al.*, 1989; Park *et al.*, 1989b). There has been a report of an acute lymphocytic leukaemia in which a translocation joins the IL-3 and immunoglobulin heavy chain genes (Grimaldi and Meeker, 1989).

SUMMARY

IL-3 functions as a link between the T lymphocytes of the immune system, that senses invasion of the body by foreign materials, and the haemopoietic system, that generates the cellular elements that mediate defence and repair responses. IL-3 stimulates the broadest range of targets within the haemopoietic system of any of the cytokines and, in addition, has the special ability to stimulate the growth of early stem cells and the progenitors of mast cells and megakaryocytes. IL-3 has no proven role in steady-state haemopoiesis, although there are preliminary data indicating an interlinking of IL-3 with the mechanisms regulating the normal production of blood cells. Evaluation of the clinical utility of IL-3 is still in progress and, in the future, antagonists of IL-3 may provide new approaches to the management of allergic and inflammatory diseases.

ACKNOWLEDGEMENTS

I thank Dr H. Ziltener and Dr V. Duronio for helpful criticism and sharing of results prior to publication. Experimental work in the author's laboratory was supported by grants from the National Cancer Institute of Canada and MRC of Canada.

REFERENCES

Abbud-Filho, M., Dy, M., Lebel, B., Luffau, G. and Hamburger, J. (1983). *Eur. J. Immunol.* **13**, 841–845.
Anderson, D.M., Lyman, S.D., Baird, A., Wignall, J.M., Eisenman, J., Rauch, C., March, C.J., Boswell, S., Gimpel, S.D., Cosman, D. and Williams, D.E. (1990). *Cell* **63**, 235–243.

Bazan, J.F. (1990). *Immunol. Today* **11**, 350–355.

Berdel, W.E., Danhauser-Riedl, S., Steinhauser, G. and Winton, E.F. (1989). *Blood* **73**, 80–83.

Budel, L.M., Touw, I.P., Delwel, R., Clark, S.C. and Lowenberg, B. (1989). *Blood* **74**, 565–571.

Burd, P.R., Rogers, H.W., Gordon, J.R. and Dorf, M. (1989a). *J. Exp. Med.* **170**, 245–258.

Burd, P.R., Rogers, H.W., Gordon, J.R., Martin, C.A. *et al.* (1989b). *J. Exp. Med.* **170**, 245–257.

Chabot, B., Stephenson, D.A., Chapman, V.M., Besmer, P. and Bernstein, A. (1988). *Nature* **335**, 88–89.

Chaikin, E., Ziltener, H.J. and Razin, E. (1990). *J. Biol. Chem.* **265**, 22109–22116.

Chan, W.-L., Ziltener, H.J. and Liew, F.Y. (1990). *Immunology* **71**, 358–363.

Chang, Y., Spicer, D.B. and Sonenshein, G.E. (1991). *Oncogene* **6**, 1979–1982.

Chen, B.D., Mueller, M. and Olencki, T. (1988). *Blood* **72**, 685–690.

Clark-Lewis, I., Kent, S.B.H. and Schrader, J.W. (1984). *J. Biol. Chem.* **259**, 7488–7494.

Clark-Lewis, I., Aebersold, R., Ziltener, H., Schrader, J.W., Hood, L.E. and Kent, S.B. (1986). *Science* **231**, 134–139.

Clark-Lewis, I., Lopez, A.F., Lo, L.B., Vadas, M., Schrader, J.W., Hood, L.E. and Kent, S.B.H. (1988). *J. Immunol.* **141**, 881–889.

Copeland, N.G., Gilbert, D.J., Cho, B.C., Donovan, P.J., Jenkins, N.A., Cosman, D., Anderson, D., Lyman, S.D. and Williams, D.E. (1990). *Cell* **63**, 175–183.

Crapper, R.M. and Schrader, J.W. (1983). *J. Immunol.* **131**, 923–928.

Crapper, R.M. and Schrader, J.W. (1986). *Immunology* **57**, 553–558.

Crapper, R.M., Clark-Lewis, I. and Schrader, J.W. (1984a). *Immunology* **53**, 33–42.

Crapper, R.M., Thomas, W.R. and Schrader, J.W. (1984b). *J. Immunol.* **133**, 2174–2179.

Crapper, R.M., Vairo, G., Hamilton, J., Clark-Lewis, I. and Schrader, J.W. (1985). *Blood* **66**, 859–865.

Donahue, R.E., Seehra, J., Metzger, M., Lefebvre, D., Rock, B., Carbone, S., Nathan, D.G., Garnick, M., Sehgal, P.K., Laston, D., La Vallie, E., McCoy, J., Schendel, P.F., Norton, C., Turner, K., Yang, Y.C. and Clark, S.C. (1988). *Science* **241**, 1820–1823.

Dunbar, C.E., Smith, D.A., Kimball, J., Garrison, L., Nienhuis, A.W. and Young, N.S. (1991). *Br. J. Hematol.* **79**, 316–321.

Duronio, V., Nip, L. and Pelech, S.L. (1989). *Biochem. Biophys. Res. Comm.* **164**, 804–808.

Duronio, V., Granleese, S.R., Clark-Lewis, I., Schrader, J.W. and Ziltener, H.J. (1991). *Cytokine* **3**, 414–420.

Duronio, V., Clark-Lewis, I., Federspiel, B., Wieler, J.S. and Schrader, J.W. (1992). *J. Biol. Chem.* **267**, 21856–21863.

Eliason, J.F., Thorens, B., Kindler, V. and Vassalli, P. (1988). *Exp. Hematol.* **16**, 307–312.

Farrar, W.L., Thomas, T. P. and Anderson, W.B. (1985). *Nature* **315**, 235–237.

Feng, Z.Y., Louis, J., Kindler, V., Pedrazzini, T. *et al.* (1988). *Eur. J. Immunol.* **18**, 1245–1251.

Ferris, D.K., Willet-Brown, J., Martensen, T. and Farrar, W.L. (1988). Biochem. *Biophys. Res. Commun.* **154**, 991–996.

Flanagan, J.G. and Leder, P. (1990). *Cell* **63**, 185–194.

Frendl, G. and Beller, D.I. (1990) *Journal of Immunology* **144**, 3392–3399.

Frendl, G., Fenton, M.J. and Beller, D.I. (1990a). *Journal of Immunology* **144**, 3400–3410.

Frendl, G., Fenton, M.J. and Beller, D.I. (1990b). *Lymphokine Research* **9**, 616 (abstract).

Fujita, J., Nakayama, H., Onoue, H., Ebi, Y., Kanakura, Y., Kuriu, A. and Kitamura, Y. (1988a). *Blood* **72**, 463–468.

Fujita, J., Nakayama, H., Onoue, H., Ebi, Y., Kanakura, Y., Nakano, T., Asai, H., Takeda, S.-I., Honjo, T. and Kitamura, Y. (1988b). *J. Cell Physiol.* **134**, 78–84.

Fung, M.C., Hapel, A.J., Ymer, S., Cohen, D.R., Johnson, R.M., Campbell, H.D. and Young, I.G. (1984). *Nature* **307**, 233–237.

Ganser, A., Lindemann, A., Seipelt, G., Ottmann, O.G., Eder, M., Falk, S., Herrmann, F., Kaltwasser, J.P., Meusers, P., Klausmann, M., Frisch, J., Schulz, G., Mertelsmann, R. and Hoelzer, D. (1990a). *Blood* **76**, 1287–1292.

Ganser, A., Lindemann, A., Seipelt, G., Ottmann, O.G., Herrmann, F., Eder, M., Frisch, J., Schulz, G., Mertelsmann, R. and Hoelzer, D. (1990b). *Blood* **76**, 666–676.

Gearing, D.P., King, J.A., Gough, N.M. and Nicola, N.A. (1989). *EMBO J.* **8**, 3667–3676.

Geissler, E.N., Ryan, M.A. and Housman, D.E. (1988). *Cell* **55**, 185–192.

Gold, M.R., Duronio, V., Saxena, S.P., Schrader, J.W. and Aebersold, R. (1994). *J. Biol. Chem.* **269**, 5403–5412.

Grau, G.E., Kindler, V., Piguet, E.-E., Lambert, P.-H. and Vassalli, P.J. (1988). *Exp. Med.* **168**, 1499–1504.

Grimaldi, J.C. and Meeker, T.C. (1989). *Blood* **73**, 2081–2085.
Halperin, D.S., Estrov, Z. and Freedman, M.H. (1989). *Blood* **73**, 1168–1174.
Hapel, A.J. and Young, I.G. (1988). In *Lymphokines 15; Interleukin 3: the Panspecific Hemopoietin* (ed. J. W. Schrader), Academic Press, San Diego, pp. 91–126.
Hapel, A.J., Lee, J.C., Farrar, W.L. and Ihle, J.M. (1981). *Cell* **25**, 179–186.
Hatakeyama, M., Kono, T., Kobayashi, N., Kawahara, A., Levin, S.D., Perlmutter, R.M. and Taniguchi, T. (1991). *Science* **252**, 1523–1528.
Hirai, K., Morita, Y., Misaki, Y., Ohta, K., Takashi, T., Suzuki, S., Motoyoshi, K. and Miyamoto, T. (1988). *J. Immunol.* **141**, 3958–3964.
Hirayama, F., Shih, J.P., Awgulewitsch, A., Warr, G.W., Clark, S.C. and Ogawa, M. (1992). *Proc. Natl. Acad. Sci. USA* **89**, 5907–5911.
Huang, E., Nocka, K., Beier, D.R., Chu, T.-Y., Buck, J., Lahm, H.-W., Wellner, D., Leder, P. and Besmer, P. (1990). *Cell* **63**, 225–233.
Ihle, J.N., Pepersack, L. and Rebar, L. (1981). *J. Immunol.* **126**, 1284–1289.
Ihle, J.M., Keller, J., Oroszlan, S., Henderson, L.E., Copeland, T.D., Fitch, F., Prystowsky, M.B., Goldwasser, E., Schrader, J.W., Palaszynski, E., Dy, M. and Lebel, B. (1983). *J. Immunol.* **131**, 282–287.
Iscove, N.N., Shaw, A.R. and Keller, G. (1989). *J. Immunol.* **142**, 2332–2337.
Isfort, R.J., Stevens, D., May, W.S. and Ihle, J.M. (1988). *Proc. Natl Acad. Sci. USA* **85**, 7982–7986.
Ishibashi, T. and Burstein, S.A. (1986). *Blood* **67**, 1512–1514.
Itoh, N., Yonehara, S., Schreurs, J., Gorman, D.M., Maruyama, K., Ishii, A., Yahara, I., Arai, K.-I. and Miyajima, A. (1990). *Science* **247**, 324–327.
Kastelein, R.A. and Shanafelt, A.B. (1993). *Oncogene* **8**, 231–236.
Kinashi, T., Inaba, K., Tsubata, T., Tashiro, K., *et al.* (1988). *Proc. Natl Acad. Sci. USA* **85**, 4473–4477.
Kindler, V., Thorens, S.B., De Kossodo, S., Allet, B., Eliason, J.F., Thatcher, D. and Vassali, P. (1985). *Proc. Natl Acad. Sci. USA* **83**, 1001–1005.
Kitamura, T. and Miyajima, A. (1992). *Blood* **80**, 84–90.
Kitamura, T., Sato, N., Arai, K. and Miyajima, A. (1991). *Cell* **66**, 1165–1174.
Kurimoto, Y., de Weck, A.L. and Dahinden, C.A. (1989). *J. Exp. Med.* **170**, 467–479.
Leslie, K.B. and Schrader, J.W. (1989). *J. Molecular and Cell Biol.* **6**, 2414–2423.
Liew, F.Y., Millot, S., Li, Y., Lelchuck, R., Chan, W.L. and Ziltener, H.J. (1989). *Eur. J. Immunol.* **19**, 1227–1232.
Lokker, N.A., Zenke, G., Fagg, B. and Movva, N.R. (1990). *Lymphokine Res.* **9**, 617 (Abstr.).
Londei, M., Verhoef, A., De Berardinis, P., Kissonerghis, M., Grubeck-Loebenstein, B. and Feldmann, M. (1989). *Proc. Natl Acad. Sci. USA* **86**, 8502–8506.
Lopez, A.F., To, L.B., Yang, Y.-C., Gamble, J.R., Shannon, M.F., Burns, G.F., Dyson, P.G., Juttner, C.A., Clark, S. and Vadas, M.A. (1987). *Proc. Natl Acad. Sci. USA* **84**, 2761–2765.
Madden, K.B., Urban, J.F. Jr., Ziltener, H.J., Schrader, J.W., Finkelman, F.D. and Katona, I.M. (1991). *J. Immunol.* **147**, 1387–1391.
Martin, F.H., Suggs, S.V., Langley, K.E., Lu, H.S., Ting, J., Okino, K.H., Morris, F., McNiece, I.K., Jacobsen, F.W., Mendiaz, E.A., Birkett, N.C., Smith, D.A., Johnson, M.J., Parker, V.P., Flores, J.C., Patel, A.C., Fisher, E.F., Erjavec, H.O., Herrera, C.J., Wypych, J., Sachdev, R.K., Pope, J.A., Leslie, I., Wen, D., Lin, C.-H., Cupples, R.L. and Zsebo, K.M. (1990). *Cell* **63**, 203–211.
Mayer, P., Valent, P., Schmidt, G., Liehl, E. and Bettelheim, P. (1989). *Blood* **74**, 613–621.
Metcalf, D. (1988). In *Lymphokines 15: Interleukin 3: The Panspecific Hemopoietin* (ed. J.W. Schrader), Academic Press, San Diego, CA, pp. 183–217.
Miyajima, A., Hayashida, K., Kitamura, T., Gorman, D., Arai, K. and Yokota, T. (1990). *Lymphokine Res.* **9**, 555 (Abstr.).
Monroy, R.L., Davis, T.A., Donahue, R.E. and MacVittie, T.J. (1990). *Lymphokine Res.* **9**, 614 (Abstr.).
Morla, A.O., Schreurs, J., Miyajima, A. and Wang, J.Y. (1988). *Mol. Cell. Biol.* **8**, 2214–2218.
Morstyn, G., Sheridan, W., Lieschke, G., Cebon, J., Layton, J. and Fox, R. (1990). In *Effects of Therapy on Biology and Kinetics of the Residual Tumor, Part B: Clinical Aspects* (eds. J. Ragaz, L. Simpson-Herren, M.E. Lippman and B. Fisher), Wiley-Liss, New York, pp. 29–36.
Mufson, R.A., Szabo, J. and Eckert, D. (1992). *J. Immunol.* **148**, 1129–1135.
Murthy, S.C., Mui, A.L.-F. and Krystal, G. (1990). *Exp. Hematol.* **18**, 11–17.
Niemeyer, C.M., Sieff, C.A., Mathey-Prevot, B., Wimperis, J.Z. *et al.* (1989). *Blood* **73**, 945–951.

O'Connor, R., Torigoe, T., Reed, J.C. and Santoli, D. (1992). *Blood* **80**, 1017–1025.

Palacios, R. and Steinmetz, M. (1985). *Cell* **41**, 727–734.

Palacios, R., Henson, G., Steinmetz, M. and McKearn, J.P. (1984). *Nature* **309**, 126–131.

Park, L.S., Friend, D., Price, V., Anderson, D., Singer, J., Prickett, K.S. and Urdal, D.L. (1989a). *J. Biol. Chem.* **264**, 5420–5427.

Park, L.S., Waldron, P.E., Friend, D., Sassenfeld, H.M. *et al.* (1989b). *Blood* **74**, 56–65.

Pelech, S.L., Paddon, H.B., Charest, D.L. and Federspiel, B.S. (1990). *J. Immunol.* **144**, 1759–1766.

Razin, E., Leslie, K. and Schrader, J. (1990). *J. Immunol*, **146**, 981–987.

Rennick, D., Jackson, J., Moulds, C., Lee, F. and Yang, G. (1989). *J. of Immunol.* **142**, 161–166.

Roberts, R., Gallagher, J., Spooncer, E., Allen, T.D. *et al.* (1988). *Nature* **332**, 376–378.

Rothenberg, M.E., Owen, W.F. Jr., Silberstein, D.S., Woods, J. *et al.* (1988). *J. Clin. Invest.* **81**, 1986–1992.

Sakamaki, K., Miyajima, I., Kitamura, T. and Miyajima, A. (1992). *EMBO J.* **11**, 3541–3549.

Satoh, T., Minami, Y., Kono, T., Yamada, K., Kawahara, A., Taniguchi, T. and Kaziro, Y. (1992). *J. Biol. Chem.* **267**, 25423–25427.

Schrader, J.W. (1981). *J. Immunol.* **126**, 452–458.

Schrader, J.W. and Crapper, R.M. (1983). *Proc. Natl Acad. Sci. USA.* **80**, 6892–6896.

Schrader, J.W. and Nossal, G.J.V. (1980). *Immunol. Rev.* **53**, 61–85.

Schrader, J.W., Battye, F. and Scollay, R. (1982). *Proc. Natl Acad. Sci. USA* **79**, 4161–4165.

Schrader, J.W., Schrader, S., Clark-Lewis, I. and Crapper, R.M. (1984). In *Long Term Bone Marrow Culture* (eds. D.G. Wright and J.S. Greenberger), Liss, New York, pp. 293–308.

Schrader, J.W., Clark-Lewis, I., Ziltener, H.J., Hood, L.E. and Kent, S.B.H. (1986b). In *Immune Regulation by Characterized Polypeptides* (eds. G. Goldstein, J.F. Bach and H. Wigzell), Liss, New York, pp. 475–484.

Schrader, J.W., Ziltener, H.J. and Leslie, K.B. (1986a). *Proc. Natl Acad. Sci. USA.* **83**, 2458–2462.

Schrader, J.W., Clark-Lewis, I., Crapper, R.M., Leslie, K.B., Schrader, S., Varigos, G. and Ziltener, H.J. (1988). In *Lymphokines 15; Interleukin 3: The Panspecific Hemopoietin* (ed. J.W. Schrader), Academic Press, San Diego, CA., pp. 281–311.

Shanafelt, A.B. and Kastelein, R.A. (1992). J. Biol. Chem. **267**, 25466–25472.

Shibata, T., Kindler, V., Chicheportiche, Y., Vassalli, P. and Izui, S. (1990). *J. Exp. Med.* **171**, 1809–1814.

Silvennoinen, O., Witthan, B.A., Quelle, F.W., Cleveland, J.L., Yi, T. and Ihle, J.N. (1993). *Proc. Natl. Acad. Sci., USA* **90**, 8429–8433.

Tavernier, J., Devos, R., Cornelis, S., Tuypens, T., Van der Heyden, J., Fiers, W. and Plaetinck, G. (1991). *Cell* **66**, 1175–1184.

Torigoe, T., O'Connor, R., Santoli, D. and Reed, J.C. (1992). *Blood* **80**, 617–624.

Uckun, F.M., Gesner, T.B., Song, C.W., Myers, D.E. and Mufson, A. (1989). *Blood* **73**, 533–542.

Wang, L.M., Keegan, A.C., Paul, W.E., Heidaran, M.A., Gutkind, J.S. and Pierce, J.H. (1992). *EMBO J.* **11** 4899–4908.

Welham, M. and Schrader, J.W. (1991). *Mol. Cell. Biol.* **11**, 2901–2904.

Welham, M.J. and Schrader, J.W. (1992). *J. Immunol.* **149**, 2772–2783.

Welham, M.J., Duronio, V., Sanghera, J., Pelech, S. and Schrader, J.W. (1992). *J. Immunol.* **149**, 1683–1693.

Welham, M.J., Duronio, V. and Schrader, J.W. (1994). *J. Biol. Chem.* **269**, 5865–5873.

Whetton, A.D., Monk, P.N., Consalvey, S.D., Huang, S.J. *et al.* (1988a). *Proc. Natl Acad. Sci. USA* **85**, 3284–3288.

Whetton, A.D., Vallance, S.J., Monk, P.N., Cragoe, E.J., Dexter, T.M. and Heyworth, C.M. (1988b). *Biochem. J.* **256**, 585–592.

Williams, D.E., Eisenman, J., Baird, A., Rauch, C., Van Ness, K., March, C.J., Park, L.S., Martin, U., Mochizuki, D.Y., Boswell, H.S., Burgess, G.S., Cosman, D. and Lyman S.D. (1990). *Cell* **63**, 167–174.

Williams, G.T., Smith, C.A., Spooncer, E., Dexter, T.M. and Taylor, D.R. (1990). *Nature* **343**, 76–79.

Wodnar-Filipowicz, A., Heusser, C.H. and Moroni, C. (1989). *Nature* **339**, 150–152.

Wong, G.H.W., Clark-Lewis, I., Hamilton, J.A. and Schrader, J.W. (1984). *J. Immunol.* **133**, 2043–2050.

Yang, Y.-C., Ciarletta, A.B., Temple, P.A., Chung, M.P., Kovacic, S., Witek-Giannotti, J.S., Leary, A.C., Kriz, R., Donahue, R.E., Wong, G.G. and Clark, S.C. (1986). *Cell* **47**, 3–10.

Yang, Y.-C., Kovacic, S., Kriz, R., Wolf, S., Clark, S., Wellems, T., Nienhuis, A. and Epstein, N. (1988). *Blood* **71**, 958–961.

Ymer, S., Tucker, W.Q., Sanderson, C.J., Hapel, A.J., Campbell, H.D. and Young, I.G. (1985). *Nature (London)* **317**, 255–258.

Yokota, T., Lee, F., Rennick, D., Hall, C., Arai, N., Mosmann, T., Nabel, G., Cantor, H. and Arai, K.-I. (1984). *Proc. Natl Acad. Sci. USA* **81**, 1070–1074.
Ziltener, H.J., Clark-Lewis, I., Hood, L.P., Kent, S.B.A. and Schrader, J.W. (1987). *J. Immunol.* **138**, 1099–1104.
Ziltener, H.J., Fazekas de St. Groth, B., Leslie, K.B. and Schrader, J.W. (1988). *J. Biol. Chem.* **263**, 14511–14517.
Zsebo, K.M., Wypych, J., McNiece, I.K., Lu, H.S., Smith, K.A., Karkare, S.B., Sachdev, R.K., Yuschenkoff, V.N., Birkett, N.C., Williams, L.R., Satyagal, V.N., Tung, W., Bosselman, R.A., Mendiaz, E.A. and Langley, K.E. (1990a). *Cell* **63**, 195–201.
Zsebo, K.M., Williams, D.A., Geissler, E.N., Broudy, V.C., Martin, F.H., Atkins, H.L., Hsu, R.-Y., Birkett, N.C., Okino, K.H., Murdock, D.C., Jacobsen, F.W., Langley, K.E., Smith, K.A., Takeishi, T., Cattanach, B.M., Galli, S.J. and Suggs, S.V. (1990b). *Cell* **63**, 213–224.

Chapter 6

Interleukin-4

Jacques Banchereau[1] and Mary Ellen Rybak[2]

[1]Schering-Plough, Laboratory for Immunological Research, Dardilly, France, and
[2]Schering-Plough Research Institute, Kenilworth, USA

INTRODUCTION

Interleukin-4 (IL-4) was identified in 1982 for its ability to induce activated mouse B lymphocytes to proliferate and to secrete IgG1. cDNAs coding for both human and murine molecules were isolated in 1986 and cDNAs coding for glycoprotein receptors binding murine and human IL-4 with high affinity were isolated in 1989–90. Studies with purified recombinant IL-4 and specific neutralizing antibodies indicated the pleiotropic nature of the molecule. Clinical trials are presently being performed aimed at determining the possible therapeutic use of this molecule as an antitumour agent. Owing to the lack of space, we will almost only refer to studies performed with human IL-4 and references on murine IL-4 can be found in the excellent recent review by W. Paul (Paul, 1991).

MOLECULAR ASPECTS OF IL-4

The principal characteristics of IL-4 are summarized in Table 1. Molecular cloning of human IL-4 cDNA revealed a single open reading frame of 153 amino acids yielding a secreted glycoprotein of 129 amino acids (Yokota et al., 1986). Expression of the recombinant protein in mammalian cells demonstrates three variants with apparent

Table 1. Properties of human and murine IL-4.

	Human	Murine
Precursor protein: amino acids	153	140
Secreted protein: amino acids	129	120
Isoelectric point	10.4	6.5
N-Glycosylation sites	2	3
Gene size (kilobase pairs)	10	6
Gene introns	3	3
Gene location: chromosome	5q23-31	11
Cell sources	T cells	T cells
	Mast cells	Mast cells

The Cytokine Handbook, 2nd ed.
ISBN 0–12–689661–5

values of 15, 18 and 19 K. The microheterogeneity of rhu IL-4 appears to be related to the nature of the N-linked oligosaccharides in the 18 and 19 K variants. Human IL-4 contains three disulphide bridges between C3-C127, C4-C65 and C46-C99 (Windsor *et al.*, 1990). X-ray diffraction of IL-4 crystals (Walter *et al.*, 1992), as well as magnetic resonance spectroscopy of IL-4 in solution (Powers *et al.*, 1992) indicate that IL-4 is a bundle of four left-handed α-helices with short stretches of β sheets. The four α-helices are situated between the residues 9–21, 45–64, 74–96 and 113–129, and the mini antiparallel β sheets are between residues 32–34 and 110–112 (Garret *et al.*, 1992). The structure of IL-4 bears a close resemblance to GM-CSF, M-CSF and growth hormone. The human IL-4 gene, composed of four exons and three introns, is localized on the long arm of chromosome 5 on bands q23–31, together with genes of other related cytokines including IL-3, IL-5, IL-9, IL-13 and GM-CSF (Asano *et al.*, 1987; Morgan *et al.*, 1992). mRNA phenotyping of cytokines recently revealed the existence of an additional IL-4 mRNA which lacks 48 bp coding for amino acid residues 22 to 37. This fragment is generated from an alternatively spliced transcript of the IL-4 gene in which exon 2 is skipped (Sorg *et al.*, 1993). Such a transcript would result in a mature protein lacking one of the cystein bridges and part of the loop connecting helices 1 and 2. The existence and the role of such a deleted IL-4 protein has not been established. An IL-4 molecule in which the tyrosine residue 124 was substituted by an aspartic acid residue was found to act as an antagonist of IL-4 (Kruse *et al.*, 1992). IL-4 displays 20% homology at the amino acid level, with the recently identified human IL-13 (McKenzie *et al.*, 1993; Minty *et al.*, 1993).

INTERLEUKIN-4 RECEPTOR

IL-4 binds to high-affinity (K_d = 40–120 pM) receptors which are expressed in low number on virtually every cell type tested, including T and B lymphocytes, monocytes, granulocytes, fibroblasts, epithelial and endothelial cells (Cabrillat *et al.*, 1987; Park *et al.*, 1987). Crosslinking studies show that IL-4 binds to three molecular species of 130, 75 and 65 kDa (Galizzi *et al.*, 1989). A specific cDNA coding for the human 130 kDa IL-4-binding protein has been isolated (Galizzi *et al.*, 1990; Idzerda *et al.*, 1990). The mature receptor is a glycoprotein composed of 800 amino acids. Its extracellular domain of 222 amino acids contains the two motifs characteristic of the cytokine receptor family (Miyajima *et al.*, 1992). A soluble form of this extracellular domain was found to bind IL-4 with high affinity and to inhibit its biological effects (Garrone *et al.*, 1991). Studies on mutants have indicated the presence of a 40 amino acid stretch in the 569 amino acid cytoplasmic domain deletion of which abrogates the transduction of a growth signal to pro-B cells (Harada *et al.*, 1992). The 75 kDa protein is unique but its present structure and function have not been established. This protein may be associated with the low-affinity IL-4 receptor (Foxwell *et al.*, 1989). Alternatively, it may be the common subunit between the receptor for IL-4 and IL-13, as determined by the inhibition of the binding of human IL-4 by murine IL-13 to the cell line TF1 which proliferates in response to IL-4 (Zurawski *et al.*, 1993). IL-4 is able to upregulate the expression of its own receptor after inducing its transient downregulation following receptor ligand internalization (Galizzi *et al.*, 1989). Following internalization, the IL-4 is degraded, most likely in lysosomes. Preliminary studies suggest a model of receptor interaction involving the formation of a ternary complex consisting of two molecules of

Table 2. Cytokines secreted by selected murine cells.

	CTL[1]	T helper-1	T helper-2	Mast cells
Interferon-γ	++	++	−	±
Interleukin-2	±	++	−	±
Lymphotoxin	+	++	−	−
GM-CSF	++	++	+	?
TNF[2]	+	++	+	+
Interleukin-3	+	++	++	++
Met-enkephalin	+	+	++	?
Interleukin-4	−	−	++	++
Interleukin-5	−	−	++	++
Interleukin-6	−	−	++	++
Interleukin-10	?	−	++	?
Interleukin-13	?	−	++	?

[1]CTL, cytotoxic T cells. [2] TNF, tumour necrosis factor.

the extracellular portion of the receptor and one molecule of IL-4 (Ramanathan *et al.*, 1993).

CELLULAR SOURCES OF IL-4

Unlike IL-1, IL-6 and IL-10, which are produced by many different cell types, IL-4, like IL-2 and IFN-γ, is secreted by restricted cell types.

T Lymphocytes

Studies with murine helper CD4$^+$ T-cell clones have indicated the presence of two cell types on the basis of their pattern of cytokine synthesis: T helper-1 cells secrete IL-2 and IFN-γ, T helper-2 cells secrete IL-4 and IL-5, and both types secrete cytokines such as GM-CSF and IL-3 (Mosmann and Coffman, 1989; Romagnani, 1992) (Table 2).

Human CD4$^+$ T cell clones specific for bacterial antigens and allergen- or helminth-specific T-cell clones have been found to exhibit T_{H1} or T_{H2}-like cytokine production profiles (Wierenga *et al.*, 1990; Del Prete *et al.*, 1991; Haanen *et al.*, 1991; Parronchi *et al.*, 1991). Both murine and human CD4$^+$ T cells with an intermediate cytokine profile T_{H0}) have been described (Paliard *et al.*, 1988; Street *et al.*, 1990). T_{H1} and T_{H2} cells may differentiate from a common precursor pool (Swain *et al.*, 1988) along differentiation pathways controlled, at least in part, by cytokines produced by lymphocytes or accessory cells. IFN-γ and IL-12 promote differentiation of T_H precursors into T_{H1} cells (Maggi *et al.*, 1992; Parronchi *et al.*, 1992; Hsieh *et al.*, 1993; Manetti *et al.*, 1993). In contrast, IL-4 induces differentiation into T_{H2} cells *in vitro* and *in vivo* (Scott, 1991; Chatelain *et al.*, 1992; Maggi *et al.*, 1992; Seder *et al.*, 1992). IL-4 involved in the differentiation of T_{H2} cells would originate from basophil/mast cells, while IFN-γ and IL-12 inducing the maturation of T_{H1} cells would originate from NK cells and macrophages, respectively.

As expected from the pattern of cytokine production, T_{H1} and T_{H2} cells regulate distinct biological functions. T_{H1} cells induce the activation of macrophages, resulting in delayed type hypersensitivity responses and the killing of intracellular parasites. In contrast, T_{H2} cells control more particularly humoral responses including the production of IgE and associated eosinophilia. An important feature of T_{H1} and T_{H2} cells is the ability of one subset to regulate the activities of the other. It occurs at the levels of the effector cells triggered by these subsets, as indicated by the inhibitory effects of IFN-γ on IL-4-induced B-cell activation or those of IL-4 on IL-2-induced T- and B-lymphocyte proliferation. It also occurs directly at the level of these subsets as the products of one subset can antagonize the activation of the other: IFN-γ inhibits proliferation of T_{H2} cells (Gajewski et al., 1989), whereas IL-4 and IL-10 inhibit cytokine production by T_{H1} cells (Fiorentino et al., 1989; Peleman et al., 1989; Vieira et al., 1991).

Other Cell Types

Both murine and human IL-4 are also produced by basophil/mast cells activated by crosslinkage of the FcεR$_I$ and FcγR$_{II}$ (Brown et al., 1987; Piccinni et al., 1991; Brunner et al., 1993). Nasal biopsy specimens from patients with allergic rhinites and bronchial biopsy specimens from patients with allergic asthma display mast cells with intracellular IL-4 (Bradding et al., 1992). Interestingly, anti-IgE induces maximum release of IL-4 within 1 h, suggesting that it is present within the cells in a preformed state similar to that reported for TNF-α.

EFFECTS OF IL-4 ON B LYMPHOCYTES

Ontogeny of B Lymphocytes

IL-4-dependent murine pro-B cell lines (which display germ-line immunoglobulin genes) can be established in the presence of stromal cells (Peschel et al., 1989a). In contrast, IL-4 inhibits stromal-cell-dependent proliferation of pre-B cells (which display rearranged μ-chain genes), possibly through the production by stromal cells of inhibitory factors (Rennick et al., 1987; Peschel et al., 1989a). Stromal cell lines producing IL-4 can induce the maturation of murine pre-B cells into mature B cells (Kinashi et al., 1988). Studies in man have also shown that IL-4 can inhibit the spontaneous proliferation of progenitor B cells, as well as that induced by IL-7 (Hofman et al., 1988; Pandrau et al., 1992). It is known that IL-4 can block the spontaneous proliferation of freshly isolated acute lymphocytic leukaemias of the pro-B-cell type.

B Lymphocyte Activation

IL-4 increases the volume of resting B cells (Vallé et al., 1989b) and induces their homotypic aggregation (Elenström and Severinson, 1989). IL-4 induces hyperexpression of MHC class II antigens on murine B cells (Noelle et al., 1984) but this effect is less pronounced on human resting B cells, which already express high levels of these surface molecules (Clark et al., 1989; Diu et al., 1990). However, human IL-4 strongly enhances HLA class II antigen expression on Burkitt lymphoma cell lines (Rousset et al., 1988) and chronic lymphocytic leukaemia cells. Furthermore, IL-4 upregulates the expression of LFA-1 and LFA-3 on Burkitt lymphoma cell lines which, unlike normal B cells, express these antigens poorly (Rousset et al., 1989).

IL-4 strongly enhances the expression of CD23 (the low-affinity receptor for IgE-$Fc\varepsilon R_{II}$) on normal and leukaemic B lymphocytes (Defrance et al., 1987; Hivroz et al., 1989). Indeed, two CD23 cDNAs, $Fc\varepsilon R_{II}a$ and $Fc\varepsilon_{II}b$, have been isolated which differ in the first few amino acids of the cytoplasmic tail, leaving identical extracellular domains (Yokota et al., 1988). In normal B cells $Fc\varepsilon R_{II}a$, but not $Fc\varepsilon R_{II}b$, is expressed spontaneously at low levels and IL-4 enhances the expression of $Fc\varepsilon R_{II}a$ and induces the expression of $Fc\varepsilon R_{II}b$. B cells isolated from atopic patients express $Fc\varepsilon R_{II}b$ mRNA, suggesting a recent encounter with IL-4. CD23 is associated with MHC class II antigens (Bonnefoy et al., 1988a) and this complex appears to play an important role in the B-cell presentation of antigen to T cells (Kehry and Hudak, 1989; Flores-Romo et al., 1990; Pirron et al., 1990). IFN-α and IFN-γ block the IL-4-dependent increase of CD23 on B cells. IL-4 also induces human B cells to produce a soluble CD23 (sCD23) molecule which binds IgE (Bonnefoy et al., 1988b). The membrane CD23 first releases 37 kDa and 33 kDa unstable molecules which subsequently yield a 25 kDa derivative through autoproteolysis (Letellier et al., 1990).

IL-4 upregulates the expression of (i) surface IgM (Shields et al., 1989), (ii) CD40 (Gordon et al., 1988a; Vallé et al., 1989a), (iii) BB1/B7 (Vallé et al., 1991; Ranheim and Kipps, 1993), a member of the immunoglobulin superfamily (Freeman et al., 1989) and the B-cell counterstructure of the T-cell CD28 and CTLA 4 (Linsley et al., 1990, 1991). Mouse IL-4 induces Thy-1 on B cells (Snapper et al., 1988) but decreases expression of $CDw32/Fc\gamma R_{II}$, which explains the IL-4-induced reversal of Fc receptor-mediated inhibition of B-lymphocyte activation (O'Garra et al., 1987).

All the above effects of IL-4 on resting B cells are suggestive of a role of IL-4 in the enhancement of antigen-presenting capacity of B cells towards T cells. More sIgM molecules permit more efficient antigen capture and more MHC class II molecules permit an enhanced presentation of processed antigen. More LFA molecules strengthen the physical association between T and B cells, thus explaining the IL-4-induced increase of T–B-cell conjugates (Sanders et al., 1987). The induced BB1/B7 can interact with CD28 whose triggering enhances T-cell cytokine production and proliferation (Lindstein et al., 1989; Ranheim and Kipps, 1993). Furthermore, sCD23 can induce T-cell proliferation and maturation (Swendeman and Thorley-Lawson, 1987; Mossalayi et al., 1990). In addition, IL-4 induces activated B cells to produce IL-6 and TNF (Smeland et al., 1989), which play an important role in the activation and expansion of activated T cells. Finally the induced expression of CD23 permits the presentation to T cells of antigen complexed to IgE. Through various means, IL-4 favours cognate T–B-cell interactions leading to enhanced antibody production. Accordingly, T_{H2} cells appear to be more efficient helpers than T_{H1} cells, for the growth and differentiation of B lymphocytes.

Effects of IL-4 on B Cell Growth

Antigen Receptor Triggering

IL-4 enhances DNA replication of B cells costimulated or preactivated with insolubilized anti-IgM antibody (Defrance et al., 1987; Clark et al., 1989). Unlike IL-2, IL-4 does not costimulate with particles of *Staphylococcus aureus* strain Cowan (SAC) (Jelinek and Lipsky, 1988), but enhances DNA replication of SAC preactivated B cells (Defrance *et al.*, 1987). The DNA replication induced by IL-4 on anti-IgM and SAC-stimulated B cells is short-lasting (up to 5 days), while that induced by IL-2 can last for up to 7–8 days. Neither IL-2 nor IL-4 can induce the expansion of viable B cells activated through their antigen receptor. PGE_2 and pharmacologic agents inducing intracellular cAMP such as cholera toxin, dibutyryl cAMP and forskolin enhance IL-4-induced DNA synthesis while they inhibit that induced by IL-2 (Vasquez *et al.*, 1991; Garrone and Banchereau, 1993).

Paradoxically, IL-4 antagonizes the IL-2-induced DNA replication of B cells costimulated through their antigen receptor (Defrance *et al.*, 1988; Jelinek and Lipsky, 1988). The inhibitory effect is particularly striking on freshly isolated leukaemic B cells, such as chronic lymphocytic leukaemia B cells (Karray *et al.*, 1988) and non Hodgkin's B-cell lymphomas (Defrance *et al.*, 1992). This antagonism may be due to an IL-4-dependent downregulation of high-affinity IL-2 receptors (Karray *et al.*, 1990; Lee *et al.*, 1990). IL-4 also inhibits TNF-α-induced proliferation of phorbol ester activated B-CLL cells. Indeed, autocrine TNF-α appears to mediate IL-2-induced B-CLL proliferation (van Kooten *et al.*, 1992). However, while blocking DNA synthesis, IL-4 protects the B-CLL cells from death by apoptosis through increased expression of the Bcl-2 protein (Dancescu *et al.*, 1992).

IL-4 allows the proliferation of antigen-activated antigen-specific B cells. It induces clonal expansion of single B cells activated by their specific antigen (Alderson *et al.*, 1987) and allows the proliferation of thymodependent antigen-specific B cells in the presence of carrier-specific T cells (Stein *et al.*, 1986). IL-4 also induces the proliferation of human TNP-specific B cells cultured in the presence of trinitrophenylpolyacrylamide beads (Llorente *et al.*, 1990).

CD40-Dependent Activation

Combinations of soluble anti-CD40 antibodies and either anti-IgM or phorbol esters have been shown to act in concert to induce DNA synthesis in B cells. IL-4 preferentially boosts the observed proliferation, while IL-2 is much less efficient (Gordon *et al.*, 1988b; Vallé *et al.*, 1989b). However, neither of these conditions results in long-term B-cell proliferation. In contrast, addition of IL-4 to B cells cultured in the CD40 system (combining irradiated fibroblastic L cells transfected with human $Fc\gamma R_{II}$/CDw32 and anti-CD40 antibody) results in their sustained proliferation (Banchereau *et al.*, 1991). The cells grow in tight clumps and within 5 weeks, the B-cell population can expand up to 1000-fold. This results in the generation of factor-dependent long-term normal B-cell lines which are negative for Epstein–Barr viral infection. These B-cell lines are dependent on the anti-CD40 antibody and IL-4, as their removal halts cell proliferation and subsequently results in cell death. B-cell clones can be generated which contain several-hundred cells. Cells cultured under these conditions express CD19, CD20 and high levels of CD23 and HLA class II antigens. A significant proportion of cells cultured for 3 weeks express sIgD, indicating that triggering of B cells with IL-4 and anti-CD40 is not sufficient to downregulate sIgD expression (Galibert *et al.*, 1993).

Whereas IL-1 and IFN-γ enhance the DNA synthesis observed in the CD40 system, they do not allow an increased recovery of viable B cells (Rousset *et al.*, 1991a). However, IL-1 and most notably IFN-γ enhance the increase of viable B cells obtained in the CD40 system with IL-4. IL-2 does not significantly alter B-cell proliferation in the CD40 system. Agents increasing intracellular cAMP strongly enhance IL-4-induced cell proliferation (Garrone and Banchereau, 1993; Garrone et al., 1994).

Both viral and human IL-10 enhance the proliferation of B cells cultured in the CD40 system (Rousset et al., 1992). IL-10 is as efficient as IL-4 for the first days of culture but proliferation subsequently slows down. The combination of IL-4 and IL-10 is additive and results in a 60–100-fold expansion of viable B cells over a 2-week period. The most powerful combination allowing growth of B cells in the CD40 system is presently that of IL-4, IL-10, IL-2 and PGE_2 because IL-10 induces functional high-affinity IL-2 receptors on anti-CD40-activated B cells (Fluckiger et al., 1993).

B-CLL cells synthesize DNA in the CD40 system and IL-4 further enhances it (Fluckiger et al., 1992). This results in the expansion of viable leukaemic cells, although its extent is lower than that obtained with normal B lymphocytes. Thus, the lack of growth-promoting activity of IL-4 on B-CLL cells activated via sIgs may be due to altered signal transduction through sIgs rather than to impaired IL-4 receptors.

Effects of IL-4 on B-Cell Differentiation

Antigen Receptor Triggering

IL-4 can induce SAC-preactivated B cells to produce IgG and IgM most likely as a consequence of induced proliferation (Defrance et al., 1988; Jelinek and Lipsky, 1988). Unlike IL-2, IL-4 is unable to induce Ig production by B cells that are costimulated rather than preactivated with SAC. IL-4 does not induce SAC-stimulated B cells to produce IgE and the IL-4-induced IgG and IgM secretion is not inhibited by IFN-γ. Moreover, IL-4 blocks IL-2-induced Ig secretion by SAC-costimulated B cells. Inhibitory effects of IL-4 on antigen-specific Ig production have also been observed. In particular, the secondary response of B cells to influenza virus, which requires both antigen and IL-2, can be inhibited by IL-4 (Callard et al., 1991). Likewise, the IL-2-dependent primary response to trinitrophenylated polyacrylamide beads is also inhibited by IL-4 (Llorente et al., 1989). However, IL-4 blocks IL-2-dependent B-cell differentiation while it stimulates antigen-dependent B-cell proliferation (Llorente et al., 1990).

CD40-Dependent Activation

Purified B cells cultured in the CD40 system produce low amounts of IgM, IgG and IgA. IL-4, which enhances proliferation, increases the production of IgM and IgG, and more strikingly, the secretion of large amounts of IgE (Rousset et al., 1991a). In contrast to long-term B-cell proliferation, the production of IgE dependent on CD40 activation does not require the presence of CDw32 L cells (Jabara et al., 1990; Gascan et al., 1991; Zhang et al., 1991; Shapira et al., 1992). Indeed, the IgE secretion dependent on the T cell-induced IL-4 production (Lundgren et al., 1989; Pène et al., 1989) results from CD40 triggering. However, to produce IgE in response to IL-4, B cells can be activated by other signals such as Epstein–Barr virus (Thyphronitis et al., 1989) or hydrocortisone (Sarfati et al., 1989; Jabara et al., 1991; Wu et al., 1991). Surprisingly, addition of IFN-γ or IFN-α to anti-CD40 activated B cells fails to inhibit IL-4-induced IgE production, thus contrasting with earlier studies in which B cells were stimulated by T cells (Pène *et al.*, 1988a,b). It is notable that TGF-β was found to totally inhibit IL-4-induced IgE production of anti-CD40-activated B cells while TNF-α was found to enhance it (de Waal Malefyt *et al.*, 1992; Gauchat *et al.*, 1992a). PGE$_2$ efficiently inhibits IL-4-induced IgE production under these culture conditions (Garrone *et al.*, 1994).

IL-4 and Isotype Switching

Many studies performed in both mouse and man have shown that IL-4-induced B cells produce IgE following isotype switching. Single sIgD$^+$ B cells cultured for 10 days in the CD40 system with IL-4, yielded B-cell clones whose isolated cells expressed the same VDJ genes coupled to different constant region genes (Lebecque *et al.*, 1993). Isotype switching is associated with a DNA recombination event in which C$_H$ genes originally lying between Sμ and the newly expressed C$_H$ gene are deleted (Esser and Radbruch, 1990). As a consequence of such a rearrangement, a circular piece of DNA is excised which has been named 'switch circle' (Matsuoka *et al.*, 1990; Yoshida *et al.*, 1990). Isotype switching is preceded by expression of transcripts that initiate 5' of the switch region specific for the constant region to be expressed and which encompass the downstream C$_H$ gene (sterile or germline transcript). Human IL-4, in a similar fashion to mouse IL-4, is able to induce purified resting B lymphocytes to express 1.8 kb germline Cε transcript (Rothman *et al.*, 1988; Gauchat *et al.*, 1990, 1992b; Jabara *et al.*, 1990; Qiu *et al.*, 1990; Shapira *et al.*, 1992). TGF-β is able to block the IL-4-dependent expression of the germline Cε transcripts thus explaining its inhibitory effects on IgE synthesis. In contrast, TNF-α is able to enhance the IL-4-dependent expression of Cε transcripts (Gauchat *et al.*, 1992b). Interestingly, IFNs and IL-6, which respectively block and stimulate IL-4 and T-cell dependent IgE synthesis, do not modify the levels of Cε germline transcripts. Further activation of B cells with anti-CD40 antibody strongly enhances the increase of germline Cε mRNA and results in the expression of a mature 2.0 kb Cε mRNA. DNA analysis of Sμ/Sε hybrid switch regions showed these fragments to result from the direct joining of Sμ to Sε. However, in another study where B cells were activated with IL-4 and EBV, fragments of Sγ were found interposed between Sμ in Sε (Mills *et al.*, 1992), as observed *in vivo* in parasite-infected mice (Yoshida *et al.*, 1990). These studies have indicated that the recombination sites in Sμ are clustered within 900 bp at the S-end of the μ switch region with some sites ('hot spots') being used preferentially. In contrast, the Sε recombination sites appear to be scattered throughout this region (Mills *et al.*, 1992; Shapira *et al.*, 1992).

IN VIVO ROLE OF IL-4 IN IgE REGULATION

Studies in mice with parasitic infections or treated with anti-IgD have confirmed the fundamental role of IL-4 in the regulation of circulating IgE levels (Finkelman *et al.*, 1990). Thus, antibodies neutralizing IL-4 or binding to the IL-4 receptor inhibit polyclonal and antigen-specific primary and secondary IgE responses (King *et al.*, 1990). Such antibodies can inhibit ongoing responses, suggesting that this should be possible in atopic patients. Anti-IL-4 suppresses the eosinophilia, hyper-IgE production and intestinal mastocytosis found in helminth infections, but not IgG1 and the protective immunity to the infection. Anti-IL-4 also reduces granuloma size in infection by *Schistosoma mansoni* (Chensue *et al.*, 1992).

The soluble extracellular domain of the IL-4 receptor represents another IL-4 antagonist (Garrone *et al.*, 1991) which also functions *in vivo*. In particular, sIL-4R inhibits the lymphoproliferative response to a localized injection of allogeneic cells and prolongs the survival of cardiac allografts (Fanslow *et al.*, 1991a; Maliszewski *et al.*, 1992). However, sIL4-R is much less efficient than anti-IL-4 antibody in inhibiting *in vivo* anti-IgD-induced IgE production. In fact, coadministration of suboptimal concentrations of anti-IL-4 antibody or sIL-4R with IL-4 can result in superinduction of IgE response (Sato *et al.*, 1993). Thus, cytokine-binding proteins can be used either as antagonists of biologic activities of endogenously produced cytokines, or as vehicles for cytokine delivery. In fact, soluble IL-4R, detected in the biological fluids of mice, was found to act as a transport protein (Fanslow *et al.*, 1990; Fernandez-Botran and Vitetta, 1990, 1991).

Inactivation of the IL-4 gene in mice through gene targeting was associated with normal T- and B-cell development but with a strong reduction of IgG1 and IgE levels (Kühn *et al.*, 1991). Conversely, IL-4 transgenic mice had increased IgE and an allergic-like disease with ocular lesions infiltrated with mast cells and eosinophils (Tepper *et al.*, 1990). Interestingly, administration of IFN-γ and (even better) IFN-α blocked the increased IgE levels induced in mice by various methods (Finkelman *et al.*, 1991).

As mice which have been induced to an hyper-IgE state display an increased production of IL-4 and a decreased production of IFN-γ through a predominance of a T_{H2} versus a T_{H1} response, studies have been performed in man attempting to correlate the IL-4 status with the IgE status. Some of these concluded that mononuclear cells from atopic patient blood display an increased capacity to produce IL-4 and/or a decreased capacity to produce IFN-γ in response to polyclonal activation (Claassen *et al.*, 1991; Rousset *et al.*, 1991b). IL-4 is not detected in the circulation of normal individuals and of most hyper-IgE patients (Chrétien *et al.*, 1989; Matsumoto *et al.*, 1991).

In hyper-IgE patients, preliminary trials have shown that IFN-α or IFN-γ can induce a decrease of IgE circulating levels (King *et al.*, 1989; Souillet *et al.*, 1989). Significant improvements were observed in patients with atopic dermatitis treated with recombinant IFN-γ and IFN-α (Boguniewicz *et al.*, 1990; Gruschwitz *et al.*, 1993), thus warranting further clinical trials. Interestingly, the *in vivo* IFN-γ treatment normalizes the diminished IL-4 response of mononuclear cells from atopic dermatitis patients (Leung *et al.*, 1991).

EFFECTS OF IL-4 ON T LYMPHOCYTES

Effects on Thymocytes

Both murine (Ziotnik *et al.*, 1987) and human (Spits *et al.*, 1987; Barcena *et al.*, 1990) thymocytes proliferate in response to IL-4 and a costimulant such as phorbol ester (PMA). In the mouse, IL-4 induces the proliferation of the most immature CD4$^-$ CD8$^-$ subset which also has the ability to produce IL-4. The intermediate CD8$^+$ CD4$^+$ subset virtually fails to proliferate under these conditions, whereas the most mature CD4$^+$ CD8$^-$ and CD4$^-$ CD8$^+$ subsets also proliferate in response to IL-4 and PMA. Fetal thymocytes also respond to IL-4 and *in situ* hybridization studies (Sideras *et al.*, 1988) have demonstrated the transcription of the IL-4 gene in fetal thymus. In addition, IL-4 can induce the maturation of thymocytes through an induction of mature T-cell antigens (CD3, CD5, T-cell receptor) and a loss of CD1. Concomitantly, the CD4$^+$ CD8$^+$ subset disappears and CD4$^-$ CD8$^-$, CD4$^+$ CD8$^-$, CD4$^-$ CD8$^+$ cells are generated (Ueno *et al.*, 1989). These data indicate that IL-4 plays an important role in T-cell ontogeny. Paradoxically, IL-4 transgenic mice were found to have involuted thymuses (Tepper *et al.*, 1990). In accordance with this finding, IL-4 inhibits early T-cell development in fetal thymus organ culture, probably during the differentiation of CD4$^-$ CD8$^-$ cells into CD4$^+$ CD8$^+$ thymocytes. The generation of TCR-$\alpha\beta$ thymocytes appears to be more impaired than that of TCR-$\gamma\delta$ thymocytes (Plum *et al.*, 1990). Likewise human IL-4 induces a preferential differentiation of TCR-γ/δ pre-T cells (Barcena *et al.*, 1990).

Effects of IL-4 on Mature T Cells

The T-cell growth promoting effects of IL-4 were initially discovered on continuous T-cell lines (Mosmann *et al.*, 1986). IL-4 can act on activated normal CD4$^+$ and CD8$^+$ T cells (Hu-Li *et al.*, 1987; Spits *et al.*, 1987) in an IL-2-independent fashion. Studies with antisense oligonucleotides showed that IL-4 and IL-2 are autocrine growth factors of T$_{H2}$ and T$_{H1}$ T-cell clones, respectively (Harel-Bellan *et al.*, 1988). Combinations of IL-2 and IL-4 result in a proliferation of activated T cells which is greater than that obtained with each cytokine alone. However, as found with B cells, IL-4 blocks the IL-2-induced proliferation of peripheral blood cells and purified T cells (Han *et al.*, 1988; Damle and Doyle, 1989; Martinez *et al.*, 1990). The inhibition is confined to the naive CD4$^+$/CD45RA$^+$ T cell subpopulation (Gaya *et al.*, 1990).

IL-4 inhibits the production of IFN-γ by activated T cells (Damle and Doyle, 1989; Peleman *et al.*, 1989; Chrétien *et al.*, 1990; Vercelli *et al.*, 1990). Since IFN-γ blocks various biological effects of IL-4 (particularly those linked to the IgE system), this observation suggests that IL-4 blocks the production of its own natural antagonist. IL-4 turns on the expression of CD8 on CD4$^+$ T-cell clones and neonate T cells (Paliard *et al.*, 1988a; Reason *et al.*, 1990). The induced CD4$^+$ CD8$^+$ neonatal cells subsequently differentiate to express only CD8. IL-4 can induce the expression of CD23 on activated T lymphocytes (Armitage *et al.*, 1989; Prinz *et al.*, 1990).

When added to mixed leukocyte cultures, IL-4 increases antigen specific cytotoxic activity against allogeneic stimulator cells (Widmer and Grabstein, 1987; Widmer *et al.*, 1987; Spits *et al.*, 1988). It also enhances the development of virus-specific cytotoxic T cells (Horohov *et al.*, 1988). The endogenous production of IL-4 in response to viral challenge is likely to play an important role in the generation of antigen-specific cytotoxic cells. T-cell clones cultured in the presence of IL-4 have been shown to display higher cytolytic ability than when cultured in IL-2. These cells grown in IL-4, but not IL-2, express a lipase that may be involved in the cytolytic process (Grusby *et al.*, 1990). Combinations of IL-2 and IL-4 have allowed the generation of cytotoxic T-cell lines starting from tumour infiltrating lymphocytes (TIL) (Kawakami *et al.*, 1988). Administration of soluble IL-4R to mice inhibits an allogenic response *in vivo* and enhances heart allograft survival, thus suggesting an *in vivo* role for IL-4 in the development of cytotoxic T cells (Fanslow *et al.*, 1991b).

Effects of IL-4 on NK Cells

CD3$^-$ NK cells proliferate in response to IL-4 provided a mitogenic stimulus is given (Spits *et al.*, 1987). Interestingly, IL-4 inhibits the IL-2-dependent proliferation of these cells and, accordingly, blocks the IL-2 dependent generation of human LAK cells (Nagler *et al.*, 1988; Spits *et al.*, 1988). The IL-4-induced suppression of IL-2 mediated nonspecific cytotoxicity is specific for the induction phase and does not affect the effector phase of cytolysis. In fact, IL-4 acts as an agonist, enhancing cell proliferation and the induction of LAK activity of preactivated cells (Kawakami *et al.*, 1989). As resting NK cells spontaneously express the intermediate affinity p70 chain of the IL-2R, it has been proposed that IL-4 blocks the IL-2-dependent induction of the p55/Tac, which permits the generation of high-affinity IL-2R. This is consistent with the fact that IL-2 preactivated cells are no longer sensitive to the inhibitory effects of IL-4 and with the lack of inhibitory effects of IL-4 on IFN-induced cytotoxicity of NK cells (Nagler *et al.*, 1988). IL-4 also inhibits the production of TNF-α and serine esterase by NK cells (Blay *et al.*, 1990). The blocking effect of IL-4 on IL-2-induced cytotoxicity appears to be linked to its ability to raise cAMP levels in NK cells. In contrast, mouse IL-4 induces mouse spleen cells to express LAK cell activity (Mulé *et al.*, 1987).

EFFECTS OF IL-4 ON MYELOMONOCYTIC CELLS

Effects of IL-4 on Haemopoiesis

IL-4 can either inhibit or enhance myelopoiesis from bone marrow progenitor cells. It blocks the development of colonies dependent on M-CSF (Jansen *et al.*, 1989) but stimulates the formation of colonies dependent on G-CSF (Rennick *et al.*, 1987; Broxmeyer *et al.*, 1988). IFN-γ and IL-4 reciprocally regulate the production of monocytes/macrophages and granulocytes. Thus, IL-4 antagonizes the stimulation by IFN-γ of monocytic colonies induced by GM-CSF or M-CSF. In contrast, IFN-γ inhibits the stimulation by IL-4 of granulocytic colonies induced by G-CSF (Snoeck *et al.*, 1993). Furthermore, in combination with IL-3, IL-4 induces the generation of basophil/mast cells from human (Favre *et al.*, 1990) and mouse (Rennick *et al.*, 1987) progenitor cells and of eosinophils (Favre *et al.*, 1990) from human progenitor cells. IL-4 also acts on the generation of eosinophils in mice, as administration of plasmacytoma expressing IL-4 results in eosinophil infiltration of tumours (Tepper *et al.*, 1989, 1992). Furthermore, IL-4 transgenic mice display eye inflammation and conjunctivitis caused by large numbers of eosinophils and mast cells (Tepper *et al.*, 1990). IL-4 is an essential growth factor for the *in vitro* growth of connective tissue-type mast cells (Hamaguchi *et al.*, 1987; Tsuji *et al.*, 1990). Combinations of erythropoietin and IL-4 induce partially purified progenitor cells to generate erythroid colonies (Peschel *et al.*, 1987; Broxmeyer *et al.*, 1988) but this may be due to an indirect effect of IL-4 on accessory cells. In contrast, IL-4 inhibits the formation of pure and mixed megakaryocyte colonies from enriched human haemopoietic progenitors (Sonoda *et al.*, 1993).

Effects on Monocytes/Macrophages

Monocytes cultured in the presence of IL-4 acquire a macrophage-like, dendritic cell morphology, as they increase in size and develop extensive processes (Te Velde *et al.*,

1988). IL-4 upregulates the expression of MHC class II antigens, of LFA-1 and CD23 (Vercelli *et al.*, 1988) but downregulates that of CD14 (Vercelli *et al.*, 1989) and of the three FcγR (FcγR$_I$ = CD64; FcγR$_{II}$ = CD32; FcγR$_{III}$ = CD16) (Te Velde *et al.*, 1990). Accordingly, it blocks the antibody-dependent cytotoxicity of macrophages without affecting their phagocytic properties. IL-4 blocks the spontaneous and induced production of IL-1, IL-6, IL-8 and TNF-α by monocytes (Essner *et al.*, 1989; Hart *et al.*, 1989; Standiford *et al.*, 1990; Miossec *et al.*, 1992). IL-4 also inhibits virus-dependent production of IFN-α and IFN-β by monocytes (Gobl and Alm, 1992). This inhibition of cytokine production is not the consequence of a general blockade of protein synthesis as IL-4 stimulates these cells to produce IL-1RA (Fenton *et al.*, 1992; Vannier *et al.*, 1992; Wong *et al.*, 1993) and the complement protein C2 (Littman *et al.*, 1989). IL-4 also inhibits the secretion of interstitial collagenase and 92 kDa type IV collagenase (Corcoran *et al.*, 1992; Lacraz *et al.*, 1992), thus reducing the ability of macrophages to degrade extracellular matrix. IL-4 has a profound inhibitory effect on the release of superoxide (Abramson and Gallin, 1990; Ho *et al.*, 1992) and the secretion of PGE$_2$ (Hart *et al.*, 1989). Taken together, these properties suggest a powerful anti-inflammatory effect of IL-4. Accordingly, *in vivo* administration of IL-4 was found to inhibit the development of an antigen-specific T-cell mediated inflammatory response in a hapten-induced model of contact sensitivity (Gautam *et al.*, 1992). *In vivo* administration of IL-4 to man also results in increased circulating levels of IL-1RA (Wong *et al.*, 1993). The induction of monocyte apoptosis may contribute to IL-4 anti-inflammatory effects (Mangan *et al.*, 1992).

The IL-4-induced inhibition of cytokine production by monocytes may be a consequence of the inhibition of *c-fos* and *c-jun* expression which constitute the transcription factor AP1 (Dokter *et al.*, 1993). IL-4 also blocks the transcription of the cellular genes *ISG-54* and *IP-10* which are upregulated by IFN-α and IFN-γ respectively (Larner *et al.*, 1993).

IL-4 inhibits the killing by macrophages of various parasites, such as *Leishmania* (Lehn *et al.*, 1989; Ho *et al.*, 1992) and asexual erythrocytic forms of *Plasmodium falciparum* (Kumaratilake and Ferrante, 1992).

Conflicting results have been reported concerning the activity of IL-4 on HIV replication in monocytes. One study showed IL-4 to be a potent enhancer of HIV infection of monocytes, yielding multinucleated giant cells (Novak *et al.*, 1990). In contrast, treatment of monocytes with IL-4 for 5 days resulted in a total inhibition of these cells' infectability with HIV, possibly because cells had differentiated into macrophages (Schuitemaker *et al.*, 1992).

Effects on Granulocytes

IL-4 was found to upregulate CD23 expression in the eosinophilic cell lines EoL 1 and 3 (Hosoda *et al.*, 1989) but this property was not confirmed in normal eosinophils (Baskar *et al.*, 1990). Normal eosinophils are nevertheless responsive to IL-4, as they express reduced levels of FcγR upon culturing with this cytokine. The downregulation of FcγR results in a decreased secretion of glucuronidase and arylsulphatase in response to IgG-coated beads, and in a reduced antibody-dependent killing of schistosomulas (Basker *et al.*, 1990).

IL-4 also acts on neutrophils by enhancing their respiratory burst and their phagocytic properties (Boey *et al.*, 1989). IL-4 also enhances the expression and secretion of membrane and soluble type II IL-1 receptor (Colotta *et al.*, 1993) by neutrophils. This may contribute to IL-4 anti-inflammatory effects by blocking IL-1 effects.

EFFECTS OF IL-4 ON OTHER CELL TYPES

IL-4 and Fibroblasts

Fibroblasts are chemoattracted by IL-4 (Postlethwaite and Seyer, 1991), IL-4 also induces dermal fibroblasts to secrete extracellular matrix proteins, such as type I and type III collagen and fibronectin (Fertin *et al.*, 1991; Gillery *et al.*, 1992; Postlethwaite *et al.*, 1992) and stimulates a fibroblast cell line to produce G-GSF and M-CSF (Tushinski *et al.*, 1991). In contrast, IL-4 blocks cytokine-induced (IL-1, PDGF) proliferation of synoviocytes (Dechanet *et al.*, 1993). Cell cycle studies have indicated a rapid and persistent blocking effect of IL-4 on the G1 phase, which is accompanied by an increased cell volume, which may explain the increase in thymidine uptake reported earlier (Monroe *et al.*, 1988; Feghali *et al.*, 1992). However, viable cell counts clearly demonstrate that IL-4 inhibits IL-1- and PDGF-induced fibroblast proliferation. Whereas IL-4 inhibits IL-6 production by monocytes, it enhances that of fibroblasts. Nevertheless, IL-4 blocks the production of PGE_2 by fibroblasts and monocytes. Treatment of dermal fibroblasts with IL-4 results in increased ICAM-1 expression which allows increased adhesion of LFA-1-bearing T lymphocytes, as well as binding of human rhinovirus (Piela-Smith *et al.*, 1992).

IL-4 and Endothelial Cells

Capillary endothelial cells are induced to proliferate in response to IL-4 (Toi *et al.*, 1992). Treatment of endothelial cells with IL-4 increases their adhesiveness for T cells, eosinophils, basophils but not for neutrophils. This results from an increased VCAM 1 expression (Masinovsky *et al.*, 1990; Thornhill *et al.*, 1991; Schleimer *et al.*, 1992). Pretreatment with IL-4 of vascular constructs, composed of endothelial cells cultivated on extracellular matrix from human fibroblasts, induces adherence and layer penetration of eosinophils but not neutrophils. For layer penetration, blood eosinophils from non-allergic donors need priming with GM-CSF, IL-3 or IL-5, whereas those from allergic donors spontaneously transmigrate (Moser *et al.*, 1992).

Cytokine-induced upregulation of ICAM-1 and ELAM-1 on endothelial cells is inhibited by IL-4. This contrasts with the IL-4-induced increase of ICAM-1 expression observed on dermal fibroblasts, macrophages and mast cells (Thornhill *et al.*, 1991; Valent *et al.*, 1991; Piela-Smith *et al.*, 1992). IL-4 synergizes with TNF or IFN-γ to cause a change of endothelial cells towards a more fibroblastic morphology (Thornhill *et al.*, 1990). These morphological changes are accompanied by a reorganization of the intracellular vimentin matrix from a diffuse pattern to a perinuclear concentration (Klein *et al.*, 1993). A synergy between IL-4 and TNF-α on VCAM-1 expression by endothelial cells is observed *in vivo*, following their injection in the skin of baboons (Briscoe *et al.*, 1992) IL-4 increases IL-6 production by endothelial cells in synergy with IL-1 and IFN-γ (Colotta *et al.*, 1992; Howells *et al.*, 1991). Finally, IL-4 counteracts the effect of LPS, IL-6 and TNF-α on the expression of procoagulant activity on endothelial cells and downregulates the thrombomodulin anticoagulation pathway (Kapiotis *et al.*, 1991). Since prothrombotic vascular changes are associated with inflammatory reactions, this illustrates a novel aspect of the anti-inflammatory effect of IL-4 (Mantovani *et al.*, 1992).

IL-4 and Epithelial Cells

IL-4 enhances the production of soluble CD23 by nasopharyngeal carcinoma, one of the human tumours associated with Epstein–Barr virus (Rousselet *et al.*, 1990). IL-4 also enhances expression of the polymeric Ig receptor by colon adenocarcinoma cell line (Phillips *et al.*, 1990). On human thymic epithelial cells, IL-4 increases IL-1-induced IL-6 production and inhibits that induced by GM-CSF (Galy and Spits, 1991).

IL-4 and Hepatocytes

IL-4 can also affect human hepatocytes in primary cultures. In particular, it decreases the spontaneous production of haptoglobin and, to a lesser extent, that of albumin and C-reactive protein while α_1-antitrypsin and fibrinogen production remain unaffected (Loyer *et al.*, 1993). Furthermore, IL-4 antagonizes the IL-6-enhanced secretion of haptoglobin, demonstrating another level of anti-inflammatory action. IL-4 also inhibits the stimulation of hepatic lipogenesis by TNF, IL-1 and IL-6 without altering that induced by IFN-α (Grunfeld *et al.*, 1991). In addition, IL-4 enhances the expression of the cytochrome P450, 2E1 in a specific manner, since levels of cytochromes P450, 1A2, 2C and 3A are not affected or weakly inhibited (Razzak *et al.*, 1993).

BIOCHEMICAL PATHWAYS OF IL-4 ACTION

B Lymphocytes

IL-4 induces the phosphorylation of B-lymphocyte membrane proteins, suggesting the activation of cellular kinases. In murine B cells, IL-4 does not induce the release of inositol triphosphate (IP3), cause Ca^{++} mobilization or protein kinase C (PKC) translocation, but synergizes with nonmitogenic concentrations of anti-Ig to provoke translocation of PKC from the cytosol to the membrane (Justement *et al.*, 1986; Mizuguchi *et al.*, 1986). IL-4 activates two distinct ion channels in B lymphocytes, inducing an inward rectifying K^+ channel and activating a large-conductance anion channel (McCann *et al.*, 1991). On quiescent human B lymphocytes, IL-4 has been found to induce increase of inositol triphosphate, Ca^{++} and cAMP (Finney *et al.*, 1990). The increase of cAMP induced by IL-4 may explain its inhibitory effect on IL-2-induced B-cell proliferation, since cAMP-inducing agents inhibit IL-2-induced B-cell proliferation without altering that of IL-4 (Vasquez *et al.*, 1991; Garrone and Banchereau, 1993). An IL-4-dependent increase of cAMP is also observed in NK cells (Blay *et al.*, 1990).

Myeloid Cells

Treatment of monocytes with IL-4 induces a significant redistribution of PKC from the cytosol to the nucleus (Arruda and Ho, 1992). IL-4 can increase the levels of cGMP in monocytes by activation of soluble guanylate cyclase (Dugas et al., submitted). This is most clearly seen when phosphodiesterase inhibitors are added because IL-4 itself is able to stimulate the phosphodiesterase activity of monocytes (Li et al., 1989). Interestingly, IL-4 induces monocytes to release nitric oxide (NO) and this stimulation of NO synthase is likely to explain the accumulation of cGMP (Dugas et al., submitted). IL-4 induces striking tyrosine phosphorylation of a 170 kDa protein, designated 4 PS, in factor-dependent myeloid cell lines (Wang et al., 1992). This molecule associates with the 85 kDa subunit of phosphoinositol-3-kinase. The expression of this enzyme correlates with cell proliferation. Interestingly, insulin and insulin-like growth factor, which also stimulate the proliferation of these cell lines, induce the tyrosine phosphorylation of 4 PS (Wang et al., 1993). IL-4-induced proliferation of human myeloid cell lines also involves the activation of a tyrosine-specific phosphatase and the dephosphorylation of an 80 kDa protein (Mire-Sluis and Thorpe, 1991).

CLINICAL ASPECTS OF IL-4

IL-4 and Neoplasia

Several independent studies have now demonstrated that IL-4 possesses potent antitumour activity in vivo in mice. When a cDNA for IL-4 is introduced into normally tumorigenic lines, the engineered lines fail to form tumours and block tumour proliferation by various other tumour lines transplanted at the same site (Tepper et al., 1989, 1992; Golumbek et al., 1991). The anti-tumour effect is clearly due to IL-4, as anti-IL-4 antibodies allow re-expression of the tumorigenic potential. Tepper's experiments carried out in nude mice, to exclude an effect of tumour-specific cytotoxic T cells, demonstrate a marked cellular infiltrate composed of eosinophils and activated macrophages at the site of tumour injection. Administration of anti-IL-5 and antigranulocyte antibodies restores the tumorigenicity of the cell lines and results in a marked reduction in the number of tumour-infiltrating eosinophils (Tepper et al., 1992). Thus, eosinophil-mediated cytotoxicity appears to be an important mechanism of action for the antitumour activity of IL-4. This finding correlates with earlier clinical observations showing that gastric and colonic malignancies infiltrated with eosinophils have an improved prognosis (Iwasaki et al., 1986).

Golumbek's experiments carried out in immunocompetent mice have indicated an important role for cytotoxic CD8$^+$ T cells, as the antitumour effect can also be transferred by T cells of mice administered with renal cancer cells transfected with IL-4 (Golumbek et al., 1991). In this study, after an early influx of macrophages and eosinophils, T cells begin infiltrating the tumour site. In addition, this study showed that the renal tumour cells engineered to secrete IL-4, induce a sufficiently strong systemic immune response to cure animals carrying small amounts of parental tumour. In addition, repeated injections of small amounts of IL-4 into tumour-draining lymph nodes result in an antitumour effect, which can be transferred with CD8$^+$ T cells (Bosco et al., 1990).

IL-4 may also display a direct antitumour effect, as shown with human colon, renal, gastric and breast carcinoma (Morisaki *et al.*, 1992; Toi *et al.*, 1992; Obiri *et al.*, 1993), lymphoma (Defrance *et al.*, 1992), acute pre-B-cell leukaemia and myelomas (Taylor *et al.*, 1990; Pandrau *et al.*, 1992), chronic lymphocytic and myelogenous leukaemias (Karray *et al.*, 1988; Akashi *et al.*, 1991) and some cases of acute myelogenous leukaemias (Akashi *et al.*, 1991; Miyauchi *et al.*, 1991).

Clinical Studies

Doses and Schedule
Phase I studies have been conducted with both recombinant *Escherichia coli*-produced human IL-4 (Schering-Plough Research Institute) and recombinant yeast-derived human IL-4 (Sterling Winthrop). The Phase I studies with rHuIL-4 (*E. coli*) were conducted with daily intravenous administration in doses of 0.25–5 μg/kg.day and daily subcutaneous dosing with 0.25–5 μg/kg.day in a single dose (Gilleece *et al.*, 1992; Markowitz *et al.*, submitted). Studies were also conducted with rHuIL-4 (yeast), with intravenous bolus injection every 8 h on days 1–5 and 15–19 in doses of 10 μg/kg–15 μg/kg per dose (Atkins *et al.*, 1992; Markowitz *et al.*, submitted).

Toxicity in Clinical Studies
Daily intravenous bolus administration 0.25–5 μg/kg.day × 10 days, rHuIL-4 was well tolerated. In 10 patients, toxicity consisted primarily of flu-like symptoms, commonly seen with cytokine treatment, including fever (<39°C in this group), rigors and myalgias. One patient did require dose reduction for a grade 3 headache. When given daily by the subcutaneous route, in doses 0.25 μg/kg.day for 28 days, again the clinical toxicity was that typically seen with cytokine treatment: specifically, a flu-like syndrome with fatigue, somnolence, fever and myalgias. Occasional abdominal and back pain, pedal and periorbital oedema, nausea and vomiting were seen. Of note, headache was an extremely common complaint in these patients, without any characteristic pattern or localization. The headache was a dose-limiting toxicity in this mode of administration. Laboratory abnormalities commonly reported included elevations in liver enzymes which were seen at all dose levels (Table 3). The severity was generally dose related, reversible and not associated with other evidence of hepatic dysfunction such as hyperbilirubinaemia or abnormalities in coagulation profile (one patient with previous hepatitis did develop hyperbilirubinaemia). Relatively little myeloid toxicity was seen and, in a number of patients, there was an increase in neutrophils while on IL-4 therapy (Gilleece *et al.*, 1992).

Glucose values were carefully monitored in these studies because of the appearance of hypoglycaemia in some animal studies of rHuIL-4. However, in patients, relatively little impact on serum glucose was noted. One patient did develop hypoglycaemia (49 μg/dl) at a dose of 5 μg/kg.day; however, no other patients developed significant hypoglycaemia.

In comparison, when rHuIL-4 (yeast) was administered by intravenous bolus at 10–15 μg/kg per dose, greater toxicity was seen. In those patients, a similar pattern of fatigue, anorexia, headache and dyspnoea was seen (Atkins *et al.*, 1992; Markowitz *et al.*, submitted). However, a greater median weight gain 6.1% (range 3.4% to 11.7%)

Table 3. Maximum clinical laboratory WHO grades recorded for patients treated with SC rhIL-4 SCH 39400.

	Number of Patients								
	0.25 μg/kg[1] (n = 10)			1 or 2 μg/kg[1] (n = 15)			4 or 5 μg/kg[1] (n = 22)		
Laboratory parameters (grade)	0 or 1	2	3 or 4	0 or 1	2	3 or 4	0 or 1	2	3 or 4
Haematology									
Decreased WBC count	10	0	0	12	2	1	21	0	1
Decreased neutrophils	10	0	0	10	4	1	17	0	4
Decreased haemoglobin	9	1	0	11	3	1	15	3	4
Decreased platelets	10	0	0	14	1	0	20	2	0
Hepatic enzyme elevation									
SGOT	8	0	2	13	1	1	17	4	1
SGPT	8	0	1	8	2	0	18	2	1
Alkaline phosphatase	6	2	2	9	2	4	11	8	3
LDH	9	0	0	15	0	0	20	0	2
Increased total bilirubin	6	2	1	14	0	0	21	0	1
Renal function									
Creatinine	10	0	0	15	0	0	21	1	0
BUN	10	0	0	14	1	0	22	0	0

[1] ECOG Score

was reported than was seen with the subcutaneous route studies. Orthostatic hypotension occurred in two patients at the 15 µg/kg dose level (Atkins *et al.*, 1992). Sustained hypotension sufficient to require pressors was not reported in that study. Decreases in lymphocyte count, sodium, albumin, fibrinogen levels, elevated partial thromboplastin time and increases in haematocrit were observed routinely in that dose and mode of administration. This was not seen in the subcutaneous studies. Increases in serum creatinine and hepatic transaminases appeared to occur less frequently than with the subcutaneous route.

Similar to the observations in the subcutaneous and intravenous dosing with the *E. coli* rHuIL-4, all side effects resolved by the follow-up visits. In the study of Markowitz *et al.* using doses of 20 to 1280 µg/M²/day yeast rHuIL-4, reversible abnormalities in liver function tests were noted, and Grade 1–2 fever was noted 6–8 h after most doses. Frequent Grade 1–2 elevations of liver function tests, rare Grade 3–4 elevations of liver function test increases in serum creatinine, the characteristic headaches, nasal congestion and a single case (1/22 patients) of Grade 2 fluid retention were seen.

Immunological and Antitumour Activity

Only limited data *in vivo* on immunological effects of rHuIL-4 are available from these Phase I studies. An increase in plasma IL-1 receptor antagonist and soluble CD23 levels were reported which were rapidly reversed following the discontinuation of IL-4 (Atkins *et al.*, 1992; Wong *et al.*, 1993). No changes in LAK or NK activity were noted. A decrease in measurable serum TNF and IL-1 levels was found in 4/4 and 3/3 patients, respectively, in whom detectable levels were present in pretreatment (Markowitz *et al.*, submitted). In the subcutaneous study, no consistent trends in changes in lymphocyte counts owing to wide interpatient variability were noted. Individual patients, however, did have evidence of elevations in CD4 and CD8 counts. There was no change in CD4:CD8 ratio as the changes tended to occur in parallel.

It was notable that, given the known *in vitro* activity of IL-4 in IgE production, there was no evidence in elevation in IgE levels in the Phase I patients. In these Phase I studies, limited antitumour activity was observed. Specifically, short-term intravenous bolus administration was not associated with any antitumour responses (Atkins *et al.*, 1992; Markowitz *et al.*, submitted). In the subcutaneous administration Phase 1 study, antitumour activity was observed, with a response in a patient with advanced refractory Hodgkin's disease, an improvement in a patient with chronic lymphocytic leukaemia, and a decrease in M-component in a patient with refractory multiple myeloma. In addition, in ongoing Phase II studies, which are too early for complete evaluation, activity has been noted in nonsmall-cell lung cancer, and Hodgkin's disease. These data, although preliminary, do suggest that IL-4 does have potential as an antitumour agent, particularly when administered over a more prolonged course, rather than short intravenous bolus. This is consistent with the known pharmacokinetics of this agent, which available data indicate has rapid clearance and a half-life of approximately 45 min (Markowitz *et al.*, submitted). The duration of immunological response following discontinuation of rHuIL-4 in patients has not yet been determined, although the data on CD23 levels in patients receiving intravenous bolus therapy suggest a relatively rapid fall-off in effect. This is in contrast to some of the animal data (Schering-Plough Research Institute, personal communication) which have shown protracted responses

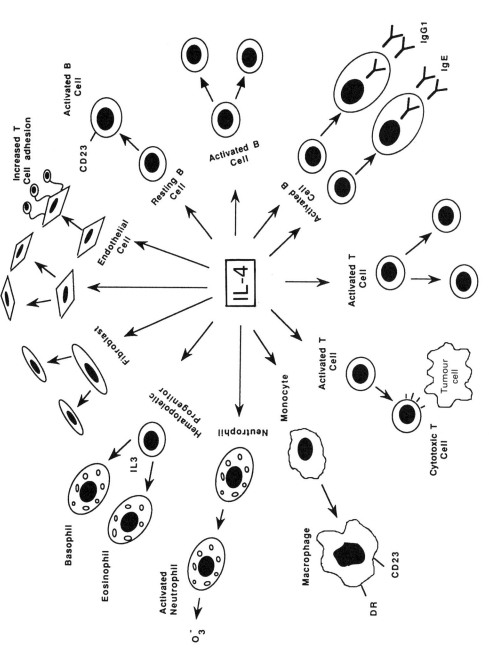

Fig. 1. Schematic representation of the multiple biological effects of IL-4.

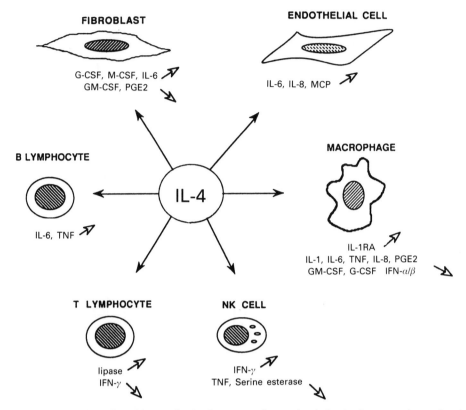

Fig. 2. IL-4 modulation of cytokine production by many cell types ($\nearrow$, induction/increase of secretion, $\searrow$, inhibition/blockade of secretion).

in animals given IL-4, particularly neutrophil activation which lasted as long as 2 weeks following discontinuation of IL-4.

CONCLUSION

In vitro studies have now shown that IL-4 can act on many cell types (Fig. 1) and that it can act at various stages of maturation of a given cell type. The biological effects of IL-4 on a given cell type depend on the surrounding cells and cytokines. Indeed, IL-4 can play an important biological role in an indirect fashion, as it modulates cytokine production by T, B and NK cells, monocytes/macrophages, endothelial cells and fibroblasts (Fig. 2) *In vivo* studies in animals have demonstrated an important antitumour effect for IL-4. Accordingly, IL-4, when administered to patients with advanced cancer, is well tolerated. This is particularly true for daily subcutaneous administration, but higher doses of intravenous bolus IL-4 were also reasonably well tolerated. There is suggestion of antitumour activity; however, the optimal dose and schedule of this molecule, in order to achieve desired immunomodulatory and antitumour effects *in vivo*, have not been determined. In addition, the tolerability of this molecule, particularly when given subcutaneously, suggests that it may be appropriate for evaluation in a variety of diseases (in addition to treatment of cancer) where its immunomodulatory/anti-inflammatory properties would be of clinical benefit. In particular, the inhibitory effects of IL-4 on the production of cytokines give a strong rationale for the use of IL-4 in chronic inflammatory diseases. The inhibitory effect of IL-4 on synoviocyte proliferation and on cytokine-induced bone resorption (Watanabe *et al.*, 1990) and its stimulatory effects on the *in vitro* mineralization of osteoblast-like cells (Ueno *et al.*, 1992) strongly support the notion of using IL-4 in the treatment of rheumatoid arthritis. Other inflammatory diseases with excess T_{H1} activity may benefit from IL-4 therapy, which may re-equilibrate the balance between T_{H1} and T_{H2} cells. In keeping with this concept, therapy may be designed in the future to counterbalance a T_{H2} overexpression observed in diseases such as allergy and possibly AIDS (Clerici *et al.*, 1993).

The near future will see many clinical trials with IL-4 itself or drugs affecting IL-4 production or IL-4 effects, such as interferons. In the long term, structural studies on IL-4, IL-4R and their complex, and studies on the intracellular pathways specifically activated by IL-4 should permit the design of chemical agents which will either inhibit or mimic part of or all the biological effects of IL-4.

ACKNOWLEDGEMENTS

The authors wish to thank Nicole Courbière for expert editorial assistance.

REFERENCES

Abramson, S.L. and Gallin, J.I. (1990). *J. Immunol.* **144**, 625–630.
Akashi, K., Harada, M., Shibuya, T., Eto, T., Takamatsu, Y., Teshima, T. and Niho, Y. (1991). *Blood* **78**, 197–204.
Alderson, M.R., Pike, B.L. and Nossal, G.J.V. (1987). *Proc. Natl Acad. Sci. USA.* **84**, 1389–1393.
Armitage, R.J., Goff, L.K. and Beverley, P.C.L. (1989). *Eur. J. Immunol.* **19**, 31–35.
Arruda, S. and Ho, J.L. (1992). *J. Immunol.* **149**, 1258–1264.
Asano, Y., Shibuya, T., Okamura, S., Yamaga, S., Otsuka, T. and Niho, Y. (1987). *Cancer Res* **47**, 5647–5648.
Atkins, M.B., Vachino, G. and Tilg, H.G. (1992). *J. Clin. Oncol.* **10**, 1802–1809.
Banchereau, J., de Paoli, P., Vallé, A., Garcia, E. and Rousset, F. (1991). *Science* **251**, 70–72.
Barcena, A., Toribio, M.L., Pezzi, L. and Martinez-A, C. (1990). *J. Exp. Med.* **172**, 439–446.
Baskar, P., Silberstein, D.S. and Pincus, S.H. (1990). *J. Immunol.* **144**, 2321–2326.
Blay, J.Y., Branellec, D., Robinet, E., Dugas, B., Gay, F. and Chouaib, S. (1990). *J. Clin. Invest.* **85**, 1909–1913.
Boey, H., Rosenbaum, R., Castracane, J. and Borish, L. (1989). *J. Allergy Clin. Immunol.* **83**, 978–984.
Boguniewicz, M., Jaffe, H.S., Izu, A., Sullivan, M.J., York, D., Geha, R. S. and Leung, D.Y.M. (1990). *Am. J. Med.* **88**, 365–370.
Bonnefoy, J.Y., Defrance, T., Péronne, C., Ménétrier, C., Rousset, F., Pène, J., de Vries, J.E. and Bancherau, J. (1988a). *Eur. J. Immunol.* **18**, 117–122.
Bonnefoy, J.Y., Guillot, O., Spits, H., Blanchard, D., Ishizaka, K. and Bancherau, J. (1988b). *J. Exp. Med.* **167**, 57–72.
Bosco, M.C., Giovarelli, M., Forni, M., Modesti, A., Scarpa, G., Masuelli, L. and Forni, G. (1990). *J. Immunol.* **145**, 3136–3143.
Bradding, P., Feather, I.H., Howarth, P.H., Mueller, R., Roberts, J.A., Britten, K., Bews, J.P.A., Hunt, T.G., Okayama, Y. and Heusser, C.H. (1992). *J. Exp. Med.* **176**, 1381–1386.
Briscoe, D.M., Cotran, R.S. and Pober, J.S. (1992). *J. Immunol.* **149**, 2954–2960.
Brown, M.A., Pierce, J.H., Watson, C.J., Falco, H., Ihle, J.N. and Paul, W.E. (1987). *Cell* **50**, 809–818.
Broxmeyer, H.E., Lu, L., Cooper, S., Tushinski, R., Mochizuki, D., Rubin, B.Y., Gillis, S. and William, D.E. (1988). *J. Immunol.* **141**, 3852–3862.

Brunner, T., Heusser, C.H. and Dahinden, C.A. (1993). *J. Exp. Med.* **177**, 605–611.
Cabrillat, H., Galizzi, J.P., Djossou, O., Arai, N., Yokota, T., Arai, K. and Banchereau, J. (1987). *Biochem. Biophys. Res. Commun.* **149**, 995–1001.
Callard, R.E., Smith, S.H. and Scott, K.E. (1991). *Int. Immunol.* **3**, 157–163.
Chatelain, R., Varkila, K. and Coffman, R.L. (1992). *J. Immunol.* **148**, 1182–1187.
Chensue, S.W., Terebuh, P.D., Warmington, K.S., Hershey, S.D., Evanoff, H.L., Kunkel, S.L. and Higashi, G.I. (1992). *J. Immunol.* **148**, 900–906.
Chrétien, I., Van Kimmenade, A., Pearce, M.K., Banchereau, J. and Abrams, J.S. (1989). *J. Immunol. Methods* **117**, 67–81.
Chrétien, I., Pène, J., Brière, F., De Waal Malefyt, R., Rousset, F. and De Vries, J.E. (1990). *Eur. J. Immunol.* **20**, 243–251.
Claassen, J.J., Levine, A.D., Schiff, S.E. and Buckley, R.H., (1991). *J. Allergy Clin Immunol.* **88**, 713–721.
Clark, E.A., Shu, G.L., Luscher, B., Draves, K.E., Banchereau, J., Ledbetter, J.A. and Valentine, M.A. (1989). *J. Immunol.* **143**, 3873–3880.
Clerici, M., Hakim, F.T., Venzon, D.J., Blatt, S., Hendrix, C.W., Wynn, T.A. and Shearer, G.M. (1993). *J. Clin. Invest.* **91**, 759–765.
Colotta, F., Sironi, M., Borrè, A., Luini, W., Maddalena, F. and Mantovani, A. (1992). *Cytokine,* **4**, 24–28.
Colotta, F., Re, F., Muzio, M., Bertini, R., Polentarutti, N., Sironi, M., Dower, S.K., Sims, J.E. and Mantovani, A. (1993). *Science* **261**, 472–475.
Corcoran, M.L., Stetler-Stevenson, W.G., Brown, P.D. and Wahl, L.M. (1992). *J. Biol. Chem.* **267**, 515–519.
Damle, N.K. and Doyle, L.V. (1989). *Lymp. Res.* **8**, 85–97.
Dancescu, M., Rubio-Trujillo, M., Biron, G., Bron, D., Delespesse, G. and Sarfati, M. (1992). *J. Exp. Med.* **176**, 1319–1326.
de Waal Malefyt, R., Yssel, H., Roncarolo, M.-G., Spits, H. and de Vries, J.E. (1992). *Curr. Opinion Immunol.* **4**, 314–320.
Dechanet, J., Briolay, J., Rissoan, M.-C., Chomarat, P., Durand, I., Banchereau, J. and Miossec, P. (1993). *J. Immunol.* **151**, 4908–4917.
Defrance, T., Vanbervliet, B., Aubry, J.P., Takebe, Y., Arai, N., Miyajima, A., Yokota, T., Lee, T., Arai, K., de Vries, J.E. and Banchereau, J. (1987). *J. Immunol.* **139**, 1135–1141.
Defrance, T., Vanbervliet, B., Aubry, J.P. and Banchereau, J. (1988). *J. Exp. Med.* **168**, 1321–1337.
Defrance, T., Fluckiger, A.C., Rossi, J.F., Magaud, J.P., Sotto, J.J. and Banchereau, J. (1992). *Blood* **79**, 990–996.
Del Prete, G.F., De Carli, M., Mastromauro, C., Biagiotti, R., Macchia, D., Falagiani, P., Ricci, M. and Romagnani, S. (1991). *J. Clin. Invest.* **88**, 346–350.
Diu, A., Fevrier, M., Mollier, P., Charron, D., Banchereau, J., Reinherz, E.L. and Theze, J. (1990). *Cell. Immunol.* **125**, 14–28.
Dokter, W.H.A., Esselink, M.T., Halie, M.R. and Vellenga, E. (1993). *Blood* **81**, 337–343.
Dugas, B., Paul-Eugène, N., Bousquet, J., Wietzerbin, J., Drapier, J.-C., Damais, C. and Kolb, J.-P. (Submitted).
Elenström, C. and Severinson, E. (1989). *Growth factors* **2**, 73–82.
Esser, C. and Radbruch, A. (1990). *Annu. Rev. Immunol.* **8**, 717–735.
Essner, R., Rhoades, K., McBride, W.H., Morton, D.L. and Economou, J.S. (1989). *J. Immunol.* **142**, 3857–3861.
Fanslow, W.C., Sims, J.E., Sassenfeld, H., Morrissey, P.J., Gillis, S., Dower, S.K. and Widmer, M. (1990). *Science* **248**, 739–742.
Fanslow, W.C., Clifford, K.N., Park, L.S., Rubin, A.S., Voice, R.F., Beckmann, M.P. and Widmer, M.B. (1991a). *J. Immunol.* **147**, 535–540.
Fanslow, W.C., Clifford, K., VandenBos, T., Teel, A., Armitage, R.J. and Beckman, M.P. (1991b). *Cytokine,* **2**, 398–404.
Favre, C., Saeland, S., Caux, C., Duvert, V. and De Vries, J.E. (1990) *Blood* **75**, 67–73.
Feghali, C.A., Bost, K.L., Boulware, D.W. and Levy, L.S. (1992). *Clin. Immunol. Immunopath.* **63**, 182–187.
Fenton, M.J., Buras, J.A. and Donnelly, R.P. (1992). *J. Immunol.* **149**, 1283–1288.
Fernandez-Botran, R. and Vitetta, E.S. (1990). *Proc. Natl Acad. Sci. USA.* **87**, 4202–4206.
Fernandez-Botran, R. and Vitetta, E.S. (1991). *J. Exp. Med.* **174**, 673–681.
Fertin, C., Nicolas, J.F., Gillery, P., Kalis, B., Banchereau, J. and Maquart, F.X. (1991). *Cell. Mol. Biol.* **37**, 823–829.

Finkelman, F.D., Holmes, J., Katona, I.M., Urban, J.F., Beckmann, M.P., Schooley, K.A., Coffman, R.L., Mosmann, T.R. and Paul, W.E. (1990). *Annu. Rev. Immunol.* **8**, 303–333.

Finkelman, F.D., Svetic, A., Gresser, I., Snapper, C., Holmes, J., Trotta, P.P., Katona, I.M. and Gause, W.C. (1991). *J. Exp. Med.* **174**, 1179–1188.

Finney, M., Guy, G.R., Michell, R.H., Gordon, J., Dugas, B., Rigley, K.P. and Callard, R.E. (1990). *Eur. J. Immunol.* **20**, 151–156.

Fiorentino, D.F., Bond, M.W. and Mosmann, T.R. (1989). *J. Exp. Med.* **170**, 2081–2095.

Flores-Romo, L., Johnson, G.D., Ghaderi, A.A., Stanworth, D.R., Veronesi, A. and Gordon, J. (1990). *Eur. J. Immunol.* **20**, 2465–2469.

Fluckiger, A.C., Rossi, J.F., Bussel, A., Bryon, P., Banchereau, J. and Defrance, T. (1992). *Blood* **80**, 3173–3181.

Fluckiger, A.-C., Garrone, P., Durand, I., Galizzi, J.P. and Banchereau, J. (1993). *J. Exp. Med.* **178**, 1473–1481.

Foxwell, B.M.J., Woerly, G. and Ryffel, B. (1989). *Eur. J. Immunol.* **9**, 1637–1641.

Freeman, G., Freedman, A.S., Segil, J.M., Le, G., Whitman, J.F. and Nadler, L.M. (1989). *J. Immunol.* **143**, 2714–2722.

Gajewski, T.F., Joyce, J. and Fitch, F.W. (1989). *J. Immunol.* **143**, 15–22.

Galibert, L., Durand, I., Rousset, F. and Banchereau, J. (1994). *J. Immunol.* **152**, 22–29.

Galizzi, J.-P., Zuber, C.E., Cabrillat, H., Djossou, O. and Banchereau, J. (1989). *J. Biol. Chem.* **264**, 6984–6989.

Galizzi, J.P., Zuber, C.E., Harada, N., Gorman, D.M., Djossou, O., Kastelein, R., Banchereau, J., Howard, M. and Miyajima, A. (1990). *Int. Immunol.* **2**, 669–675.

Galy, A.H. and Spits, H. (1991). *J. Immunol.* **147**, 3823–3830.

Garret, D.S., Powers, R., March, C.J., Frieden, E.A., Clore, G.M. and Gronenborn, A.M. (1992). *Biochemistry* **31**, 4347.

Garrone, P. and Banchereau, J. (1993). *Mol. Immunol.* **30**, 627–635.

Garrone, P., Djossou, O., Galizzi, J.P. and Banchereau, J. (1991). *Eur. J. Immunol.* **21**, 1365–1369.

Garrone, P., Galibert, L., Rousset, F. and Banchereau, J. (1994). *J. Immunol.* (in press).

Gascan, H., Gauchat, J.-F., Roncarolo, M.-G., Yssel, H., Spits, H. and de Vries, J.E. (1991). *J. Exp. Med.* **173**, 747–750.

Gauchat, J.-F., Lebman, D.A., Coffman, R.L., Gascan, H. and de Vries, J.E. (1990). *J. Exp. Med.* **172**, 463–473.

Gauchat, J.-F., Aversa, G., Gascan, H. and de Vries, J.E. (1992a). *Int. Immunol.* **4**, 379.

Gauchat, J.F., Gascan, H., de Waal Malefyt, R. and de Vries, J.E. (1992b). *J. Immunol.* **148**, 2291–2299.

Gautam, S.C., Chikkala, N.F. and Hamilton, T.A. (1992). *J. Immunol.* **148**, 1411–1415.

Gaya, A., Alsinet, E., Martorell, J., Places, L., De La Calle, O., Yagüe, J. and Vives, J. (1990). *Int. Immunol.* **2**, 685–689.

Gilleece, M.H., Scarffe, J.H. and Ghosh, A. (1992). *Br. J. Cancer.* **66**, 204–210.

Gillery, P., Fertin, C., Nicolas, J.F., Chastang, F., Kalis, B., Banchereau, J. and Maquart, F.X. (1992). *FEBS L.* **302**, 231–234.

Gobi, A.E. and Alm, G.V. (1992). *Scand. J. Immunol.* **35**, 167–175.

Golumbek, P.T., Lazenby, A.J., Levitsky, H.I., Jaffee, L.M., Karasuyama, H., Baker, M. and Pardoll, D.M. (1991). *Science* **254**, 713–716.

Gordon, J., Cairns, J.A., Millsum, M.J., Gillis, S. and Guy, G.R. (1988a). *Eur. J. Immunol.* **18**, 1561–1565.

Gordon, J., Millsum, M.J., Guy, G.R. and Ledbetter, J.A. (1988b). *J. Immunol.* **140**, 1425–1430.

Grunfeld, C., Soued, M., Adi, S., Moser, A.H., Fiers, W., Dinarello, C.A. and Feingold, K.R. (1991). *Cancer Res.* **51**, 2803–2807.

Grusby, M.J., Nabavi, N., Wong, H., Dick, R.F., Bluestone, J.A., Schotz, M.C. and Glimcher, L.H. (1990). *Cell.* **60**, 451–459.

Gruschwitz, M.S., Peters, K.-P., Heese, A., Stosiek, N., Koch, H.U. and Hornstein, O.P. (1993). *Int. Arch. Allergy Immunol.* **101**, 20–30.

Haanen, J.B.A.G., de Waal Malefyt, R., Res, P.C.M., Kraakman, E.M., Ottenhoff, T.H.M., de Vries, R.R.P. and Spits, H. (1991). *J. Exp. Med.* **174**, 583–592.

Hamaguchi, Y., Kanakura, Y., Fusita, J., Takeoa, S.I., Nakano, T., Tarui, S., Honjo, T. and Kitamura, Y. (1987). *J. Exp. Med.* **165**, 268–273.

Han, X., Itoh, H., Balch, C.M. and Pellis, N.R. (1988). *Lymphokine Res.* **7**, 227–235.
Harada, N., Yang, G., Miyajima, A. and Howard, M. (1992). *J. Biol. Chem.* **267**, 22752–22758.
Harel-Bellan, A., Durum, S., Muegge, K., Abbas, A.K. and Farrar, W.L. (1988). *J. Exp. Med.* **168**, 2309–2318.
Hart, P.H., Vitti, G.F., Burgess, D.R., Whitty, G.A., Piccoli, D.S. and Hamilton, J.A. (1989). *Proc. Natl Acad. Sci. USA.* **86**, 3803–3807.
Hivroz, C., Vallé, A., Brouet, J.C., Banchereau, J. and Grillot-Courvalin, C. (1989). *Eur. J. Immunol.* **19**, 1025–1030.
Ho, J.L., He, S.H., Rios, M.J. and Wick, E.A. (1992). *J. Inf. Dis.* **165**, 344–351.
Hofman, F.M., Brock, M., Taylor, C.R. and Lyons, B. (1988). *J. Immunol.* **141**, 1185–1190.
Horohov, D.W., Crim, J.A., Smith, P.L. and Siegel, J.P. (1988). *J. Immunol.* **141**, 4217–4223.
Hosoda, M., Makino, S., Kawabe, T., Maeda, Y., Satoh, S., Takami, M., Mayumi, M., Arai, K.I., Saitoh, H. and Yodoi, J. (1989). *J. Immunol.* **143**, 147–152.
Howells, G., Pham, P., Taylor, D., Foxwell, B. and Feldman, M. (1991). *Eur. J. Immunol.* **21**, 97–101.
Hsieh, C.-S., Macatonia, S.E., Tripp, C.S., Wolf, S.F., O'Garra, A. and Murphy, K.M. (1993). *Science* **260**, 547–550.
Hu-Li, J., Shevach, E.M., Mizuguchi, J., Ohara, J., Mosmann, T. and Paul, W.E. (1987). *J. Exp. Med.* **165**, 157–172.
Idzerda, R.L., March, C.J., Mosley, B., Lyman, S.D., Vanden Bos, T., Gimpel, S.D., Din, W.S., Grabstein, K.H., Widmer, M.B., Park, L.S., Cosman, D. and Beckmann, M.P. (1990). *J. Exp. Med.* **171**, 861–873.
Iwasaki, K., Torisu, M. and Fujimura, T. (1986). *Cancer Res.* **58**, 1321–1327.
Jabara, H.H., Fu, S.M., Geha, R.S. and Vercelli, D. (1990). *J. Exp. Med.* **172**, 1861–1864.
Jabara, H.H., Ahern, D.J., Vercelli, D. and Geha, R.S. (1991). *J. Immunol.* **147**, 1557–1560.
Jansen, J.H., Wientjens, G.-J.H.M., Fibbe, W.E., Willemze, R. and Kluin-Nelemans, H.C. (1989) *J. Exp. Med.* **170**, 577–582.
Jelinek, D.F. and Lipsky, P.E. (1988). *J. Immunol.* **141**, 164–173.
Justement, L., Chen, Z.Z., Harris, L.K., Ransom, J.T., Sandoval, V.S., Smith, C., Rennick, D., Roehm, N. and Cambier, J. (1986). *J. Immunol.* **137**, 3664–3670.
Kapiotis, S., Besemer, J., Bevec, D., Valent, P., Bettelheim, P., Lechner, K. and Speiser, W. (1991). *Blood* **78**, 410–415.
Karray, S., Dautry-Varsat, A., Tsudo, M., Merle-Beral, H., Debré, P. and Galanaud, P. (1990). *J. Immunol.* **145**, 1152–1158.
Karray, S., Defrance, T., Merle-Béral, H., Banchereau, J., Debré, P. and Galanaud, P. (1988). *J. Exp. Med.* **168**, 85–94.
Kawakami, Y., Rosenberg, S.A. and Lotze, M.T. (1988). *J. Exp. Med.* **168**, 2183–2191.
Kawakami, Y., Custer, M.C., Rosenberg, S.A. and Lotze, M.T. (1989). *J. Immunol.* **142**, 3452–3461.
Kehry, M. and Hudak, S.A. (1989). *Cell. Immunol.* **118**, 504–515.
Kinashi, T., Inaba, K., Tsubata, T., Tashiro, K., Palacios, R. and Honjo, T. (1988). *Proc. Natl Acad. Sci. USA.* **85**, 4473–4477.
King, C.L., Gallin, J.I., Malech, H.L., Abramson, S.T. and Nutman, T.B. (1989). *Proc. Natl Acad. Sci. USA.* **86**, 10085–10089.
King, C.L., Ottesen, E.A. and Nutman, T.B. (1990). *J. Clin. Invest.* **85**, 1810–1815.
Klein, N.J., Rigley, K.P. and Callard, R.E. (1993). *Intern. Immunol.* **5**, 293–301.
Kruse, N., Tony, H.P. and Sebald, W. (1992). *EMBO J.* **11**, 3237–3244.
Kühn, R., Rajewsky, K. and Müller, W. (1991). *Science* **254**, 707–710.
Kumaratilake, L.M. and Ferrante, A. (1992). *J. Immunol.* **149**, 194–199.
Lacraz, S., Nicod, L., Galve-de-Rochemonteix, B., Baumberger, C., Dayer, J.-M. and Welgus, H.G. (1992). *J. Clin. Invest.* **90**, 382–388.
Larner, A.C., Petricoin, E.F., Nakagawa, Y. and Finbloom, D.S. (1993). *J. Immunol.* **150**, 1944–1950.
Lebecque, S., Galibert, L., van Dooren, J., Jefferis, R., Martinez-Valdez, H., Rousset, F. and Banchereau, J. (1993). *J. Cell Biochem.* **17 B**, 181.
Lee, H.K., Xia, X. and Choi, Y.S. (1990) *J. Immunol.* **144**, 3431–3436.
Lehn, M., Weiser, W.Y., Engelhorn, S., Gillis, S. and Remold, H.G. (1989). *J. Immunol.* **143**, 3020–3024.
Letellier, M., Nakajima, T., Pulido-Cejudo, G., Hofstetter, H. and Delespesse, G. (1990) *J. Exp. Med.* **172**, 693–700.
Leung, D.Y.M., Or, R., Boguniewicz, M., Milgrom, H., Gelfans, E.W. and Renz, H. (1991). *Proc. 27th Ann. Meet. Am. Soc. Clin. Onc.* **10**, 235 (Abs.).

Li, Y.S., Kouassi, E. and Revillard, J.-P. (1989). *Eur. J. Immunol.* **19**, 1721–1725.

Lindstein, T., June, C.H., Ledbetter, J.A., Stella, G. and Thompson, C.B. (1989). *Science* **244**, 339–343.

Linsley, P.S., Clark, E.A. and Ledbetter, J.A. (1990). *Proc. Natl Acad. Sci. USA.* **87**, 5031–5035.

Linsley, P.S., Brady, W., Urnes, M., Grosmaire, L.S., Damie, N.K. and Ledbetter, J.A. (1991). *J. Exp. Med.* **174**, 561–569.

Littman, B.H., Dastvan, F.F., Carlson, P.L. and Sanders, K.M. (1989). *J. Immunol.* **142**, 520–525.

Llorente, L., Crevon, M.L., Karray, S., Defrance, T., Banchereau, J. and Galanaud, P. (1989). *Eur. J. Immunol.* **19**, 765–769.

Llorente, L., Mitjavila, F., Crevon, M.C. and Galanaud, P. (1990). *Eur. J. Immunol.* **20**, 1887–1892.

Loyer, P., Ilyin, G., Razzak, Z.A., Dézier, J.-F., Banchereau, J., Campion, J.-P., Guguen-Guillouzo, C. and Guillouzo, A. (1993) *Febs Lett.* **336**, 215–220.

Lundgren, M., Persson, U., Larsson, P., Magnusson, C., Smith, C.I.E., Hammarström, L. and Severinson, E. (1989). *Eur. J. Immunol.* **19**, 1311–1315.

McCann, F.V., McCarthy, D.C. and Noelle, R.J. (1991). *Cel. Signalling.* **3**, 483–490.

McKenzie, A.N.J., Culpepper, J.A., de Waal Malefyt, R., Brière, F., Punnonen, J., Aversa, G., Sato, A., Dang, W., Cocks, B.G., Menon, S., de Vries, J.E., Banchereau, J. and Zurawski, G. (1993). *Proc. Natl Acad. Sci. USA.* **90**, 3735–3739.

Maggi, E., Parronchi, P., Manetti, R., Simonelli, C., Piccinni, M.-P., Rugiu, F.S., De Carli, M., Ricci, M. and Romagnani, S. (1992). *J. Immunol.* **148**, 2142–2147.

Maliszewski, C.R., Morrissey, P.J., Fanslow, W.C., Sato, T.A., Willis, C. and Devison, B. (1992). *Cell. Immunol.* **143**, 434–448.

Manetti, R., Parronchi, P., Giudizi, M.G., Piccinni, M.-P., Maggi, E., Trinchieri, G. and Romagnani, S. (1993). *J. Exp. Med.* **177**, 1199–1204.

Mangan, D.F., Robertson, B. and Wahl, S.M. (1992). *J. Immunol.* **148**, 1812–1816.

Mantovani, A., Bussolino, F. and Dejana, E. (1992). *FASEB J.* **6**, 2591–2599.

Markowitz, A., Jakubowski, A. and Rybak, M.E. (Submitted).

Markowitz, A.B., Hudson, M.M. and Itoh, K. (Submitted).

Martinez, O.M., Gibbons, R.S., Garovoy, M.R. and Aronson, F.R. (1990). *J. Immunol.* **144**, 2211–2215.

Masinovsky, B., Urdal, D., and Gallatin, M.W. (1990). *J. Immunol.* **145**, 2886–2895.

Matsumoto, T., Miike, T., Yamaguchi, K., Murakami, M., Kawabe, T. and Yodoi, J. (1991). *Clin. Exp. Immunol.* **85**, 288–292.

Matsuoka, M., Yoshida, K., Maeda, T., Usuda, S. and Sakano, H. (1990). *Cell.* **62**, 135–142.

Mills, F.C., Thyphronitis, G., Finkelman, F.D. and Max, E.E. (1992). *J. Immunol.* **149**, 1075–1085.

Minty, A., Chalon, P., Derocq, J.-M., Dumont, X., Guillemot, J.-C., Kaghad, M., Labit, C., Leplatois, P., Liauzun, P., Miloux, B., Minty, C., Casellas, P., Loison, G., Lupker, J., Shire, D., Ferrara, P. and Caput, D. (1993). *Nature* **362**, 248–250.

Miossec, P., Briolay, J., Dechanet, J., Wijdenes, J., Martinez-Valdez, H. and Banchereau, J. (1992). *Arthritis and Rheum.* **35**, 874–883.

Mire-Sluis, A.R. and Thorpe, R. (1991). *J. Biol. Chem.* **266**, 18113–18118.

Miyajima, A., Kitamura, T., Harada, N., Yokota, T. and Arai, K. (1992). *Annu. Rev. Immunol.* **10**, 295–331.

Miyauchi, J., Clark, S.C., Tsunematsu, Y., Shimizu, K., Park, J.W., Ogawa, T. and Toyama, K. (1991). *Leukemia,* **5**, 108–115.

Mizuguchi, J., Beaven, M.A., O'Hara, J. and Paul, F.E. (1986). *J. Immunol.* **137**, 2215–2219.

Monroe, J.G., Haldar, S., Prystowsky, M.B. and Lammie, P. (1988). *Clin. Immunol. & Immunopath.* **49**, 292–298.

Morgan, J.G., Dolganov, G.M., Robbins, S.E., Hinton, L.M. and Lovett, M. (1992). *Nucleic Acids Res.* **20**, 5173–5179.

Morisaki, T., Yuzuki, D.H., Lin, R.T., Foshag, L.J., Morton, D.L. and Hoon, D.S.B. (1992). *Cancer Res.* **52**, 6059–6065.

Moser, R., Fehr, J. and Bruijnzeel, P.L.B. (1992). *J. Immunol.* **149**, 1432–1438.

Mosmann, T.R. and Coffman, R.L. (1989). *Annu. Rev. Immunol.* **7**, 145–173.

Mosmann, T.R., Bond, M.W., Coffman, R.L., Ohara, J. and Paul, W.E. (1986). *Proc. Natl Acad. Sci. USA.* **83**, 5654–5658.

Mossalayi, M.D., Lecron, J.C., Dalloul, A.H., Sarfati, M., Bertho, J.M., Hofstetter, H., Delespesse, G. and Debré, P. (1990). *J. Exp. Med.* **171**, 959–964.

Mulé, J.J., Smith, C.A. and Rosenberg, S.A. (1987). *J. Exp. Med.* **166**, 792–797.
Nagler, A., Lanier, L.L. and Phillips, J.H. (1988). *J. Immunol.* **141**, 2349–2351.
Noelle, R., Krammer, P.H., Ohara, J., Uhr, J.W. and Vitetta, E.S. (1984). *Proc. Natl Acad. Sci. USA.* **81**, 6149–6153.
Novak, R.M., Holzer, T.J., Kennedy, M.M., Heynen, C.A. and Dawson, G. (1990). *Aids Res. Human Retroviruses.* **6**, 973–976.
O'Garra, A., Rigley, K.P., Holman, M., McLaughlin, J.B. and Klaus, G.G.B. (1987). *Proc. Natl Acad. Sci. USA.* **84**, 6254–6258.
Obiri, N.I., Hillman, G.G., Haas, G.P., Sud, S. and Puri, R.K. (1993). *J. Clin. Invest.* **91**, 88–93.
Paliard, X., de Waal Malefijt, R., de Vries, J.E. and Spits, H. (1988a). *Nature* **335**, 642–644.
Paliard, X., de Waal Malefijt, R., Yssel, H., Blanchard, D., Chretien, I., Abrams, J., de Vries, J.E. and Spits, H. (1988b). *J. Immunol.* **141**, 849–855.
Pandrau, D., Saeland, S., Duvert, V., Durand, I., Manel, A.M., Zabot, M.T., Philippe, N. and Banchereau, J. (1992). *J. Clin. Invest.* **90**, 1697–1706.
Park, L.S., Friend, D., Sassenfeld, H.M. and Urdal, D.L. (1987). *J. Exp. Med.* **166**, 476–488.
Parronchi, P., Macchia, D., Piccini, M.P., Biswas, P., Simonelli, C., Maggi, E., Ricci, M., Ansari, A.A. and Romagnani, S. (1991). *Proc. Natl Acad. Sci. USA.* **88**, 4538–4542.
Parronchi, P., De Carli, M., Manetti, R., Simonelli, C., Sampognaro, S., Piccinni, M.-P., Macchia, D., Maggi, E., Del Prete, G.F. and Romagnani, S. (1992). *J. Immunol.* **149**, 2977–2983.
Paul, W.E. (1991). *Blood* **77**, 1859.
Peleman, R., Wu, J., Fargeas, C. and Delespesse, G. (1989). *J. Exp. Med.* **170**, 1751–1756.
Pène, J., Rousset, F., Brière, F., Chrétien, I., Paliard, X., Banchereau, J., Spits, H. and De Vries, J.E. (1988a). *J. Immunol.* **141**, 1218–1224.
Pène, J., Rousset, F., Brière, F., Chrétien, I., Wideman, J., Bonnefoy, J.Y. and De Vries, J.E. (1988b). *Eur. J. Immunol.* **18**, 929–935.
Pène, J., Chrétien, I., Rousset, F., Brière, F., Bonnefoy, J.Y. and De Vries, J.E. (1989). *J. Cell. Biochem.* **39**, 253–264.
Peschel, C., Paul, W.E., Ohara, J. and Green, I. (1987), *Blood* **70**, 254–263.
Peschel, C., Green, I. and Paul, W.E. (1989a). *Blood* **73**, 1130–1141.
Peschel, C., Green, I. and Paul, W.E. (1989b). *J. Immunol.* **142**, 1558–1568.
Phillips, J.O., Everson, M.P., Moldoveanu, Z., Lue, C. and Mestecky, J. (1990). *J. Immunol.* **145**, 1740–1744.
Piccinni, M.P., Macchia, D., Parronchi, P., Giudizi, M.G., Bani, D., Alternini, R., Grossi, A., Ricci, M., Maggi, E. and Romagnani, S. (1991). *Proc. Natl Acad. Sci. USA.* **88**, 8656–8660.
Piela-Smith, T.H., Broketa, G., Hand, A. and Korn, J.H. (1992). *J. Immunol.* **148**, 1375–1381.
Pirron, U., Schlunck, T., Prinz, J.C. and Rieber, E.P. (1990). *Eur. J. Immunol.* **20**, 1547–1551.
Plum, J., De Smedt, M., Leclercq, G. and Tison, B. (1990). *J. Immunol.* **145**, 1066–1073.
Postlethwaite, A.E. and Seyer, J.M. (1991). *J. Clin. Invest.* **87**, 2147–2152.
Postlethwaite, A.E., Holness, M.A., Katai, H. and Raghow, R. (1992). *J. Clin. Invest.* **90**, 1479–1485.
Powers, R., Garrett, D.S., March, C.J., Frieden, E.A., Gronenborn, A.M. and Clore, G.M. (1992). *Science* **256**, 1673–1677.
Prinz, J.C., Baur, X., Mazur, G. and Rieber, E.P. (1990). *Eur. J. Immunol.* **20**, 1259–1264.
Qiu, G., Gauchat, J.-F., Vogel, M., Mandallaz, M., De Weck, A.L. and Stadler, B.M. (1990). *Eur. J. Immunol.* **20**, 2191–2199.
Ramanathan, L., Ingram, R., Sullivan, L., Greenberg, R., Reim, R., Trotta, P.P. and Le, H.V. (1993). *Biochemistry* **32**, 3549–3556.
Ranheim, E.A. and Kipps, T.J. (1993). *J. Exp. Med.* **177**, 925–939.
Razzak, Z.A., Loyer, P., Fautrel, A., Gautier, J.-C., Corcos, L., Turlin, B., Beaune, P. and Guillouzo, A. (1993). *Molec. Pharm.* **44**, 707–715.
Reason, D.C., Ebisawa, M., Saito, H., Nagakura, T. and Likura, Y. (1990). *Biochem Biophys. Res. Commun.* **168**, 830–836.
Rennick, D., Yang, G., Muller-Sieburg, C., Smith, C., Arai, N., Takabe, Y. and Gemmell, L. (1987). *Proc. Natl Acad. Sci. USA* **84**, 6889–6893.
Romagnani, S. (1992). *Int. Arch. Allergy Imunol.* **98**, 279–285.
Rothman, P., Lutzker, S., Cook, W., Coffman, R. and Alt, F.W. (1988). *J. Exp. Med.* **168**, 2385–2389.
Rousselet, G., Busson, P., Billaud, M., Guillon, J.M., Scamps, C., Wakasugi, H., Lenoir, G. and Tursz, T. (1990). *Int. Immunol.* **2**, 1159–1166.

Rousset, F., de Waal Malefijt, R., Slierendregt, B., Aubry, J.P., Bonnefoy, J.Y., Defrance, T., Banchereau, J. and de Vries, J.E. (1988). *J. Immunol.* **140**, 2625–2632.

Rousset, F., Billaud, M., Blanchard, D., Figdor, C., Lenoir, G.M., Spits, H. and de Vries, J.E. (1989). *J. Immunol.* **143**, 1490–1498.

Rousset, F., Garcia, E. and Banchereau, J. (1991a). *J. Exp. Med.* **173**, 705–710.

Rousset, F., Robert, J., Andary, M., Bonnin, J.P., Souillet, G., Chrétien, I., Brière, F., Pène, J. and de Vries, J.E. (1991b). *J. Allergy Clin. Immunol.* **87**, 58–69.

Rousset, F., Garcia, E., Defrance, T., Péronne, C., Vezzio, N., Hsu, D.H., Kastelein, R., Moore, K.W. and Banchereau, J. (1992). *Proc. Natl Acad. Sci. USA.* **89**, 1890–1893.

Sanders, V.M., Fernandez-Botran, R., Uhr, J.W. and Vitetta, E.S. (1987). *J. Immunol.* **139**, 2349–2354.

Sarfati, M., Luo, H. and Delespesse, G. (1989). *J. Exp. Med.* **170**, 1775–1780.

Sato, T.A., Widmer, M.B., Finkelman, F.D., Madani, H., Jacobs, C.A., Grabstein, K.H. and Maliszewski, C.R. (1993). *J. Immunol.* **150**, 2717–2723.

Schleimer, R.P., Sterbinsky, S.A., Kaiser, J., Bickel, C.A., Klunk, D.A., Tomioka, K., Newman, W., Luscinskas, F.W., Gimbrone, M.A., McIntyre, B.W. and Bochner, B.S. (1992). *J. Immunol.* **148**, 1086–1092.

Schuitemaker, H., Kootstra, N.A., Koppelman, M.H.G.M., Bruisten, S.M., Huisman, H.G., Tersmette, M. and Miedema, F. (1992). *J. Clin. Invest.* **89**, 1154–1160.

Scott, P. (1991). *J. Immunol.* **147**, 3149–3155.

Seder, R.A., Boulay, J.-L., Finkelman, F., Barbier, S., Ben-Sasson, S.Z., Le Gros, G. and Paul, W.E. (1992). *J. Immunol.* **148**, 1652–1656.

Shapira, S.K., Vercelli, D., Jabara, H.H., Fu, S.M. and Geha, R.S. (1992). *J. Exp. Med.* **175**, 289–292.

Shields, J.G., Armitage, R.J., Jamieson, B.N., Beverley, P.C.L. and Callard, R.E. (1989). *Immunol.* **66**, 224–227.

Sideras, P., Funa, K., Zalcberg-Quintana, I., Xanthopoulos, K.G., Kisielow, P. and Palacios, R. (1988). *Proc. Natl Acad. Sci. USA.* **85**, 218–221.

Smeland, E.B., Blomhoff, H.K., Funderud, S., Shalaby, M.R. and Espevik, T. (1989). *J. Exp. Med.* **170**, 1463–1468.

Snapper, C.M., Hornbeck, P.V., Atasoy, U., Pereira, G.M.B. and Paul, W.E. (1988). *Proc. Natl Acad. Sci. USA* **85**, 6107–6111.

Snoeck, H.-W., Lardon, F., Lenjou, M., Nys, G., Van Bockstaele, D.R. and Peetermans, M.E. (1993). *Eur. J. Immunol.* **23**, 1072–1077.

Sonoda, Y., Kuzuyama, Y., Tanaka, S., Yokota, S., Maekawa, T., Clark, S.C. and Abe, T. (1993). *Blood* **81**, 624–630.

Sorg, R.V., Enczmann, J., Sorg, U.R., Schneider, E.M. and Wernet, P. (1993). *Exp. Hematol.* **21**, 560–563.

Souillet, G., Rousset, F. and de Vries, J.E. (1989). *Lancet* **i**, 1384–1384.

Spits, H., Yssel, H., Takebe, Y., Arai, N., Yokota, T., Lee, F., Arai, K., Banchereau, J. and de Vries, J.E. (1987). *J. Immunol.* **135**, 1142–1147.

Spits, H., Yssel, H., Paliard, X., Kastelein, R., Figdor, D. and de Vries, J.E. (1988). *J. Immunol.* **141**, 29–36.

Standiford, T.J., Strieter, R.M., Kasahara, K. and Kunkel, S.L. (1990). *Biochem. Biophys. Res. Commun.* **171**, 531–536.

Stein, P., Dubois, P., Greenblatt, D. and Howard, M. (1986). *J. Immunol.* **136**, 2080–2089.

Street, N.E., Schumacher, J.H., Fong, T.A.T., Bass, H., Fiorentino, D.F., Leverah, J.A. and Mosmann, T.R. (1990). *J. Immunol.* **144**, 1629–1639.

Swain, S.L., McKenzie, D.T., Dutton, R.W., Tonkonogy, S.L. and English, M. (1988). *Immunol. Rev.* **102**, 77–105.

Swendeman, S. and Thorley-Lawson, D.A. (1987). *EMBO J.* **6**, 1637–1642.

Taylor, C.W., Grogan, T.M. and Salmon, S.E. (1990). *Blood* **75**, 1114–1118.

Te Velde, A.A., Klomp, J.P.G., Yard, B.A., de Vries, J.E. and Figdor, C.G. (1988). *J. Immunol.* **140**, 1548–1554.

Te Velde, A.A., Huybens, R.J.F., de Vries, J.E. and Figdor, C.G. (1990). *J. Immunol.* **144**, 3046–3051.

Tepper, R.I., Pattengale, P.K. and Leder, P. (1989). *Cell.* **57**, 503–512.

Tepper, R.I., Levinson, D.A., Stanger, B.Z., Campos-Torres, J., Abbas, A.K. and Leder, P. (1990). *Cell.* **62**, 457–467.

Tepper, R.I., Coffman, R.L. and Leder, P. (1992). *Science,* **257**, 548–551.

Thornhill, M.H., Kyan-Aung, U. and Haskard, D.O. (1990). *J. Immunol.* **144**, 3060–3065.

Thornhill, M.H., Wellicome, S.M., Mahiouz, D.L., Lanchbury, J.S.S., Kyan-Aung, U. and Haskard, D.O. (1991). *J. Immunol.* **146**, 592–598.

Thyphronitis, G., Tsokos, G.C., June, C.H., Levine, A.D. and Finkelman, F.D. (1989). *Proc. Natl Acad. Sci. USA.* **86**, 5580–5584.

Toi, M., Bicknell, R. and Harris, A.L. (1992). *Cancer Res.* **52**, 275–279.

Tsuji, K., Nakahata, T., Takagi, M., Kobayashi, T., Ishiguro, A., Kikuchi, T., Naganuma, K., Koike, K., Miyajima, A., Arai, K. and Akabane, T. (1990). *Blood* **75**, 421–427.

Tushinski, R.J., Larsen, A., Park, L.S. and Spoor, E. (1991). *Exp. Hematol.* **19**, 238–244.

Ueno, Y., Boone, T. and Uittenbogaart, C.H. (1989). *Cell. Immunol.* **118**, 382–393.

Ueno, K., Katayama, T., Muyamoto, T. and Koshihara, Y. (1992). *Biochem. Bioph. Res. Commun.* **189**, 1521–1526.

Valent, P., Bevec, D., Maurer, D., Besemer, J., Di Padova, F., Butterfield, J.H., Speiser, W., Majdic, O., Lechner, K. and Bettelheim, P. (1991). *Immunol.* **88**, 3339–3342.

Vallé, A., Garrone, P., Aubry, J.P. and Banchereau, J. (1989a). In *Leukocyte Typing IV. White Cell Differentiation Antigens.* (ed. W. Knapp), Oxford University Press, Oxford, p. 510.

Vallé, A., Zuber, C.E., Defrance, T., Djossou, O., De Rie, M. and Banchereau, J. (1989b). *Eur. J. Immunol.* **19**, 1463–1467.

Vallé, A., Aubry, J.-P., Durand, I. and Banchereau, J. (1991). *Int. Immunol.* **3**, 229–235.

van Kooten, C., Rensink, I., Aarden, L. and van Oers, R. (1992). *Blood* **80**, 1299–1306.

Vannier, E., Miller, L.C. and Dinarello, C.A. (1992). *Proc. Natl Acad. Sci. USA.* **89**, 4076–4080.

Vasquez, A., Auffredou, M.T., Chaouchi, N., Taib, J., Sharma, S., Galanaud, P. and Leca, G. (1991). *Eur. J. Immunol.* **21**, 2311–2316.

Vercelli, D., Jabara, H.H., Lee, W., Woodland, N., Geha, R.S. and Leung, D.Y.M. (1988). *J. Exp. Med.* **167**, 1406–1416.

Vercelli, D., Jabara, H.H., Arai, K. and Geha, R.S. (1989). *J. Exp. Med.* **169**, 1295–1307.

Vercelli, D., Jabara, H.H., Lauener, R.P. and Geha, R.S. (1990). *J. Immunol.* **144**, 570–573.

Vieira, P., de Waal-Malefyt, R., Dang, M.N., Johnson, K.E., Kastelein, R., Fiorentino, D.F., de Vries, J.E., Roncarolo, M.G., Mossmann, T.R. and Moore, K.W. (1991). *Proc. Natl Acad. Sci. USA.* **88**, 1172–1176.

Walter, M.R., Cook, W.J., Zhao, B.G., Cameron, R.P., Ealick, S.E., Walter, R.L., Reichert, P., Nagabhushan, T.L., Trotta, P.P. and Bugg, C.E. (1992). *J. Biol. Chem.* **267**, 20371–20376.

Wang, L.-M., Keegan, A.D., Paul, W.E., Heidaran, M.A., Gutkind, J.S. and Pierce, J.H. (1992). *EMBO J.* **11**, 4899–4908.

Wang, L.-M., Keegan, A.D., Li, W., Lienhard, G.E., Pacini, S., Gutkind, J.S., Myers, M.G., Sun, X.-J., White, M.F., Aaronson, S.A., Paul, W.E. and Pierce, J.H. (1993). *Proc. Natl. Acad. Sci. USA* **90**, 4032–4036.

Watanabe, K., Tanaka, Y., Morimoto, I., Yahata, K., Zeki, K., Fujihara, T., Yamashita, U. and Eto, S. (1990). *Biochem. Biophys. Res. Commun.* **172**, 1035–1041.

Widmer, M.B. and Grabstein, K.H. (1987). *Nature* **326**, 795–798.

Widmer, M.B., Acres, R.B., Sassenfeld, H.M. and Grabstein, K.H. (1987). *J. Exp. Med.* **166**, 1447–1455.

Wierenga, E.A., Snoek, M., de Groot, C., Chrétien, I., Bos, J.D., Hansen, H.M. and Kapsenberg, M.L. (1990). *J. Immunol.* **144**, 4651–4656.

Windsor, W.T., Syto, R., Durkin, J., Das, P., Reichert, P., Pramanik, B., Tindall, S., Le. H.V., Labdon, J., Nagabhushan, T.L. and Trotta, P.P. (1990). *Biophys. J.* **57**, 423A.

Wong, H.L., Costa, G.L., Lotze, M.T. and Wahl, S.M. (1993). *J. Exp. Med.* **177**, 775–781.

Wu, Q., Li, L., Cooper, M.D., Pierres, M. and Gorvel, J.P. (1991). *Proc. Natl Acad. Sci. USA.* **88**, 676–680.

Yokota, A., Kikutani, H., Tanaka, T., Sato, R., Barsumian, E.L., Suemura, M. and Kishimoto, T. (1988). *Cell.* **55**, 611–618.

Yokota, T., Otsuka, T., Mosmann, T., Banchereau, J., Defrance, T., Blanchard, D., de Vries, J.E., Lee, F. and Arai, K. (1986). *Proc. Natl Acad. Sci. USA.* **83**, 5894–5898.

Yoshida, K., Matsuoka, M., Usuda, S., Mori, A. and Ishizaka, K. (1990). *Proc. Natl Acad. Sci. USA.* **87**, 7829–7833.

Zhang, X., Werner-Favre, C., Tang, H., Brouwers, N., Bonnefoy, J.-Y. and Zubler, R.H. (1991). *J. Immunol.* **147**, 3001–3004.

Zlotnik, A., Ramsom, J., Franck, G., Fischer, M. and Howard, M. (1987). *Proc. Natl Acad. Sci. USA.* **84**, 3856–3860.

Zurawski, S.M., Vega, Jr., F., Huyghe, B. and Zurawski, G. (1993). *EMBO J.* **12**, 2663–2670.

Chapter 7

Interleukin-5

Colin J. Sanderson

Institute for Child Health Research, Perth, Western Australia

INTRODUCTION

Interleukin-5 (IL-5) is produced by T lymphocytes as a glycoprotein with an M_r of 40 000–45 000 and is unusual among the T-cell-produced cytokines in being a disulphide-linked homodimer. It is the most highly conserved member of a group of evolutionarily related cytokines, including also IL-3, IL-4 and granulocyte/macrophage colony stimulating factor (GM-CSF), which are closely linked on human chromosome 5.

Historically, two lines of research converged when it was demonstrated that two very different biological activities were properties of this molecule. In the early 1970s a number of different factors were emerging which showed activity on mouse B cells *in vitro*. These preparations were mixtures of cytokines, particularly IL-4 and IL-5, and the assays available did not distinguish between the two molecules. It was not until the early 1980s that a group of high-molecular-weight activities emerged which were clearly based on IL-5, although in published reviews in 1984 the identity of the activities was not appreciated (Howard *et al.*, 1984; Vitetta *et al.*, 1984). Three main groups were working with this molecule: Takatsu in Japan who considered the activity to be various forms of T-cell replacing factor (TRF) (Takatsu *et al.*, 1988), Swain and Dutton in California, who used the term B-cell growth factor II (BCGFII) (Swain *et al.*, 1988), and Vitetta in Texas, who called it B-cell differentiation factor μ (BCDFμ) (Vitetta *et al.*, 1984). In 1985 Takatsu's group purified TRF and showed that it was identical to BCGF-II (Harada *et al.*, 1985).

In the early 1970s, work on the colony stimulating factors (CSFs) by Metcalf's group in Australia had also demonstrated the production of eosinophilic colonies from mouse bone marrow in the presence of crude spleen-cell-conditioned medium (Metcalf *et al.*, 1974). It is now clear that this medium contained IL-5 because it was shown to produce a selective stimulation of human eosinophil colonies (Metcalf *et al.*, 1983) and IL-5 is the only eosinophil haematopoietic growth factor that crossreacts between man and mouse. This line of work culminated in the identification of murine eosinophil differentiation factor in the laboratory of the author and his colleagues in the mid-1980s. This was done using a liquid assay system that, in the mouse, is a much more sensitive assay than the colony assay (Sanderson *et al.*, 1985; Warren and Sanderson, 1985). However, as is

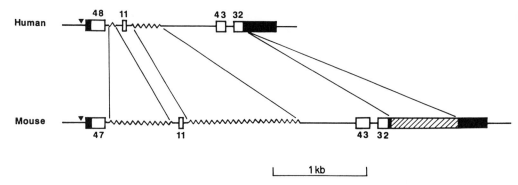

Fig. 1.   Maps of the human and mouse IL-5 genomic genes. Exons are shown as boxes and the open boxes show the coding regions. The numbers indicate the number of amino acids encoded by each exon. The shaded area indicates the insert in the 3'-untranslated region of the mouse gene (▼, TATA box; -, parts of introns showing significant homology; ∧∧∧, parts of introns not showing homology) (from Sanderson *et al.*, 1988, with permission).

discussed in detail in this review, IL-5 is a colony stimulating factor for which the name Eo-CSF would have been appropriate.

These two lines of research came together in 1986, when our group purified eosinophil differentiation factor (EDF) and showed that it was identical to BCGFII (Sanderson *et al.*, 1986). It is interesting to note that the observations on the identity of TRF, BCGFII and EDF were made before the cloning of IL-5, which confirmed the biochemical data.

There are two intriguing aspects of these dual biological activities of IL-5. First, although there is a well-known association between eosinophilia and IgE levels, IL-5 does not appear to be involved in the IgE response, where IL-4 is the major controlling cytokine. Second, although the activity on murine B cells *in vitro* is well characterized (see below), hIL-5 is not active in assays on human B cells analogous to those used in the mouse system.

The role of IL-5 in eosinophilia, coupled with a better understanding of the part played by eosinophils in the development of tissue damage in chronic allergy, suggests that IL-5 will be a major target for a new generation of anti-allergy drugs.

GENE STRUCTURE AND EXPRESSION

Sequence information is available for both the human and mouse genomic genes (Campbell *et al.*, 1987, 1988). There appears to be only a single copy of the gene per haploid genome. The coding sequence of the IL-5 gene forms four exons (Fig. 1). The introns show areas of similarity between the mouse and human sequences, although the mouse has a considerable amount of sequence (including repeat sequences) which are not present in the human gene. Interestingly, the mouse gene includes a 738-bp segment in the 3'-untranslated region which is not present in the human gene. Each of the exons contains the codons for an exact number of amino acids, and in each case begins with GT and ends in AG. These features of gene structure are also shared by IL-3, IL-4 and GM-CSF. All four cytokine genes are located in tandem on chromosome 5 in man

(Sutherland *et al.*, 1988; Van Leeuwen *et al.*, 1989; Chandrasekharappa *et al.*, 1990) and chromosome 11 in the mouse (Lee *et al.*, 1989). Although there is no overall sequence homology, at either the nucleotide or amino acid level, between any of these four cytokines, the localization and structural similarities suggest a common evolutionary origin (Sanderson *et al.*, 1988). In addition, they are all produced by T cells and show an overlap in some of their biological activities; thus, they may be regarded as members of a gene family.

Transcription in T cells is induced by antigen, mitogens and phorbol esters and occurs for about 24 h, before the gene becomes silent again (Tominaga *et al.*, 1988). Studies with T-cell clones *in vitro* indicate that IL-4 and IL-5 are often co-expressed in clones designated T_{H2} (Coffman *et al.*, 1988). However, anti-CD3 induces the expression of IL-4, IL-5 and GM-CSF mRNA in mouse T cells, whereas treatment with IL-2 induced IL-5 mRNA expression but did not induce detectable IL-4 or GM-CSF (Bohjanen *et al.*, 1990). The fact that eosinophilia can occur without increases in other leukocytes suggests an independent control for IL-5 expression, while the association between high levels of IgE antibody and eosinophilia, suggests coordinate expression of IL-4 and IL-5 in these cases.

Corticosteroids inhibit IL-5 production both *in vivo* (Corrigan *et al.*, 1993) and *in vitro* (Rolfe *et al.*, 1992; Wang *et al.*, 1993). This may be an important mechanism of corticosteroid activity in asthma. Both progesterone and testosterone induce IL-5 transcription, which can be inhibited by dexamethasone but not by cylosporine (Wang *et al.*, 1993). These observations suggest complex mechanisms of IL-5 gene expression which are not yet understood.

PROTEIN STRUCTURE

IL-5 is unusual among the T-cell-produced cytokines in being a disulphide-linked homodimeric glycoprotein that is highly homologous between species (Fig. 2), and with cross reactivity of the protein across a variety of mammalian species. Studies with mouse IL-5 indicate that the monomer has no biological activity and has no inhibitory activity, suggesting that it does not form high affinity interactions with the IL-5 receptor (McKenzie *et al.*, 1991). The dimer exists in an antiparallel (head to tail) configuration (Minamitake *et al.*, 1990; McKenzie *et al.*, 1991; Proudfoot *et al.*, 1991).

Mature human IL-5 monomer comprises 115 amino acids (M_r of 12 000 and 24 000 for the dimer). The secreted material has a M_r of 40 000 to 45 000; nearly half the native material consists of carbohydrate. Human IL-5 has one *N*-linked carbohydrate chain at position Asn-28, and one *O*-linked carbohydrate at position Thr-3 (Minamitake *et al.*, 1990). Mouse IL-5 has an additional *N*-linked carbohydrate at Asn-55 (Kodama *et al.*, 1992); this site does not exist in hIL-5. The potential *N*-linked site at Asn-71 is apparently not glycosylated in either species. Deglycosylated IL-5 has been reported to have full (Tominaga *et al.*, 1990) activity or increased activity (Kodama *et al.*, 1993) *in vitro*.

The crystal structure of human IL-5 (Milburn *et. al.*, 1993) shows it to be similar to the structures of other cytokines and most closely resembles IL-4 and GM-CSF, which consist of a bundle of four α helices (A,B,C,D from the *N*-terminus) with two overconnecting loops. The dimer structure of IL-5 forms an elongated ellipsoidal disk, made up of two domains about a twofold axis (Fig. 3). Remarkably each domain is

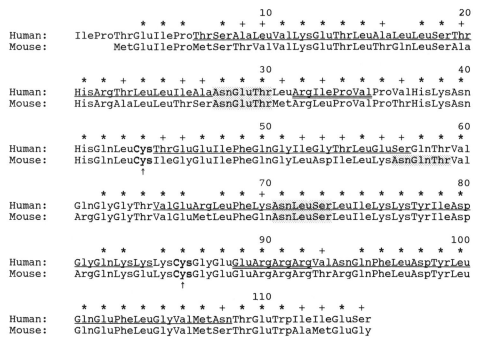

Fig. 2. Alignment of human and mouse mature IL-5 amino acid sequences. The numbering is based on the human sequence. *Indicates identity, + indicates a conservative change; ↑, cysteines. Predicted *N*-linked glycosylation sites are shown with a shaded background. Residues forming α helices are underlined. Residues involved in anti-parallel β sheets are double underlined.

made up of three helices from one monomer (A,B,C) and one helix (D′) from the other. The two monomers are held together by two sulphide bridges connecting Cys-44 of one molecule with Cys-86 of the other. In addition residues 32 to 35 form an anti-parallel β sheet with residues 89 to 92 of the other monomer. A large proportion of the monomer surface is at the interface of the two monomers. It is possible that the lack of biological activity in the monomer results from instability owing to exposure of hydrophilic residues normally concealed in the dimer.

IL-5 RECEPTORS

The receptors for each of the three cytokines, IL-3, IL-5 and GM-CSF consist of an α chain which is different for each ligand, and a β chain which is common to each receptor complex (Lopez *et al.*, 1992a). The α chain forms the low-affinity interaction with its ligand, and the β chain serves to increase the affinity to give the high-affinity interaction (Tavernier *et al.*, 1991; Tominaga *et al.*, 1991). The β chain appears not to form a measurable interaction with any of the ligands in the absence of the α chain. It seems likely that the cross-inhibition exhibited within the group results from numbers of β chains (Lopez *et al.*, 1989, 1990; Nicola and Metcalf, 1991).

Murine eosinophils have been calculated to express approximately 50 high-affinity receptors for IL-5, and approximately 5000 low-affinity receptors (Barry *et al.*, 1991). A

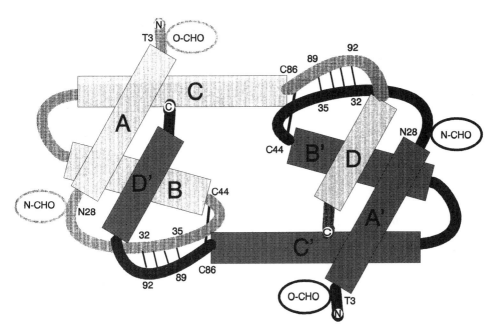

Fig. 3. Diagram based on the crystal structure (Milburn *et al.*, 1993) of hIL-5 showing the main structural features. One monomer is shown in light grey and the other in dark grey. Helices are indicated A–D, and A′–D′ respectively starting at the *N*-terminus (N). The disulphide bridges connecting cysteines at positions 44 and 86 are shown as black lines. The interactions between anti-parallel β sheets are shown by fine black lines (residues 32–35 and 89–92). The attachment positions of *O*-linked carbohydrate (*O*-CHO) attached to residue 3 and *N*-linked carbohydrate (*N*-CHO) attached to residue 28 are indicated.

number of murine cell lines have been established which require the presence of IL-5 for growth, these are all of B-cell origin, and have relatively high numbers of IL-5 receptors. They represent an important tool in the study of the IL-5 receptor in the mouse, but no analogues of these B-cell lines have been described from human tissues. Initial work on the human receptor utilized a clone of the human promyelocytic leukaemia cell line HL-60 (Plaetinck *et al.*, 1990). These cells express only a single population of high-affinity IL-5-binding sites. Similarly, only a single high-affinity receptor population has been identified on human eosinophils (Ingley and Young, 1991; Lopez *et al.*, 1991; Migita *et al.*, 1991).

Both the α and the β subunits share a number of features with other receptors which has led to their classification as members of the cytokine/haemopoietin superfamily. They have a modular structure build-up of fibronectin-III-like domains, a number of conserved amino acids, and exist in a number of isoforms generated by alternative splicing. In each case the membrane bound isoform results from splicing which retains a transmembrane domain (Tavernier *et al.*, 1991). The other isoforms lack the transmembrane domain, resulting in soluble forms of the receptor. The possibility that the soluble forms of these receptors act as antagonists of the membrane-bound form to provide a negative control on haemopoiesis has been widely discussed. The soluble form of the hIL-5R α chain is antagonistic *in vitro* (Tavernier *et al.*, 1991) but there is not yet any evidence that it is active *in vivo*.

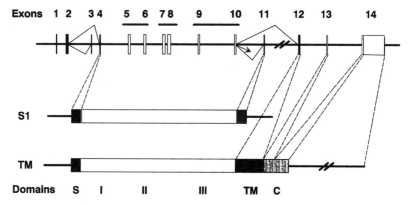

Fig. 4. Diagram showing the exon structure (not to scale) of hIL-5R α chain (top) and two of the alternatively spliced transcripts. S1 indicates the major transcript in human eosinophilic cells; a soluble form formed by splicing in exon 11 causing transcription to end before the exon encoding the transmembrane domain. TM indicates the transcript of the active form of the receptor formed by splicing out exon 11. Exon numbers are indicated at the top. Alternative splicing events are indicated by fine lines (the arrow indicates no splicing at this donor site, forming the soluble S2 transcript — see text). The structural domains of the protein are indicated at the bottom: S, signal peptide; I, II, and III, the three fibronectin type III-like domains derived from exons 5 and 6, 7 and 8, and 9 and 10, respectively; TM, transmembrane domain; C, intracytoplasmic tail. Adapted from Tuypens *et al.* (1992) with permission.

The cloning of cDNAs for both the human and mouse IL-5Rα chain revealed different isoforms. Remarkably, in man, the major transcript is a soluble isoform. The structure of the IL-5Rα gene provides an explanation for the isotypes observed (Tavernier *et al.*, 1992; Tuypens *et al.*, 1992). Figure 4 shows a map of the gene, and illustrates the transmembrane (TM) and soluble (S1) transcripts. The gene contains 14 exons. Three introns are located in the 5' untranslated region, alternative splicing leads to skipping of exon 3 in some transcripts. Exon 4 corresponds to the signal peptide (S), and each of the three FN-III-like domains is encoded by exons 3 and 4, 5 and 6, 7 and 8, respectively. Exon 11 encodes four amino acids followed by a stop codon and a polyadenylation site. Exon 12 encodes a transmembrane domain, and the two remaining exons encode an intracytoplasmic tail. Three alternative events can occur at the 3' end of exon 10.

(1) No splicing. Translation continues adding two amino acids before a stop codon. This gives rise to one soluble isoform (S2).
(2) Normal splicing leads to the inclusion of exon 11, and gives rise to a transcript truncated by the polyA site at the 3' end of the exon. This soluble isoform (S1) is the most abundant transcript in HL60 cells and cultured eosinophils.
(3) Alternative splicing skips exon 11, and gives rise to the functional membrane-bound form of the receptor (TM).

Based on cDNA sequences, the situation in the mouse is different. The soluble isoforms are formed by alternative splicing which skips the exon encoding the transmembrane domain (exon 12 in man), or both this exon and the next (exons 12 and 13 in man). As the structure of the murine gene has not yet been reported it is not known whether there is an exon analogous to the human exon 11.

Interaction Between IL-5 and the Receptor

There is an area of sequence similarity, determined using Dayhoff mutation indices, at the *C*-terminal region of a number of different cytokines including IL-5 (Sanderson *et al.*, 1988). This region lies in helix D of IL-5, IL-4 and GM-CSF. Making use of the 100-fold lower specific activity of hIL-5 when tested in a mouse assay system, a series of human–mouse hybrid IL-5 molecules were constructed and tested for biological activity and receptor displacement. The *C*-terminal one-third of the molecule was found to determine the species specificity (McKenzie *et al.*, 1991). This region contains eight residues which differ between human and mouse, two at the end of the C helix, three in the D helix and the remaining three in the *C*-terminal tail. Determination of the residue(s) involved in species specificity will locate the region of interaction with the α chain of the receptor more accurately. Despite the twofold symmetry of the IL-5 dimer, which suggests two potential binding sites for the receptor, the α chain of the receptor appears to bind to IL-5 in a 1:1 ratio (Devos *et al.*, 1993).

Experiments with GM-CSF suggest that the β chain may bind in the region of residue 21 (Lopez *et al.*, 1992b) and a series of mouse–human GM-CSF hybrids identified residue 20 as important in the interaction with the β chain. Furthermore, a hybrid in which the *N*-terminal region of GM-CSF was substituted by the analogous region from IL-5, showed strong biological activity. This very important approach demonstrated that IL-5 uses the same β-receptor subunit as GM-CSF, and implies an interaction between the β chain and the *N*-terminal region of the cytokine molecule (Scanafelt *et al.*, 1991). A comparison of the structure of IL-5 and GM-CSF suggests that the interaction site between IL-5 and the β chain in the complex is Glu-13 (Lopez *et al.*, 1992b).

EOSINOPHILIA

T-Cell Dependence

Eosinophilia is T-cell-dependent and therefore it is not surprising that the controlling factor is a T-cell-derived cytokine (Sanderson *et al.*, 1985). It is characteristic of a limited number of disease states, most notably parasitic infections and allergy. Clearly, as eosinophilia is not characteristic of all immune responses, it is obvious that the factors controlling eosinophilia must not be produced by all T cells. Similarly, as it is now clear that IL-5 is the main controlling cytokine for eosinophilia (see below), then if IL-5 has other biological activities, it is likely that these will coincide with the production of eosinophils.

Biological Specificity of Eosinophilia

One of the features of eosinophilia, which has attracted the curiosity of haematologists for several decades, is the apparent independence of eosinophil numbers on the numbers of other leukocytes. Thus, eosinophils are present in low numbers in normal individuals but can increase dramatically and independently of the number of neutrophils. Such changes are common during the summer months in individuals with allergic rhinitis (hay fever), or in certain parasitic infections. Clearly, such conditions will result in more broadly based leukocytosis when complicated by other infections. Although this specificity has been known for many years, it is, somewhat surprisingly, not easy to find clear examples in the early literature. More recently, in experimental infection of volunteers with hookworms (*Necator americanus*), it was noted that an increase in eosinophils was the only significant change (Maxwell *et al.*, 1987), and our own work with *Mesocestoides corti* in the mouse demonstrated massive increases in eosinophils, independent of changes in neutrophils (Strath and Sanderson, 1986). This biological specificity suggests a mechanism of control which is independent of the control of other leukocytes. This, coupled with the normally low numbers of eosinophils, provides a useful model for the study of the control of haemopoiesis by the immune system.

Eosinophil Production *In Vitro*

In the mouse system, IL-5 induces the production of eosinophils in liquid bone-marrow cultures. This is lineage-specific, as only eosinophil numbers are increased in these cultures (Sanderson *et al.*, 1985, 1988; Sanderson, 1990. In contrast, both IL-3 and GM-CSF induce eosinophils as well as other cell types, most notably neutrophils and macrophages in bone-marrow cultures (Campbell *et al.*, 1988). The production of eosinophils is considerably higher when the bone marrow is taken from mice infected with *M. corti* than it is from normal marrows. This suggests that marrow from infected mice contains more eosinophil precursors than marrow from normal mice (Sanderson *et al.*, 1985). However, when tested in a colony assay with semisolid agar, both normal and parasitized mice have similar, relatively small numbers of eosinophil colonies (Warren and Sanderson, 1985). We have interpreted this as indicating a low sensitivity of the mouse colony assay for eosinophil precursor cells (eosinophil colony forming cells). The technical basis for this is not clear, as similar conditions give rise to large numbers of eosinophil colonies from human bone-marrow cells (Lopez *et al.*, 1986; Clutterbuck and Sanderson, 1988; Strath *et al.*, 1990).

Liquid bone-marrow cultures produce neutrophils for extended periods of time without exogenous factors (Dexter *et al.*, 1977). It appears that the microenvironment of these cultures maintains the production of neutrophil precursors. In contrast, no eosinophils are seen in the absence of exogenous factors. IL-5 induces a production of eosinophils that reaches a peak at about 3 weeks, and continues until about 6–8 weeks. This transient production of eosinophils suggests that IL-5 is unable to stimulate the production of eosinophil precursors at least in these bone-marrow cultures. This had led to the concept of IL-5 as a late-acting factor in eosinophil haemopoiesis (Sanderson *et al.*, 1985, 1988; Sanderson, 1993).

To study the production of the eosinophil progenitor we have used human bone-marrow cultures. This has the advantage that these cells can be quantified in a colony assay in semisolid medium. Both IL-3 and GM-CSF stimulate a greater number of eosinophil colonies than IL-5 (Clutterbuck *et al.*, 1989). As all the cells in these colonies were morphologically mature and there was no obvious difference in colony size, this surprising result suggests that either IL-3 or GM-CSF would be capable of inducing eosinophilia without the action of IL-5. In addition, it suggests that there must be a large pool of eosinophil precursors that are unresponsive to IL-5. Similar experiments were carried out with human bone marrow in liquid cultures, where the total number of eosinophils produced, rather than the number of colonies, could be assessed. In these experiments there was a marked difference from the results in the colony assay, in that IL-5 induced a larger number of eosinophils than IL-3 or GM-CSF. There are two possible explanations. First, there is the trivial possibility that IL-5 is simply a poor stimulant of eosinophils in semisolid cultures. Second, it is possible that IL-5 is capable of inducing a larger number of eosinophils from a smaller pool of precursors (Clutterbuck *et al.*, 1989). There is increasing evidence that the trivial explanation is the more plausible (see below).

To assess the role of IL-3 in the development of eosinophil precursors, a two-step culture system was utilized. Human bone-marrow cells were cultured in liquid medium in the first step, then these cells were set up in semisolid cultures to assay the number of eosinophil precursors. It was quite clear from these experiments that IL-5 did not influence the number of eosinophil colonies when included in the primary culture (Clutterbuck and Sanderson, 1990), thus confirming our earlier suggestion that IL-5 is a late-acting factor. However, both GM-CSF and IL-3 gave a significant increase in eosinophil colonies compared with control or IL-5-containing cultures. This represented a four- to sixfold increase in colonies compared with controls.

Except for this relatively modest increase in precursors, IL-3 appeared to increase the proportion of precursors that were responsive to IL-5. In the primary bone marrow less than 30% of the total (that is, IL-3 responsive) precursors responded to IL-5, whereas after incubation with IL-3 about 90% of the precursors were IL-5 responsive, suggesting that IL-3 induces IL-5 responsiveness (Clutterbuck and Sanderson, 1990).

If IL-3 is capable of amplifying eosinophil precursors *in vitro* it would be expected that IL-3 would induce a more sustained production of eosinophils in liquid cultures than IL-5. This is not the case. In experiments with human marrow both IL-3 and GM-CSF produce a transient peak of eosinophils similar to that seen with IL-5. To date, no combination of cytokines has been able to induce the long-term production of eosinophils in either mouse or human cultures.

Yamaguchi *et al.* (1988a) confirmed that IL-5 is active only at a late stage of eosinophil differentiation, and showed that either IL-3 or G-CSF but not GM-CSF is able to induce IL-5-responsive eosinophil progenitors. However, in comparison with the total number of other colony types induced by IL-3 or G-CSF the number of eosinophil colonies was small, raising some doubts about the significance of the system. In contrast to these results, Warren and Moore (1988) reported that preincubation of normal bone marrow with IL-3 and GM-CSF, but not G-CSF or M-CSF, induces an increase in IL-5-responsive eosinophil progenitors. Again in contrast to the results of Yamaguchi *et al.* (1988a) these authors reported that IL-3 had no effect in a preincubation experiment with cells from mice treated with 5-fluorouracil. A combination of IL-1 and IL-3 was active in this system.

Thus, the interpretation of these experiments carried out *in vitro* is not straightforward. While it is possible to build a hypothesis around an involvement of IL-3 and other cytokines in eosinophil progenitor production or maintenance *in vitro*, there remain unresolved differences between studies from different laboratories. More important is the conceptual problem: if IL-3 is involved in the induction of the eosinophil precursor, it is difficult to understand how eosinophilia could occur in the absence of a concurrent neutrophilia.

Eosinophil Production *In Vivo*

Few experiments have been carried out in which IL-5 is administered to mice. This is probably because of the limited amounts of material available. In our own (unpublished) experiments in which purified rmIL-5 was administered, an increase in eosinophil numbers was observed, which rapidly returned to normal. However, because of the short time-course of these experiments it was not possible to determine whether there was an increase in eosinophil precursors or whether this represented a maturation of existing precursors.

An alternative approach to understanding the role of IL-5 *in vivo* is to alter the expression of IL-5 in transgenic mice. As IL-5 is normally a T-cell product and the gene is transcribed for only a relatively short period of time after antigen stimulation, transgenic mice in which IL-5 is constitutively expressed by all T cells have been produced (Dent *et al.*, 1990). These mice have detectable levels of IL-5 in the serum. They show a profound and life-long eosinophilia, with large numbers of eosinophils in the blood, spleen and bone marrow. This indicates that the expression of IL-5 is sufficient to induce the full pathway of eosinophil differentiation. If other cytokines are required for the development of eosinophilia, then either they must be expressed constitutively, or their expression is secondary to the expression of the IL-5 gene. This clear demonstration that the expression of the IL-5 gene in transgenic animals is sufficient for the production of eosinophilia, provides an explanation for the biological specificity of eosinophilia. It therefore seems likely that because eosinophilia can occur without a concomitant neutrophilia or monocytosis, a mechanism must exist by which IL-5 is the dominant haemopoietic cytokine produced by the T-cell system in natural eosinophilia.

Another important aspect of these transgenic animals is that despite their massive long-lasting eosinophilia the mice remained normal. This illustrates that an increased number of eosinophils is not, itself, harmful, and that the tissue damage seen in allergic reactions and other diseases must be due to agents that trigger the eosinophils to degranulate.

The observation that IL-5 in transgenic mice is capable of inducing the full pathway of eosinophil production leaves unresolved the question of why IL-5 appears to be unable to induce the production of eosinophil progenitors *in vitro*. One possibility is that the action of IL-5 is uniquely dependent on stromal cells for the production of the progenitor cells. Although there is no direct evidence for this, there are a number of factors that suggest that IL-5 may be at least partly dependent on stromal cells, even in the later stages of eosinophil differentiation. For example, in the mouse system few eosinophil colonies form in semisolid medium, whereas large numbers of eosinophils are produced in the adherent layer of stromal cells in liquid culture (Warren and Sanderson, 1985; Sanderson *et al.*, 1985). Second, in human liquid-bone-marrow cultures more eosinophils are produced in round-bottomed vessels than in flat-bottomed vessels, possibly owing to better cell–cell interactions (Clutterbuck and Sanderson, 1988). Third, although in contrast to the mouse, human eosinophil colonies are produced in semisolid cultures, the number is significantly lower in the presence of IL-5 compared with either IL-3 or GM-CSF. However, in liquid cultures the situation is reversed and IL-5 stimulates the production of more eosinophils than either IL-3 or GM-CSF. This is again consistent with a requirement for stromal cells by IL-5.

Another important approach to the understanding of the biological role of IL-5, comes from the administration of neutralizing antibody. Mice infected with *Trichinella spiralis* develop eosinophilia and have increased levels of IgE; however, when treated with an anti-IL-5 antibody, no eosinophils are observed (Coffman *et al.*, 1989). Indeed, the number of eosinophils is lower than that seen in control animals. These experiments illustrate the unique role of IL-5 in the control of eosinophilia in this parasite infection. They also show that the apparent redundancy seen *in vitro*, where both IL-3 and GM-CSF are also able to induce eosinophil production, does not operate in these infections. Furthermore, IL-5 plays no role in the development of IgE antibody (this activity is controlled by IL-4), or in the development of the granuloma seen surrounding schistosomes in the tissues (Sher *et al.*, 1990).

Mechanism of Control of Eosinophilia

Although it has become clear that IL-5 is the controlling factor in eosinophilia (Sanderson, 1992, 1993), the mechanisms which allow a selective production of IL-5 and thus provide a selective increase in eosinophils remain unknown. Furthermore, in other diseases eosinophils are not observed in significant numbers, suggesting that the expression of IL-5 is not induced in these cases. The cellular pathology typical of particular diseases may reflect the induction of different cytokines by the immune system, in response to different antigenic exposure.

It has been suggested that murine helper T-cells fall into two groups (T_{H1} and T_{H2}), the former producing predominantly IFN-γ and IL-2, and the latter producing IL-4 and IL-5 (Coffman *et al.*, 1988). This hypothesis provides an explanation for the frequently observed association between high levels of IgE antibody and eosinophilia, but does not provide an explanation for many of the complexities seen in the pathology of different diseases. For example, in the mouse IL-4 and IL-5 are thought to be the two major lymphokines in the control of antibody production; thus, this classification leaves open the question of how antibody responses are controlled in the absence of eosinophilia. While the variety of cellular and antibody responses in different infections suggests some form of selection for T cells producing different patterns of cytokines, no clear mechanism has emerged to explain this selective response. The association between eosinophilia and helminth infections or allergic reactions could result from either features in common between the antigens involved in these reactions, or features in common between the tissues in which the immune system encounters these antigens. For example, differences have been observed in the subsets of T cells migrating into mucosal lymphoid organs (Kraal *et al.*, 1983), and T cells expressing the $\gamma\delta$ receptor are associated with epithelia (Bonneville *et al.*, 1990). Clearly, understanding these processes will be an important step forward in our understanding of the immune system, and these preliminary attempts to understand functional subsets in T cells are a basis for future studies.

Activation of Eosinophils

The ability of eosinophils to perform in functional assays can be increased markedly by incubation with a number of different agents, including IL-5. The phenomenon of activation is apparently independent of differentiation. It appears to have a counterpart *in vivo*, as eosinophils from different individuals vary in functional activity. It has been demonstrated that the ability of eosinophils to kill schistosomula increases in proportion to the degree of eosinophilia (David *et al.*, 1980; Hagan *et al.*, 1985). This is consistent with a common control mechanism for both the production and activation of eosinophils in these cases.

The first observations on selective activation of human eosinophils by IL-5 showed that the ability of purified peripheral-blood eosinophils to lyse antibody-coated tumour cells, was increased when IL-5 was included in the assay medium (Lopez *et al.*, 1986). Similarly, the phagocytic ability of these eosinophils towards serum-opsonized yeast particles was increased in the presence of IL-5. There was a 90% increase in surface C3bi complement receptors, as well as an approximately 50% increase in the granulocyte functional antigens GFA1 and GFA2. Later studies demonstrated that IL-5 increases 'polarization', including membrane ruffling and pseudopod formation, which appear to reflect changes in the cytoskeletal system. IL-5 also induces a rapid increase in superoxide anion production by eosinophils (Lopez *et al.*, 1988). In addition, IL-5 increases the survival of peripheral-blood eosinophils (Begley *et al.*, 1986).

A further interesting observation in this context was the demonstration that IL-5 is a potent inducer of Ig-induced eosinophil degranulation, as measured by the release of eosinophil-derived neurotoxin (EDN). IL-5 increased EDN release by 48% for secretory IgA and 136% for IgG. This enhancing effect appeared by 15 min and reached a maximum by 4 h (Fujisawa *et al.*, 1990). The finding that secretory IgA can induce eosinophil degranulation is particularly important because eosinophils are frequently found at mucosal surfaces where IgA is the most abundant immunoglobulin.

Tissue Localization

Another aspect of the pathology of diseases characterized by eosinophilia, is the preferential accumulation of eosinophils in tissues. As the blood contains both eosinophils and neutrophils, there must exist a specific mechanism which allows the eosinophils to pass preferentially from the blood vessels to the tissues. A number of factors, including IL-5, are reported to have a specific chemotactic activity for eosinophils (Yamaguchi *et al.*, 1988b; Wang *et al.*, 1989).

The different tissue distribution of eosinophils in the two transgenic mice systems probably results from the different tissue expression of IL-5. Using the metallothionein promoter, transgene expression was demonstrated in the liver and skeletal muscle, and eosinophils were observed in these tissues (Murata *et al.*, 1992). In contrast the CD2-IL5 mice with IL-5 expression in T cells did not have eosinophils in the liver or skeletal muscle (Dent *et al.*, 1990). This suggests that eosinophils migrate into tissues where IL-5 is expressed. While IL-5 is reported to be chemotactic for eosinophils (Yamaguchi *et al.*, 1988a; Wang *et al.*, 1989), the activity is relatively weak, and it is not clear what role this could play *in vivo*.

An alternative mechanism of extravasation of eosinophils is suggested by experiments in which IL-5 has been shown to upregulate adhesion molecules. Thus, it was demonstrated that IL-5 increased the expression of the integrin CD11b on human eosinophils (Lopez *et al.*, 1986), and this increased expression was accompanied by an increased adhesion to endothelial cells (Walsh *et al.*, 1990). Adhesion was inhibited by antibody to CD11b or CD18, suggesting that the integrins are involved in eosinophil adhesion to endothelial cells (Walsh *et al.*, 1990). More recently it has been shown that eosinophils can use the integrin VLA-4 (CD49d/CD29) in adherance to endothelial cells. In this case the ligand is VCAM-1. In contrast, neutrophils do not express VLA-4 and do not use this adherance mechanism (Walsh *et al.*, 1991).

ACTIVITIES ON OTHER CELL TYPES

Human Tissues

The most pronounced effect of IL-5 on cells other than eosinophils in man, is the effect on basophils. While our studies suggested that IL-5 induced only eosinophils, a detailed study by electron microscopy of cells produced in human cord blood cultures revealed a small number of basophils (Dvorak *et al.*, 1989). Other studies have shown that IL-5 primes basophils for increased histamine production and leukotriene generation (Bischoff *et al.*, 1990; Hirai *et al.*, 1990), and basophils in the blood clearly express the IL-5 receptor (Lopez *et al.*, 1990). Thus, while the effect of IL-5 on the production of basophils may be minor, the priming effect on mature basophils may be of significance in the allergic response.

In view of the well-characterized activity of IL-5 on mouse B cells it was surprising that no activity could be demonstrated in a wide range of human B-cell assay systems (Clutterbuck *et al.*, 1987). This lack of activity of human IL-5 has been confirmed in many different systems (Bende *et al.*, 1992), although a recent report (Bertolini *et al.*, 1993) of activity in one human assay has reopened this question. Until the true biological role of IL-5 in the mouse B-cell system is understood it is unlikely that the human activity will be clarified.

An intriguing observation that both IL-4 and IL-5 regulate nerve growth factor production by astrocytes suggests a possible role in the regulation of the neural system (Awatsuji *et al.*, 1993).

Mouse B Cells

As discussed in the Introduction the characterization of the activities of IL-5 on mouse B cells developed around several different *in vitro* assay systems. In the TRF assay, IL-5 induces specific antibody production by B cells primed with antigen *in vivo* (Takatsu *et al.*, 1988). The BCGFII assay was based on the ability of IL-5 to induce DNA synthesis in normal splenic B cells in the presence of dextran sulphate, and later on the ability of IL-5 to increase DNA synthesis in the BCL1-cell (a mouse B-cell tumour) line (Swain *et al.*, 1988). The BCDFn assay depends on the ability of IL-5 to induce BCL1 cells to secrete IgM (Vitetta *et al.*, 1984).

IL-5 is a late-acting factor in the differentiation of primary B cells, requiring a priming stimulus to make resting B cells responsive. This stimulus can be either polyclonal stimulants such as dextran sulphate, bacterial lipopolysaccharide (LPS), anti-immunoglobulin or specific antigen. Large splenic B cells, presumed to have been activated *in vivo*, when cultured with IL-5 for 7 days show markedly enhanced numbers of IgM- and IgG-producing cells (O'Garra *et al.*, 1986). IL-5, in combination with antigen, is sufficient to induce growth and differentiation of B cells at the single cell level

(Alderson *et al.*, 1987). Combinations of IL-2, IL-4 and IL-5 appear to regulate the amount of IgG1 isotype secreted by B cells (Purkerson *et al.*, 1988; McHeyzer-Williams 1989). Neutralizing antibody to IL-5 was found to inhibit the polyclonal antibody response induced by T-cell clones on B cells, suggesting a critical role for IL-5 in this system (Rasmussen *et al.*, 1988).

A possible role for IL-5 in the development of autoimmunity in mice was suggested by the observation that this cytokine stimulates B cells from NZB mice to produce high levels of IgM anti-DNA antibody (Howard *et al.*, 1984). In another study the B cells from autoimmune NZB/W mice were found to be hyper-responsive to IL-5, whereas two other strains of mice which are prone to autoimmunity did not show this response. As NZB/W mice have elevated numbers of Ly-1-positive B cells, these were tested and found to show a higher response to IL-5 than the negative cells, suggesting that the increased responsiveness to IL-5 in these mice may be due to the increased numbers of Ly-1 B cells (Umland *et al.*, 1989). In support of this, freshly isolated peritoneal Ly-1 B cells express high levels of IL-5 receptor, and IL-5 increases the frequency of cells that produce autoantibodies (Wetzel, 1989). As these effects concern mainly the production of IgM, whereas autoimmune disease appears to be caused mainly by IgG, the significance of these findings for autoimmunity are unclear. However, these experiments point to the possible restriction of IL-5 activity to the Ly-1 subpopulation of B cells.

A potentially interesting observation was the demonstration that IL-5 appears preferentially to enhance IgA production. When added to cultures in the presence of LPS, the highest increase over background occurs with the IgA-producing cells, with significant increases in IgM and IgG1 as well (Bond *et al.*, 1987; Yokota *et al.*, 1987). The interpretation of these experiments is not straightforward, as the LPS also induces a large effect and the activity on IgA and IgG1 was small in comparison with the total levels of IgM produced. In a study of B cells from gut-associated lymphoid tissue (Peyer's patches), IL-5 increased the production of IgA but maximum enhancement of IgA in these cultures required IL-4 (Murray *et al.*, 1987; Lebman and Coffman, 1988). This effect of IL-5 was shown to be due to the induction of a high rate of IgA synthesis in cells positive for surface IgA expression. No IgA secretion was induced in the surface-IgA-negative cells (Murray *et al.*, 1987; Harriman *et al.*, 1988; Kunimoto *et al.*, 1988). This suggests that IL-5 does not induce switching to IgA production, but acts after switching to enhance the production of IgA.

In contrast to these studies, which suggest a key role for IL-5 in the production of IgA, more recent studies have indicated that its effect is minor compared with the activity of other cytokines, and that it may only augment these activities. For example, IL-5 was shown to enhance IgA secretion from B cells isolated from Peyer's patches, but the effect was small compared with the effect of IL-6 (Beagley *et al.*, 1989). A combination of IL-5 and IL-6 had a greater effect than either cytokine alone (Kunimoto *et al.*, 1989). It has been shown that TGF-β has an important activity in the switching to IgA production in LPS-stimulated B cells, and while IL-5 enhances this effect it is less active than IL-2 (Sonoda *et al.*, 1989a). TGF-β is required early while IL-5 appears only to act late in these cultures (Sonoda *et al.*, 1989b).

Important developments towards understanding the mechanism of action of IL-5 in the production of antibody have shown an increase in μ-chain mRNA in both B cells and BCL1 cells (Webb *et al.*, 1989). More recently it has been shown that IL-5 induces CL-3 (a B-cell line) cells into the IgM-secretory state, and this is accompanied by an increase in the secretory form of μ-chain mRNA. The action of IL-5 allows the cells to respond to IL-2 by amplification of J-chain mRNA. Thus, IL-5 and IL-2 are both necessary for IgM secretion (Matsui *et al.*, 1989). A possible mechanism for the effect of IL-2 on B cells is suggested by the observation that IL-5 increases the expression of the IL-2R (Loughnan *et al.*, 1988; Nakanishi *et al.*, 1988).

The significance of these activities remains unclear. While transgenic mice expressing IL-5 on a metallothionein promoter were shown to develop autoimmunity (Tominaga *et al.*, 1991), no effects on B cells or antibody levels were detected in transgenic mice expressing IL-5 under control of the CD2 locus control region (Sanderson *et al.*, 1993). Similarly, treatment of mice with anti-IL-5 antibody completely blocked eosinophil production but had no effect on antibody levels (Finkelman *et al.*, 1990). This question of the biological role of IL-5 on the mouse antibody system will probably only be resolved by IL-5 gene 'knock-out' studies.

SOURCES OF IL-5

All of the original reports on the characterization, purification and cloning of murine IL-5 utilized T-cell lines or lymphomas as the source of material, suggesting that T cells are an important source of the cytokine. The demonstration that IL-5 as well as other cytokine mRNAs are produced by mast-cell lines opens the possibility that these cells may serve to induce or amplify the development of eosinophilia (Burd *et al.*, 1989; Plaut *et al.*, 1989). Similarly, the observation that human Epstein–Barr virus-transformed B cells produce IL-5 raises the possibility that B cells may be an additional source of this cytokine (Paul *et al.*, 1990). Furthermore, eosinophils have been demonstrated to produce IL-5 (Broide *et al.*, 1992). It is not clear whether the non-T-cell derived IL-5 plays a significant biological role in the development of eosinophilia.

Eosinophilia has been observed in a significant proportion of a wide range of human tumours. In many cases the presence of eosinophils has been found to be of positive prognostic significance (reviewed by Sanderson, 1992). Clearly, it is important to understand the mechanism of production of these eosinophils. In a study of Hodgkin's disease with associated eosinophilia all 16 cases examined gave a positive signal for IL-5 mRNA by *in situ* hybridization (Samoszuk and Nansen, 1990). This suggests that IL-5 may be responsible for the production of eosinophils in these cases, and raises the possibility that eosinophilia in other tumours may also be caused by production of IL-5 by the tumour cells.

REFERENCES

Alderson, M.R., Pike, B.L., Harada, N., Tominaga, A., Takatsu, K. and Nossal, G.J. (1987). *J. Immunol.* **139**, 2656–2660.

Awatsuji, H., Furukawa, Y., Hirota, M., Murakami, Y., Nii, S., Furukawa, S. and Hayashi, K. (1993). *J. Neurosci. Res.* **34**, 539–545.

Barry, S.C., McKenzie, A.N., Strath, M. and Sanderson, C.J. (1991). *Cytokine* **3**, 339–344.

Beagley, K.W., Eldridge, J.H., Lee, F., Kiyono, H., Everson, M.P., Koopman, W.J., Hirano, T., Kishimoto, T. and McGhee, J.R. (1989). *J. Exp. Med.* **169**, 2133–2148.

Begley, C.G., Lopez, A.F., Nicola, N.A., Warren, D.J., Vadas, M.A., Sanderson, C.J. and Metcalf, D. (1986). *Blood* **68**, 162–166.

142 C.J. Sanderson

Bende, R.J., Jochems, G.J., Frame, T.H., Klein, M.R., Van Eijk, R.V.W., Van Lier, R.A.W. and Zeijlemaker, W.P. (1992). *Cell. Immunol.* **143**, 310–323.

Bertolini, J.W., Sanderson, C.J. and Benson, E.M., (1993). *Eur. J. Immunol.* **23**, 398–402.

Bischoff, S.C., Brunner, T., De Weck, A.L. and Dahinden, C.A. (1990). *J. Exp. Med.* **172**, 1577–1582.

Bohjanen, P.R., Okajima, M. and Hodes, R.J. (1990). *Proc. Natl Acad. Sci. USA.* **87**, 5283–5287.

Bond, M.W., Shrader, B., Mosmann, T.R. and Coffman, R.L. (1987). *J. Immunol.* **139**, 3691–3696.

Bonneville, M., Itohara, S., Krecko, E.G., Mombaerts, P., Ishida, I., Katsuki, M., Berns, A., Ferr, A.G., Janeway, C.A. and Tonegawa, S. (1990). *J. Exp. Med.* **171**, 1015–1026.

Broide, D.H., Paine, M.M. and Firestein, G.S., (1992). *J. Clin. Invest.* **90**, 1414–1424.

Burd, P.R., Rogers, H.W., Gordon, J.R., Martin, C.A., Jayaraman, S., Wilson, S.D., Dvorak, A.M., Galli, S.J. and Dorf, M.E. (1989). *J. Exp. Med.* **170**, 245–257.

Campbell, H.D., Tucker, W.Q., Hort, Y., Martinson, M.E., Mayo, G., Clutterbuck, E.J., Sanderson, C.J. and Young, I.G. (1987). *Proc. Natl Acad. Sci. USA* **84**, 6629–6633.

Campbell, H.D., Sanderson, C.J., Wang, Y., Hort, Y., Martinson, M.E., Tucker, W.Q., Stellwagen, A., Strath, M. and Young, I.G. (1988). *Eur. J. Biochem.* **174**, 345–352.

Chandrasekharappa, S.C., Rebelsky, M.S., Firak, T.A., Le-Beau, M.M. and Westbrook, C.A. (1990). *Genomics,* **6**, 94–99.

Clutterbuck, E.J. and Sanderson, C.J. (1988). *Blood* **71**, 646–651.

Clutterbuck, E.J. and Sanderson, C.J. (1990). *Blood* **75**, 1774–1779.

Clutterbuck, E., Shields, J.G., Gordon, J., Smith, S.H., Boyd, A., Callard, R.E., Campbell, H.D., Young, I.G. and Sanderson, C.J. (1987). *Eur. J. Immunol.* **17**, 1743–1750.

Clutterbuck, E.J., Hirst, E.M. and Sanderson, C.J. (1989). *Blood* **73**, 1504–1512.

Coffman, R.L., Seymour, B.W.P., Lebman, D.A., Hiraki, D.D., Christiansen, J.A., Shrader, B., Cherwinski, H.M., Savelkoul, H.F.J., Finkelman, F.D., Bond, M.W. and Mosmann, T.R. (1988). *Immunol. Rev.* **102**, 5–28.

Coffman, R.L., Seymour, B.W., Hudak, S., Jackson, J. and Rennick, D. (1989). *Science* **245**, 308–310.

Corrigan, C.J., Haczku, A., Gemou-Engesaeth, V., Doi, S., Kikuchi, Y., Takatsu, K., Durham, S.R. and Kay, A.B. (1993). *Am. Rev. Respir. Dis.* **147**, 540–547.

David, J.R., Vadas, M.A., Butterworth, A.E., de Brito, P.A., Carvalho, E.M., David, R.A., Bina, J.C. and Andrade, Z.A. (1980). *N. Engl. J. Med.* **303**, 1147–1152.

Dent, L.A., Strath, M., Mellor, A.L. and Sanderson, C.J. (1990). *J. Exp. Med.* **172**, 1425–1431.

Devos, R., Guisez, Y., Cornelis, S., Verhee, A., Van der Heyden, J., Manneberg, M., Lahm, H.-W., Fiers, W., Tavernier, J. and Plaetinck, G. (1993). *J. Biol. Chem.* **268**, 6581–6587.

Dexter, T.M., Allen, T.D. and Lajtha, L.G. (1977). *J. Cell. Physiol.* **91**, 335–344.

Dvorak, A.M., Saito, H., Estrella, P., Kissell, S., Arai, N. and Ishizaka, T. (1989). *Lab. Invest.* **61**, 116–132.

Finkelman, F.D., Holmes, J., Katona, I.M., Urban, J.F., Beckmann, M.P., Park, L.S., Schooley, K.A., Coffman, R.L., Mosmann, T.R. and Paul, W.E., (1990). *Annu. Rev. Immunol.* **8**, 303–333.

Fujisawa, T., Abu-Chazaleh, R., Kita, H., Sanderson, C.J. and Gleich, G.J. (1990). *J. Immunol.* **144**, 642–646.

Hagan, P., Moore, P.J., Adjukiewicz, A.B., Greenwood, B.M. and Wilkins, H.A. (1985). *Parasite Immunol.* **7**, 617–624.

Harada, N., Kikuchi, Y., Tominaga, A., Takaki, S. and Takatsu, K. (1985). *J. Immunol.* **134**, 3944–3951.

Harriman, G.R., Kunimoto, D.Y., Elliott, J.F., Paetkau, V. and Strober, W. (1988). *J. Immunol.* **140**, 3033–3039.

Hirai, K., Yamaguchi, M., Misaki, Y., Takaishi, T., Ohta, K., Morita, Y., Ito, K. and Miyamoto, T., (1990). *J. Exp. Med.* **172**, 1525–1528.

Howard, M., Nakanishi, K. and Paul, W.E. (1984). *Immunol. Rev.* **78**, 185–210.

Ingley, E. and Young, I.G., (1991). *Blood* **78**, 339–344.

Kodama, S., Endo, T., Tsujimoto, M. and Kobata, A. (1992). *Glycobiology* **2**, 419–427.

Kodama, S., Tsujimoto, M., Tsuruoka, N., Sugo, T., Endo, T. and Kobata, A., (1993). *Eur. J. Biochem.* **211**, 903–908.

Kraal, G., Weissman, I.L. and Butcher, E.C. (1983). *J. Immunol.* **130**, 1097–1102.

Kunimoto, D.Y., Harriman, G.R. and Strober, W. (1988). *J. Immunol.* **141**, 713–720.

Kunimoto, D.Y., Nordan, R. P. and Strober, W. (1989). *J. Immunol.* **143**, 2230–2235.

Lebman, D.A. and Coffman, R.L. (1988). *J. Immunol.* **141**, 2050–2056.

Lee, J.S., Campbell, H.D., Kozak, C.A. and Young, I.G. (1989). *Somat. Cell Mol. Genet.* **15**, 143–152.

Lopez, A.F., Begley, C.G., Williamson, D.J., Warren, D.J., Vadas, M.A. and Sanderson, C.J. (1986). *J. Exp. Med* **163**, 1085–1099.

Lopez, A.F., Sanderson, C.J., Gamble, J.R., Campbell, H.D., Young, I.G. and Vadas, M.A. (1988). *J. Exp. Med.* **167**, 219–224.

Lopez, A.F., Eglinton, J.M., Gillis, D., Park, L.S., Clark, S. and Vadas, M.A. (1989). *Proc. Natl Acad. Sci. USA.* **86**, 7022–7026.

Lopez, A.F., Eglinton, J.M., Lyons, A.B., Tapley, P.M., To, L.B., Park, L.S., Clark, S.C. and Vadas, M.A. (1990). *J. Cell. Physiol.* **145**, 69–77.

Lopez, A.F., Vadas, M.A., Woodcock, J.M., Milton, S.E., Lewis, A., Elliott, M.J., Gillis, D., Ireland, R., Olwell, E. and Park, L.S. (1991). *J. Biol. Chem.* **267**, 24741–24747.

Lopez, A.F., Elliott, M.J., Woodcock, J. and Vadas, M.A., (1992a). *Immunol. Today* **13**, 495–500.

Lopez, A.F., Shannon, M.F., Hercus, T., Nicola, N.A., Camareri, B., Dottore, M., Layton, M.J., Eglinton, L. and Vadas, M.A. (1992b). *EMBO J.* **11**, 901–916.

Loughnan, M.S., Sanderson, C.J. and Nossal, G.J. (1988). *Proc. Natl Acad. Sci. USA.* **85**, 3115–3119.

McHeyzer-Williams, M.G. (1989). *Eur. J. Immunol.* **19**, 2025–2030.

McKenzie, A.N.J., Barry, S.C., Strath, M. and Sanderson, C.J. (1991a). *EMBO J.* **10**, 1193–1199.

McKenzie, A.N.J., Ely, B. and Sanderson, C.J., (1991b). *Molec. Immunol.* **28**, 155–158.

Matsui, K., Nakanishi, K., Cohen, D.I., Hada, T., Furuyama, J., Hamaoka, T. and Higashino, K. (1989). *J. Immunol.* **142**, 2918–2923.

Maxwell, C., Hussian, R., Nutman, T.B., Poindexter, R.W., Little, M.D., Schad, G.A. and Ottesen, E.A. (1987). *Am. J. Trop. Med. Hyg.* **37**, 126–134.

Metcalf, D., Parker, J.W., Chester, H.M. and Kincade, P.W. (1974). *J. Cell. Physiol.* **84**, 275–290.

Metcalf, D., Cutler, R.L. and Nicola, N.A. (1983). *Blood* **61**, 999–1005.

Migita, M., Yamaguchi, N., Mita, S., Higuchi, S., Hitoshi, Y., Yoshida, Y., Tominaga, M., Matsuda, F., Tominaga, A. and Takatsu, K. (1991). *Cell. Immunol.* **133**, 484–497.

Milburn, M., Hassell, A.M., Lambert, M.H., Jordan, S.R., Proudfoot, A.E.I., Grabar, P. and Wells, T.N.C. (1993). *Nature* **363**, 172–176.

Minamitake, Y., Kodama, S., Katayama, T., Adachi, H., Tanaka, S. and Tsujimoto, M. (1990). *J. Biochem. Tokyo.* **107**, 292–297.

Murata, Y., Takaki, S., Migita, M., Kikuchi, Y., Tominaga, A. and Takatsu, K., (1992). *J. Exp. Med.* **175**, 341–351.

Murray, P.D., McKenzie, D.T., Swain, S.L. and Kagnoff, M.F. (1987). *J. Immunol.* **139**, 2669–2674.

Nakanishi, K., Yoshimoto, T., Katoh, Y., Ono, S., Matsui, K., Hiroishi, K., Noma, T., Honjo, T., Takatsu, K., Higashino, K. *et al.* (1988). *J. Immunol.* **140**, 1168–1174.

Nicola, N.A. and Metcalf, D. (1991). *Cell* **67**, 1–4.

O'Garra, A., Warren, D.J., Holman, W., Popham, A.M., Sanderson, C.J. and Klaus, G.G.B. (1986). *Proc. Natl Acad. Sci. USA.* **83**, 5228–5232.

O'Garra, A., Barbis, D., Wu, J., Hodgkin, P.D., Abrams, J. and Howard, M. (1989). *Cell. Immunol.* **123**, 189–200.

Paul, C.C., Keller, J.R., Armpriester, J.M. and Baumann, M.A. (1990). *Blood* **75**, 1400–1403.

Plaetinck, C., der Heyden, J.V., Tavernier, J., Fache, I., Tuypens, T., Fischkoff, S., Fiers, W. and Devos, R. (1990). *J. Exp. Med.* **172**, 683–691.

Plaut, M., Pierce, J.H., Watson, C.J., Hanley-Hyde, J., Nordan, R.P. and Paul, W.E. (1989). *Nature* **339**, 64–67.

Proudfoot, A.E., Davies, J.G., Turcatti, G. and Wingfield, P.T. (1991). *FEBS Lett.* **283**, 61–64.

Purkerson, J.M., Newberg, M., Wise, G., Lynch, K.R. and Isakson, P.C. (1988). *J. Exp. Med.* **168**, 1175–1180.

Rasmussen, R., Takatsu, K., Harada, N., Takahashi, T. and Bottomly, K. (1988). *J. Immunol.* **140**, 705–712.

Rolfe, F.G., Hughes, J.M., Armour, C.L. and Sewell, W.A. (1992). *Immunology* **77**, 494–499.

Samoszuk, M. and Nansen, L. (1990). *Blood* **75**, 13–16.

Sanderson, C.J. (1990). In: *Colony Stimulating Factors: Molecular and Cellular Biology* (eds T.M. Dexter, J.M. Garland and N.G. Testa), Marcel Dekker, Inc., New York, pp. 231–256.

Sanderson, C.J. (1992). *Blood* **79**, 3101–3109.

Sanderson, C.J. (1993). In: *Immunopharmacology of Eosinophils*, (eds H. Smith and R.M. Cook), Academic Press Ltd., London, pp. 11–24.

Sanderson, C.J., Warren, D.J. and Strath, M. (1985). *J. Exp. Med.* **162**, 60–74.

Sanderson, C.J., O'Garra, A., Warren, D.J. and Klaus, G.G.B. (1986). *Proc. Natl Acad. Sci. USA.* **83**, 437–440.

Sanderson, C.J., Campbell, H.D. and Young, I.G. (1988). *Immunol Rev.* **102**, 29–50.

Sanderson, C.J., Strath, M., Mudway, I. and Dent, L.A. (1993) In: *Eosinophils: Immunological and Clinical Aspects.* (eds Gleich, G.J. and Kay, A.B.) Marcel Dekker Inc., New York.

Scanafelt, A.B., Miyajima, A., Kitamura, T. and Kastelelein, R.A., (1991). *EMBO J.* **10**, 4105–4112.

Sher, A., Coffman, R.L., Hieny, S., Scott, P. and Cheever, A.W. (1990). *Proc. Natl Acad. Sci. USA.* **87**, 61–65.

Sonada, Y., Arai, N. and Ogawa, M. (1989a). *Leukemia* **3**, 14–18.

Sonada, E., Matsumoto, R., Hitoshi, Y., Ishii, T., Sugimoto, M., Araki, S., Tominaga, A., Yamaguchi, N. and Takatsu, K. (1989b). *J. Exp. Med.* **170**, 1415–1420.

Strath, M. and Sanderson, C.J. (1986). *Exp. Hematol.* **14**, 16–20.

Strath, M., Clutterbuck, E.J. and Sanderson, C.J. (1990). In: *Methods in Molecular Biology, Vol. 5. Animal Cell Culture* (eds J.W. Pollard and J.M. Walker), The Humana Press Inc., Clifton, NJ, pp. 361–378.

Sutherland, G.R., Baker, E., Callen, D.F., Campbell, H.D., Young, I.G., Sanderson, C.J., Garson, O.M., Lopez, A.F. and Vadas, M.A. (1988). *Blood,* **71**, 1150–1152.

Swain, S.L., McKenzie, D.T., Dutton, R.W., Tonkonogy, S.L. and English, M. (1988). *Immunol. Rev.* **102**, 77–105.

Takatsu, K., Tominaga, A., Harada, N., Mita, S., Matsumoto, M., Takashi, T., Kikuchi, Y and Yamaguchi, N. (1988). *Immunol. Rev.* **102**, 107–135.

Tavernier, J., Devos, R., Cornelis, S., Tuypens, T., Van der Heyden, J., Fiers, W. and Plaetinck, G. (1991). *Cell* **66**, 1175–1184.

Tavernier, J., Tuypens, T., Plaetinck, G., Verhee, A., Fiers, W. and Devos, R. (1992). *Proc. Natl Acad. Sci. USA.* **89**, 7041–7045.

Tominaga, A., Matsumoto, M., Harada, N., Takahashi, T., Kikuchi, Y. and Takatsu, K. (1988). *J. Immunol.* **140**, 1175–1181.

Tominaga, A., Takahashi, T., Kikuchi, Y., Mita, S., Noami, S., Harada, N., Yamaguchi, N. and Takatsu, K. (1990). *J. Immunol.* **144**, 1345–1352.

Tominaga, A., Takaki, S., Koyama, N., Katoh, S., Matsumoto, R., Migita, M., Hitoshi, Y., Hosoya, Y., Yamauchi, S., Kanai, Y., Miyazaki, J.-I., Usuku, G., Yamamura, K.-I. and Takatsu, K. (1991). *J. Exp. Med.* **173**, 429–437.

Tuypens, T., Plaetinck, G., Baker, E., Sutherland, G., Brusselle, G., Fiers, W., Devos, R. and Tavernier, J. (1992). *Eur. Cytokine. Netw.* **3**, 451–459.

Umland, S.P., Go, N.F., Cupp, J.E. and Howard, M. (1989). *J. Immunol.* **142**, 1528–1535.

Van Leeuwen, B.H., Martinson, M.E., Webb, G.C. and Young, I.G. (1989). *Blood* **73**, 1142–1148.

Vitetta, E.S., Brooks, K., Chen, Y.-W., Isakson, P., Jones, S., Layton, J., Mishra, G.C., Pure, E., Weiss, E., Word, C., Yuan, D., Tucker, P., Uhr, J.W. and Krammer, P.H. (1984). *Immunol. Rev.* **78**, 137–157.

Walsh, G.M., Hartnell, A., Wardlaw, A.J., Kurihara, K., Sanderson, C.J. and Kay, A.B. (1990). *Immunology* **71**, 258–265.

Walsh, G.M., Mermod, J.-J., Hartnell, A., Kay, A.B. and Wardlaw, A.J. (1991). *J. Immunol.* **146**, 3419–3423.

Wang, J.M., Rambaldi, A., Biondi, A., Chen, Z.G., Sanderson, C.J. and Mantovani, A. (1989). *Eur. J. Immunol.* **19**, 701–705.

Wang, Y., Campbell, H.D. and Young, I.G., (1993). *J. Steroid Biochem. Mol. Biol.* **44**, 203–210.

Warren, D.J. and Moore, M.A. (1988). *J. Immunol.* **140**, 94–99.

Warren, D.J. and Sanderson, C.J. (1985). *Immunology* **54**, 615–623.

Webb, G.C., Lee, J.S., Campbell, H.D. and Young, I.G. (1989). *Cytogenet. Cell. Genet.* **50**, 107–110.

Wetzel, G.D. (1989). *Eur. J. Immunol.* **19**, 1701–1707.

Yamaguchi, Y., Suda, T., Suda, J., Eguchi, M., Miura, Y., Harada, N., Tominaga, A. and Takatsu, K. (1988a). *J. Exp. Med.* **167**, 43–56.

Yamaguchi, Y., Hayashi, Y., Sugama, Y., Miura, Y., Kasahara, T., Kitamura, S., Torisu, M., Mita, S., Tominaga, A. and Takatsu, K. (1988b). *J. Exp. Med.* **167**, 1737–1742.

Yokota, T., Coffman, R.L., Hagiwara, H., Rennick, D.M., Takebe, Y., Yokota, K., Gemmell, L., Shrader, B., Yang, G., Meyerson, P., Luh, J., Hoy, P., Pene, J., Briere, F., Spits, H., Banchereau, J., de Vries, J., Lee, F.D., Aria, N. and Aria, K. (1987). *Proc. Natl Acad. Sci. USA.* **84**, 7388–7392.

Chapter 8

Interleukin-6

Toshio Hirano

Division of Molecular Oncology, Biomedical Research Center,
Osaka University Medical School, Osaka, Japan

INTRODUCTION

Interleukin-6 (IL-6) is a multifunctional cytokine which is produced by both lymphoid and nonlymphoid cells and regulates immune responses, acute-phase reactions and haemopoiesis (Sehgal *et al.*, 1989; Hirano and Kishimoto, 1990; Hirano, 1992a). IL-6 has been called by a variety of names, such as IFN-$\beta 2$ (Weissenbach *et al.*, 1980; May *et al.*, 1986; Zilberstein *et al.*, 1986), TRF-like factor (Teranishi *et al.*, 1982), B-cell differentiation factor (BCDF) (Okada *et al.*, 1983), BCDF2 (Hirano *et al.*, 1984a,b), 26-kDa protein (Haegeman *et al.*, 1986), B-cell stimulatory factor 2 (BSF-2) (Hirano *et al.*, 1985, 1986), hybridoma/plasmacytoma growth factor (HPGF or IL-HP1) (Aarden *et al.*, 1985; Nordan and Potter, 1986; Van Damme *et al.*, 1987a; Van Snick *et al.*, 1988), hepatocyte stimulating factor (HSF) (Andus *et al.*, 1987; Gauldie *et al.*, 1987), and monocyte granulocyte inducer type 2 (MGI-2) (Shabo *et al.*, 1988). However, the molecular cloning of IFN-$\beta 2$ (May *et al.*, 1986; Zilberstein *et al.*, 1986), 26-kDa protein (Haegeman *et al.*, 1986) and BSF-2 (Hirano *et al.*, 1986) revealed that all these molecules are identical (Sehgal *et al.*, 1987a), and it was proposed that this molecule be referred to as IL-6 at the end of 1988 (Sehgal *et al.*, 1989; Hirano and Kishimoto, 1990; Le and Vilček, 1989; Heinrich *et al.*, 1990; Van Snick, 1990; Hirano, 1992a). In the following sections, the structure and function of IL-6 and its receptor, the regulatory mechanisms governing IL-6 gene expression, signal transduction mechanisms and the possible involvement of IL-6 in a variety of diseases are described.

STRUCTURE OF IL-6 AND ITS GENE

IL-6 is a glycoprotein with a molecular mass ranging from 21 to 28 kDa. Post-translational modifications include *N*- and *O*-linked glycosylations and phosphorylations (May *et al.*, 1988; Santhanam *et al.*, 1989). Human IL-6 consists of 212 amino acids, including a hydrophobic signal sequence of 28 amino acids (Hirano *et al.*, 1986). Human IL-6 shows a homology with those of mouse and rat by 65% and 68% at the DNA level and 42% and 58% at the protein level, respectively (Van Snick *et al.*, 1988; Northemann *et al.*, 1989). The mouse and rat protein sequences are 93% identical (Van

Snick *et al.*, 1988; Northemann *et al.*, 1989). Both *C*-terminus and *N*-terminus play a critical role for its biological functions (Brakenhoff *et al.*, 1989; Ida *et al.*, 1989; Krüttgen *et al.*, 1990). Recent studies based on a computer-aided structural analysis have predicted that IL-6 consists of four anti-parallel α helices with two long and one short loop connections, like other cytokines, including growth hormone prolactin, erythropoietin, IL-2, IL-4, G-CSF and GM-CSF, leukaemia inhibitory factor (LIF), oncostatin M (OSM) and CNTF (Bazan, 1992). The evidence suggests an evolutionary relationship between these molecules acting in the immune, haemopoietic, endocrine and nerve systems. The human and mouse IL-6 genes are approximately 5 and 7 kb in length, respectively, and both consist of five exons and four introns (Yasukawa *et al.*, 1987; Tanabe *et al.*, 1988). The genomic genes for human and murine IL-6 have been mapped to chromosomes 7 and 5, respectively (Sehgal *et al.*, 1986; Mock *et al.*, 1989). The human IL-6 gene has been further localized to 7p21 (Bowcock *et al.*, 1988). The sequence similarity in the coding region of human and mouse IL-6 genes is about 60%, whereas the 3'-untranslated region and the first 300 bp of the 5' flanking region are highly conserved (80%) (Tanabe *et al.*, 1988). The production of IL-6 is regulated by a variety of stimuli. IL-6 production is induced in T cells or T-cell clones by T-cell mitogens or antigenic stimulation (Van Snick *et al.*, 1987; Horii *et al.*, 1988; Hodgkin *et al.*, 1988; Espevik *et al.*, 1990). LPS enhances IL-6 production in monocytes and fibroblasts, whereas glucocorticoids inhibit it (Helfgott *et al.*, 1987, Sehgal, 1992). Various viruses induce IL-6 production in fibroblasts (Sehgal *et al.*, 1988; Van Damme *et al.*, 1989) or in the central nervous system (Frei *et al.*, 1988). Human immuno-deficiency virus also induces IL-6 production (Nakajima *et al.*, 1989; Breen *et al.*, 1990; Emilie *et al.*, 1990). A variety of peptide factors, such as IL-1, TNF, IL-2, IFN-β and PDGF (Content *et al.*, 1985; May *et al.*, 1986; Wong and Goeddel, 1986; Zilberstein *et al.*, 1986; Kohase *et al.*, 1987; Van Damme *et al.*, 1987a, b; Kasid *et al.*, 1989), protein kinase C (Hirano *et al.*, 1986; Sehgal *et al.*, 1987b), calcium ionophore A23187 (Sehgal *et al.*, 1987b) and various agents causing elevation of intracellular cAMP levels (Zhang *et al.*, 1988a, b) also induce IL-6 production. In contrast to these, IL-4 and IL-13 inhibit IL-6 production in monocytes (Gibbons *et al.*, 1990; Velde *et al.*, 1990; Minty *et al.*, 1993).

Several potential transcriptional control elements, such as glucocorticoid-responsive elements, an AP-1 binding site, a c-fos serum-responsive element homology (c-fos SRE), c-fos retinoblastoma control element (RCE) homology, a cAMP-responsive element (CRE) and an NF-κB binding site have been identified within the conserved region of the IL-6 promoter (Ray *et al.*, 1988, 1989; Tanabe *et al.*, 1988; Sehgal, 1992), as shown in Fig. 1. Among them, c-fos SRE and AP-1-like elements appear to contain the major *cis*-acting regulatory elements which confer responsiveness to several reagents (including serum, forskolin, and phorbol ester) upon the heterologous herpes virus thymidine kinase (TK) promoter (Ray *et al.*, 1989). The 23-bp oligonucleotide designated MRE within the IL-6-enhancer region (173 to 151), which contains a CGTCA motif, binds nuclear proteins. A single copy of MRE inserted upstream of the herpes virus TK promoter renders this heterologous promoter inducible by IL-1α, tumour necrosis factor and serum, as well as by activators of protein kinase A (forskolin) and protein kinase C (phorbol ester). The IL-1-responsive element was also mapped within the region from 180 to 111 bp of the IL-6 gene and a nuclear factor, NF-IL-6,was identified which was also called C/EBP-β that binds specifically to a 14-bp

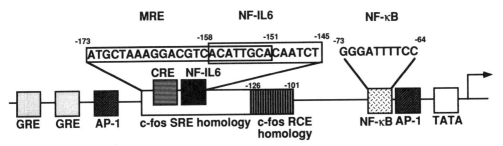

Fig. 1. *Cis*-regulatory elements in the 5′-flanking region of the IL-6 gene. GRE, glucocorticoid-responsive elements; CRE, cAMP-responsive element; SRE, serum responsive element; RCE, retinoblastoma control element.

palindrome (Akira *et al.*, 1990; Isshiki *et al.*, 1990). Shimizu *et al.* (1990) showed that the NF-κB binding motif located between 73 to 63 bp relative to the mRNA cap site is required for IL-1/TNF-α-induced expression of the IL-6 gene. Libermann and Baltimore (1990) and Zhang *et al.* (1990) also demonstrated the involvement of an NF-κB-like molecule in IL-6 gene expression. In fact, antisense oligonucleotide of NF-κB inhibits the expression of IL-6 mRNA in tumour cells derived from HTLV-1 tax transgenic mice (Kitajima *et al.*, 1992) and p40tax induces IL-6 mRNA through the NF-κB binding site concomitantly inducing NF-κB-binding protein (Muraoka *et al.*, 1993). Although NF-κB site functions as a potent IL-1/TNF-responsive element in nonlymphoid cells, its activity is repressed in lymphoid cells and NF-κB-binding factor containing c-Rel seems to act as repressor in lymphoid cells (Nakayama *et al.*, 1992). p53 and RB also repress the IL-6 gene promoter, although the biological significance has not been evaluated (Sehgal, 1992).

IL-6 RECEPTORS

The Cytokine Receptor Family

The IL-6 receptor consists of at least two molecules, one is a 80 kDa IL-6-binding protein (α chain) and the other 130 kDa signal transducer, gp 130 (β chain) (Taga *et al.*, 1989; Hibi *et al.*, 1990) as illustrated in Fig. 2. Human IL-6Rα consists of 468 amino acids, including a putative signal peptide of 19 amino acids, a transmembrane domain of 28 amino acids and cytoplasmic domain of 82 amino acids (Yamasaki *et al.*, 1988). Mature IL-6Rα is a glycoprotein with a molecular mass of 80 kDa that binds IL-6 with low affinity. The first domain of the IL-6Rα, consisting of 90 amino acid residues, is similar to an immunoglobulin domain. Murine IL-6Rα consists of 460 amino acids with essentially the same structure as human IL-6R (Sugita *et al.*, 1990). The overall homology between murine and human IL-6Rα is 69% and 54% at DNA and protein levels, respectively. The second and third domains of IL-6Rα show distinct similarity with many receptors, including the receptors for growth hormone, CNTF, IL-2, erythropoietin, G-CSF and IL-5, all of which belong to a newly identified superfamily of cytokine receptors. The most striking features of these receptors are the conservation of

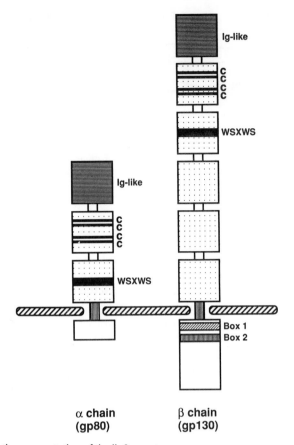

Fig. 2. Schematic representation of the IL-6 receptor.

four cysteine residues and a tryptophan-serine-X-tryptophan-serine (W–S–X–W–S) motif (WS motif) located just outside the transmembrane domain (Bazan, 1990). The evidence indicates that not only the ligands acting in the immune, haemopoietic, endocrine and nerve systems but also their receptors show structural similarity, suggesting that the signal transduction system of these systems may have a common, or very similar, mechanism.

In almost all receptors, the cytoplasmic domain is necessary for signal transduction. However, the cytoplasmic domain of the IL-6Rα is not required for IL-6-mediated signal transduction (Taga *et al.*, 1989; Hibi *et al.*, 1990). Insertion of the intracisternal A particle gene (IAP-LTR) in the cytoplasmic domain of murine IL-6Rα was found in some mouse plasmacytoma. This plasmacytoma abundantly expresses an abnormal but functional IL-6Rα whose cytoplasmic domain is replaced with IAP sequence (Sugita *et al.*, 1990). Furthermore, even the complex of IL-6 and soluble IL-6Rα could generate IL-6-mediated signal transduction (Taga *et al.*, 1989; Hibi *et al.*, 1990), indicating the presence of an additional cell surface molecule. The binding of IL-6 to its receptor triggered the association of IL-6Rα with a second membrane glycoprotein with a molecular mass of 130 kDa (gp130) (Taga *et al.*, 1989). The complex of IL-6 and

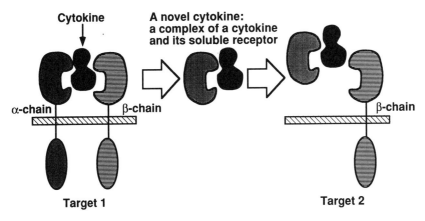

Fig. 3. A novel mechanism generating cytokine diversity.

soluble IL-6Rα could also associate with gp130 (Hibi *et al.*, 1990). Human gp130 consists of an extracellular domain of 597 amino acids, a transmembrane domain of 22 amino acids, and a cytoplasmic domain of 277 amino acids; it encodes a protein belonging to the cytokine receptor family, having a WS motif and a contactin-like sequence and significant homology with the G-CSF receptor (G-CSF-R) (Hibi *et al.*, 1990) (Fig. 2). Murine gp130 showed 76.8% homology with human gp130 at the amino acid level (Saito *et al.*, 1992). Murine gp130 is ubiquitously expressed in murine tissues, embryonic stem cells and embryos as early as day 6 of gestation, suggesting that gp130 acts not only as IL-6 receptor subunit but also as a subunit of the other receptors. gp130 by itself cannot bind IL-6, but IL-6Rα together with gp130 forms a high-affinity IL-6 binding site (Hibi *et al.*, 1990). The human gp130 cDNA that was expressed in mouse IL-3-dependent cells confers proliferative potential in the presence of human IL-6 and the soluble form of IL-6Rα (Hibi *et al.*, 1990).

A Novel Mechanism Generating Cytokine Diversity

Investigations of the IL-6R system have provided evidence that a complex of IL-6 and a soluble form of IL-6Rα could act on the cells which express gp130 but not IL-6Rα (Fig. 3). The other molecule that acts in a similar manner to soluble IL-6Rα–IL-6 complexes is natural killer cell stimulating factor (NKSF), which is also called IL-12. IL-12 consists of disulphide heterodimer of 40 kDa (p40) and 35 kDa (p35) subunits (Wolf *et al.*, 1991). p35 is a helical cytokine and p40 shows a similarity to the soluble form of IL-6Rα (Gearing and Cosman, 1991). IL-12 is therefore a complex of a cytokine and a soluble form of its presumed receptor. Thus, the p40–p35 heterodimer can act through a gp130-type molecule as its receptor. Based on these facts, I propose a novel mechanism by which the diversity of cytokines could be generated (Fig. 3). A complex of a soluble cytokine receptor and its corresponding cytokine could be converted to a novel cytokine with functions distinct from the original cytokine because it has a different target specificity from the original one. In this respect, it is noteworthy that mRNA encoding a soluble form of the IL-6Rα is expressed in normal lymphocytes, trans-formed B-cell lines and myeloma cells (Lust *et al.*, 1992) and soluble IL-6Rα is present in urine and serum (Novic *et al.*, 1989; Honda *et al.*, 1992). Furthermore, there are many cells or tissues which express gp130 but not IL-6Rα (Hibi *et al.*, 1990; Saito *et al.*, 1992). In support of this model, the soluble form of CNTF-Rα, together with CNTF, can act on cells not normally responsive to CNTF (Davis *et al.*, 1993). Furthermore, soluble CNTF-Rα is present in cerebrospinal fluid and is released from skeletal muscle in response to peripheral nerve injury, suggesting potential physiological roles of soluble CNTF-Rα (Davis *et al.*, 1993).

gp130 is a Common Signal Transducer Involved in the Immune, Haemopoietic and Nervous Systems

The redundancy of activity is another feature of cytokines. For example, IL-6, LIF and OSM induce macrophage differentiation in a myeloid leukaemic cell line, M1 (Miyaura *et al.*, 1988; Shabo *et al.*, 1988; Metcalf, 1989; Rose *et al.*, 1991; Oritani *et al.*, 1992) and acute phase protein synthesis in hepatocytes (Andus *et al.*, 1987; Baumann *et al.*, 1987, 1989; Gauldie *et al.*, 1987; Richards *et al.*, 1992). One of the important findings on cytokine receptors is that one constituent of a certain cytokine receptor is shared among several other cytokine receptors, as first demonstrated for GM-CSF, IL-3 and IL-5 receptor systems (Miyajima *et al.*, 1992). Another example is gp130 that acts as a subunit not only for IL-6 receptor but also for LIF, OSM and CNTF receptors and plays a role in signalling (Gearing *et al.*, 1992; Hibi *et al.*, 1990; Ip *et al.*, 1992; Taga *et al.*, 1992). This fact may explain one of the mechanisms of functional redundancy of cytokine activity.

CNTF-Rα is a member of the cytokine receptor family and most closely resembles IL-6Rα (Davis *et al.*, 1991). CNTF-Rα is anchored to the cell surface by a glycosyl-phosphatidylinositol linkage. The lack of a cytoplasmic domain in the CNTF-Rα chain and its sequence similarity to IL-6Rα suggest that the signal transduction of CNTF may be through a gp130-type molecule. In fact, CNTF-R consists of CNTF-specific α chain, LIF-R and gp130 and tyrosine residues of LIF-R and gp130 are phosphorylated upon the stimulation with CNTF-R, indicating that CNTF-R-mediated signals could be generated, at least in part, through gp130 (Ip *et al.*, 1992). LIF-R cDNA confers low-affinity binding when expressed in COS7 cells and high-affinity binding when expressed in murine B9 cells, suggesting the presence of the additional chains required for the formation of a high-affinity binding site (Gearing *et al.*, 1991). The binding of radiolabelled LIF and OSM to M1 cells was inhibited by both unlabelled OSM and LIF. However, OSM was a less effective competitor than LIF. The soluble form of cloned LIF-R could bind LIF with low affinity but not OSM at all. Thus, OSM could bind to the high-affinity LIF-R but not the low affinity LIF-R (Gearing and Bruce, 1992). The cDNA for the high-affinity converting subunit of the LIF-R was cloned by a screening for binding of radiolabelled OSM, which does not bind to the low-affinity LIF-R. After the molecular cloning, IL-6 signal transducer, gp130, was found to be an affinity converter for LIF-R and the low-affinity OSM-R (Gearing *et al.*, 1992). Thus, gp130 was found to be a common subunit of the cytokine receptor for IL-6, OSM, LIF/CDF and CNTF and to play a role in transmitting the signals for all these receptors. It is now known that anti-gp130 can inhibit the activity of IL-6, LIF and CNTF (Taga *et al.*,

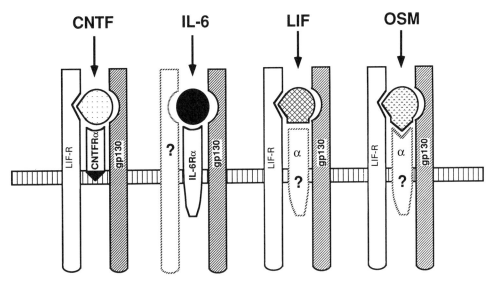

Fig. 4. gp130 is a common subunit among the receptors for IL-6, LIF, CNTF and OSM.

1992). The tentative model of these receptors is schematically presented in Fig. 4, where the possible presence of a ligand specific α-chain for LIF and OSM is also shown.

Signal Transduction Through the IL-6 Receptor Complex

Many cytokines induce a rapid and transient tyrosine phosphorylation, but the cytokine receptor family lacks the intrinsic protein tyrosine domain, indicating that a non-receptor type tyrosine kinase, such as an src family may closely associate with cytokine receptors, as in the case of p56 lck which associates with IL-2Rβ (Hatakeyama *et al.*, 1991). IL-6 induces a rapid and transient tyrosine phosphorylation of a 160 kDa molecule in a murine IL-6-dependent hybridoma MH60. BSF2 (Nakajima and Wall, 1991) and increases tyrosine kinase activity in a variety of cell lines, including myeloma, T lymphoma, hepatoma and myeloleukaemic cell lines (Matsuda *et al.*, 1993). IL-6 also induces a rapid and transient phosphorylation of the cytoplasmic domain of gp130 (Murakami *et al.*, 1991). Both tyrosine kinase and H7-sensitive protein kinase appear to be required for the activation of *junB* and *tis11* gene transcription (Nakajima and Wall, 1991).

In the 277-amino-acid cytoplasmic region of gp130, a 61-amino-acid region proximal to the transmembrane domain was sufficient to generate the growth signal (Murakami *et al.*, 1991). In this region two segments that were highly conserved in the cytokine receptor family were identified (Fig. 2). One (Box 1) is conserved in almost all members of the cytokine receptor family, and the other (Box 2) is conserved among G-CSFR, IL-2Rβ, IL-3Rα and IL-3Rβ (Fukunaga *et al.*, 1991; Murakami *et al.*, 1991). Furthermore, a mutation with two prolines in the highly conserved consensus sequence resulted in the loss of tyrosine phosphorylation of the cytoplasmic domain of gp130 upon IL-6 stimulation (Murakami *et al.*, 1991).

The induction of the *junB* gene by IL-6 was observed in a wide range of cells, including human myeloma cell lines (unpublished observation), hepatoma cell lines

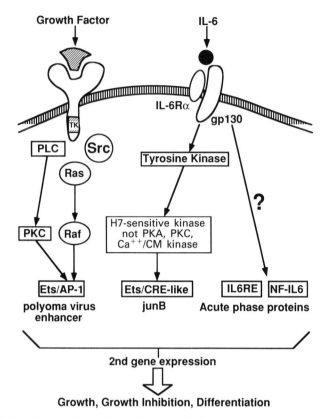

Fig. 5.   A novel signal transduction pathway through gp130.

(Nakajima *et al.*, 1993) and myeloleukaemic cell lines (Lord *et al.*, 1991; Oritani *et al.*, 1992). The IL-6-responsive element of the *junB* gene, designated JRE-IL6, contains an ETS binding site (CAGGAAGC) and a CRE-like site (TGACGCGA) and both sites are required for IL-6-induced activation of JRE-IL6. The signal transduction pathway activating the JRE-IL6 does not utilize well-characterized signal transduction molecules such as C-kinase, A-kinase, calcium/calmodulin-dependent kinase, ras, raf-1 or MAP kinase (Nakajima *et al.*, 1993). Therefore, one may predict that a H7-sensitive novel protein kinase may be involved in the IL-6-induced signal transduction pathway (Fig. 5).

   IL-6 response elements other than the JRE-IL6 have been characterized in regulatory regions of a large set of genes encoding the acute-phase proteins. These genes are considered to be regulated by tissue-specific (liver-specific) transcription factors and IL-6- and/or IL-1-inducible transcription factors (Toniatti *et al.*, 1990). Two types of IL-6 response elements have been identified. Type 1 elements found in the CRP, haemopexin A, haptoglobin genes have a consensus sequence TT/GNNGNAAT and have been shown to be a binding site for NF-IL6/IL-6DBP/LAP/C/EBP-β (Akira *et al.*, 1990; Poli *et al.*, 1990a; Cao *et al.*, 1991; De Groot *et al.*, 1991) whose binding activity is induced by IL-6 (Poli *et al.*, 1989; Majello *et al.*, 1990). Type II elements found in the fibrinogen, α-2-macroglobulin and α-1-acid glycoprotein genes have a consensus

Table 1. Biological activities of IL-6.

Immune response
B-cell differentiation
Cytotoxic T-cell differentiation
Induction of IL-2 production and IL-2 receptor expression in T cells
T-cell growth

Haemopoiesis
Haemopoietic stem cell growth
Maturation of megakaryocytes

Acute-phase reaction
Induction of acute-phase protein synthesis

Malignancies
Hybridoma/plasmacytoma/myeloma growth
Lennert's T-cell lymphoma growth
EBV-transformed B-cell growth
Renal carcinoma-cell growth
Myeloid leukaemic cell-line growth inhibition
Breast carcinoma cell-line growth inhibition

Others
Neural cell differentiation
Induction of ACTH synthesis
Activation of osteoclast
Mesangial cell growth
Keratinocyte growth
Hepatitis B virus envelope protein binding activity

sequence, CTGGGAA, and the elements (IL-6 REs) in the promoter of rat α-2-macroglobulin gene were shown to be responsive to IL-6 in HepG2 cells (Hocke *et al.*, 1992). The activation of a nuclear factor requires ongoing protein synthesis (Hocke *et al.*, 1992), occurs in the cytoplasm and involves phosphorylation (Wegenka *et al.*, 1993).

BIOLOGICAL ACTIVITY

IL-6 acts on a variety of cells and exerts a number of activities, as summarized in Table 1.

IL-6 and Immune Responses

B cells stimulated with antigen proliferate and differentiate into antibody-forming cells under the control of a variety of cytokines produced by T cells and macrophages (Kishimoto and Hirano, 1988). IL-6 was identified as one of the factors acting on B cells in the culture supernatants of PHA- or antigen-stimulated peripheral mononuclear cells which induce Ig production in B cell lines transformed with Epstein–Barr virus (EBV) (Teranishi *et al.*, 1982). Furthermore, it was demonstrated that IL-6 functions in the late phase of *Staphylococcus aureus* Cowan 1 (SAC) stimulation of normal B cells (Hirano *et al.*, 1984a; Teranishi *et al.*, 1984), or leukaemic B cells (Yoshizaki *et al.*, 1982), inducing

Ig production when other factors such as IL-2 are available. Further effects of IL-6 on B cells have been demonstrated utilizing recombinant human IL-6. The original observation that IL-6 acts on B-cell lines at the mRNA level and induces biosynthesis of secretory-type Ig (Kikutani *et al.*, 1985) was confirmed and it was demonstrated that transcriptional activation is the primary mechanism for the quantitative increase of secretory immunoglobulin mRNAs (Raynal *et al.*, 1989). Furthermore, IL-6 was found to activate Ig heavy-chain enhancer (Eμ) in large, but not unstimulated small B-cells obtained from transgenic mice carrying the Eμ and κ light-chain promoter-driving CAT gene (Miller *et al.*, 1992). IL-6 acts on B cells activated with SAC or pokeweed mitogen (PWM) to induce IgM, IgG and IgA production, but not on resting B cells (Muraguchi *et al.*, 1988). Anti-IL-6 antibody inhibits PWM-induced Ig production, indicating that IL-6 is essential for PWM-induced Ig production. An essential role of IL-6 was also demonstrated in IL-4-dependent IgE synthesis (Vercelli *et al.*, 1989) and in polysaccharide-specific antibody production (Ambrosino *et al.*, 1990) in human B cells, and in the influenza A virus-specific primary response in murine B cells (Hilbert *et al.*, 1989). Anti-IL-6 antibody inhibits IL-4-driven IgE production, suggesting that endogenous IL-6 plays an obligatory role in the IL-4 dependent induction of IgE (Vercelli *et al.*, 1989); it has been demonstrated that IL-4 induces IL-6 production in normal human B cells (Smeland *et al.*, 1989). An obligatory role for IL-6 in antibody production has also been shown in IL-2-induced Ig production in SAC-stimulated B cells (Xia *et al.*, 1989). In this case IL-2 does not induce IL-6 production but may induce the IL-6 responsiveness in SAC-activated B cells, which produce IL-6 spontaneously. The dependence on IL-2 of the action of IL-6 in B cells was demonstrated utilizing partly purified IL-6 (Teranishi *et al.*, 1984) and this has since been confirmed utilizing recombinant IL-6 (Splawski *et al.*, 1990) indicating that, in addition to antigenic stimulation, additional signals provided by growth factors such as IL-2 are required for B cells to acquire IL-6 responsiveness. IL-6 has been demonstrated to be required differentially for antigen-specific antibody production by primary and secondary murine B cells. The former response is dependent on IL-6 but the latter is not (Hilbert *et al.*, 1989). IL-6 and IL-1 synergistically stimulate the growth and differentiation of murine B cells activated with anti-Ig or dextran sulphate (Vink *et al.*, 1988). In addition, IL-6 increases IgA production in murine Peyer's patch B cells (Beagley *et al.*, 1989; Kunimoto *et al.*, 1989) or human appendix B cells that express IL-6 receptor (Fujihashi *et al.*, 1991). This effect of IL-6 is not the result of isotype switching, since membrane-bound IgA-negative B cells were not induced to secrete IgA by IL-6 (Beagley *et al.*, 1989). These facts indicate that IL-6 plays a role in mucosal immune response (Fujihashi *et al.*, 1992). IL-6 is also reported to augment the *in vivo* production of anti-SRBC antibodies in mice (Takatsuki *et al.*, 1988).

IL-6 is involved in T-cell activation, growth and differentiation (see the review by Van Snick, 1990; Houssiau and Van Snick, 1992). IL-6 induces IL-2 receptor (Tac antigen) expression in one T-cell line (Noma *et al.*, 1987) and in thymocytes (Le *et al.*, 1988), and functions as a second signal for IL-2 production by T cells (Garman *et al.*, 1987). IL-6 promotes the growth of human T cells stimulated with PHA (Houssiau *et al.*, 1988; Lotz *et al.*, 1988) or mouse peripheral T cells (Uyttenhove *et al.*, 1988). It also acts on murine thymocytes to induce proliferation (Helle *et al.*, 1988; Le *et al.*, 1988; Uyttenhove *et al.*, 1988). The effects of IL-6 are synergistic with IL-1 and TNF (Le *et al.*, 1988). IL-6 enhances the proliferative response of thymocytes to IL-4 and PMA

(Hodgkin *et al.*, 1988). Since IL-6 stimulates thymocyte proliferation and IL-1 can induce IL-6 production in thymocytes (Helle *et al.*, 1989), the effect of IL-1 on thymocyte proliferation is possibly mediated by induced IL-6. After the removal of thymocytes with low buoyant density, which are capable of producing IL-6 upon stimulation with IL-1, IL-1 cannot induce cell proliferation but IL-6 or IL-2 is still comitogenic; the IL-1-induced proliferation of thymocytes thus seems to be dependent on endogenous IL-6 production (Helle *et al.*, 1989). A part of the effect of IL-6 on T-cell growth is mediated by endogenously produced IL-2. Anti-IL-2R α chain (Tac) antibody generally inhibits IL-6-induced T-cell proliferation (Garman *et al.*, 1987; Le *et al.*, 1988; Helle *et al.*, 1989; Kawakami *et al.*, 1989; Tosato *et al.*, 1990). IL-1 and IL-6 synergistically induce IL-2 production (Holsti and Raulet, 1989; Houssiau *et al.*, 1989) and IL-2R α-chain expression in T cells (Houssiau *et al.*, 1989). IL-6 also induces the differentiation of cytotoxic T lymphocytes (CTLs) in the presence of IL-2 from murine, as well as from human, thymocytes and splenic T cells (Okada *et al.*, 1988; Takai *et al.*, 1988; Uyttenhove *et al.*, 1988). Utilizing purified murine T cells, both IL-1 and IL-6 were demonstrated to be required for the generation of CTLs and, in this case, induction of the IL-2R α chain and IL-2 production by IL-1 and IL-6 were critical for CTL generation (Renauld *et al.*, 1989). IL-6 also induces serine esterase and perforin, required for mediating target-cell lysis in the granules of CTLs (Takai *et al.*, 1988; Liu *et al.*, 1990), which suggests a critical role in the differentiation and expression of cytotoxic T-cell function.

IL-6 and Haemopoiesis

IL-6 and IL-3 induce synergistically the proliferation of murine pluri-potential haemo-poietic progenitors *in vitro* (Ikebuchi *et al.*, 1987). The combination of IL-6 and IL-3 acts on blast-cell colony-forming cells to cause them to leave G0 earlier. IL-6 appears to trigger the entry into cell cycle of the dormant progenitor cells, whereas IL-3 can support continued proliferation of progenitors after they exit from the G0 phase (Ogawa, 1992). The colony-forming units in spleen (CFU-S) were increased by culturing bone-marrow cells in the presence of both IL-6 and IL-3 (Bodine *et al.*, 1989; Okano *et al.*, 1989a). Those bone-marrow cells cultured with IL-3 and IL-6 for 6 days had a much higher capacity to rescue lethally irradiated mice than did cells cultured with IL-3 alone. These data indicate that the combination of IL-6 and IL-3 stimulates haemopoietic stem cells *in vitro* and therefore could be applied in bone-marrow transplantation. IL-6 synergizes with MCSF in the stimulation of CFU-M with respect to both the number and size of macrophage colonies (Bot *et al.*, 1989). IL-6 has also been found to act synergistically with GM-CSF (Caracciolo *et al.*, 1989). Colony-forming units in culture (CFU-C) in the spleen and femur of mice that had been exposed to 7.50 Gy and reconstituted with bone-marrow cells were increased when IL-6 was injected (Okano *et al.*, 1989b). Furthermore, the survival rate of lethally irradiated mice transplanted with 5×10^4 bone marrow cells was increased with IL-6 treatment from 20% to 75% at day 21. The effect of IL-6 was more pronounced if it was administered as a continuous perfusion through an osmotic minipump (Suzuki *et al.*, 1989). One interesting report on IL-6 and haemopoietic system is that the defect in differentiation of the haemopoiesis in Fanconi anaemia may be caused by a deficiency in IL-6 production (Rosselli *et al.*, 1992).

In vitro megakaryopoiesis is supported by several haemopoietic colony stimulating factors such as IL-3, GM-CSF and erythropoietin. IL-6 was found to induce the maturation of megakaryocytes synergistically with IL-3 (Ishibashi *et al.*, 1989a); IL-6 promoted marked increments in megakaryocyte size and acetylcholinesterase activity. Furthermore, IL-6 induced a significant shift towards higher ploidy classes. These effects of IL-6 on megakaryocytes have subsequently been confirmed (Lotem *et al.*, 1989; Williams *et al.*, 1990). Consistent with these facts, thrombopoietin purified from the conditioned medium of TNK-01 cell line established from a liposarcoma was identical to IL-6 (Nagasawa *et al.*, 1990). The obligatory role of IL-6 in megakaryocyte development is further demonstrated by the fact that anti-mouse IL-6 monoclonal antibody inhibits megakaryocyte development in mouse bone-marrow cultures in both the absence and presence of IL-3 (Lotem *et al.*, 1989). Human megakaryocytes were demonstrated to express IL-6 receptor and produce IL-6, which suggests that IL-6 may regulate terminal maturation of megakaryocytes by autocrine activity (Hegyi *et al.*, 1990); IL-6 can also function *in vivo*. The number of mature megakaryocytes in the bone marrow was increased in IL-6 transgenic mice (Suematsu *et al.*, 1989). Moreover, it was found that administration of IL-6 increased platelet numbers in both mice (Ishibashi *et al.*, 1989b) and monkeys (Asano *et al.*, 1990). The additive or synergistic effect of IL-3 and IL-6 on megakaryocytopoiesis was further demonstrated in mice (Carrington *et al.*, 1991) and monkey (Geissler *et al.*, 1992).

Human and mouse myeloid leukaemic cell lines, such as human histiocytic U937 cells and mouse myeloid M1 cells, can be induced to differentiate into macrophages and granulocytes *in vitro* by several synthetic and natural products. Several factors have been identified which can induce differentiation of leukaemic cells, such as G-CSF (Nicola *et al.*, 1983), MGI-2 (Sachs, 1987) which was found to be identical to IL-6 (Shabo *et al.*, 1988), D factor (Tomida *et al.*, 1984) and LIF (Gearing *et al.*, 1987). In addition to these molecules, IL-6 has been found to inhibit the growth of several human and murine myeloid leukaemic cell lines (Miyaura *et al.*, 1988; Shabo *et al.*, 1988; Onozaki *et al.*, 1989; Oritani *et al.*, 1992; Revel, 1992).

Acute-phase Reactions

The biosynthesis of acute-phase proteins by hepatocytes is regulated by several factors, including IL-1, TNF and HSF. It was found that recombinant IL-6 can function as HSF (Gauldie *et al.*, 1987) and that the activity of crude HSF can be neutralized by anti-IL-6 (Andus *et al.*, 1987), indicating that HSF activity is exerted by the IL-6 molecule (see the review by Heinrich *et al.*, 1990; Gauldie *et al.*, 1992). IL-6 can induce a variety of acute-phase proteins, such as fibrinogen, α-1-antichymotrypsin, α-1-acid glycoprotein and haptoglobin, in the human hepatoma cell line HepG2. In addition to these proteins, it induces serum amyloid A, C-reactive protein (CRP) and α-1-antitrypsin in human primary hepatocytes (Castell *et al.*, 1988). The proteins induced in rats by IL-6 are fibrinogen, cysteine proteinase inhibitor, α-2-macroglobulin and α-1-acid glycoprotein (Andus *et al.*, 1987; Gauldie *et al.*, 1987; Heinrich *et al.*, 1990). *In vivo* administration of IL-6 in rats induces typical acute-phase reactions similar to those induced by turpentine; the IL-6-induced expression of mRNAs for acute-phase proteins is more rapid than that induced by turpentine (Geiger *et al.*, 1988). These results confirm the *in vivo* effect of IL-6 in the acute-phase reaction. It has also been reported that serum levels of IL-6 correlate well with that of CRP and with fever in patients with severe burns (Nijstein *et al.*, 1987). An increase in serum IL-6 has been observed prior to an increase in serum CRP in patients undergoing surgical operations (Nishimoto *et al.*, 1989; Shenkin *et al.*, 1989), supporting a causal role of IL-6 in the acute-phase response.

Other Activities

Stimulation of glioblastoma cells or astrocytoma cells with IL-1 was found to induce the expression of IL-6 mRNA (Yasukawa *et al.*, 1987). Both virus-infected microglial cells and astrocytes were also found to produce IL-6 (Frei *et al.*, 1989), indicating the possible involvement of IL-6 in nerve cell functions. It has been shown that IL-6 induces the typical differentiation of PC12 cells into neural cells (Satoh *et al.*, 1988). It has further been demonstrated that human IL-6 can support the survival of cultured cholinergic neurons (Hama *et al.*, 1989). IL-6 has been shown to stimulate the secretion of adrenocorticotropic hormone either through the corticotropin-releasing hormone (Naitoh *et al.*, 1988) or directly (Fukata *et al.*, 1989). IL-6 also stimulates the release of a variety of anterior pituitary hormones, such as PRL, GH and LH (Spangelo *et al.*, 1989). Anterior pituitary cells produce IL-6 spontaneously (Spangelo *et al.*, 1990). Trophoblast was also found to produce IL-6 *in vivo*, although the biological significance of IL-6 in the placenta is not known (Kameda *et al.*, 1990). Because IL-6 was demonstrated to stimulate hepatic lipogenesis in mice, and IL-6 is induced by TNF, the lipogenic effects of TNF may be mediated, in part, by IL-6 (Grunfeld *et al.*, 1990). IL-6 is produced by vascular smooth muscle cells (Loppnow and Libby, 1990) and may induce their growth (Nabata *et al.*, 1990), suggesting the possible involvement of IL-6 in arteriosclerosis. IL-6 may directly or indirectly affect osteoclast development and play a role in postmenopausal osteoporosis as it has been observed that osteoclast development was enhanced in ovariectomized mice which were released from the estrogen-induced suppression of IL-6 gene expression. Furthermore, enhanced osteoclast development in ovariectomized mice was prevented by administration of anti-IL-6 antibody (Jilka *et al.*, 1992). IL-6 is a growth factor for various cells, including plasmacytoma, myeloma, hybridoma, renal cell carcinoma, Kaposi's sarcoma and keratinocyte (see IL-6 and Disease). Conversely, IL-6 acts as a growth inhibitor for a number of carcinoma and leukaemia cell lines, including breast carcinoma, ovarian carcinoma and myeloleukaemic cell lines (Revel, 1992). Cell surface-associated IL-6 functions as a hepatitis B virus (HBV) receptor and may play a role in the entry of this virus into cells (Neurath *et al.*, 1992).

IL-6 AND DISEASE

A possible involvement of deregulated expression of the IL-6 gene in polyclonal B cell abnormalities was first demonstrated in a patient with cardiac myxoma (Hirano *et al.*, 1987). Since then, much evidence has been accumulated to indicate that deregulated production of IL-6 could be involved in a variety of diseases, including inflammations, autoimmune diseases and malignancies. Considering the possible involvement of IL-6 in such diseases, it might be worth noting that IL-6 was identified as virus-induced IFN-β_2 (Weissenbach *et al.*, 1980) and was found in the culture supernatants of infiltrating cells in the pleural effusion of patients with tuberculous pleurisy (Teranishi *et al.*,

Table 2. IL-6 and diseases.

Polyclonal B-cell abnormalities or autoimmune diseases	
Cardiac myxoma	Hirano *et al.* (1987)
Rheumatoid arthritis	Hirano *et al.* (1988)
Castleman's disease	Yoshizaki *et al.* (1989)
Alcoholic liver cirrhosis	Deviere *et al.* (1989)
Type 1 diabetes	Campbell *et al.* (1989)
Thyroiditis	Bendtzen *et al.* (1989)
Chronic proliferative diseases	
Mesangial proliferative glomerulonephritis	Horii *et al.* (1989)
Psoriasis	Grossman *et al.* (1989)
Kaposi's sarcoma	Miles *et al.* (1990)
Malignancies	
Plasmacytoma and myeloma	Kawano *et al.* (1988)
	Suematsu *et al.* (1992)
Lymphoma and leukaemia	Shimizu *et al.* (1988)
	Bauer and Herrmann (1991)
Renal cell carcinoma	Miki *et al.* (1989)
Others	
AIDS	Nakajima *et al.* (1989)
	Poli *et al.* (1990b)
Sepsis	Waage *et al.* (1989)
Osteoporosis	Jilka *et al.* (1992)
Fanconi anaemia	Rosselli *et al.* (1992)
Hepatitis type B	Neurath *et al.* (1992)

1982) which also contained factor(s) capable of inducing Ig production in activated human B cells (Hirano *et al.*, 1981). Diseases in which deregulated production of IL-6 was observed are summarized in Table 2.

IL-6 and B-cell Abnormalities in Chronic Inflammation

Patients with cardiac myxoma show a variety of autoimmune symptoms, such as hypergammaglobulinaemia, presence of autoantibodies and an increase in acute-phase proteins, all of which disappear after the resection of the tumour cells. Involvement of IL-6 in B-cell abnormalities was first demonstrated in myxoma cells which produced IL-6 (Hirano *et al.*, 1987; Jourdan *et al.*, 1990). Before this finding, it was demonstrated that pleural effusion cells of patients with pulmonary tuberculosis (TB) when stimulated with purified protein derivative produced large quantities of factors capable of inducing Ig production in activated normal B cells (Hirano *et al.*, 1981) — one of these factors was identified as IL-6 (previously called either TRF-like factor, BCDFII or BSF-2). (Teranishi *et al.*, 1982; Hirano *et al.*, 1984a,b, 1985, 1986). It is noteworthy that patients with pulmonary TB often have a wide range of autoantibodies (Shoenfeld and Isenberg, 1988) and, in certain cases, a significant diffuse hypergammaglobulinaemia has been reported (Sela *et al.*, 1987). Taken together, the evidence led us to speculate that overproduction of IL-6 may play a critical role in autoimmune diseases (Hirano *et al.*, 1987). Abnormal IL-6 production was further observed in patients with

Castleman's disease (Yoshizaki *et al.*, 1989) and rheumatoid arthritis (Hirano *et al.*, 1988; Houssiau *et al.*, 1988; Bhardwaj *et al.*, 1989). IL-6 production was also observed in type II collagen-induced arthritis in mice (Takai *et al.*, 1989) and MRL/lpr mice (Tang *et al.*, 1993) which develop autoimmune disease with proliferative glomerulonephritis, and arthritis. IL-6 was also found to be produced by pancreatic islet *B* cells and thyroid (Bendtzen *et al.*, 1989; Campbell *et al.*, 1989), suggesting that by enhancing the response of autoreactive T cells, IL-6 may be involved in type I diabetes (Campbell *et al.*, 1990). The evidence suggests that IL-6 plays a critical role in autoimmune diseases, although IL-6 alone may not be sufficient for the generation of autoimmune disease (Hirano, 1992b). The observation that anti-IL-6 antibody inhibits the development of insulin-dependent diabetes in NOD/Wehi mice may support a role of IL-6 in autoimmune disease (Campbell *et al.*, 1991). Furthermore, the critical role of IL-6 in T-cell activation (Van Snick, 1990) also supports a role of IL-6 in autoimmune disease. Other interesting evidence is that a striking, increased prevalence of agalactosyl IgG has been observed in a variety of autoimmune and/or IL-6-related diseases, such as pulmonary TB, rheumatoid arthritis, Crohn's disease, sarcoidosis, leprosy, Castleman's disease, Takayasu's arteritis, multiple myeloma and pristane-induced arthritis (Nakao *et al.*, 1991; Rook *et al.*, 1991; Rook and Stanford, 1992). In accordance with these facts, IL-6 transgenic mice showed an increase in agalactosyl IgG (Rook *et al.*, 1991), further strengthening the relationship between IL-6 and certain autoimmune diseases.

Chronic Inflammatory Proliferative Diseases

Glomerulonephritis is commonly accompanied with a variety of autoimmune diseases and several growth factors have been suggested as candidates which induce the pathological growth of mesangial cells, but none has yet been determined to contribute to its pathogenesis. IL-6 was demonstrated to be a possible autocrine growth factor for rat mesangial cells (Horii *et al.*, 1989; Ruef *et al.*, 1990). Furthermore, IL-6 was found to be produced by renal mesangial cells in patients with mesangial proliferative glomerulonephritis (Horii *et al.*, 1989). IL-6 could be detected in urine samples from patients with mesangial proliferative glomerulonephritis, but not from patients with other types of glomerulonephritis. Moreover, there was a correlation between the levels of urine IL-6 and the progressive stage of mesangial proliferative glomerulonephritis.

Other chronic inflammatory proliferative diseases that may be related to IL-6 are psoriasis (Grossman *et al.*, 1989) and Kaposi's sarcoma (Miles *et al.*, 1990), in which IL-6 is considered as one of the growth factors for keratinocytes and Kaposi's sarcoma cells. Because mesangial cell proliferative glomerulonephritis, psoriasis and Kaposi's sarcoma are diseases where abnormal cell growth and inflammatory and/or immunological reactions are occurring, one may categorize them as chronic inflammatory proliferative disease (CIPD). From this point of view, rheumatoid arthritis is also considered in the same disease category, because one of the prominent features of this disease is a chronic expansion of synovial cells.

Plasma Cell Neoplasias

IL-6 is a potent growth factor for murine plasmacytoma cells (Aarden *et al.*, 1985; Van Damme *et al.*, 1987a; Van Snick *et al.*, 1988) and human myeloma cells (Kawano *et al.*,

1988), which suggests a possible involvement of IL-6 in the generation of plasmacytoma/myeloma (Hirano, 1991). A significant association of the occurrence of plasma cell neoplasias and chronic inflammations has been found (Isobe *et al.*, 1971; Isomaki *et al.*, 1978). Plasmacytomas could be induced in BALB/c mice by mineral oil or pristane, both of which are potent inducers of chronic inflammation and IL-6 biosynthesis (Potter and Boyce, 1962; Nordan and Potter, 1986). The *in vitro* growth of the primary mouse plasmacytoma induced by the above was found to be dependent on IL-6 (Namba *et al.*, 1972). IL-6 was further found to be a possible autocrine growth factor for human myeloma cells (Kawano *et al.*, 1988). Freeman *et al.* (1989) demonstrated that myelomas and plasma cell leukaemias expressed IL-6 mRNA. Cytoplasmic IL-6 was detected in myeloma cells of the bone marrow by light and electron microscopy (Ohtake *et al.*, 1990). It was reported that the growth-inducing activity of IL-1 or TNF on freshly isolated myeloma cells could be due to an IL-6-mediated autocrine mechanism (Carter *et al.*, 1990). The rearrangement of the IL-6 gene was reported in certain myeloma cells that expressed the IL-6 gene (Fiedler *et al.*, 1990). Constitutive IL-6 production in a murine plasmacytoma cell line owing to the insertion of an intracisternal A particle retrotransposon in the IL-6 gene has also been reported (Blankenstein *et al.*, 1990). The expression of the IL-6 gene in an IL-6-dependent murine plasmacytoma cell line made the cells proliferate in an autocrine manner (Tohyama *et al.*, 1990; Vink *et al.*, 1990). These cells displayed greatly enhanced tumorigenicity and monoclonal antibodies capable of blocking the binding of IL-6 to its receptor inhibited their growth *in vivo*. (Vink *et al.*, 1990). IL-6 was also demonstrated to be an autocrine growth factor for EBV-transformed B-cell lines (Yokoi *et al.*, 1990) and expression of an exogenous IL-6 gene in these B-cell lines conferred growth advantage and *in vivo* tumorigenicity (Scala *et al.*, 1990). However, there is controversy whether all myeloma cells produce IL-6, because only some myeloma cell lines were found to produce IL-6 (Kawano *et al.*, 1988; Klein *et al.*, 1989; Shimizu *et al.*, 1989; Hata *et al.*, 1990) and bone-marrow adherent cells rather than bone-marrow nonadherent cell populations containing myeloma cells were demonstrated to be major producers of IL-6 (Klein *et al.*, 1989). Data indicate that IL-6 plays an important role in *in vivo* growth of myeloma cells and generation of plasma cell neoplasias in either an autocrine or paracrine manner. This was further supported by the following findings. The *in vitro* IL-6 responsiveness of myeloma cells obtained from patients with multiple myeloma was directly correlated with the *in vivo* labelling index of these tumours (Zhang *et al.*, 1989) and increased serum IL-6 levels correlated well with disease severity in multiple myelomas and plasma cell leukaemias (Bataille *et al.*, 1989). Finally, administration of anti-IL-6 antibody suppresses myeloma cell growth in patients (Klein *et al.*, 1991).

However, IL-6 alone is not enough for the generation of plasmacytoma. Plasma cells generated in the IL-6 transgenic mice were not transplantable to syngeneic animals, indicating that additional factors may be required for malignant transformation. Interestingly, C57BL/6 IL-6 transgenic mice, when backcrossed to BALB/c mice, showed a progression from polyclonal plasmacytosis to fully transformed monoclonal plasmacytoma which contained chromosomal translocation with *c-myc* gene rearrangement (Suematsu *et al.*, 1992). The evidence strongly supports the hypothesis that deregulated expression of the IL-6 gene can trigger polyclonal plasmacytosis, resulting in the generation of malignant monoclonal plasmacytoma (Hirano, 1991).

CONCLUSIONS

IL-6 has been found to play a central role in defence mechanism(s), the immune response, haemopoiesis and acute-phase reactions. Conversely, deregulated expression of the IL-6 gene has been implicated in the pathogenesis of a variety of diseases, especially autoimmune diseases, plasmacytoma/myeloma and several chronic proliferative diseases. Future studies on the regulation of IL-6 gene expression and the mechanisms of IL-6 action through its receptor, and development of inhibitors for IL-6 action could provide critical information on the molecular mechanisms of a variety of diseases and allow development of new therapeutic strategies.

NOTE ADDED IN PROOF

A novel Ras-independent signal transduction pathway through gp130 illustrated in Fig. 5 has been found to be mediated by Jak tyrosine kinase and Stat family factors (Lutticken et al., 1993; Stahl et al., 1993; Sadowski et al., 1993; Bonni et al., 1993; Matsuda et al., 1994a; Matsuda et al., 1994b; Nakajima et al., manuscript submitted and also see a review by Hirano et al., 1994). The studies on IL-6 deficient mice showed that IL-6 is not essential for normal development of lymphoid cells. However, IL-6-deficient mice showed impairment of T cell-dependent antibody response, cytotoxic T lymphocyte generation, macrophage function and acute phase response (Kopf et al., 1994). Furthermore, IL-6-deficient mice are protected from osteoporosis induced by estrogen depletion, showing the involvement of IL-6 in the generation of post menopausal osteoporosis (Poli et al., 1994).

ACKNOWLEDGEMENTS

The author thanks Ms R. Masuda and Ms M. Tsuda for their excellent secretarial assistance.

REFERENCES

Aarden, L., Lansdorp, P. and De Groot, E. (1985). *Lymphokines 10*, 175–185.
Akira, S., Isshiki, H., Sugita, T., Tanabe, O., Kinoshita, S., Nishio, Y., Nakajima, T., Hirano, T. and Kishimoto, T. (1990). *EMBO J.* **9**, 1897–1906.
Ambrosino, D.M., Delaney, N.R. and Shamberger, R.C. (1990). *J. Immunol.* **144**: 1221–1226.
Andus, T., Geiger, T., Hirano, T., Northoff, H., Ganter, U., Bauer, J., Kishimoto, T. and Heinrich, P.C. (1987). *FEBS Lett.* **221**, 18–22.
Asano, S., Okano, A., Ozawa, K., Nakahata, T., Ishibashi, T., Koike, K., Kimura, H., Tanioka, Y., Shibuya, A., Hirano, T., Kishimoto, T., Takaku, F. and Akiyama, Y. (1990). *Blood* **75**, 1602–1605.
Bataille, R., Jourdan, M., Zhang, X.-G. and Klein, B. (1989). *J. Clin Invest* **84**, 2008–2011.
Bauer, J. and Herrmann, F. (1991). *Ann Hematol.* **62**, 203–210.
Baumann, H., Onorato, V., Gauldie, J., Jahreis, G.P. (1987). *J. Biol. Chem.* **262**, 9756–9768.
Baumann, H., Wong, G.G. (1989). *J. Immunol.* **143**, 1163–1167.
Bazan, J.F. (1990). *Immunol. Today* **11**, 350–354.
Bazan, J.F. (1992). *Neuron* **7**, 1–12.
Beagley, K.W., Eldridge, J.H., Lee, F., Kiyono, H., Everson, M.P., Koopman, W.J., Hirano, T., Kishimoto, T. and McGhee, J.R. (1989). *J. Exp. Med.* **169**, 2133–2148.
Bendtzen, K., Buschard, K., Diamant, M., Horn, T. and Svenson, M. (1989). *Lymphokine Res.* **8**, 335–340.
Bhardwaj, N., Santhanam, U., Lau, L.L., Tatter, S.B., Ghrayeb, J., Rivelis, M., Steinman, R.M., Sehgal, P.B. and May, L.T. (1989). *J. Immunol.* **143**, 2153–2159.

162   T. Hirano

Blankenstein, T., Qin, Z., Li, W. and Diamanstein, T. (1990). *J. Exp. Med.* **171**, 965–970.
Bodine, D.M., Karlsson, S. and Nienhuis, A.W. (1989). *Proc. Natl Acad. Sci. USA.* **86**, 8897–8901.
Bonni, A., Frank, D.A., Schindler, C. and Greenberg, M.E. (1993). *Science* **262**, 1575–1579.
Bot, F.J., Van Eijk, L., Broeders, L., Aarden, L.A. and Lowenber, B. (1989). *Blood* **73**, 435–437.
Bowcock, A.M., Kidd, J.R., Lathrop, M., Danshvar, L., May, L.T., Ray, A., Sehgal, P.B., Kidd, K.K. and Cavallisforza, L.L. (1988). *Genomics* **3**, 8–16.
Brakenhoff, J.P., Hart, M. and Aarden, L.A. (1989). *J. Immunol.* **143**, 1175–1182.
Breen, E.C., Rezai, A.R., Nakajima, K., Beall, G.N., Mitsuyasu, R.T., Hirano, T., Kishimoto, T. and Martinez-Maza, O. (1990). *J. Immunol.* **144**, 480–484.
Campbell, I.L., Cutri, A., Wilson, A. and Harrison, L.C. (1989). *J. Immunol.* **143**, 1188–1191.
Campbell, I.L. and Harrison, C. (1990). *J. Autoimmunity,* **3**, 53–62.
Campbell, I.L., Kay, T.W., Oxbrow, L., Harrison, L.C. (1991). *J. Clin. Invest.* **87**, 739–742.
Cao, Z., R.M. Umek and S.L. Mcknight. (1991). *Genes Dev.* **5**, 1538–1552.
Caracciolo, D., Clark, S.C. and Rovera, G. (1989). *Blood* **73**, 666–670.
Carrington, P.A., Hill, R.J., Stenberg, P.E., Levin, J., Corash, L., Schreurs, J., Baker, G. and Levin, F.C. (1991). *Blood* **77**, 34–41.
Carter A., Merchav, S. Silvian Draxler, I. and Tatarsky, I. (1990). *Br. J. Haematol.* **74**, 424–431.
Castell, J.V., Gomez-Lechon, M.J., David, M., Hirano, T., Kishimoto, T. and Heinrich, P.C. (1988). *FEBS Lett.* **232**, 347–350.
Content, J., De Wit, L., Poupart, P., Opdenakker, G., Van Damme, J. and Billiau, A. (1985). *Eur. J. Biochem.* **152**, 253–257.
Davis, S., Aldrich, T.H., Valenzula, D.M., Wong, V., Furth, M.E., Squinto, S.P. and Yancopoulos, G.D. (1991). *Science* **253**, 59–63.
Davis, S., Aldrich, T.H., Ip, N.Y., Stahl, N., Scherer, S., Farrugella, T., DiStefano, P.S., Curtis, R., Panayotatos, N., Gascan, H., Chevalier, S. and Yancopoulos, G.D. (1993). *Science* **259**, 1736–1739.
De Groot, R.P., J. Auwerx, M., Karperien, B., Staels and W. Kruijer. (1991). *Nucl. Acids Res.* **19**, 775–781.
Deviere, J., Content, J., Denys, C., Vandenbussche, P., Schandene, L., Wybran, J. and Dupont, E. (1989). *Clin. Exp. Immunol.* **77**, 221–225.
Emilie, D., Peuchmaur, M., Malillot, M.C., Crevon, M.C., Brousse, N., Delfraissy, J.F., Dormont, J. and Galanaud, P. (1990). *J. Clin. Invest.* **86**, 148–159.
Espevik, T., Waage, A., Faxvaag, A. and Shalaby, M.R. (1990). *Cell. Immunol.* **126**, 47–56.
Fiedler, W., Weh H.J., Suciu, E. Wittlief, C., Stocking, C., Hossfeld DK. (1990). *Leukemia* **4**, 462–465.
Freeman, G.J., Freedman, A.S., Rabinowe, S.N., Segil, J.M., Horowitz, J., Rosen, K., Whitman, J.F. and Nadler, L.M. (1989). *J. Clin. Invest.* **83**, 1512–1518.
Frei, K., Leist, T.P., Meager, A., Gallo, P., Leppert, D., Zinkernagel, R.M. and Fontana, A. (1988). *J. Exp. Med.* **168**, 449–453.
Frei, K., Malipiero, U.V., Leist, T.P., Zinkernagel, R.M., Schwab, M.E. and Fontana, A. (1989). *Eur. J. Immunol.* **19**, 689–694.
Fukata, J., Usui, T., Naitoh, Y., Nakai, Y. and Imura, H. (1989). *J. Endocrinol.* **122**, 33–39.
Fujihashi, K., McGhee, J.R., Lue, C., Beagley, K.W., Taga, T., Hirano, T., Kishimoto, T., Mestecky, J. and Kiyono, H. (1991). *J. Clin. Invest.* **88**, 248–252.
Fujihashi, K., Kono, Y. and Kiyono, H. (1992). *Res. Immunol.* **143**, 744–749.
Fukunaga, R., Ishizaka-Ikeda, E., Pan, C-X., Seto, Y. and Nagata, S. (1991). *EMBO J.* **10**, 2855–2865.
Garman, R.D., Jacobs, K.A., Clark, S.C. and Raulet, D.H. (1987). *Proc. Natl Acad. Sci. USA.* **84**, 7629–7633.
Gauldie, J., Richards, C., Harnish, D., Lansdorp, P. and Baumann, H. (1987). *Proc. Natl Acad. Sci. USA* **84**, 7251–7255.
Gauldie, J., Richards, C. and Baumann, H. (1992). *Res. Immunol.* **143**, 755–759.
Gearing, D.P., Bruce, A.G. (1992). *New Biol.* **4**, 61–65.
Gearing, D.P., Cosman, D. (1991). *Cell.* **66**, 9–10.
Gearing, D., Gough, N.M., King, J.A., Hilton, D.J., Nicola, N.A., Simpson, R.J., Nice, E.C., Kelso, A. and Metcalf, D. (1987). *EMBO J.* **6**, 3995–4002.
Gearing, D.P., Thut, C.J., VandenBos, T., Gimpel, S.D., Delaney, P.B., King, J., Price, V., Cosman, D. and Beckman, M.P. (1991). *EMBO J.* **10**, 2839–2848.
Gearing, D.P., Comeau, M.R., Friend, D.J., Gimpel, S.D., Thut, C.J., Mcgourty, J., Brasher, K.K., King, J.A., Gills, S., Mosley, B., Ziagler, S.F. and Cosman, D. (1992). *Science* **255**, 1434–1437.

Geissler, K., Valent, P., Bettelheim, P., Sillaber, C., Wagner, B., Kyrle, P., Hinterberger, W., Lechner, K., Liehl, E. and Mayer, P. (1992) *Blood,* **79**, 1155–1160.

Geiger, T., Andus, T., Klapproth, J., Hirano, T., Kishimoto, T. and Heinrich, P.C. (1988). *Eur. J. Immunol.* **18**, 717–721.

Gibbons, R., Martinez, O., Matli, M., Heinzel, F., Bernstein, M. and Warren, R. (1990). *Lymphokine Res.* **9**, 283–293.

Grossman, R.M., Krueger, J., Yourish, D., Granelli-Piperno, A., Murphy, D.P., May, L.T., Kupper, T.S., Sehgal, P.B. and Gottlieb, A.B. (1989). *Proc. Natl Acad. Sci. USA.* **86**, 6367–6371.

Grunfeld, C., Adi, S., Soued, M., Moser, A., Fiers, W. and Feingold, K.R. (1990). *Cancer Res.* **50**, 4233–4238.

Haegeman, G., Content, J., Volckaert, G., Derynck, R., Tavernier, J. and Fiers, W. (1986). *Eur. J. Biochem.* **159**, 625–632.

Hama, T., Myamoto, M., Tsukui, H., Nishio, C. and Hatanaka, H. (1989). *Neurosci. Lett.* **104**, 340–344.

Hirano, T., Matsuda, T. and Nakajima, K. (1994). *Stem Cell* (in press).

Hata H., Matsuzaki, H. and Takatsuki, K. (1990). *Acta. Haematol Basel.* **83**, 133–136.

Hatakeyama, M., Kono, T., Kobayashi, N., Kawahara, A., Levin, S.D., Perlmutter, R.M. and Taniguchi, T. (1991). *Science* **252**, 1523–1528.

Hegyi E., Navarro, S., Debili, N., Mouthon, M.A., Katz, A., Breton-Gorius, J. and Vainchenker, W. (1990). *Int. J. Cell Cloning* **8**, 236–244.

Heinrich, P.C., Castell, J.V. and Andus, T. (1990). *Biochem. J.* **265**, 621–636.

Helfgott, D.C., May, L.T., Sthoeger, Z., Tamm, I. and Sehgal, P.B. (1987). *J. Exp. Med.* **186**, 1300–1309.

Helle, M., Brakenhoff, J.P.J., De Groot, E.R. and Aarden, L.A. (1988). *Eur. J. Immunol.* **18**, 957–959.

Helle, M., Boeije, L. and Aarden, L.A. (1989). *J. Immunol.* **142**, 4335–4338.

Hibi, M., Murakami, M., Saito, M., Hirano, T., Taga, T. and Kishimoto, T. (1990). *Cell* **63**, 1149–1157.

Hilbert, D.M., Cancro, M.P., Scherle, P.A., Nordan, R.P., Van-Snick, J., Gerhard, W. and Rudikoff, S. (1989). *J. Immunol.* **143**, 4019–4024.

Hirano, T. (1991). *Int. J. Cell Cloning* **9**, 166–184.

Hirano, T. (1992a). *Chem. Immunol.* **51**, 153–180.

Hirano, T. (1992b). *Res. Immunol.* **143**, 759–763.

Hirano, T. and Kishimoto, T. (1990) In *Handbook of Experimental Pharmacology Peptide Growth Factors and Their Receptors* vol. 95/I (ed. M.B. Sporn and A.B. Roberts), Springer, Berlin, pp. 633–665.

Hirano, T., Teranishi, T., Toba, T., Sakaguchi, N., Fukukawa, T. and Tsuyuguchi, I. (1981). *J. Immunol.* **126**, 517–522.

Hirano, T., Teranishi, T., Lin, B.H. and Onoue, K. (1984a). *J. Immunol.* **133**, 798–802.

Hirano, T., Teranishi, T. and Onoue, K. (1984b). *J. Immunol.* **132**, 229–234.

Hirano, T., Taga, T., Nakano, N., Yasukawa, K., Kashiwamura, S., Shimizu, K., Nakajima, K., Pyun, K.H. and Kishimoto, T. (1985). *Proc. Natl. Acad. Sci. USA.* **82**, 5490–5494.

Hirano, T., Yasukawa, K., Harada, H., Taga, T., Watanabe, Y., Matsuda, T., Kashiwamura, S., Nakajima, K., Koyama, K., Iwamatsu, A., Tsunasawa, S., Sakiyama, F., Matsui, H., Takahara, Y., Taniguchi, T. and Kishimoto, T. (1986). *Nature* **324**, 73–76.

Hirano, T., Taga, T., Yasukawa, K., Nakajima, K., Nakano, N., Takatsuki, F., Shimizu, M., Murashima, A., Tsunasawa, S., Sakiyama, F. and Kishimoto, T. (1987). *Proc. Natl Acad. Sci. USA.* **84**, 228–231.

Hirano, T., Matsuda, T., Turner, M., Miyasaka, N., Buchan, G., Tang, B., Sato, K., Shimizu, M., Maini, R., Feldman, M. and Kishimoto, T. (1988). *Eur. J. Immunol.* **18**, 1797–1801.

Hocke, G., Barry, D. and Gey, G.H. (1992). *Mol. Cell Biol.* **12**, 2282–2294.

Hodgkin, P.D., Bond, M.W., O'Garra, A., Frank, G., Lee, F., Coffman, R.L., Zlotnik, A. and Howard, M. (1988). *J. Immunol.* **141**, 151–157.

Holsti, M.A. and Raulet, D.H. (1989). *J. Immunol.* **143**, 2514–2519.

Honda, M., Yamamoto, S., Cheng, M., Yasukawa, K., Suzuki, H., Saito, T., Osugi, Y., Tokunaga, T. and Kishimoto, T. (1992). *J. Immunol.* **148**, 2175–2180.

Horii, Y., Muraguchi, A., Suematu, S., Matsuda, T., Yoshizaki, K., Hirano, T. and Kishimoto, T. (1988). *J. Immunol.* **141**, 1529–1535.

Horii, Y., Muraguchi, A., Iwano, M., Matsuda, T., Hirayama, T., Yamada, H., Fujii, Y., Dohi, K., Ishikawa, H., Ohmoto, Y., Yoshizaki, K., Hirano, T. and Kishimoto, T. (1989). *J. Immunol.* **143**, 3949–3955.

Houssiau, F. and Van Snick, J. (1992). *Res. Immunol.* **143**, 740–743.

Houssiau, F.A., Coulie, P.G., Olive, D. and Van Snick, J. (1988). *Eur. J. Immunol.* **18**, 653–656.

Houssiau, F.A., Coulie, P.G. and Van Snick, J. (1989). *J. Immunol.* **143**, 2520–2524.

164   T. Hirano

Ida, N., Sakurai, S., Hosaka, T., Hosoi, K., Kunitomo, T., Shimazu, T., Maruyama, Y. and Kahase, M. (1989). *Biochem. Biophys. Res. Commun.* **165**, 728–734.

Ikebuchi, K., Wong, G.G., Clark, S.C., Ihle, J.N., Hirai, Y. and Ogawa, M. (1987). *Proc. Natl Acad. Sci. USA.* **84**, 9035–9039.

Ip, N.Y., Nye, S.H., Boulton, T.G., Davis, S., Taga, T., Li, Y., Birren, S.J., Yasukawa, K., Kishimoto, T., Anderson, D.J. Stahl, N. and Yancopoulos, G.D. (1992). *Cell* **69**, 1121–1132.

Ishibashi, T., Kimura, H., Uchida, T., Kariyone, S., Friese, P. and Burstein, S.A. (1989a). *Proc. Natl Acad. Sci. USA.* **86**, 5953–5957.

Ishibashi, T., Kimura, H., Shikama, Y., Uchida, T., Kariyone, S., Hirano, T., Kishimoto, T., Takasuki, F. and Akiyama, Y. (1989b). *Blood* **74**, 1241–1244.

Isobe, T. and Osserman, E.F. (1971). *Ann. NY. Acad. Sci.* **190**, 507–517.

Isomaki, H.A., Hakulinen, T. and Joutsenlahti, U. (1978). *J. Chronic Dis.* **31**, 691–696.

Isshiki, H., Akira, S., Tanabe, O., Nakajima, T., Shimamoto, T., Hirano, T. and Kishimoto, T. (1990). *Mol. Cell. Biol.* **10**, 2757–2764.

Jilka, R.L., Hangoc, G., Girasole, G., Passeri, G., Williams, D.C., Abrams, J.S., Boyce, B., Broxmeyer, H. and Manolagas, S.C. (1992). *Science* **257**, 88–91.

Jourdan, M., Bataille, R., Seguin, J., Zhang, X.G., Chaptal, P.A. and Klein, B. (1990). *Arthritis Rheum.* **33**, 398–402.

Kameda, T., Matsuzaki N., Sawai, K., Okada, T., Saji, F., Matsuda, T., Hirano, T., Kishimoto, T. and Tanizawa, O. (1990). *Placenta.* **11**, 205–213.

Kasid, A., Director, E.P. and Rosenberg, S.A. (1989). *J. Immunol.* **143**, 736–739.

Kawakami, K., Kakimoto, K., Shinbori, T. and Onoue, K. (1989). *Immunology* **67**, 314–320.

Kawano, M., Hirano, T., Matsuda, T., Taga, T., Horii, Y., Iwato, K., Asaoku, H., Tang, B., Tanabe, O., Tanaka, H., Kuramoto, A. and Kishimoto, T. (1988). *Nature* **332**, 83–85.

Kikutani, H., Taga, T., Akira, S., Kishi, H., Miki, Y., Saiki, O., Yamamura, Y. and Kishimoto, T. (1985). *J. Immunol.* **134**, 990–995.

Kishimoto, T. and Hirano, T. (1988). *Annu. Rev. Immunol.* **6**, 485–512.

Kitajima, I., Shinohara, T., Bilakovics, J., Brown, D.A., Xu, X. and Nerenberg, M. (1992). *Science* **258**, 1792–1794.

Klein, B., Zhang, X.G., Jourdan, M., Content, J., Houssiau, F., Aarden, L., Piechaczyk, M. and Bataille, R. (1989). *Blood* **73**, 517–526.

Klein, B., Wijdenes, J., Zhang, X.G., Jourdan, M., Boiron, J.M., Brochier, J., Liautard, J., Merlin, M., Clement, C., Morel-Fournier, B., Lu, Z.Y., Mannoni, P., Sany, J. and Bataille, R. (1991). *Blood* **5**, 1198–1204.

Kohase, M., May, L.T., Tamm, I., Vilček, J. and Sehgal, P.B. (1987). *Mol. Cell. Biol.* **7**, 273–280.

Kopf, M., Baumann, H., Freer, G., Frudenberg, M., Lamers, M., Kishimoto, T., Zinkernagel, R., Bluethmann, H. and Kohler, G. (1994). *Nature* **368**, 339–342.

Krüttgen, A., Rosejohn, S., Môller, C., Wroblowski, B., Wollmer, A., Müllberg, J., Hirano, T., Kishimoto, T. and Heinrich, P.C. (1990). *FEBS Lett.* **262**, 323–326.

Le, J. and Vilček, J. (1989). *Lab. Invest.* **61**, 588–602.

Le, J., Fredrickson, G., Reis, L.F.L., Diamantstein, T., Hirano, T., Kishimoto, T. and Vilček, J. (1988). *Proc. Natl Acad. Sci. USA.* **85**, 8643–8647.

Libermann, T.A. and Baltimore, D. (1990). *Mol. Cell Biol.* **10**, 2327–2334.

Liu, C.C., Joag, S.V., Kwon, B.S. and Young, J.D. (1990). *J. Immunol.* **144**, 1196–1201.

Loppnow, H. and Libby, P. (1990) *J. Clin. Invest.* **85**, 731–738.

Lord, F.A., Abdollahi, A., Thomas, S.M., DeMarco, M., Brugge, J.S., Hoffman-Liebermann, B. and Liebermann, D.A. (1991). *Mol. Cell Biol.* **11**, 4371–4379.

Lotem, J., Shabo, Y. and Sachs, L. (1989). *Blood* **74**, 1545–1551.

Lotz, M., Jirik, F., Kabouridis, R., Tsoukas, C., Hirano, T., Kishimoto, T. and Carson, D.A. (1988). *J. Exp. Med.* **167**, 1253–1258.

Lust, J.A., Donovan, K.A., Kline, M.P., Greipp, P.R., Kyle, R.A. and Maihle, N.J. (1992). *Cytokine* **4**, 96–100.

Lutticken, C., Wegenka, U.M., Yuan, J., Buschmann, J., Schindler, C., Ziemiecki, A., Harpur, A.G., Wilks, A.F., Yasukawa, K., Taga, T., Kishimoto, T., Barbieri, G., Pellegrini, S., Sendtner, M., Heinrich, P.C. and Horn, F. (1993). *Science* **263**, 89–92.

Majello, B., Arcone, R., Toniatti, C. and Ciliberto, G. (1990). *EMBO J.* **9**, 457–465.

Matsuda, T., Nakajima, T., Kaisho, T., Nakajima, K. and Hirano, T. (1994). *Adv. Biochem. Biol. Membrane*, in press.

Matusda, T. and Hirano, T. (1994b). *Blood* (in press).

May, L.T., Helfgott, D.C. and Sehgal, P.B. (1986). *Proc. Natl Acad. Sci. USA.* **83**, 8957–8961.

May, L.T., Grayeb, J., Santhanam, U., Tatter, S.B., Sthoeger, Z., Helfgott, D.C., Chiorazzi, N., Grieninger, G. and Sehgal, P.B. (1988). *J. Biol. Chem.* **263**, 7760–7766.

Miki, S., Iwano, M., Miki, Y., Yamamoto, M., Tang, B., Yokokawa, K., Sonoda, T., Hirano, T. and Kishimoto, T. (1989). *FEBS Lett.* **250**, 607–610.

Miles, S.A., Rezai, A.R., Salazar-Gonzalez, J.F., Meyden, M.V., Stevens, R.H., Logan, D.M., Mitsuyasu, R.T., Taga, T., Hirano, T., Kishimoto, T. and Martinez-Maza, O. (1990). *Proc. Natl Acad. Sci. USA.* **87**, 4068–4072.

Miyajima, A., Kitamura, T., Harada, N., Yokota, T. and Arai, K. (1992). *Annu. Rev. Immunol.* **10**, 295–331.

Metcalf, D. (1989). *Leukemia* **3**, 349–355.

Miller, A.E., Ennist, D.L., Ozatao, K. and Westphal, H. (1992) *Immunogenetics,* **35**, 24–32.

Minty, P., Chalon, P., Derocq, J.-M., Dumont, X., Guillemont, J.-C., Kaghad, M., Labit, C., Leplatois, P., Liauzum, P., Miloux, B., Minty, C., Casellas, P., Loison, G., Lupker, J., Shire, D., Ferrara, P. and Caput, D. (1993). *Nature,* **362**, 248–250.

Miyaura, C., Onozaki, K., Akiyama, Y., Taniyama, T., Hirano, T., Kishimoto, T. and Suda, T. (1988). *FEBS Lett.* **234**, 17–21.

Mock, B.A., Nordan, R.P., Justice, M.J., Kozak, C., Jenkins, N.A., Copeland, N.G., Clask, S.C., Wong, G.G. and Rudikoff, S. (1989). *J. Immunol.* **142**, 1372–1376.

Murakami, M., Narazaki, M., Hibi, M., Yawata, H., Yasukawa, K., Hamaguchi, M., Taga, T. and Kishimoto, T. (1991). *Proc. Natl Acad. Sci. USA.* **88**, 11349–11353.

Muraguchi, A., Hirano, T., Tang, B., Matsuda, T., Horii, Y., Nakajima, K. and Kishimoto, T. (1988). *J. Exp. Med.* **67**, 332–344.

Muraoka, O., Kaisho, T., Tanabe, M. and Hirano, T. (1993). *Immunol. Lett.* **37**, 159–165.

Nabata, T., Morimoto, S., Koh, E., Shiraishi, T. and Ogihara, T. (1990). *Biochem. Int.* **20**, 445–453.

Nagasawa, T., Orita, T., Matsushita, J., Tsuchiya, M., Neichi, T., Imazeki, I., Imai, N., Ochi, N., Kanma, H. and Abe, T. (1990). *FEBS Lett.* **260**, 176–178.

Nakao, H., Nishikawa, A., Nishiura, T., Kanayama, Y., Tarui, S. and Taniguchi, N. (1991). *Clin. Chim. Acta.* **197**, 221–228.

Nakayama, K., Shimizu, H., Mitomo, K., Watanabe, T., Okamoto, S. and Yamamoto, K. (1992). *Mol. Cell Biol.* **12**, 1736–1746.

Naitoh, Y., Fukata, J., Tominaga, T., Nakai, Y., Tamai, S., Mori, K. and Imura, H. (1988). *Biochem. Biophys. Res. Commun.* **155**, 1459–1463.

Nakajima, K. and Wall. R. (1991). *Mol. Cell Biol.* **11**, 1409–1418.

Nakajima, K., Martinez-Maza, O., Hirano, T., Nishanian, P., Salazar-Gonzalez, J.F., Fahey, J.L. and Kishimoto, T. (1989). *J. Immunol.* **142**, 144–147.

Nakajima, K., Kusafuka, T., Takeda, T., Fujitani, Y., Nakae, K. and Hirano, T. (1993). *Mol. Cell Biol.* **13**, 3027–3041.

Namba, Y. and Hanaoka, M. (1972). *J. Immunol.* **109**, 1193–1200.

Neurath, A.R., Strick, N. and Li, Y.-Y. (1992). *J. Exp. Med.* **176**, 1561–1569.

Nicola, N.A., Metcalf, D., Matsumoto, M. and Johnson, G.R. (1983). *J. Biol. Chem.* **258**, 9017–9023.

Nijstein, M.W.N., De Groot, E.R., Ten Duis, H.J., Klasen, H.J., Hack, C.E. and Aarden, L.A. (1987). *Lancet* **ii**, 921.

Nishimoto, N., Yoshizaki, K., Tagoh, H., Monden, M., Kishimoto, S., Hirano, T. and Kishimoto, T. (1989). *Clin. Immunol. Immunopathol.* **50**, 399–401.

Noma, T., Mizuta, T., Rosen, A., Hirano, T., Kishimoto, T. and Honjo, T. (1987). *Immunol. Lett.* **15**, 249–253.

Nordan, R.P. and Potter, M. (1986). *Science* **233**, 566–569.

Northemann, W., Braciak, T.A., Hattori, M., Lee, F. and Fey, G.H. (1989). *J. Biol. Chem.* **264**, 16072–16082.

Novick, D., Engelmann, H., Wallach, D. and Rubinstein, M. (1989). *J. Exp. Med.* **170**, 1409–1414.

Ogawa, M. (1992). *Res. Immunol.* **143**, 749–751.

Ohtake, K., Yano, T., Kameda, K. and Ogawa, T. (1990). *Am. J. Hematol.* **35**, 84–87.

Okada, M., Sakaguchi, N., Yoshimura, N., Hara, H., Shimizu, K., Yoshida, H., Yoshizaki, K., Kishimoto, S., Yamamura, Y. and Kishimoto, T. (1993). *J. Exp. Med.* **157**, 583–590.

Okada, M., Kitahara, M., Kishimoto, S., Matsuda, T., Hirano, T. and Kishimoto, T. (1988). *J. Immunol.* **141**, 1543–1549.

Okano, A., Suzuki, C., Takatsuki, F., Akiyama, Y., Koike, K., Ozawa, K., Hirano, T., Kishimoto, T., Nakahata, T. and Asano, S. (1989a). *Transplantation* **48**, 495–498.

Okano, A., Suzuki, C., Takatsuki, F., Akiyama, Y., Koike, K., Nakahata, T., Hirano, T., Kishimoto, T., Ozawa, K. and Asano, S. (1989b). *Transplantation* **47**, 738–740.

Onozaki, K., Akiyama, Y., Okano, A., Hirano, T., Kishimoto, T., Hashimoto, T., Yoshizawa, K. and Taniyama, T. (1989). *Cancer Res.* **49**, 3602–3607.

Oritani, K., Kaisho, T., Nakajima, K., Hirano, T. (1992). *Blood* **80**, 2298–2305.

Poli, V. and Cortese, R. (1989). *Proc. Natl Acad. Sci. USA.* **86**, 8202–8206.

Poli, V., Mancini, F.P. and Cortese, R. (1990a). *Cell* **63**, 643–653.

Poli, V., Bressler, P., Kinter, A., Duh, E., Timmer, W.C., Rabson, A., Justerment, J.S., Stanley, S. and Fauci, A.S. (1990b). *J. Exp. Med.* **172**, 151–158.

Poli, V., Balenna, R., Fattori, E., Markatos, A., Yamamoto, M., Tanaka, H., Ciliberto, F., Rodan, G.A. and Costantini, F. (1994). *EMBO J.* **13**, 1189–1196.

Potter, M. and Boyce, C. (1962). *Nature* **193**, 1086–1087.

Ray, A., Tatter, S.B., May, L.T. and Sehgal, P.B. (1988). *Proc. Natl Acad. Sci. USA.* **85**, 6701–6705.

Ray, A., Sassone Corsi, P. and Sehgal, P.B. (1989). *Mol. Cell Biol.* **9**, 5537–5547.

Raynal, M.C., Liu, Z.Y., Hirano, T., Mayer, L., Kishimoto, T. and Chen Kiang, S. (1989). *Proc. Natl Acad. Sci. USA.* **86**, 8024–8028.

Renauld, J.C., Vink, A. and Van Snick, J. (1989). *J. Immunol.* **143**, 1894–1898.

Revel, M. (1992). *Res. Immunol.* **143**, 769–773.

Richards, C.D., Brown, T.J., Shoyab, M., Baumann, H. and Gauldie, J. (1992). *J. Immunol.* **148**, 1731–1736.

Rook, G.A.W., Thompson, S., Buckley, M., Elson, C., Brealey, R., Lambert, C., White, T. and Rademacher, T. (1991). *Eur. J. Immunol.* **21**, 1027–1032.

Rook, G.A.W. and Stanford, J.L. (1992). *Immunol. Today,* **13**, 160–164.

Rose, T.M. and Bruce, A.G. (1991). *Proc. Natl Acad. Sci. USA.* **88**, 8641–8645.

Rosselli, F., Sanceau, J., Wietzerbin, J. and Moustacchi, E. (1992). *Hum. Genet.* **89**, 42–48.

Ruef, C., Budde, K., Lacy, J., Northemann, W., Baumann, M., Sterzel, R.B. and Coleman, D.L. (1990). *Kidney Int.* **38**, 249–257.

Sachs, L. (1987). *Science* **238**, 1374–1379.

Sadowski, H.B., Shuai, K., Darnell Jr, J.E. and Gilman, M.Z. (1993). *Science* **261**, 1739–1744.

Santhanam, U., Ghrayeb, J., Sehgal, P.B. and May, L.T. (1989). *Arch. Biochem. Biophys.* **274**, 161–170.

Saito, M., Yoshida, K., Hibi, M., Taga, T. and Kishimoto, T. (1992). *J. Immunol.* **148**, 4066–4071.

Satoh, T., Nakamura, S., Taga, T., Matsuda, T., Hirano, T., Kishimoto, T. and Kaziro, Y. (1988). *Mol. Cell. Biol.* **8**, 3546–3549.

Scala, G., Quinto, I., Ruocco, M.R., Arcucci, A., Mallardo, M., Caretto, P., Forni, G. and Venuta, S. (1990). *J. Exp. Med.* **172**, 61–68.

Sehgal, P.B. (1992). *Res. Immunol.* **143**, 724–734.

Sehgal, P.B., Zilberstein, A., Ruggieri, R.M., May, L.T., Ferguson Smith, A., Slate, D.L., Revel, M. and Ruddle, F. (1986). *Proc. Natl Acad. Sci. USA.* **83**, 5219–5222.

Sehgal, P.B., May, L.T., Tamm, I. and Vilček, J. (1987a). *Science* **235**, 731–732.

Sehgal, P.B., Walther, Z. and Tamm, I. (1987b). *Proc. Natl Acad. Sci. USA.* **84**, 3663–3667.

Sehgal, P.B., Helfgott, D.C., Santhanam, U., Tatter, S.B., Clarick, R.H., Ghrayeb, J. and May, L.T. (1988). *J. Exp. Med.* **167**, 1951–1956.

Sehgal, P.B., Grienger, G. and Tosata, G. (1989). *Ann. NY. Acad. Sci.* **557**, 1–583.

Sela, O., El-Roeiy, O., Isenberg, D.A. (1987). Arthritis Rheum. **30**, 50–56.

Shabo, Y., Lotem, J., Rubinstein, M., Revel, M., Clark, S.C., Wolf, S.F., Kamen, R. and Sachs, L. (1988). *Blood* **72**, 2070–2073.

Shenkin, A., Fraser, W.D., Series, J., Winstanley, F.P., McCartney, A.C., Burns, H.J. and Van Damme, J. (1989). *Lymphokine Res.* **8**, 123–127.

Shimizu, S., Hirano, T., Yoshioka, K., Sugai, S., Matsuda, T., Taga, T., Kishimoto, T. and Konda, S. (1988). *Blood* **72**, 1826–1828.

Shimizu, S., Yoshioka, R., Hirose, Y., Sugai, S., Tachibana, J. and Konda, S. (1989). *J. Exp. Med.* **169**, 339–344.

Shimizu, H., Mitomo, K., Watanabe, T., Okamoto, S. and Yamamoto, K. (1990). *Mol. Cell Biol.* **10**, 561–568.

Shoenfeld, Y. and Isenberg, D.A. (1988). *Immunol. Today* **9**, 178–182.
Smeland, E.B., Blomhoff, H.K., Funderud, S., Shalaby, M.R. and Espevik, T. (1989). *J. Exp. Med.* **170**, 1463–1468.
Spangelo, B.L., Judd, A.M., Isakson, P.C. and MacLeod, R.M. (1989). *Endocrinology* **125**, 575–577.
Spangelo, B.L., MacLeod, R.M. and Isakson, P.C. (1990). *Endocrinology* **126**, 582–586.
Splawski, J.B., McAnally, L.M. and Lipsky, P.E. (1990). *J. Immunol.* **144**, 562–569.
Stahl, N., Boulton, T.G., Farruggella, T., Ip, N.Y., Davis, S., Witthuhn, B.A., Quelle, F.W., Silvernnoinen, O., Barbieri, G., Pellgrini, S., Ihle, J.N. and Yancopoulos, G.D. (1993). *Science* **263**, 92–95.
Suematsu, S., Matsuda, T., Aozasa, K., Akira, S., Nakano, N., Ohno, S., Miyazaki, J., Yamamura, K., Hirano, T. and Kishimoto, T. (1989). *Proc. Natl Acad. Sci. USA.* **86**, 7547–7551.
Suematsu, S., Matsusaka, T., Matsuda, T., Ohno, S., Miyazaki, J., Yamamura, K., Hirano, T. and Kishimoto, T. (1992). *Proc. Natl Acad. Sci. USA.* **89**, 232–235.
Sugita, T., Totsuka, T., Saito, M., Yamasaki, K., Taga, T., Hirano, T. and Kishimoto, T. (1990). *J. Exp. Med.* **171**, 2001–2009.
Suzuki, C., Okano, A., Takatsuki, F., Miyasaka, Y., Hirano, T., Kishimoto, T., Ejima, D. and Akiyama, Y. (1989). *Biochem. Biophys. Res. Commun.* **159**, 933–938.
Taga, T., Hibi, M., Hirata, Y., Yamasaki, K., Yasukawa, K., Matsuda, T., Hirano, T. and Kishimoto, T. (1989). *Cell* **58**, 573–581.
Taga, T., Narazaki, M., Yasukawa, K., Saito, T., Miki, D., Hamaguchi, M., Davis, S., Shoyab, M., Yancopoulos, G.D. and Kishimoto, T. (1992). *Proc. Natl Acad. Sci. USA.* **89**, 10998–11001.
Takai, Y., Wong, G.G., Clark, S.C., Burakoff, S.J. and Herrmann, S.H. (1988). *J. Immunol.* **140**, 508–512.
Takai, Y., Seki, N., Senoh, H., Yokota, T., Lee, F., Hamaoka, T. and Fujiwara, H. (1989). *Arthritis Rheum.* **32**, 594–600.
Takatsuki, F., Okano, A., Suzuki, C., Chieda, R., Takahara, Y., Hirano, T., Kishimoto, T., Hamuro, J. and Akiyama, Y. (1988). *J. Immunol.* **141**, 3072–3077.
Tanabe, O., Akira, S., Kamiya, T., Wong, G.G., Hirano, T. and Kishimoto, T. (1988). *J. Immunol.* **41**, 3875–3881.
Tang, B., Matsuda, T., Akira, S., Nagata, N., Ikehara, S., Hiranio, T. and Kishimoto, T. (1993). *International Immunol.* **3**, 273–278.
Teranishi, T., Hirano, T., Arima, N. and Onoue, K. (1982). *J. Immunol.* **128**, 1903–1908.
Teranishi, T., Hirano, T., Lin, B.H. and Onoue, K. (1984). *J. Immunol.* **133**, 3062–3067.
Tohyama, N., Karasuyama, H. and Tada, T. (1990). *J. Exp. Med.* **171**, 389–400.
Tomida, M., Yamamoto-Yamaguchi, Y. and Hozumi, M. (1984). *J. Biol. Chem.* **259**, 10978–10982.
Toniatti, C., Demartis, A., Monaci, P., Nicosia, A. and Ciliberto, G. (1990). *EMBO J.* **9**, 4467–4475.
Tosato, G., Seamon, K.B., Goldman, N.D., Sehgal, P.B., May, L.T., Washington, G.C., Jones, K.D. and Pike, S.E. (1988). *Science* **239**, 502–504.
Uyttenhove, C., Coulie, P.G. and Van Snick, J. (1988). *J. Exp. Med.* **167**, 1417–1427.
Van Damme, J., Opdenakker, G., Simpson, R.J., Rubira, M.R., Cayphas, S., Vink, A., Billiau, A. and Snick, J.V. (1987a). *J. Exp. Med.* **165**, 914–919.
Van Damme, J., Cayphas, S., Opdenakker, G., Billiau, A. and Van Snick, J. (1987b). *Eur. J. Immunol.* **17**, 1–7.
Van Damme, J., Schaafsma, M.R., Fibbe, W.E., Falkenburg, J.H., Opdenakker, G. and Billiau, A. (1989). *Eur. J. Immunol.* **19**, 163–168.
Van Snick, J. (1990). *Ann. Rev. Immunol.* **8**, 253–278.
Van Snick, J., Vink, A., Cayphas, S. and Uyttenhove, C. (1987). *J. Exp. Med.* **165**, 641–649.
Van Snick, J., Cayphas, S., Szikora, J.-P., Renauld, J.-C., Van Roost, E., Boon, T. and Simpson, R.J. (1988). *Eur. J. Immunol.* **18**, 193–197.
Vercelli, D., Jabara, H.H., Arai, K., Yokota, T. and Geha, R.S. (1989). *Eur. J. Immunol.* **19**, 1419–1424.
Velde, A., Huijbens, R.J., Heije, K., Varies, J. and Figdor, C.G. (1990). *Blood* **76**, 1392–1397.
Vink, A., Coulie, P.G., Wauters, P., Nordan, R.P. and Van Snick, J. (1988). *Eur. J. Immunol.* **18**, 607–612.
Vink, A., Coulie, P., Warnier, G., Renauld, J.C., Stevens, M., Donckers, D. and Van Snick, J. (1990). *J. Exp. Med.* **172**, 997–1000.
Waage, A., Brandtzaeg, P., Halstensen, A., Kierulf, P. and Espevik, T. (1989). *J. Exp. Med.* **169**, 333–338.
Wegenka, U.M., Buschmann, J., Lutticken, C., Heinrich, P.C. and Horn, F. (1993). *Mol. Cell Biol.* **13**, 276–288.

Weissenbach, J., Chernajovsky, Y., Zeevi, M., Shulman, L., Soreq, H., Nir, U., Wallach, D., Perricaudet, M., Tiollais, P. and Revel, M. (1980). *Proc. Natl Acad. Sci. USA.* **77**, 7152–7156.

Williams, N., De Giorgio, T., Banu, N., Withy, R., Hirano, T. and Kishimoto, T. (1990). *Exp. Hematol.* **18**, 69–72.

Wolf, S.F., Temple, P.A., Kobayashi, M., Young, D., Dicig, M., Lowe, L., Dzialo, R., Fitz, L., Ferenz, C., Hewick, R.M., Kelleher, K., Herrmann, S.H., Clark, S., Azzoni, L., Chan, S., Trinchieri, G. and Perussia, B. (1991). *J. Immunol.* **146**, 3074–3081.

Wong, G.H.W. and Goeddel, D.V. (1986). *Nature* **323**, 819–822.

Xia, X., Lee, H.K., Clark, S.C. and Choi, Y.S. (1989). *Eur. J. Immunol.* **19**, 2275–2281.

Yamasaki, K., Taga, T., Hirata, Y., Yawata, H., Kawanishi, Y., Seed, B., Taniguchi, T., Hirano, T. and Kishimoto, T. (1988). *Science* **241**, 825–828.

Yasukawa, K., Hirano, T., Watanabe, Y., Muratani, K., Matsuda, T. and Kishimoto, T. (1987). *EMBO J.* **6**, 2939–2945.

Yoshizaki, K., Nakagawa, T., Kaieda, T., Muraguchi, A., Yamamura, Y. and Kishimoto, T. (1982). *J. Immunol.* **128**, 1296–1301.

Yokoi, T., Miyawaki, T., Yachie, A., Kato, K., Kasahara, Y. and Taniguchi, N. (1990). *Immunology* **70**, 100–105.

Yoshizaki, K., Matsuda, T., Nishimoto, N., Kuritani, T., Taeho, L., Aozasa, K., Nakahata, T., Kawai, H., Tagoh, H., Komori, T., Kishimoto, S., Hirano, T. and Kishimoto, T. (1989). *Blood* **74**, 1360–1367.

Zhang, Y., Lin, J.-X. and Vilček, J. (1988a). *J. Biol. Chem.* **263**, 6177–6182.

Zhang, Y., Lin, J.-X., Yip, Y.K. and Vilček, J. (1988b). *Proc. Natl Acad. Sci. USA.* **85**, 6802–6805.

Zhang, X.-G., Klein, B. and Bataille, R. (1989). *Blood* **74**, 11–13.

Zhang, Y., Lin, J.-X. and Vilček, J. (1990). *Mol. Cell Biol.* **10**, 3818–3823.

Zilberstein, A., Ruggieri, R., Korn, J.H. and Revel, M. (1986). *EMBO J.* **5**, 2529–2537.

Chapter 9

Interleukin-7

Howard Edington and Michael T. Lotze

Departments of Surgery, Molecular Genetics and Biochemistry, University of Pittsburgh
Medical Center and the Biological Therapeutics Division of the Pittsburgh Cancer Center,
Pittsburgh, PA, USA

INTRODUCTION

The steps governing the development and maturation of lymphoid cell subsets (lympho-poietins) are not completely understood. Interleukin-7 (IL-7) appears to be at least one factor acting during early development of lymphoid cells. IL-7 was first identified as a factor derived from bone-marrow stroma. The development of a method of *in vitro* study of marrow lymphopoiesis by Whitlock and Witte in 1984 — the Whitlock–Witte cultures — represented a major advance, enabling investigators to dissect further the regulatory microenvironment of the bone marrow (Whitlock and Witte, 1982; Whitlock *et al.*, 1984). B-cell proliferation and maturation from early progenitors requires a fairly complex orchestration of signals mediated by cytokines including IL-7 and other signals by stromal cells which may involve cytokines or direct cell–cell interaction. IL-7 plays a major role in B-cell development and maturation. In addition, IL-7 is a T-cell growth factor and stimulates growth of both mature peripheral T cells and fetal T cells. IL-7 also activates NK precursors, inducing cytolytic activity. Its role in NK cell ontogeny from bone-marrow cells is not understood. Further clarification of the other factors influencing lymphopoiesis and their interaction with IL-7/IL-7R signalling will significantly advance our understanding of a number of diverse pathological states, including immunodeficiency disorders and malignancies facilitating a number of therapeutic endeavours including bone marrow and organ transplantation, as well as cancer immunotherapy.

CLONING AND PURIFICATION

Following the development of techniques for studying bone-marrow cultures, it was apparent that B-cell maturation required the presence of bone-marrow stromal cells, suggesting the existence of a growth and/or maturation-enhancing cytokine (Hunt *et al.*, 1987). Namen and associates demonstrated that conditioned medium from stromal cell cultures stimulated the growth of B-cell precursors. They immortalized a stromal cell line by transfecting it with the plasmid pSV3neo (encoding both the large and small

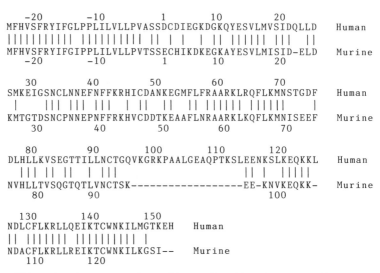

```
      -20         -10           1          10          20
      MFHVSFRYIFGLPPLILVLLPVASSDCDIEGKDGKQYESVLMVSIDQLLD    Human
      ||||||||||| ||||||||||| || |  |  | || ||||||| ||| ||
      MFHVSFRYIFGIPPLILVLLPVTSSECHIKDKEGKAYESVLMISID-ELD    Murine
      -20         -10           1          10          20


       30          40          50          60          70
      SMKEIGSNCLNNEFNFFKRHICDANKEGMFLFRAARKLRQFLKMNSTGDF    Human
      |    ||| ||| ||| | ||  ||  || ||||||| ||||||    |
      KMTGTDSNCPNNEPNFFRKHVCDDTKEAAFLNRAARKLKQFLKMNISEEF    Murine
       30          40          50          60          70


       80          90         100         110         120
      DLHLLKVSEGTTILLNCTGQVKGRKPAALGEAQPTKSLEENKSLKEQKKL    Human
      ||| || ||  | | |||                        || |  |||||
      NVHLLTVSQGTQTLVNCTSK------------------EE-KNVKEQKK-    Murine
       80          90                              100


      130         140         150
      NDLCFLKRLLQEIKTCWNKILMGTKEH    Human
      || |||||||| |||||||||||| |
      NDACFLKRLLREIKTCWNKILKGSI--    Murine
      110         120
```

Fig. 1. Amino acid homology between murine and human IL-7. (From Goodwin, R.G. and Namen, A.E. (1991). In: *The Cytokine Handbook* (Ed. A. Thomson), Academic Press with permission.)

T antigens of SV40) and isolated a clone (I×N/A6) which produced a factor initially called lymphopoietin-1 (LP-1) that stimulated the growth of B-cell precursors. Conditioned medium from the growth of this clone was then purified. High-performance liquid chromatography (HPLC) column fractions containing LP-1 bioactivity were isolated. A single unit of LP-1 activity is that causing half-maximal ^{3}H-TdR incorporation in a culture of precursor B cells (LP-1 bioassay). At this stage of purification it was clear that several proteins were present in the fraction that could account for the biological activity. Additional sodium dodecyl sulphate-polyacrylamide gel electrophoresis (SDS-PAGE) analysis associated bioactivity with a protein of 25×10^3 Da. This observation was substantiated by ^{125}I-labelled LP-1 binding experiments. The purified protein has a specific activity of approx 4×10^6 U/μg of protein and is active at a half-maximal concentration of 10^{-13} M (Namen *et al.*, 1988). The same murine stromal cell clone provided a cDNA library which was screened for LP-1 activity following expression in COS-7 cells. A clone (1046) was identified that was associated with a high biological activity. The nucleotide sequence was determined (see Fig. 1). The sequence contains a 548 bp 5′ noncoding region which may be involved in expression regulation, since its removal results in increased COS cell production of protein. The sequence includes a 462 bp coding sequence and a 579 bp 3′ noncoding region containing a consensus polyadenylation signal and terminating in 15 adenine residues. Purified protein was subjected to *N*-terminal analysis. Results suggested that the nucleotide sequence from clone 1046 codes for the same protein identified in the biological assay: the protein was named IL-7. The mature protein has a 25-amino-acid leader sequence followed by 129 amino acids with two N-linked glycosylation sites and six cysteine residues, which may be involved with intramolecular disulphide-bond formation. Biological activity is lost following treatment with 2-mercaptoethanol which breaks disulphide bonds. The calculated molecular weight of IL-7 is 14.9 kDa. The disparity between calculated molecular weight and that predicted by migration of the native protein (25 kDa) may be accounted for by external glycosylation. Two such N-linked glycosylation sites in murine IL-7 are located at amino acids 69 and 90 (Namen *et al.*, 1988). IL-7 mRNA has been detected in murine thymus, spleen, kidney and liver. IL-7 mRNA has been detected in both human and murine keratinocytes (Heufler *et al.*, 1993). Keratinocyte elaborated IL-7 may promote survival and proliferation of dendritic epidermal T cells and play a role in the cutaneous immune response (Matsue, *et al.*, 1993). In the human, the IL-7 message has been detected in the spleen and thymus (Namen *et al.*, 1990; Goodwin and Namen, 1991). Various sized transcripts are present, suggesting the use of alternative splicing and/or polyadenylation sites.

Goodwin and colleagues identified and isolated the human IL-7 gene by hybridization with the murine gene. There is considerable homology between the two IL-7 nucleotide sequences (81% in the coding region). Human IL-7 overall has a 60% amino-acid homology with murine IL-7 (Goodwin *et al.*, 1989). The human IL-7 gene contains six exons over 33 kbp. There is an 18-amino-acid insert in the human IL-7 protein (coded for by exon 5 in the human genome) which does not exist in murine IL-7. In murine IL-7, synthesis transcription is initiated at multiple sites within a 200 bp region (Lupton *et al.*, 1990). Bovine IL-7 has also been sequenced. cDNA from a bovine leukaemia virus induced B-cell lymphosarcoma was used to isolate a clone and the IL-7 sequence was determined. Bovine IL-7 is 176 amino acids long and shows 75% homology with human IL-7 and 65% homology with murine IL-7 (Cludts *et al.*, 1992).

THE IL-7 RECEPTOR

A cell line absolutely dependent on IL-7 for growth (I × N/2b) was used to characterize the IL-7 receptor. Equilibrium binding studies and ^{125}I-IL-7 studies are consistent with the presence of two classes of IL-7R. Receptors having affinity K_a values of 1×10^{10} M and 4×10^8 M have been defined. Dissociation of ^{125}I-radiolabelled IL-7 suggests the presence of a receptor population displaying negative cooperativity. Crosslinking studies are consistent with a receptor size of 75–79 kDa and a second species approximately twice as large (159–162 kDa). The IL-7R may form dimers in the membrane. A variety of other cytokines and growth factors failed to block binding of IL-7 to its receptor (Park *et al.*, 1990).

cDNA clones encoding human and murine IL-7R have been expressed in COS-7 cells (Goodwin *et al.*, 1990). Binding studies in this system have also demonstrated curvilinear Scatchard plots consistent with both a high- and low-affinity IL-7R. Sequence homology in the extracellular domain to other cytokine receptors was noted making this a member of the cytokine receptor superfamily which includes IL-2, IL-4, GM-CSF, IL-5, IL-6, erythropoietin, prolactin and growth hormone (Goodwin *et al.*, 1990). The presence of a soluble form of the receptor has been noted (Goodwin *et al.*, 1990). A differential splicing event results in mRNA encoding for the secreted form of IL-7 (Pleiman *et al.*, 1991). The IL-7 receptor gene maps to 5p13 (Lynch *et al.*, 1992).

IL-7R has been detected on pre-B cells, thymocytes, and other T-lineage cells as well as bone-marrow-derived macrophages but not on mature B cells (Park *et al.*, 1990; Rich *et al.*, 1993). The lack of IL-7R on mature B cells is consistent with observations showing the lack of effect of IL-7 on mature B cells (see below). There appears to be a differential expression of IL-7R on T cells according to their state of activation. Resting T cells express an IL-7 receptor characterized as a cross-linked protein of 107 kDa, whereas activated T cells express an IL-7 cross-linked product of 93 kDa (Foxwell *et al.*, 1992, 1993). Expression of the 93 kDa receptor is associated with IL-7-induced proliferation. Expression of the 93 kDa receptor is stimulated by IL-7, ionomycin and phorbol esters and is inhibited by cyclosporin A and FK506 (Foxwell *et al.*, 1993). Expression of the IL-7R by freshly isolated human T cells was not increased with PHA, Con A or CD3 (Armitage *et al.*, 1991). Interestingly, activation of PBMCs with anti-CD3 results in a fourfold downregulation of IL-7 receptors (high and low affinity) (Foxwell *et al.*, 1992). Studies by Page and associates have shown that the p76 IL7-R (93 kDa complex) is detected on PBMCs 24 hours following mitogen stimulation and the presence of p76 IL-7R correlates with the proliferative response of activated T cells to IL-7. Interestingly, unstimulated thymocytes which proliferate in response to IL-7 without co-stimulation seem to express the p76 IL-7R. Preliminary data suggests that the two IL-7 receptors – p76 (93 kDa complex) and p90 (107 kDa cross-linked complex) – are products of separate genes and not simply variant glycosylated isoforms of a single receptor (Page *et al.*, 1993).

Following receptor binding, human rIL-7 induces tyrosine phosphorylation (five major proteins — 175, 155, 135, 110, and 85 kDa — and five minor proteins). IL-7 did not induce tyrosine phosphorylation of phospholipase C-γ. IL-7 stimulation does not increase phosphatidylinositol turnover. IL-7 binding does not induce a rise in cytosolic free Ca^{++} in thymocytes, mature T cells or pre-B cells. Thus, IL-7R mediates activation of the tyrosine phosphorylation pathway but does not activate the phosphatidylinositol-phospholipase C pathway (Roifman *et al.*, 1992) leading to DNA synthesis and clonal proliferation (Rich *et al.*, 1993).

IL-7 IS A LYMPHOPOIETIN

Following the initial characterization of IL-7 as a growth factor for B-cell progenitors, a number of studies have demonstrated the growth-promoting activity of IL-7 on immature cells of other lineages. IL-7 exerts significant effects on both T and B cells (see Fig. 2). Monoclonal antibodies that recognize the IL-7R inhibit the *in vitro* proliferation of B-precursor cell lines. *In vivo* administration of antibody results in a decrease in the number of both B-precursor cells and thymocytes. These studies suggest a significant role is played by IL-7 in the normal maturation of both B and T cells (Sudo *et al.*, 1993; Grabstein *et al.*, 1993).

Details regarding the effects of IL-7 on myeloid and erythroid cell lineages are less clear than for B and T cells. IL-7 has no direct effect on human myeloid cells expressing CD15 and does not stimulate proliferation of granulocyte precursors (Williams *et al.*, 1990; Tushinski *et al.*, 1991). IL-7 does not support the *in vitro* growth of cells of the granulocytic/monocytic or erythroid lineage but does stimulate eosinophil colony formation. This activity can be abolished by anti-IL-5 antibody treatment, which suggests that IL-7 acts by stimulating release of IL-5 or potentially that IL-5 is an obligate cofactor (Vellenga *et al.*, 1992). IL-7 stimulates the growth of purified mature NK cells ($CD56^+$) although it is clearly less potent in this effect than IL-2 (8–15-fold less activity). IL-7 synergizes with suboptimal levels of IL-2 to support NK-cell proliferation. Antibodies to IL-2 do not abrogate the proliferative or LAK-generating activities of IL-7 (Naume and Espevik, 1991). Both IL-2 and IL-7 induce low-level expression of TNFR. IL-7 also induces low levels of TNF production at day 5 compared with a 50-fold

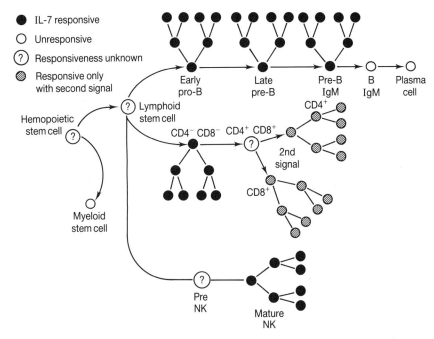

Fig. 2. Maturation of B and T cells. (Modified from Henney, C. S. (1989) *Immunology Today* **10**, 170–173 with permission.)

higher TNF production induced by IL-2 (Naume and Espevik, 1991). The most compelling evidence that IL-7 represents an important lymphopoietin and possibly one of clinical importance comes from a number of *in vivo* investigations. IL-7 administration to normal mice (5μg twice daily for 4–7 days) results in a two- to fivefold increase in the number of peripheral and splenic white cells without any significant change in bone-marrow cellularity. Analysis of the bone-marrow showed an increase in B-cell precursors (B220$^+$, sIg$^-$) with a concurrent decrease in 8C5 and MAC-1 cells (myelo-monocytic markers) (Damia *et al.*, 1992). In mice rendered neutropenic/lymphopenic by either radiation or cyclophosphamide administration, exogenous IL-7 administration accelerates cellular recovery. In irradiated mice given IL-7 the population showing greatest expansion was the B-cell population, with increases in the number of both precursor and mature B cells. In addition a significant T-cell population expansion occurred, particularly within the CD8$^+$ population. There was a more rapid normalization of the CD4/CD8 ratios in those animals receiving IL-7. Exogenous IL-7 administration also increased the white blood cell count in the peripheral blood and spleen of normal mice. Minor stimulatory effects on granulocytes and megakaryocytes were seen in irradiated mice given IL-7 (Faltynek *et al.*, 1992). Similar results were seen in a separate study in mice rendered neutropenic by cyclophosphamide administration and given IL-7. IL-7 promoted regeneration of spleen and node cellularity without signifi-cantly changing bone-marrow and thymus cellularity. A significant expansion of the pre-B-cell population was seen as in the radiation experiments. IL-7 did not seem to accelerate myeloid recovery. IL-7 stimulated recovery of CD4$^+$ and CD8$^+$ cells in the spleen and node and doubled the number of CD8$^+$ cells (Morrissey *et al.*, 1991).

Although IL-7 does not seem to have significant independent myeloproliferative effects, it does enhance the myeloid colony formation (Lin− Sca− 1+ murine progenitor cells) activity of colony stimulating factor (Jacobsen *et al.*, 1993). The recent observation that IL-7 stimulates maturation of embryonic hippocampal progenitor cells in culture suggests that IL-7 may also effect the proliferation and differentiation of immature cells of non-haemopoietic origin (Mehler *et al.*, 1993).

EFFECTS ON B CELLS

A general schema for B-cell maturation is outlined in Fig. 2. The earliest committed B cell is the pro-B cell (pre-pre B cell). The B220 antigen is not expressed and the Ig light- and heavy chains are in the germline configuration. Pre-B cells are B220$^+$ and rearrange and express the IgM heavy chain within the cytoplasm. Light chains rearrange and mature B cells expressing surface Ig are produced (Henney, 1989). Regulatory steps involving proliferation and differentiation through these stages remain incompletely defined; however, the growth and differentiation of early B cells appears to depend on the availability of IL-7 in conjunction with other stromal-cell-related factors or alternatively requires direct cell–cell contact.

The transition from the pro-B stage to pre-B stage of development appears to require the presence of stromal cells; IL-7 alone is not sufficient (Gunji *et al.*, 1991). Pro-B cells as one do not grow in response to IL-7 or Steel locus factor, although they do have receptors for both factors. Interestingly, no growth occurs when cells are separated from the stromal layer by a porous membrane, suggesting that cell–cell contact is necessary (Faust *et al.*, 1993). A working model of B-cell development follows: pro-B cells which do not express Ig heavy- or light-chain protein develop into B220 and c-μ expressing pre-B cells in response to a low molecular weight stromal cell factor with little or no associated proliferation (Dorshkind *et al.*, 1992). A number of genes and surface antigens appear to be expressed following IL-7 incubation, including N-myc and c-myc, which are induced in normal pre-B cells (Dorshkind *et al.*, 1992; Morrow *et al.*, 1992). Incubation with IL-7 is associated with an increase in 6C3Ag expression by pre-B cells but not mature B cells (Sherwood and Weissman, 1990). IL-7 incubation induces expression of B7/BB1 and increased ICAM-1 (CD54) expression by pre B cells (NALM-6) in culture. These phenotypic changes are correlated with increased co-stimulation of T cell proliferation (Dennig and O'Reilly, 1994). The BP-1/6C3 molecule is expressed by early B-lineage cells and some stromal cells. Expression of BP-1 coincided with B-cell precursor proliferation. IL-7 appears to induce expression of BP-1 by B-cell precursors. The source of IL-7 is presumably stromal cells, since they express high levels of IL-7 transcript and stromal cell supernatant is able to induce antigen expression (Sherwood *et al.*, 1990). Differentiation from B220$^-$ cells to B220$^+$ apparently requires stromal cell factors other than IL-7 (Gunji *et al.*, 1991). It is known that this maturation step can be mediated by stromal cell clones that do not produce IL-7 (Cumano *et al.*, 1990). Although these stromal factors are not yet well characterized, it has been suggested that SCF might represent one stromal-cell-derived factor responsible for B-cell maturation (McNiece *et al.*, 1991). IL-7, in conjunction with SCF, did not stimulate the expansion or differentiation of B220$^-$ lymphoid precursors but did stimulate synergistically the proliferation of B220$^+$ cells (Funk *et al.*, 1993). The *in vivo* role of SCF in B-cell maturation remains unclear. While the administration of c-kit blocking antibodies does not block B-cell lymphopoiesis in normal animals, the ability of bone marrow cells from c-kit deficient mice (W/W^v) to regenerate B-cell populations in irradiated normal mice is depressed (Landreth *et al.*, 1984; Opstelten *et al.*, 1985; Ogawa *et al.*, 1991). Insulin like growth factor (IGF-1) seems also to enhance the proliferative effects of pro B cells in mixed culture (Gibson *et al.*, 1993).

Human pro-B cells but not pre-B cells respond to IL-7 — this is in contrast to the data for murine cells, suggesting that some species-specific differences in mode of action exist between humans and mice (Tushinski *et al.*, 1991). This human/rodent dichotomy exists for other cytokines, perhaps most notably for IL-4.

The second step in the development of B cells involves proliferation of B220$^+$, IgM$^-$ cells with expression of cytoplasmic IgM. This step is IL-7 responsive and can occur in the absence of stromal cells, as long as IL-7 is provided (Gunji *et al.*, 1991; Dorshkind *et al.*, 1992). The next step is one where the cells become unresponsive to IL-7 and express surface Ig (see Fig. 2). In summary, the sequence of development suggests, first, a cellular dependence on stromal cells, second, a cellular dependence on stromal cells and IL-7, third, an IL-7-dependent stage, and finally, an IL-7-independent stage. Progression through these stages is associated with Ig gene rearrangement (Hayashi *et al.*, 1990). Once cells have completed rearrangement and express their Ig heavy-chain genes on the cell surface, they are no longer sensitive to IL-7 and KL (kit ligand or SCF) (Dorshkind *et al.*, 1992). The link between rearrangement and maturation is further developed by observations involving transgenic animals. Era and associates have proposed a model of B-cell development using an IL-7-deficient stromal-cell line, PA6. By adding either IL-7 and/or the PA6 stromal-cell line to cultures of developing B cells, the relative importance of each signal in development can be inferred. A complete arrest in the transition from the second to the third stage was noted in *SCID* mice, suggesting that expression of a functional heavy-chain gene was necessary for B-cell transition to the next stage of maturation. While proliferation of B-cell precursors was driven by stromal cell factors such as IL-7, differentiation is regulated by intracellular events related to Ig expression (Hayashi *et al.*, 1990; Era *et al.*, 1991). In μ-chain transgenic animals there is a reduction in the IL-7- and stromal-cell-dependent cell population. In animals with a κ-chain transgene there is an increase in the IL-7-dependent cell population. Expression of cytosolic μ-chain promotes differentiation to an IL-7-dependent stage. The μ-chain-positive cells with a functional light-chain gene become IL-7 unresponsive. These results suggest that B-cell precursors are driven to the next stage of maturation by functional Ig molecules provided by the transgene (Era *et al.*, 1991). IL-6 induces the terminal differentiation to plasma cells in the absence of IL-7 (Herrod, 1989).

IL-7 EFFECTS ON T CELLS

In addition to its importance as a B-cell growth factor, IL-7 has been found to also promote the growth and maturation of T cells both *in vitro* and *in vivo*.

Effects on Fetal T-cells

IL-7 added to murine fetal thymic organ cultures (at day 13) causes a preferential expansion of immature cells of the phenotype CD4$^-$, CD8$^-$ CD3$^-$, CD2$^-$, SCA-1$^+$.

Cells expressing TCR-γ/β are increased and the numbers expressing TCR-α/β are decreased. Neutralizing anti-IL-7 antibody inhibits growth of fetal thymocytes (Leclercq et al., 1992; Plum et al., 1993). In vitro culture of human fetal thymocytes in rIL-7 results in the proliferation of CD4$^+$ and CD8$^+$ thymocytes and partial differentiation of thymocytes with preferential expansion of the CD4$^+$ CD8$^-$ population (Uckun et al., 1991). IL-7 promotes the growth of pre-T cells from fetal liver (at day 14) and promotes the expression of TCR-γ, TCR-α and TCR-β genes. Culture of fetal liver cells in IL-7 is associated with the appearance of Thy-1 and Pgp-1 positive phenotypes, as occurs normally in day 14 fetal thymus (Appasamy, 1992). Culture of murine fetal liver cells in IL-7 caused the re-arrangement and expression of specific TCR gamma variable genes (V gamma 4 and V gamma 6) as well as induction of RAG-1 and RAG-2 mRNA expression (Appasamy and Kenniston, 1993). In murine embryonic thymocyte cultures incubation with IL-7 uniquely induced V(D) J gene re-arrangement and RAG-1 and RAG-2 gene expression (Muegga et al., 1993). IL-7 incubation promotes the growth of gamma delta + thymocytes in both human and murine thymocyte cultures (He and Kabelitz, 1993; Tomana et al., 1993). IL-7 mRNA can be detected in the fetal thymus as early as day 12 and peaks at day 15 (Wiles et al., 1992). IL-7 stimulates the generation of CD3$^+$ cells from human bone-marrow cultures with the production of both CD4$^+$ and CD8$^+$ populations (Tushinski et al., 1991). Reconstitution of lethally irradiated mice with bone marrow transfected with the mIL-7 gene results in marked alteration in T cell subsets in extrathymic sites (spleen and nodes) of many animals. There appears to be an expansion of immature thymocyte populations. These changes were not well tolerated with 23% of animals becoming moribund (Fraser et al., 1993). These observations suggest that IL-7 may be produced locally in the thymic and bone-marrow microenvironments and that IL-7 plays a role in the proliferation and, potentially, in the differentiation of immature T cells (Watanabe et al., 1992).

Effects on Thymocytes and Mature T Cells

Intrathymic T-cell maturation represents an orchestrated interaction between maturing T cells and the thymic microenvironment. This microenvironment is perceived as a combination of both stromal cells and other cells influencing the developing T cell either through the action of cytokines and/or through mechanisms requiring direct cell–cell contact. The role played by IL-7 in intrathymic development is not yet understood. T-cell maturation involves coordinated signals for both differentiation and proliferation, which often seem to be mutually exclusive. These signals include IL-7 as well as other stromal-cell-derived factors — presumably cytokines that are still undefined.

IL-7 is directly mitogenic for thymocytes. Proliferation is not abrogated by neutralizing antibodies to IL-2, IL-2R, IL-1 (α, β), TNF, IL-4, IL-6, or IL-2R (p55, p70). IL-2, IL-6 and TNF synergize to increase IL-7 induced proliferation (Murray et al., 1989; Okazaki et al., 1989; Everson et al., 1990). IL-7-driven proliferation of both adult and fetal murine thymocytes is enhanced by IL-10 (MacNeil et al., 1990).

Incubation of CD4$^-$ CD8$^-$ thymocytes in IL-7 resulted in the appearance of both CD8$^+$ and CD4$^+$ cells after 1 day and CD3$^+$ cells after 2 days. When triple-negative T cells are separated according to IL-2R expression, differential effects of IL-7 are observed. Generation of CD4$^+$ and CD8$^+$ cells occurs only in the IL-2R$^-$ group. IL-7 appears to act as a survival factor for triple negative (CD3$^-$ CD4$^-$ CD8$^-$) cells.

Lifespan is prolonged without induction of proliferation (Vissinga *et al.*, 1992). IL-7 does, however, promote the proliferation of CD3$^+$ double-negative cells (Suda and Zlotnick, 1991). Circulating human T cells also proliferate when incubated in IL-7. Both CD4$^+$ and CD8$^+$ subsets proliferate to a similar degree in response to IL-7 incubation; however, when T cells are separated on the basis of reactivity with an antibody (anti-CD45) that reacts with the 220 kDa isoform (CD45RA) of the common leukocyte antigen, memory T cells (CD45R$^-$) respond more readily than naive T cells (CD45R$^+$). IL-7 incubation is associated with upregulation of receptors for IL-2, transferrin and increased levels of the 4F2 activation antigen. These effects are not abrogated by antibodies to IL-2 or IL-2R (Welch *et al.*, 1989). These studies suggest a potential role for IL-7 in the maturation of a T-cell response. The differential activity of IL-7 on primed T cells suggests a possible mechanism for amplifying T-cell reactivity. IL-7 stimulates Con-A-induced murine T-cell proliferation, IL-2 release and IL-2R expression. Proliferation occurs via both an IL-2-dependent and IL-2-independent pathway and is not abrogated by antibodies to IL-4 nor IL-6 (Armitage *et al.*, 1990; Grabstein *et al.*, 1990). IL-7 induces B7/BB1 expression on peripheral and cloned human T cells (Yesel *et al.*, 1993). Proliferation and cytokine secretion (TNF-alpha, IL-4 and GMCSF) by human peripheral blood T-cells is induced by IL-7 incubation with CD2 and CD28 co-stimulation suggesting that IL-7 may facilitate interactions between T-lymphocytes and thymic stromal cells (Costello *et al.*, 1993).

While it seems clear that IL-7 can exert significant effects on circulating T cells, the source of IL-7 *in vivo* and its *in vivo* role in immune regulation remain uncertain. The fact that the message for IL-7 is found in abundance in the spleen and has recently been found in epidermal keratinocytes supports an *in vivo* role for IL-7 (Welch *et al.*, 1989).

Cyclosporine suppresses IL-2 and IL-4 gene expression but not IL-7, suggesting that IL-7 may promote the generation of memory cells in the absence of IL-2 (Motta *et al.*, 1991). IL-4 production by activated T cells is enhanced by IL-7 (Dokter *et al.*, 1993b).

Interactions with other T-cell Cytokines

As with other cytokines, the pleiotropic effects of IL-7 make it very difficult to predict effects occurring in concert with other cytokines or growth factors. IL-7 has been found to synergize with a number of other cytokines on T cells, B cells and NK cells.

Although IL-7 alone does not stimulate human T cells to generate mRNA for IL-3 or GM-CSF, it acts to stabilize the mRNA for IL-3 and GM-CSF that is produced in response to Con-A stimulation (Dokter *et al.*, 1993).

IL-7 enhances IL-1-induced proliferation of murine thymocytes and these IL-1-driven effects are abrogated by anti-IL-7 antibody treatment, suggesting that IL-1 effects on murine thymocytes are mediated more proximally by IL-7 (Herbelin *et al.*, 1992) One would guess that such interdependencies will become even more complex as additional knowledge is accrued regarding cytokine networks.

EFFECTS OF IL-7 ON MONOCYTES

A variety of effects of IL-7 on monocytes have been reported. mRNA for both IL-8 and human macrophage inflammatory protein-1 β gene is induced directly in monocytes by IL-7 (Ziegler *et al.*, 1991; Standiford *et al.*, 1992). Monocytes incubated in IL-7 are also stimulated to secrete IL-6 as well as IL-1α, IL-1β and TNF-α. Interestingly, this response was abrogated by the provision of IL-4. Activation of monocytes with IL-7 results in the lysis of a sensitive melanoma tumour target in an 18-h [51]chromium release assay (Alderson *et al.*, 1991). Treatment of murine macrophages infected with *Leishmania major* with IL-7 resulted in a dose-dependent reduction of cellular amastigote burden. This activity was accompanied by nitric oxide production and was abrogated by N-omega-monomethyl-L-arginine acetate or anti-TNF antibodies (Gessner *et al.*, 1993).

EFFECTS OF IL-7 ON NK CELLS

IL-7 mediates a number of NK cell effects. IL-7 upregulates CD56 expression and induces the production of low levels of TNF-α but not TNF-β by NK cells (Naume and Espevik, 1990; Naume *et al.*, 1992). IL-7 can generate LAK activity both alone and in conjunction with low dose IL-2 from cultures of NK cells. Neither proliferation nor LAK generation were abrogated by antibodies to IL-2 (Naume and Espevik, 1991). However, both TGF-β and IL-4 downregulate IL-7-induced LAK generation (Stotter and Lotze, 1991; Stotter *et al.*, 1991). IL-7 induced low levels of TNF production at day 5 compared with a 50-fold higher TNF production by IL-2. Both cytokines induced low levels of TNF-R expression (Naume and Espevik, 1991). *In vivo* activity of IL-7 on NK cells has also been demonstrated. Administration of IL-7 significantly prolonged the survival of mice infected with the Friend leukaemia virus complex. IL-7 appeared to normalize lowered NK-cell activity and restored IL-6 and IFN-γ levels in such infected mice (Lu *et al.*, 1992). IL-7 may function as a survival factor for NK cell precursors preserving their viability and IL-2 responsiveness (Pollack and Tsuji, 1993).

OBSERVATIONS ON IL-7 TRANSGENIC ANIMALS

A transgene created by fusing the IL-7 gene with an immunoglobulin heavy-chain promoter and enhancer has been introduced into mice. The transgene is expressed in thymus, spleen, bone-marrow, lymph nodes and skin. T-cell development is abnormal with a reduction of double-positive thymocytes. The transgenic animals develop a skin disorder characterized by hyperkeratosis, alopecia and exfoliation. This is accompanied by an infiltration of T-cell lineage cells into the skin which, interestingly, occurs also in athymic nude mice. Both B- and T- cell lymphomas occur in these animals during the first 4 months of life (Rich *et al.*, 1993). The occurrence of lymphomas in these animals along with the observation that IL-7 stimulates the growth of a number of human malignancies (see below) suggests that IL-7 may play an important role in the biology of certain haematologic malignancies.

IL-7 AND ANTI-TUMOUR IMMUNOTHERAPY

Cytokine-based approaches to the immunotherapy of cancer seek to upregulate the immune response to a patient's own tumour. Considerable clinical experience has been accrued using a number of biological response modifiers, including IL-2. Unsolved problems, including lack of specificity, unpredictable anti-tumour responses and toxicity associated with current regimens has encouraged the evaluation of other cytokines, including IL-7. IL-7 has both *in vitro* and *in vivo* effects, which suggest potential clinical applications. IL-7 generates LAK activity from thymocytes and peripheral blood mononuclear cells. In comparison with IL-2, IL-7 appears to be a relatively weak LAK inducer. IL-2 stimulates fivefold more LAK precursors than IL-7 (Alderson *et al.*, 1990). Thymocytes from cultures grown in IL-2 were highly cytolytic compared with cultures grown in IL-7, which exhibited minimal cytolytic activity. Cytolytic activity, however, was increased when cells were incubated secondarily in IL-2. In a similar manner IL-7 induced significant LAK activity from *in vitro* cultures of PBNCs harvested from patients treated with bone marrow transplants (both syngeneic and allogeneic) and systemic IL-2 (Pavletic *et al.*, 1993). The addition of IL-4 does not induce cytolytic activity of the cells grown in IL-7 but rather downregulated IL-2-induced proliferation and cytolytic activity (Widmer *et al.*, 1990). IL-7 can generate human LAK activity from cultures of peripheral blood mononuclear cells in the absence of IL-2 and induces or upregulates expression of CD25, CD54, Mic β-1 and CD69. LAK generation is negatively influenced by TGF-β and IL-4. Anti-IL-4 antibody and IL-4 antisense enhances IL-7-induced LAK activity (Stotter and Lotze, 1991; Stotter *et al.*, 1991). IL-7 promotes the secretion of TNF but not IFN-γ (Stotter and Lotze, 1991). The nature of the LAK precursor for IL-7-induced LAK is not totally clear. One study showed that LAK activity (comparable with IL-2) could be generated from a population of NK cells (CD56$^+$), whereas no LAK activity was generated in PBMCs (Naume and Espevik, 1991). Another study using murine cells compared IL-7-induced LAK with IL-2-induced LAK. IL-7-induced LAK peaked at days 6–8. IL-7 was more effective at maintaining cytotoxic activity over longer periods of time than IL-2 and IL-7 LAK was induced from secondary lymphoid tissue (spleen and nodes) but not from primary lymphoid tissue (thymus and bone marrow). LAK activity in these studies was abrogated by anti-CD8 or anti-Thy-1$^+$C and unaffected by anti-CD4, anti-asialo GM1 or anti-NK1.1$^+$C, suggesting that IL-7 LAK activity is not mediated by NK cells but rather by T cells (Lynch and Miller, 1990). We have been unable to confirm a T-cell origin for IL-7-induced LAK. The anti-tumor activity of systemically administered IL-7 has been disappointing. However, in numerous animal models (see below) systemic IL-7 when combined with adoptive transfer of sensitized cells has resulted in apparent tumor regression. IL-7 combined with hyperthermia prolonged the survival of mice bearing a B16 amelanoma (Wu *et al.*, 1993).

IL-7 Enhances the Generation of CTL and Proliferative Activity of T-cells in Tumour-bearing Mice

Various cytokines, including IL-2 and IL-4, are active in promoting the clonal expansion of T cells *in vitro* while maintaining their tumour-lytic activity. IL-7 appears to have similar properties. IL-7 alone generates modest CTL activity, which is augmented by IL-2, IL-6, or IL-4 (Bertagnolli and Herrmann 1990; Hickman *et al.*, 1990). Removal of CD8$^+$ cells resulted in decreased killing, whereas removal of CD4$^+$ cells enhanced the CTL response. IL-7 enhanced cell proliferation and duration of growth more than IL-2. Allospecific cytotoxicity was maintained for at least 60 days in these cultured cells (Bertagnolli and Herrman 1990; Jicha *et al.*, 1992). Addition of anti-IL-4, anti-IL-2 or anti-IL-6 decreased the proliferation of CTL in culture (Bertagnolli and Herrman, 1990).

CTLs harvested from draining nodes of tumour-bearing animals and incubated in IL-7 were four-fold more effective than CTL grown in media alone in adoptive transfer experiments (Lynch *et al.*, 1991). Interestingly IL-7 seems to promote long term CTL cultures without the requisite CD4$^+$ cell stimulation required by IL-2 driven cultures. Antigen specificity and *in vivo* reactivity of transfered cells is retained (Lynch and Miller, 1994). CTLs incubated in IL-7 and adoptively transferred to mice bearing 3-day pulmonary metastases (MCA tumour) were effective in mediating tumour regression (Jicha *et al.*, 1991). Systemic administration of IL-7 did not effect survival of nude mice bearing a human colon cancer xenograft. However, survival was prolonged when human peripheral T cells were adoptively transfered in additon to the systemic IL-7 therapy (Murphy *et al.*, 1993).

IL-7 stimulates proliferation of human TIL derived from renal cell carcinoma but only if the TILs are first incubated in either IL-2 alone or in combinations of IL-2 + IL-7. IL-7 stimulated proliferations of CD4$^+$ or CD8$^+$ TIL lines specific for renal cell carcinoma and synergized with anti-CD3 in the induction of IFN-γ from short-term TIL cultures (Sica *et al.*, 1993). As noted earlier, IL-7 seems to have an effect in upregulating late responses following activation. Cytolytic activity in memory cells to a sensitizing influenza A antigen occurs when the cell is stimulated by IL-2 and antigen. This IL-2 requirement may be replaced by exogenous IL-7 (Kos and Mullbacher, 1992, 1993).

Human T cells harvested from peripheral blood and incubated in IL-7 when restimulated with phorbol ester and ionomycin secrete IL-2, IL-4, IL-6 and IFN-γ. This effect was not seen so readily in cultures initiated with either IL-2 or IL-4. Both CD4$^+$ and CD8$^+$ subsets responded with cytokine secretion. Almost all the potential to secrete IL-4 and IL-6 in response to IL-7 incubation resides within the memory subset in contrast to the naive population (Armitage *et al.*, 1992).

The data suggests that IL-7 either alone or in conjunction with IL-2 acts to stimulate both proliferation and tumour-lytic activity in sensitized T cells and therefore may be useful clinically in the immunotherapy of malignancy and possibly some infectious diseases.

IL-7 Transfection of Tumour

Transfection of cytokine genes into tumour-cell lines has been developed as a strategy to increase the local–regional anti-tumour response and, hopefully, enhance a systemic response to nontransfected tumour. IL-7 transfection experiments have yielded provocative results. Transfection of IL-7 into a murine tumour line (J5581) leads to rejection of the tumour. Although CD8$^+$ cells are required for long-term tumour eradication, short-term regression may occur in the absence of CD8$^+$ cells implying that CD4$^+$ cells are central for the response. While tumour transfected with IL-2, IL-4, TNF, or IFN-γ regressed when placed in nude or *SCID* mice, regression of IL-7 transfected tumour required the presence of CD4$^+$ cells. No tumour regression was observed in nude mice bearing tumour transfected with IL-7. IL-7-transfected tumours contained an infiltrate of macrophages and eosinophils (Hock *et al.*, 1993). Similar results were noted using a murine glioma model (Aoki *et al.*, 1992).

IL-7 was transfected into a murine fibrosarcoma. The tumour grew slowly in normal animals with a high rate of spontaneous regression but grew at a normal rate in T-cell-deficient mice. After tumour regression, animals were specifically immune to further tumour challenge. Tumours were heavily infiltrated with T cells, predominantly CD8$^+$ cells but also some CD4$^+$ cells, eosinophils, and basophils. Direct injection of IL-7 into tumours (20 μg BID for 10 days) also mediated tumour regression and resulted in specific immunity (McBride *et al.*, 1992).

IL-7 and Haematological Malignancy

The growth-promoting activity of IL-7 suggests that growth of some malignancies might be accelerated by IL-7 or, alternatively, that exogenous IL-7 might be able to induce differentiation of cells transformed to the malignant phenotype.

The IL-7 gene was transfected into an IL-7-dependent murine pre-B cell line via a retroviral vector. Vectors were based on the Moloney murine leukaemia virus (MoMLV) having, in addition, a simian virus 40 (SV40) early promoter-*neo* cassette placed downstream from the IL-7 cDNA. Transfection resulted in transformation to IL-7 independence. Cell proliferation could be inhibited by coincubation with anti-IL-7 antibody. The transfected cells were tumorigenic. It is unlikely that this autocrine growth stimulation represents a common end point for all B-cell malignancies, since two murine pre-B-cell lines transformed by Abelson murine leukaemia virus failed to express any detectable IL-7 mRNA and cell proliferation was not affected by anti-IL-7 antibody (Overell *et al.*, 1991). Co-transfection of a murine pre-B cell line with both V-Ha-*ras* and IL-7 increases the malignant transformation rate compared with either transfection alone (Chen *et al.*, 1993).

A number of leukaemia and lymphoma cells isolated from patients have been screened for their growth responses and/or dependence on IL-7. Many, but not all, proliferate when exposed to IL-7. Both B- and T-cell malignancies appear to respond to exogenous IL-7, including a cutaneous Sézary cell malignancy (Eder *et al.*, 1990; Touw *et al.*, 1990; Makrynikola *et al.*, 1991; Shand and Betlach, 1991; Skjonsberg *et al.*, 1991; Lu *et al.*, 1992; Yoshioka *et al.*, 1992). Evidence of lymphoid maturation of the tumour cells in response to IL-7 incubation was not seen (Eder *et al.*, 1990).

In leukaemic cells isolated from patients with chronic lymphocytic leukaemia (CLL), the IL-7 coding sequence is transcribed as well as an alternatively spliced IL-7 mRNA. These transcripts are not found in lymphocytes from normal patients nor in non-leukaemic cells from patients with leukaemia. Some cells from CLL patients also expressed the IL-7 receptor and bound IL-7 whereas T-cell-depleted populations from healthy patients do not normally express the IL-7R. The IL-7R$^+$ cells in the leukaemic patients included the CLL cells themselves. Abnormal IL-7 and IL-7R expression and regulation may play a role not only in the growth kinetics of CLL but also, perhaps, in the genesis of the disease (Frishman *et al.*, 1993). In a separate study, pre-B cells transformed by a variety of oncogenes were tested for IL-7 production. None produced any IL-7 bioactivity. Some V-abl but none of the BCR/ABL, v-src, v-fms, v-myc, v-ras or v-raf contained elevated IL-7 transcripts. IL-7 overexpression achieved by removing portions of the 5′ flanking region did not cause dramatic colony formation in agar and most clones were not tumorigenic *in vivo* (syngeneic mice) (Young *et al.*, 1991). It seems therefore that production of IL-7 does not represent a final common step in the malignant transformation of lymphoid cells, but in selected malignancies may represent a target for therapeutic intervention. An additional role for IL-7 in the malignant progression has been suggested by the observation that IL-7 upregulates ICAM expression by melanoma cells — a phenotype correlated with metastatic behaviour (Kimbauer *et al.*, 1992).

SUMMARY

IL-7 is a potent lymphopoietin which appears to play a critical role in the early stages of both B- and T-cell maturation. IL-7 stimulates the growth of a number of mature T cells, as well as T- and B-cell malignancies. IL-7 shares a number of properties with IL-2, including the *in vitro* expansion of T cells having anti-tumour reactivity, which suggests a potential for clinical application in cancer diagnosis and treatment. Although there are much *in vitro* data available, it remains unclear exactly what role IL-7 plays in the *in vivo* immune response and both normal and pathological lymphoid maturation and its association with other cytokines to enhance lymphopoiesis has still to be defined.

REFERENCES

Alderson, M.R., Sassenfeld, H.M. and Widmer, M.B. (1990). *J. Exp. Med.* **172**, 577.

Alderson, M.R., Tough, T.W., Ziegler, S.F. and Grabstein, K.H. (1991). *J. Exp. Med.* **173**, 923.

Aoki, T., Tashiro, K., Miyatake, S., Kinashi, T., Nakano, Y, Oda, Y., Kikuchi, H. and Honjo, T. (1992). *Proc. Nat. Acad. Sci. USA.* **89**, 3850.

Appasamy, P.M. (1992) *J. Immunol.* **149**, 1649.

Armitage, R.J., Namen, A.E., Sassenfeld, H.M. and Grabstein, K.H. (1990). *J. Immunol.* **41**, 938.

Armitage, R.J., Ziegler, S.F., Beckmann, M.P., Idzerda, R.L., Park, L.S. and Fanslow, W.C. (1991). *Adv. Exp. Med. Biol.* **292**, 121.

Armitage, R.J., Macduff, B.M. Ziegler, S.F. and Grabstein, K.H. (1992). *Cytokine* **41**, 461.

Bertagnolli, M. and Herrmann, S. (1990). *J. Immunol.* **145**, 1706.

Cludts, I., Droogmans, L., Cleuter, Y., Kettmann, R. and Burny, A. (1992). *DNA Sequ.* **3**, 55.

Cumano, A., Dorshkind, K., Gillis, S. and Paige, C.J. (1990). *Eur. J. Immunol.* **20**, 2183.

Damia, G., Komschlies, K.L., Faltynek, C.R., Ruscetti, F.W. and Wiltrout, R.H. (1992). *Blood* **79**, 1121.

Dokter, W.H., Sierdsema, S.J., Esselink, M.T., Halie, M.R. and Vellenga, E. (1993). *J. Immunol.* **150**, 2584.

Dorshkind, K., Narayanan, R. and Landreth, K.S. (1992). *Adv. Exp. Med. Biol.* **323**, 119.

Eder, M., Ottmann, O.G., Hansen-Hagge, T.E., Bartram, C.R., Gillis, S., Hoelzer, D. and Ganser, A. (1990). *Leukemia* **4**, 533.

Era, T., Ogawa, M., Nishikawa, S., Okamoto, M., Honjo, T., Akagi, K., Miyazaki, J. and Yamamura, K. (1991). *EMBO J.* **10**, 337.

Everson, M.P., Eldridge, J.H. and Koopman, W.J. (1990). *Cell. Immunol.* **127**, 470.

Faltynek, C.R., Wang, S., Miller, D., Young, E. Tiberio, L., Kross, K., Kelley, M. and Kloszewski, E. (1992). *J. Immunol.* **149**, 1276.

Faust, E.A., Saffran, D.C., Toksoz, D., Williams, D.A. and Witte, O.N. (1993). *J. Exp. Med.* **177**, 915.

Foxwell, B.M., Taylor-Fishwick, D.A., Simon, J.L., Page, T.H. and Londei, M. (1992). *Int. Immunol.* **4**, 277.

Foxwell, B.M., Willcocks, J.L., Taylor-Fishwick, D.A., Kulig, K., Ryffel, B. and Londei, M. (1993). *Eur. J. Immunol.* **23**, 85.

Frishman, J., Long, B., Knospe, W., Gregory, S. and Plate, J. (1993) *J. Exp. Med.* **177**, 955.

Funk, P.E., Varas, A. and Witte, P.L. (1993). *J. Immunol.* **150**, 748.

Goodwin, R.G. and Namen, A.E. (1991). In *The Cytokine Handbook* (ed. A. V. Thomson), Academic Press, London, p. 191–200.

Goodwin, R.G., Lupton, S., Schmier, A., Hjerrild, K.L., Jerzy, R., Clevenger, W., Gillis, S., Cosman, D. and Namen, A.E. (1989). *Proc. Natl. Acad. Sci. USA* **86**, 302–306.

Goodwin, R.G., Friend, D., Ziegler, S.F., Jerzy, R., Falk, B.A., Gimpel, S., Cosman, D., Dower, S.K., March, C.J., Namen, A.E. *et al.* (1990). *Cell* **60**, 941.

Grabstein, K.H., Namen, A.E., Shanebeck, K., Voice, R.F., Reed, S.G. and Widmer, M.B. (1990). *J. Immunol.* **144**, 3015.

Gunji, Y., Sudo, T., Suda, J., Yamaguchi, Y., Nakauchi, H., Nishikawa, S., Yanai, N., Obinata, M., Yanagisawa, M., Miura, Y. *et al.* (1991). *Blood* **77**, 2612.

Hayashi, S., Kunisada, T., Ogawa, M., Sudo, T., Kodama, H., Suda, T. and Nishikawa, S. (1990). *J. Exp. Med.* **171**, 1683.

Henney, C.S. (1989). *Immunol. Today* **10**, 170.

Herbelin, A., Machavoine,F., Schneider, E., Papiernik, M. and Dy. M. (1992). *J. Immunol.* **148**, 99.

Herrod, H.G. (1989). *Ann. Allergy* **63**, 269.

Hickman, C.J., Crim, J.A., Mostowski, H.S. and Siegel, J.P. (1990). *J. Immunol.* **145**, 2415.

Hock, H., Dorsch, M., Kunzendorf, U., Qin, Z., Diamantstein, T. and Blankenstein, T. (1993). *Proc. Natl Acad. Sci. USA.* **90**, 2774.

Hunt, P.A., Weiss, D., Rennick, D., Lee, F. and Witte, O.N. (1987). *Cell* **48**, 997.

Jicha, D.L., Mule, J.J. and Rosenberg, S.A. (1991). *J. Exp. Med.* **174**, 1511.

Jicha, D.L., Schwarz, S., Mule, J.J. and Rosenberg, S.A. (1992). *Cell. Immunol.* **141**, 71.

Kirnbauer, R., Charvat, B., Schauer, E., Kock, A., Urbanski, A., Forster, E., Neuner, P., Assmann, I., Luger, T.A. and Schwarz, T. (1992). *J. Invest. Dermatol.* **98**, 320.

Kos, F.J. and Mullbacher, A. (1992). *Eur. J. Immunol.* **22**, 3183.

Kos, F.J. and Mullbacher, A. (1993). *J. Immunol.* **150**, 387.

Landreth, K.S., Kincade, P.W., Lee, G. and Harrison, D.E. (1984). *J. Immunol.* **132**, 2724.

Leclercq, G., De Smedt, M. and Plum, J. (1992). *Eur. J. Immunol.* **22**, 2189.

Lu, L., Zhou, Z., Wu, B., Xiao, M., Shen, R.N., Williams, D.E., Kim, Y.J., Kwon, B.S., Ruscetti, S. and Broxmeyer, H.E. (1992). *Int. J. Cancer* **52**, 261.

Lupton, S.D., Gimpel, S., Jerzy, R., Brunton, L.L., Hjerrild, K.A., Cosman, D. and Goodwin, R.G. (1990). *J. Immunol.* **144**, 3592.

Lynch, D.H. and Miller, R.E. (1990). *J. Immunol.* **145**, 1983.

Lynch, D.H., Namen, A.E. and Miller, R.E. (1991). *Eur. J. Immunol.* **21**, 2977.

Lynch, M., Baker, E., Park, L.S., Sutherland, G.R. and Goodwin, R.G. (1992). *Human Genet.* **89**, 566.

McBride, W.H., Thacker, J.D., Comora, S., Economou, J.S., Kelley, D., Hogge, D., Dubinett, S.M. and Dougherty, G.J. (1992). *Cancer Res.* **52**, 3931.

MacNeil, I.A., Suda, T., Moore, K., Mosmann, T.R. and Zlotnik, A. (1990) *J. Immunol.* **145**, 4167.

McNiece, I.K., Langley, K.E. and Zsebo, K.M. (1991). *J. Immunol.* **146**, 3785.

Makrynikola, V., Kabral, A. and Bradstock, K.F. (1991). *Exp. Hematol.***19**, 674.

Mehler, M.F., Rozental, R., Dougherty, M., Spray, D.C. and Kessler, J.A. (1993). *Nature* **362**, 62.

Morrissey, P.J., Conlon, P., Braddy, S., Williams, D.E., Namen, A.E. and Mochizuki, D.Y. (1991). *J. Immunol.* **146**, 1547.

Morrow, M.A., Lee, G., Gillis, S., Yancopoulous, G.D. and Alt, F.W. (1992). *Genes Devel.* **6**, 61.

Motta, I., Colle, J.H., Shidani, B. and Truffa-Bachi, P. (1991). *Eur. J. Immunol.* **21**, 551.

Murray, R., Suda, T., Wrighton, N., Lee, F. and Zlotnik, A. (1989). *Int. Immunol.* **1**, 526.

Namen, A.E., Lupton, S. and Hjerrild, K. *et al.* (1988a). *Nature* **333**, 571.

Namen, A.E., Schmierer, A.E., March, C.J., Overell, R.W., Park, L., Urdal, D.L. and Mochizuki, D.Y. (1988b). *J. Exp. Med.* **167**, 988.

Namen, A.E., Williams, D.E. and Goodwin, R.G. (1990). In *Hematopoietic Growth Factors in Transfusion Medicine.* (ed. Anonymous), Wiley–Liss, New York.

Naume, B. and Espevik, T. (1991). *J. Immunol.* **147**, 2208.

Naume, B., Gately, M. and Espevik, T. (1992). *J. Immunol.* **148**, 2429.

Ogawa, M., Matsuzaki, Y., Nishikawa, S., Hayashi, S., Kunisada, T., Sudo, T., Kina, T. and Nakauchi, H. (1991). *J. Exp. Med.* **174**, 63.

Okazaki, H., Ito, M., Sudo, T., Hattori, M., Kano, S., Katsura, Y. and Minato, N. (1989). *J. Immunol.* **143**, 2917.

Opstelten, D. and Osmond, D.G. (1985) *Eur. J. Immunol.* **15**, 599.

Overell, R.W., Clark, L., Lynch, D., Jerzy, R., Schmierer, A., Weisser, K.E., Namen, A.E. and Goodwin, R.G. (1991). *Mol. Cell. Biol.* **11**, 1590.

Pandrau, D., Frances, V., Martinez-Valdez, H., Pages, M.P., Manel, A.M., Philippe, N., Banchereau, J. and Saeland, S. (1993). *Leukemia* **7**, 635.

Park, L.S., Friend, D.J., Schmierer, A.E., Dower, S.K. and Namen, A.E. (1990). *J. Exp. Med.* **171**, 1073.

Pleiman, C.M., Gimpel, S.D., Park, L.S., Harada, H., Taniguchi, T. and Ziegler, S.F. (1991). *Mol. Cell. Biol.* **11**, 3052.

Plum, J., De Smedt, M. and Leclercq, G. (1993). *J. Immunol.* **150**, 2706.

Rich, B.E., Campos-Torres, J., Tepper, R.I., Moreadith, R.W. and Leder, P. (1993). *J. Exp. Med.* **177**, 305.

Roifman, C.M., Wang, G.X., Freedman, M. and Pan, Z.Q. (1992). *J. Immunol.* **148**, 1136.

Shand, R.F. and Betlach, M.C. (1991). *J. Bacteriol.* **173**, 4692.

Sherwood, P.J. and Weissman, I.L. (1990). *Int. Immunol.* **2**, 399.

Sica, D., Rayman, P., Stanley, J., Edinger, M., Tubbs, R.R., Klein, E., Bukowski, R. and Finke, J.H. (1993). *Int. J. Cancer* **53**, 941.

Skjonsberg, C., Erikstein, B.K., Smeland, E.B., Lie, S.O., Funderud, S., Beiske, K. and Blomhoff, H.K. (1991). *Blood* **77**, 2445.

Standiford, T.J., Strieter, R.M., Allen, R.M., Burdick, M.D. and Kunkel, S.L. (1992). *J. Immunol.* **149**, 2035.

Stotter, H., Custer, M.C., Bolton, E.S., Guedez, L. and Lotze, M.T. (1991). *J. Immunol.* **146**, 150.

Stotter, H. and Lotze, M.T. (1991). *Arch. Surgery* **126**, 1525.

Suda, T. and Zlotnik, A. (1991). *J. Immunol.* **146**, 3068.

Touw, I., Pouwels, K., van Agthoven, T., van Gurp, R., Budel, L., Hoogerbrugge, H., Delwel, R., Goodwin, R., Namen, A. and Lowenberg, B. (1990). *Blood* **75**, 2097.

Tushinski, R.J., McAlister, I.B., Williams, D.E. and Namen, A.E. (1991). *Exp. Hematol.* **19**, 749.

Uckun, F.M., Tuel-Ahlgren, L., Obuz, V., Smith, R., Dibirdik, I., Hanson, M., Langlie, M.C. and Ledbetter, J.A. (1991). *Proc. Natl Acad. Sci. USA.* **88**, 6323.

Vellenga, E., Esselink, M.T., Straaten, J., Stulp, B.K., De Wolf, J.T., Brons, R., Giannotti, J., Smit, J.W. and Halie, M.R. (1992). *J. Immunol.* **149**, 2992.

Vissinga, C.S., Fatur-Saunders, D.J. and Takei, F. (1992). *Exp. Hematol.* **20**, 998.

Watanabe, Y., Mazda, O., Aiba, Y., Iwai, K., Gyotoku, J., Ideyama, S., Miyazaki, J. and Katsura, Y. (1992). *Cell. Immunol.* **142**, 385.

Welch, P.A., Namen, A.E., Goodwin, R.G., Armitage, R. and Cooper, M.D. (1989). *J. Immunol.* **143**, 3562.

Whitlock, C.A. and Witte, O.N. (1982). *Proc. Natl Acad. Sci. USA.* **79**, 3608.

Whitlock, C.A., Robertson, D. and Witte, O.N. (1984). *J. Immunol. Methods* **6**, 353.

Widmer, M.B., Morrissey, P.J., Namen, A.E., Voice, R.F. and Watson, J.D. (1990). *Int. Immunol.* **2**, 1055.

Wiles, M.V., Ruiz, P. and Imhof, B.A. (1992). *Eur. J. Immunol.* **22**, 1037.

Williams, D.E., Namen, A.E., Mochizuki, D.Y. and Overell, R.W. (1990). *Blood* **75**, 1132.

Yoshioka, R., Shimizu, S., Tachibana, J., Hirose, Y., Fukutoku, M., Takeuchi, Y., Sugai, S., Takiguchi, T. and Konda, S. (1992). *J. Clin. Immunol.* **12**, 101.

Young, J.C., Gishizky, M.L. and Witte, O.N. (1991). *Mol. Cell. Biol.* **11**, 854.

Ziegler, S.F., Tough, T.W., Franklin, T.L., Armitage, R.J. and Alderson, M.R. (1991) *J. Immunol.* **147**, 2234.

Chapter 10

Interleukin-8 and related chemotactic cytokines

Jo Van Damme

Rega Institute for Medical Research, Leuven, Belgium

INTRODUCTION

IL-8 has been characterized as a neutrophil-activating protein (NAP-1) with biological effects similar to known chemotactic substances such as the plasma-derived anaphylatoxin C5a, the cell-derived chemotaxins leukotriene B_4 (LTB_4) and platelet activating factor (PAF), and bacterial- or synthetic formylmethionyl peptides (e.g. FMLP). The amino acid sequence of this cytokine was disclosed first by Schmid and Weissmann (1987), but these authors could not indicate a biological function for their putative protein.

The identification of biologically active IL-8/NAP-1 originates from studies with IL-1 to which neutrophil activating effects were ascribed both *in vitro* (Luger *et al.*, 1983; Sauder *et al.*, 1984) and *in vivo* (Dinarello, 1984; Van Damme *et al.*, 1985a). These *in vitro* functional effects of IL-1 on neutrophils could not be reproduced with pure IL-1 (Georgilis *et al.*, 1987), indicating that a contaminating factor was responsible for the chemotactic effect. As a consequence, several laboratories independently isolated a novel cytokine that was designated monocyte-derived neutrophil chemotactic factor (MDNCF; Yoshimura *et al.*, 1987), monocyte-derived neutrophil-activating peptide (MONAP; Schröder *et al.*, 1987), neutrophil activating factor (NAF; Walz *et al.*, 1987) or granulocyte chemotactic protein (GCP; Van Damme *et al.*, 1988). Its sequence had no structural similarity with that of IL-1, but showed identity with the cDNA-derived protein sequence described by Schmid and Weissmann (1987). GCP/IL-8 caused *in vivo* neutrophil activation (granulocytosis, skin reactivity) with the same histology, but dissimilar in kinetics when compared with IL-1 (Van Damme *et al.*, 1988). This suggested an indirect chemotactic effect of the latter.

NAP-1/IL-8 was isolated first from stimulated leukocytes, but the molecule can be produced by a wide variety of cell types in response to cytokine inducers. NAP-1/IL-8 is also active on cell types other than neutrophils (Larsen *et al.*, 1989a). The protein fulfilled the criteria to be considered as an interleukin. In this review the molecule will therefore be referred to as IL-8 (Westwick *et al.*, 1989). In view of the increasing number of newly discovered chemotactic proteins, that are structurally related to IL-8, these cytokines are now designated 'chemokines' (Baggiolini *et al.*, 1993). The hallmark for this family of proinflammatory proteins is the conservation of four cysteine

The Cytokine Handbook, 2nd ed.
ISBN 0–12–689661–5

Table 1.   Cellular sources of human IL-8.

Designation	Cell type	Stimulus	Reference
3-10C	Leukocytes	SEA	Schmid & Weissmann 1987
MDNCF	Monocytes/macrophages	LPS	Yoshimura *et al.*, (1987)
MONAP		LPS,PMA	Schröder *et al.* (1987)
NAF		LPS,ConA,PHA	Peveri *et al.* (1988)
GCP		LPS,ConA	Van Damme *et al.* (1988)
MDNCF		IL-1, TNF	Matsushima *et al.* (1988)
IL-8		Virus	Becker *et al.* (1991)
IL-8		Phagocytosis	Friedland *et al.* (1992)
IL-8		IL-7	Standiford *et al.* (1992)
IL-8		Oxygen stress	Metinko *et al.* (1992)
LYNAP	Lymphocytes	ConA,PHA	Gregory *et al.* (1988)
LYNAP			Schröder *et al.* (1988)
IL-8		PMA+PHA	Smyth *et al.* (1991)
IL-8	Neutrophils	LPS	Strieter *et al.* (1990)
IL-8		Phagocytosis	Bazzoni *et al.* (1991)
IL-8		FMLP	Cassatella *et al.* (1992)
IL-8		GM-CSF	Takahashi *et al.* (1993)
IL-8		IL-1, TNF	Fujishima *et al.* (1993)
IL-8	Eosinophils	Ca^{++} ionophore	Braun *et al.* (1993)
IL-8	Myeloid precursors	LPS	Dibb *et al.* (1992)
GCP/IL-8	Fibroblasts	IL-1,virus,dsRNA	Van Damme *et al.* (1989a)
NCF		IL-1,TNF	Strieter *et al.* (1989b)
FINAP		IL-1,TNF	Schröder *et al.* (1990b)
IL-8		Leukoregulin	Mauviel *et al.* (1992)
NCF	Synovial cells	IL-1	Golds *et al.* (1989)
IL-8		IL-1,TNF,LPS	Koch *et al.* (1991)
ENAP	Endothelial cells	LPS	Schröder and Christophers (1989)
NCF		LPS,IL-1,TNF	Strieter *et al.* (1989a)
LAI/IL-8		IL-1	Gimbrone *et al.* (1989)
IL-8		IL-1	Sica *et al.* (1990a)
IL-8		Membrane IL-1	Kaplanski *et al.* (1993)
IL-8	Smooth muscle cells	IL-1,TNF,LPS	Wang *et al.* (1991)

residues that are important for the tertiary structure. The chemokines can be divided into two subfamilies depending on whether the first two cysteines are adjacent (C–C chemokines) or not (C–X–C chemokines). A number of human genes for the C–X–C and C–C chemokines have been located on chromosomes 4 and 17, respectively. In contrast to classical chemotactic agents (such as PAF, LTB4 and C5a), the chemokines selectively attract and activate distinct leukocyte populations. Since all these chemokines have related biological effects, this review will focus mainly on IL-8 which represents, at present, the best-characterized member of this family. Further extensive coverage of the chemokines can be found in chapter 22 of this volume.

PRODUCTION OF IL-8: CELL SOURCES AND INDUCERS

Certain cytokines, e.g. IL-2 and IFN-γ are produced by specific cell types i.e. T-lymphocytes. In contrast, other cytokines such as IL-6 and IL-8 can be released by a variety of cells, including leukocytes, fibroblasts, endothelial cells, epithelial cells, chondrocytes, keratinocytes, etc. Table 1 describes the cell sources of IL-8 and the

Table 1. *continued.*

Designation	Cell type	Stimulus	Reference
NCF/IL-8	Epithelial cells	IL-1,TNF	Elner*et al.* (1990)
IL-8		IL-1,TNF	Standiford *et al.* (1992)
IL-8		Virus	Choi and Jacoby, (1992)
IL-8		Elastase	Nakamura *et al.* (1992)
IL-8	Keratinocytes	IL-1,	Larsen *et al.* (1989b)
IL-8		IFN-γ+TNF	Barker *et al.* (1990)
GCP/IL-8	Chondrocytes	IL-1,TNF,dsRNA	Van Damme *et al.* (1990a)
IL-8			Lotz *et al.* (1992)
IL-8			Recklies and Golds, (1992)
NAP-1/IL-8	Mesothelial cells	TNF,IL-1,IFN-γ	Goodman *et al.* (1992)
IL-8		Asbestos	Boylan *et al.* (1992)
IL-8		TNF	Jonjic *et al.* (1992)
IL-8	Amnion cells (placenta)	–	Shimoya *et al.* (1992)
IL-8			Trautman *et al.* (1992)
IL-8	Endocrine cells	IL-1	Weetman *et al.* (1992)
IL-8	Astrocytes	IL-1,TNF	Aloisi *et al.* (1992)
IL-8	Choriodecidual cells	IL-1,TNF	Kelly *et al.* (1992)
IL-8			Dudley *et al.* (1993)
IL-8	Mesangial cells	IL-1,TNF	Brown *et al.* (1991)
IL-8			Zoja *et al.* (1991)
GCP/IL-8	Hepatocytes, hepatoma	IL-1,TNF,virus	Van Damme *et al.* (1989b)
NCF/IL-8			Thornton *et al.* (1990)
LUCT	Carcinoma	–	Suzuki *et al.* (1989b)
IL-8		IL-1,TNF	Abruzzo *et al.* (1992)
GCP/IL-8	Osteosarcoma	IL-1,virus	Van Damme *et al.* (1989a)
LECT/IL-8	Myelomonocyte	PMA	Suzuki *et al.* (1993)
MONAP	Promyelocyte	PMA,DMSO	Kowalski and Denhardt, (1989)

Abbreviations to Table 1
LPS, lipopolysaccharide; Con A, concanavalin A; PHA, phytohaemagglutinin; PMA, phorbol 12-myristate 13-acetate; dsRNA, double-stranded RNA; polyrl:rC, polyriboinosinic.polyribocytidilic acid; DMSO, dimethyl sulphoxide; TNF, tumour necrosis factor α; IFN, interferon; SEA, staphylococcus enterotoxin A; FMLP, formyl-methionyl-leucyl-phenylalanine.

inducers used as well as the corresponding references from the literature. This Table is illustrative for the increase of literature data during the last 3 years (see review by Van Damme, 1991). Most researchers originally isolated the molecule from peripheral blood monocytes stimulated with lipopolysaccharide or mitogen. Fibroblasts, endo-thelial cells, epithelial cells, smooth muscle cells, and a variety of more specialized cell types, can produce IL-8 in response to the primary cytokines IL-1 and TNF-α. In addition, viruses such as measles and rubella virus, as well as the double-stranded RNA polyrI.polyrC can act as inducers of IL-8, e.g. in fibroblasts. Since IL-8 can also be produced by neutrophils under specific circumstances it should be considered as an autocrine chemotactic factor. Finally, IL-8 has been isolated from different tumour cell lines, including carcinoma and sarcoma cells (Table 1).

Comparison of the conditions to induce IL-6 and IL-8 in human monocytes and fibroblasts reveals striking parallels (Fig. 1). In fibroblasts, IL-1, double-stranded RNA and virus are the best inducers whereas virus, lipopolysaccharide and mitogen are

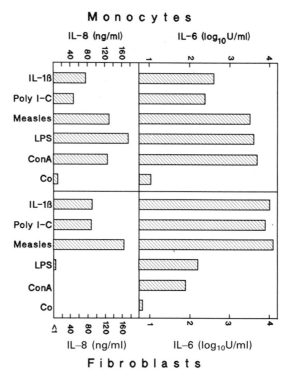

Fig. 1. Production of IL-8 (radioimmunoassay, Rampart *et al.*, 1992) and IL-6 (hybridoma growth factor; Van Snick *et al.*, 1986) by human monocytes and fibroblasts stimulated with IL-1β (100 U/ml), poly rI:rC (100 μg/ml), Measles virus ($10^{4.6}$ TCID$_{50}$/ml), LPS (50 μg/ml) or Con A (10 μg/ml) for 48 h (abbreviations: see footnote of Table 1). Co = control o.

superior inducers in monocytes. Although these two inflammatory cytokines can be produced by a variety of different cell types, the immunological response retains its specificity by the nature of stimulus to trigger the cells. Indeed, after bacterial infection, IL-6 and IL-8 are efficiently produced by peripheral blood monocytes, whereas fibroblasts respond better during the course of a viral infection. Furthermore, endogeneous IL-1 from monocytes can efficiently stimulate the release of the secondary cytokines IL-6 and IL-8. Antibodies against the IL-1 type I receptor inhibit IL-6 and IL-8 induction by monocytes. However, antibodies against the IL-1 type II receptor augmented cytokine production, indicating that the latter is acting as a decoy target for IL-1 (Colotta *et al.*, 1993). This parallel secretion of IL-6 and IL-8 in response to IL-1 and other cytokine inducers can be explained through common responsive elements as possible sites of gene transactivation. These include the NF-κB consensus motif and the NF/IL-6-like motif (Hirano *et al.*, 1990; Mukaida *et al.*, 1990).

BIOCHEMICAL CHARACTERIZATION OF IL-8 PROTEIN

Natural IL-8 has been purified from different cell sources, including monocytes (Schröder *et al.*, 1987; Walz *et al.*, 1987; Yoshimura *et al.*, 1987; Van Damme *et al.*,

Table 2. Purification procedure for IL-8.

Purification step	Volume (ml)	Protein (mg)	IL-8 (U/ml)	Specific Activity (U/mg)	Purific. (fold)	Yield (%)
1. Crude material*	6500	9750	3.51	2.34	1	100
2. Silicic acid	270	81	52.6	175	75	62
3. Heparin-sepharose	15	0.82	644	11 800	5040	42
4. Cation-exchange FPLC	2	0.10	4130	82 600	35 300	36

*IL-8 produced on human monocytes and purified as described by Van Damme *et al.* (1989c).

1988), lymphocytes (Gregory *et al.*, 1988), fibroblasts (Golds *et al.*, 1989; Van Damme *et al.*, 1989a) and endothelial cells (Gimbrone *et al.*, 1989; Schröder and Christophers, 1989). The molecule has originally been reported as a 10 kDa protein upon gel filtration or SDS–PAGE, but careful determinations have demonstrated that natural IL-8 occurs as a 6–8 kDa doublet (Van Damme *et al.*, 1989c). The low M_r of IL-8 has served as a criterion to distinguish it from other cytokines, such as IL-1 and TNF, that were reported to activate neutrophils *in vitro* or *in vivo* (Van Damme *et al.*, 1985a; Wang *et al.*, 1987).

IL-8 is heat-stable and resistant to extremes of pH (Schröder *et al.*, 1987; Peveri *et al.*, 1988). These properties have been helpful for the development of an efficient purification strategy. However, the use of heat stability can also be disadvantageous because possible contamination of IL-8 preparations with lipopolysaccharide cannot be excluded by heat inactivation of the protein.

The purification method that was originally used in our laboratory allowed us to purify IL-8 to homogeneity in three steps (Table 2). Silicic acid or controlled pore glass are nonspecific adsorbants, that are useful in concentrating simultaneously several cytokines (IFN-β, INF-γ, IL-1, IL-6) from large volumes of cell culture supernatant (Van Damme *et al.*, 1985a, 1987). IL-8 can then be separated from these cytokines by its affinity for heparin and by FPLC or HPLC. Homogeneous natural IL-8 has a specific activity of 10^5 to 10^6 U/mg, depending on the assay system used (Schröder *et al.*, 1987; Yoshimura *et al.*, 1987; Van Damme *et al.*, 1988; Gimbrone *et al.*, 1989; Proost *et al.*, 1993a).

Sequence analysis of mature IL-8 has shown that it occurs in multiple forms that differ in truncation at the *N*-terminus (Table 3). The composition of IL-8 preparations depends on the cell source used to produce IL-8, rather than on the purification method (Van Damme *et al.*, 1989a; Schröder *et al.*, 1990b). Different *N*-terminal truncation forms of natural IL-8 have also been observed in other laboratories (Gregory *et al.*, 1988; Lindley *et al.*, 1988; Yoshimura *et al.*, 1989a; Schröder *et al.*, 1990b). There is evidence that specific proteases (e.g. those secreted by the stimulated producer cells) are responsible for this phenomenon (Hébert *et al.*, 1990; Nakagawa *et al.*, 1991). This could explain why fibroblasts predominantly produce less processed *N*-terminal forms of IL-8, whereas IL-8 from leukocytes occurs in shorter forms (Table 3). This *N*-terminal processing is important for the biological activity of IL-8 *in vitro*, since the 72-amino-acid protein (form III, Table 3) is more potent than the 77 residue IL-8 (form II, Table 3) (Tanaka *et al.*, 1988; Suzuki *et al.*, 1989a; Hébert *et al.*, 1990; Nourshargh *et*

Table 3. Different *N*-terminal truncation forms of natural IL-8 and platelet basic protein (PBP)-derived peptides.

Description	Form	*N*-terminus*	Relative amount (%)	
			leukocytes	fibroblasts
IL-8/NAP-1	I	EGAVLPRSAKELRCQCIKTYS	1	0
	II	AVLPRSAKELRCQCIKTYS	14	62
	III	SAKELRCQCIKTYS	64	35
	IV	AKELRCQCIKTYS	4	3
	V	KELRCQCIKTYS	12	0
	VI	ELRCQCIKTYS	5	0
			thrombocytes	thrombocytes + leukocytes
PBP	I	SSTKSQTKRNLAKGKEESLDSDLYAELRCMCIKTTS	5	0
	II	RNLAKGKEESLDSDLYAELRCMCIKTTS	2	0
CTAP-III	III	NLAKGKEESLDSDLYAELRCMCIKTTS	56	26
	IV	AKGKEESLDSDLYAELRCMCIKTTS	3	0
β-TG	V	GKEESLDSDLYAELRCMCIKTTS	15	3
	VI	EESLDSDLYAELRCMCIKTTS	1	0
NAP-2	VII	AELRCMCIKTTS	18	71

*N-termini determined by automated protein sequence analysis (Van Damme *et al.* 1989c).

al., 1992). In contrast, *in vivo* both IL-8 forms are equipotent. This is possibly owing to proteolytic cleavage of the 77-amino-acid protein (Nourshargh *et al.*, 1992). Similarly, the structurally related platelet basic protein (PBP, see Similarity of IL-8 with other chemokines) is also processed in multiple *N*-terminal truncation forms. As documented in Table 3, the relative amount of these forms also differs depending on the cell substrate used. If platelets are cocultivated with leukocytes, inactive PBP is processed predominantly to its shortest *N*-terminal form, which is also a neutrophil-activating peptide (NAP-2) (Walz *et al.*, 1989; Van Damme *et al.*, 1990b). PBP can be converted to shorter forms by exposure to proteases (Holt and Niewiarowski, 1980; Brandt *et al.*, 1990; Walz and Baggiolini, 1990). Remarkably, IL-8 and PBP only show sequence similarity starting at the *N*-terminal residue of their ultimately processed forms (Van Damme *et al.*, 1989c). The importance of these *N*-terminal residues for receptor binding and biological activity has been demonstrated using chemically synthesized analogues (Clark-Lewis *et al.*, 1991a,b; Moser *et al.*, 1993) or scanning mutagenesis (Hébert *et al.*, 1991).

PROTEIN AND GENE STRUCTURE OF IL-8

The cDNA for human IL-8 has been cloned independently in several laboratories (Schmid and Weissmann, 1987; Matsushima *et al.*, 1988; Kowalsky and Denhardt, 1989). The sequence encodes a precursor protein of 99 residues, including a highly hydrophobic *N*-terminal region, representing a typical signal peptide. The natural protein is probably not glycosylated and there are no potential N-glycosylation sites present in its sequence. The mature protein of 72 to 77 residues (Table 3; Fig. 3) has also been completely sequenced (Lindley *et al.*, 1988). Synthetic as well as recombinant IL-8 have been shown to be biologically active (Lindley *et al.*, 1988; Furuta *et al.*, 1989). Synthesized, biologically active IL-8 forms two intramolecular disulphide bridges, which are important for its activity (Tanaka *et al.*, 1988). Determination of the secondary and three-dimensional structure of IL-8 by nuclear magnetic resonance spectroscopy and by X-ray crystallography indicates that, in solution, the molecule occurs as a dimer of two identical subunits (Clore *et al.*, 1989; Clore *et al.*, 1990; Baldwin *et al.* 1990, 1991). Differences related to the relative orientation of these subunits were detected when comparing the quaternary structures of IL-8 in solution and in the crystal (Clore and Gronenborn, 1991).

Cloning of the genomic DNA has shown that the human IL-8 gene consists of 4 exons and 3 introns (Mukaida *et al.*, 1989; Hotta *et al.*, 1990). Although expression of IL-8 and IL-6 genes seems to be parallel-regulated (Fig. 1), no overall sequence similarity could be observed between their 5'-flanking regions. This region contains potential binding sites for several nuclear factors, indicative for their role as possible regulatory sequences for IL-8 expression (Mukaida *et al.*, 1989). There exists evidence that a cooperative interaction between two such *cis*-elements may be required for induction of IL-8 gene expression by IL-1 and TNF (Mukaida *et al.*, 1990).

The gene for IL-8 is located on the q12–21 region of human chromosome 4 (Modi *et al.*, 1990). This locus also contains the genes of structurally and functionally related inflammatory proteins (see Similarity of IL-8 with other chemokines). This is indicative for origin of the superfamily by a mechanism of gene duplication (Matsushima and Oppenheim, 1989; Wolpe and Cerami, 1989).

IL-8 RECEPTOR, SIGNAL TRANSDUCTION AND POSTRECEPTOR EVENTS

Cross-desensitization experiments using IL-8 and other neutrophil chemotactic substances (C5a, FMLP, LTB4 and PAF) have shown that IL-8 does not crossreact with these chemotaxins. This indicates that the cellular responses elicited by this cytokine are transmitted via specific receptors (Schröder *et al.*, 1987; Peveri *et al.*, 1988). High-affinity receptors (67 kDa and 59 kDa) have been identified on the surface of human neutrophils (20 000/cell) that bind IL-8 but not IL-1 or TNF-α (Samanta *et al.*, 1989). Lower numbers of IL-8 receptors were found on various types of leukocytes, including T lymphocytes and monocyte cell lines (Matsushima and Oppenheim, 1989; Grob *et al.*, 1990). IL-8 rapidly downregulates its own receptor expression on neutrophils, a process that is associated with internalization of the ligand–receptor complex (Samanta *et al.*, 1990). The receptors rapidly reappear on the cell surface probably not through *de novo* synthesis but through recycling. The existence of two classes of receptors for IL-8 was shown by binding competition assays, crosslinking studies and cross-desensitization experiments using the related chemokines GRO and NAP-2 (Schröder *et al.*, 1990a; Leonard *et al.*, 1991a; Moser *et al.*, 1991; Oppenheim *et al.*, 1991).

More recently, two cDNAs have been isolated from human neutrophils that encode functional IL-8 receptors (Holmes *et al.*, 1991; Murphy and Tiffany 1991). The corresponding proteins show 77% structural similarity and are both members of the superfamily of receptors that are coupled to guanine-nucleotide-binding proteins (G-proteins). These serpentine-like receptors are characterized by seven transmembrane domains. The two types of receptors bind IL-8 with high affinity, but one also binds NAP-2 and GRO at high affinity, whereas the other binds GRO with low affinity (Lee *et al.*, 1992; Schumacher *et al.*, 1992; Cerretti *et al.*, 1993). Using chimaeric receptors the differential binding of IL-8 and GRO was found to reside in the *N*-terminal heterogeneity of the IL-8 receptors (LaRosa *et al.*, 1992; Gayle *et al.*, 1993). At least two conformationally vicinal free reactive sulphydryl groups located in the binding domain of the IL-8 receptor are essential for biological activity (Samanta *et al.*, 1993). The genes for the two IL-8 receptors, as well as an IL-8 receptor pseudogene were assigned to human chromosome 2Q35 (Morris *et al.*, 1992; Lloyd *et al.*, 1993; Mollereau *et al.*, 1993). Recently, a 39 kDa binding protein for IL-8 has been characterized on erythrocytes (Horuk *et al.*, 1993b). Multiple chemokines were able to cross-compete with IL-8 for binding to this promiscuous receptor, which was discovered to be a receptor for the malaria parasite *Plasmodium vivax* (Horuk *et al.*, 1993a).

Transmembrane signal transduction of IL-8 in neutrophils occurs by a mechanism that implies a direct role for guanosine triphosphate binding proteins (Kupper *et al.*, 1992; Barnett *et al.*, 1993; Wu *et al.*, 1993). IL-8 induces a rapid rise in cytosolic free Ca^{++} that could be inhibited by *Bordetella pertussis* toxin, whereas the respiratory burst elicited by IL-8 was blocked by inhibitors of protein kinase C (Thelen *et al.*, 1988). This indicates that IL-8 activates neutrophils via a GTP-binding protein by a process that is dependent on Ca^{++} and protein kinase C. The Ca^{++} influx is initiated via production of inositol triphosphate after stimulation by IL-8 (Pike *et al.*, 1992). Lymphocyte migration induced by IL-8 is also specifically inhibited by Ca^{++} channel antagonists (Bacon *et al.*, 1989). Evidence has also been provided for the production of inositol phosphate metabolites during IL-8 receptor-mediated signal transduction in lymphocytes (Bacon *et al.*, 1993). IL-8 was also found to specifically induce phosphorylation of intracellular 48 kDa and 64 kDa proteins (Suzuki *et al.*, 1989a; Oppenheim *et al.*, 1991). Finally, it was found that IL-8 activates kinases resulting in protein phosphorylation (Van Lint *et al.*, 1993).

BIOLOGICAL ACTIVITIES OF IL-8

In vitro Effects

IL-8 stimulates neutrophils to directed migration, as measured under agarose or in the Boyden chamber (Schröder *et al.*, 1987; Yoshimura *et al.*, 1987; Van Damme *et al.*, 1988). The protein also induces neutrophil degranulation measurable by the release of granule constituents such as β-glucuronidase, elastase, myeloperoxidase, gelatinase B, vitamin B_{12}-binding protein and lactoferrin (Schröder *et al.*, 1987; Peveri *et al.*, 1988; Willems *et al.*, 1989; Masure *et al.*, 1991). In addition, IL-8 elicits a rapid increase of cytoplasmic-free Ca^{++} (Thelen *et al.*, 1988), but induces only a weak respiratory burst through formation of superoxide and hydrogen peroxide (Schröder *et al.*, 1987; Peveri *et al.*, 1988; Kownatski and Uhrich, 1990). Like C5a, FMLP and PAF, it activates arachidonate-5-lipoxygenase with release of LTB_4 from neutrophils in the presence of exogenous arachidonic acid (Schröder, 1989). PAF can be synthesized by neutrophils stimulated with IL-8 (Bussolino *et al.*, 1992). IL-8 stimulates phagocytosis of opsonized particles (Detmers *et al.*, 1991) and enhances the growth-inhibitory activity of neutrophils to *Candida albicans* (Djeu *et al.*, 1990). This antifungal effect of IL-8 is not direct, nor mediated by stimulation of superoxide production by neutrophils.

IL-8 is identical to leukocyte adhesion inhibitor (LAI) that inhibits neutrophil adhesion to cytokine-activated endothelial monolayers, thereby protecting the blood vessel cells from neutrophil-mediated damage (Gimbrone *et al.*, 1989). This effect is complex since high doses of IL-8 stimulate neutrophil adhesion to unactivated endothelial cells (Carveth *et al.*, 1989; Gimbrone *et al.*, 1989). Furthermore, others have shown that IL-8 is essential for the invasion of neutrophils across endothelial cell monolayers or a blood-vessel wall construct (Huber *et al.*, 1991; Smith *et al.*, 1991; Kuijpers *et al.*, 1992). Neutrophil binding in response to IL-8 involves rapid shedding of neutrophil L-selectin (LECAM-1) and altered expression of the leukocyte CD11/CD18 β_2 integrins (Carveth *et al.*, 1989; Huber *et al.*, 1991). Increased expression of CD11/ CD18 on the neutrophil cell surface appears also to correlate with the IL-8 mediated release of specific granules and with the LAI effect of IL-8 (Detmers *et al.*, 1990; Luscinkas *et al.*, 1992).

Compared with other chemotaxins (C5a,PAF,FMLP,LTB_4), activation of neutrophils by IL-8 seems to be more selective in that eosinophils and monocytes are not responsive (Schröder *et al.*, 1987; Yoshimura *et al.*, 1987). In addition, IL-8 is only a poor inducer of cytosolic free Ca^{++} changes in monocytes and lymphocytes (Thelen *et al.*, 1988; Walz *et al.*, 1991b). However, IL-8 is chemotactic for T lymphocytes when measured by adherence of migrating cells to collagen-coated filters in Boyden chambers (Larsen *et al.*, 1989a). Although only a small percentage of small T-cells respond, lymphocytes are approximately 10 times more sensitive to IL-8 than neutrophils. Other studies confirm that IL-8 is chemotactic for activated T lymphocytes and basophils, but show that lymphocytes and neutrophils are equally sensitive to IL-8 (Leonard *et al.*,

1990; Wilkinson and Newman, 1992). Furthermore, after exposure to IL-3, basophils were originally reported to release histamine and leukotrienes in response to IL-8 (Dahinden *et al.*, 1989). However, more detailed studies revealed that IL-8 inhibits release of histamine and leukotriene from basophils (Bischoff *et al.*, 1991; Kuna *et al.*, 1991; Alam *et al.*, 1992a). Circulating eosinophils from patients with atopic dermatitis and allergic asthma show an increased migratory response toward IL-8 (Bruijnzeel *et al.*, 1993; Warringa *et al.*, 1993). In addition, IL-8 induces chemokinesis of IL-2-activated NK cells (Sebok *et al.*, 1993). IL-8 also induces haptotactic migration of neutrophils and melanoma cells (Wang *et al.*, 1990; Rot, 1993) and stimulates chemotaxis of endothelial cells (Koch *et al.*, 1992). Binding to heparan sulphate or to heparin enhances the neutrophil responses to IL-8 (Webb *et al.*, 1993). Finally, IL-8 selectively inhibits IgE production induced by IL-4 in human B cells (Kimata *et al.*, 1992) as well as nitric oxide induction in peritoneal neutrophils (McCall *et al.*, 1992).

In vivo Effects

Human IL-8 has initially been studied in our laboratory as a factor, different from IL-1, that provokes early skin reactivity in rabbits (Van Damme *et al.*, 1985b; Van Damme and Opdenakker 1990). Since the effect of IL-8 is more rapid than with its physiological inducer IL-1, it is likely that skin reaction caused by IL-1 is, in part, mediated by IL-8 production. More detailed experiments have shown that intradermal injection of IL-8 induces plasma leakage and neutrophil accumulation in the skin (Foster *et al.*, 1989; Rampart *et al.*, 1989). In the presence of the vasodilator substance PGE_2, pmol amounts of IL-8 induce neutrophil infiltration and plasma protein extravasation (Rampart *et al.*, 1989). Both effects are fast in onset and relatively short in duration (Fig. 2). These effects could be inhibited by antibodies against leukocyte integrins (Forrest *et al.*, 1992). The oedema formation by IL-8 is neutrophil-dependent. Histology of IL-8-induced lesions has also demonstrated intravascular neutrophil accumulation, aggregate formation and venular wall damage (Colditz *et al.*, 1989; Foster *et al.*, 1989). The effects of IL-8 in the skin are comparable to those observed with FMLP and C5a. Intradermal injection of IL-8 in rats causes an increase in accumulation of both lymphocytes and neutrophils in the connective tissue (Larsen *et al.*, 1989a). In contrast, injection of IL-8 into the lymphatic drainage areas of rat lymph nodes results in an accelerated emigration of only lymphocytes in high endothelial venules of the draining lymph nodes (Larsen *et al.*, 1989a). The predominant effect of intradermal injection of IL-8 in human subjects was neutrophil accumulation in proximity to dermal blood vessels (Leonard *et al.*, 1991b). Introduction of IL-8 in canine tracheal luminal fluid results in neutrophil accumulation (Jorens *et al.*, 1992a). During the late phase of an acute inflammatory reaction in the peritoneal cavity of rabbits, IL-8 was found to be responsible for neutrophil infiltration and plasma protein leakage (Beaubien *et al.*, 1990).

Intraveneous injection of IL-8 in animals leads to an immediate leukopenia followed by a profound neutrophilia (Van Damme *et al.*, 1988; Matsushima and Oppenheim, 1989; Jagels and Hugli, 1992; Van Zee *et al.*, 1992). Such neutrophilia is accompanied by release of nonsegmented neutrophils from the bone-marrow reservoir (Jagels and Hugli, 1992). The systemic vascular effect of IL-8 also results from its interference with neutrophil adhesion to endothelial cells (Hechtman *et al.*, 1991). Induction of

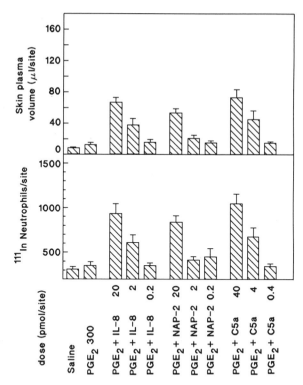

Fig. 2. Induction of skin reactivity (neutrophil accumulation and plasma leakage) in rabbit skin by IL-8, NAP-2 and C5a (Rampart *et al.*, 1989; Van Damme *et al.*, 1990b).

neutrophilia by IL-8 might be important of nonspecific resistance to infection (Vogels *et al.*, 1993).

IL-8 has been reported as a mediator for sympathetic pain using a rat paw pressure test (Cunha *et al.*, 1991). In addition to its proinflammatory effect, IL-8 exerts growth-regulatory effects since it is angiogenic when implanted in the rat cornea and induces neovascularization in a rabbit corneal pocket model (Koch *et al.*, 1992; Strieter *et al.*, 1992). Finally, it promotes epidermal cell proliferation (Tuschil *et al.*, 1992) and enhances neuronal survival (Araujo and Cotman, 1993).

SIMILARITY OF IL-8 TO OTHER CHEMOKINES

The neutrophil-activating protein IL-8/NAP-1 is recognized to belong to a superfamily of inflammatory and growth-regulatory proteins (Schmid and Weissmann, 1987; Yoshimura *et al.*, 1987; Van Damme *et al.*, 1989c; Westwick *et al.*, 1989; Wolpe *et al.*, 1989). The structural similarity between these different chemokines is based mainly on the conservation of four cysteines in all proteins (Fig. 3). Depending on the arrangement of the two *N*-terminal cysteines, the chemokine family is divided in two subfamilies: C–X–C and C–C chemokines.

```
                  5    10   15   20   25   30   35   40   45   50   55   60   65   70   75   80
                  .    .    .    .    .    .    .    .    .    .    .    .    .    .    .    .      % Identity

C-X-C CHEMOKINES

IL-8    EGAVLPRSAKELRCQCIKTYSKPFHPKFIKELRVIESGPHCANTEIIVKLSD GRELCLDPKENWVQRVVEKFLKRAENS     (100)
NAP-2       AELRCMCIKTTSG IHPKNIQSLEVIGKGTHCNQVEVIATLKD GRKICLDPDAPRIKIVQKKLAGDESAD          (48)
PF-4    EAEEDGDLQCLCVKTTSQ VRPRHITSLEVIKAGPHCPTAQLIATLKN GRKICLDLQAPLYKKIIKKLLES             (34)
GROα    ASVATELRCQCLQTLQG IHPKNIQSVNVKSPGPHCAQTEVIATLKN GRKACLNPASPIVKKIIEKMLNSDKSN          (42)
GROβ    APLATELRCQCLQTLQG IHLKNIQSVKVKSPGPHCAQTEVIATLKN GQKACLNPASPMVKKIIEKMLKNGKSN          (41)
GROγ    ASVVTELRCQCLQTLQG IHLKNIQSVNVRSPGPHCAQTEVIATLKN GKKACLNPASPMVQKIIEKILNKGSTN          (40)
IP-10   VPLSRTVRCTCISISNQPVNPRSLEKLEIIPASQFCPRVEIIATMKKKGEKRCLNPESKAIKNLLKAVSKEMSKRSP         (23)
ENA-78  AGPAAAVLRELRCVCLQTTQG VHPKMISNLQVFAIGPQCSKVEVVASLKN GKEICLDPEAPFLKKVIQKILDGGNKEN      (34)
GCP-2   GPVSAVLTELRCTCLRVTLR VNPKTIGKLQVFPAGPQCSKVEVVASLKN GKQVCLDPEAPFLKKVIQKILDSGNK         (31)
MIG     TPVVRKGRCSCISTNQGTIHLQSLKDLKQFAPSPSCEKIEIIATLKN GVQTCLNPDSADVKELIKKWEKQVSQKKKQK....   (28)

C-C CHEMOKINES

MCP-1   QPDAINAPVTCCYNFTNRKISVQRLASYRRITSSKCPKEAVIFKTIVAKEICADPKQKWVQDSMDHLDKQTQTPKT          (100)
MCP-2   QPDSVSIPITCCFNVINRKIPIQRLESYTRITNIQCPKEAVIFKTKRGKEVCADPKERWVRDSMKHLDQIFQNLKP          (62)
MCP-3   QPVGINTSTTCCYRFINKKIPKQRLESYRRTTSSHCPREAVIFKTKLDKEICADPTQKWVQDFMKHLDKKTQTPKL          (71)
MIP-1α  SLAADTPTACCFSYTSRQIPQNFIADY FETSSQCSKPGVIFLTKRSRQVCADPSEEWVQKYVSDLELSA                (38)
MIP-1β  APMGSDPPTACCFSYTARKLPRNFVVDY YETSSLCSQPAVVPQTKRSKQVCADPSESWVQEYVYDLELN                (36)
RANTES  SPYSSDTTPCCFAYIARPLPRAHIKEY FYTSGKCSNPAVVFVTRKNRQVCANPEKKWVREYINSLEMS                (28)
I-309   SKSMQVPFSRCCFSFAEQEIPLRAILCY RNTSSICSNEGLIPFLKRGKEACALDTVGWVQRHRKMLRHCPSKRK           (31)
```

Fig. 3. Amino acid sequence alignment of IL-8 and related human chemokines.

C–X–C Chemokines

In addition to IL-8, this subfamily includes the human platelet-derived factors, platelet factor 4 (PF4) (Deuel *et al.*, 1977) and β-thromboglobulin (β-TG) (Begg *et al.*, 1978). As shown in Table 3, β-TG is an *N*-terminally processed form of PBP (Holt *et al.*, 1986) and connective tissue activating peptide III (CTAP-III) (Castor *et al.*, 1983). CTAP-III has previously been designated low-affinity platelet factor-4 (LA-PF4) (Rucinski *et al.*, 1979) in order to illustrate the higher affinity of PF4 for heparin. LA-PF4 can be converted to β-TG by plasmin and trypsin (Holt and Niewiarowski, 1980). Similarly, the molecule can be further processed to its shortest form (Van Damme *et al.*, 1989c; Table 3), designated by others as NAP-2 (Walz and Baggiolini, 1990). Multiple biological effects have been ascribed to these platelet products. These include chemotactic, mitogenic, immunoregulatory and angiogenesis-inhibitory activities (Deuel *et al.*, 1981; Castor *et al.*, 1983; Senior *et al.*, 1983; Katz *et al.*, 1986; Brandt *et al.*, 1989; Maione *et al.*, 1990). Some of these activities, such as the mitogenic effect of CTAP-III could result from contamination with other molecules (Holt *et al.*, 1986). The mitogenic effect of CTAP-III has been confirmed with recombinant material (Mullenbach *et al.*, 1986). *N*-terminal processing of β-TG is important, since only the shorter forms (NAP-2) of the molecule appear to induce *in vitro* neutrophil activation (Walz *et al.*, 1989; Brandt *et al.*, 1990). In general, NAP-2 has a lower specific activity than IL-8 for both its *in vitro* and *in vivo* effects on neutrophils (Fig. 2 and Van Damme *et al.*, 1990b; Van Osselaer *et al.*, 1991).

A melanoma growth-stimulatory activity (MGSA) has been isolated for human melanoma cells (Richmond *et al.*, 1988) and found to be identical to the gene product of a cDNA, designated GRO, which is overexpressed in transformed fibroblasts (Anisowicz *et al.*, 1987). This molecule is structurally related to IL-8 and can be induced in normal fibroblasts and synovial cells by IL-1 (Anisowicz *et al.*, 1988; Golds *et al.*, 1989; Schröder *et al.*, 1990b). Furthermore, GRO/MGSA is functionally related to IL-8 in that it induces chemotaxis and degranulation of neutrophils (Moser *et al.*, 1990; Schröder *et al.*, 1990a). GRO/MGSA is reported to decrease collagen expression in human fibroblasts (Unemori *et al.*, 1993). Two additional highly related genes, designated GRO-β and, GRO-γ, have been identified (Haskill *et al.*, 1990; Iida and Grotendorst, 1990). Macrophage inflammatory protein-2 (MIP-2) is a molecule isolated from murine LPS-stimulated macrophages. It shares several biological characteristics with human IL-8. These include neutrophil chemotactic activity and induction of local skin reactivity (Wolpe *et al.*, 1989). Cloning and characterization of cDNAs for human MIP-2 revealed three related genes identical to those encoding for MGSA/GRO (Tekamp-Olson *et al.*, 1990).

Treatment of human mononuclear cells, fibroblasts or endothelial cells with IFN-γ results in the production of an induced protein, IP-10, which also belongs to the IL-8 superfamily (Luster *et al.*, 1985). The molecule is expressed during delayed immune responses in human skin (Kaplan *et al.*, 1987) and is detectable in psoriatic plaques (Gottlieb *et al.*, 1988). Human IP-10 is chemotactic for monocytes and T lymphocytes and promotes T-cell adhesion to endothelial cells (Taub *et al.*, 1993b). Murine IP-10 elicits a powerful host-mediated antitumour response *in vivo*, but has no effect on tumour cells *in vitro* (Luster and Leder, 1993). This antitumour activity appears to be mediated by the recruitment of lymphocytes, neutrophils and monocytes. In the presence of growth factors, IP-10 can inhibit colony formation of early human haemopoietic progenitors (Sarris *et al.*, 1993). IFN-γ can induce in monocytes other C–X–C chemokines, such as the newly described human MIG (Farber, 1993).

Recently, two additional human neutrophil activating factors have been identified, designated ENA-78 (Walz *et al.*, 1991a) and GCP-2 (Proost *et al.*, 1993a). The last two proteins show 77% similarity and could be classified as a subgroup (cf. GRO-α, β, γ) within the CXC chemokine family (Proost *et al.*, 1993b).

C–C Chemokines

Most C–X–C chemokines are active on neutrophils, whereas C–C chemokines predominantly stimulate monocytes. The human macrophage chemoattractant and activating factor (MCAF) or monocyte chemotactic protein-1 (MCP-1) has been isolated and identified from normal or tumour cells (Furutani *et al.*, 1989; Graves *et al.*, 1989; Robinson *et al.*, 1989; Van Damme *et al.*, 1989b; Yoshimura *et al.*, 1989b; Decock *et al.*, 1990; Leonard and Yoshimura, 1990). In contrast to IL-8, the gene of MCP-1 is localized on human chromosome 17 (Mehrabian *et al.*, 1991; Rollins *et al.*, 1991). Human MCP-1 is, nevertheless, coinduced with IL-8 in diploid fibroblasts and endothelial cells in response to various stimuli, such as IL-1, TNF, double-stranded RNA and virus (Larsen *et al.*, 1989c; Strieter *et al.*, 1989c; Van Damme *et al.*, 1989b; Sica *et al.*, 1990b). MCP-1 is considered as the human homologue of the *JE* gene identified in murine fibroblasts after stimulation with PDGF (Rollins *et al.*, 1988) and of a monocyte chemotactic factor from primate vascular cells (Valente *et al.*, 1988). In addition to MCP-1, two highly related human monocyte chemotactic proteins (designated MCP-2 and MCP-3) have recently been identified (Van Damme *et al.*, 1992).

Macrophage inflammatory protein-1 (MIP-1), another member of the C–C chemokine family consisting of two distinct mouse proteins (MIP-1α and MIP-1β), has originally been characterized by its neutrophil chemokinetic activity and by footpad inflammation (Davatelis *et al.*, 1988; Wolpe and Cerami, 1989). The human homologues of MIP-1α and MIP-1β were independently isolated from various cell types by cDNA cloning (for review see Schall, 1991). Activities other than chemotaxis have been assigned to MIP-1. These include costimulation (Broxmeyer *et al.*, 1989), as well as inhibition (Graham *et al.*, 1990) of haemopoietic colony formation, prostaglandin independent pyrogenicity (Davatelis *et al.*, 1989) and T-cell chemotaxis and adhesion (Taub *et al.*, 1993a; Schall *et al.*, 1993; Tanaka *et al.*, 1993). Another C–C chemokine, RANTES, has been reported to act as a chemoattractant for human monocytes and a subset of memory T lymphocytes (Schall *et al.*, 1990; Schall, 1991). The T-cell-derived human I-309 was shown to be a monocyte chemoattractant (Miller and Krangel, 1992).

A number of C–C chemokines, such as MCP-1, RANTES and MIP-1α are able to induce basophil histamine release (Alam *et al.*, 1992b,c; Kuna *et al.*, 1992), whereas RANTES and MIP-1α induce the migration and activation of eosinophils (Kameyoshi *et al.*, 1992; Rot *et al.*, 1992). Recently, a receptor that binds MCP-1, MIP-1 and RANTES has been cloned and found to be a member of the G-protein-coupled receptor superfamily. It shows about 33% amino acid identity with the receptors for IL-8 (Gao *et al.*, 1993; Neote *et al.*, 1993).

ROLE OF IL-8 IN PATHOLOGY

Since its discovery there has been a rapidly increasing number of reports on the *in vivo* release of IL-8 during infection or inflammation. IL-8 was first demonstrated in skin lesions of psoriasis patients (Camp *et al.*, 1986, 1990; Schröder and Christophers, 1986; Fincham *et al.*, 1988; Gearing *et al.*, 1990; Nickoloff *et al.*, 1991; Sticherling *et al.*, 1991; Schröder *et al.*, 1992). It might also play a role in the hyperproliferation and chemotaxis of keratinocytes (Tuschil *et al.*, 1992; Michel *et al.*, 1992). Induction of IL-8 by *in vitro* cultured chondrocytes (Van Damme *et al.*, 1990a) and synovial cells (Watson *et al.*, 1988; Golds *et al.*, 1989) by IL-1 corresponds with the presence of IL-8 in synovial fluids and subsequent cartilage degradation during rheumatoid arthritis (Brennan *et al.*, 1990; Elford and Cooper, 1991; Peichl *et al.*, 1991; Rampart *et al.*, 1992). IL-8 could be an important mediator in lung pathology since increased levels have been detected in bronchoalveolar lavage from patients with adult respiratory distress syndrome, idiopathic pulmonary fibrosis, sarcoidosis and metal fume fever (Carré *et al.*, 1991; Jorens *et al.*, 1992b; Lynch *et al.*, 1992; Miller *et al.*, 1992; Blanc *et al.*, 1993). Bronchial epithelium from asthma and cystic fibrosis patients shows increased IL-8 expression (Marini *et al.*, 1992; Nakamura *et al.*, 1992). Furthermore, IL-8 is thought to be involved in neutrophil-mediated vessel-wall injury, as observed after cardiopulmonary bypass and during atherosclerotic disease (Finn *et al.*, 1993; Koch *et al.*, 1993).

Induction of IL-8 is also demonstrated after IL-1 or TNF infusion, sublethal endotoxaemia, septic shock, microbial invasion of the amniotic cavity, Jarisch–Herxheimer reaction of relapsing fever, infectious diseases of the central nervous system, acute pancreatitis, ulcerative colitis, empyaema, haemolytic uraemic syndrome, meningococcal disease, gastric infection, pertussis and peritonitis (Martich *et al.*, 1991; Redl *et al.*, 1991; Romero *et al.*, 1991; Van Zee *et al.*, 1991; Broaddus *et al.*, 1992; Fitzpatrick *et al.*, 1992; Gross *et al.*, 1992; Mahida *et al.*, 1992; Negussie *et al.*, 1992; Sheron and Williams, 1992; Torre *et al.*, 1992; Van Meir *et al.*, 1992; Crabtree *et al.*, 1993; Halstensen *et al.*, 1993; Lin *et al.*, 1993; Van Deventer *et al.*, 1993). During inflammatory reactions, the biological effects of its production and release can be limited by IL-1 receptor antagonist (DeForge *et al.*, 1992b; Porat *et al.*, 1992), by adsorption to red blood cells (Darbonne *et al.*, 1991) and by free anti-IL8 antibody in serum (Sylvester *et al.*, 1992; Reitamo *et al.*, 1993). Furthermore, cytokines, hormones, cyclooxygenase products, antioxidants and immunosuppressive agents can provide a negative feedback for IL-8 production (Standiford *et al.*, 1990b; Larsen *et al.*, 1991; Martich *et al.*, 1993; Zipfel *et al.*, 1991; DeForge *et al.*, 1992a; Cassatella *et al.*, 1993; Mulligan *et al.*, 1993). Finally, IL-8 can exert beneficial effects during noninflammatory pathologies, e.g. by improving neutrophil functions in myelodysplastic syndromes (Zwierzina *et al.*, 1993).

Research on IL-8 and related chemokines appears to be in an exponential phase. The molecular heterogeneity of the C–X–C and C–C chemokine families is intriguing. Future research should be directed to characterize their specific receptors and to unravel their individual and common impact under pathological conditions.

ACKNOWLEDGEMENTS

The author thanks G. Opdenakker for the critical reading of the manuscript. The accurate editorial help of D. Brabants, P. Proost, W. Put and R. Conings is gratefully acknowledged.

REFERENCES

Abruzzo, L.V., Thornton, A.J., Liebert, M., Grossman, H.B., Evanoff, H., Westwick, J., Strieter, R.M. and Kunkel, S.L. (1992). *Am. J. Pathol.* **140**, 365–373.

Alam, R., Forsythe, P.A., Lett-Brown, M.A. and Grant, J.A. (1992a). *Am. J. Respir. Cell Mol. Biol.* **7**, 427–433.

Alam, R., Forsythe, P.A., Stafford, S., Lett-Brown, M.A. and Grant, J.A. (1992b). *J. Exp. Med.* **176**, 781–786.

Alam, R., Lett-Brown, M.A., Forsythe, P.A., Anderson-Walters, D.J., Kenamore, C., Kormos, C. and Grant, J.A. (1992c). *J. Clin. Invest.* **89**, 723–728.

Aloisi, F., Caré, A., Borsellino, G., Gallo, P., Rosa, S., Bassani, A., Cabibbo, A., Testa, U., Levi, G. and Peschle, C. (1992). *J. Immunol.* **149**, 2358–2366.

Anisowicz, A., Bardwell, L. and Sager, R. (1987). *Proc, Natl Acad. Sci. USA* **84**, 7188–7192.

Anisowicz, A., Zajchowski, D., Stenman, G. and Sager, R. (1988). *Proc. Natl Acad. Sci. USA* **85**, 9645–9649.

Araujo, D.M. and Cotman, C.W. (1993). *Brain Res.* **600**, 49–55.

Bacon, K.B., Westwick, J. and Camp, R.D.R. (1989). *Biochem. Biophys Res. Commun.* **165**, 349–354.

Bacon, K.B., Quinn, D.G., Aubry, J.-P. and Camp, R.D.R. (1993). *Blood* **81**, 430–436.

Baggiolini, M., Dahinden, C., Kunkel, S.L., Leonard, E., Lindley, I.J.D., Mantovani, A., Matsushima, K., Oppenheim, J.J., Rot, A., Schall, T., Schröder, J.M., Strieter, R., Van Damme, J., Walz, A. and Westwick, J. (1993) *Immunol. Today* **14**, 24.

Baldwin, E.T., Franklin, K.A., Appella, E., Yamada, M., Matsushima, K., Wlodawer, A. and Weber, I.T. (1990). *J. Biol. Chem.* **265**, 6851–6853.

Baldwin, E.T., Weber, I.T., Charles, R.St., Xuan, J.-C., Appella, E., Yamada, M., Matsushima, K., Edwards, B.F.P., Clore, G.M., Gronenborn, A.M. and Wlodawer, A. (1991). *Proc. Natl Acad. Sci, USA* **88**, 502–506.

Barker, J.N.W.N., Sarma, V., Mitra, R.S., Dixit, V.M. and Nickoloff, B.J. (1990). *J. Clin. Invest.* **85**, 605–608.

Barnett, M.L., Lamb, K.A., Costello, K.M. and Pike, M.C. (1993). *Biochim. Biophys. Acta* **1177**, 275–282.

Bazzoni F., Cassatella, M.A., Rossi, F., Ceska, M., Dewald, B. and Baggiolini, M. (1991). *J. Exp. Med.* **173**, 771–774.

Beaubien, B.C., Collins, P.D., Jose, P.J., Totty, N.F., Hsuan, J., Waterfield, M.D. and Williams, T.J. (1990). *Biochem. J.* **271**, 797–801.

Becker, S., Quay, J. and Soukup, J. (1991). *J. Immunol.* **147**, 4307–4312.

Begg, G.S., Pepper, D.S., Chesterman, C.N. and Morgan, F.J. (1978). *Biochemistry* **17**, 1739–1744.

Bischoff, S.C., Baggiolini, M., de Weck, A.L. and Dahinden, C.A. (1991). *Biochem. Biophys. Res. Commun.* **179**, 628–633.

Blanc, P.D., Boushey, H.A., Wong, H., Wintermeyer, S.F. and Bernstein, M.S. (1993). *Am. Rev. Respir. Dis.* **147**, 134–138.

Boylan, A.M., Rüegg, C., Kim, K.J., Hébert, C.A., Hoeffel, J.M., Pytela, R., Sheppard, D., Goldstein, I.M. and Broaddus, V.C. (1992). *J. Clin. Invest.* **89**, 1257–1267.

Brandt, E., Ernst, M. and Flad, H.-D. (1990). In *The Molecular and Cellular Aspects of Cytokines* (eds. J.J. Oppenheim, C.A. Dinarello, M. Kluger and M. Powanda), Wiley–Liss Inc., New York, pp. 357–362.

Brandt, E., Ernst, M., Loppnow, H. and Flad, H.-D. (1989). *Lymphokine Res.* **8**, 281–287.

Braun, R.K., Franchini, M., Erard, F., Rihs, S., De Vries, I.J.M., Blaser, K., Hansel, T.T. and Walker, C. (1993). *Eur. J. Immunol.* **23**, 956–960.

Brennan, F.M., Zachariae, C.O.C., Chantry, D., Larsen, C.G., Turner, M., Maini, R.N., Matsushima, K. and Feldman, M. (1990). *Eur. J. Immunol.* **20**, 2141–2144.

Broaddus, V.C., Hébert, C.A., Vitangcol, R.V., Hoeffel, J.M., Bernstein, M.S. and Boylan, A.M. (1992). *Am. Rev. Respir. Dis.* **146**, 825–830.

Brown, Z., Strieter, R.M., Chensue, S.W., Ceska, M., Lindley, I., Neild, G.H., Kunkel, S.L. and Westwick, J. (1991). *Kidney International*, **40**, 86–90.

Broxmeyer, H.E., Sherry, B., Lu, L., Cooper, S., Carow, C., Wolpe, S.D. and Cerami, A. (1989). *J. Exp. Med.* **170**, 1583–1594.

Bruijnzeel, P.L.B., Kuijper, P.H.M., Rihs, S., Betz, S., Warringa, R.A.J. and Koenderman, L. (1993). *J. Invest. Dermatol.* **100**, 137–142.

Bussolino, F., Sironi, M., Bocchietto, E. and Mantovani, A. (1992). *J. Biol. Chem.* **267**, 14598–14603.

Camp, R.D.R., Fincham, N.J., Cunningham, F.M., Greaves, M.W., Morris, J. and Chu, A. (1986). *J. Immunol.* **137**, 3469–3474.

Camp, R.D.R., Fincham, N.J., Ross, J.S., Bacon, K.B. and Gearing, A.J.H. (1990). *J. Invest. Dermatol.* **95**, 108S–110S.

Carré P.C., Mortenson, R.L., King, T.E., Noble, P.W., Sable, C.L. and Riches, D.W.H. (1991). *J. Clin. Invest.* **88**, 1802–1810.

Carveth, H.J., Bohnsack, J.F., McIntyre, T.M., Baggiolini, M., Prescott, S.M. and Zimmerman, G.A. (1989). *Biochem. Biophys. Res. Commun.* **162**, 387–393.

Cassatella, M.A., Bazzoni, F., Ceska, M., Ferro, I., Baggiolini, M. and Berton, G. (1992). *J. Immunol.* **148**, 3216–3220.

Cassatella, M.A., Guasparri, I., Ceska, M., Bazzoni, F. and Rossi, F. (1993). *Immunology* **78**, 177–184.

Castor, C.W., Miller, J.W. and Walz, D.A. (1983). *Proc. Natl Acad. Sci. USA* **80**, 765–769.

Cerretti, D.P., Kozlosky, C.J., Vanden Bos, T., Nelson, N., Gearing, D.P. and Beckmann, M.P. (1993). *Mol. Immunol.* **30**, 359–367.

Choi, A.M.K. and Jacoby, D.B. (1992). *FEBS Lett.* **309**, 327–329.

Clark-Lewis, I., Moser, B., Walz, A., Baggiolini, M., Scott, G.J. and Aebersold, R. (1991a). *Biochemistry* **30**, 3128–3135.

Clark-Lewis, I., Schumacher, C., Baggiolini, M. and Moser, B. (1991b). *J. Biol. Chem.* **266**, 23128–23134.

Clore, G.M. and Gronenborn, A.M. (1991). *J. Mol. Biol.* **217**, 611–620.

Clore, G.M., Appella, E., Yamada, M., Matsushima, K. and Gronenborn, A.M. (1989). *J. Biol. Chem.* **264**, 18907–18911.

Clore, G.M., Appella, E., Yamada, M., Matsushima, K. and Gronenborn, A.M. (1990). *Biochemistry* **29**, 1689–1696.

Colditz, I., Zwahlen, R., Dewald, B. and Baggiolini, M. (1989). *Am. J. Pathol.* **134**, 755–760.

Colotta, F., Re, F., Muzio, M., Bertini, R., Polentarutti, N., Sironi, M., Giri, J.G., Dower, S.K., Sims, J.E., and Mantovani, A. (1993). *Science* **261**, 472–475.

Crabtree, J.E., Peichl, P., Wyatt, J.I., Stachl, U. and Lindley, I.J.D. (1993). *Scand. J. Immunol.* **37**, 65–70.

Cunha, F.Q., Lorenzetti, B.B., Poole, S. and Ferreira, S.H. (1991). *Br. J. Pharmacol.* **104**, 765–767.

Dahinden, C.A., Kurimoto, Y., De Weck, A.L., Lindley, I., Dewald, B. and Baggiolini, M. (1989). *J. Exp. Med.* **170**, 1787–1792.

Darbonne, W.C., Rice, G.C., Mohler, M.A., Apple, T., Hébert, C.A., Valente, A.J. and Baker, J.B. (1991). *J. Clin. Invest.* **88**, 1362–1369.

Davatelis, G., Tekamp-Olson, P., Wolpe, S.D., Hermsen, K., Luedke, C., Gallegos, C., Goit, D., Merryweather, J. and Cerami, A. (1988). *J. Exp. Med.* **167**, 1939–1944.

Davatelis, G., Wolpe, S.D., Sherry, B., Dayer, J.-M., Chicheportiche, R. and Cerami, A. (1989). *Science* **243**, 1066–1068.

Decock, B., Conings, R., Lenaerts, J.-P., Billiau, A. and Van Damme, J. (1990). *Biochem. Biophys. Res. Commun.* **167**, 904–909.

DeForge, L.E., Fantone, J.C., Kenney, J.S. and Remick, D.G. (1992a). *J. Clin. Invest.* **90**, 2123–2129.

DeForge, L.E., Tracey, D.E., Kenney, J.S. and Remick, D.G. (1992b). *Am. J. Pathol.* **140**, 1045–1054.

Detmers, P.A., Lo, S.K., Olsen-Egbert, E., Walz, A., Baggiolini, M. and Cohn, Z.A. (1990). *J. Exp. Med.* **171**, 1155–1162.

Detmers, P.A., Powell, D.E., Walz, A., Clark-Lewis, I., Baggiolini, M. and Cohn, Z.A. (1991). *J. Immunol.* **147**, 4211–4217.

Deuel, T.F., Keim, P.S., Farmer, M., Heinrikson, R.L. (1977). *Proc. Natl Acad. Sci. USA* **74**, 2256–2258.

Deuel, T.F., Senior, R.M., Chang, D., Griffin, G.L., Heinrikson, R.L. and Kaiser, E.T. (1981). *Proc. Natl Acad. Sci.* **78**, 4584–4587.

Dibb, C.R., Strieter, R.M., Burdick, M. and Kunkel, S.L. (1992). *Infection and Immunity* **60**, 3052–3058.

Dinarello, C.A. (1984). *Rev. Inf. Dis.* **6**, 51–95.

Djeu, J.Y., Matsushima, K., Oppenheim, J.J., Shiotsuki, K. and Blanchard, D.K. (1990). *J. Immunol.* **144**, 2205–2210.

Dudley, D.J., Trautman, M.S. and Mitchell, M.D. (1993). *J. Clin. Endocrinol. Metabolism* **76**, 404–410.

Elford, P.R. and Cooper, P.H. (1991). *Arthritis and Rheumatism* **34**, 325–332.

Elner, V.M., Strieter, R.M., Elner, S.G., Baggiolini, M., Lindley, I. and Kunkel, S.L. (1990). *Am. J. Pathol.* **136**, 745–750.

Farber, J.M. (1993). *Biochem. Biophys. Res. Commun.* **192**, 223–230.

Fincham, N.J., Camp, R.D.R., Gearing, A.J.H., Bird, C.R. and Cunningham, F.M. (1988). *J. Immunol.* **140**, 4294–4299.

Finn, A., Naik, S., Klein, N., Levinsky, R.J., Strobel, S. and Elliott, M. (1993). *J. Thorac. Cardiovasc. Surg.* **105**, 234–241.

Fitzpatrick, M.M., Shah, V., Trompeter, R.S., Dillon, M.J. and Barratt, T.M. (1992). *Kidney Int.* **42**, 951–956.

Forrest, M.J., Eiermann, G.J., Meurer, R., Walakovits, L.A. and MacIntyre, D.E. (1992). *Br. J. Pharmacol.* **106**, 287–294.

Foster, S.J., Aked, D.M., Schröder, J.-M. and Christophers, E. (1989). *Immunology* **67**, 181–183.

Friedland, J.S., Remick, D.G. Shattock, R. and Griffin, G.E. (1992). *Eur. J. Immunol.* **22**, 1373–1378.

Fujishima, S., Hoffman, A.R., Vu, T., Kim, K.J., Zheng, H., Daniel, D., Kim, Y., Wallace, E.F., Larrick, J.W. and Raffin, T.A. (1993). *J. Cell. Physiol.* **154**, 478–485.

Furuta, R., Yamagishi, J., Kotani, H., Sakamoto, F., Fukui, T., Matsui, Y., Sohmura, Y., Yamada, M., Yoshimura, T., Larsen, C.G., Oppenheim, J.J. and Matsushima, K. (1989). *J. Biochem.* **106**, 436–441.

Furutani, Y., Nomura, H., Notake, M., Oyamada, Y., Fukui, T., Yamada, M., Larsen, C.G., Oppenheim, J.J. and Matsushima, K. (1989). *Biochem. Biophys. Res. Comm.* **159**, 249–255.

Gao, J.-L., Kuhns, D.B., Tiffany, H.L., McDermott, D., Li, X., Francke, U. and Murphy, P.M. (1993). *J. Exp. Med.* **177**, 1421–1427.

Gayle, R.B. III., Sleath, P.R., Srinivason, S., Birks, C.W., Weerawarna, K.S., Cerretti, D.P., Kozlosky, C.J., Nelson, N., Vanden Bos, T. and Beckmann, M.P. (1993). *J. Biol. Chem.* **268**, 7283–7289.

Gearing, A.J.H., Fincham, N.J., Bird, C.R., Wadhwa, M., Meager, A., Cartwright, J.E. and Camp, R.D.R. (1990). *Cytokine* **2**, 68–75.

Georgilis, K., Schaefer, C., Dinarello, C.A. and Klempner, M.S. (1987). *J. Immunol.* **138**, 3403–3407.

Gimbrone, M.A. Jr., Obin, M.S., Brock, A.F., Luis, E.A., Hass, P.E., Hébert, C.A., Yip, Y.K., Leung, D.W., Lowe, D.G., Kohr, W.J., Darbonne, W.C., Bechtol, K.B. and Baker, J.B. (1989). *Science* **246**, 1601–1603.

Golds, E.E., Mason, P. and Nyirkos, P. (1989). *Biochem. J.* **259**, 585–588.

Goodman, R.B., Wood, R.G., Martin, T.R., Hanson-Painton, O. and Kinasewitz, G.T. (1992). *J. Immunol.* **148**, 457–465.

Gottlieb, A.B., Luster, A.D., Posnett, D.N. and Carter, D.M. (1988). *J. Exp. Med.* **168**, 941–948.

Graham, G.J., Wright, E.G., Hewick, R., Wolpe, S.D., Wilkie, N.M., Donaldson, D., Lorimore, S. and Pragnell, T.B. (1990). *Nature* **344**, 442–444.

Graves, D.T., Jiang, Y.L., Williamson, M.J., Valente, A.J. (1989). *Science* **245**, 1490–1493.

Gregory, H., Young, J., Schröder, J.-M., Mrowietz, U. and Christophers, E. (1988). *Biochem. Biophys. Res. Commun.* **151**, 883–890.

Grob, P.M., David, E., Warren, T.C., DeLeon, R.P., Farini, P.R. and Homon, C.A. (1990). *J. Biol. Chem.* **265**, 8311–8316.

Gross, V., Andreesen, R., Leser, H.-G., Ceska, M., Liehl, E., Lausen, M., Farthmann, E.H. and Schölmerich, J. (1992). *Eur. J. Clin. Invest.* **22**, 200–203.

Halstensen, A., Ceska, M., Brandtzaeg, P., Redl, H., Naess, A. and Waage, A. (1993). *J. Infect. Dis.* **167**, 471–475.

Haskill, S., Peace, A., Morris, J., Sporn, S.A., Anisowicz, A., Lee, S.W., Smith, T., Martin, G., Ralph, P. and Sager, R. (1990). *Proc. Natl Acad. Sci. USA* **87**, 7732–7736.

Hébert C.A., Luscinskas, F.W., Kiely, J.-M., Luis, E.A., Darbonne, W.C., Bennett, G.L., Liu, C.C., Obin, M.S., Gimbrone, M.A. Jr and Baker, J.B. (1990). *J. Immunol.* **145**, 3033–3040.

Hébert, C.A., Vitangcol, R.V. and Baker, J.B. (1991). *J. Biol. Chem.* **266**, 18989–18994.

Hechtman, D.H., Cybulsky, M.I., Fuchs, H.J., Baker, J.B. and Gimbrone, M.A. Jr (1991). *J. Immunol.* **147**, 883–892.

Hirano, T., Akira, S., Taga, T. and Kishimoto, T. (1990). *Immunology Today* **11**, 443–449.

Holmes, W.E., Lee, J., Kuang, W.-J., Rice, G.C., Wood, W.I. (1991). *Science* **253**, 1278–1280.

Holt, J.C. and Niewiarowski, S. (1980). *Biochem. Biophys. Acta* **632**, 284–289.

Holt, J.C., Harris, M.E., Holt, A.M., Lange, E., Henschen, A. and Niewiarowski, S. (1986). *Biochemistry* **25**, 1988–1996.

Horuk, R., Chitnis, C.E., Darbonne, W.C., Colby, T.J., Rybicki, A., Hadley, T.J. and Miller, L.H. (1993a). *Science* **261**, 1182–1184.

Horuk, R., Colby, T.J., Darbonne, W.C., Schall, T.J. and Neote, K. (1993b). *Biochemistry* **32**, 5733–5738.

Hotta, K., Hayashi, K., Ishikawa, J., Tagawa, M., Hashimoto, K., Mizuno, S. and Suzuki, K. (1990). *Immunology Letters* **24**, 165–170.

Huber, A.R., Kunkel, S.L., Todd, R.F., III and Weiss, S.J. (1991). *Science* **254**, 99–102.

Iida, N. and Grotendorst, G.R. (1990). *Mol. Cell. Biol.* **10**, 5596–5599.

Jagels, M.A. and Hugli, T.E. (1992). *J. Immunol.* **148**, 1119–1128.

Jonjic, N., Peri, G., Bernasconi, S., Sciacca, F.L., Colotta, F., Pelicci, P.G., Lanfrancone, L. and Mantovani, A. (1992). *J. Exp. Med.* **176**, 1165–1174.

Jorens, P.G., Richman-Eisenstat, J.B.Y., Housset, B.P., Graf, P.D., Ueki, I.F., Olesch, J. and Nadel, J.A. (1992a). *Am. J. Physiol.* **263**, L708–L713.

Jorens, P.G., Van Damme, J., De Backer, W., Bossaert, L., De Jongh, R.F., Herman, A.G. and Rampart, M. (1992b). *Cytokine* **4**, 592–597.

Kameyoshi, Y., Dörschner, A., Mallet, A.I., Christophers, E. and Schröder, J.-M. (1992). *J. Exp. Med.* **176**, 587–592.

Kaplan, G., Luster, A.D., Hancock, G. and Cohn, Z.A. (1987). *J. Exp. Med.* **166**, 1098–1108.

Kaplanski, G., Porat, R., Aiura, K., Erban, J.K., Gelfand, J.A. and Dinarello, C.A. (1993). *Blood* **81**, 2492–2495.

Katz, I.R., Thorbecke, G.J., Bell, M.K., Yin, J.-Z., Clarke, D. and Zucker, M.B. (1986). *Proc. Natl Acad. Sci. USA* **83**, 3491–3495.

Kelly, R.W., Leask, R. and Calder, A.A. (1992). *Lancet* **339**, 776–777.

Kimata, H., Yoshida, A., Ishioka, C., Lindley, I. and Mikawa, H. (1992). *J. Exp. Med.* **176**, 1227–1231.

Koch, A.E., Kunkel, S.L., Burrows, J.C., Evanoff, H.L., Haines, G.K., Pope, R.M. and Strieter, R.M. (1991). *J. Immunol.* **147**, 2187–2195.

Koch, A.E., Polverini, P.J., Kunkel, S.L., Harlow, L.A., DiPietro, L.A., Elner, V.M., Elner, S.G. and Strieter, R.M. (1992). *Science* **258**, 1798–1801.

Koch, A.E., Kunkel, S.L., Pearce, W.H., Shah, M.R., Parikh, D., Evanoff, H.L., Haines, G.K., Burdick, M.D. and Strieter, R.M. (1993). *Am. J. Pathol.* **142**, 1423–1431.

Kowalski, J. and Denhardt, D.T. (1989). *Mol. Cell. Biol.* **9**, 1946–1957.

Kownatzki, E. and Uhrich, S. (1990). *Int. Arch. Allergy Appl. Immunol.* **93**, 344–349.

Kuijpers, T.W., Hakkert, B.C., Hart, M.H.L. and Roos, D. (1992). *J. Cell Biol.* **117**, 565–572.

Kuna, P., Reddigari, S.R., Kornfeld, D. and Kaplan, A.P. (1991). *J. Immunol.* **147**, 1920–1924.

Kuna, P., Reddigari, S.R., Schall, T.J., Rucinski, D., Viksman, M.Y. and Kaplan, A.P. (1992). *J. Immunol.* **149**, 636–642.

Kupper, R.W., Dewald, B., Jakobs, K.H., Baggiolini, M. and Gierschik, P. (1992). *Biochem. J.* **282**, 429–434.

LaRosa, G.J., Thomas, K.M., Kaufmann, M.E., Mark, R., White, M., Taylor, L., Gray, G., Witt, D. and Navarro, J. (1992). *J. Biol. Chem.* **267**, 25402–25406.

Larsen, C.G., Anderson, A.O., Appella, E., Oppenheim, J.J. and Matsushima, K. (1989a). *Science* **243**, 1464–1466.

Larsen, C.G., Anderson, A.O., Oppenheim, J.J. and Matsushima, K. (1989b). *Immunology* **68**, 31–36.

Larsen, C.G., Zachariae, C.O.C., Oppenheim, J.J. and Matsushima, K. (1989c). *Biochem. Biophys. Res. Comm.* **160**, 1403–1408.

Larsen, C.G., Kristensen, M., Paludan, K., Deleuran, B., Thomsen, M.K., Zachariae, C., Kragballe, K., Matsushima, K. and Thestrup-Pedersen, K. (1991). *Biochem. Biophys. Res. Commun.* **176**, 1020–1026.

Lee, J., Horuk, R., Rice, G.C., Bennett, G.L., Camerato, T. and Wood, W.I. (1992). *J. Biol. Chem.* **267**, 16283–16287.

Leonard, E.J. and Yoshimura, T. (1990). *Immunol. Today* **11**, 97–101.

Leonard, E.J., Skeel, A., Yoshimura, T., Noer, K., Kutvirt, S. and Van Epps, D. (1990). J. Immunol. **144**, 1323–1330.

Leonard, E.J., Yoshimura, T., Rot, A., Noer, K., Walz, A., Baggiolini, M., Walz, D.A., Goetzl, E.J. and Castor, C.W. (1991a). *J. Leukocyte Biol.* **49**, 258–265.

Leonard, E.J., Yoshimura, T., Tanaka, S. and Raffeld, M. (1991b). *J. Invest. Dermatol.* **96**, 690–694.

Lin, C.-Y., Lin, C.-C. and Huang, T.-P. (1993). *Nephron* **63**, 404–408.

Lindley, I., Aschauer, H., Seifert, J.-M., Lam, C., Brunowsky, W., Kownatzki, E., Thelen, M., Peveri, P., Dewald, B., von Tscharner, V., Walz, A. and Baggiolini, M. (1988). *Proc. Natl Acad. Sci. USA* **85**, 9199–9203.

Lloyd, A., Modi, W., Sprenger, H., Cevario, S., Oppenheim, J. and Kelvin, D. (1993). *Cytogenet. Cell Genet.* **63**, 238–240.

Lotz, M., Terkeltaub, R. and Villiger, P.M. (1992). *J. Immunol.* **148**, 466–473.

Luger, T.A., Charon, J.A., Colot, M., Micksche, M. and Oppenheim, J.J. (1983). *J. Immunol.* **131**, 816–820.

Luscinskas, F.W., Kiely, J.-M., Ding, H., Obin, M.S., Hébert, C.A., Baker, J.B. and Gimbrone, M.A., Jr (1992). *J. Immunol.* **149**, 2163–2171.

Luster, A.D., Unkeless, J.C., Ravetch, J.V. (1985). *Nature* **315**, 672–676.

Luster, A.D. and Leder, P. (1993). *J. Exp. Med.* **178**, 1057–1065.

Lynch, J.P., III, Standiford, T.J., Rolfe, M.W., Kunkel, S.L. and Strieter, R.M. (1992). *Am. Rev. Respir. Dis.* **145**, 1433–1439.

McCall, T.B., Palmer, R.M.J. and Moncada, S. (1992). *Biochem. Biophys. Res. Commun.* **186**, 680–685.

Mahida, Y.R., Ceska, M., Effenberger, F., Kurlak, L., Lindley, I. and Hawkey, C.J. (1992). *Clin. Science* **82**, 273–275.

Maione, T.E., Gray, G.S., Petro, J., Hunt, A.J., Donner, A.L., Bauer, S.I., Carson, H.F. and Sharpe, R.J. (1990). *Science* **247**, 77–79.

Marini, M., Vittori, E., Hollemborg, J. and Mattoli, S. (1992). *J. Allergy Clin. Immunol.* **89**, 1001–1009.

Martich, G.D., Danner, R.L., Ceska, M. and Suffredini, A.F. (1991). *J. Exp. Med.* **173**, 1021–1024.

Masure, S., Proost, P., Van Damme, J. and Opdenakker, G. (1991). *Eur. J. Biochem.* **198**, 391–398.

Matsushima, K. and Oppenheim, J.J. (1989). *Cytokine* **1**, 2–13.

Matsushima, K., Morishita, K., Yoshimura, T., Lavu, S., Kobayashi, Y., Lew, W., Appella, E., Kung, H.F., Leonard, E.J. and Oppenheim, J.J. (1988). *J. Exp. Med.* **167**, 1883–1893.

Mauviel, A., Reitamo, S., Remitz, A., Lapière, J.-C., Ceska, M., Baggiolini, M., Walz, A., Evans, C.H. and Uitto, J. (1992). *J. Immunol.* **149**, 2969–2976.

Mehrabian, M., Sparkes, R.S., Mohandas, T., Fogelman, A.M. and Lusis, S.J. (1991). *Genomics* **9**, 200–203.

Metinko, A.P., Kunkel, S.L., Standiford, T.J. and Strieter, R.M. (1992). *J. Clin. Invest.* **90**, 791–798.

Michel, G., Kemény, L., Peter, R.U., Ried, C., Arenberger, P. and Ruzicka, T. (1992). *FEBS Lett.* **305**, 241–243.

Miller, M.D. and Krangel, M.S. (1992). *Proc. Natl Acad. Sci. USA* **89**, 2950–2954.

Miller, E.J., Cohen, A.B., Nagao, S., Griffith, D., Maunder, R.J., Martin, T.R., Weiner-Kronish, J.P., Sticherling, M., Christophers, E. and Matthay, M.A. (1992). *Am. Rev. Respir. Dis.* **146**, 427–432.

Modi, W.S., Dean, M., Seuanez, H.N., Mukaida, N., Matsushima, K. and O'Brien, S.J. (1990). *Hum. Genet.* **84**, 185–187.

Mollereau, C., Muscatelli, F., Mattei, M.-G., Vassart, G. and Parmentier, M. (1993). *Genomics* **16**, 248–251.

Morris, S.W., Nelson, N., Valentine, M.B., Shapiro, D.N., Look, A.T., Kozlosky, C.J., Beckmann, M.P. and Cerretti, D.P. (1992). *Genomics* **14**, 685–691.

Moser, B., Clark-Lewis, I., Zwahlen, R. and Baggiolini, M. (1990). *J. Exp. Med.* **171**, 1797–1802.

Moser, B., Schumacher, C., von Tscharner, V., Clark-Lewis, I. and Baggiolini, M. (1991). *J. Biol. Chem.* **266**, 10666–10671.

Moser, B., Dewald, B., Barella, L., Schumacher, C., Baggiolini, M. and Clark-Lewis, I. (1993). *J. Biol. Chem.* **268**, 7125–7128.

Mukaida, N., Shiroo, M. and Matsushima, K. (1989). *J. Immunol.* **143**, 1366–1371.

Mukaida, N., Mahe, Y. and Matsushima, K. (1990). *J. Biol. Chem.* **265**, 21128–21133.

Mullenbach, G.T., Tabrizi, A., Blacher, R.W. and Steimer, K.S. (1986). *J. Biol. Chem.* **261**, 719–722.

Mulligan, M.S., Jones, M.L., Bolanowski, M.A., Baganoff, M.P., Deppeler, C.L., Meyers, D.M., Ryan, U.S. and Ward, P.A. (1993). *J. Immunol.* **150**, 5585–5595.

Murphy, P.M. and Tiffany, H.L. (1991). *Science* **253**, 1280–1283.

Nakagawa, H., Hatakeyama, S., Ikesue, A. and Miyai, H. (1991). *FEBS Lett.* **282**, 412–414.

Nakamura, H., Yoshimura, K., McElvaney, N.G. and Crystal, R.G. (1992). *J. Clin. Invest.* **89**, 1478–1484.

Negussie, Y., Remick, D.G., DeForge, L.E., Kunkel, S.L., Eynon, A. and Griffin, G.E. (1992). *J. Exp. Med.* **175**, 1207–1212.

Neote, K., DiGregorio, D., Mak, J.Y., Horuk, R. and Schall, T.J. (1993). *Cell* **72**, 415–425.

Nickoloff, B.J., Karabin, G.D., Barker, J.N.W.N., Griffiths, C.E.M., Sarma, V., Mitra, R.S., Elder, J.T., Kunkel, S.L. and Dixit, V.M. (1991). *Am. J. Pathol.* **138**, 129–140.

Nourshargh, S., Perkins, J.A., Showell, H.J., Matsushima, K., Williams, T.J. and Collins, P.D. (1992). *J. Immunol.* **148**, 106–111.

Oppenheim, J.J., Zachariae, C.O.C., Mukaida, N. and Matsushima, K. (1991). *Annu. Rev. Immunol.* **9**, 617–648.

Peichl, P., Ceska, M., Effenberger, F., Haberhauer, G., Broell, H. and Lindley, I.J.D. (1991). *Scand. J. Immunol.* **34**, 333–339.

Peveri, P., Walz, A., Dewald, B. and Baggiolini, M. (1988). *J. Exp. Med.* **167**, 1547–1559.

Pike, M.C., Costello, K.M. and Lamb, K.A. (1992). *J. Immunol.* **148**, 3158–3164.

Porat, R., Poutsiaka, D.D., Miller, L.C., Granowitz, E.V. and Dinarello, C.A. (1992). *FASEB J.* **6**, 2482–2486.

Proost, P., De Wolf-Peeters, C., Conings, R., Opdenakker, G., Billiau, A. and Van Damme, J. (1993a). *J. Immunol.* **150**, 1000–1010.

Proost, P., Wuyts, A., Conings, R., Lenaerts, J.-P., Billiau, A., Opdenakker, G. and Van Damme, J. (1993b). *Biochemistry,* **32**, 10170–10171.

Rampart, M., Van Damme, J., Zonnekeyn, L. and Herman, A.G. (1989). *Am. J. Pathol.* **135**, 21–25.

Rampart, M., Herman, A.G., Grillet, B., Opdenakker, G. and Van Damme, J. (1992). *Laboratory Investigation* **66**, 512–518.

Recklies, A.D. and Golds, E.E. (1992). *Arthritis and Rheumatism* **35**, 1510–1519.

Redl, H., Schlag, G., Bahrami, S., Schade, U., Ceska, M. and Stütz, P. (1991). *J. Inf. Dis.* **164**, 383–388.

Reitamo, S., Remitz, A., Varga, J., Ceska, M., Effenberger, F., Jimenez, S. and Uitto, J. (1993). *Arch. Dermatol.* **129**, 189–193.

Richmond, A., Balentien, E., Thomas, H.G., Flaggs, G., Barton, D.E., Spiess, J., Bordoni, R., Francke, U. and Derynck, R. (1988). *EMBO J.* **7**, 2025–2033.

Robinson, E.A., Yoshimura, T., Leonard, E.J., Tanaka, S., Griffin, P.R., Shabanowitz, J., Hunt, D.F. and Appella, E. (1989). *Proc. Natl Acad. Sci. USA* **86**, 1850–1854.

Rollins, B.J., Morrison, E.D. and Stiles, C.D. (1988). *Proc. Natl Acad. Sci. USA* **85**, 3738–3742.

Rollins, B.J., Morton, C.C., Ledbetter, D.H., Eddy, R.L. Jr. and Shows, T.B. (1991). *Genomics* **10**, 489–492.

Romero, R., Ceska, M., Avila, C., Mazor, M., Behnke, E. and Lindley, I. (1991). *Am. J. Obstet. Gynecol.* **165**, 813–820.

Rot, A. (1993). *Eur. J. Immunol.* **23**, 303–306.

Rot, A., Krieger, M., Brunner, T., Bischoff, S.C., Schall, T.J. and Dahinden, C.A. (1992). *J. Exp. Med.* **176**, 1489–1495.

Rucinski, B., Niewiarowski, S., James, P., Walz, D.A. and Budzynski, A.Z. (1979). *Blood* **53**, 47–62.

Samanta, A.K., Oppenheim, J.J. and Matsushima, K. (1989). *J. Exp. Med.* **169**, 1185–1189.

Samanta, A.K., Oppenheim, J.J. and Matsushima, K. (1990). *J. Biol. Chem.* **265**, 183–189.

Samanta, A.K., Dutta, S. and Ali, E. (1993). *J. Biol. Chem.* **268**, 6147–6153.

Sarris, A.H., Broxmeyer, H.E., Wirthmueller, U., Karasavvas, N., Cooper, S., Lu, L., Krueger, J. and Ravetch, J.V. (1993). *J. Exp. Med.* **178**, 1127–1132.

Sauder, D.N., Mounessa, N.L., Katz, S.I., Dinarello, C.A. and Gallin, J.I. (1984). *J. Immunol.* **132**, 828–832.

Schall, T.J. (1991). *Cytokine* **3**, 165–183.

Schall, T.J., Bacon, K., Toy, K.J. and Goeddel, D.V. (1990). *Nature* **347**, 669–671.

Schall, T.J., Bacon, K., Camp, R.D.R., Kaspari, J.W. and Goeddel, D.V. (1993). *J. Exp. Med.* **177**, 1821–1825.

Schmid, J. and Weissmann, C. (1987). *J. Immunol.* **139**, 250–256.

Schröder, J.-M. (1989). *J. Exp. Med.* **170**, 847–863.

Schröder, J.-M. and Christophers, E. (1986). *J. Invest. Dermatol.* **87**, 53–58.

Schröder, J.-M. and Christophers, E. (1989). *J. Immunol.* **142**, 244–251.

Schröder, J.-M., Mrowietz, U., Morita, E. and Christophers, E. (1987). *J. Immunol.* **139**, 3474–3483.

Schröder, J.-M., Mrowietz, U. and Christophers, E. (1988). *J. Immunol.* **140**, 3534–3540.

Schröder, J.-M., Persoon, N.L.M. and Christophers, E. (1990a). *J. Exp. Med.* **171**, 1091–1100.

Schröder, J.-M., Sticherling, M., Henneicke, H.H., Preissner, W.C. and Christophers, E. (1990b). *J. Immunol.* **144**, 2223–2232.

Schröder, J.-M., Gregory, H., Young, J. and Christophers, E. (1992). *J. Invest. Dermatol.* **98**, 241–247.

Schumacher, C., Clark-Lewis, I., Baggiolini, M. and Moser, B. (1992). *Proc. Natl Acad. Sci. USA* **89**, 10542–10546.

Sebok, K., Woodside, D., Al-Aoukaty, A., Ho, A.D., Gluck, S. and Maghazachi, A.A. (1993). *J. Immunol.* **150**, 1524–1534.

Senior, R.M., Griffin, G.L., San Huang, J., Walz, D.A. and Deuel, T.F. (1983). *J. Cell Biol.* **96**, 382–385.

Sheron, N. and Williams, R. (1992). *Clin. Exp. Immunol.* **89**, 100–103.

Shimoya, K., Matsuzaki, N., Taniguchi, T., Kameda, T., Koyama, M., Neki, R., Saji, F. and Tanizawa, O. (1992). *Biol. Reproduction* **47**, 220–226.

Sica, A., Matsushima, K., Van Damme, J., Wang, J.M., Polentarutti, N., Dejana, E., Colotta, F. and Mantovani, A. (1990a). *Immunology* **69**, 548–553.

Sica, A., Wang, J.-M., Colotta, F., Dejana, E., Mantovani, A., Oppenheim, J.J., Larsen, C.G., Zachariae, C.O.C. and Matsushima, K. (1990b). *J. Immunol.* **144**, 3034–3038.

Smith, W.B., Gamble, J.R., Clark-Lewis, I. and Vadas, M.A. (1991). *Immunology* **72**, 65–72.

Smyth, M.J., Zachariae, C.O.C., Norihisa, Y., Ortaldo, J.R., Hishinuma, A. and Matsushima, K. (1991). *J. Immunol.* **146**, 3815–3823.

Standiford, T.J., Kunkel, S.L., Basha, M.A., Chensue, S.W., Lynch, J.P., III, Toews, G.B., Westwick, J. and Strieter, R.M. (1990a). *J. Clin. Invest.* **86**, 1945–1953.

Standiford, T.J., Strieter, R.M., Chensue, S.W., Westwick, J., Kashara, K. and Kunkel, S.L. (1990b). *J. Immunol.* **145**, 1435–1439.

Standiford, T.J., Strieter, R.M., Allen, R.M., Burdick, M.D. and Kunkel, S.L. (1992). *J. Immunology* **149**, 2035–2039.

Sticherling, M., Bornscheuer, E., Schröder, J.-M. and Christophers, E. (1991). *J. Invest. Dermatol.* **96**, 26–30.

Strieter, R.M., Kunkel, S.L., Showell, H.J., Remick, D.G., Phan, S.H., Ward, P.A. and Marks, R.M. (1989a). *Science* **243**, 1467–1469.

Strieter, R.M., Phan, S.H., Showell, H.J., Remick, D.G., Lynch, J.P., Genord, M., Raiford, C., Eskandari, M., Marks, R.M. and Kunkel, S.L. (1989b). *J. Biol. Chem.* **264**, 10621–10626.

Strieter, R.M., Wiggins, R., Phan, S.H., Wharram, B.L., Showell, H.J., Remick, D.G., Chensue, S.W. and Kunkel, S.L. (1989c). *Biochem. Biophys. Res. Comm.* **162**, 694–700.

Strieter, R.M., Kasahara, K., Allen, R., Showell, H.J., Standiford, T.J. and Kunkel, S.L. (1990). *Biochem. Biophys. Res. Commun.* **173**, 725–730.

Strieter, R.M., Kunkel, S.L., Elner, V.M., Martonyi, C.L., Koch, A.E., Polverini, P.J. and Elner, S G. (1992). *Am. J. Pathol.* **141**, 1279–1284.

Suzuki, K., Koshio, O., Ishida-Okawara, A., Shibata, M., Yamakawa, Y., Tagawa, M., Ota, H., Kuramoto, A. and Mizuno, S. (1989a). *Biochem. Biophys. Res. Commun.* **163**, 1298–1305.

Suzuki, K., Miyasaka, H., Ota, H., Yamakawa, Y., Tagawa, M., Kuramoto, A. and Mizuno, S. (1989b). *J. Exp. Med.* **169**, 1895–1901.

Suzuki, K., Yamakawa, Y., Matsuo, Y., Kamiya, T., Minowada, J. and Mizuno, S. (1993). *Immunol. Lett.* **36**, 71–82.

Sylvester, I., Yoshimura, T., Sticherling, M., Schröder, J.-M., Ceska, M., Peichl, P. and Leonard, E.J. (1992). *J. Clin. Invest.* **90**, 471–481.

Takahashi, G.W., Andrews D.F., III, Lilly, M.B., Singer, J.W. and Alderson, M.R. (1993). *Blood* **81**, 357–364.

Tanaka, Y., Robinson, E.A., Yoshimura, T., Matsushima, K., Leonard, E.J. and Appella, E. (1988). *FEBS Lett.* **236**, 467–470.

Tanaka, S., Adams, D.H., Hubscher, S., Hirano, H., Siebenlist, U. and Shaw, S. (1993). *Nature* **361**, 79–82.

Taub, D.D., Conlon, K., Lloyd, A.R., Oppenheim, J.J. and Kelvin, D.J. (1993a). *Science* **260**, 355–358.

Taub, D.D., Lloyd, A.R., Conlon, K., Wang, J.M., Ortaldo, J.R., Harada, A., Matsushima, K., Kelvin, D.J. and Oppenheim, J.J. (1993b). *J. Exp. Med.* **177**, 1809–1814.

Tekamp-Olson, P., Gallegos C., Bauer, D., McClain, J., Sherry, B., Fabre, M., van Deventer, S. and Cerami, A. (1990). *J. Exp. Med.* **172**, 911–919.

Thelen, M., Peveri, P., Kernen, P., von Tscharner, V., Walz, A. and Baggiolini, M. (1988). *FASEB J.* **2**, 2702–2706.

Thornton, A.J., Strieter, R.M., Lindley, I., Baggiolini, M. and Kunkel, S.L. (1990). *J. Immunol.* **144**, 2609–2613.

Torre, D., Zeroli, C., Giola, M., Fiori, G.P., Nespoli, L., Daverio, A., Ferrario, G. and Martegani, R. (1992). *Am. J. Dis. Child.* **147**, 27–29.

Trautman, M.S., Dudley, D.J., Edwin, S.S., Collmer, D. and Mitchell, M.D. (1992). *J. Cell. Physiol.* **153**, 38–43.

Tuschil, A., Lam, C., Haslberger, A. and Lindley, I. (1992). *J. Invest. Dermatol.* **99**, 294–298.

Unemori, E.N., Amento, E.P., Bauer, E.A. and Horuk, R. (1993). *J. Biol. Chem.* **268**, 1338–1342.

Valente, A.J., Graves, D.T., Vialle-Valentin, C.E., Delgado, R. and Schwart, C.J. (1988). *Biochemistry* **27**, 4162–4168.

Van Damme, J. (1991). *The Cytokine Handbook*, (ed. A. W. Thomson), Academic Press, London, pp. 201–214.

Van Damme, J. and Opdenakker, G. (1990). *J. Invest. Dermatol.* **95**, 90S–93S.

Van Damme, J., De Ley, M., Opdenakker, G., Billiau, A., De Somer, P. and Van Beeumen, J. (1985a). *Nature* **314**, 266–268.

Van Damme, J., De Ley, M., Van Beeumen, J., Opdenakker, G., Dayer, J.-M., Billiau, A. and De Somer, P. (1985b). *Brit. J. Rheum.* **24**, (Suppl.1), 72–76.

Van Damme, J., Cayphas, S., Van Snick, J., Conings, R., Put, W., Lenaerts, J.-P., Simpson, R.J. and Billiau, A. (1987). *Eur. J. Biochem.* **168**, 543–550.

Van Damme, J., Van Beeumen, J., Opdenakker, G. and Billiau, A. (1988). *J. Exp. Med.* **167**, 1364–1376.

Van Damme, J., Decock, B., Conings, R., Lenaerts, J.-P., Opdenakker, G. and Billiau, A. (1989a). *Eur. J. Immunol.* **19**, 1189–1194.

Vam Damme, J., Decock, B., Lenaerts, J.-P., Conings, R., Bertini, R., Mantovani, A. and Billiau, A. (1989b). *Eur. J. Immunol.* **19**, 2367–2373.

Van Damme, J., Van Beeumen, J., Conings, R., Decock, B. and Billiau, A. (1989c). *Eur. J. Biochem.* **181**, 337–344.

Van Damme, J., Bunning, R.A.D., Conings, R., Russell, G.G. and Opdenakker, G. (1990a). *Cytokine* **2**, 106–111.

Van Damme, J., Rampart, M., Conings, R., Decock, B., Van Osselaer, N., Willems, J. and Billiau, A. (1990b). *Eur. J. Immunol.* **20**, 2113–2118.

Van Damme, J., Proost, P., Lenaerts, J.-P. and Opdenakker, G. (1992). *J. Exp. Med.* **176**, 59–65.

van Deventer, S.J.H., Hart, M., van der Poll, T., Hack, C.E. and Aarden, L.A. (1993). *J. Inf. Dis.* **167**, 461–464.

Van Lint, J., Van Damme, J., Billiau, A., Merlevede, W. and Vandenheede, J.R. (1993). *Mol. Chem. Biochem,* **127/128**, 171–177.

Van Meir, E., Ceska, M., Effenberger, F., Walz, A., Grouzmann, E., Desbaillets, I., Frei, K., Fontana, A. and de Tribolet, N. (1992). *Cancer Res.* **52**, 4297–4305.

Van Osselaer, N., Van Damme, J., Rampart, M. and Herman, A.G. (1991). *Am. J. Pathol.* **138**, 23–27.

Van Snick, J., Cayphas, S., Vink, A., Uyttenhove, C., Coulie, P.G., Rubira, M.R. and Simpson, R.J. (1986). *Proc. Natl Acad. Sci. USA* **83**, 9679–9683.

Van Zee, K.J., DeForge, L.E., Fischer, E., Marano, M.A., Kenney, J.S., Remick, D.G., Lowry, S.F. and Moldawer, L.L. (1991). *J. Immunol.* **146**, 3478–3482.

Van Zee, K.J., Fischer, E., Hawes, A.S., Hébert, C.A., Terrell, T.G., Baker, J.B., Lowry, S.F. and Moldawer, L.L. (1992). *J. Immunol.* **148**, 1746–1752.

Vogels, M.T.E., Lindley, I.J.D., Curfs, J.H.A.J., Eling, W.M.C. and van der Meer, J.W.M. (1993). *Antimicrob. Agents Chemother.* **37**, 276–280.

Walz, A. and Baggiolini, M. (1990). *J. Exp. Med.* **171**, 449–454.

Walz, A., Peveri, P., Aschauer, H. and Baggiolini, M. (1987). *Biochem. Biophys. Res. Commun.* **149**, 755–761.

Walz, A., Dewald, B., von Tscharner, V. and Baggiolini, M. (1989). *J. Exp. Med.* **170**, 1745–1750.

Walz, A., Burgener, R., Car, B., Baggiolini, M., Kunkel, S.L. and Strieter, R.M. (1991a). *J. Exp. Med.* **174**, 1355–1362.

Walz, A., Meloni, F., Clark-Lewis, I., von Tscharner, V. and Baggiolini, M. (1991b). *J. Leukocyte Biol.* **50**, 279–286.

Wang, J.M., Bersani, L. and Mantovani, A. (1987). *J. Immunol.* **138**, 1469–1474.

Wang, J.M., Taraboletti, G., Matsushima, K., Van Damme, J. and Mantovani, A. (1990). *Biochem. Biophys. Res. Commun.* **169**, 165–170.

Wang, J.M., Sica, A., Peri, G., Padura, M.I., Libby, P., Ceska, M., Lindley, I., Colotta, F. and Mantovani, A. (1991). *Arteriosclerosis* **11**, 1166–1174.

Warringa, R.A.J., Mengelers, H.J.J., Raaijmakers, J.A.M., Bruijnzeel, P.L.B. and Koenderman, L. (1993). *J. Allergy Clin. Immunol.* **91**, 1198–1205.

Watson, M.L., Westwick, J., Fincham, N.J. and Camp, R.D.R. (1988). Biochem. Biophys. Res. Commun. **155**, 1154–1160.

Webb, L.M.C., Ehrengruber, M.U., Clark-Lewis, I., Baggiolini, M. and Rot, A. (1993). *Proc. Natl Acad. Sci. USA* **90**, 7158–7162.

Weetman, A.P., Bennett, G.L. and Wong, W.L.T. (1992). *J. Clin. Endocrinol. and Metabolism* **75**, 328–330.

Westwick, J., Li, S.W. and Camp, R.D. (1989). *Immunol. Today* **10**, 146–147.

Wilkinson, P.C. and Newman, I. (1992). *J. Immunol.* **149**, 2689–2694.

Willems, J., Joniau, M., Cinque, S. and Van Damme, J. (1989). *Immunology* **67**, 540–542.

Wolpe, S.D. and Cerami, A. (1989). *FASEB J.* **3**, 2565–2573.

Wolpe, S.D., Sherry, B., Juers, D., Davatelis, G., Yurt, R.W. and Cerami, A. (1989). *Proc. Natl Acad. Sci. USA* **86**, 612–616.

Wu, D., LaRosa, G.J. and Simon, M.I. (1993). *Science* **261**, 101–103.

Yoshimura, T., Matsushima, K., Tanaka, S., Robinson, E.A., Appella, E., Oppenheim, J.J. and Leonard, E.J. (1987). *Proc. Natl Acad. Sci. USA* **84**, 9233–9237.

Yoshimura, T., Robinson, E.A., Appella, E., Matsushima, K., Showalter, S.D., Skeel, A. and Leonard, E.J. (1989a). *Mol. Immunol.* **26**, 87–93.

Yoshimura, T., Robinson, E.A., Tanaka, S., Appella, E. and Leonard, E.J. (1989b). *J. Immunol.* **142**, 1956–1962.

Yoshimura, T., Yuhki, N., Moore, S.K., Appella, E., Lerman, M.I. and Leonard, E.J. (1989c). *FEBS Lett.* **244**, 487–493.

Zipfel, P.F., Bialonski, A. and Skerka, C. (1991). *Biochem. Biophys. Res. Commun.* **181**, 179–183.

Zoja, C., Wang, J.M., Bettoni, S., Sironi, M., Renzi, D., Chiaffarino, F., Abboud, H.E., Van Damme, J., Mantovani, A., Remuzzi, G. and Rambaldi, A. (1991). *Am. J. Pathol.* **138**, 991–1003.

Zwierzina, H., Holzinger, I., Gaggl, S., Wolf, H., Schöllenberger, S., Lam, C., Bammer, T., Geissler, D. and Lindley, I. (1993). *Scand. J. Immunol.* **37**, 322–328.

Chapter 11

Interleukin-9

Jean-Christophe Renauld and Jacques Van Snick

Ludwig Institute for Cancer Research, Brussels Branch and Experimental Medicine Unit,
Catholic University of Louvain, Brussels, Belgium

INTRODUCTION

Interleukin-9 (IL-9) shares some typical features with an ever-growing number of molecules that regulate multiple functions in the immune system. Produced preferentially by T_{H2} lymphocytes, IL-9 is a 30–40 kDa glycoprotein active on various cell subsets in the immune and haemopoietic systems. Its gene is located on human chromosome 5, in the near vicinity of other cytokine genes such as IL-3, IL-4, IL-5, GM-CSF and IL-13, and its receptor is structurally related to the haemopoietic receptor superfamily.

Originally described as a T-cell growth factor present in the supernatant of murine activated T-cell clones, this molecule was characterized by a narrow specificity for some T-helper clones and by its ability to sustain long-term growth in the absence of feeder cells and antigen. Taking advantage of such factor-dependent cell lines, the protein was purified to homogeneity, provisionally designated P40, and molecularly cloned (Uyttenhove et al., 1988; Van Snick et al., 1989).

Independently, Hültner and coworkers observed that the proliferation of mast cell lines in response to IL-3 or IL-4 could be enhanced by a factor produced by activated splenocytes (Hültner et al., 1989; Moeller et al., 1989). This activity was partially purified and called mast cell growth-enhancing activity (MEA). High levels of MEA were also found in the supernatant from a murine Mls-reactive T_H-cell line derived by Schmitt and colleagues, who had observed that these cells produced a T-cell growth factor distinct from IL-2 and IL-4, which was called TCGF-III (Moeller et al., 1990). The molecular cloning of a murine P40 cDNA and the availability of recombinant protein led to the demonstration that the same factor, now termed IL-9, was responsible for all these biological activities (Hültner et al., 1990).

Human IL-9 cDNA was identified by expression cloning of a factor stimulating the proliferation of a human megakaryoblastic leukaemia (Yang et al., 1989) and by cross-hybridization with a mouse probe (Renauld et al., 1990a). More recently, IL-9 activities were described on normal haemopoietic progenitors (Donahue et al., 1990), human T cells (Houssiau et al., 1993), B cells (Dugas et al., 1993; Petit-Frère et al., 1993), fetal thymocytes (Suda et al., 1990a) and thymic lymphomas (Vink et al., 1993).

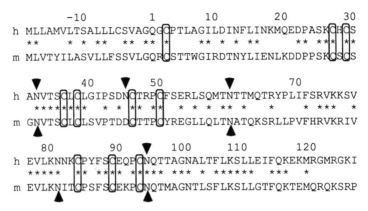

Fig. 1. Alignment of human and mouse IL-9 protein sequences. Amino acids are indicated in one-letter code. The 10 cysteine residues of the mature protein are boxed and arrows indicate the potential N-linked glycosylation sites. Amino acid number 1 refers to the *N*-terminus of the mature mouse protein.

Taken together, these observations suggest that IL-9 is a T_{H2} factor interacting with many other cytokines and potentially involved in mast cell responses and T-cell oncogenesis.

IDENTIFICATION AND CLONING OF MOUSE AND HUMAN IL-9

The purification of mouse IL-9 from the supernatants of activated helper T cells was made possible by the use of stable factor-dependent T-cell lines, derived from normal antigen-dependent clones. The purified protein, originally designated P40 on the basis of its apparent size in gel filtration, was characterized by an elevated pI ($\approx$10) and a high level of glycosylation (Uyttenhove *et al.*, 1988). Partial amino acid sequences obtained after cyanogen bromide treatment allowed the cloning of a full-length cDNA encoding the murine IL-9 protein (Van Snick *et al.*, 1989). In parallel with the cDNA cloning, a complete sequencing of the purified protein has been achieved (Simpson *et al.*, 1989), confirming the deduced amino acid sequence of the mature protein. A cDNA encoding the human homologue of mouse IL-9 was cloned independently by expression cloning of a factor stimulating the growth of a human megakaryoblastic leukaemia (Yang *et al.*, 1989) and by cross-hybridization with the mouse gene (Renauld *et al.*, 1990a). A comparison of the mouse and human IL-9 sequences is shown in Fig. 1. Both deduced protein sequences contain 144 residues, with a typical signal peptide of 18 amino acids. The overall identity reached 69% at the nucleotide level and 55% at the protein level. In accordance with the heavy glycosylation observed with the natural murine protein, four potential N-linked glycosylation sites were noticed in both sequences. This glycosylation is probably responsible for the discrepancy observed between the predicted relative molecular mass (14 150) and the M_r measured for native IL-9. The sequence is also characterized by the presence of 10 cysteines that are perfectly matched in both mature proteins and a strong predominance of cationic residues, which explains the elevated pI ($\approx$10) measured with purified natural IL-9.

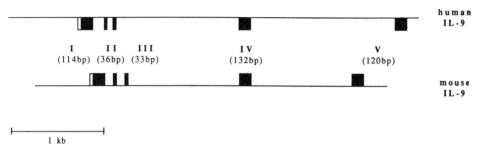

Fig. 2. Map of the human and murine IL-9 genes. Closed boxes represent the coding regions and open boxes correspond to the 5′ untranslated sequence. Exons are numbered and their respective size is indicated; homology levels are 56, 67, 64, 73 and 74% respectively.

THE IL-9 GENE: STRUCTURE AND EXPRESSION

Genomic Organization

The human IL-9 gene is a single-copy gene and was mapped on chromosome 5, in the 5q31–>q35 region (Modi *et al.*, 1991). Interestingly, this region also contains various growth factor- and growth factor receptor-genes such as IL-3, IL-4, IL-5, CSF-1 and CSF-1R and has been shown to be deleted in a series of haematological disorders. Radiation hybrid mapping analysis has recently located the IL-9 gene between the IL-3- and the EGR-1 (early growth response-1) genes (Warrington *et al.*, 1992). However, in the mouse, the IL-9 gene does not appear to be linked to the same gene cluster, as it has been localized on mouse chromosome 13 (Mock *et al.*, 1990) while the IL-3, IL-4, IL-5 and GM-CSF genes are located on chromosome 11.

As shown in Fig. 2, the human and murine IL-9 genes share a similar structure with 5 exons and 4 introns stretching over about 4 kb (Renauld *et al.*, 1990b). The 5 exons are identical in size for both species and show homology levels ranging from 56 to 74%. In contrast, no significant sequence homology was found in the introns (except for intron 2, which is also the smallest), although their size is roughly conserved. However, 3′ and 5′ untranslated regions show a high level of identity, supporting a possible involvement of these sequences in the transcriptional or post-transcriptional regulation of IL-9 expression. In particular, numerous ATTTA motifs were found in the 3′ untranslated region of both genes. These sequences, frequently seen in cytokine mRNAs, are thought to influence the short half-life of these messengers by modulating their stability.

The transcription start has been mapped by S1 nuclease protection 22 to 24 nucleotides downstream from a classical TATA box sequence. The promoter of the IL-9 gene contains potential recognition sites for several TPA-inducible transcription factors such as AP-1 and AP-2, which could provide a structural basis for the induction of IL-9 expression by phorbol esters. A consensus sequence for IRF-1 (interferon regulatory factor-1) was also identified in both promoters, but its physiological relevance remains more elusive (Renauld *et al.*, 1990b). Recently, Kelleher and coworkers identified other consensus sequences in the 5′ untranslated region of the human gene (SP1, NF-κB, Octamer, AP-3, AP-5, glucocorticoid responsive element, cAMP response element among others...) and suggested that the NF-κB site and cAMP response element could be involved in the constitutive expression of IL-9 by HTLV-1-transformed T cells (Kelleher *et al.*, 1991). Functional analysis using deletion or substitution mutants of the IL-9 promoter are still required to clarify the regulatory mechanisms underlying IL-9 expression.

Regulation of IL-9 Expression

The regulation of human IL-9 expression has been studied at the RNA level using freshly isolated peripheral blood mononuclear cells (PBMC). No IL-9 message could be detected in these cells in the absence of any stimulation or after activation of B cells or monocytes. In contrast, T-cell mitogens such as phytohaemagglutinin (PHA) or anti-CD3 mAb induced a substantial IL-9 expression that was further enhanced by addition of PMA. Sorting experiments confirmed that IL-9 was preferentially produced by T-cell-enriched lymphocyte populations and, more specifically, by $CD4^+$ T cells (Renauld et al., 1990b).

Regarding the kinetics of induction, the IL-9 mRNA expression appeared in the late stages of T-cell activation, with a peak at 28 h. Moreover, it was completely abrogated by cycloheximide, an inhibitor of protein synthesis, indicating the involvement of secondary signals in this process. Further experiments identified IL-2 as a required mediator for IL-9 induction in T cells, as anti-IL-2R mAb blocked IL-9 expression after stimulation with PMA and anti-CD3 mAb (Houssiau et al., 1992). However, these experiments do not exclude the possibility that other cytokines could be involved in this process as IL-2 seems to induce many T-cell derived cytokines in this experimental system.

The central role played by IL-2 for IL-9 expression in freshly isolated human T cells was also confirmed in the mouse, as IL-2 was capable of inducing IL-9 in fresh murine splenocytes co-stimulated with PMA (Monteyne, P., personal communication). However, other regulatory mechanisms could be involved in IL-9 expression by some T-cell lines and tumours. It was reported that IL-1, and not IL-2, serves as a secondary signal for IL-9 expression in murine T cell lines (Schmitt et al., 1991) and that HTLV-I-transformed T cells produce IL-9 constitutively (Yang et al., 1989; Kelleher et al., 1991).

BIOASSAYS FOR IL-9

The original bioassay for murine IL-9 is based on the proliferation of a factor-dependent T-cell line called TS1, the half-maximal proliferation being obtained with 15 pg/ml of purified IL-9 (Uyttenhove et al., 1988). These cells are not responsive to IL-2 but proliferate in response to IL-4 (Fig. 3). Most of the IL-9-dependent lines have lost the α chain of the IL-2 receptor as well as the capacity to proliferate in the presence of IL-2, with one exception, the ST2.K9 line which is responsive to IL-2 and IL-9 but not to IL-4 (Schmitt et al., 1989). Recently, LIF was found to stimulate the proliferation of some IL-9-responsive T-cell lines (Van Damme et al., 1992). Murine mast-cell lines such as MC9 also respond to IL-9 in addition to IL-3, IL-4 and IL-10.

Human IL-9 was identified as having a growth-promoting activity for the Mo7E cell line, isolated from a child with acute megakaryoblastic leukaemia (Yang et al., 1989). This cell line is also responsive to Steel factor, GM-CSF and IL-3, which are more potent stimulators of these cells (Fig. 4 and Hendrie et al., 1991) and render the measurement of IL-9 in mixtures of cytokines difficult. While human and mouse IL-9

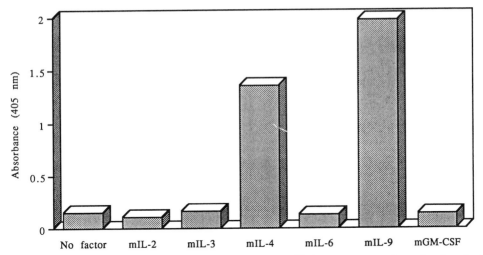

Fig. 3. Factor-dependent proliferation of the TS1 cell line. The TS1 bioassay was performed as described by Uyttenhove *et al.* (1988), in the presence or absence of the indicated cytokines at a concentration of 100 U/ml.

are equally active in a Mo7E proliferation assay, human IL-9 is not active on murine cells. However, a new bioassay for human IL-9 was recently described using murine TS1 cells transfected with the human IL-9 receptor cDNA (Renauld *et al.*, 1992). Among the human factors described to date only LIF/HILDA and insulin were shown to promote the proliferation of this transfected murine cell line.

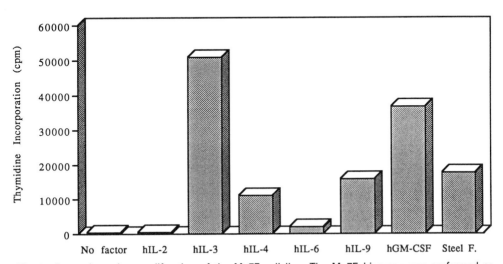

Fig. 4. Factor-dependent proliferation of the Mo7E cell line. The Mo7E bioassay was performed as described by Yang *et al.* (1989). Thymidine incorporations were measured after 24 h in the presence or absence of hIL-2 (20 U/ml), hIL-3 (3 ng/ml), hIL-4 (1/100 of crude baculovirus supernatant), hIL-6 (1000 U/ml), hIL-9 (100 U/ml), hGM-CSF (0.1 ng/ml) and hSteel Factor (1/100 of transfected COS-cells supernatant).

BIOLOGICAL ACTIVITIES OF IL-9

Mast Cells

IL-9 and Mast-cell Lines in vitro

Murine mast-cell lines can be established from bone-marrow haemopoietic progenitors in the presence of lectin-activated T-cell supernatants. Originally, IL-3 was identified as the growth factor required by these cells, which are phenotypically and functionally related to mucosal mast cells (Ihle *et al.*, 1983). Another mast-cell growth factor present in these supernatants was identified as IL-4 (Mossman *et al.*, 1986). Subsequently, Hültner and colleagues observed that a third factor, present in spleen-cell conditioned medium, was able to synergize with IL-3 for the proliferation of permanent bone-marrow-derived mast-cell lines (BMMC) such as L138.8A (Hültner *et al.*, 1989). This factor, provisionally designated MEA, was finally identified as IL-9, since the activity of semi-purified MEA was inhibited by an anti-IL-9 rabbit antiserum and recombinant IL-9 displayed a similar growth-factor activity for L138.8A (Hültner *et al.*, 1990). The proliferative activity of IL-9 alone, or in synergy with IL-3, was confirmed on other permanent mast-cell lines such as MC-6, H7 and MC-9 (Williams *et al.*, 1990; our unpublished data).

Responses of BMMC to IL-9 are highly dependent on the time spent *in vitro*. When primary BMMC are derived from haemopoietic progenitors, IL-9 alone is not sufficient to sustain mast-cell growth, but synergistically enhances the proliferation induced by IL-3 or the combination of IL-3 and IL-4. Moreover, in the absence of other factors, IL-9 significantly increases the survival of these primary BMMC. After more time *in vitro*, when stable mast-cell lines are obtained, IL-9 alone becomes capable of inducing proliferation without the need for additional factors. Finally, autonomous cells, which induce tumours in syngeneic animals, can be derived from factor-dependent cell lines (Hültner and Moeller, 1990).

In addition to its proliferative activity, IL-9 also appears to be a potent regulator of mast-cell effector molecules. It was shown to induce IL-6 secretion by mast-cell lines (Hültner and Moeller, 1990; Hültner *et al.*, 1990) and the recent identification of genes specifically induced by IL-9 has shown that protease genes belonging to the granzyme family are efficiently expressed and produced in response to IL-9. Moreover, expression of the α chain of the high-affinity IgE receptor is also upregulated by IL-9, indicating that this factor could be a key mediator of mast-cell differentiation (Louahed *et al.* manuscript in preparation).

IL-9 and Mastocytosis in vivo

In vivo, infections by helminth parasites typically induce an immune response characterized by strong IgE production and a massive mucosal mastocytosis resulting from T_{H2} cytokine production. During infection with *Trichinella spiralis*, IL-9 production is induced in mesenteric lymph nodes, like other T_{H2} cytokines such as IL-3, IL-4 and IL-5 (Grencis *et al.*, 1991). The protective potential of a T_{H1}-like or T_{H2}-like response appears to vary depending on the parasites so that a T_{H2} response may be harmful in some helminth infections but protective for others. For instance, resistance to *Trichuris muris* was found to correlate with the production of IL-5 and IL-9 in mesenteric lymph nodes (Else *et al.*, 1992).

The cytokine responses induced by *Heligmosomiodes polygyrus* or *Nippostrongylus brasiliensis*, two gastrointestinal nematode parasites, have been investigated by Urban *et al.* (1992). Interestingly, strong T_{H2} cytokine inductions were noted during these infections, but with considerable differences between the kinetics and level of induction of these factors (Svetic *et al.*, 1992). *H. polygyrus* has a strictly enteral life cycle, invading the intestinal mucosa less than 24 h after ingestion and developing there into mature adults. Within 3–6 h after oral inoculation of *H. polygyrus* larvae, IL-9 mRNA levels increased considerably in Peyer's patches and remained elevated for several days.

Similarly, when *N. brasiliensis* larvae were inoculated subcutaneously, IL-9 mRNA induction was found in the lungs by 24 h, and in mesenteric lymph nodes after 4 days. Since the larvae reached the lungs within 1 day and the gut after 3–4 days, IL-9 expression appears to be an early event in the immune response that actually precedes the production of other cytokines such as IL-4. In contrast, the IL-9 expression was substantially decreased from its peak level by day 6 after inoculation, while expression of IL-3, IL-4 and IL-5 genes was maintained at least to day 12 (Madden *et al.* 1991; and Finkelman, F., personal communication).

The role of IL-3 and IL-4 in *Nippostrongylus*-induced mastocytosis was demonstrated by the observation that either anti-IL-3 or anti-IL-4 antibodies partially (40–50%) inhibit the mucosal mast cell response. As the combination of both anti-IL-3 and anti-IL-4 antibodies failed to block more than 85% of the mastocytosis, a third factor was possibly involved in the mast-cell response (Madden *et al.*, 1991). Although an anti-IL-9 antiserum did not by itself influence mast-cell hyperplasia, addition of such antibodies to anti-IL-3 and anti-IL-4 antibodies increased the suppression of the mast-cell response from 85% to 95%. Moreover, when mice received suboptimal doses of anti-IL-3 plus anti-IL-4 antibodies, the suppression of mastocytosis was raised from 60% to 94% after injection of an anti-IL-9 antiserum (Finkelman, F., personal communication), demonstrating that IL-9 may contribute to the development of mucosal mast-cell hyperplasia induced by worm infections, particularly under conditions where IL-3 and IL-4 are limiting.

B Cells

The involvement of IL-9 in mast-cell activation and proliferation as well as in IL-9 production during parasite infections raised the hypothesis of a potential role of this factor in IgE-mediated responses. The ability of IL-9 to modulate IgE production by mouse B cells has been recently investigated by Petit-Frère *et al.* (1993). Their results indicated that IL-9 synergized with suboptimal doses of IL-4 for IgE and IgG1 production by LPS-activated semi-purified B cells but did not induce IgE or IgG1 production in the absence of IL-4. The IL-9 activity on the IL-4-induced IgG1 production correlated with an increase in the number of IgG1 secreting cells. In contrast, IL-9 did not affect the IL-4-induced CD23 expression by LPS-activated B cells, indicating that its activity did not consist in a simple upregulation of the IL-4 responsiveness by the B cells. Moreover, these experiments have not eliminated the possibility that the effect of IL-9 observed on murine B cells would be mediated by accessory cells.

In the human, very similar observations have been recently reported by Dugas and coworkers using semi-purified B cells (Dugas *et al.*, 1993). In this experimental system,

IL-9 synergized with IL-4 for IgE and IgG production but not for that of IgM. Moreover, IL-9 also potentiated IL-4-induced IgE production by sorted CD20$^+$ cells upon costimulation by irradiated EL4 murine T cells, thereby suggesting a direct activity on the B cells.

T Cells

IL-9 and Mouse T Cells: a Model of T Cell Oncogenesis

Initially, the response of murine T cells seemed to be restricted to a small number of T-helper clones. However, it appeared that the responsiveness to IL-9 was not a characteristic of a particular T-cell subpopulation but is gradually acquired by long-term *in vitro* culture. Interestingly, this process is reminiscent of, and eventually leads to, some kind of tumoral transformation.

T-helper clones can be derived from lymph nodes of mice immunized with proteins and maintained *in vitro* by repeated stimulation with antigen and syngeneic antigen-presenting cells. After stimulation, the T cells go through a stage of blastic activation and proliferate intensively before undergoing a considerable size reduction. A quiescent period of 1 or 2 weeks is then needed before restimulation of the cells, otherwise no stable T-cell clones can be maintained in culture.

In this experimental system, responses to IL-9 varied not only between different clones but also for a single clone depending on the total number of *in vitro* stimulations. Early T-cell clones, like freshly isolated T cells, were not responsive to IL-9, although significant proliferations were induced by IL-2. After a few passages *in vitro*, T-helper clones responded to IL-9 by blast formation, IL-6 secretion and enhanced survival but no significant proliferation. After more weeks in culture, short-term proliferation could be observed, but only in synergy with another factor like IL-4 or IL-3. After months of culture, IL-9 alone induced significant proliferation.

During this progressive transition, major changes appeared in the phenotype of the corresponding cultures. Cells remained blastic during the complete culture period and required more frequent passages. At this stage, cultures could be maintained by addition of IL-9 and permanent IL-9-dependent cell lines could be derived. An increase in cell size was noted, as well as an accelerated growth rate. Progressively, all T-cell markers such as Thy-1, CD4, CD3 and TCR expression were totally lost. Most of these IL-9-dependent lines also lost the α chain of the IL-2 receptor as well as the capacity to proliferate in the presence of IL-2 but usually remained IL-4-responsive. Recently, LIF/HILDA and insulin have also been shown to support the long-term proliferation of some of these IL-9-dependent lines but the significance of this latter observation is not known (Lehmann *et al.* unpublished data; Van Damme *et al.*, 1992).

The progressive deregulation undergone by T cells during acquisition of IL-9 responsiveness raised the possibility that some form of tumorigenic transformation occurred in these cell lines. To address this question, we transfected an IL-9-dependent T-cell line with IL-9 cDNA and obtained transfected cells secreting IL-9 and growing autonomously *in vitro*. Most interestingly, when these cells were injected into syngeneic mice, a very high tumour incidence was observed and animals died in 3–4 months as a result of widespread lymphoma development (Uyttenhove *et al.*, 1991).

To assess further the *in vivo* relevance of these observations, we generated transgenic mice expressing high levels of IL-9 constitutively (Renauld *et al.*, 1994). About 5%

of these mice spontaneously developed lymphoblastic lymphomas. Moreover, the IL-9 transgenic mice were highly susceptible to chemical mutagenesis as all transgenic animals developed such tumours after injection of doses of a mutagen (N-methyl-N-nitroso-Urea) that were totally innocuous in control mice.

The growth-promoting activity of IL-9 for T-cell tumours was further investigated *in vitro* using other models of thymic lymphomas. In these experiments, it has been found recently that IL-9 significantly stimulates the *in vitro* proliferation of primary lymphomas induced either by chemical mutagenesis in DBA/2 mice or by X-ray radiation in B6 mice (Vink *et al.*, 1993). Moreover, these studies have demonstrated a strong synergy between IL-9 and IL-2 for several lymphomas; a synergy reminiscent of the activity of IL-9 on murine fetal thymocytes (Suda *et al.*, 1990a).

In the human, an association between dysregulated IL-9 expression and lymphoid malignancies has been initially suggested by the observation that lymph nodes from patients with Hodgkin- and large-cell anaplastic lymphomas constitutively produce IL-9 (Merz *et al.*, 1991). Constitutive IL-9 expression was also detected in HTLV-1 transformed T cells (Kelleher *et al.*, 1991) and in Hodgkin cell lines (Merz *et al.*, 1991; Gruss *et al.*, 1992). Moreover, the recent demonstration of an autocrine loop for the *in vitro* growth of one of these Hodgkin cell lines (Gruss *et al.*, 1992) suggests a potential involvement of IL-9 in this disease.

IL-9 and Human T Cells: Requirement for Preactivation

A different aspect of the T-cell growth factor activity of IL-9 has been recently unravelled using human peripheral T cells (Houssiau *et al.*, 1993). It was found that all T-cell lines derived by weekly stimulation with PHA, IL-2 and irradiated allogeneic PBMC as feeders, strongly expressed IL-9 receptor message and proliferated in response to IL-9, after only 2–3 weekly passages. By contrast, unlike other T-cell growth factors such as IL-2, IL-4 or IL-7, IL-9 did not induce any proliferation of freshly isolated T cells, neither alone nor in synergy with other cytokines or T-cell costimuli. Interestingly, significant proliferations could be induced by IL-9 when PBMC were activated for only 10 days with PHA, IL-2 and irradiated allogeneic feeder cells, thereby indicating that responses to IL-9 might require previous activation. The importance of a state of activation was further reinforced by the observation that responses to IL-9, unlike those elicited by IL-2, varied depending on the time after restimulation of the cultures; this was optimal when the cells were in a fully blastic stage and rapidly decreased when the cells underwent a size reduction. These observations suggested that the response to IL-9 varies according to the stage of cell activation.

In order to characterize further the IL-9 responsive T cells, clones were derived either from established PHA-stimulated T-cell lines or by direct cloning from freshly isolated purified T cells. It was found that most of these clones proliferated in response to IL-9, irrespective of their CD4 or CD8 phenotype. In addition, tumour-specific cytolytic T-cell clones responded to IL-9 by proliferation or increased survival.

The results obtained with human T cells differ in several ways from those initially reported in the murine model (Uyttenhove *et al.*, 1988; Schmitt *et al.*, 1989). Murine T cells require months of *in vitro* culture before responding to IL-9. Moreover, when murine T cells become responsive to IL-9, factor-dependent lines are readily derived that grow independently of their antigen and feeder cells, while no such long-term proliferation has yet been obtained in the human system. However, these discrepancies could be related to the distinct experimental systems used, and in particular, to the differences in the stimulation procedures. Human IL-9-responsive T cells are strongly activated with PHA, IL-2 and feeder cells on a weekly basis and this strong stimulation was found to be crucial for IL-9 responses. In contrast, a much less potent antigen-specific stimulation is used in the murine model. This difference could explain why freshly raised murine T-cell clones do not respond to IL-9. Alternatively the acquisition of IL-9 responsiveness by murine T cells is linked to a cryptic *in vitro* transformation process. The fact that no permanent IL-9-dependent human T-cell lines or clones have been derived to date, suggests that such an *in vitro* transformation process does not take place under the conditions used in the human model. Taken together these results indicate that different mechanisms may render T cells responsive to IL-9: potent activation of freshly isolated cells, as observed in the human model, or progressive dysregulation resulting from long-term *in vitro* culture, as observed in the mouse model.

IL-9 AND HAEMOPOIETIC PROGENITORS

The identification of human IL-9 as a factor promoting the growth of a megakaryoblastic leukaemia line Mo7E (Yang *et al.*, 1989) raised the question of the activity of IL-9 on haemopoietic progenitors. The Mo7E cells display early markers of haemopoietic differentiation, such as CD33 and CD34, and markers for bipotent erythro-megakaryoblastic haemopoietic precursors. However, IL-9 did not seem to be active on megakaryoblastic precursors but was found to support erythroid colony formation in the presence of erythropoietin using progenitors from human peripheral blood or bone marrow (Donahue *et al.*, 1990). This activity appeared to reflect a direct effect of IL-9 on erythroid progenitors since it was not blocked by a neutralizing antiserum against IL-3 or GM-CSF and the effect was observed with highly purified progenitors after selecting for CD34$^+$ cells and T-cell depletion (Birner *et al.*, 1992; Lu *et al.*, 1992). In contrast, granulocyte or macrophage colony formation (CFU-GM, CFU-G or CFU-M) was not influenced by IL-9, suggesting that, within the adult haemopoietic system, IL-9 is a specific regulator of erythropoiesis. A similar erythroid-burst-promoting activity has been described with murine bone-marrow progenitors but this effect was unexpectedly abolished by T-cell depletion (Williams *et al.*, 1990).

   Subsequent studies have shown that IL-9 is more effective on fetal cells than on adult progenitors, suggesting that it supports the maturation of a primitive subset of fetal BFU-E. Moreover, when combined to IL-3 or GM-CSF, IL-9 induced the maturation of CFU-Mix and CFU-GM in cultures of fetal progenitors, an activity that is not detected in adult cultures (Holbrook *et al.*, 1991). The observation that murine 15-day fetal thymocytes (Suda *et al.*, 1990a), but not adult thymocytes (Suda *et al.*, 1990b), responded synergistically to IL-9 and IL-2, further indicates that the spectrum of activities of IL-9 is larger on fetal progenitors.

THE IL-9 RECEPTOR

A single class of high-affinity binding sites for IL-9 ($K_d \approx 100$ pM) have been detected on various IL-9-responsive murine cells. Crosslinking data indicated that IL-9 binds to a single-chain receptor consisting in a 64 kDa glycoprotein (Druez *et al.*, 1990). The murine IL-9 receptor cDNA has been identified by expression cloning in COS cells (Renauld *et al.*, 1992). The deduced protein is a 468-amino-acid polypeptide with two hydrophobic regions corresponding to the signal peptide and the transmembrane domain. The extracellular domain, composed of 233 amino acids, contains a W–S–E–W–S motif and six cysteine residues, whose position indicates that the IL-9 receptor is a member of the haemopoietin receptor superfamily (Idzerda *et al.*, 1990). The human IL-9 receptor cDNA, which was isolated by cross-hybridization with a mouse probe, encodes a 522-amino-acid protein with a 53% identity with the mouse molecule. The cytoplasmic domain, which is less conserved than the extra-cellular region, is significantly larger in the human receptor (231 versus 177 residues).

The mechanisms of signal transduction through the IL-9 receptor are still unclear. In the human Mo7E cells, at least four unidentified tyrosine-phosphorylated bands have been detected by Western blot analysis after IL-9 stimulation. However, IL-9 did not induce nor enhance the phosphorylation of the serine–threonine kinases raf-1 or MAP (Miyazawa *et al.*, 1992). Sequence analysis of the cytoplasmic domain of the IL-9 receptor did not provide any significant information regarding signal transduction, except for a high percentage of serine and proline residues, as already observed for most cytokine receptors. In addition, some sequence homology with other receptors was noted proximally to the transmembrane domain. As previously shown for many cytokine receptors (IL-4R, IL-7R, IL-3R, EPOR, IL-2Rβ, G-CSFR), a Pro–X–Pro sequence was found upstream from a cluster of hydrophobic residues that partially fits a recently described consensus sequence (Murakami *et al.*, 1991). Downstream from this motif, a striking homology was observed with the β chain of the IL-2 receptor and with the erythropoietin receptor. Interestingly, these two receptors interact with the cytokines that have been shown to synergize with IL-9 for the proliferation of fetal thymocytes and erythroid progenitors, respectively.

As previously observed for many cytokine receptors, IL-9 receptor messenger RNAs encoding a putative soluble receptor have been identified as a result of alternative splicing. This phenomenon, as well as the use of alternative polyadenylation signals, is responsible for the multiple bands observed in Northern blot, particularly in human cells, and raises intriguing questions regarding the post-transcriptional regulation of IL-9 receptor expression.

CONCLUSIONS

Since its discovery as a growth factor for T-helper cell clones, IL-9 has been found to be involved in various other biological systems. Its role in mast-cell activation and differentiation, as well as its ability to enhance IgE production *in vitro*, suggest possible implication of this cytokine in allergic reactions. Its physiological function regarding T-cell responses is still far from clear. Besides its oncogenic potential, which has been well established in the mouse and suggested in human Hodgkin's disease, IL-9 could affect normal T-cell responses by further stimulating preactivated T cells. Finally, the activity of IL-9 on haemopoiesis could represent an important aspect of the biology of this cytokine, but further *in vivo* studies are required to assess its clinical relevance.

REFERENCES

Birner, A., Hültner, L., Mergenthaler, H.G., Van Snick, J. and Dörmer, P. (1992). *Exp. Hematol.* **20**, 541–545.
Donahue, R.E., Yang, Y.C. and Clark, S.C. (1990). *Blood* **75**, 2271–2275.
Druez, C., Coulie, P., Uyttenhove, C. and Van Snick, J. (1990). *J. Immunol.* **145**, 2494–2499.
Dugas, B., Renauld, J-C., Bonnefoy, J.Y., Petit-Frère, C., Braquet, P., Van Snick, J. and Mencia-Huerta, J.M. (1993). *Eur. J. Immunol.* **23**, 1687–1692.
Else, K., Hültner, L. and Grencis, R. (1992). *Immunology* **75**, 232–237.
Grencis, R.K., Hültner, L. and Else, K.J. (1991). *Immunology* **74**, 329–332.
Gruss, H.J., Brach, M.A., Drexler, H.G., Bross, K.J. and Herrman, F. (1992). *Cancer Res.* **52**, 1026–1031.
Hendrie, P., Miyazawa, K., Yang, Y.C., Langefeld, C. and Broxmeyer, H. (1991). *Exp. Hematol.* **19**, 1031–1037.
Holbrook, S.T., Ohls, R.K., Schribler, K.R., Yang, Y.C. and Christensen, R.D. (1991). *Blood* **77**, 2129–2134.
Houssiau, F., Renauld, J-C., Fibbe, W. and Van Snick, J. (1992). *J. Immunol.* **148**, 3147–3151.
Houssiau, F., Renauld, J-C., Stevens, M., Lehmann, F., Coulie, P.G. and Van Snick, J. (1993). *J. Immunol.* **150**, 2634–2640.
Hültner, L. and Moeller, J. (1990). *Exp. Hematol.* **18**, 873–877.
Hültner, L., Moeller, J., Schmitt, E., Jäger, G., Reisbach, G., Ring, J. and Dörmer, P. (1989). *J. Immunol.* **142**, 3440–3446.
Hültner, L., Druez, C., Moeller, J., Uyttenhove, C., Schmitt, E., Rüde, E., Dörmer, P. and Van Snick, J. (1990). *Eur. J. Immunol.* **20**, 1413–1416.
Idzerda, R.J., March, C.J., Mosley, B., Lyman, S.D., Vanden Bos, T., Gimpel, S.D., Din, W.S., Grabstein, K.H., Widmar, M.B., Park, L., Cosman, D. and Beckman, M.P. (1990). *J. Exp. Med.* **171** 861–873.
Ihle, J., Keller, J., Oroszlan, S., Henderson, L., Copeland, T., Fitch, F., Prystowsky, M., Goldwasser, E., Schrader, J., Palaszynski, E., Dy, M. and Lebel, B. (1983). *J. Immunol.* **131**, 282–287.
Kelleher, K., Bean, K., Clark, S.C., Leung, W.Y., Yang-Feng, T.L., Chen, J.W., Lin, P.F., Luo, W. and Yang, Y.C. (1991). *Blood* **77**, 1436–1441.
Lu, L., Leemhuis, T., Srour, E. and Yang, Y.C. (1992). *Exp. Hematol.* **20**, 418–424.
Madden, K., Urban, K., Ziltener, H., Schrader, J., Finkelman, F. and Katona, I. (1991). *J. Immunol.* **147**, 1387–1391.
Merz, H., Houssiau, F., Orscheschek, K., Renauld, J-C., Fliedner, A., Herin, M., Noël, H., Kadin, M., Meuller-Hermelink, K.H., Van Snick, J. and Feller, A.C. (1991). *Blood* **78**, 1311–1317.
Miyazawa, K., Hendrie, P., Kim, Y.J., Mantel, C., Yang, Y.C., Se Kwon, B. and Broxmeyer, H. (1992). *Blood* **80**, 1685–1692.
Mock, B.A., Krall, M., Kozak, C.A., Nesbitt, M.N., McBride, O.W., Renauld, J-C. and Van Snick, J. (1990). *Immunogenetics* **31**, 265–270.
Modi, W.S., Pollock, D.D., Mock, B.A., Banner, C., Renauld, J-C. and Van Snick, J. (1991). *Cytogenet. Cell. Genet.* **57**, 114–116.
Moeller, J., Hültner, L., Schmitt, E. and Dörmer, P. (1989). *J. Immunol.* **142**, 3447–3451.
Moeller, J., Hültner, L., Schmitt, E., Breuer, M. and Dörmer, P. (1990). *J. Immunol.* **144**, 4231–4234.
Mossman, T., Bond, M., Coffman, R., Ohara, J. and Paul, W. (1986). *Proc. Natl Acad. Sci. USA* **83**, 5654–5658.
Murakami, M., Narazaki, M., Hibi, M., Yawata, H., Yasukawa, K., Hamaguchi, M., Taga, T. and Kishimoto, T. (1991). *Proc. Natl Acad. Sci. USA* **88**, 11349–11353.
Petit-Frère, C., Dugas, B., Braquet, P. and Mencia-Huerta, J.M. (1993). *Immunology* **79**, 146–151.
Renauld, J-C., Goethals, A., Houssiau, F., Van Roost, E. and Van Snick, J. (1990a). *Cytokine* **2**, 9–12.
Renauld, J-C., Goethals, A., Houssiau, F., Merz, H., Van Roost, E. and Van Snick, J. (1990b). *J. Immunol.* **144**, 4235–4241.
Renauld, J-C., Druez, C., Kermouni, A., Houssiau, F., Uyttenhove, C., Van Roost, E. and Van Snick, J. (1992). *Proc. Natl Acad. Sci. USA* **89**, 5690–5694.
Renauld, J-C., van der Lugt, N., Vink, A., Van Roon, M., Godfraind, C., Warnier, G., Merz, H., Feller, A., Berns, A. and Van Snick, J. (1994). *Oncogene* (in press).
Schmitt, E., van Brandwijk, R., Van Snick, J., Siebold, B. and Rüde, E. (1989). *Eur. J. Immunol.* **19**, 2167–2170.
Schmitt, E., Beuscher, H.U., Huels, C., Monteyne, P., van Brandwijk, R., Van Snick, J. and Rüde, E. (1991). *J. Immunol.* **147**, 3848–3854.

Simpson, R.J., Moritz, R.L., Gorman, J.J. and Van Snick, J. (1989). *Eur. J. Biochem.* **183**, 715–722.

Suda, T., Murray, R., Fischer, M., Tokota, T. and Zlotnik, A. (1990a). *J. Immunol.* **144**, 1783–1787.

Suda, T., Murray, R., Guidos, C. and Zlotnik, A. (1990b). *J. Immunol.* **144**, 3039–3045.

Svetic, A., Madden, K.B., Katona, I.M., Finkelman, F.D., Urban J.F. and Gause, W.C. (1992). *FASEB J.* **6**, A1688.

Urban, J.F., Madden, K.B., Svetic, A., Cheever, A., Trotta, P.P., Gause, W.C., Katona, I.M. and Finkelman, F.D. (1992). *Immunol. Rev.* **127**, 205–220.

Uyttenhove, C., Simpson, R.J. and Van Snick, J. (1988). *Proc. Natl Acad. Sci. USA* **85**, 6934–6938.

Uyttenhove, C., Druez, C., Renauld, J-C., Herin, M., Noel, H. and Van Snick, J. (1991). *J. Exp. Med.* **173**, 519–522.

Van Damme, J., Uyttenhove, C., Houssiau, F., Put, W., Proost, P. and Van Snick, J. (1992). *Eur. J. Immunol.* **22**, 2801–2808.

Van Snick, J., Goethals, A., Renauld, J-C., Van Roost, E., Uyttenhove, C., Rubira, M.R., Moritz, R.L. and Simpson, R.J. (1989). *J. Exp. Med.* **169**, 363–368.

Vink, A., Renauld, J-C., Warnier, G. and Van Snick, J. (1993). *Eur. J. Immunol.* **23**, 1134–1138.

Warrington, J., Bailey, S., Armstrong, E., Aprelikova, O., Alitalo, K., Dolganov, G., Wilcox, A., Sikela, J., Wolfe, S., Lovett, M. and Vasmuth, J. (1992). *Genomics* **13**, 803–808.

Williams, D.E., Morrissey, P.J., Mochizuki, D.Y., de Vries, P., Anderson, D., Cosman, D., Boswell, H.S., Cooper, S., Grabstein, K.H., and Broxmeyer, H.E. (1990). *Blood* **76**, 906–911.

Yang, Y., Ricciardi, S., Ciarletta, A., Calvetti, J., Kelleher, K. and Clark, S.C. (1989). *Blood* **74**, 1880–1884.

Chapter 12

Interleukin-10

Tim R. Mosmann

Department of Immunology, University of Alberta, Edmonton, Alberta, Canada

INTRODUCTION

IL-10 was originally discovered during a search for a cross-regulatory cytokine that would be produced by T_{H2} cells and inhibit the functions of T_{H1} cells. We found that T_{H2} supernatants contained an activity that inhibited cytokine production in cocultures of T_{H1} cells, antigen-presenting cells (APCs) and antigen (Fiorentino *et al.*, 1989). This effect was specific for T_{H1} cells since T_{H2} cells responded normally in the presence or absence of the T_{H2} supernatant factor, which was named cytokine synthesis inhibitory factor (CSIF). After immunochemical and biochemical analysis indicated that CSIF was likely to be a novel cytokine, a cDNA clone encoding CSIF was isolated by expression cloning (Moore *et al.*, 1990). Characterization of the recombinant cytokine revealed that additional activities of CSIF were being analysed in other laboratories. These activities included stimulation of proliferation of mast cells (Thompson Snipes *et al.*, 1991) and thymocytes (Suda *et al.*, 1990). The name 'Interleukin-10' was then proposed (Moore *et al.*, 1990). The mouse cDNA sequence was used to isolate a human homologue from a human T-cell cDNA library (Vieira *et al.*, 1991), and the biological activities of the human recombinant IL-10 were found to be similar to those of the mouse cytokine. As observed for many other cytokines, IL-10 mediates several functions on multiple cell types. IL-10 inhibits several macrophage functions, including presentation of antigen to T_{H1} cells, cytokine synthesis and some microbicidal activities. In contrast, IL-10 generally enhances or stimulates mast cells and B cells. IL-10 is produced by macrophages and other cell types, in addition to the T cells from which it was originally identified, and so IL-10, in common with several other cytokines, has a much more complex role in the immune system than could be inferred from the original activity.

BIOCHEMICAL PROPERTIES OF IL-10

Mouse IL-10 has an approximate molecular mass of 35 kDa (Fiorentino *et al.*, 1989) and is a non-disulphide-linked homodimer. The monomer polypeptide chains migrate during SDS–gel electrophoresis in two major bands corresponding to apparent molecular masses of 17 kDa and 21 kDa. Treatment with N-glycanase, or synthesis in the presence of tunicamycin, results in nonglycosylated IL-10 that migrates at 17 kDa

Table 1. Functions of IL-10.

Macrophages
Inhibition of cytokine production in response to LPS and T cells (IL-1, IL-6, IL-8, IL-10, IL-12, TNF)
Inhibition of NO production
Reduction of APC function for T_{H1} cells.

NK cells
Inhibition of cytokine production

T cells
Inhibition of cytokine synthesis by T_{H1} and CD8 cells (indirect, when macrophages are APC).
Enhancement of mouse CTL differentiation

B cells
Enhancement of proliferation (human).
Enhancement of antibody secretion (human)
Enhancement of MHC II expression (mouse)

Mast cells
Enhancement of proliferation
Enhancement of protease expression

In vivo
Inhibition of DTH induction
Inhibition of DTH effector function

(Moore *et al.*, 1990). In contrast, human IL-10 has little or no glycosylation and migrates as a single band at about 18 kDa. Glycosylated and nonglycosylated mouse IL-10 appear to have similar activities, at least *in vitro*. Chromatography on a hydrophic interaction column separates three components, corresponding to glycosylation of two, one or neither of the polypeptides. All three species have similar specific bioactivities (Bond, Fiorentino and Mosmann, unpublished data). Mouse and human IL-10 are very labile in acid solutions and activity is lost rapidly below pH 5.5. Monoclonal antibodies specific for mouse IL-10 revealed that, as for many other cytokines, some IL-10 molecules appear to be nonfunctional and antigenically different, since two monoclonal antibodies were isolated that bound IL-10 but did not recognize any biologically active molecules (Mosmann *et al.*, 1990). Four other monoclonal antibodies recognized active IL-10, but did not cross-absorb the IL-10 molecules recognized by the other two antibodies.

RECOMBINANT CLONING OF IL-10

An IL-10 cDNA clone was isolated by expression cloning. Pools of a cDNA library from an activated T_{H2} clone (D10) in the pcDSR-α cloning vector (Takebe *et al.*, 1988) were screened for their ability to direct the synthesis of CSIF activity in COS cells. A full-length cDNA clone encoding CSIF activity was isolated, and the sequence of the open reading frame was not related to any of the known cytokines. A cDNA clone for human IL-10 was isolated from a human T-cell cDNA library by cross-hybridization with mouse IL-10 oligonucleotide probes (Vieira *et al.*, 1991). Conserved regions of the mouse and human clones were used to design PCR primers for the amplification of rat IL-10 cDNA from RNA extracted from Con-A-stimulated T cells from a parasite-infected rat (Goodman *et al.*, 1992). The amplified product was then cloned. Human and rat IL-10 nucleotide sequences are both 90% homologous to mouse IL-10. Mouse and human cDNA clones have been expressed as secreted proteins in monkey COS cells and the *N*-terminal 18 amino acids of the open reading frame are consistent with the presence of a secretion-leader sequence. The *N*-termini of recombinant mouse and human IL-10 are Gln-22 ad Ser-19, respectively. Mouse IL-10 has two potential N-linked glycosylation sites, and one of these is present in human IL-10, although human IL-10 appears to be unglycosylated. The mature human IL-10 polypeptide has four cysteines and mouse has five, although both proteins are noncovalent homodimers (Fiorentino *et al.*, 1989; Moore *et al.*, 1993). The 3' untranslated region of the mRNA contains AT-rich regions, similar to those that lead to messenger RNA instability in other cytokines.

Recombinant DNA clones for the IL-10 gene were also isolated from mouse cells (Kim *et al.*, 1992). The IL-10 gene contains 5 exons spread over approximately 5.1 kb of the genome. The noncoding upstream regions of the IL-10 gene share sequences with the upstream regulatory regions of several other cytokine genes. Mouse and human IL-10 genes are both found on chromosome 1 in their respective genomes (Kim *et al.*, 1992).

IL-10-RELATED GENES IN HERPES VIRUSES

Surprisingly, the open reading frame of mouse IL-10 cDNA had high sequence homology to a previously uncharacterized open reading frame (BCRF1) in the Epstein–Barr virus (EBV) genome (Baer *et al.*, 1984; Moore *et al.*, 1990). Human IL-10 (Vieira *et al.*, 1991) is homologous to these two sequences and BCRF1 is more homologous to human than mouse IL-10. The BCRF1 homology is present in the open reading frame but not in flanking or leader sequences and the amino acid sequence homology (84%) is higher than the nucleotide sequence homology (71%) suggesting that the sequence has been conserved owing to selection at the protein level. Since the mouse IL-10 gene contains introns whereas BCRF1 does not, it appears that the IL-10 gene has been acquired from a mammalian genome by EBV, possibly via a step involving reverse transcriptase provided by a retrovirus since the lack of introns in BCRF1 is consistent with its derivation from mRNA rather than genomic DNA. When BCRF1 was subcloned into an expression vector (Hsu *et al.*, 1990) it encoded a secreted protein similar in size to human and mouse IL-10. The BCRF1 protein exhibits IL-10 activity on both mouse and human cells, particularly in assays involving macrophages and human B cells (Hsu *et al.*, 1990; de Waal Malefyt *et al.*, 1991b; Rousset *et al.*, 1992; Niiro *et al.*, 1992). Thus, EBV appears to have captured a mammalian IL-10 gene and maintained this gene for the purpose of interfering with the immune response. An additional herpes virus, equine herpes virus (EHV), also carries a gene with sequence homology to IL-10 (Rode *et al.*, 1993).

The expression of viral IL-10-like cytokines by EBV and EHV may be advantageous to the viruses because IL-10 inhibits the synthesis of macrophage- and T-cell cytokines that would otherwise contribute to the antiviral immune response. These cytokines include IFN-γ, LT and TNF. Thus, the production of viral IL-10 in the late phase of lytic infection (Hudson *et al.*, 1985) should reduce the synthesis of these cytokines in the vicinity of the infected B cell, thus inhibiting local immune attack. In addition to this effect of weakening antiviral immune responses, the B-cell proliferation-enhancing activity of IL-10 (Rousset *et al.*, 1992) may also benefit the virus since EBV infects human B cells and IL-10/BCRF1 would induce an increased number of activated B cells that would be targets for viral infection. EBV may further bias the local immune response by inducing expression of the endogenous IL-10 gene, since EBV-transformed B cells express human IL-10 (Benjamin *et al.*, 1992; Burdin *et al.*, 1993).

Other viruses have also acquired mammalian cytokine-related genes that could be used to interfere with immune responses. In addition to the two herpesvirus IL-10 homologues, poxviruses carry genes homologous to the mammalian receptors for TNF (Smith *et al.*, 1990) and IFN-γ (Upton *et al.*, 1992). Both of these genes have been modified from the original mammalian genes by deletion of the transmembrane region, resulting in small secreted molecules that still bind the relevant cytokine. These viral

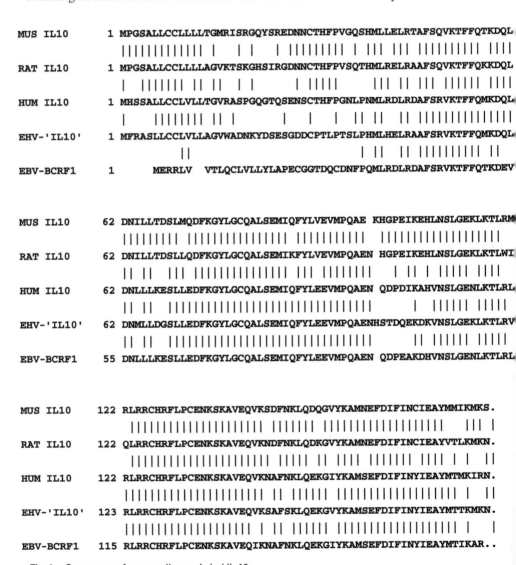

Fig. 1. Sequences of mammalian and viral IL-10s.

molecules may be advantageous to the virus since they can neutralize IFN-γ or TNF in solution before the cytokines can interact with the genuine receptors on infected cells and induce death of the cells.

THE IL-10 RECEPTOR

Mouse and human cDNA clones for IL-10-binding proteins have been isolated (Moore, K.W., personal communication). These two clones are about 75% homologous at both protein and DNA levels and the open reading frames encode 570 amino acids, including a transmembrane domain and an extracellular domain of about 220 amino acids. The IL-10 receptor is expressed on a wide variety of cells, consistent with the response of many cell types to IL-10. It is likely that this component represents at least part of the IL-10 receptor, and there is some evidence that suggests additional component(s). Mouse IL-10 binds to COS cells expressing either the human or mouse recombinant IL-10 receptor chains, whereas human cells, presumably expressing complete IL-10 receptors, bind only human IL-10. This differential specificity of binding suggests that the human receptor polypeptide expressed in COS cells is not identical to the natural receptor expressed on human cells.

CELL TYPES PRODUCING IL-10

IL-10 is produced by mouse T_{H2} and T_{H0} subsets of helper (CD4$^+$) T-cell clones but not by T_{H1} cells or CD8$^+$ T-cell clones (Fiorentino et al., 1989; Moore et al., 1990; Mosmann et al., 1990). In all cases, T cells only produce IL-10 after stimulation with antigen or polyclonal activators. Many but not all human T-cell clones produce IL-10 (Yssel et al., 1992; Barnes et al., 1993), including T_{H2}-like clones and T_{H1}-like cells that produce IFN-γ but little or no IL-4 (Del Prete et al., 1993). This suggests that the production of IL-10 may not be limited to the same T-cell subsets in humans as in mice, or alternatively, human clones expressing the true T_{H1} cytokine pattern may be less frequently isolated. IL-10 is also produced by rat T cells (Goodman et al., 1992).

In addition to T cells, IL-10 is expressed by mouse mast-cell lines (Moore et al., 1990) and normal mouse B-cell populations after stimulation (O'Garra et al., 1990). The Ly-1 B-cell subset appears to be the major mouse B-cell source of IL-10 (O'Garra et al., 1992). Human B cells also produce IL-10, especially after EBV transformation (Benjamin et al., 1992; Burdin et al., 1993). Macrophages produce substantial amounts of IL-10 (de Waal Malefyt et al., 1991a) and other cytokines such as IL-1, TNF and IL-6 in response to activation by, for example LPS. Keratinocytes and keratinocyte cell lines also produce IL-10 (Enk and Katz, 1992; Rivas and Ullrich, 1992), particularly after exposure to ultraviolet light.

FUNCTIONS OF IL-10

Inhibition of Macrophages

IL-10 inhibits the synthesis of several cytokines that are normally secreted by both human and mouse monocytes/macrophages in response to activation by LPS. These cytokines include IL-1, GM-CSF, TNF, IL-6, IL-8, IL-10 and IL-12 (de Waal Malefyt et *al.*, 1991a; Fiorentino *et al.*, 1991a). IL-10 is secreted by activated macrophages, and this is also inhibited by IL-10 (de Waal Malefyt *et al.*, 1991a). IL-10 is secreted relatively late compared with other cytokines, which may explain why macrophages are able to secrete substantial amounts of various cytokines before IL-10 inhibition occurs. IFN-γ also inhibits macrophage secretion of IL-10 (Chomarat *et al.*, 1993). Thus IL-10 and IFN-γ can each inhibit the synthesis of the other cytokine resulting in direct cross-inhibition.

IL-10-mediated inhibition of macrophage cytokine synthesis has a number of indirect effects. IFN-γ induces macrophage TNF-α synthesis, which in turn induces killing activity against larvae of *Schistosoma mansoni* (Gazzinelli *et al.*, 1992c). IL-10 inhibits this killing, presumably by blocking the synthesis of TNF-α, since supplementation of the cultures with TNF-α restored the ability to kill (Oswald *et al.*, 1992b). One of the cytotoxic mechanisms induced by TNF-α may be the induction of nitric oxide synthesis, which is also inhibited by IL-10 (Cunha *et al.*, 1992; Gazzinelli *et al.*, 1992b,c). IL-10 inhibits macrophage cytotoxic activity by a mechanism distinct from the pathways used by IL-4 and TGF-β since both of these cytokines synergize with IL-10 to inhibit macrophage killing (Oswald *et al.*, 1992a). This is consistent with the enhancement of cytokine mRNA degradation in macrophages by IL-10, in contrast to the translational inhibition mediated by TGF-β (Bogdan *et al.*, 1992).

IL-10 also inhibits expression of MHC Class II antigens on certain classes of monocytes/macrophages (de Waal Malefyt *et al.*, 1991b), but stimulates the expression of FcγRI on human monocytes (Te Velde *et al.*, 1992). This stimulatory effect is unusual especially since IFN-γ has a similar effect, in contrast to the antagonistic effects of IL-10 and IFN-γ in most situations.

The inhibition of cytokine synthesis by T_{H1} cells, which is the assay used originally to characterize IL-10, is also caused at least partly by inhibition of macrophage cytokine synthesis. T_{H1} cells stimulated by cell-free stimuli (Fiorentino *et al.*, 1989) or by nonmacrophage APC (e.g. B cells) are resistant to the effects of IL-10 (Fiorentino *et al.*, 1991b). However, when T_{H1} cells are stimulated by antigen presented by whole-spleen cell populations or macrophages, IL-10 partially blocks the secretion of cytokines by the T cells (Fiorentino *et al.*, 1989). IL-10 pretreatment of macrophages, but not T cells, reduces the subsequent secretion of IFN-γ (Fiorentino *et al.*, 1991b). At least part of this effect appears to be mediated via the ability of IL-10 to inhibit the synthesis of IL-12, which is identical to T-cell stimulating factor, a costimulator required for T_{H1} cytokine production in response to macrophage APCs (Germann *et al.*, 1990; Germann, Gately, Schoenhaut, Lohoff, Fischer, Jin, Schmitt and Rüde, unpublished data). IL-12 is synthesized by macrophages during a T_{H1}–macrophage interaction. IL-10 inhibits IL-12 synthesis, and the synthesis of IFN-γ can be partially restored by exogenous recombinant IL-12 (Germann, Rüde and Mosmann, unpublished data: O'Garra, A., personal communication). Inhibition of IL-12 secretion is not the only mechanism whereby IL-10 reduces cytokine synthesis by T_{H1} cells, as saturating amounts of IL-12 do not fully restore the cytokine response of the T_{H1} cells.

Selective Inhibition/Enhancement of T cells

IL-10 strongly inhibits the synthesis of cytokines by T_{H1} clones, by an indirect mechanism as described above. The synthesis of IFN-γ is also inhibited in mixed populations of cells from animals infected with parasites. Spleen cells from mice infected with *Nippostrongylus brasiliensis* or *S. mansoni* produced large amounts of IL-4 and IL-5 after stimulation, but secreted very little IFN-γ (Street *et al.*, 1990; Sher *et al.*, 1991). Anti-IL-10 antibodies enhanced the production of IFN-γ in response to Con A or antigen, which suggests that IL-10 was synthesized at sufficiently high levels to inhibit the expression of a cryptic T_{H1} response. This effect is also likely to be mediated indirectly, via effects on the APCs.

IL-10 also inhibits IFN-γ synthesis by cytotoxic T cells, but has no effect on killing of tumour target cells by $CD8^+$ T cell-clones or allospecific normal $CD8^+$ populations (Fong and Mosmann, unpublished data). It is not yet known whether the inhibition of CD8 cytokine secretion is mediated via the APC as is the case for $CD4^+$ cells.

IL-10 reduces IL-2 production (Fiorentino *et al.*, 1989; Taga and Tosato, 1992), which causes inhibition of T-cell proliferation if IL-2 production is limiting (Ding and Shevach, 1992). In one study, IL-10 inhibited cytokine synthesis by T cells responding to either macrophages or dendritic cells, but proliferation was only inhibited by IL-10 if macrophages were used as APCs (Macatonia *et al.*, 1993). Since IL-10 normally causes partial inhibition of cytokine synthesis, it is possible that the dendritic cells were more efficient APCs, and that even the reduced levels of IL-2 induced by dendritic cells in the presence of IL-10 were sufficient to support proliferation. IL-10 does not appear to have directly inhibitory effects on T-cell proliferation, as exogenous IL-2 can normally reverse any inhibitory effects.

IL-10 effectively inhibits cytokine secretion by mature T_{H1} cell clones or during T_{H1}-like responses in normal T-cell populations, but may have less effect on the differentiation of T cells from precursor cells. Uncommitted T-helper precursors initially secrete only IL-2 (Salmon *et al.*, 1989; Street *et al.*, 1990; Swain *et al.*, 1990a) and then differentiate into mature effector cells secreting T_{H1}, T_{H2}, T_{H0} or other cytokine patterns (Sad and Mosmann, unpublished data). IL-4 and IFN-γ each induce the differentiation of more cells producing the same cytokine (Le Gros *et al.*, 1990; Swain *et al.*, 1990a) (Sad and Mosmann, unpublished data). In one study using TCR-transgenic mice, IL-10 induced the production of more T_{H2}-like cells (Hsieh *et al.*, 1992), whereas in another study, IL-10 or anti-IL-10 had little effect on the differentiation of T cells into T_{H1} or T_{H2} phenotypes (Seder *et al.*, 1992).

In contrast to these inhibitory effects, IL-10 stimulates the proliferation of peripheral and particularly thymic T cells. IL-2 and IL-4 induce a moderate level of thymocyte proliferation, which is enhanced by the addition of IL-10 (MacNeil *et al.*, 1990). IL-10 is a proliferation and differentiation factor for $CD8^+$ cells, increasing both the precursor frequency and also the cytolytic activity of the expanded clones in limiting dilution cultures (Chen and Zlotnik, 1991) in synergy with IL-2. This appears to be a differentiative effect since IL-10 did not enhance $CD8^+$ cytotoxic T cells that had been initially grown only in IL-2.

Inhibition of Natural Killer (NK) Cells

The major producers of IFN-γ are T_{H1}, CD8 and NK cells. In addition to inhibiting IFN-γ production by T cells, IL-10 also inhibits the production of IFN-γ by NK cells responding to IL-2 in the presence of accessory cells. This does not mean that IL-10 always inhibits IFN-γ synthesis – for example, when T_{H1} cells are stimulated by B cells as APCs, the resulting IFN-γ synthesis is not inhibited by IL-10. The synthesis of cytokines by NK cells is inhibited by both IL-4 and IL-10, but by different mechanisms, as IL-4 is directly inhibitory for purified NK cells, whereas the effect of IL-10 requires macrophage–monocytes (Hsu *et al.*, 1992). As described above, IL-12 is an important costimulus for both T_{H1} and NK stimulation (Kobayashi *et al.*, 1989; Chan *et al.*, 1991), and IL-10 also inhibits the synthesis of IL-12 in a mouse NK-cell stimulation system (Germann, Rüde and Mosmann, unpublished data). Recombinant IL-12 almost completely restored the levels of IFN-γ, suggesting that the major mechanism of action of IL-10 on NK cells may be indirect, via inhibition of macrophage IL-12 synthesis.

Stimulation of Mast Cells

Continuous lines of mouse mast cells can be grown *in vitro*, and these respond to many cytokines such as IL-3, IL-4, IL-9 and SCF. IL-10 also enhances the proliferation of mast-cell lines (Thompson Snipes *et al.*, 1991), in synergy with other cytokines such as IL-3 or IL-4. The synergy indicates that IL-10 acts on the mast cell by an independent mechanism. It is not yet known if human mast cells also show enhancement of proliferation in response to IL-10, of if this mast-cell growth-enhancing activity of IL-10 is important *in vivo* in mice. IL-10 also activates transcription of the genes for two mast-cell proteases MMCP1 and MMCP2 in bone-marrow-derived mast-cell lines (Ghildyal *et al.*, 1992a, b).

Stimulation of B Cells

IL-10 induces expression of MHC Class II antigens but not CD23 (the Fc-ε receptor) on resting B cells (Go *et al.*, 1990). Since IL-4 induces expression of both proteins, this indicates that IL-10 does not act through induction of IL-4. IL-10 also increases the survival of small resting B cells in culture (Go *et al.*, 1990). IL-10 causes strong proliferation of human B cells that have been activated by anti-CD40 antibodies or crosslinking of the antigen receptor (Rousset *et al.*, 1992). The stimulatory effects of IL-10 are additive with those of IL-4. IL-10 also induces differentiation of human B cells (Rousset *et al.*, 1992). In the presence of IL-10, activated B cells secrete larger amounts of IgG, IgA and IgM and some anti-CD40-activated B cells acquire a plasma-cell-like morphology. IL-10 appears to synergize with TGF-β to induce human IgA production (Defrance *et al.*, 1992). TGF-β may induce switching to IgA, whereas IL-10 probably amplifies the switched cells, as TGF-β generally inhibits the synthesis or secretion of all immunoglobulin isotypes, including IgA, by cells that have already switched. TGF-β also induces an IgA switch in mouse B cells, but IL-10 does not appear to be required as a cofactor (Lebman *et al.*, 1990). In contrast to these stimulatory effects on mouse and human B cells, IL-10 inhibits antibody secretion by mouse B cells that have been activated by TNP-Ficoll and IL-5 (Pecanha *et al.*, 1992).

T_{H1} AND T_{H2} SUBSETS OF T CELLS

Two major patterns of cytokine synthesis have been identified in panels of both mouse (Mosmann *et al.*, 1986b) and human (Del Prete *et al.*, 1991) T-cell clones. After stimulation via the T-cell receptor, T_{H1} cells secrete IL-2, (IFN-γ) and LT (Mosmann *et al.*, 1986b; Cherwinski *et al.*, 1987; Mosmann and Coffman, 1989a, b), provide limited help for B-cell responses (Coffman *et al.*, 1988) and strongly activate cell-mediated responses such as delayed type hypersensitivity (DTH) (Cher and Mosmann, 1987). IFN-γ is a major macrophage-activating factor (Murray *et al.*, 1983, 1985; Nathan *et al.*, 1983), TNF and IFN-γ activate granulocytes (van Strijp *et al.*, 1991; Stevenhagen and van Furth, 1993), and the T_{H1} cytokine pattern is often associated with strong DTH reactions *in vivo*. These cytotoxic-enhancing functions of T_{H1} cells are particularly effective against intracellular pathogens. In contrast, T_{H2} cells secrete IL-4, IL-5, IL-6, IL-9, IL-10 and P600 (IL-13) (Cherwinski *et al.*, 1987; Brown *et al.*, 1989). T_{H2} cells stimulate antibody responses but inhibit macrophage activation and DTH responses. Strong T_{H2} responses cause an allergic reaction because IL-4 induces switching to IgE (Coffman *et al.*, 1986; Del Prete *et al.*, 1988). IL-5 is the major growth and differentiation factor for eosinophils (Sanderson *et al.*, 1986; Enokihara *et al.*, 1988; Lopez *et al.*, 1988) and, at least in the mouse, IL-3, IL-4, IL-9 and IL-10 stimulate mast-cell proliferation and activation (Ihle *et al.*, 1983; Mosmann *et al.*, 1986a; Moeller *et al.*, 1990; Thompson Snipes *et al.*, 1991). Thus, the secretion of different patterns of cytokines contributes strongly to the major functional differences between these subtypes. Many strong immune responses tend to involve either mainly DTH or mainly antibody secretion, and there is considerable evidence that these two responses are often mutually exclusive (Parish, 1972; Katsura, 1977). This may be explained, in part, by cross-regulation of T_{H1} and T_{H2} cells and their cytokines during an immune response. IFN-γ is produced by T_{H1} cells and inhibits the proliferation of T_{H2} clones (Gajewski and Fitch, 1988; Fernandez-Botran *et al.*, 1988), whereas IL-4 and IL-10 are produced by T_{H2} cells and inhibit differentiation and cytokine synthesis, respectively, of T_{H1} cells (Fiorentino *et al.*, 1989; Le Gros *et al.*, 1990; Swain *et al.*, 1990b). Although IL-10 is produced by a number of cell types in addition to T_{H2} cells, the expression of IL-10 during *in vivo* responses often correlates with T_{H2}-like responses.

EXPRESSION OF IL-10 DURING IMMUNE RESPONSES

IL-10 Expression in Mice

IL-10 production is generally enhanced in cells derived from mice responding to a variety of infectious agents and treatments that induce T_{H2}-like responses. These include the responses to infection by *N. brasiliensis* (Fiorentino *et al.*, 1989), *S. mansoni* (Sher *et al.*, 1991), or the retrovirus causing MAIDS (Gazzinelli *et al.*, 1992a), or treatment of tissue culture keratinocytes or whole mice with ultraviolet light (Rivas and Ullrich, 1992). There are several experimental models of infection in which resistant and susceptible strains of mice differ in their cytokine expression patterns. In at least three infections that require a cell-mediated immune response for resistance, IL-10 is produced at higher levels by cells from susceptible than resistant mice. These infectious agents include *Leishmania major* (Locksley *et al.*, 1987; Heinzel *et al.*, 1991), *Candida* (Romani *et al.*, 1993), and *Trypanosoma cruzi* (Silva *et al.*, 1992). Cells from infected animals produce higher IL-10 levels, either spontaneously or after stimulation in tissue culture, and for *Schistosoma* and *Trypanosoma* infections the endogenous IL-10 inhibits the synthesis of IFN-γ (Sher *et al.*, 1991; Silva *et al.*, 1992) and/or downregulates macrophages (Silva *et al.*, 1992).

IL-10 and other T_{H2} cytokine levels are elevated during a chronic GVH reaction (De Wit *et al.*, 1993) whereas T_{H1} cells may be involved in acute GVH (Antin and Ferrara, 1992). However, IL-10 and other T_{H2} cytokines are associated with tolerance to heart allografts rather than chronic rejection (Takeuchi *et al.*, 1992). Some tissues may be more susceptible to attack by T_{H2} cells, but in neither case does a T_{H2} response lead to acute allogeneic attack.

IL-10 Expression in Humans

As in mice, IL-10 expression by human cells is often correlated with a T_{H2}-like response and susceptibility to an infection that may be more effectively dealt with by a DTH-like response. During the early stages of HIV infection, when the patient's immune system begins to deteriorate, but before CD4 T cell counts drop, peripheral blood cells produce increased levels of IL-10 in response to stimulation in tissue culture (Clerici and Shearer, 1993). High levels of IgE and T_{H2} cytokines, including IL-10, are expressed in Ommen's syndrome (Schandene *et al.*, 1993). During immune responses against basal cell carcinoma, high levels of mRNA for IL-10 and other T_{H2} cytokines were found in the basal cell carcinoma lesion (Yamamura *et al.*, 1993). In contrast, T_{H1}-like cytokines, including IL-2, IFN-γ and lymphotoxin, were expressed at higher levels in a benign growth of epidermis, seborrhoeic keratosis. IL-10 mRNA is expressed more strongly in lesions of lepromatous leprosy, which involves high levels of antibody production, than in tuberculoid leprosy, which involves more DTH-like reactions (Yamamura *et al.*, 1991). During the erythema nodosum leprosum reaction, which involves immediate hypersensitivity, levels of mRNA for IL-10 and other T_{H2} cytokines were elevated, whereas IL-10 expression was reduced in lesions of patients undergoing the DTH-like reversal reaction (Yamamura *et al.*, 1992).

From these examples, it can be seen that IL-10 is often expressed in association with poor or absent responses against infections or tumours that would be most effectively eliminated by a cell-mediated response. This correlation, and the known functions of IL-10 in inhibiting macrophage activation and IFN-γ production, suggest that IL-10 may inhibit the development of strong T_{H1}-like cell-mediated responses. During immune responses against cancer and many intracellular pathogens, IL-10 may therefore inhibit the development of an appropriate immune response. Conversely, during autoimmunity or transplant rejection, T_{H2} responses may result in minimal or chronic attack as opposed to more acute rejection or damage caused by T_{H1} mechanisms, and so excess production of IL-10 may be beneficial. IL-10 may thus have therapeutic potential for inhibition of cell-mediated responses.

Although the expression of IL-10 during immune responses often correlates with overall T_{H2}-like responses, this is not always the case, as might be expected from the number of cell types that are able to synthesize IL-10. Even among T cells, additional cytokine patterns have been identified among mouse and human T-cell clones (Gajewski and Fitch, 1988; Paliard *et al.*, 1988; Firestein *et al.*, 1989; Street *et al.*, 1990), and so the extreme T_{H1} and T_{H2} dichotomy does not account for all immune responses. In a model of experimental autoimmune encephalitis, several cytokines, including both IL-4 and IFN-γ, are produced during the acute phase of the disease. As the disease begins to resolve, there is a rise in IL-10 mRNA and a concurrent rapid decline in the mRNA for IL-2, IL-4, IL-6, and IFN-γ (Kennedy *et al.*, 1992). During infection of mice with *Eimeria*, cells from both resistant and susceptible strains produce both T_{H1}- and T_{H2}-specific cytokines, but IL-10 is expressed only by cells from the resistant BALB/c strain (Wakelin *et al.*, 1993).

IL-10 Expression During Pregnancy

During pregnancy the maternal immune response shows enhanced antibody responses but reduced DTH (T_{H1}-like) responses. Possibly as a result, pregnant women and mice are more susceptible to several intracellular pathogens and have reduced symptoms for rheumatoid arthritis, a cell-mediated inflammatory disease (reviewed by Wegmann *et al.* (1993). Recently, we have found that IL-10 and other T_{H2} cytokines are expressed constitutively at high levels in placental tissues (Lin, Guilbert, Mosmann, Wegmann, unpublished data). IL-10 mRNA has been localized by *in situ* hybridization to the interface area between maternal and fetal tissues. We have suggested (Wegmann *et al.*, 1993) that this local T_{H2} response may be important to protect the fetus from the known damaging effects of NK cells and T_{H1}-like responses. A less desirable side effect of this local T_{H2} bias may be a systemic inhibition of the mother's immune system, resulting in increased susceptibility to intracellular pathogens.

IL-10 EFFECTS *IN VIVO*

Injection of IL-10

Endotoxin-induced toxicity is thought to be caused by the release of macrophage mediators, particularly TNF. As IL-10 inhibits macrophage activation and cytokine synthesis, it has been tested *in vivo* for its ability to reduce TNF production and toxicity in mice injected with LPS. Circulating TNF levels induced by LPS were reduced by prior IL-10 treatment, which also inhibited the hypothermia induced by larger amounts of LPS (Gérard *et al.*, 1993). After LPS challenge at a dose normally toxic for 50% of the mice, IL-10 completely prevented mortality. These effects are all consistent with IL-10-mediated inhibition of cytokine secretion by activated macrophages.

Because IL-10 inhibits activation of T_{H1} cells and macrophages, it has been tested for its effects on DTH reactions. We have measured the effect of injecting IL-10 during the effector phase of the DTH reaction induced by injecting T_{H1} clones plus antigen into mouse footpads. IL-10 causes moderate inhibition (20–50% of swelling) of the DTH reaction (Li, Elliott and Mosmann, unpublished data). A strong DTH reaction is also generated during *Leishmania* infection in resistant mice, and injection of IL-10 modestly inhibits this antigen-induced DTH response (Coffman, R.L., personal communication). IL-4 also inhibits moderately and the combination of IL-4 and IL-10 is more effective than either cytokine alone.

In other studies examining the induction of DTH rather than the effector phase, injection of supernatants of ultraviolet-treated keratinocyte cultures inhibited the generation of a subsequent DTH reaction (Rivas and Ullrich, 1992). Since anti-IL-10 antibodies prevented the ability of the supernatants to inhibit DTH, IL-10 was at least partly responsible. Thus, the effects of IL-10 injected *in vivo* are, so far, consistent with the *in vivo* ability of IL-10 to inhibit macrophage and T_{H1} cell function.

IL-10-minus Mice and Anti-IL-10 Treatment

IL-10-deficient mice have been constructed by disruption of the IL-10 gene by homologous recombination (Kuhn *et al.*, 1992). These mice do not express IL-10, and do not show major alterations in the populations of B cells, T cells, macrophages, etc. indicating that IL-10 does not have an essential role in haemopoiesis. Interestingly, the IL-10-minus mice have normal Ly-1 B-cell populations.

In contrast, treatment of mice from birth with anti-IL-10 antibody causes severe depletion of peritoneal Ly-1 B cells, without other obvious effects (Ishida *et al.*, 1992). The depletion of Ly-1 B cells by anti-IL-10 can be prevented by treatment with anti-IFN-γ antibodies, which suggests that the depletion of Ly-1 B cells is a result of increased levels of IFN-γ produced in the absence of IL-10. Although at first sight this appears to conflict with the IL-10-minus mouse results, it is possible that repeated injections of rat IgM anti-IL-10 antibody during the life of the animal induce an anti-rat immune response, including higher levels of IFN-γ because of the absence of IL-10. In contrast, in IL-10-minus mice there may not be a strong immune response, resulting in less IFN-γ and hence no Ly-1 B-cell depletion.

CONCLUSIONS

IL-10 now appears to have a variety of functions, particularly those involving the inhibition of macrophage activation and function. Although a number of cell types can produce IL-10, the *in vivo* production of IL-10 is often associated with T_{H2}-like responses and suppression of cell-mediated immunity. The pattern of IL-10 production *in vivo* and the results of IL-10 interventions suggest that IL-10 is deleterious when a DTH response is required, for example during infections by many intracellular pathogens. In contrast, the inhibition of DTH responses by IL-10 may be advantageous during autoimmunity and transplantation, as strong T_{H1} responses may cause acute damage whereas T_{H2} responses may cause less damage and be better tolerated by the patients.

REFERENCES

Antin, J.H. and Ferrara, J.L. (1992). *Blood* **80**, 2964–2968.
Baer, R., Bankier, A.T., Biggin, M.D., Deininger, P.L., Farrell, P.J., Gibson, T.J., Hatfull, G., Hudson, G.S., Satchwell, S.C., Seguin, C., Tuffnell, P.S. and Barrell, B.G. (1984). *Nature* **310**, 207–211.
Barnes, P.F., Abrams, J.S., Lu, S., Sieling, P.A., Rea, T.H. and Modlin, R.L. (1993). *Infect. Immun.* **61**, 197–203.
Benjamin, D. Knobloch, T.J. and Dayton, M.A. (1992). *Blood* **80**, 1289–1298.
Bogdan, C., Paik, J., Vodovotz, Y. and Nathan, C. (1992). *J. Biol. Chem.* **267**, 23301–23308.
Brown, K.D., Zurawski, S.M., Mosmann, T.R. and Zurawski, G. (1989). *J. Immunol.* **142**, 679–687.
Burdin, N., Pérone, C., Banchereau, J. and Rousset, F. (1993). *J. Exp. Med.* **177**, 295–304.
Chan, S.H., Perussia, B., Gupta, J.W., Kobayashi, M., Pospisil, M., Young, H.A., Wolf, S.F., Young, D., Clark, S.C. and Trinchieri, G. (1991). *J. Exp. Med.* **173**, 869–879.
Chen, W.F. and Zlotnik, A. (1991). *J. Immunol.* **147**, 528–534.
Cher, D.J. and Mosmann, T.R. (1987). *J. Immunol.* **138**, 3688–3694.

Cherwinski, H.M., Schumacher, J.H., Brown, K.D. and Mosmann, T.R. (1987). *J. Exp. Med.* **166**, 1229–1244.

Chomarat, P., Rissoan, M.-C., Banchereau, J. and Miossec, P. (1993). *J. Exp. Med.* **177**, 523–527.

Clerici, M. and Shearer, G.M. (1993). *Immunol. Today* **14**, 107–111.

Coffman, R.L., Ohara, J., Bond, M.W., Carty, J., Zlotnik, A. and Paul, W.E. (1986). *J. Immunol.* **136**, 4538–4541.

Coffman, R.L., Seymour, B.W., Lebman, D.A., Hiraki, D.D., Christiansen, J.A., Shrader, B., Cherwinski, H.M., Savelkoul, H.F., Finkelman, F.D., Bond, M.W. and Mosmann, T.R. (1988). *Immunol. Rev.* **102**, 5–28.

Cunha, F.Q., Moncada, S. and Liew, F.Y. (1992). *Biochem. Biophys. Res. Commun.* **182**, 1155–1159.

Defrance, T., Vanbervliet, B., Briere, F., Durand, I., Rousset, F. and Banchereau, J. (1992). *J. Exp. Med.* **175**, 671–682.

Del Prete, G.F., Maggi, E., Parronchi, P., Chretien, I., Tiri, A., Macchia, D., Ricci, M., Banchereau, J., de Vries, J.E. and Romagnani, S. (1988). *J. Immunol.* **140**, 4193–4198.

Del Prete, G.F., De Carli, M., Mastromauro, C., Biagiotti, R., Macchia, D., Falagiani, P., Ricci, M. and Romagnani, S. (1991). *J. Clin. Invest.* **88**, 346–350.

Del Prete, G.F., De Carli, M., Almerigogna, F., Giudizi, M.G., Biagiotti, R. and Romagnani, S. (1993). *J. Immunol.* **150**, 353–360.

de Waal Malefyt, R., Abrams, J., Bennett, B., Figdor, C.G. and de Vries, J.E. (1991a). *J. Exp. Med.* **174**, 1209–1220.

de Waal Malefyt, R., Haanen, J., Spits, H., Roncarolo, M.G., te Velde, A., Figdor, C., Johnson, K., Kastelein, R., Yssel, H. and de Vries, J.E. (1991b). *J. Exp. Med.* **174**, 915–924.

De Wit, D., Van Mechelen, M., Zanin, C., Doutrelepont, J.M., Velu, T., Gerard, C., Abramowicz, D., Scheerlinck, J.P., De Baetselier, P., Urbain, J., Oberdan, L., Goldman, M. and Moser, M. (1993). *J. Immunol.* **150**, 361–366.

Ding, L. and Shevach, E.M. (1992). *J. Immunol.* **148**, 3133–3139.

Enk, A.H. and Katz, S.I. (1992). *J. Immunol.* **149**, 92–95.

Enokihara, H., Nagashima, S., Noma, T., Kajitani, H., Hamaguchi, H., Saito, K., Furusawa, S., Shishido, H. and Honjo, T. (1988). *Immunol. Lett.* **18**, 73–76.

Fernandez-Botran, R., Sanders, V.M., Mosmann, T.R. and Vitetta, E.S. (1988). *J. Exp. Med.* **168**, 543–558.

Fiorentino, D.F., Bond, M.W. and Mosmann, T.R. (1989). *J. Exp. Med.* **170**, 2081–2095.

Fiorentino, D.F., Zlotnik, A., Mosmann, T.R. Howard, M. and O'Garra, A.O. (1991a). *J. Immunol.* **147**, 3815–3822.

Fiorentino, D.F., Zlotnik, A., Vieira, P., Mosmann, T.R., Howard, M., Moore, K.W. and O'Garra, A. (1991b) *J. Immunol.* **146**, 3444–3451.

Firestein, G.S., Roeder, W.D., Laxer, J.A., Townsend, K.S., Weaver, C.T., Hom, J.T., Linton, J., Torbett, B.E. and Glasebrook, A.L. (1989). *J. Immunol.* **143**, 518–525.

Gajewski, T.F. and Fitch, F.W. (1988). *J. Immunol.* **140**, 4245–4252.

Gazzinelli, R.T., Makino, M., Chattopadhyay, S.K., Snapper, C.M., Sher, A., Hugin, A.W. and Morse, H.C. (1992a). *J. Immunol.* **148**, 182–188.

Gazzinelli, R.T., Oswald, I.P., Hieny, S., James, S.L. and Sher, A. (1992b). *Eur. J. Immunol.* **22**, 2501–2506.

Gazzinelli, R.T., Oswald, I.P., James, S.L. and Sher, A. (1992c). *J. Immunol.* **148**, 1792–1796.

Germann, T., Partenheimer, A. and Rude, E. (1990). *Eur. J. Immunol.* **20**, 2035–2040.

Ghildyal, N., McNeil, H.P., Gurish, M.F., Austen, K.F. and Stevens, R.L. (1992a). *J. Biol. Chem.* **267**, 8473–8477.

Ghildyal, N., McNeil, H.P., Stechschulte, S., Austen, K.F., Silberstein, D., Gurish, M.F., Somerville, L.L. and Stevens, R.L. (1992b). *J. Immunol.* **149**, 2123–2129.

Go, N.F., Castle, B.E., Barrett, R., Kastelein, R., Dang, W., Mosmann, T.R., Moore, K.W. and Howard, M. (1990). *J. Exp. Med.* **172**, 1625–1631.

Goodman, R.E., Oblak, J. and Bell, R.G. (1992). *Biochem. Biophys. Res. Commun.* **189**, 1–7.

Gérard, C., Bruyns, C., Marchant, A., Abramowicz, D., Vandenabeele, P., Delvaux, A., Fiers, W., Goldman, M. and Velu, T. (1993). *J. Exp. Med.* **177**, 547–550.

Heinzel, F.P., Sadick, M.D., Mutha, S.S. and Locksley, R.M. (1991). *Proc. Natl Acad. Sci. USA* **88**, 7011–7015.

Hsieh, C.S., Heimberger, A.B., Gold, J.S., O'Garra, A. and Murphy, K.M. (1992). *Proc. Natl Acad. Sci. USA* **89**, 6065–6069.

Hsu, D.H., de Waal Malefyt, R., Fiorentino, D.F., Dang, M.N., Vieira, P., De Vries, J., Spits, H., Mosmann, T.R. and Moore, K.W. (1990). *Science* **250**, 830–832.

Hsu, D.H., Moore, K.W. and Spits, H. (1992). *Int. Immunol.* **4**, 563–569.

Hudson, G.S., Bankier, A.T., Satchwell, S.C. and Barrell, B.G. (1985). *Virol.* **147**, 81–98.

Ihle, J.N., Keller, J., Oroszlan, S., Henderson, L.E., Copeland, T.D., Fitch, F., Prystowsky, M.B., Goldwasser, E., Schrader, J.W., Palaszynski, E., Dy, M. and Lebel, B. (1983). *J. Immunol.* **131**, 282–287.

Ishida, H., Hastings, R., Kearney, J. and Howard, M. (1992). *J. Exp. Med.* **175**, 1213–1220.

Katsura, Y. (1977). *Immunology* **32**, 227–235.

Kennedy, M.K., Torrance, D.S., Picha, K.S. and Mohler, K.M. (1992). *J. Immunol.* **149**, 2496–2505.

Kim, J.M., Brannan, C.I., Copeland, N.G., Jenkins, N.A., Khan, T.A. and Moore, K.W. (1992). *J. Immunol.* **148**, 3618–3623.

Kobayashi, M., Fitz, L., Ryan, M., Hewick, R.M., Clark, S.C., Chan, S., Loudon, R., Sherman, F., Perussia, B. and Trinchieri, G. (1989). *J. Exp. Med.* **170**, 827–845.

Kuhn, R., Rajewsky, K. and Muller, W. (1992). *8th Int. Cong. Imm.* p. 203.(Abstr.)

Le Gros, G., Ben Sasson, S.Z., Seder, R., Finkelman, F.D., and Paul, W.E. (1990). *J. Exp. Med.* **172**, 921–929.

Lebman, D.A., Lee, F.D. and Coffman, R.L. (1990). *J. Immunol.* **144**, 952–959.

Locksley, R.M., Heinzel, F.P., Sadick, M.D., Holaday, B.J. and Gardner, K.D., Jr. (1987). *Ann. Inst. Pasteur. Immunol.* **138**, 744–749.

Lopez, A.F., Sanderson, C.J., Gamble, J.R., Campbell, H.D., Young, I.G. and Vadas, M.A. (1988). *J. Exp. Med.* **167**, 219–224.

Macatonia, S.E., Doherty, T.M., Knight, S.C. and O'Garra, A. (1993). *J. Immunol.* **150**, 3755–3765.

MacNeil, I.A., Suda, T., Moore, K.W., Mosmann, T.R. and Zlotnik, A. (1990). *J. Immunol.* **145**, 4167–4173.

Moeller, J., Hultner, L., Schmitt, E., Breuer, M. and Dormer, P. (1990). *J. Immunol.* **144**, 4231–4234.

Moore, K.W., Vieira, P., Fiorentino, D.F., Trounstine, M.L., Khan, T.A. and Mosmann, T.R. (1990). *Science* **248**, 1230–1234.

Moore, K.W., O'Garra, A., de Waal Malefyt, R., Vieira, P. and Mosmann, T.R. (1993). *Annu. Rev. Immunol.* **11**, 165–190.

Mosmann, T.R., Bond, M.W., Coffman, R.L., Ohara, J. and Paul, W.E. (1986a). *Proc. Natl Acad. Sci. USA* **83**, 5654–5658.

Mosmann, T.R., Cherwinski, H., Bond, M.W., Giedlin, M.A. and Coffman, R.L. (1986b). *J. Immunol.* **136**, 2348–2357.

Mosmann, T.R. and Coffman, R.L. (1989a). *Annu. Rev. Immunol.* **7**, 145–173.

Mosmann, T.R. and Coffman, R.L. (1989b). *Adv. Immunol.* **46**, 111–147.

Mosmann, T.R., Schumacher, J.H., Fiorentino, D.F., Leverah, J., Moore, K.W. and Bond, M.W. (1990). *J. Immunol.* **145**, 2938–2945.

Murray, H.W., Rubin, B.Y. and Rothermel, C.D. (1983). *J. Clin. Invest.* **72**, 1506–1510.

Murray, H.W., Spitalny, G.L. and Nathan, C.F. (1985). *J. Immunol.* **134**, 1619–1622.

Nathan, C.F., Murray, H.W., Wiebe, M.E. and Rubin, B.Y. (1983). *J. Exp. Med.* **158**, 670–689.

Niiro, H., Otsuka, T., Abe, M., Satoh, H., Ogo, T., Nakano, T., Furukawa, Y. and Niho, Y. (1992). *Lymphokine. Cytokine. Res.* **11**, 209–214.

O'Garra, A., Stapleton, G., Dhar, V., Pearce, M., Schumacher, J., Rugo, H., Barbis, D., Stall, A., Cupp, J., Moore, K., Vieira, P., Mosmann, T.R., Whitmore, A., Arnold, L., Haughton, G. and Howard, M. (1990). *Int. Immunol.* **2**, 821–832.

O'Garra, A., Chang, R., Go, N., Hastings, R., Haughton, G. and Howard, M. (1992). *Eur. J. Immunol.* **22**, 711–717.

Oswald, I.P., Gazzinelli, R.T., Sher, A. and James, S.L. (1992a). *J. Immunol.* **148**, 3578–3582.

Oswald, I.P., Wynn, T.A., Sher, A. and James, S.L. (1992b). *Proc. Natl Acad. Sci. USA* **89**, 8676–8680.

Paliard, X., de Waal Malefijt, R., Yssel, H., Blanchard, D., Chretien, I., Abrams, J., de Vries, J.E. and Spits, H. (1988). *J. Immunol.* **141**, 849–855.

Parish, C.R. (1972). *Transplant. Rev.* **13**, 35–66.

Pecanha, L.M., Snapper, C.M., Lees, A. and Mond, J.J. (1992). *J. Immunol.* **148**, 3427–3432.

Rivas, J.M. and Ullrich, S.E. (1992). *J. Immunol.* **149**, 3865–3871.

Rode, H.-J., Janssen, W., Rösen-Wolff, A., Bugert, J.J., Thein, P., Becker, Y. and Darai, G. (1993). *Virus Genes* **7**, 111–116.

Romani, L., Mencacci, A., Cenci, E., Spaccapelo, R., Mosci, P., Puccetti, P. and Bistoni, F. (1993). *J. Immunol.* **150**, 925–931.

Rousset, F., Garcia, E., Defrance, T., Peronne, C., Vezzio, N., Hsu, D.H., Kastelein, R., Moore, K.W. and Banchereau, J. (1992). *Proc. Natl Acad. Sci. USA* **89**, 1890–1893.

Salmon, M., Kitas, G.D. and Bacon, P.A. (1989). *J. Immunol.* **143**, 907–912.

Sanderson, C.J., O'Garra, A., Warren, D.J. and Klaus, G.G. (1986). *Proc. Natl Acad. Sci. USA* **83**, 437–440.

Schandene, L., Ferster, A., Mascart Lemone, F., Crusiaux, A., Gerard, C., Marchant, A., Lybin, M., Velu, T., Sariban, E. and Goldman, M. (1993). *Eur. J. Immunol.* **23**, 56–60.

Seder, R.A., Paul, W.E., Davis, M.M. and Fazekas de St.Groth, B. (1992). *J. Exp. Med.* **176**, 1091–1098.

Sher, A., Fiorentino, D., Caspar, P., Pearce, E. and Mosmann, T. (1991). *J. Immunol.* **147**, 2713–2716.

Silva, J.S., Morrissey, P.J., Grabstein, K.H., Mohler, K.M., Anderson, D. and Reed, S.G. (1992). *J. Exp. Med.* **175**, 169–174.

Smith, C.A., Davis, T., Anderson, D., Solam, L., Beckmann, M.P., Jerzy, R., Dower, S.K., Cosman, D. and Goodwin, R.G. (1990). *Science* **248**, 1019–1023.

Stevenhagen, A. and van Furth, R. (1993). *Clin. Exp. Immunol.* **91**, 170–175.

Street, N.E., Schumacher, J.H., Fong, T.A.T., Bass, H., Fiorentino, D.F., Leverah, J.A. and Mosmann, T.R. (1990). *J. Immunol.* **144**, 1629–1639.

Suda, T., O'Garra, A., MacNeil, I., Fischer, M., Bond, M. and Zlotnik, A. (1990). *Cell Immunol.* **129**, 228–240.

Swain, S.L., Weinberg, A.D. and English, M. (1990a). *J. Immunol.* **144**, 1788–1799.

Swain, S.L., Weinberg, A.D., English, M. and Huston, G. (1990b). *J. Immunol.* **145**, 3796–3806.

Taga, K. and Tosato, G. (1992). *J. Immunol.* **148**, 1143–1148.

Takebe, Y., Seiki, M., Fujisawa, J., Hoy, P., Yokota, K. Arai, K., Yoshida, M. and Arai, N. (1988). *Mol. Cell Biol.* **8**, 466–472.

Takeuchi, T., Lowry, R.P. and Konieczny, B. (1992). *Transplantation* **53**, 1281–1294.

Te Velde, A.A., de Waal Malefijt, R., Huijbens, R.J., de Vries, J.E. and Figdor, C.G. (1992). *J. Immunol.* **149**, 4048–4052.

Thompson Snipes, L., Dhar, V., Bond, M.W., Mosmann, T.R., Moore, K.W. and Rennick, D.M. (1991). *J. Exp. Med.* **173**, 507–510.

Upton, C., Mossman, K. and McFadden, G. (1992). *Science* **258**, 1369–1372.

van Strijp, J.A., van der Tol, M.E., Miltenburg, L.A., van Kessel, K.P. and Verhoef, J. (1991). *Immunology* **73**, 77–82.

Vieira, P., de Waal Malefyt, R., Dang, M.N., Johnson, K.E., Kastelein, R., Fiorentino, D.F., DeVries, J.E., Roncarolo, M.G., Mosmann, T.R. and Moore, K.W. (1991). *Proc. Natl Acad. Sci. USA* **88**, 1172–1176.

Wakelin, D., Rose, M.E., Hesketh, P., Else, K.J. and Grencis, R.K. (1993). *Parasite Immunol.* **15**, 11–19.

Wegmann, T.G., Lin, H., Guilbert, L.J. and Mosmann, T.R. (1993). *Immunol. Today* **14**, 353–356.

Yamamura, M., Uyemura, K., Deans, R.J., Weinberg, K., Rea, T.H., Bloom, B.R. and Modlin, R.L. (1991). *Science* **254**, 277–279.

Yamamura, M., Wang, X.H., Ohmen, J.D., Uyemura, K., Rea, T.H., Bloom, B.R. and Modlin, R.L. (1992). *J. Immunol.* **149**, 1470–1475.

Yamamura, M., Modlin, R.L., Ohmen, J.D. and Moy, R.L. (1993). *J. Clin. Invest.* **91**, 1005–1010.

Yssel, H., de Waal Malefyt, R., Roncarolo, M.G., Abrams, J.S., Lahesmaa, R., Spits, H. and de Vries, J.E. (1992). *J. Immunol.* **149**, 2378–2384.

Chapter 13

Interleukin-12

Herbert J. Zeh III, Hideaki Tahara and Michael T. Lotze

Departments of Surgery, Molecular Genetics and Biochemistry, University of Pittsburgh, Pittsburgh, PA, USA

INTRODUCTION

Interleukin-12 (IL-12) was originally identified by two groups: one group (Gately *et al.* 1986; Wong *et al.*, 1988) described a factor that they called cytotoxic lymphocyte maturation factor (CLMF). It synergized with IL-2 to enhance generation of LAK cell activity in PBMC as well as induced the proliferation of PHA-activated PBMC. The other group (Kobayashi *et al.*, 1989) described natural killer cell stimulatory factor (NKSF), a factor capable of enhancing the lytic activity and inducing INF-γ secretion from NK cells. The cloning and characterization of these two factors showed them to be identical, and the conventional name of IL-12 was proposed (Gubler *et al.*, 1991; Wolf *et al.*, 1991). IL-12 is a 75 kDa heterodimeric cytokine consisting of disulphide-linked 35 kDa and 40 kDa subunits. Two distinct genes encode these subunits, and coexpression of each gene in the same cell is required for the production of a biologically active protein. Sequence homology studies have revealed a distant but significant relationship between the p35 subunit of IL-12 and the IL-6/G-CSF gene families. The p40 subunit shares homology with the extracellular domain of the IL-6 receptor. Thus, IL-12 appears to belong to the extended family of haemopoietin molecules. Originally identified as a product of activated EBV-transformed B cells, it now appears that the principal source of IL-12 *in vivo* is activated macrophages. IL-12 receptor expression is evidently limited to activated T and NK cells through which IL-12 modulates their cytolytic and proliferative activity. In addition, IL-12 is a potent inducer of IFN-γ and to a lesser extent TNF-α production in peripheral blood mononuclear cells. *In vitro* studies indicate that IL-12 directs naive T-helper cells towards a T_{H1} pattern of cytokine release. *In vivo* studies have shown that the exogenous administration of IL-12 is able to modulate T and NK cell function, stimulate extramedullary haemopoiesis and mediate potent anti-tumour effects. The characterization and specific biological functions of IL-12 are discussed in the following sections.

The Cytokine Handbook, 2nd ed.
ISBN 0–12–689661–5

MOLECULAR CHARACTERIZATION AND CLONING OF IL-12

Wong *et al.* (1987) identified CLMF in the IL-2 depleted supernatants of PHA-stimulated PBMC. This factor synergized with IL-2 (in the presence of hydrocortisone) to induce LAK activity from PBMC, as well as cause the IL-2-independent proliferation of PHA-activated T cells. Levels of this factor were initially insufficient to allow for its purification to homogeneity. Therefore, human lymphoid cell lines were screened for the production of cytokines which could mediate CLMF-like activity. In 1990 Stern *et al.* isolated and characterized a 70 kDa glycoprotein, consisting of 35 kDa and 40 kDa disulphide-linked subunits, from the supernatant of phorbol diester activated NC-37 B cells. CLMF activity was quantified using a PHA blast proliferation assay (Stern *et al.*, 1990). Concurrently, Kobayashi *et al.* (1989) found that the RPMI 8866 B-cell line, when stimulated with phorbol diester, produced a cytokine capable of mediating three activities not accountable for by other known B-cell cytokines. This novel cytokine when used to treat PBL (1) induced IFN-γ production from PBL, (2) augmented the spontaneous lytic activity of PBL against a variety of targets, and (3) enhanced the proliferation of PBL activated with PHA. Subsequently, based on its ability to induce PBL secretion of IFN-γ a heterodimeric 70 kDa glycoprotein was isolated (NKSF). One unit of NKSF per milliliter was defined as the amount necessary to induce one-half the maximal IFN-γ production from PBL. The cloning of NKSF (Wolf *et al.*, 1991) and CLMF (Gubler *et al.*, 1991) showed these two factors to be identical. NKSF and CLMF were given the provisional designation interleukin-12, based on their pleotropic effects on both T and NK cells.

Sequencing of the human genes encoding IL-12 by Wolf *et al.* (1991) and Gubler *et al.* (1991) has aided in the further characterization of the biological activity of IL-12 (Fig. 1). The mature p40 subunit cDNA contains a single long open reading frame encoding a 328-amino-acid polypeptide. The amino acid sequence includes a characteristic hydrophobic signal peptide (residues 1–22) and a cleavage site immediately preceding the *N*-terminal sequence of the natural p40 protein, characteristic of a secreted protein. The mature protein (calculated M_r 34 700) contains 10 cysteine residues, four consensus sequences for asparagine-linked glycosylation (Asn X–Ser/Thr) and one theoretical heparin-binding site (Wolf *et al.*, 1991). Chemical and enzymatic deglycosylation of the heterodimer has demonstrated that the p40 subunit contains approximately 10% carbohydrate (Podlaski *et al.*, 1992). The p35 cDNA sequence contains a single long open reading frame encoding a 253-amino-acid polypeptide. The mature protein (calculated M_r = 27 500) contains seven cysteine residues, and three consensus *N*-linked glycosylation sites. The p35 subunit contains approximately 20% carbohydrate (Podlaski *et al.*, 1992). The p35 sequence contains two potential initiation codons (residues 1 and 35) 5' to the amino-terminal sequence determined from the natural p35 protein. The peptide sequence from the second methionine encodes a typical hydrophobic signal peptide (residues 35–56) with a consensus cleavage site immediately adjacent to the *N*-terminal sequence of the mature p35 protein. From the characteristics of the sequence and preliminary transfection data using cDNA lacking the methionine at position 1, Wolf *et al.* (1991) concluded that the second methionine is sufficient for expression of the p35 IL-12 subunit. We have constructed a retroviral vector encoding human p35 cDNA initiated from the second methionine start site at the position 35. Transfection of NIH3T3 cells using this vector and a vector encoding the p40 subunit gene results in the production of bioactive IL-12 (Zitvogel, unpublished results). Interestingly, sequences similar to sequence 1–34 of the p35 cDNA are found linked to signal peptides in other membrane-associated proteins. This suggests that an alternative membrane form of the p35 molecule may be generated (Wolf *et al.*, 1991). The 3' noncoding region of both the p35 and p40 subunits contains multiple copies of ATTTA mRNA destabilizing sequences similar to those found in many cytokines. These sequences are thought to enhance message degradation, thereby limiting mRNA longevity.

In order to better characterize the role of IL-12 in the immune response, we have constructed a single retroviral vector which can express the genes for both subunits of IL-12 with similar efficiency (Tahara and Zitvogel, unpublished results). Genes for mIL-12 (provided by Gubler, U.) and hIL-12 (provided by Wolf, S.F.) were cloned into the recombinant retroviral vector termed MFG (Dranoff *et al.*, 1993). An internal ribosome entry site (IRES) sequence of the encephalomyocarditis (EMC) virus (Novagen®, Wisconsin, USA) was subcloned into the vector to increase the efficiency of translation of the second gene (Fig. 2). The efficacy of these retroviral vectors (termed DFG-mIL-12 and hIL-12) was examined by infecting NIH3T3 cells and various tumour-cell lines, harvesting the resultant supernatant 48 h after the infection of NIH3T3 cells and measuring IL-12 bioactivity. IL-12 expression by transfected cells was determined to be 480 U/1 × 106 cells/48 h, as measured in PHA blast assay. We are currently using these vectors (*in vitro* and *in vivo*) to elucidate the role of IL-12 in the immune response.

Since human IL-12 has not been found to be biologically active in murine systems, cloning of the genes encoding murine p35 and p40 subunits was necessary to obtain recombinant protein for murine studies (Schoenhaut *et al.*, 1992). Comparison of the murine and human sequences demonstrated the p40 subunit to be highly conserved: 70% identical in cDNA sequence and 79% similarity in amino acid composition. The murine p35 subunit was found to have 60% identity with its human counterpart (Fig. 3). Analysis of human genomic DNA by Southern hybridization revealed that the gene encoding p40 and that encoding p35 are most likely single copy (Wolf *et al.*, 1991). Chromosomal location of these genes was determined by polymerase chain reaction (PCR) analysis of DNA from rodent–human hybrids. The p40 gene is located at 5q31–q33, and p35 maps to 3p12–3q13.2 (Sieburth *et al.*, 1992). Computer searches of sequence databases have shown that the two subunit sequences of IL-12 are unique (Gubler *et al.*, 1991; Wolf *et al.*, 1991). Interestingly, the murine and human p40 subunit have been shown to have a significant level of homology with the genes that encode IL-6R and cilliary neurotrophic factor receptor (CFNTR) (Gearing and Cosman, 1991; Gubler *et al.*, 1991). Conserved regions between these molecules include two cysteine residues of the Ig superfamily, three cysteines and several fibronectin type II residues within the haemopoietin receptor domain. Similarly, the p35 subunit has been shown to have structural similarities to the IL-6 and G-CSF gene families (Merberg *et al.*, 1992). Collectively, these data demonstrate that IL-12 is a unique protein with properties and structural homology linking it to the extended family of haemopoietin molecules.

PRODUCTION OF IL-12

D'Andrea *et al.* (1992) have recently examined production of IL-12 by radioimmunoassays specific for either the p35, p40, or p70 heterodimer. In this study, nine out of nine

A.

```
   1  GGCCCAGAGC AAGATGTGTC ACCAGCAGTT GGTCATCTCT TGGTTTTCCC
  51  TGGTTTTTCT GGCATCTCCC CTCGTGGCCA TATGGGAACT GAAGAAAGAT
 101  GTTTATGTCG TAGAATTGGA TTGGTATCCG GATGCCCCTG GAGAAATGGT
 151  GGTCCTCACC TGTGACACCC CTGAAGAAGA TGGTATCACC TGGACCTTGG
 201  ACCAGAGCAG TGAGGTCTTA GGCTCTGGCA AAACCCTGAC CATCCAAGTC
 251  AAAGAGTTTG GAGATGCTGG CCAGTACACC TGTCACAAAG GAGGCGAGGT
 301  TCTAAGCCAT TCGCTCCTGC TGCTTCACAA AAAGGAAGAT GGAATTTGGT
 351  CCACTGATAT TTTAAAGGAC CAGAAAGAAC CCAAAAATAA GACCTTTCTA
 401  AGATGCGAGG CCAAGAATTA TTCTGGACGT TTCACCTGCT GGTGGCTGAC
 451  GACAATCAGT ACTGATTTGA CATTCAGTGT CAAAAGCAGC AGAGGCTCTT
 501  CTGACCCCCA AGGGGTGACG TGCGGAGCTG CTACACTCTC TGCAGAGAGA
 551  GTCAGAGGGG ACAACAAGGA GTATGAGTAC TCAGTGGAGT GCCAGGAGGA
 601  CAGTGCCTGC CCAGCTGCTG AGGAGAGTCT GCCCATTGAG GTCATGGTGG
 651  ATGCCGTTCA CAAGCTCAAG TATGAAAACT ACACCAGCAG CTTCTTCATC
 701  AGGGACATCA TCAAACCTGA CCCACCCAAC AACTTGCAGC TGAAGCCATT
 751  AAAGAATTCT CGGCAGGTGG AGGTCAGCTG GGAGTACCCT GACACCTGGA
 801  GTACTCCACA TTCCTACTTC TCCCTGACAT TCTGCGTTCA GGTCCAGGGC
 851  AAGAGCAAGA GAGAAAAGAA AGATAGAGTC TTCACCGACA AGACCTCAGC
 901  CACGGTCATC TGCCGCAAAA ATGCCAGCAT TAGCGTGCGG GCCCAGGACC
 951  GCTACTATAG CTCATCTTGG AGCGAATGGG CATCTGTGCC CTGCAGTTAG
1001  GTTCTGATCC AGGATGAAAA TTTGGAGGAA AAGTGGAAGA TATTAAGCAA
1051  AATGTTTAAA GACACAACGG AATAGACCCA AAAAGATAAT TTCTATCTGA
1101  TTTGCTTTAA AACGTTTTTT TAGGATCACA ATGATATCTT TGCTGTATTT
1151  GTATAGTTCG ATGCTAAATG CTCATTGAAA CAATCAGCTA ATTTATGTAT
1201  AGATTTTCCA GCTCTCAAGT TGCCATGGGC CTTCATGCTA TTTAAATATT
1251  TAAGTAATTT ATGTATTTAT TAGTATATTA CTGTTATTTA ACGTTTGTCT
1301  GCCAGGATGT ATGGAATGTT TCATACTCTT ATGACCTGAT CCATCAGGAT
1351  CAGTCCCTAT TATGCAAAAT GTGAATTTAA TTTTATTTGT ACTGACAACT
1401  TTTCAAGCAA GGCTGCAAGT ACATCAGTTT TATGACAATC AGGAAGAATG
1451  CAGTGTTCTG ATACCAGTGC CATCATACAC TTGTGATGGA TGGGAACGCA
1501  AGAGATACTT ACATGGAAAC CTGACAATGC AAACCTGTTG AGAAGATCCA
1551  GGAGAACAAG ATGCTAGTTC CCATGTCTGT GAAGACTTCC TGGAGATGGT
1601  GTTGATAAAG CAATTTAGGG CCACTTACAC TTCTAAGCAA GTTTAATCTT
1651  TGGATGCCTG AATTTTAAAA GGGCTAGAAA AAAATGATTG ACCAGCCTGG
1701  GAAACATAAC AAGACCCCGT CTCTACAAAA AAAATTTAAA ATTAGCCAGG
1751  CGTGGTGGCT CATGCTTGTG GTCCCAGCTG TTCAGGAGGA TGAGGCAGGA
1801  GGATCTCTTG AGCCCAGGAG GTCAAGGCTA TGGTGAGCCG TGATTGTGCC
1851  ACTGCATACC AGCCTAGGTG ACAGAATGAG ACCCTGTCTC AAAAAAAAAA
1901  ATGATTGAAA TTAAAATTCA GCTTTAGCTT CCATGGCAGT CCTCACCCCC
1951  ACCTCTCTAA AAGACACAGG AGGATGACAC AGAAACACCG TAAGTGTCTG
2001  GAAGGCAAAA AGATCTTAAG ATTCAAGAGA GAGGACAAGT AGTTATGGCT
2051  AAGGACATGA AATTGTCAGA ATGGCAGGTG GCTTCTTAAC AGCCATGTGA
2101  GAAGCAGACA GATGCAAAGA AAATCTGGAA TCCCTTTCTC ATTAGCATGA
2151  ATGAACCTGA TACACAATTA TGACCAGAAA ATATGGCTCC ATGAAGGTGC
2201  TACTTTTAAG TAATGTATGT GCGCTCTGTA AAGTGATTAC ATTTGTTTCC
2251  TGTTTGTTTA TTTATTTATT TATTTTTGCA TTCTGAGGCT GAACTAATAA
2301  AAACTCTTCT TTGTAATC
```

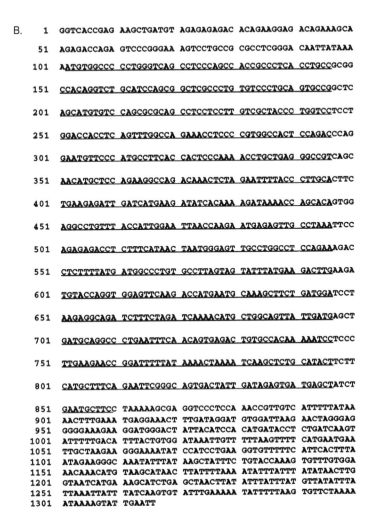

B.
```
   1  GGTCACCGAG AAGCTGATGT AGAGAGAGAC ACAGAAGGAG ACAGAAAGCA

  51  AGAGACCAGA GTCCCGGGAA AGTCCTGCCG CGCCTCGGGA CAATTATAAA

 101  AATGTGGCCC CCTGGGTCAG CCTCCCAGCC ACCGCCCTCA CCTGCCGCGG

 151  CCACAGGTCT GCATCCAGCG GCTCGCCCTG TGTCCCTGCA GTGCCGGCTC

 201  AGCATGTGTC CAGCGCGCAG CCTCCTCCTT GTCGCTACCC TGGTCCTCCT

 251  GGACCACCTC AGTTTGGCCA GAAACCTCCC CGTGGCCACT CCAGACCCAG

 301  GAATGTTCCC ATGCCTTCAC CACTCCCAAA ACCTGCTGAG GGCCGTCAGC

 351  AACATGCTCC AGAAGGCCAG ACAAACTCTA GAATTTTACC CTTGCACTTC

 401  TGAAGAGATT GATCATGAAG ATATCACAAA AGATAAAACC AGCACAGTGG

 451  AGGCCTGTTT ACCATTGGAA TTAACCAAGA ATGAGAGTTG CCTAAATTCC

 501  AGAGAGACCT CTTTCATAAC TAATGGGAGT TGCCTGGCCT CCAGAAAGAC

 551  CTCTTTTATG ATGGCCCTGT GCCTTAGTAG TATTTATGAA GACTTGAAGA

 601  TGTACCAGGT GGAGTTCAAG ACCATGAATG CAAAGCTTCT GATGGATCCT

 651  AAGAGGCAGA TCTTTCTAGA TCAAAACATG CTGGCAGTTA TTGATGAGCT

 701  GATGCAGGCC CTGAATTTCA ACAGTGAGAC TGTGCCACAA AAATCCTCCC

 751  TTGAAGAACC GGATTTTTAT AAAAACTAAAA TCAAGCTCTG CATACTTCTT

 801  CATGCTTTCA GAATTCGGGC AGTGACTATT GATAGAGTGA TGAGCTATCT

 851  GAATGCTTCC TAAAAAGCGA GGTCCCTCCA AACCGTTGTC ATTTTTATAA
 901  AACTTTGAAA TGAGGAAACT TTGATAGGAT GTGGATTAAG AACTAGGGAG
 951  GGGGAAAGAA GGATGGGGACT ATTACATCCA CATGATACCT CTGATCAAGT
1001  ATTTTTGACA TTTACTGTGG ATAAATTGTT TTTAAGTTTT CATGAATGAA
1051  TTGCTAAGAA GGGAAAAATAT CCATCCTGAA GGTGTTTTTC ATTCACTTTA
1101  ATAGAAGGGC AAATATTTAT AAGCTATTTC TGTACCAAAG TGTTTGTGGA
1151  AACAAACATG TAAGCATAAC TTATTTTAAA ATATTTATTT ATATAACTTG
1201  GTAATCATGA AAGCATCTGA GCTAACTTAT ATTTATTTAT GTTATATTTA
1251  TTAAATTATT TATCAAGTGT ATTTGAAAAA TATTTTTAAG TGTTCTAAAA
1301  ATAAAAGTAT TGAATT
```

Fig. 1. cDNA sequences of IL-12 p40 (A) and p35 (B) subunits.

EBV-transformed B-cell lines examined produced biologically active p70 heterodimer upon stimulation with the phorbol diester PDBu. IL-12 production was not observed from the Burkitt lymphoma cell lines Daudi and Raji T cell lines Jurkat and J32 or several myeloid leukaemic cell lines (HL-60, U937, Ml-3, THP-2). No solid tumour-cell lines (including melanoma and colon carcinoma) were found to produce IL-12. As has been previously described by Stern *et al.* (1990), most IL-12 producer cell lines examined in this study secreted excess free p40 subunit upon stimulation with phorbol diester. Secretion of free p35 protein was not detected from any cell lines examined under any condition.

Examination of freshly isolated peripheral blood mononuclear cells revealed constitutive secretion of low levels of both free p40 subunit and the biologically active p70 heterodimer (p40 ≫ p70). In contrast to established B-cell lines, secretion of IL-12 by PBMC was not significantly enhanced by phorbol ester stimulation. However, stimulation with *Staphylococcus aureus* Cowan strain I (SAC) greatly increased production

A

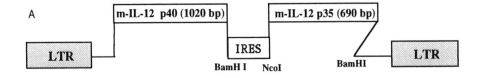

B

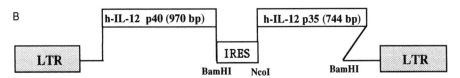

Fig. 2.   Diagram of retroviral vectors containing p35, p40 and IRES sequence. (A) DFG-m (B) DFG-hIL-12.

of both free p40 and the p70 heterodimer. SAC was shown to be the most powerful inducer of p40 and p70 production. Other inducers of IL-12 production included LPS and *Mycobacterium tuberculosis*. More recently, monocytes infected with *Toxoplasma gondi* or *Listeria monocytogenes* have also been shown to produce IL-12 (Hsieh *et al.*, 1993). Interestingly, no cytokines, including IL-1α or IL-1β, IL-2, IL-4, IL-6, IFN-γ, IFN-β, TNF-α, TNF-β, or GM-CSF, were found to induce IL-12 production. Fractionation of PBMC showed that both the nonadherent (mostly B and T cells) and adherent cell subset (>90% monocytes) were capable of secreting p40 and/or p70 heterodimer. Neither p35, p40 nor p70 production was detected in the supernatants of PHA blasts (activated T cells) or purified NK cells. Removal of CD19[+] CD20[+] B cells partly abrogated IL-12 production from the nonadherent PBMC subset. These data suggest that the chief producers of IL-12 are macrophages and B cells.

Differential expression of the p35 and p40 subunits of IL-12 has been described by Wolf *et al.* (1991) and Schoenhaut *et al.* (1992). The latter authors showed, by RNA blot analysis of murine tissues, that the p40 subunit is constitutively expressed in all lymphoid tissues including thymus, spleen and lymph nodes. Interestingly, mRNA encoding the p35 subunit was found to be expressed in lung and brain tissues as well as lymphoid tissue (Schoenhaut *et al.*, 1992). Additionally, Wolf *et al.* (1991) have examined, by PCR, a large panel of human cell lines for presence of mRNA for the individual subunits of IL-12. Virtually all cell types examined, with the notable exceptions of the NCI-H128 (small-cell carcinoma), the Molt-4 (T-cell line), and the HL60 (leukaemic myeloid line) screened as IL-12 p35[+], suggesting that p35 expression is essentially ubiquitous. In contrast, p40 expression was found to have a limited range of expression. Among the human cell types found to be positive for the presence of p40 and mRNA were B cells, monocytes and, to a much lesser extent, T cells (Wolf, S., personal communication). Differential expression of the two subunits may reflect favourable kinetics for heterodimer formation, or it may be that the p40 subunit is a carrier molecule for a family of as yet uncharacterized p35-like molecules. Alternatively, the p40 subunit could have a biological activity distinct from the p70 heterodimer. However, p40 has not been shown to be biologically active in any system

A.

```
Human P40    1 MCHQQLVISWFSLVFLASPLVAIWELKKDVYVVELDWYPDAPGEMVVLTC 50
               ||.|.|.||||.:|:|.|||:|:|||.|||||||:||  |||||| | |||
Mouse P40    1 MCPQKLTISWFAIVLLVSPLMAMWELEKDVYVVEVDWTPDAPGETVNLTC 50

Human P40   51 DTPEEDGITWTLDQSSEVLGSGKTLTIQVKEFGDAGQYTCHKGGEVLSHS 100
               ||||||:|||| ||.  :|:|||||||||| |||| ||||||||| ||||
Mouse P40   51 DTPEEDDITWTSDQRHGVIGSGKTLTITVKEFLDAGQYTCHKGGETLSHS 100

Human P40  101 LLLLHKKEDGIWSTDILKDQKEPKNKTFLRCEAKNYSGRFTCWWLTTIST 150
               |||||||:|||||:|||:       ||||||:|||.||||||||||.||.
Mouse P40  101 HLLLHKKENGIWSTEILKN...FKNKTFLKCEAPNYSGRFTCSWLVQRNM 147

Human P40  151 DLTFSVKSSRGSSDPQGVTCGAATLSAERVRGDNKEYE.YSVECQEDSAC 199
               ||.|.:|||.:|.|..:|||| |.||||:| |.:|| |||.||||| .|
Mouse P40  148 DLKFNIKSSSSSPDSRAVTCGMASLSAEKVTLDQRDYEKYSVSCQEDVTC 197

Human P40  200 PAAEESLPIEVMVDAVHKLKYENYTSSFFIRDIIKPDPPNNLQLKPLKNS 249
               |.|||.||||: ::| :. ||||||..||||||||||||||.|||:||||||
Mouse P40  198 PTAEETLPIELALEARQQNKYENYSTSFFIRDIIKPDPPKNLQMKPLKNS 247

Human P40  250 RQVEVSWEYPDTWSTPHSYFSLTFCVQVQGKSKREK........KDRVFT 291
               ||||||||||.||||||||||||.| |.:| |..: |       |: .:.
Mouse P40  248 .QVEVSWEYPDSWSTPHSYFSLKFFVRIQRKKEKMKETEEGCNQKGAFLV 296

Human P40  292 DKTSATVICRKNASISVRAQDRYYSSSWSEWASVPCS... 328
               :|||..| | |.:.::|.|||||.|| |.||:|||.
Mouse P40  297 EKTSTEVQC.KGGNVCVQAQDRYYNSSCSKWACVPCRVRS 335
```

B.

```
Human P35    1 MWPPGSASQPPPSPAAATGLHPAARPVSLQCRLSMCPARSLLLVATLVLL 50
                                                 ||..| ||::|||.||
Mouse P35    1 ..............................MCQSRYLLFLATLALL 16

Human P35   51 DHLSLARNLPVATPDPGMFPCLHHSQNLLRAVSNMLQKARQTLEFYPCTS 100
               :|||||| :||..|.  .|| :|.|||:...:|:..||:.|. |.||.
Mouse P35   17 NHLSLARVIPVSGPA....RCLSQSRNLLKTTDDMVKTAREKLKHYSCTA 62

Human P35  101 EEIDHEDITKDKTSTVEACLPLELTKNESCLNSRETSFITNGSCLASRKT 150
               |:|||||||:|.|||.|||||||||||||| ||||. .|.||||...:||
Mouse P35   63 EDIDHEDITRDQTSTLKTCLPLELHKNESCLATRETSSTTRGSCLPPQKT 112

Human P35  151 SFMMALCLSSIYEDLKMYQVEFKTMNAKLLMDPKRQIFLDQNMLAVIDEL 200
               |:||.||||||||||||||:||  |.  ..||:||:||..||.||||||
Mouse P35  113 SLMMTLCLGSIYEDLKMYQTEFQAINAALQNHNHQQIILDKGMLVAIDEL 162

Human P35  201 MQALNFNSETVPQKSSLEEPDFYKTKIKLCILLHAFRIRAVTIDRVMSYL 250
               ||.|| |:||:.||..::|:| |:.|:|||||||||..|.|||:|||:||
Mouse P35  163 MQSLNHNGETLRQKPPVGEADPYRVKMKLCILLHAFSTRVVTINRVMGYL 212

Human P35  251 NAS 253
               ...
Mouse P35  213 SSA 215
```

Fig. 3. Comparison of predicted amino acid composition of human p40 and murine p40, and human p35 and murine p35.

examined to date. The significance of ubiquitous expression of p35 is not yet known, although it has been suggested that IL-12 may be produced by 'non-professional APC' following viral infection (Zitvogel, L., Wolf, S., personal communication).

In summary, production of IL-12 appears to be limited chiefly to professional APCs. Antigen-stimulated macrophages and B cells were found to be the chief producers of IL-12 in peripheral blood mononuclear cells. Other cytokines examined were not able to induce the secretion of IL-12. Collectively, these data suggest that IL-12 may be crucial early in the development of an immune response.

IL-12 RECEPTOR

The receptor for IL-12 (IL-12R) was characterized using highly purified ^{125}I-labelled IL-12 on 4-day PHA-activated lymphoblasts (Chizzonite *et al.*, 1992). Neutralizing anti-IL-12 antibodies were found to block ^{125}I-IL-12 binding to lymphoblasts and neutralize IL-12 bioactivity. Scatchard analysis of steady-state binding identified a single receptor with approximately 1000 to 9000 sites per lymphoblast, with an equilibrium dissociation constant of 100 to 600 pM. Affinity crosslinking of surface-bound ^{125}I-IL-12 to PHA-activated lymphoblasts at 4°C identified a complex of approximately 210 to 280 kDa. Cleavage of this complex with a reducing agent identified one radiolabelled protein of approximately 110 kDa. Thus, the IL-12 binding site on PHA-activated lymphoblasts was suggested to be composed of a single protein of approximately 110 kDa. IL-12R expression on lymphocytes was observed to be dependent upon activation by PHA or IL-2 (Desai *et al.*, 1992). Expression of IL-12R on PHA-activated lymphocytes peaked between days 2 and 4 following stimulation. In contrast, lymphocytes activated with IL-2 showed maximal IL-12R expression between days 6 and 8. Screening studies of a variety of cell types and cell lines revealed that IL-12R expression was apparently limited to activated T and NK cells (Desai *et al.*, 1992).

Monoclonal antibodies specific for the p40 subunit have yielded information pertinent to IL-12/IL-12R interaction (Chizzonite *et al.*, 1991). Only antibodies specific for the p40 subunit (or the p70 heterodimer) have been shown to have the capacity to neutralize IL-12. These results suggest that localized determinants on the 40-kDa subunit may be necessary for binding of IL-12 to its cognate receptor. However, additional evidence by Schoenhaut *et al.* (1992), using murine-human hybrid IL-12, has indicated that the p35 subunit does play some role in determining IL-12 specificity for its receptor. A hybrid heterodimer consisting of murine p35 and human p40 subunits was found to be active on murine cells; however, the combination of human p35 and murine p40 was completely inactive on murine cells. Both hybrid factors were active on human cells.

EFFECTS OF IL-12 ON NK CELLS

Early studies of IL-12 found it to be a potent modulator of the *in vitro* functions of NK cells. IL-12 has been shown to: (1) generate LAK cell activity from PBMC and purified NK cells; (2) enhance the spontaneous lytic activity of NK cells following overnight incubation; (3) inhibit the IL-2-driven proliferation of NK cells; (4) upregulate a variety of cell surface molecules on NK cells, as well as enhance the migration and binding of these cells to a tumour-cell monolayer; and (5) enhance NK cell secretion of IFN-γ and, to lesser extent, TNF-α.

Cytolytic Activity

The phenomenon of LAK cell activity was originally described by the ability of IL-2 to generate nonMHC restricted killing from human PBMC against a wide variety of fresh tumour targets (Lotze *et al.*, 1981). The population responsible for IL-2 LAK activity was subsequently found to largely reside in the CD56[+] NK subset of human PBMC (Roberts *et al.*, 1987). IL-12 was originally identified as a factor that synergized with IL-2 in the presence of hydrocortisone to generate LAK activity from human PBMC

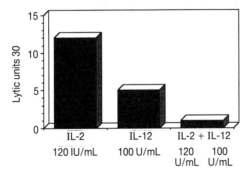

Fig. 4. IL-12 inhibits IL-2-generated LAK when added concurrently to culture. Fresh PBMC were harvested from volunteer donors and incubated in the presence of IL-2 (120 IU/ml), IL-12 (100 U/ml), or a combination of IL-2 (120 IU/ml) and IL-12 (100 U/ml). Effectors were then harvested and tested for their ability to lyse K562 and Daudi labelled targets. (From Zeh *et al.*, 1993.)

(Gately *et al.*, 1986). These initial studies indicated that IL-12, when used alone, was inactive. Subsequently, we and others have shown that IL-12 is able to generate low levels of LAK activity from unfractionated PBMC in the absence of hydrocortisone (Kobayashi *et al.*, 1989; Gately *et al.*, 1991; Chehimi *et al.*, 1992; Zeh *et al.*, 1993). Maximal IL-12 induced LAK activity in these studies has been reported to be from 10 to 40% of that generated with optimal levels of IL-2. The effective concentration of IL-12 found to induce 50% (EC_{50}) of its LAK-generating capacity was 6–35 pM; in comparison, the EC_{50} of IL-2 was 16 pM (Gately *et al.*, 1991). IL-12-induced LAK activity, similar to IL-2-induced LAK, was found to be dependent upon $CD56^+$ NK cells. IL-12 has not been shown to generate MHC nonrestricted killing from T cells (Gately *et al.*, 1991; Chehimi *et al.*, 1992).

Neutralizing antibodies to TNF-α inhibit IL-12 generated LAK activity from high-density peripheral blood lymphocytes by up to 70%. Similarly, antibodies to IFN-γ were found to inhibit IL-12 generation of LAK by 18–64%. However, the total inhibition observed with combinations of these two antibodies was never found to be greater than inhibition observed by neutralization of TNF-α alone. Neutralization of IL-2 was not able to inhibit IL-12 generation of LAK activity. Interestingly, neutralizing antibodies to IL-12 were observed to inhibit the ability of IL-2 to generate LAK activity from certain donors. Moreover, combinations of neutralizing antibodies to TNF and IL-12 caused additive inhibitory effects on IL-2-generated LAK (Gately *et al.*, 1991).

Studies of combinations of IL-12 and IL-2 on LAK generation have yielded synergistic, additive, or inhibitory results, depending on the system examined. We have recently reported that in a 5-day LAK generation assay, IL-12 inhibited the ability of IL-2 to generate LAK activity from PBMC. In contrast, IL-12 enhanced the LAK activity generated from PBMC preactivated with IL-2 (Fig. 4; Zeh *et al.*, 1993). Similar studies have also demonstrated such results. IL-12 has been shown (in a 4-day culture) to inhibit high-dose IL-2 generation of LAK activity from low-density peripheral blood lymphocytes. Conversely, it was found to synergize with low-dose IL-2 in this activity (Gately *et al.*, 1991). PBL incubated for shorter periods of time (18 h) with combinations of IL-2 and IL-12 have also resulted in less than additive or additive enhancement of cytotoxicity (Chehimi *et al.*, 1992).

Naume *et al.* (1992) have also described the ability of IL-12 to generate LAK activity from highly purified populations of NK cells. When compared with other LAK-inducing cytokines (IL-2 and IL-7), IL-12 was found to have intermediate efficacy. IL-12 was able to induce 50% of the maximal LAK activity observed with 120 U/ml of IL-2. IL-7 was found to induce 60% of the maximal IL-12 response. Again, neutralizing antibodies to TNF-α were able to partially abrogate the effects of IL-12 on purified NK cells. However, unlike unfractionated PBMC, inhibition of IFN-γ did not significantly inhibit IL-12 generation of LAK from purified NK cells. This is consistent with the studies of Chan *et al.* (1991) which indicate that $CD56^+$ NK cells require the presence of $HLA-DR^+$ accessory cells in order to produce IFN-γ in response to IL-12.

IL-12 also enhances the cytolytic activity of purified NK cells following a brief (18 h) incubation (Kobayashi *et al.*, 1989; Robertson *et al.*, 1992). Concentrations ranging from 0.29–35 pM enhanced the ability of NK cells to lyse the NK-resistant Colo, RDMC, and Daudi targets. In contrast, IL-2 enhancement of spontaneous lytic activity of NK cells required nanomolar concentrations. However, optimal concentrations of IL-2 consistently produced greater enhancement of NK lytic function than optimal concentrations of IL-12. IL-12 enhanced the lytic activity of both $CD56^{bright}$ and $CD56^{dim}$ subpopulations (Robertson *et al.*, 1992). Various other studies have shown that IL-12 is able to increase the cytolytic activity of PBL derived from HIV-infected individuals (Chehimi *et al.*, 1992) as well as enhance ADCC mediated activity against a colon carcinoma cell line (Lieberman *et al.*, 1991).

Collectively, these data demonstrate the ability of IL-12 to enhance spontaneous lytic activity as well as generate LAK activity from NK cells. IL-12 enhances lytic activity from NK cells at much lower concentrations than IL-2, although IL-12 alone is never more effective than IL-2. The ability of IL-12 to augment the lytic activity of NK cells appears to be partly dependent upon the *in situ* production of TNF-α, and IFN-γ, but not IL-2. In contrast, antibody-blocking studies have shown IL-2 LAK induction to be dependent upon IL-12. Studies of combinations of these two cytokines on LAK induction has yielded mixed results. The timing and relative doses of the two cytokines appear to be crucial to the final development of LAK activity. IL-2 and IL-12 may induce LAK activity from NK cells through distinct but overlapping pathways. Additional studies are necessary to elucidate the mechanism of interaction between these two potent cytokines.

Proliferation

IL-12 is a weak inducer of proliferation from NK cells (Chehimi *et al.*, 1992; Naume *et al.*, 1992; Robertson *et al.*, 1992). IL-12 induces low levels of proliferation in immuno-magnetically purified NK cells, producing 10% of IL-2 and 50% of the IL-7-induced response (Naume *et al.*, 1992). Robertson *et al.* (1992) have also reported the inability of IL-12 to effectively drive the proliferation of $CD56^{bright}$ or $CD56^{dim}$ NK cells. Moreover, IL-12 was observed to completely abrogate the IL-2-driven proliferation of NK cells. Addition of neutralizing antibodies to IFN-γ to cultures was not able to reverse this inhibition. However, consistent with previously published reports (Gately *et al.*, 1991), IL-12 was found to enhance the proliferation of NK cells preactivated by IL-2. The addition of IL-12 to NK cells preactivated with IL-2 either *in vitro* or *in vivo* resulted in a lower proliferation than observed with IL-2 alone (Robertson *et al.*, 1992).

Thus, it appears that in contrast to its ability to enhance lytic activity of NK cells, IL-12 does not serve as a particularly effective growth factor for these cells.

Cell Surface Phenotypic Modulation

IL-12 is a potent modulator of certain cell-surface markers on purified NK cells. IL-12 upregulates IL-2Rα, TNF-R and CD56 expression on the surface of highly purified NK cells (Naume et al., 1992). Other studies have demonstrated the ability of IL-12 to upregulate the NK cell adhesion molecules and activation markers CD2, CD11a, CD54, CD25, HLA-DR, CD69, and CD71 (Robertson et al., 1992; Rabinowich et al., 1993). Functionally, IL-12 has been shown to increase the level of NK conjugate formation with K562 tumour targets, as well as increase the binding of NK cells to a monolayer of squamous cell carcinoma (Rabinowich et al., 1993).

Induction of Other Cytokines

IL-12 alone, and in synergy with IL-2, is a potent inducer of IFN-γ, and to a lesser extent TNF-α, secretion by NK cells. The ability of IL-12 to enhance the secretion of IFN-γ from peripheral blood mononuclear cells was initially described by Kobayashi et al. (1989). Subsequently, Chan et al. (1991) have shown it to synergize in the induction of IFN-γ production from PBMC with IL-2, PHA, phorbol esters, anti-CD3 antibodies and alloantigens. IL-12 enhanced production of IFN-γ at the transcriptional level by directly increasing the amount of detectable IFN-γ mRNA (Chan et al., 1992). IFN-γ production by PBL in response to IL-12 was found to be dependent upon the presence of HLA-DR$^+$ accessory cells (Chan et al., 1991). IL-12 has also been found to increase IFN-γ production by PBL isolated from individuals infected with HIV (Chehimi et al., 1992). Other studies have shown that IL-12 induces the production of TNF-α from purified NK cells (Naume et al., 1992). Maximal secretion of TNF-α in response to IL-12 peaked at 72 h. IL-12 was found to stimulate 10% of the IL-2 and 50% of the IL-7-induced TNF-α production by NK cells. Interestingly, unlike IL-2, IL-12 and IL-7 were not found to induce secretion of appreciable levels of TNF-β.

EFFECTS OF IL-12 ON T CELLS

Early studies of the effects of IL-12 on T cells have shown it to be a potent inducer of proliferation and enhancer of cytotoxicity in both naive and memory T cells. More recent evidence suggests that IL-12 plays a crucial role in the ontogeny of a T_{H1} type immune response, directing T cells to produce more IFN-γ (a T_{H1}-associated cytokine) and less IL-4 (a T_{H2}-associated cytokine).

Proliferation

Recombinant IL-12 was first shown to be an effective inducer of proliferation of activated T cells by Stern et al. (1990). This activity was later extensively characterized by Gately et al. (1991). In these latter studies, IL-12 consistently induced proliferation of PBMC that had been preactivated with PHA. These PHA blasts were shown to be >90% CD3$^+$ T cells. PHA blast responsiveness to IL-12 began on day 2, peaked at day

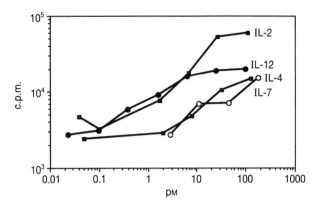

Fig. 5. IL-12 induces proliferation of PBMC preactivated with PHA. PBMC were harvested and incubated in the presence of 0.1% PHA for 4 days. Cells were washed and incubated in varying concentrations of IL-2, IL-4, IL-7 and IL-12 for an additional 48 h. Cells were pulsed incubated with ^{3}H-labelled thymidine for the final 24 h of culture. (From Zeh *et al.*, 1993.)

4 and disappeared by day 6 following stimulation. These 'windows of responsiveness' were later shown to be dependent upon the upregulation of specific IL-12 receptors on T cells in response to PHA (Chizzonite *et al.*, 1992). Maximal proliferation of PHA blasts induced by IL-12 was 30–70% of that observed with optimal doses of IL-2. However, IL-12 was found to be the most potent inducer of proliferation in PHA blasts, (EC_{50} = 8.5 pM) greater than IL-2 (EC_{50} = 52 pM), IL-7 (EC_{50} = 80 pM) and IL-4 (EC_{50} = 189 pM). Figure 5 demonstrates the ability of IL-12 to induce proliferation of PHA-activated lymphocytes. Enrichment of PHA blasts for CD4$^+$ or CD8$^+$ cells yielded similar results, which suggests that IL-12 is equally effective on both of these subsets. In contrast to its inhibitory effect on IL-2-driven proliferation of NK cells, IL-12 was found to synergize with IL-2 to induce proliferation of PHA-activated T cells. IL-12 was unable to induce proliferation of naive/unstimulated PBMC in these studies, consistent with the prerequisite activation-associated expression of the IL-12R (Desai *et al.*, 1992).

This requirement for T-cell activation for IL-12 responsiveness has been demonstrated to be true for both polyclonally induced peripheral blood T cells and for antigen-specific T cells (Bertagnolli *et al.*, 1992; Zeh *et al.*, 1993). We have recently reported that T-cell clones, isolated from a metastatic melanoma and initially grown in IL-2, were able to proliferate in response to IL-12 following restimulation with appropriate antigen. In the absence of tumour restimulation, little or no effect of IL-12 was demonstrated. This contrasts with our experience with IL-2, which is able to support the proliferation of tumour-infiltrating lymphocytes (TIL) in the absence of tumour restimulation for greater than 90 days. IL-12 induced 10–30% of the maximal proliferation observed with IL-2 stimulation of these TIL. However, IL-12 was effective at 10–20 fold lower molar concentrations. Bertagnolli *et al.* (1992) have similarly demonstrated that IL-12 is an effective mitogen for both allospecific and influenza peptide-specific T cells. Response to IL-12 was observed to be optimal 3–7 days following exposure to specific antigens. T cells cultured for >7 days in the absence of appropriate antigen gradually lost their ability to respond to IL-12 alone. However, addition of low doses of IL-2 to resting T cells restored their capacity to subsequently proliferate in response to IL-12. Combinations of IL-12 and IL-2 synergized to drive the proliferation of memory T cells.

In summary, these data demonstrate that IL-12 is able to, alone and in concert with IL-2, serve as a potent comitogen for antigen-activated T cells. Unlike IL-2, which is able to induce proliferation of resting T cells, IL-12 appears to be specific for those T cells that have been activated through ligation of their T-cell receptors. IL-12 may function *in vivo* to focus and amplify the immune response by selectively inducing the outgrowth of those T cells that have been preactivated by appropriate antigen.

Cytolytic Activity

IL-12 enhances the generation of alloreactive T cells and augments the specific lytic activity of tumour-infiltrating T lymphocytes. Evidence of the ability of IL-12 to enhance the lytic activity of T cells was first described by Gately *et al.* (1986). In these studies, IL-12 enhanced the generation of specific effector T cells from primary cultures of high-density peripheral blood lymphocytes stimulated with γ-irradiated allogeneic HT144 melanoma. Specific cytolytic activity was demonstrated as the ability of CD3$^+$ effectors from these cultures to preferentially lyse HT144 melanoma targets over class-I-deficient Daudi and K562 targets. IL-12 enhanced generation of specific CTL at 10-fold lower concentration than that observed with IL-2. Furthermore, higher concentrations of IL-2, but not IL-12, resulted in increased levels of nonspecific LAK activity from these cultures. Neutralizing antibodies to IL-2 were found to inhibit IL-12-mediated generation of CTL, indicating that IL-2 must be present in these cultures in order for IL-12 to mediate this activity.

We have recently reported that IL-12 augmented the cytolytic activity of an HLA-A2 restricted CD8$^+$ melanoma-specific TIL clone. In these experiments, IL-12 enhanced, in a dose-dependent manner, the lytic activity of the clone against autologous but not allogeneic targets. When IL-2 was allowed to remain in culture, the addition of IL-12 augmented the lytic activity of the T-cell clone over that typically observed with maximal doses of IL-2 (6000 IU/ml) (Fig. 6). Apparently, in addition to inducing proliferation of activated T cells, IL-12 is also able to enhance the lytic potential of these cells. These data raise the possibility that IL-12 may be a potent adjunct to the adoptive transfer of cytolytic cells. IL-12 could be coadministered with effector cells or added briefly *in vitro* before administration in order to enhance their cytolytic activity.

T$_{H1}$ Stimulation

Perhaps the most important description of the role of IL-12 in the immune response has been the recent finding that IL-12 directs the development of a T$_{H1}$-type immune response. It has been known for some time now that mature, murine T$_H$ cells fall into one of several cytokine secretion patterns, T$_{H1}$ versus T$_{H2}$ (Mosmann *et al.*, 1986). Further, these differential cytokine production patterns play an essential role in regulating the nature of the immune response. Specifically in the mouse, T$_H$ cells that produce high levels of IFN-γ, lymphotoxin, and IL-2 (T$_{H1}$) are associated with the development of strong cellular immunity (Cher and Mosmann, 1987), while those producing high levels of IL-4 and IL-5 (T$_{H2}$) result in predominantly humoral immunity (Mosmann *et al.*,

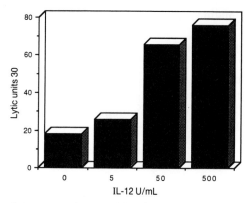

Fig. 6.   IL-12 augments IL-2 supported cytotoxicity of melanoma TIL clone 2.46.1. Melanoma TIL clone 2.46.1 was restimulated with autologous tumour and grown in (6000 IU/ml) IL-2 for 2 days. TIL was then washed, harvested and incubated for an additional 24 h in IL-2 (6000 IU/ml) and 0, 5, 50, or 500 U/ml of IL-12. Cytotoxicity was then measured against autologous and allogeneic tumour. Lysis of allogeneic tumour was less than 10% in all experimental groups (data not shown). IL-12 augmented, in a dose-dependent manner, the IL-2-driven cytoxicity of TIL clone 2.46.1. (From Zeh *et al.*, 1993.)

1986). Functionally, the ability of the immune response to generate a predominantly cellular (T_{H1}) or humoral (T_{H2}) immune response has been associated with enhanced elimination of certain pathogens. Three recent papers have outlined the ability of IL-12 to induce a predominantly T_{H1}-type response. Kiniwa *et al.* (1992) have shown that IL-12 is a potent inhibitor of IL-4-induced IgE synthesis from peripheral blood mononuclear cells. IL-12 inhibited IgE synthesis both at the transcriptional and translational level. IL-12 is postulated to mediate this effect through both an IFN-γ-dependent and -independent mechanism. Manetti *et al.* (1993) have shown that dust mite, Der p I-specific T helper cells derived in the presence of IL-12 have a reduced capacity to produce IL-4 and an increased ability to secrete IFN-γ. Furthermore, clones derived from these lines showed a higher propensity to develop T_{H0} or T_{H1} cytokine secretion profiles. Purified protein derivative (PPD)-specific T-cell clones in this study, which were derived in the presence of neutralizing IL-12 antibodies, showed an increase in the ability to produce IL-4 and a decreased tendency towards developing into T_{H1} clones. Macatonia *et al.* (1993) have demonstrated that macrophages treated with heat-killed *L. monocytogenes* direct the development of a T_{H1} type response both *in vitro* and *in vivo*. More recently they have shown that the ability of macrophages to induce production of T_{H1} CD4$^+$ cells could be reproduced by addition of exogenous IL-12. Moreover IL-12 alone was found to be sufficient for the induction of the T_{H1} phenotype in naïve T cells. Neutralization of a variety of alternative cytokines produced by macrophages was unable to inhibit T_{H1} development. However, the presence of IFN-γ was found to be required, but not sufficient for *L. monocytogenes*-treated macrophage induction of T_{H1} phenotypic T cells. Interestingly, also in this study, IL-10 was found to inhibit the *L. monocytogenes*-treated macrophages' ability to induce a T_{H1} phenotypic response. IL-10, however, did not block IL-12 induction of T_{H1} T cells. This suggests that IL-10 suppresses the development of T_{H1} response by blocking macrophage production of IL-12. Figure 7 demonstrates a scenario for the development of either a predominantly T_{H1} or T_{H2} immune response.

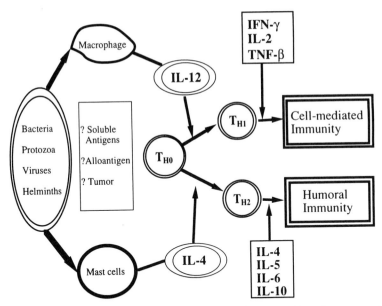

Fig. 7. Depiction of T-helper-cell differentiation. Interaction of antigen with antigen-presenting cell leads to the release of IL-12 or IL-4, leading to preferential development of either T_{H1} or T_{H2}-type response. (Figure adapted from Scott P. (1993) *Science* **260**, 496–497 with permission).

In summary IL-12 has been found to be a powerful comitogen for naïve and antigen-specific T cells. IL-12 is also able to enhance the production of specific allogenic responses, as well as directly augment the cytolytic potential of $CD8^+$ TIL clones. IL-12 also appears to be a crucial factor in the development of T_{H1} response.

IN VIVO EFFECTS OF IL-12

The cloning of the murine IL-12 genes and the subsequent production of highly purified recombinant murine IL-12 has made it possible to investigate the *in vivo* effects of IL-12 (Schoenhaut *et al.*, 1992). Preliminary data examining IL-12 administration has shown it to (1) augment NK lytic function, (2) induce IFN-γ secretion, (3) promote extramedullary haemopoiesis, (4) enhance generation of an allogeneic response, and (5) mediate potent anti-tumour effects *in vivo*.

Gately *et al.* (1993) have recently examined the effects of daily administration of 1 ng to 1 μg of recombinant mIL-12 to normal mice. IL-12 was shown to cause enhancement of lytic activity in NK cells (as measured against Yac-1 targets) isolated from the liver and spleen of treated animals. IL-12-mediated enhancement peaked on day 2 of adminstration and decreased thereafter. IL-12 was also observed to cause focal mononuclear cell infiltrates in the liver of treated animals. Flow cytometric examination of lymphoid cells recovered from the livers of IL-12-treated animals revealed an increase in the proportion of NK-1.1$^+$, NK/T and $CD8^+$T cells. Liver lymphoid cells recovered from treated, but not untreated, animals were also observed to spontaneously produce IFN-γ. Interestingly, IL-12 induced splenomegaly in treated animals

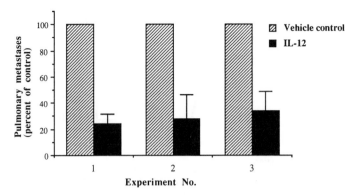

Fig. 8. Reduction in pulmonary metastases following systemic IL-12 therapy. IL-12 was administered by daily IP injection of 0.5–1.0 mg. Treatment was begun 7–10 days following intravenous administration of 3–5×10^5 MC38 adenocarcinoma tumour cells. Number of macroscopic pulmonary metastases were counted on days 21–24. IL-12 consistently decreased the number of pulmonary metastases over three independent experiments. (C. Nastala unpublished results.)

which upon histologic examination proved to be largely a result of increased extramedullary haemopoiesis. Erythroid, myeolid and megakaryocytic lineages were all represented. Lastly, exogenous administration of IL-12 was shown to enhance the generation of Lyt2$^+$ anti-allogenic specific T cells by approximately 14-fold. Enhancement of these T-cell-mediated allogenic responses (in contrast to enhancement of NK function which peaked on day 2 of therapy) peaked on day 5 following immunization. In these experiments administration of IL-12 up to 1 μg of IL-12 per day resulted in only minor side effects (fur ruffling and mild lethargy). No IL-12-associated mortality was observed (Gately *et al.*, submitted for publication).

Early data regarding the administration of IL-12 to tumour-bearing mice has yielded promising results. We have recently shown that the daily intratumoural administration of 0.008 to 1 μg of IL-12 is able to partially inhibit or completely eradicate (at higher doses) MC-38 adenocarcinoma or MCA-105 sarcoma growth. IL-12 therapy was most effective when initiated on days 0–5 following tumour inoculation. However, remarkable anti-tumour effects were observed with treatment begun as late as day 14. Interestingly, contralateral sentinel tumours were also noted to regress, indicating that the effects of IL-12 administration are systemic. Neutralizing antibodies to IFN-γ but not TNF-α were able to abrogate the anti-tumour effects of IL-12. IFN-γ levels (but not TNF-α) were noted to be elevated in experimental animals in days 3 and 4 following IL-12 therapy. Interestingly, in this same study, serum nitrite and nitrate levels were also found to be elevated in IL-12-treated animals, indicating that NO production might be an important component of IL-12 anti-tumour efficacy (Nastala *et al.*, manuscript in preparation). Figure 8 demonstrates IL-12's anti-tumour effects on experimental pulmonary metastases. Similar anti-tumour properties of IL-12 have also been demonstrated against several other murine tumour models including B16F10 melanoma, M5076 reticulum sarcoma, X5563 B cell lymphoma and the Renca renal cell carcinoma (Brunda, M., *et al.*, personal communication).

We have also found IL-12 to have anti-tumour properties in a murine gene therapy model. Utilizing NIH3T3 cells genetically altered to secrete IL-12, we have demonstrated that local production of IL-12 is able to inhibit the establishment of the poorly immunogenic BL-6 melanoma in B6 mice. Animals were inoculated subcutaneously with a mixture of NIH3T3 cells secreting 100–300 U IL-12/10^6 cells/48 h or NIH3T3 cells transfected with the gene for neomycin resistance and BL-6 murine melanoma cells and followed for establishment of tumour. Day of emergence of tumour was significantly delayed in animals that received inocula containing NIH3T3 cells secreting IL-12. In a parallel model, we have also shown that vaccines consisting of a mixture of irradiated tumour cells and IL-12 secreting tumour cells were able to enhance anti-tumour immunity as measured by the ability of treated animals to inhibit the establishment of a subsequent live tumour challenge (Tahara *et al.*, manuscript in preparation).

CONCLUSION

IL-12 is a novel cytokine, produced by professional APCs, and capable of inducing the outgrowth and enhancing the cytolytic activity of T and NK cells. IL-12 is active at extremely low concentrations (pM quantities). Furthermore, unlike IL-2, IL-12 responsiveness is limited to those T and NK cells that have been pre- or coactivated. IL-12 appears to preferentially induce a T_{H1}-type immune response. Preliminary *in vivo* studies have demonstrated that the systemic administration of doses of IL-12 capable of eliciting potent anti-tumour responses are not associated with significant toxicity. Collectively, these data suggest that IL-12 may have great potential as an immunotherapeutic agent against a wide variety of human diseases. Further elucidation of the precise role of IL-12 in directing the immune response and evaluation of its chemical utility, including genetherapy approach, are currently being pursued.

ACKNOWLEDGEMENTS

We thank Dr Walt Storkus for his helpful comments and Drs M. Gately, S. Wolf, M. Brunda, C. Nastala and D. Geller for their valuable input.

REFERENCES

Bertagnolli, M.M., Lin, B.-Y. and Hermann, S.H. (1992). *J. Immunol.* **149**, 3778–3783.
Chan, S.H., Perussia, B., Gupta, J.W., Kobayashi, M., Pospisil, M., Young, H., Wolf, S.F., Young, D., Clark, S.C. and Trinchieri, G. (1991). *J. Exp. Med.* **173**, 869–879.
Chan, S.H., Koabayashi, M., Santoli, D., Perussia, B. and Trinchieri, G. (1992). *J. Immunol.* **148**, 92–98.
Chehimi,J., Starr, S., Frank, I., Rengaraju, M., Jackson, S., Llanes, C., Kobayashi, M., Perussi, B. and Young, D. (1992). *J. Exp. Med.* **175**, 789–796.
Cher, D.J. and Mosmann, T.R. (1987). *J. Immunol.* **138**, 3688.
Chizzonite, R., Truitt, T., Podlaski, F.J., Wolitzky, A.G., Quinn, P.M., Nunes, P., Stern, A.S. and Gately, M.K. (1991). *J. Immunol.* **147**, 1548–1556.
Chizzonite, R., Truitt, T., Desai, B., Nunes, P., Podlaski, F.J., Stern, A. and Gately, M.K. (1992). *J. Immunol.* **148**, 3117–3124.
D'Andrea, A., Rengaraju, M., Valiante, Nm, Chehimi, J., Kubin, M., Aste, M., Chan, S.H., Kobayashi, M., Young, D., Nickbarg, E., Chizzonite, R., Wolf, S., Trinchieri, G. (1992). *J. Exp. Med.* **176(5)**, 1387–1398.
Desai, B.B., Quinn, P.M., Wolitzky, A.G., Mongini, P.K., Chizzonite, R. and Gately, M.K. (1992). *J. Immunol.* **148**, 3125–3132.
Dranoff, G., Jaffe, E., Lazenby, A., Golumbek, P., Levitsky, H., Brose, K., Jackson, V., Hamada, H., Pardoll, D. and Mulligan, R.C. (1993). *Proc. Natl Acad. Sci. USA* **90**, 3539–3543.
Gately, M., Wilson, D. and Wong, H. (1986). *J. Immunol.* **136**, 1274–1281.

Gately, M.K., Desai, B.B., Wolitzky, A.G., Quinn, P.M., Dwyer, C.M., Podlaski, F.J., Familletti, P.C., Sinigaglia, F., Chizonnite, R. and Gubler, U. (1991). *J. Immunol.* **147**, 874–882.

Gately, M., Wolitzky, A., Quinn, P. and Chizzonite, R. (1992). *Cell. Immunol.* **143**, 127–142.

Gately, M.K., Warrier, R., Honasoge, S., Faherty, D., Connaughton, S., Anderson, T., Sarmiento, U., Hubbard, B. and Murphy, M. (1994). *Int. Immunology* **6**(1), 157–167.

Gately, M.K., Wolitzky, A., Quinn, P. and Chizzonite, R. Submitted for publication.

Gearing, D.P. and Cosman, D. (1991). *Cell* **66**, 9–10.

Gubler, U., Chua, A.O., Gately, M.K., Schoenhaut, D.S., Dwyer, C.M., McComas, W., Motyka, R., Nabavi, N., Wolitzky, A.G., Quinn, P.M. and Familletti, P.C. (1991). *Proc. Natl Acad. Sci. USA* **88**(10), 4143–4147.

Hsieh, C.-S., Macatonia, S., Tripp. C., Wolf, S., O-Garra, A. and Murphy, K. (1993). *Science* **260**, 547–549.

Kiniwa, M., Gately, M.K., Gubler, U., Chizzonite, R., Fargeas, C. and Delespesse G. (1992). *J. Clin. Invest.* **90**, 262–266.

Kobayashi, M., Fitz, L., Ryan, M., Hewick, R.M., Clark, S.C., Chang, S., Loudon, R., Sherman, F., Perussia and Trinchieri, G. (1989). *J. Exp. Med.* **170**, 827–845.

Lieberman, M.D., Sigal, R.K., Williams, N. and Daly, J.M. (1991). *J. Surg. Res.* **50**, 410–415.

Lotze, M.T., Grimm, E., Mazumder, A., Strausser, J. and Rosenburg, S.A. (1981). *Cancer Res.* **41**, 4420–4425.

Macatonia, S.E., Hsieh, C.-S., O'Gara, A. and Murphy, K.M. (1993). *Int Immunology* **5**(9), 1119–1128.

Manetti, R., Parronchi, P., Giudizi, M., Piccinni, M.P., Maggi, E., Trinchieri, G. and Romagnani S. (1993). *J. Exp. Med.* **177**, 1199–1204.

Merberg, Dm., Wolf, Sf. and Clark, S.C. (1992). *Immunology Today* **13**(2), 77–78.

Mosmann, T.R. and Coffman, R.L. (1987). *Immunology Today* **8**, 223.

Mosmann, T.R., Cherwinski, W.M., Bond, M.W., Giedlin, M.A. and Coffman, R.L. (1986). *J. Immunol.* **136**, 2348.

Naume, B., Gately, M.K. and Espevik, T. (1992). *J. Immunol.* **148**, 2429–2436.

Perusia, B., Chan, S., D'Andrea, A., Tsuji, K., Santoli, D., Pospisil, M., Young, D., Wolf, S.F. and Trinchieri, G. (1992). *J. Immunol.* **149**, 3495–3502.

Podlaski, F.J., Nanduri, V.B., Hulmes, J.D., Pan, Y.E., Levin, W., Danho, W., Chizzonite, R., Gately, M.K. and Stern, A.S. (1992). *Archiv. Biochem. Biophys.* **294**, 230–237.

Rabinowich, H., Herberman, R. and Whiteside, T. (1993). *Cell. Immunol.* **152**(2), 481–498.

Roberts, K., Lotze, M.T. and Rosenburg, S.A. (1987). *Cancer Res.* **47**, 4366–4371.

Robertson, M.J., Soiffer, R.J., Wolf, S.F., Manley, T.J., Donahue, C., Young, D., Herrmann, S.H. and Ritz, J. (1992). *J. Exp. Med.* **175**, 779–788.

Schoenhaut, D.S., Chua, A.O., Wolitzky, A.G., Quinn, P.M., Dwyer, C.M., McComas, W., Familletti, P.C., Gately, M.K. and Gubler, U. (1992). *J. Immunol.* **148**, 3433–3440.

Scott, P. (1993). *Science* **260**, 496–497.

Sieburth, D., Jabs, E.W., Warrington, J.A., Li, X., Lasota, J., LaForgia, S., Kelleher, K., Huebner, K., Wasmuth, J.J. and Wolfe, S.F. (1992). *Genomics* **14**, 59–62.

Stern, A.S., Podlaski, F.J., Hulmes, J.D., Pan, Y.C., Quinn, P.M., Wolitzky, A.G., Familletti, P.C., Stremlo, D.L., Truitt, T., Chiszzonite, R. and Gately, M. (1990). *Proc. Natl Acad. Sci. USA* **87**, 6808–6812.

Tahara, H., Zeh, H.J.III, Storkus, W.J., Pappo, I., Watkins, S.C., Gubler, U., Wolf, S.F., Robbins, P.D. and Lotze, M. (1994). *Cancer Res.* **54**, 182–189.

Wolf, S.F., Temple, P.A., Kobayashi, M., Young, D., Dicig, M., Zlowe, L., Dzialo, R., Fitz, L., Ferenz, C., Hewick, R.M., Keller, K., Herrmann, S.H., Clark, S.C., Azzoni, L., Chan, S.H., Trinchieri, G. and Perussia, B. (1991). *J. Immunol.* **146**, 3074–3081.

Wong, H.L., Wilson, D.E., Jenson, J., Familletti, P., Stremlo, D. and Gately, M.K. (1987). *Cell. Immunol.* **111**, 39–54.

Zeh, H.J. III, Hurd, S., Storkus, W.J. and Lotze, M.T. (1993). *J. Immunother.* **14**, 155–161.

Chapter 14

Interleukins 13, 14 and 15

Angus W. Thomson and Michael T. Lotze

Departments of Surgery and Molecular Genetics and Biochemistry, University of Pittsburgh
Medical Center, Pittsburgh, Pennsylvania 15261, USA

INTRODUCTION

There are at least three more recently described cytokines (interleukins 13, 14 and 15) that were detailed well after writing assignments for the interleukins described in the preceding chapters had been completed. We have provided an overview below of each of these cytokines with the relevant recent literature citations.

INTERLEUKIN-13 (IL-13)

IL-13 is a recently described, pleiotropic cytokine produced primarily by activated Th2 cells in the mouse and human. It was formerly designated P600 (Cherwinski *et al.*, 1987; Brown *et al.*, 1989). P600 mRNA is expressed in the Th2 mouse lymphocyte subset, which also expresses mRNA for IL-3, IL-4, GM-CSF and IL-10. The IL-13 gene is inducible in a number of murine Th2 clones, but only in a few Th1 clones and is not inducible in fibroblasts (Brown *et al.*, 1989). IL-13 is secreted as mainly an unglycosylated protein of 132 amino acids with an Mr of 10 000 (McKenzie *et al.*, 1993a). The genomic structure of IL-13 has been determined both for mouse and human genes (McKenzie *et al.*, 1993b). Both loci contain 4 exons that comprise the entire coding region of each gene (Fig. 1). The IL-13 gene shares about 30% homology with the sequence for murine IL-4 but has no homology with other known cytokines. A 4.3-kb DNA fragment of the mouse IL-13 gene has been sequenced and occurs as a single copy mapping to chromosome 11. In the human, a 4.6-kb DNA segment of the IL-13 gene occurs as a single copy and maps to chromosome 5 (McKenzie *et al.*, 1993b). Potential recognition sequences for transcription factors in the 5′-flanking region that are conserved between the mouse and human genes include IFN-γ response elements, binding sites for AP-1, -2 and -3, and NF-IL-6 site and a TATA-like sequence. The clustering of genes encoding IL-13, IL-3, IL-4, IL-5 and GM-CSF to the same regions of murine chromosome 11 and human chromosome 5, respectively, suggests that IL-13 is another member of this cytokine gene family that may have arisen by gene duplication.

Both mouse and human IL-13 induce proliferation of the human premyeloid cell line TF-1. IL-13 also induces changes in the morphology of human monocytes and in the

The Cytokine Handbook, 2nd ed.
ISBN 0–12–689661–5

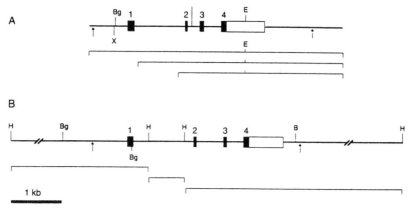

Fig. 1. Schematic representation and partial restriction map of the human (A) and mouse (B) IL-13 genes. ■ Represent exons 1 to 4; □ indicate untranslated sequences. Restriction fragments that were subcloned are indicated by bars below the diagram. Regions between the arrows were sequenced completely. E, EcoRI; B, BamHI; Bg, BgIII; H, HindIII; X, XhoI. Reproduced from McKenzie et al. (1993b) with permission of the authors and publishers of the Journal of Immunology.

phenotype both of human monocytes and B cells by upregulating expression of MHC class II and inducing expression of the low affinity receptor for IgE (Fc$_\varepsilon$ RII; CD23) (McKenzie et al., 1993a; Punnonen et al., 1993). IL-13 induces B-cell proliferation, affecting predominantly virgin sIgD$^+$ B cells (Defrance et al., 1994) and also induces IgE switching (Cocks et al., 1993). Its IgE-inducing activity suggests that IL-13 like IL-4, may be a regulator of IgE synthesis in atopic individuals. IL-13 also induces IL-4 independent IgG4 and IgE synthesis in the presence of T cell clones or CD40 ligand (Cocks et al., 1993; Punnonen et al., 1993). Thus IL-13 shares many of the activities of IL-4. One activity distinguishing the function of IL-13 and IL-4 is that whereas IL-4 antagonizes the human B cell response to IL-2, IL-13 potentiates the DNA synthesis elicited by this cytokine (Defrance et al., 1994). Further, it has been suggested that IL-13 stimulates IFN-γ release whereas IL-4 suppresses it.

It appears that IL-14 may be a potent and critical regulator of inflammatory and immune responses, particularly with regard to monocyte/macrophage function. Thus, treatment of activated murine macrophages or human monocytes with recombinant IL-13 inhibits the production of inflammatory cytokines (including IL-1 α/β, IL-6, IL-8, IL-10, IL-12 p35, IL-12 p40, MIP-1α, GM-CSF, IFN-α and TNFα) in response to IFN-γ or LPS (de Waal Malefyt et al., 1993; Doherty et al., 1993; Minty et al., 1993). In contrast, IL-13 (like IL-4 and IL-10) enhances the production of IL-1ra by LPS-activated human monocytes (de Waal Malefyt et al., 1993). Moreover, IL-13 decreases the production of nitric oxide by activated murine macrophages, leading to impaired parasiticidal activity (Doherty et al., 1993). It also strongly inhibits spontaneous, and IFN-γ- or IL-10-induced cytotoxic (ADCC) activity of human monocytes against anti-D-coated Rh$^+$ red blood cells. These effects of IL-13 on mononuclear phagocytes are similar to those of IL-4. No additive or synergistic effects of the two cytokines on human monocytes have been observed (de Waal Malefyt et al., 1993), suggesting that IL-13 and IL-4 may share common receptors. Human (h) IL-13 competitively inhibits binding of hIL-4 to functional hIL-4 receptors expressed on TF-1 cells that respond to both IL-4 and IL-13 (Zurawski *et al.*, 1993). This raises the possibility that IL-4R and IL-13R on TF-1 cells are the same. This is unlikely, however, as high levels of IL-13 do not inhibit binding of IL-4 to an IL-4 responsive cloned CD4$^+$T cell line (SP-B21) that does not respond to IL-13. These findings show that IL-13R and IL-4R are different but that the two receptors share a novel component that is important in signal transduction. IL-13 may bind to the common γ chain—a functional component shared by the IL-4 and IL-2 receptors (Russell *et al.*, 1993).

By blocking the production of proinflammatory cytokines and by inducing IL-1ra, IL-13 may (like IL-4 and IL-10) exert powerful anti-inflammatory activity. Moreover, inhibition of IL-10 and IL-12 by IL-13 could affect cross-regulation of Th1 and Th2 subsets, as IL-10 has been shown to be a suppressor of inflammatory (Th1) cytokines, whereas IL-12 has recently been shown to play a role in the development of Th1 cells.

Minty *et al.* (1993) have reported that IL-13 synergizes with IL-2 in upregulating IFN-γ synthesis in large granular lymphocytes (LGL), thus resembling in its action IL-12 rather than IL-4, which strongly inhibits IFN-γ synthesis by LGL. Thus, IL-13 is a highly pleiotropic cytokine that potently inhibits proinflammatory cytokine production by macrophages, stimulates antibody production and plays a 'Th2-type' role together with IL-4 and IL-10.

An inhibitory effect of human rIL-13 on HIV replication in primary tissue culture-derived human macrophages, but not blood lymphocytes, has been reported (Montaner *et al.*, 1993). This effect was not mediated by altered viral entry, reverse transcription or viral release. Conceivably, IL-13 treatment of HIV$^+$ subjects could inhibit viral dissemination and be of therapeutic value in combination with other forms of anti-viral treatment.

INTERLEUKIN-14 (IL-14)

IL-14 is a 53 kDa secreted protein with three potential N-linked glycosylation sites (Ambrus *et al.*, 1993) and evidenced sequence homology with the complement protein Bb. It was initially identified as a high molecular weight B cell growth factor (HMW-BCGF) derived from the human Burkitt's B lymphoma cell line, Namalva, and the human T-cell line, T-ALL (Ambrus and Fauci, 1985), but also found in supernatants derived from T-cell clones, T-T hybridomas, or mitogen-stimulated unfractionated peripheral lymphocytes. Like IL-4, this factor induces B cell proliferation activated by anti-μ, inhibits immunoglobulin secretion and expands certain B cell subpopulations selectively. It has an alkaline isoelectric point (6.7–7.8) when isolated by isoelectric focusing. A lower peak of biologic activity with a higher molecular mass of 200 kDa migrates at 4.8–5.9 and may represent a complex of the molecule with albumin (Ambrus *et al.*, 1985). IL-14 was prepared from Namalva cells stimulated with phytohaemagglutinin with mRNA reverse transcribed and a cDNA library screened with a monoclonal antibody (Ambrus *et al.*, 1985) to the factor. IL-14 appears to be produced by malignant B cells as well as normal and malignant T cells. Interestingly, this factor is unable to stimulate resting B cells and, unlike any of the other B cell factors (Clark *et al.*, 1989), is unable to induce antibody synthesis or secretion. It appears that only B lineage cells (Uckun *et al.*, 1989), including B cell precursor acute lymphoblastic leukaemia, hairy cell leukaemia cells, prolymphocytic leukaemia cells and chronic lymphocytic leukaemia (CLL) cells, have receptors for this factor. Approximately

```
        10        20        30        40        50                          10        20        30        40        50
1234567890 1234567890 1234567890 1234567890 1234567890           1234567890 1234567890 1234567890 1234567890 1234567890
CAACACCTTC AGAAATAATC CTTTGGGTGA TCTCTTGTCA ATCATTTGTG    50      AGCACTCAGG TCCTGTACCC TCTTGTTCAG GTCATTGCGC TCTGTCTGCA   1000
                                                                  A  L  R  S  C  T  L  L  F  R  S  L  R  S  V  C  S

CAGGCTAGAG AGGCACCTGT GAATGATAAG GCTACTGAGA AGCATCATTG   100      GTGCCCGGCA CAGCTTCTCC AGCCGGTTGGA TTTTTACCTG CAGGCCCTCC   1050
           M  I  R  L  L  R  S  I  I  G                            A  R  H  S  F  S  S  R  W  I  F  T  C  R  P  S

GCCTGGTTCCT GGCACTACCA AAGGGCAGGG GAAGGGATGC CAAGGGGCTC  150      AGTTCTTTAT CCCGGACTGT TTTCTCCTCA GCCATCTCAA GCAGGGCCTT   1100
 L  V  L  A  L [P  K  G  R  G  S  D  A  K  G  L]                   S  S  L  S  R  T  V  F  S  S  A  I  S  S  R  A  L

CTGACCAGCA CATCATCCCA CGCAAAAACA TTCTCCAGGT CCCTTGTTTC   200      GTTGCTGCTC TCCCACCGGG ACCGGTACAT GGTGGTTTCT TTCTCCAGGT   1150
 L  T  S  T  S  S  H  A  K  T  F  S [R  S  L  V] S                 L  L  L  S  H  R  D  R  Y  M  V  V  S  P  S  S  F

CAGGCAGGAA ATCCCCAGCT CTGAGCCCCC TGCCAGGCTC TGCCTAGGGA   250      TCTTGATCTT CTTAGTCATC TTTTCCATCT CCTGCTTGAA TGTGGTGAAT   1200
 R  Q  E  I  P  S  S  E  R  P  A  R  L  C  L  G  T                 L  I  F  L  V  I  F  S  I  S  C  L  N  V  V  N

CACCTTTTCT CAGGTCTAGA GAAGTCAAAG TGAGCCTGCC AGAGCAGCTA   300      ACCTCGCTGC TTTTGGAAAG TGTGTTCTGG AACTCCTCCA ACTTCTCTGT   1250
 P  F  L  R  S  R  E  V  K  V  S  L  P  E  Q  L                    T  S  L  L  L  E  S  V  F  W  N  S  S  N  F  S  V

GGAGGGCCTG AGCTGGAACCT AAGCAAGCCC TGCTCATCAA GACAAATGCA  350      GTATAGGGCA AGCTGTTGCT TCAGGTGGGT CTCTTGCTGC TTCATCAGCT   1300
 G  G  P  E  L  D  L  S  K  P  C  S  S  R  Q  M (Q                 Y  R  A  S  C  C  F  R  W  V  S  C  C  F  I  S  S

GTTCAATGAC CTGGGTGTAT TACTTGTCGT GAGCTCTGAA GGGCAGGGAG   400      CACACATCCT CTGGGACTGT ACTGCCTCTT TCAGGAGAAA ATCCTTCTCC   1350
 F  N  D  L  G  V  L  L) V  L  S  S  E  G  Q  G  G                 H  I  L  W  D  S  T  A  S  F  R  R  K  S  F  S

GGGTCATGGA GCCTCAAAGT CAGACAGAGA AATGCTCAAG TCACTTCTGC   450      CGCTGGTGCC GCTCTTCTGC CTCCTTTAGC ATCTCCTGGG CCTGCTGGAG   1400
 V  I  E  P  Q  S  Q  T  E  K  C  S  S  H  F  C                    R  W  C  R  S  S  A  S  F  S  I  S  W  A  C  W  S

CAACTCACTG TGATGGCAAC TACAGATGAC AGCCCCTCTC AAGACTCTTC   500      CTTGGCATCC ACCAGCTGCT GTTGTAGGTC CTTGTGTTTG AAGACTTTGT   1450
 Q  L  T  V  M (A  A  T  D  D  S  P  S) Q  D  S  S                 L  A  S  T  S  C  C  C  R  S  L  C  L  K  T  L  S

AGCTCACAGA CAAGCCACTG ACTTCATCTG TACACACCCC CATCCCCAAT   550      CGATATGCTC CTCGCGCAGC TCATACTGCT CAATCAGCTT CTTGAGCCTC   1500
 A  H  R  Q  A  T  D  F  I  C  T  H  P  H  P  Q  C                 I  C  S  S  R  S  S  Y  C  S  I  S  F  L  S  L

GCAAGCTCCA CTGTACACTT ACAGGTATAA ATGCATTTGC AAGGCCTTGC   600      TCAGCCAGCT CCATGTTCTC TTGGCGCAGC TTGGAGTTGC GCTCATTGTG   1550
 K  L  H  C  T  L  T  G  I  N  A  F  A  R  P  C                    S  A  S  S  M  F  S  W  R  S  L  E  L  R  S  L  C

AAAATGCCCT ATGTACGTAA AACTGACCCA CAAAAGTGCC AAAATTGCAA   650      CTGTTCCATC TGCAGCTGAA TGTCATTCAG TGTCACCTGG AAGTGCGAGG   1600
 K  M [P  Y  V  R  K  T  D  P  Q  K] C  Q  N  C  K                 C  S  I  C  S

GTGCCAGATG CCAGCCAGGT CAGAACGTGC CTGGCTTCAG CAATGGGCTG   700      TCACCTCCTT GGGCTTCTCC TCCTCCTCCC GGGCCCGCTG CACACCTTCT   1650
 C  Q  M  P  A  R  S  E  H  A  W  L  Q  Q  W  A  A

CTCAGCATGG GAGCCTTTTA TGGGCCAGGC TGGCTGGGCT GCGGCTCCCT   750      TCCTTGAGGG AGCGGTTGTG CCCGTGCAGC TCACGGCATA GGCTCTCAAG   1700
 Q  H  G  S  L  L  W  A  R  L  A  G  L  P  L  P

TCCCAGCATG ACCCAACACC AGGCTCTCTA GGCCCTGGGG GAGGTGGGCT   800      CTTGCTGCGG GCCAGGACGG CTTGCTGTGC TCACGCGGCA GGTGGTCCTT   1750
 S  Q  H  D  P  T  P  G  S  L  G  P  G  G  G  G  L

CTTGAGCCCA GTCTGGCCTG ATGCTTCTGT GCTCGGTTGC TCCTGGGTAG   850      CTCTTGCACC AGCTGGCTCT GCTTTTTCTG TAGGAGCTTC ATCTGCTTAC   1800
 L  R  P  V  W  P  D  A  S  V  L  G  C  S  W  V  A

CAAGGGGCTT CTGGTGACCCT GGGGAGCTG GGTGCTTGAT GCCCCAGTGC   900      ACATCCTCTG GGACTCTACT GCCTCTTTCA GGAGAAAATC CTTCTCCCGC   1850
 R  R  F  C  D  P  G  G  A  G  C  L  M (P  Q  C

CCCTCTGGCC TCCTCTCAGG GCCACTGTCA GTGAGGGGAGC CCTGGCCACC  950      TGATTTCCAT                                              1860
 P  S  G  L  L  S) G  P  L  S  V  R  E  P  W  P  P
```

Fig. 2. cDNA sequence from the pI 7.8-HMW-BCGF clone 210B. The signal peptide is underlined. Amino acid sequence that is consistent with sequence from native HMW-BCGF in brackets; amino acid sequence that is consistent with sequence from recombinant HMW-BCGF is in parentheses. In both cases, deduced amino acids that do not agree with amino acids from sequencing MHW-BCGF protein are underlined twice. Potential N-linked glycosylation sites are indicated with arrowheads. Reproduced from Ambrus *et al.* (1993) with permission of the authors and publishers of *Proc. Natl. Acad. Sci. USA.*

60% of CLL cells express the receptor for IL-14 and proliferate in response to it. Approximately 3000 receptors exist on the surface of CLL cells with an apparent K_a of 4.6×10^7 M^{-1} and a molecular mass of 90 kDa. Receptor/ligand binding is associated with a modest increase in intracellular calcium (Ambrus *et al.*, 1991). It may be that the major role of IL-14 is to select or expand a subpopulation of memory B cells. The sequence shown in Fig. 2 is in the GenBank data base (accession no. L15344).

INTERLEUKIN-15 (IL-15)

There are now several T-cell growth factors, many of which have activity on the murine CTLL line originally isolated by Steve Gillis and colleagues. IL-15, another factor capable of inducing proliferation of CTLL, is produced by a large number of different cell types and shares many of the activities of IL-2. A major exception is its inability to bind to the α chain of the IL-2 receptor. Like the other major T-cell (IL-2, IL-4, IL-7, IL-13) growth factors (Aversa et al., 1993; Kondo et al., 1993; Noguchi et al., 1993; Russell et al., 1993;) it appears likely that the γ chain of the IL-2 receptor is utilized by this cytokine. IL-15 was originally identified in the supernatants of a kidney epithelial cell line, CV1/EBNA (a predecessor to COS) and found to induce proliferation of CTLL cells (Grabstein et al., 1994). The protein was partially purified and found to have a molecular mass of 14 to 15 kDa. Amino terminal sequencing was performed and then degenerate oligonucleotide primers used to PCR amplify a 92 base pair cDNA fragment. This was subsequently used to probe a plasmid library prepared from the CV1 EBNA and finally a full length of cDNA clone was isolated encoding a 162 amino

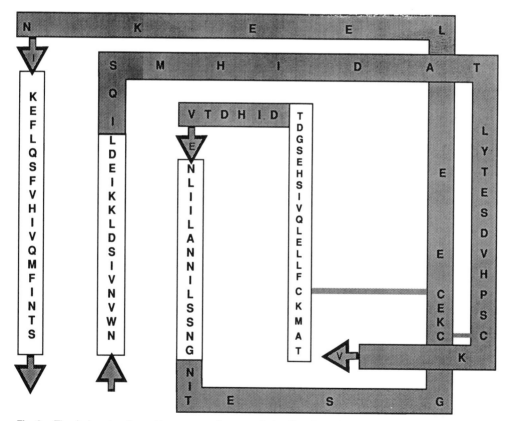

Fig. 3. The deduced amino acid sequence of mature simian IL-15 in a schematic representing its predicted folding topology, with four helices (▭) in an up-up-down-configuration, three loops connecting the helices (←), with two disulphide crosslinks (▬) as suggested by homology modelling of IL-15 built with the crystal structure of IL-2 as template using FOLDER. (Reproduced with permission from Grabstein et al., 1994.)

acid precursor polypeptide with an extremely long 48 amino acid leader sequence. The protein has no significant homology to other proteins in Genbank or EMBL. Analysis of the predicted secondary structure of IL-15 reveals that, like IL-2, it is a member of the helical cytokine family with four helical bundles. Two disulphide cross-links are incorporated at Cys42-Cys88 (homologous to IL-2) and Cys35-Cys91 (Fig. 3). The simian IL-15 cDNA was used to probe a human library and a human cDNA containing a 316 base pair 5′ noncoding region, an open reading frame of 486-bp and a 400-bp 3′ noncoding region. Surprisingly, Northern blot studies revealed widespread expression of IL-15, most abundantly in placenta and skeletal muscle but also in kidney, lung, liver and heart. IL-15 message was observed in PBMC enriched in monocytes cultured for 4 h in LPS as well as freshly isolated peripheral blood mononuclear cells. It appears that the predominant sources of IL-15 are monocytes and epithelial cells.

Recombinant IL-15 produced in yeast demonstrated that IL-15 stimulated CTLL and that this was inhibited by antibody to the β chain of the IL-2 receptor. The nonglycosylated recombinant protein is 2–3 fold more active than the fully glycosylated molecule (Grabstein, K., personal communication). It enhances the cytolytic activity of antigen-specific T cells and lymphokine-activated killer cells but does not stimulate the proliferation of 32D, an IL-3 dependent cell line which normally responds very well to IL-2. The sequence for simian IL-15 has been submitted to GenBank EMBL with the accession number U03099.

REFERENCES

Ambrus, J.L., Chesky, L., McFarland, P., Young, K.R., Mostowski, H., August, A. and Chused, T.M. (1991). Cell Immunol. 134, 314–324.

Ambrus, J.L. and Fauci, A.S. (1985) J. Clin. Invest. 75, 732–739.

Ambrus, J.L., Jurgenssen, C.H., Brown, E.J. and Fauci, A.S. (1985). J. Exp. Med. 162, 1319–1335.

Ambrus, J.L., Pippin, J., Joseph, A., Xu, C., Blumenthal, D., Tamayo, A., Claypool, K., McCourt, D., Srikiatchatochorn, A. and Ford, R.J. (1993). Proc. Natl. Acad. Sci. USA 90, 6330–6334.

Aversa, G., Punnonen, J., Cocks, B.G., de Waal Malefyt, R., Vega, F., Zurawski, S.M., Zurawski, G. and de Vries, J.E. (1993). J. Exp. Med. 178, 2213–2218.

Brown, K.D., Zurawski, S.M., Mosmann, T.R. and Zurawski, G. (1989). J. Immunol. 142, 679–687.

Cherwinski, H.M., Schumacher, J.H., Brown, K.D. and Mossmann, T.R. (1987). J. Exp. Med. 166, 1229–1244.

Clark, E.A., Shu, G.L., Luscher, B., Draves, D.E., Banchereau, J., Ledbetter, J.A. and Valentine, M.A. (1989). J. Immunol. 143, 3873–3880.

Cocks, B.G., de Waal Malefyt, R., Galizzi, J.P., de Vries, J.E. and Aversa, G. (1993). International Immunology 5, 657–663.

Defrance, T., Carayon, P., Billian, G., Guillemot, J.-C., Minty, A., Caput, D. and Ferrara, P. (1994). J. Exp. Med. 179, 135–143.

de Waal Malefyt, R., Figdor, C.G., Huijbens, R., Mohan-Peterson, S., Bennett, B., Culpepper, J., Dang, W., Zurawski, G. and de Vries, J.E. (1993) J. Immunol. 151, 6370–6381.

Doherty, T.M., Kastelein, R., Menon, S., Andrade, S. and Coffman, R.L. (1993). J. Immunol. 151, 7151–7160.

Grabstein, K., Shanebeck, K., Rauch, C., Srinivasan, S., Fung, V., Beers, C., Richardson, J., Schoenborn, M.A., King, J., Johnson, L., Giri, J.G., Alderson, M.R., Watson, J.D., Anderson, D.M. and Eisenman, J. (1994). Science In press.

Kondo, M., Takeshita, T., Ishii, N., Nakamura, M., Watanabe, S., Arai, K. and Sugamura, K. (1993). Science 262, 1874–1877.

McKenzie, A.N.J., Culpepper, J.A., de Waal Malefyt, R., Briere, F., Punnonen, J., Aversa, G., Sato, A., Dang, W., Cocks, B.G., Menon, S., De Vries, J.E., Banchereau, J. and Zurawski, G. (1993a). Proc. Natl. Acad. USA 90, 3735–3739.

McKenzie, A.N.J., Li, X., Largaespada, D.A., Sato, A., Kaneda, A., Zurawski, S.M., Doyle, E.L., Milatovich, A., Francke, U., Copeland, N.G., Jenkins, N.A. and Zurawski, G. (1993b). *J. Immunol.* **150**, 5436–5444.

Minty, A., Chalon, P., Derocq, J.M., Dumont, X., Guillemont, J.C., Kaghad, M., Labit, C., Leplatois, P., Liauzun, P., Miloux, B., Monty, C., Casellas, P., Loison, G., Lupker, J., Shire, D., Ferrara, P. and Caput, D. (1993). *Nature* **362**, 248–250.

Montaner, L.J., Doyle, A.G., Collins, M., Herbein, G., Illei, P., James, W., Minty, A., Caput,, D., Ferrara, P. and Gordon, S. (1993). *J. Exp. Med.* **178**, 743–747.

Noguchi, M., Nakamura, Y., Russell, S.M., Ziegler, S.F., Tsang, M., Cao, X. and Leonard, W.J. (1993). *Science* **262**, 1877–1880.

Punnonen, J., Aversa, G., Cocks, B.G., McKenzie, A.N.J., Menon, S., Zurawski, G., de Waal Malefyt, R. and de Vries, J.E. (1993). *Proc. Natl. Acad. Sci. USA* **90**, 3730–3734.

Russell, S.M., Keegan, A.D., Harada, N., Nakamura, Y., Noguchi, M., Leland, P., Friedmann, M.C., Miyajima, A., Puri, R.K., Paul, W.E. and Leonard, W.J. (1993). *Science* **262**, 1880–1883.

Uckun, F.M., Fauci, A.S., Chandan-Langlie, M., Myers, D.E. and Ambrus, J.L. (1989). *J. Clin. Invest.* **84**, 1595–1608.

Zurawski, S.M., Vega, Jr., F., Huyghe, B. and Zurawski, G. (1993). *EMBO J.* **12**, 2663–2670.

Chapter 15

Interferons

Edward De Maeyer and Jaqueline De Maeyer-Guignard

CNRS-URA 1343, Institut Curie, Université de Paris-Sud, Orsay, France

INTRODUCTION

Interferons (IFNs) are major contributors to the first line of antiviral defence, which by itself is sufficient to make them of great interest, but they exert many other important effects on cells in addition to inhibiting virus replication. They belong to the network of cytokines that are involved in the control of cellular function and replication and that become actively engaged in host defence during an infection. Since the first edition of this chapter, considerable progress has been made in our knowledge of the IFN receptors and our understanding of the molecular mechanisms of IFN induction and of signal transduction in IFN-activated cells.

STRUCTURE OF INTERFERONS

Type I IFNs are all derived from the same ancestral gene and have still sufficient structural homology to act via the same cell-surface receptor. They comprise IFN-α, IFN-ω, IFN-β and IFN-τ (trophoblast IFN) (see Table 1). The latter species has only been described in cattle and sheep. Type II IFN- or IFN-γ is a lymphokine that displays no molecular homology with type I IFNs, but shares some important biologic activities.

IFN-α, IFN-ω and IFN-β

The Human IFN-α, IFN-ω and IFN-β Gene Cluster
There are at least 13 nonallelic genes coding for structurally different forms of human IFN-α. The IFN-α genes encode mature proteins of 165 or 166 amino acids, and the IFN-ω gene encodes a mature protein of 172 amino acids. IFN-ω shares about 60% of its amino acid sequence with the various species of IFN-α, and only about 30% with IFN-β. Unlike the majority of structural genes in the human genome, including the genes for all other cytokines, the IFN-α, IFN-ω and IFN-β genes lack introns, a feature they share with all other known mammalian IFN-α and IFN-β genes. It has been estimated that IFN-α and IFN-ω genes diverged more than 100 million years ago, prior to the mammalian radiation.

The Cytokine Handbook, 2nd ed.
ISBN 0–12–689661–5

Table 1. Characteristics of human and murine IFN-α, ω and β genes.

	IFN-α	IFN-ω	IFN-β
Human			
Number of amino acids	165 or 166	172	166
Number of structural genes coding for active proteins	At least 13	1	1
Gene designation and chromosomal localization	IFNA 9p21-pter	IFNW 9p21-pter	IFNB 9p21-pter
Murine			
Number of amino acids	166 or 167 (IFN-α_4: 161)	No IFN-ω genes described	161
Number of structural genes coding for active proteins	At least 12		1
Gene designation and chromosomal localization	Ifa 4		Ifb 4

In bovines and sheep, in addition to IFN-α/β and ω, a fourth class, IFN-τ, has been described. The genes coding for these four IFN species belong to the same gene cluster.

In contrast to the many genes coding for the different IFN-α species, there is only a single gene coding for human IFN-β. The mature peptide contains 166 amino acids and the significant degree of homology between human IFN-α and IFN-β—about 30% at the amino acid and 45% at the nucleotide level—suggests that the genes are derived from a common ancestor by gene duplication.

The human IFN-α, IFN-ω and IFN-β genes are clustered in the same chromosomal region, on the short arm of chromosome 9. The IFN-α and IFN-ω genes are interspersed, and the IFN-β gene is situated distal from the IFN-α/ω cluster (Owerbach *et al.*, 1981; Shows *et al.*, 1982; Slate *et al.*, 1982; Trent *et al.*, 1982; Weissmann and Weber, 1986; De Maeyer and De Maeyer-Guignard, 1988).

The Murine IFN-α/β Gene Cluster

At least 12 nonallelic intronless genes have been identified in the murine IFN-α gene family. Eleven different genes have been cloned and expressed into biologically active proteins. Murine IFN-ω genes have not yet been described.

The general structure of the murine IFN-α genes is comparable to that of the corresponding human genes. The mature proteins contain 166 or 167 amino acids (except for murine IFN-α4, which has a five-codon deletion between codons 102 and 108), and the maximum divergence for replacement sites is about 13% (Kelley and Pitha, 1985a,b; Le Roscouet *et al.*, 1985; Ryals *et al.*, 1985; Seif and Maeyer-Guignard, 1986).

The single-copy, intronless murine IFN-β gene codes for a mature protein consisting of 161 residues, with three potential N-glycosylation sites at position 29, 69 and 76, which explains the difference between the 17 kDa molecular mass calculated from the amino acid sequence and the apparent molecular mass of about 28–35 kDa for natural murine IFN-β. The amino acid sequence displays 48% homology with that of human IFN-β.

Like the human IFN genes, the murine IFN-α genes and the IFN-β gene are clustered on murine chromosome 4, with the IFN-β gene distal from the IFN-α cluster (Dandoy *et al.*, 1984; De Maeyer and Dandoy, 1987).

IFN-τ

In sheep and cattle, a novel type I IFN, called trophoblast IFN or IFN-τ, has been identified. These IFNs are the major secretory products of the trophoblast of ruminant ungulates during pregnancy, in the period immediately preceding attachment and implantation of the fertilized ovum. Trophoblast IFNs share most of the biologic activities of other type I IFNs but are poorly responsive to viral induction; their major function is to create the conditions for efficient implantation of the ovum. Bovine trophoblast IFN shows more homology with bovine IFN-ω than with bovine IFN-α (Roberts *et al.*, 1991).

IFN-γ

Human IFN-γ

The single-copy human IFN-γ gene differs significantly from the human IFN-α and IFN-β structural genes, with which it shares no obvious sequence homology and no obvious evolutionary relationship. The gene, situated on chromosome 12, contains three introns; the four exons code for a polypeptide of 166 amino acids, 20 of which constitute the signal peptide (Devos *et al.*, 1982; Gray and Goeddel, 1982; Gray *et al.*, 1982; Naylor *et al.*, 1983).

Murine IFN-γ

Like the human IFN-γ gene, the murine IFN-γ gene contains four exons and three introns. The coding part of the gene displays an overall nucleotide homology with the human gene of about 65%; the overall protein homology is 40%. Mature murine IFN-γ has 136 amino acids (Gray and Goeddel, 1982). The murine IFN-γ structural gene (Ifg locus) is on chromosome 10 (Naylor *et al.*, 1984).

INDUCTION OF IFN SYNTHESIS

Induction of IFN-α and IFN-β

The production of IFN-α and IFN-β is not a specialized cell function, and probably all cells of the organism are capable of producing these IFNs. Most cells, whether in the organism or in culture, do not release measurable amounts of IFN-α/β. However, spontaneous IFN production has frequently been observed in cultures of cells derived from the haemopoietic system (as reviewed in De Maeyer and De Maeyer-Guignard, 1988), and there is a low level of constitutive IFN synthesis in murine BALB/c 3T3 cells (Seif *et al.*, 1991). Since growth factors and other cytokines can induce IFN-α and IFN-β, it is possible that very low levels of some IFN species are made by many cells during a certain period of the cell cycle. Indeed, low levels of human IFN-α1 and IFN-α2 mRNA are constitutively transcribed in spleen, liver, kidney and peripheral-blood lymphocytes of normal individuals, and *in situ* hybridization has shown that IFN-α and IFN-β genes are actively transcribed in normal murine bone marrow and peritoneal cells (Friedman-Einat *et al.*, 1982; Tovey *et al.*, 1987; Proietti *et al.*, 1992).

If cells either do not normally produce, or at the most produce a very low level of IFN-α/β, exposure to a variety of agents triggers the production and secretion of IFN-α or IFN-β, or of a mixture of both. IFN was discovered during the study of viral interference (Isaacs and Lindenmann, 1957), and viruses are the most efficient natural inducers of IFN-α/β, but other infectious agents can also induce IFN. Many bacteria, especially those that replicate inside animal cells such as *Listeria monocytogenes*, induce IFN-α/β during systemic infection of the host. Endotoxin, the lipopolysaccharide derived from the cell walls of Gram-negative bacteria, and the M proteins of group A Streptococci are also IFN inducers; IFN induction by bacterial endotoxin takes place mainly in macrophages.

Induction by Double-stranded RNA and Viruses
Both natural and synthetic double-stranded RNAs (dsRNAs) induce IFN-α/β with high efficiency (Field *et al.*, 1967). Of the synthetic polynucleotides, the homopolymer pair polyrI:rC is the most active and the most widely used for induction studies.

Despite their differences in structure and mode of replication, all animal viruses can induce IFN production under appropriate conditions and a unifying hypothesis would be the formation of dsRNA as a common pathway for induction. For RNA viruses, there are many arguments in favour of dsRNA as an essential intermediate for IFN induction; one of the most compelling is the demonstration with vesicular stomatitis virus particles that viral dsRNA generated within the cell is the actual trigger for IFN production. Theoretical considerations suggest that a single molecule of dsRNA is sufficient for induction (Sekellick and Marcus, 1982).

DNA viruses, as a rule, are less efficient IFN inducers than are RNA viruses, and although the formation of dsRNA has been demonstrated during the replication of vaccinia virus and adenovirus (Colby and Duesberg, 1969; Petterson and Philipson, 1974), for many other DNA viruses there is no direct evidence for the formation of dsRNA during their replicative cycle. It is therefore quite possible that other, as yet uncharacterized, molecules generated during virus replication are involved in stimulating the transcription of IFN genes.

Induction by Growth Factors and Other Cytokines
Several growth factors and cytokines have been shown to induce the synthesis of IFN-α and IFN-β. For example, stimulation of murine bone-marrow cells with CSF-1 results in the production of murine IFN-α/β (Moore *et al.*, 1984). Two other cytokines, IL-1 and TNF, induce the synthesis of human IFN-β in human diploid fibroblasts, and IL-2 can induce the production of murine IFN-α/β in mouse bone-marrow cells (Reis *et al.*, 1989). IFN-γ can also sometimes act as an inducer of IFN-α or of IFN-β (Hughes and Baron, 1987; Gessani *et al.*, 1989).

Induction of IFN-γ

In contrast to IFN-α and IFN-β synthesis, which can occur in any cell, production of IFN-γ is a function of T cells and of NK cells. All IFN-γ inducers activate T cells either in a polyclonal (mitogens or antibodies) or in a clonally restricted, antigen-specific, manner.

Cells of the Cytotoxic/Suppressor Phenotype (Human CD8 or Murine Ly-2 Phenotype)
Both in humans and in mice, IFN-γ synthesis has been observed in T cells of the cytotoxic/suppressor phenotype, bearing either the CD8 or the Ly-2 antigen, respectively. T cells expressing the CD8 antigen, isolated from individuals after an infection with influenza virus or after immunization against rabies virus, are stimulated to release IFN-γ when exposed to the corresponding viral antigens *in vitro* (Celis *et al.*, 1986; Yamada *et al.*, 1986). Similarly, cells from a line of cytotoxic T cells derived from BALB/c mice immunized with influenza virus, react specifically against influenza virus-infected target cells in an MHC-restricted way and release IFN-γ (Morris *et al.*, 1982; Taylor *et al.*, 1985).

Cells of the T-Helper Phenotype (Human CD4 or Murine L3T4 Phenotype)
IFN-γ is produced during infection, since antigen specific IFN-γ-producing circulating T cells of the helper phenotype are found in patients with recurrent herpes labialis (Cunningham *et al.*, 1985). Similarly, rabies virus-specific, MHC class II restricted, IFN-γ-producing T-helper cells are present in rabies vaccine recipients (Celis *et al.*, 1986).

Based on the array of lymphokines secreted, two different subsets of mouse Th cells have been described. Th1 cells secrete IL-2, IL-3, TNF-β and IFN-γ, whereas Th2 cells mainly produce IL-3, IL-4, IL-5 and IL-10, but little or no IFN-γ (Mosmann *et al.*, 1986). IFN-γ preferentially inhibits the proliferation of Th2 but not Th1 cells, indicating that the presence of IFN-γ during an immune response will result in the preferential proliferation of Th1 cells (Gajewski and Fitch, 1988). Evidence that IFN-γ is one of the natural regulators that limit proliferation of T-cell clones has been provided by a comparison of the rate of proliferation of mitogen-stimulated splenocytes derived from normal and from gene knock-out mice lacking a functional IFN-γ gene (Dalton *et al.*, 1993).

Distinction between self and nonself is one of the major operating principles of the immune system and the two major mechanisms involved in self-tolerance are intrathymic deletion and peripheral inactivation of naive T cells. Recently, a third mechanism, involving IFN-γ production, has been proposed, based on the observation that, in Th1 cells, ligation of the T-cell receptor in the absence of costimulatory signals from accessory cells can lead to cell death via IFN-γ production (Liu and Janeway, 1990).

The Molecular Mechanism of IFN-α/β Induction

Like the expression of many other genes, production of IFN-α and IFN-β is controlled both at the transcriptional and the post-transcriptional levels. Upon induction, transcription starts rapidly, reaches a peak and is then terminated, despite the continuous presence of the inducer. The cause of the shut-off of IFN synthesis is unknown: it is unlikely that a negative feedback by IFN is responsible for the arrest of transcription, since treatment of cells, even with very high doses of IFN-α/β, increases rather than decreases polyI-C-induced IFN synthesis (De Maeyer-Guignard *et al.*, 1980).

Although very often IFN-α and IFN-β are induced coordinately, cell-determined selective induction of either IFN-α or IFN-β can occur. Such cell-determined selective induction could be due to differential transcription of the IFN genes, to differential post-transcriptional processing of mRNA, or to a combination of both. There is good evidence that differential transcription is involved, since the ratio of IFN-α to IFN-β mRNA transcripts, as well as the proportion of individual IFN-α mRNAs, varies significantly with cell type as well as with the inducer (Hiscott *et al.*, 1985; Raj *et al.*, 1991), but post-transcriptional mechanisms can also be operative (Mosca *et al.*, 1992). The comparative analysis of the promoter regions of the IFN-β gene and the different IFN-α genes and their corresponding positive and negative transcriptional regulators which is presently being carried out in several laboratories shows that there can be significant differences between the various promoters that regulate the expression of IFN genes (MacDonald *et al.*, 1990). The extreme example of this is the promoter of the bovine trophoblast IFNs (IFN-τ), which, although still virus-inducible, is functionally quite distinct from other IFN-ω genes and contains a region that directs trophoblast-specific expression (Cross and Roberts, 1991; Hansen *et al.*, 1991).

Regulation of Human IFN-α/β Gene Expression

Several sequences of the IFN-α1 and IFN-β gene-promoter regions responsible for induction have been delineated, and transcriptional activators and repressors specific for these regions have been characterized. The same transcriptional factors are sometimes designated by different names, depending on the group that described them.

The regulatory region of the IFN-β gene spans about 200 bp immediately upstream from the transcription start site. A minimal sequence, necessary for virus induction and called IRE (IFN-response element) or VRE (virus-response element) has been described by Goodbourn and Maniatis (1988). The complete viral induction region spans the region from -125 to -38. This region contains an array of overlapping positive and negative regulatory domains, comprising at least four positive regulatory domains (PRDI to IV). Each domain contains binding sites for one or several transcriptional regulators, and at least two of the domains are also implicated in post-transcriptional shut-off (Goodbourn and Maniatis, 1988; Fan and Maniatis, 1989; Lenardo *et al.*, 1989). PRDI contains two copies of the hexamer sequence AAGTG(A/G), and the PRDII domain contains a recognition site GGGAAATTCC for the NF-κB transcription factor which probably explains why many agents that can activate NFκB are IFN-inducers (Hiscott *et al.*, 1989; Lenardo and Baltimore, 1989; Xanthoudakis *et al.*, 1989). Two negative regulatory domains, NRDI (-79 to -39) and NRDII (-168 to -94) are possibly implicated in the normal repression of IFN gene expression, but this remains to be unequivocally established (Zinn and Maniatis, 1986).

Several transcriptionally regulatory proteins that interact with the PRDI have been characterized. Of these, IRF-1 (also called ISGF2) acts as a transcriptional activator, and IRF-2 can function as a repressor of IRF-1-activated expression. IRF-2 is probably involved in pre- and postinduction silencing of the IFN-β gene. The gene coding for IRF-1 is not only inducible by viruses or dsRNA, but its expression is also stimulated by TNF, IL-1 and by IFN-β (Goodbourn *et al.*, 1985; Miyamoto *et al.*, 1988; Fujita *et al.*, 1989a,b,c; Harada *et al.*, 1989; Price *et al.*, 1990; Palombella and Maniatis, 1992; Sims *et al.*, 1993). Interestingly, constitutive expression of the IRF-1-/ISGF2 gene, obtained in cells transfected with this gene, causes resistance to infection with several different viruses (Pine, 1992). Another protein that interacts with PRDI, PRDI-BF1, has been identified as a postinduction repressor (Keller and Maniatis, 1991).

The analysis of the molecular mechanisms of IFN-β gene regulation is thus revealing a multitude of transcriptional activators and repressors, and the complexity of their interaction is, for the time being, only partly understood. Many of the factors characterized are also involved in the expression control of other genes, and the knowledge gained from the study of IFN gene regulation has implications for the understanding of gene regulation in general.

INTERFERON RECEPTORS

IFN-α and IFN-β Receptors

The existence of specific cell-surface receptors for IFN-α and IFN-β has been demonstrated in mice and in humans. In both species, IFN-α and IFN-β compete for the same binding sites whereas IFN-γ has a separate binding site (Aguet *et al.*, 1982). In humans, IFN-ω also binds to the α/β receptor (Flores *et al.*, 1991).

There are sufficient structural homologies between IFN-α, IFN-ω and IFN-β to allow for common receptor-binding domains, and nothing is unusual in the fact that they share a common receptor since these IFN species evolved from the same ancestral gene. Competitive receptor-binding experiments using several human IFN-α subspecies also indicate that they share the same receptors, but that they can have significantly different binding affinities (Aguet *et al.*, 1984; Uzé *et al.*, 1990).

The IFN-α/β Receptor

The cDNA coding for the human IFN-α/β receptor codes for a 590-amino-acid protein, corresponding to a size of about 66 kDa. The extracellular N-terminal part of the molecule contains two distinct 200-amino-acid domains, which suggests that it belongs to the cytokine receptor family, possibly derived from an ancestor gene common with the immunoglobulin superfamily. Binding studies carried out with different IFN-α subtypes as well as an analysis using anti-receptor monoclonal antibodies strongly suggest that, to ensure complete binding activity, accessory proteins have to associate with the receptor chain. The exact position of the IFNAR locus is on the distal part of the long arm of chromosome 21, in the 21q22.1 band; it contains 11 exons and is one of the more polymorphic loci of this chromosomal region (Lutfalla *et al.*, 1990; Uzé *et al.*, 1990; Benoît *et al.*, 1993).

A cDNA sequence coding for the 590-amino-acid murine IFN-α/β receptor has been isolated and expressed. The overall organization of the human and murine IFN receptor protein appears similar, in that the putative extracellular domain of the murine receptor also appears to be organized in two 200-amino-acid domains. As is the case for other receptors of the cytokine receptor family, accessory intracytoplasmic proteins are probably required for a full activity of the receptor (Uzé *et al.*, 1992).

Downregulation of the IFN-α/β receptor occurs after interaction of IFNs with their receptors as has been described, for example, after the binding of human IFN-β to Daudi cells (Branca and Baglioni, 1982; Lau *et al.*, 1986). When the receptor is bypassed by micro-injecting IFN-α or IFN-β directly into the cytoplasm or into the nucleus, no antiviral state is induced (Huez *et al.*, 1983; Rivière and De Maeyer-Guignard, 1990).

The IFN-γ Receptor

IFN-γ binds to a species-specific glycoprotein cell-surface receptor consisting, both in humans and mice, of a 228-amino-acid extracellular domain, a single transmembrane domain, and an intracellular domain of 222 amino acids for the human receptor and 200 amino acids for the murine receptor. To be functionally active, the human IFN-γ receptor requires the presence of at least two other components, the IFN-γ-binding protein, whose structural gene is on a different chromosome, and a species-specific signal-transducing factor, encoded by a gene on chromosome 21 in humans and on chromosome 16 in mice. Studies using various combinations of chimaeric human–mouse hybrid receptors show that the intracellular species-specific factor must interact with the extracellular domain of the receptor to generate an internal signal after ligand binding (Gray *et al.*, 1989; Hemmi *et al.*, 1989; Kumar *et al.*, 1989; Farrar *et al.*, 1991; Gibbs *et al.*, 1991; Hibino *et al.*, 1991, 1992; Kalina *et al.*, 1993).

   Recently, mice with a disrupted IFN-γ receptor gene that have no longer a functional IFN-γ receptor have been obtained. These mice have no overt anomalies, and their immune system appears to develop normally. However, the animals showed decreased resistance when challenged with an intercellular parasite such as *L. monocytogenes* and also after infection with vaccinia virus, the latter despite an apparently normal development of cell-mediated immunity against this virus (Huang *et al.*, 1993).

THE IFN SIGNALLING PATHWAY

Many genes are transcriptionally activated in IFN-treated cells, and a short summary of some important IFN-induced genes and of some important biologic activities is given in Tables 2 and 3. A *cis*-acting DNA element, called ISRE (IFN-stimulated response element), common to the promoters of IFN-α, IFN-β and of some IFN-γ-stimulated genes, mediates the transcriptional response. The core ISRE is 13 bp long and is highly conserved among the many IFN-induced genes, but there is no obvious homology in the sequences flanking them. Over the past 2 years, great progress has been made towards our understanding of gene activation by IFN-α. Several transcriptional activators involved in the signal transduction from the IFN receptor to the IFN-induced genes have been characterized and cloned; the best characterized of these is ISGF3 (IFN-stimulated gene factor 3). The activated ISGF3 is a complex of four distinct polypeptides; three of these, with a molecular mass of 113, 91 and 84 kDa, respectively, are already present in the cytoplasm of non-IFN treated cells and, after IFN-receptor binding, become very rapidly activated, in a matter of minutes, by phosphorylation of tyrosine residues. The activated proteins then form a complex, termed ISGF3α, that immediately translocates to the nucleus and binds to the fourth component, a 48 kDa protein, called the ISGF3γ protein. This 48 kDa nuclear protein, which is probably the major subunit that binds to the ISRE, normally displays some ISRE-binding activity, which is boosted 20-fold in the active ISGF3 complex. The 84 kDa and 91 kDa proteins are products of the same gene; amino acid sequence analysis has shown that the ISGF3 proteins belong to a new family of tyrosine-kinase-activated signal transducers (Levy *et*

Table 2. Some important proteins induced by IFN-α and IFN-β in humans.

Protein	Size in kDa	Chromosomal localization	Principal activity
2-5 A synthetases	100 69 46 40	– – 12 12	Antiviral, and antitumoral; a role in splicing has also been suggested
P1/eIF2 Kinase	68	2	Inhibition of translation of viral mRNA
MxA	76	21	Inhibition of orthomyxovirus replication
MxB	73	21	?
GBP-1	67	–	Guanylate binding protein
17 kDa protein	17	–	Inhibition of cellular replication
MHC-class I	45	6	Antigen processing and immune regulation
β-2 microglobulin	12	15	Antigen processing and immune regulation
MHC-class II	24 to 33	6	Antigen processing and immune regulation
Metallothionein II	–	16	Heavy metal binding

al., 1989; Fu *et al.*, 1990, 1992; Imam *et al.*, 1990; Kessler *et al.*, 1990; McKendry *et al.*, 1991; Fu, 1992; Schindler *et al.*, 1992a,b; Veals *et al.*, 1992). The tyrosine kinase that activates the ISGF3α subunits after binding of IFN-α to its receptor, has been cloned and characterized as tyk 2, a kinase that had been previously identified but whose function was unknown. This IFN-tyk kinase is probably in close physical contact with the IFN receptor, since its presence has been demonstrated in cell-membrane extracts. It is possible that another tyrosine kinase, different from tyk 2, is involved in signal transduction after binding of IFN-β (Velazquez *et al.*, 1992). The signal transduction pathway thus activated by IFN provides the first example of a very rapid and direct route from the cell surface to the promoter regions of genes transcriptionally activated as a result of ligand–receptor binding; no intervention of secondary messengers such as, for example, cyclic AMP is needed. It is likely that in the near future other cytokines will be found to use comparable direct signalling pathways.

INTERFERONS AS ANTIVIRAL AGENTS

IFN-α and IFN-β play an important role in host resistance to virus infections since they occupy the first line of defence, before immune mechanisms come into play. During viral infection, IFN-γ is produced only after T cells have been sensitized to viral antigens and, although its key function then resides in the activation of antiviral immune

Table 3. A synopsis of the principal biological activities of IFN-α/β.

Antiviral effect	Broad-spectrum antiviral activity, owing to a variety of mechanisms that, depending on the virus involved, can act at different stages of the infectious cycle. Some viruses have developed more or less efficient ways of escaping the antiviral effect.
	Clinical use: IFN-β is used to treat infection with hepatitis C virus.
Effect on cell growth and division	Inhibition of the replication of normal and tumour cells. IFN-α and β prolong G1, reduce rate of entry into the S-phase, and lengthen S and G2, resulting in a slower replication rate. Cells show highly different sensitivities to this activity.
Modulation of the expression of the MHC I, and to a lesser extent, of MHC-II cell surface molecules	This is one of the mechanisms responsible for the immunomodulatory activities of IFN-α/β. Modulation of MHC class II antigens is more specifically a function of IFN-γ.
Stimulation of macrophage activity	Stimulation of receptor- and nonreceptor-mediated phagocytosis (the major macrophage activator is IFN-γ).
Stimulation of NK cell activity	Contributes to the antitumour activity, but treatment of target cells with IFN-α/β sometimes results in protection against NK activity
Up- or downregulation of delayed-type hypersensitivity	DTH is an important immune mechanism which can be up- or downregulated by IFN-α/β, depending on timing of action.
Antitumoral activity	The mechanism of the antitumour activity is complex, and only partly understood. Stimulation of macrophages, T cells and NK cells are involved, as is sometimes the direct antiproliferative activity.
	Clinical use: for example, renal carcinoma, hairy-cell leukaemia.

reactions, it has also been shown to exert direct antiviral effects that contribute to host defence (see for example Huang *et al.*, 1993).

The production of IFN-α/β has been demonstrated in humans during viral disease and in mouse models using a wide variety of different viruses. The kinetics of the appearance of IFN-α/β stand out as an important factor in determining the efficacy of endogenous IFN action: early IFN production is instrumental in limiting infection, whereas late IFN production generally has a much less apparent protective effect. This is explained by the time required to mount a specific antiviral immune response; during this interval, IFN-α/β production is the only known active defence mechanism.

Treatment of mice with anti-IFN-α/β globulin markedly enhances the severity of infection with many different viruses (Gresser, 1984). Moreover, mice that are normally resistant to infection with some viruses can become susceptible as a result of treatment with anti-IFN globulin. For example, C3H/He mice resistant to infection with mouse hepatitis virus (MHV-3) become fully susceptible when treated with anti-IFN globulin, and die a few days after injection (Virelizier and Gresser, 1978). It is clear from mouse model studies that the antiviral activity of IFN-α/β *in vivo* results not only from an induction of the antiviral state in cells, but also from a wide variety of other IFN effects on host defence mechanisms, such as stimulation of NK cells and of cell-mediated immunity, and activation of macrophages. This is discussed in later sections of this chapter.

Multiple Mechanisms of the Antiviral State

The interaction of IFNs with their specific cell-surface receptors is followed by the rapid activation of DNA-binding factors which stimulate the transcription of a set of genes containing IFN-response sequences (IRSs) homologous to the prototypic sequence GGGAAANNGAAACT (Cohen et al., 1988; Hug et al., 1988; Levy et al., 1988; Shirayoshi et al., 1988; Dale et al., 1989a,b; Reich and Darnell, 1989). Several IFN-stimulated genes code for proteins responsible for the antiviral state, such as the dsRNA-dependent P1/eIF-2a kinase, the (2′-5′)oligo-adenylate synthetase, and the Mx proteins. In addition to these, many other proteins are induced in IFN-treated cells (see De Maeyer and De Maeyer-Guignard, 1988, for an extensive review), but we will limit our discussion to those whose contribution to the antiviral state has been well established.

Oligo-adenylate Synthetase

This enzyme, also called $(2′-5′)A_n$ synthetase or (2′-5′)oligo(A) adenyltransferase, is constitutively present in many cells, but at very low levels; its concentration can increase by several orders of magnitude after IFN-treatment. IFN-γ is a less efficient inducer of $(2′-5′)A_n$ synthetase than are IFN-α or IFN-β (Baglioni and Maroney, 1980; Verhaegen-Lewalle et al., 1982). When activated by dsRNA, $(2′-5′)A_n$ synthetase polymerizes ATP into a series of 2′-5′-linked oligomers $(ppp(A2′p)_n)$ of which the trimer is the most abundant. These oligomers, collectively called 2-5A, then activate a latent cellular endoribonuclease, designated RNase L, which is responsible for the antiviral activity. The third enzyme of this system, which is present in both untreated and IFN-treated cells, is a 2′-5′ phosphodiesterase that catalyses the degradation of 2-5A. The dsRNA required to activate the $(2′-5′A)_n$ synthetases are most likely intermediates or by-products of viral RNA replication (Gribaudo et al., 1991).

Functional mRNAs of different sizes, 1.65 and 1.85 kb in human and 1.8 and 3.6 kb in murine cells, have been described for this enzyme. The human 1.6 and 1.8 kb mRNAs are transcribed from the same gene but are spliced differently (Merlin et al., 1983; St Laurent et al., 1983; Benech et al., 1985a,b; Saunders et al., 1985), and the 40- and 46-kDa synthetases derived from them are identical in their first 346 residues but differ at their C-terminal ends (Benech et al., 1985b; Wathelet et al., 1986). The structural gene is located on human chromosome 12; it contains six exons, spread over 12 kb of DNA (Williams et al., 1986; Wathelet et al., 1987). Altogether, human cells contain four different $(2′-5′)A_n$ synthetases, all antigenically related, with sizes of 40, 46, 67 and 100 kDa. The last two forms are in all likelihood encoded by genes different from the one encoding the 40 kDa and 46 kDa forms. These four enzymes differ in their preferential intracellular localization and in their optimal conditions for activity (Chebath et al., 1987; Hovanessian et al., 1987).

In the mouse, a 40, 75 and 100 kDa form have been described (Hovanessian et al., 1987). The murine 42-kDa $(2′-5′)A_n$ synthetase displays 62% homology at the amino acid level and 73% homology at the nucleotide level with the human 46 kDa enzyme

(Ichii *et al.*, 1986). Two different genes, closely linked and each encoding $(2'-5')A_n$ synthetase have been identified in mice (Rutherford *et al.*, 1991).

The best documented function of the 2-5A oligomers made by the $(2'-5')A_n$ synthetase is activation of a latent endonuclease, ribonuclease L, resulting in the degradation of viral RNA. *In vitro*, however, degradation is not limited to viral RNA, and cellular mRNA and ribosomal RNA are also degraded by ribonuclease L (Nilsen *et al.*, 1981; Silverman *et al.*, 1983). A role for the 2-5A system in RNA splicing has recently been proposed, but this interesting possibility remains subject to further investigation (Sperling *et al.*, 1991).

Protein Kinase

Activation of the protein kinase P1/eIF2 (a serine–threonine kinase) is the second pathway of IFN-induced translational control that is dependent on the presence of dsRNA. P1/eIF2 kinase, when activated in IFN-treated cells by low levels of dsRNA, first autophosphorylates and then phosphorylates the α subunit of eIF2, the eukariotic protein synthesis initiation factor. As a result, the recycling of the α subunit is inhibited and the initiation of translation cannot take place (Lengyel, 1982; Samuel *et al.*, 1984). When expressed in the yeast *Saccharomyces,* the human P1/eIF2 kinase has growth-suppressing activity, which correlates with phosphorylation of yeast eIF2α (Chong *et al.*, 1992).

In addition to its role in the IFN-activated antiviral, and probably also antiprolifera-tive, mechanism, the possibility has been raised that the P1/eIF2 kinase plays a role in normal cells as a homeostatic regulator, whose aberrant expression can lead to malignant transformation. This is based on the observation that expression of a functionally defective mutant in NIH 3T3 cells, acting as a dominant negative mutation, leads to malignant transformation (Koromilas *et al.*, 1992; Meurs *et al.*, 1993).

The human P1/eIF2 kinase is 68 kDa polypeptide, and the murine P1/eIF2 kinase a 65 kDa polypeptide; the corresponding cDNAs have been isolated, and the dsRNA binding domains of the protein have been identified. The dsRNA required to activate the enzyme is usually of viral origin; for example, in the case of HIV, efficient binding and activation of the kinase is a result of the interaction with the TAT-responsive sequence of the virus (Hovanessian *et al.*, 1988; Meurs *et al.*, 1989; Roy *et al.*, 1991; Feng *et al.*, 1992).

Several viruses have developed strategies to counter the effects of the P1 kinase, and we will cite only two examples. In the case of adenovirus, small viral RNA transcripts bind to the protein kinase in such a way that subsequent interaction with activating dsRNA is prevented (Galabru *et al.*, 1989). In poliovirus infected cells, the P1 kinase is degraded by a cellular protease that somehow becomes activated in poliovirus-infected cells (Black *et al.*, 1993).

Mx Protein

Mx proteins constitute a family of IFNα/β-inducible GTPases that display antiviral activity against specific viruses. The murine Mx protein causes an antiviral state that is specifically directed against influenza virus replication. It is a 72 kDa nuclear protein that is induced by IFN-α/β, but not by IFN-γ, in cells from mice with the Mx^+ genotype. Mice of $Mx1^-$ strains that are genetically susceptible to influenza virus infection carry a defective *Mx* gene, with deletions in the coding exons. The *Mx1* gene maps to murine chromosome 16. A corresponding gene, *MxA*, has been found in humans; it maps to chromosome 21. The human IFN-induced *MxA* protein, however, is a cytoplasmic protein that confers resistance not only to influenza virus but also to vesicular stomatitis virus (for a review of this interesting system, see Staeheli, 1990).

Other Antiviral Mechanisms

There are abundant indications that IFNs can increase the antiviral resistance of cells— for example against retroviral infection, including infection with HIV—by a mechanism other than the above-mentioned, but the molecular basis for these activities remains to be elucidated.

Conclusion

The study of the antiviral state in specific virus–host-cell systems has provided examples of interference with virus production at virtually every stage of the infectious cycle in cells treated with IFN-α or IFN-β. The main mechanism is inhibition of translation, with involvement of the 2-5A and the protein kinase pathways, but other mechanisms are activated and have still to be resolved.

The molecular mechanisms of the antiviral action of IFN-γ have received less attention. This IFN can also activate the 2-5A pathway and the dsRNA-dependent protein kinase, but to a lesser extent than IFN-α or IFN-β. However, and in contrast to IFN-α and IFN-β, an important exception to the usual antiviral activity of IFN-γ has recently been observed, in that the expression of HIV is stimulated after IFN-γ treatment of promonocytic cells chronically infected with this virus (Biswas *et al.*, 1992).

MODULATION OF THE EXPRESSION OF THE MAJOR HISTOCOMPATIBILITY ANTIGENS

The modulation of the expression of the cell-surface antigens of the MHC is one of the major mechanisms by which all three IFN species can influence the immune system. MHC modulation is, furthermore, implicated in the antiviral activity of IFNs, since a successful antiviral cell-mediated immune response depends on the ability of the target cells to present the antiviral antigens in conjunction with class I antigens (Zinkernagel and Doherty, 1974). It has been shown, for example, that by increasing the expression of MHC class I antigens, murine IFN-α/β enhances the susceptibility of Vaccinia or lymphocytic choriomeningitis virus-infected fibroblasts to lysis by cytotoxic T cells (Bukowski and Welsh, 1985).

Modulation of MHC Antigen Expression by IFN-γ

Monocytes/Macrophages

By inducing or augmenting the expression of class II antigens on many different accessory cells, and thus stimulating the interaction of these cells with T cells, IFN-γ promotes antibody formation and the development of cytotoxic T cells. Intravenous administration of recombinant murine IFN-γ to mice results in an increased expression of these antigens on macrophages and on many other cells. In the lymphatic– haemopoietic system, the most significant increase of both class I and class II antigens is observed in bone-marrow cells (Skoskiewicz *et al.*, 1985; Momburg *et al.*, 1986). The final demonstration that endogenous IFN-γ production is of paramount importance in augmenting MHC class II expression has recently been provided by the use of gene knock-out mice lacking a functional IFN-γ gene: in such animals, class II expression on macrophages from BCG-infected mice is significantly reduced compared with normal mice (Dalton *et al.*, 1993).

T and B Cells

Enhanced expression of class II antigens after IFN-γ treatment also takes place on cells of T and B lineage. For example, addition of human IFN-γ to adult T cells or to T cells derived from human cord blood, significantly increase the expression of HLA-DR antigens. Similarly, cells belonging to various murine and human B-cell lines can be stimulated by IFN-γ to enhanced expression of class I and class II antigens (Kim *et al.*, 1983; Wong *et al.*, 1983; Capobianchi *et al.*, 1985).

Tumour Cells

MHC class II antigen expression is important for the antigen-presenting ability of tumour cells: for example, melanoma cells expressing HLA-DR induce the proliferation of autologous T cells, and this T-cell stimulation is abolished by treatment of the tumour cells with anti-HLA-DR antibodies (Guerry *et al.*, 1984). Stimulation or expression of class II antigens has been observed with both IFN-α and IFN-γ. Cells belonging to established lines derived from many different types of human tumours, such as melanomas, malignant glioma, breast cancer, bladder cancer, can be induced to express class II antigens by IFN-γ (Basham and Merigan, 1983; Houghton *et al.*, 1984; Takiguchi *et al.*, 1985; Balkwill *et al.*, 1987). However, this is not a general property of all malignant cells, as some tumour-cell lines are resistant to this effect.

Modulation of MHC Antigen Expression by IFN-α and IFN-β

IFN-α/β and Class II Antigen Expression

As described above, IFN-γ is one of the prime inducers of class II antigens but IFN-α and IFN-β are also capable of doing so (Basham and Merigan, 1983; Kim *et al.*, 1983; Virelizier *et al.*, 1984; Capobianchi *et al.*, 1985). Differential effects of individual IFN-α subspecies have been observed: human IFN-α_1 increases class II but not class I antigen expression on human monocytes, whereas human IFN-α_2 increases class I but not class II (Sztein *et al.*, 1984; Rhodes *et al.*, 1986). The observation that the effects of IFN-α can vary with the molecular subspecies could explain some contradictory findings with IFN preparations, since different proportions of the IFN-α subspecies can be found in leukocyte and lymphoblastoid IFN preparations.

Modulation of Class I Antigen Expression by IFN-α/β

Although IFN-α and IFN-β can stimulate the expression of class II antigens, their major effect on MHC expression is induction of class I antigens. These effects have been observed *in vitro* and also *in vivo* after systemic administration of IFN to animals, which means that they can occur as a result of IFN production during viral infection. Increased expression of MHC class I antigens induced by murine IFN-α/β on malignant cells significantly reduces the tumorigenicity of these cells in immunocompetent hosts, which shows the importance of class I antigens for the anti-tumour effect of IFN (Hayashi *et al.*, 1985).

STIMULATION OF MACROPHAGE ACTIVITY BY INTERFERONS

IFN-α, IFN-β and more especially IFN-γ play an important role in macrophage activation, mainly as a result of effects on the expression and activity of cell-surface receptors.

Fc Receptor-mediated Phagocytosis

Binding of antibodies to macrophages and monocytes via receptors to the constant regions (Fc receptors) is the first step leading to phagocytosis and antibody-coated infectious agents. The Fc receptor proteins are members of the immunoglobulin supergene family, displaying homology with the major histocompatibility antigens.

Treatment with murine IFN-β enhances the expression of Fc receptors at the surface of macrophages. For example, phagocytosis via Fc receptor is defective in macrophages from C3H/HeJ mice owing to the presence of Lps^d allele, and this decreased expression can be partly corrected by IFN treatment (Vogel *et al.*, 1983).

Murine IFN-α and IFN-β are capable of boosting the binding and phagocytosis of antibody-coated sheep erythrocytes by cells of a murine macrophage-like cell line, with very similar kinetics and dose dependence. Both IFN species, induce a two- to fivefold increase in Fc receptors; this is an active process, requiring RNA and protein synthesis (Yoshie *et al.*, 1982).

Phagocytosis Mediated via the Receptor for the Third Complement Component

The receptor for the inactivated complement component C_{3bi} corresponds to the cellular adhesion glycoprotein Mac-1 (Beller *et al.*, 1983). The expression of Mac-1 is influenced by IFN-γ, which can induce transcription of the Mac-1 α-subunit mRNA (Sastre *et al.*, 1986). However, in addition to stimulating its expression, IFN-γ also influences the function of the C_3 receptor in mature cells, by decreasing its affinity for the C_{3b} protein. Indeed, in human monocytes exposed to human IFN-γ, a significant decrease in the binding of C_{3b} occurs, although the number of C_{3b} receptors is not diminished. The capacity of these monocytes to bind C_{3b}-coated erythrocytes is restored to normal levels if the cells are allowed to spread on a surface coated with fibronectin (Wright *et al.*, 1986).

Tumoricidal Activity

Lymphokines released by activated T cells are capable of priming macrophages for tumoricidal activity. This activity, called macrophage activating factor (MAF), is at least partly due to IFN-γ, since it is inactivated by highly specific antibodies to IFN-γ and can be reproduced by recombinant murine IFN-γ (Le *et al.*, 1983; Nathan *et al.*, 1983; Svedersky *et al.*, 1984). Activation of cell killing by macrophages is an important function of IFN-γ, since tumour-cell lysis by activated macrophages is, in all likelihood, part of the mechanism of natural resistance to cancer. Although IFN-γ is undoubtedly a major macrophage priming agent, it shares this function with other lymphokines that also prime or activate macrophages to kill tumour cells by releasing reactive oxygen intermediates and by producing other cytotoxic molecules such as TNF-α (Urban *et al.*, 1986). IFN-γ induces the formation and release of TNF by macrophages (Philip and Epstein, 1986).

Although most attention has been focused on macrophage activation by IFN-γ, it should be stressed that IFN-α and IFN-β are also capable of boosting the tumoricidal activity of macrophages. For example, phagocytosis of tumour cells by macrophages in the peritoneal cavity of mice is enhanced by treatment with IFN-α/β (Gresser and Bourali, 1970), and *in vitro* treatment of mouse peritoneal macrophages or human monocytes with IFN-α or IFN-β induces cytolytic activity against malignant target cells (Dean and Virelizier, 1983; Blasi *et al.*, 1984).

Destruction of Parasites by IFN-activated Macrophages

Intracellular parasite killing is significantly activated when infected macrophages are exposed to IFN-γ, for example, in IFN-γ-treated suspensions of human monocytes infected with *Leishmania donovani*. The effect can be either preventive or curative, since parasite killing is also enhanced when previously infected monocytes are treated subsequently with IFN-γ (Hoover *et al.*, 1985). Production of reactive oxygen intermediates and secretion of hydrogen peroxide are correlated with the capacity of macrophages to kill intracellular parasites (Murray, 1981). For example, in human and murine macrophages, exposure for a few hours to recombinant IFN-γ leads to substantial activation of hydrogen-peroxide-releasing capacity that can last for several days, and is accompanied by a stimulation of intracellular killing of *Toxoplasma gondii*. Stimulation of the secretion of reactive oxygen intermediates seems to be an exclusive function of IFN-γ. It has not been found for IFN-α, IFN-β, CSF-1, TNF or IL-2 (Murray *et al.*, 1985; Nathan *et al.*, 1985; Nathan and Tsunawaki, 1986). Moreover, in human monocytes recombinant human IFN-α_2 and IFN-β antagonize the hydrogen-peroxide-stimulating activity of IFN-γ (Garotta *et al.*, 1986).

MODULATION OF T-, B- AND NK-CELL ACTIVITY BY IFNs

Effects on T-cell Function

T cells with Cytolytic Activity
Cytotoxic T cells react with target cells in the context of class I MHC antigens, and both IFN-α/β and IFN-γ stimulate the expression of these antigens, as a result of which the cytotoxic activity of T cells is boosted. Thus, virus-induced IFNs restrict infection not only by inducing the antiviral state but also by conditioning infected cells for destruction by cytotoxic T cells (Blackman and Morris, 1985; Bukowski and Welsh, 1985). Moreover, IFN-α/β enhances the specific cytotoxicity of sensitized lymphocytes against allogeneic tumour cells.

T cells with Suppressive Activity
The effects of IFNs on T-suppressor cells can result in either the boosting or downregulation of suppression. IFN-γ is capable of stimulating accessory cells to induce

T-suppressor cells, and stimulation by IFN-γ of MHC class II antigen expression on macrophages is followed by an increase in the ability of these macrophages to induce the generation of T-suppressor cells (Noma and Dorf, 1985). The effect of IFNs on suppressor-cell generation is not always stimulatory, and under certain conditions suppressor-cell formation is inhibited. Frequently, T-suppressor cells have been found to be particularly sensitive to inhibition by IFNs in delayed hypersensitivity and in other immune reactions. For example, human leukocyte IFN added to mixed lymphocyte cultures causes a marked decrease in suppressor-cell activity, as a result of inhibition of the differentiation of presuppressor cells into active suppressor cells (Fradelizi and Gresser, 1982). Similarly, the stimulatory effect of IFN-α/β on the expression of delayed hypersensitivity is a result of specific inhibition of either the generation or the expansion of T-suppressor cells (Knop et al., 1982, 1987).

Effects on Antibody Formation and B-cell Differentiation

IFNs affect B-cell differentiation in various ways; whether the effect is up- or downregulation depends on the Ig isotype and on the lymphokines present in the supernatants from the activated T cells that are used in these experiments.

IFN-α and IFN-β

IFN-α of various origins and compositions influences immunoglobulin secretion by B cells. When human peripheral-blood cell suspensions are pretreated with human leukocyte IFN before stimulation with pokeweed mitogen, IgG synthesis by B cells is significantly enhanced. The degree of stimulation varies from donor to donor, indicating the existence of individual differences in the capacity to respond to this particular effect of human IFN-α (Härfast et al., 1981). Human IFN-β stimulates immunoglobulin synthesis by B cells as efficiently as IFN-α (Siegel et al., 1986).

IFN-γ

Human IFN-γ promotes proliferation of activated human B cells and, in cultures of human B cells, can act synergistically with IL-2 to enhance immunoglobulin light-chain synthesis (Bich-Thuy et al., 1986; Romagnani et al., 1986). IFN-γ is one of the natural B-cell differentiation factors, since the addition of anti-IFN-γ antibodies to activated T-cell supernatants abrogates the capacity of these supernatants to stimulate B cells into production of antibody-forming cells (Sidman et al., 1984; Brunswick and Lake, 1985). Studies in gene knock-out mice lacking a functional IFN-γ receptor have unequivocally shown that IFN-γ is essential for the generation of normal IgG2a and, to a lesser extent, IgG3 response (Huang et al., 1993). IFN-γ is, furthermore, a potent inhibitor of the action of IL-4 and appears as a natural downregulator of the autocrine IL-4-induced pathway of T-helper cells, in that it blocks the response of all resting B cells to this growth factor (Noelle et al., 1984; Rabin et al., 1986).

Effects on NK Cells

NK cells can be activated without previous sensitization and they are, therefore, like macrophages, in the first line of defence against tumour cells and infectious agents. NK-cell activity is boosted by IFN-α, IFN-β, and IFN-γ, with an optimal IFN dosage above which NK activity is often decreased instead of being enhanced (Herberman et al., 1982; Brunda and Rosenbaum, 1984; Edwards et al., 1985).

IFNs of all three species can protect target cells against NK activity, as shown for example in HeLa cells, which can be protected by human IFN-α, IFN-β or IFN-γ (Wallach, 1983).

EFFECTS OF INTERFERONS ON TUMOUR CELLS

The first cytokines to have found large-scale clinical use were the IFNs, and Hu IFN-α and IFN-β are currently used as therapeutic agents in patients with, among others, different forms of carcinoma, metastatic melanoma, myeloma, ovarian cancers and hairy-cell leukaemia. The effects of IFNs on tumours *in vivo* can result either from a direct action of IFN on the tumour cell, or indirectly, via the activation of several, not completely defined, effector mechanisms. These include stimulation of MHC antigen expression, macrophage activation, and stimulation of T cells and NK-cell activity. Many murine model studies have shown tumour inhibition as a result of IFN treatment. Recently, however, we have found that host genes can up- or downregulate the anti-tumour activity of IFN-α/β in the mouse and that, on some genetic backgrounds, IFN treatment has no effect or even enhances tumour development. This may help to explain the apparent discordance between mouse model studies showing inhibition of tumour formation by IFN, and the clinic in which only a limited percentage of individuals show tumour regression (De Maeyer-Guignard et al., 1993). Some of the direct effects of IFNs on tumour cells that have been reported are discussed below.

Antiproliferative Effects

IFNs slow down the growth and proliferation of normal and of tumour cells by prolonging the cell cycle. Some tumour cells are extremely sensitive to this effect, whereas others can be totally resistant. Mutants resistant to the antiproliferative effect can be isolated from IFN-sensitive tumour-cell lines (Gresser et al., 1974); such mutants can retain their sensitivity to antiviral activity (Lin et al., 1982). On freshly isolated tumour cells, the antiproliferative activity of human IFNs ranges from complete inhibition of cell replication to total resistance, with no obvious correlation between tumour-cell type and degree of inhibition (Bradley and Ruscetti, 1981; Epstein and Marcus, 1981; Ludwig et al., 1983). Evidence for a direct cytostatic effect of IFNs on the growth and development of tumour cells *in vivo* is provided by the inhibition of human tumour growth in nude mice treated with human IFNs of various origins (Balkwill et al., 1983).

Effects on Oncogene Expression

IFNs have various effects on oncogene expression. They can, for example, down-regulate c-*myc* expression in malignant cells. In Burkitt's lymphoma Daudi cells have been treated with IFN-β, a reduction in c-*myc* mRNA levels occurs as early as 3 h after the addition of IFN and precedes the inhibition of cell growth, suggesting a correlation between inhibition of c-*myc* expression and cessation of cell proliferation (Jonak et al., 1987).

Like the expression of c-*myc*, the expression of the *ras* oncogene, either endogenous or transfected, can be influenced by IFNs. When murine 3T3 cells transformed with the human Ha-*ras*1 gene are cultured in the continuous presence of murine IFN-α/β, revertant colonies arise that no longer give rise to tumours in nude mice. In the revertant cells, there is a significant reduction in c-Ha-*ras*-specific mRNA and of the c-Has-*ras* p21 protein (Samid *et al.*, 1984).

Effects on Differentiation

IFNs can cooperate with other agents to stimulate differentiation of malignant cells. A good example of this capacity is provided by the effects of murine IFN-α/β on Friend erythroleukaemic cells, which become more responsive to a differentiation-inducing chemical after IFN treatment (Rossi, 1985). Moreover, even in the absence of any other differentiation-inducing agent, IFNs have the potential to redirect tumour cells towards a more differentiated state. A pertinent example of this is the plasmacytoid differentiation and refractoriness to growth factor that occurs in Daudi cells after IFN treatment. This is a result of the capacity of IFN-α to act sometimes as a B-cell differentiation factor, which may also explain the success of IFN-α treatment in hairy-cell leukaemia (Quesada *et al.*, 1984; Chebath *et al.*, 1987; Exley *et al.*, 1987).

CONCLUSION

In this short overview, we have summarized some important properties and activities of IFNs, a family of cytokines that have a truly impressive broad range of activities, with a much wider spectrum than it has been possible to discuss here. By virtue of their broad-spectrum antiviral activity, IFNs stand out from the other cytokines in that they play a unique role in host response to viral infection. But IFNs also belong to the cytokine network and many of the other cytokines discussed in this book influence the production and action of IFNs, and have their own production and activity influenced by IFNs. Unravelling the intricacy, complexity and biological significance of these interactions is of prime importance for the clinical application of these substances.

REFERENCES

Aguet, M., Belardelli, F., Blanchard, B., Marcucci, F. and Gresser, I. (1982). *Virology* **117**, 541–544.
Aguet, M., Grobke, M. and Dreiding, P. (1984). *Virology* **132**, 211–216.
Baglioni, C. and Maroney, P.A. (1980). *J. Biol. Chem.* **255**, 8390–8393.
Balkwill, F.R., Stevens, M.H., Griffin, D.B., Thomas, J.A. and Bodmer, J.G. (1987). *Eur. J. Cancer Clin. Oncol.* **23**, 101–106.
Balkwill, F.R., Moodie, E.M., Freedman, V., Lane, E.B. and Fantes, K.H. (1983). *J. Interferon Res.* **3**, 319–326.
Basham, T.Y. and Merigan, T.C. (1983). *J. Immunol.* **130**, 1492–1494.
Beller, D.I., Springer, T.A. and Schreiber, R.D. (1983). *J. Exp. Med.* **156**, 1000–1009.
Benech, P., Merlin, G., Revel, M. and Chebath, J. (1985a). *Nucleic Acids Res.* **13**, 1267–1281.
Benech, P., Mory, Y., Revel, M. and Chebath, J. (1985b). *EMBO J.* **4**, 2249–2256.
Benoît, P., Maguire, D., Plavec, I., Kocher, H., Tovey, M. and Meyer, F. (1993). *J. Immunol.* **150**, 707–716.
Bich-Thuy, L.T., Queen, C. and Fauci, A.S. (1986). *Eur. J. Immunol.* **16**, 547–550.
Biswas, P., Poli, G., Kinter, A.L., Justement, J.S., Stanley, S.K., Maury, W.J. Bressler, P., Orenstein, J.M. and Fauci, A.S. (1992). *J. Exp. Med.* **176**, 739–750.
Black, T.L., Barber, G.N. and Katze, M.G. (1993). *J. Virol.* **67**, 791–800.
Blackman, M.J. and Morris, A.G. (1985). *Immunology* **56**, 451–457.
Blasi, E., Herberman, R.B. and Varesio, L. (1984). *J. Immunol.* **132**, 3226–3228.

Bradley, E.C. and Ruscetti, F.W. (1981). *Cancer Res.* **41**, 244–249.
Branca, A.A. and Baglioni, C. (1982). *J. Biol. Chem.* **257**, 13197–13200.
Brunda, J.M. and Rosenbaum, D. (1984). *Cancer Res.* **44**, 597–601.
Brunswick, M. and Lake, P. (1985). *J. Exp. Med.* **161**, 953–971.
Bukowski, J.F. and Welsh, R.M. (1985). *J. Exp. Med.* **161**, 257–262.
Capobianchi, M.R., Facchini, J., Di Marco, P., Antonelli, G. and Dianzani, F. (1985). *Proc. Soc. Exp. Biol. Med.* **178**, 551–556.
Celis, E., Miller, R.W., Wiktor, T.J., Dietzschold, B. and Koprowski, H. (1986). *J. Immunol.* **136**, 692–697.
Chebath, J., Benech, P., Hovanessian, A., Galabru, J. and Revel, M. (1987). *J. Biol. Chem.* **262**, 3852–3857.
Chong, K.L., Schappert, K., Meurs, E., Feng, F., Donahue, T.F., Friesen, J.D., Hovanessian, A.G. and Williams, B.R.G. (1992). *EMBO J.* **11**, 1553–1562.
Cohen, B., Peretz, D., Vaiman, D., Benech, P. and Chebath, J. (1988). *EMBO J.* **7**, 1411–1419.
Colby, C. and Duesberg, P.H. (1969). *Nature* **222**, 940–944.
Cross, J.C. and Roberts, M.R. (1991). *Proc. Natl Acad. Sci. USA* **88**, 3817–3821.
Cunningham, A.L., Nelson, P.A., Fathman, C.G. and Merigan, T.C. (1985). *J. Gen. Virol.* **66**, 249–258.
Dale, T.C., Imam, A.M.A., Kerr, I.M. and Stark, G.R. (1989a). *Proc. Natl. Acad. Sci. USA* **86**, 1203–1207.
Dale, T.C., Rosen, J.M., Guille, M.J., Lewin, A.R., Porter, A.G.C., Kerr, I.M. and Stark, G.R. (1989b). *EMBO J.* **8**, 831–839.
Dalton, D., Pitts-Meek, S., Keshav, S., Figari, I.S., Bradley, A. and Stewart, T.A. (1993). *Science* **259**, 1739–1742.
Dandoy, F., Kelley, K.A., De Maeyer-Guignard, J., De Maeyer, E. and Pitha, P.M. (1984). *J. Exp. Med.* **160**, 294–302.
Dean, R.T. and Virelizier, J.L. (1983). *Clin. Exp. Immunol.* **51**, 501–510.
De Maeyer, E. and Dandoy, F. (1987). *J. Hered.* **78**, 143–146.
De Maeyer, E. and De Maeyer-Guignard, J. (1988). *Interferons and Other Regulatory Cytokines*, Wiley, New York.
De Maeyer-Guignard, J., Cachard, A. and De Maeyer, E. (1980). *Virology* **102**, 222–225.
De Maeyer-Guignard, J., Lauret, E., Eusèbe, L. and De Maeyer, E. (1993). *Proc. Natl Acad. Sci, USA* **90**, 5708–5712.
Devos, R., Cheroutre, H., Taya, Y., Degrave, W., Van Heuverswyn, H. and Fiers, W. (1982). *Nucl. Acids Res.* **10**, 2487–2501.
Edwards, B.S., Merrin, J.A., Fuhlbridge, R.C. and Borden, E.C. (1985). *J. Clin. Invest.* **75**, 1908–1913.
Epstein, L.B. and Marcus, S.G. (1981). *Cancer Chemother. Pharmacol.* **6**, 273–277.
Exley, R., Nathan, P., Walker, L., Gordon, J. and Clemens, M.J. (1987). *Int. J. Cancer* **40**, 53–57.
Fan, C.-M. and Maniatis, T. (1989). *EMBO J.* **8**, 101–110.
Farrar, M.A., Fernandez-Luna, J. and Schreiber, R.D. (1991). *J. Biol. Chem.* **266**, 19626–19635.
Feng, G.S., Chong, K., Kumar, A. and Williams, B.R.G. (1992). *Proc. Natl Acad. Sci. USA* **89**, 5447–5451.
Field, A.K., Tytell, A.A., Lampson, G.P. and Hilleman, M.R. (1967). *Proc. Natl Acad. Sci. USA* **58**, 1004–1010.
Flores, I., Mariano, T.M. and Pestka, S. (1991). *J. Biol. Chem.* **266**, 19875–19877.
Fradelizi, D. and Gresser, I. (1982). *J. Exp. Med.* **155**, 1610–1622.
Friedman-Einat, M., Revel, M. and Kimchi, A. (1982). *Mol. Cell. Biol.* **2**, 1472–1480.
Fu, X.Y. (1992). *Cell* **70**, 323–335.
Fu, X.Y., Kessler, D.S., Veals, S.A., Levy, D.E. and Darnell, J.E., Jr. (1990). *Proc. Natl. Acad. Sci. USA* **87**, 8555–8559.
Fu, X.Y., Schindler, C., Improta, T., Aebersold, R. and Darnell, J.E., Jr. (1992). *Proc. Natl. Acad. Sci. USA* **89**, 7840–7843.
Fujita, T., Onno, S., Yasumitsu, H. and Taniguchi, T. (1985). *Cell* **41**, 489–496.
Fujita, T., Kimura, Y., Miyamoto, M., Barsoumian, E.L. and Taniguchi, T. (1989a). *Nature* **337**, 270–272.
Fujita, T., Miyamoto, M., Kimura, Y., Hammer, J. and Taniguchi, T. (1989b). *Nucl. Acids Res.* **17**, 3335–3346.
Fujita, T., Reis, L.F.L., Watanabe, N., Kimura, Y., Taniguchi, T. and Vilček, J. (1989c). *Proc. Natl Acad. Sci. USA* **86**, 9936–9940.
Gajewski, T.F. and Fitch, F.W. (1988). *J. Immunol.* **140**, 4245–4252.
Galabru, J., Katze, M.G., Robert, N. and Hovanessian, A.G. (1989). *Eur. J. Biochem.* **178**, 581–589.
Garotta, G., Talmadge, K.W., Pink, J.R.L., Dewald, B. and Aggiolini, M. (1986). *Biochem. Biophys. Res. Commun.* **140**, 948–954.

Gessani, S., Belardelli, F., Pecorelli, A., Puddu, P. and Baglioni, C. (1989). *J. Virol.* **63**, 2785–2789.

Gibbs, V.C., Williams, S.R., Gray, P.W., Schreiber, R.D., Pennica, D., Rice, G. and Goeddel, D.V. (1991). *Mol. Cell. Biol.* **11**, 5860–5866.

Goodbourn, S. and Maniatis, T. (1988). *Proc. Natl Acad. Sci. USA* **85**, 1447–1451.

Goodbourn, S., Zinn, K. and Maniatis, T. (1985). *Cell* **41**, 509–520.

Gray, P.W. and Goeddel, D.V. (1982). *Nature* **298**, 859–863.

Gray, P.W., Leung, D.W., Pennica, D., Yelverton, E., Najarian, R., Simonsen, C.C., Derynck, R., Sherwood, P.J., Wallace, D.M., Berger, S.L., Levinson, A.D. and Goeddel, D.V. (1982). *Nature* **295**, 503–508.

Gray, P.W., Leong, S., Fennie, E.H., Farrar, M.A., Pingel, J.T., Fernandez-Luna, J. and Schreiber, R.D. (1989). *Proc. Natl Acad. Sci. USA* **86**, 8497–8501.

Gresser, I. (1984). In: *Interferon 2. Interferons and the Immune System* (eds J. Vilček and E. De Maeyer), Elsevier Science Publishers, Amsterdam, pp. 221–247.

Gresser, I., Bandu, M.T. and Brouty-Boye, D. (1974). *J. Natl. Cancer Inst.* **52**, 553–559.

Gribaudo, G., Lembo, D., Cavallo, G., Landolfo, S. and Lengyel, P. (1991). *J. Virol.* **65**, 1748–1757.

Guerry, D.P., Alexander, M.A., Herlyn, M.F., Zehngebot, L.M., Mitchell, K.F., Zmijewski, C.M. and Lusk, E.J. (1984). *J. Clin. Invest.* **73**, 267–271.

Hansen, T.R., Leaman, D.W., Cross, J.C., Mathialagan, N., Bixby, J.A. and Roberts, R.M. (1991). *J. Biol. Chem.* **266**, 3060–3067.

Harada, H., Fujita, T., Miyamoto, M., Kimura, Y., Maruyama, M., Furia, A., Miyata, T. and Taniguchi, T. (1989). *Cell* **58**, 729–739.

Härfast, B., Huddlestone, J.R., Casali, P., Merigan, T.C. and Oldstone, M.B.A. (1981). *J. Immunol.* **127**, 2146–2150.

Hayashi, H., Tanaka, K., Jay, F., Khoury, G. and Jay, G. (1985). *Cell* **43**, 263–267.

Hemmi, S., Peghini, P., Metzler, M., Merlin, G., Dembic, Z. and Aguet, M. (1989). *Proc. Natl. Acad. Sci. USA* **86**, 9901–9905.

Herberman, R.B., Ortaldo, J.R., Mantovani, A., Hobbs, D.S., Kung, H.F. and Pestka, S. (1982). *Cell Immunol.* **67**, 160–167.

Hibino, Y., Mariano, T.M., Kumar, C.S., Kozak, C.A. and Pestka, S. (1991). *J. Biol. Chem.* **266**, 6948–6951.

Hibino, Y., Kumar, C.S., Mariano, T.M., Lai, D. and Pestka, S. (1992). *J. Biol. Chem.* **267**, 3748–3749.

Hiscott, J., Alper, D., Cohen, L., Leblanc, J.F., Sportza, L., Wong, A. and Xanthoudakis, S. (1989). *J. Virol.* **63**, 2557–2566.

Hiscott, J., Cantell, K. and Weissmann, C. (1984). *Nucleic Acids Res.* **12**, 3727–3746.

Hoover, D.L., Nacy, C.A. and Meltzer, M.S. (1985). *Cell Immunol.* **94**, 500–511.

Houghton, A.N., Thompson, T.M., Gross, D., Oettgen, H.F. and Old, L.J. (1984). *J. Exp. Med.* **160**, 255–269.

Hovanessian, A.G., Laurent, A.G., Chebath, J., Galabru, J., Robert, N. and Svab, J. (1987). *EMBO J.* **6**, 1273–1280.

Hovanessian, A.G., Svab, J., Marie, I., Robert, N., Chamaret, S. and Laurent, A.G. (1988). *J. Biol. Chem.* **263**, 4945–4949.

Huang, S., Hendriks, W., Althage, A., Hemmi, S., Bluethmann, H., Kamijo, R., Vilček, J., Zinkernagel, R.M. and Aguet, M. (1993). *Science* **259**, 1742–1745.

Huez, G., Silhol, M. and Lebleu, B. (1983). *Biochem. Biophys. Res. Commun.* **110**, 155–160.

Hug, H., Costa, M., Staeheli, P., Aebi, M. and Weissmann, C. (1988). *Mol.Cell. Biol.* **8**, 3065–3079.

Hughes, T.K. and Baron, S.A. (1987). *J. Biol. Regul. Homeostatic Agents* **1**, 29–32.

Ichii, Y, Fukunaga, R., Shiojiri, S. and Sokawa, Y. (1986). *Nucleic Acids Res.* **14**, 10117.

Imam, A.M.A., Ackrill, A.M., Dale, T.C., Kerr, I.M. and Stark, G.R. (1990). *Nucl. Acids Res.* **18**, 6573–6580.

Isaacs, A. and Lindenmann, J. (1957). *Proc. R. Soc. (London), Ser. B.* **147**, 258–273.

Jonak, G.J., Friedland, B.K., Anton, E.D. and Knight, E., Jr. (1987). *J. IFN Res.* **7**, 41–52.

Kalina, U., Ozmen, L., Di Padova, K., Gentz, R. and Garotta, G. (1993). *J. Virol.* **67**, 1702–1706.

Keller, A.D. and Maniatis, T. (1991). *Genes Dev.* **5**, 868–879.

Kelley, K.A. and Pitha, P.M. (1985a). *Nucl. Acids Res.* **13**, 805–823.

Kelley, K.A. and Pitha, P.M. (1985b). *Nucl. Acids Res.* **13**, 825–839.

Kessler, D.S., Veals, S.A., Fu, X.Y. and Levy, D.E. (1990). *Genes & Development* **4**, 1753–1765.

Kim, K.J., Chaouat, G., Leiserson, W.M., King, J. and De Maeyer, E. (1983). *Cell. Immunol.* **75**, 253–267.

Knop, J., Stremmer, R., Neumann, C., De Maeyer, E. and Macher, E. (1982). *Nature* **296**, 775–776.

Knop, J., Taborksi, B. and De Maeyer-Guignard, J. (1987). *J. Immunol.* **138**, 3684–3687.

Koromilas, A.E., Roy, S., Barber, G.N., Katze, M.G. and Sonenberg, N. (1992). *Science* **257**, 1685–1689.

Kumar, C.S., Muthukumaran, G., Frost, L.J., Noe, M., Ahn, Y.H., Mariano, T.M. and Pestka, S. (1989). *J. Biol. Chem.* **264**, 17939–17946.

Lau, A.S., Hannigan, G.E., Freedman, M.H. and Williams, B.R.G. (1986). *J. Clin. Invest.* **77**, 1632–1638.

Le, J., Prensky, W., Yip, Y.K., Chang, Z., Hoffmann, T., Stevenson, H.C., Balazs, I., Sadlick, J.R. and Vilček, J. (1983). *J. Immunol.* **131**, 2821–2826.

Le Roscouet, D., Vodjdani, G., Lemaigre-Dubreuil, Y., Tovey, M.G., Latta, M. and Doly, J. (1985). *Mol. Cell. Biol.* **5**, 1343–1348.

Lenardo, M.J. and Baltimore, D. (1989). *Cell* **58**, 227–229.

Lenardo, M.J., Fan, C.-M., Maniatis, T. and Baltimore, D. (1989). *Cell* **57**, 287–294.

Lengyel, P. (1982). *Ann. Rev. Biochem.* **51**, 251–282.

Levy, D.E., Kessler, D.S., Pine, R., Reich, N. and Darnell, J.E., Jr. (1988). *Genes Development* **2**, 383–393.

Levy, D.E., Kessler, D.S., Pine, R. and Darnell, J.E., Jr. (1989). *Genes & Development* **3**, 1362–1371.

Lin, S.L., Greene, J.J., Ts'O, P.O.P. and Carter, W.A. (1982). *Nature* **297**, 417–419.

Liu, Y. and Janeway, C.A., Jr. (1990). *J. Exp. Med.* **172**, 1735–1739.

Ludwig, C.U., Durie, B.G.M., Salmon, S.E. and Moon, T.E. (1983). *Eur. J. Cancer* **19**, 1625–1632.

Lutfalla, G., Roeckel, N., Mogensen, K.E., Mattei, M.-G. and Uzé, G. (1990). *J. Interferon Res.* **10**, 515–517.

Lutfalla, G., Gardiner, K., Proudhon, D., Vielh, E. and Uzé, G. (1992). *J. Biol. Chem.* **267**, 2802–2809.

MacDonald, N.J., Kuhl, D., Maguire, D., Naf, D., Gallant, P., Goswamy, A., Hug, H., Bueler, H., Chaturvedi, M., de la Fuente, J., Ruffner, H., Meyer, F. and Weissmann, C. (1990). *Cell* **60**, 767–779.

McKendry, R., John, J., Flavell, D., Müller, M., Kerr, I.M. and Stark, G.R. (1991). *Proc. Natl Acad. Sci. USA* **88**, 11455–11459.

Merlin, G., Chebath, J., Benech, P., Metz, R. and Revel, M. (1983). *Proc. Natl Acad. Sci. USA* **80**, 4904–4908.

Meurs, D.F., Galabru, J., Barber, G.N, Katze, M.G. and Hovanessian, A.G. (1993). *Proc. Natl Acad. Sci. USA* **90**, 232–236.

Meurs, E., Galabru, J., Chong, K., Thomas, S.B., Robert, N., Svab, J., Brown, R.E., Kerr, I.M., Williams, B.R.G. and Hovanessian, A.G. (1989). *J. Interferon Res.* **9**, (Suppl. 2), S94.

Miyamoto, M., Fujita, T., Kumura, Y., Maruyama, M., Harada, H., Sudo, Y., Miyata, T. and Taniguchi, T. (1988). *Cell* **54**, 903–913.

Momburg, F., Koch, N., Moller, P., Moldenhauer, G. and Hammerling, G.J. (1986). *Eur. J. Immunol.* **16**, 551–557.

Moore, R.N., Larsen, H.S., Horohov, D.W. and Rouse, B.T. (1984). *Science* **223**, 178–181.

Morris, A.G., Lin, Y.L. and Askonas, B.A. (1982). *Nature* **295**, 150–152.

Mosca, J.D., Pitha, P.M. and Hayward, G.S. (1992). *J. Virol.* **66**, 3811–3822.

Mosmann, T.R., Cherwinski, H., Bond, M.W., Giedlin, M.A. and Coffman, R.L. (1986). *J. Immunol.* **136**, 2348–2357.

Murray, H.W. (1981). *J. Exp. Med.* **153**, 1302–1315.

Murray, H.W., Spitalny, G.L. and Nathan, C.F. (1985). *J. Immunol.* **134**, 1619–1622.

Nathan, C.F. and Tsunawaki, S. (1986). In: *Biochemistry of Macrophages* (eds O. Evered, J. Nugent and M. O'Connor), Pitman, London, *Ciba Foundation Symposium* **118**, 211–230.

Nathan, C.F., Horowitz, C.R., De La Harpe, J., Vadhan-Raj, S., Sherwin, S.A., Orttgen, H.F and Krown, S.E. (1985). *Proc. Natl Acad. Sci, USA* **82**, 8686–8690.

Nathan, C.F., Murray, H.W., Wiebe, M.E. and Rubin, B.Y. (1983). *J. Exp. Med.* **158**, 670–689.

Naylor, S.L., Gray, P.W. and Lalley, P.A. (1984). *Somat. Cell Mol. Genet.* **10**, 531–534.

Naylor, S.L., Sakaguchi, A.Y., Shows, T.B., Law, M.L., Goeddel, D.V. and Gray, P.W. (1983). *J. Exp. Med.* **57**, 1020–1027.

Nilsen, T.W., Maroney, P.A. and Baglioni, C. (1981). *J. Biol. Chem.* **256**, 7806–7811.

Noelle, R., Krammer, P.H., Ohara, J., Uhr, J.W. and Vitetta, E.S. (1984). *Proc. Natl. Acad. Sci. USA* **81**, 6149–6153.

Noma, T. and Dorf, M.E. (1985). *J. Immunol.* **135**, 3655–3660.

Owebach, D., Rutter, W.J., Shows, T.B., Gray, P., Goeddel, D.V. and Lawn, R.M. (1981). *Proc. Natl. Acad. Sci. USA* **78**, 3123–3127.

Palombella, V.J. and Maniatis, T. (1992). *Mol. Cell. Biol.* **12**, 3325–3336.

Petterson, U. and Philipson, R. (1974). *Proc. Natl Acad. Sci. USA* **71**, 4887–4889.

Philip, R. and Epstein, L.B. (1986). *Nature* **33**, 86–89.

Pine, R. (1992). *J. Virol.* **66**, 4470–4478.

Pine, R., Decker, T., Kessler, D.S., Levy, D.E. and Darnell, J.E., Jr. (1990). *Mol. Cell. Biol.* **10**, 2448–2457.

Proietti, E., Vanden Broecke, C., Di Marzio, P., Gessani, S., Gresser, I. and Tovey, M.G. (1992). *J. Interferon Res.* **12**, 27–34.

Quesada, J.R., Reuben, J., Manning, J.T., Hersh, E.M. and Gutterman, J.U. (1984). *N. Engl. J. Med.* **310**, 15–18.

Rabin, E.M., Mond, J.J. Ohara, J. and Paul, W.E. (1986). *J. Immunol.* **137**, 1573–1576.

Raj, N.B., An, W.C. and Pitha, P.M. (1991). *J. Biol. Chem.* **266**, 11360–11365.

Reich, N.C. and Darnell, J.E., Jr. (1989). *Nucl. Acids Res.* **17**, 3415–3424.

Reis, L.F.L., Lee, T.H. and Vilček, J. (1989). *J. Biol. Chem.* **264**, 16351–16354.

Rivière, I. and De Maeyer-Guignard, J. (1990). *J. Virol.* **64**, 2430–2432.

Roberts, M.R., Cross, J.C. and Leaman, D.W. (1991). *Pharmac. Ther.* **51**, 329–345.

Romagnani, S., Giudizi, M.G., Biagiotti, R., Almerigogna, F., Mingari, C., Maggi, E., Liang, C.M. and Moretta, L. (1986). *J. Immunol.* **136**, 3513–3516.

Rossi, G.B. (1985). In: *Interferon 6* (ed. I. Gresser), Academic Press, London, pp. 31–68.

Roy, S., Agy, M., Hovanessian, H.G., Sonenberg, N. and Katze, M.G. (1991). *J. Virol.* **65**, 632–640.

Rutherford, M.N., Kumar, A., Nissim, A., Chebath, J. and Williams, B.R.G. (1991). *Nucl. Acids Res.* **19**, 1917–1924.

Ryals, J., Dierks, P., Ragg, H. and Weissmann, C. (1985). *Cell* **41**, 497–507.

Samid, D., Chang, E.H. and Friedman, R.M. (1984). *Biochem. Biophys. Res. Commun.* **119**, 21–28.

Samuel, C.E., Duncan, G.S., Knutson, G.S. and Hershey, J.W.B. (1984). *J. Biol. Chem.* **259**, 13451–13457.

Sastre, L., Roman, J.M., Teplow, D.B., Dreyer, W.J., Gee, C.E., Larson, S., Roberts, T.M. and Springer, T.A. (1986). *Proc. Natl Acad. Sci. USA* **83**, 5644–5648.

Saunders, M.E., Gewert, D.R., Tugwell, M.E., McMahon, M. and Williams, B.R.G. (1985). *EMBO J.* **4**, 1761–1768.

Schindler, C., Fu, X.Y., Improta, T., Aebersold, R. and Darnell, J.E., Jr. (1992a). *Proc. Natl Acad. Sci. USA* **89**, 7836–7839.

Schindler, C., Shuai, K., Prezioso, V.R. and Darnell, J.E., Jr. (1992b). *Science* **257**, 809–813.

Seif, I. and De Maeyer-Guignard, J. (1986). *Gene* **43**, 111–121.

Seif, I., De Maeyer, E., Rivière, I. and De Maeyer-Guignard, J. (1991). *J. Virol.* **65**, 664–671.

Sekellick, M.J. and Marcus, P.I. (1982). *Virology* **117**, 280–285.

Shirayoshi, Y., Burke, P.A., Appella, E. and Ozato, K. (1988). *Proc. Natl. Acad. Sci. USA* **85**, 5884–5888.

Shows, T.B., Sakaguchi, A.Y., Naylor, S.L., Goeddel, D.G. and Lawn, R.M. (1982). *Science* **218**, 373–374.

Sidman, C.L., Marshall, J.D., Shultz, L.D., Gray, P.W. and Johnson, H.M. (1984). *Nature* **309**, 801–803.

Siegel, D.S., Le, J. and Vilček, J. (1986). *Cell Immunol.* **101**, 380–390.

Silverman, R.H., Skehel, J.J., James, T.C., Wreschner, D.H. and Kerr, I.M. (1983). *J. Virol.* **46**, 1051–1055.

Sims, S.H., Cha, Y., Romine, M.F., Gao, P.Q., Gottlieb, K. and Deisseroth, A.B. (1993). *Mol. Cell. Biol.* **13**, 690–702.

Skoskiewicz, M.J., Colvin, R.B., Schneeberger, E.E. and Russell, P.S. (1985). *J. Exp. Med.* **162**, 1645–1664.

Slate, D.L., D'Eustachio, P., Pravtcheva, D., Cunningham, A.C., Nagata, S., Weissmann, C. and Ruddle, F.H. (1982). *J. Exp. Med.* **155**, 1019–1024.

Sperling, J., Chebath, J., Arad-Dann, H., Offen, D., Spann, P., Lehrer, R., Goldblatt, D., Jolles, B. and Sperling, R. (1991). *Proc. Natl. Acad. Sci. USA* **88**, 10377–10381.

St Laurent, G., Yoshie, O., Floyd-Smith, G., Samanta, H., Sehgal, P. and Lengyel, P. (1983). *Cell* **33**, 95–102.

Staeheli, P. (1990). In: *Advances in Virus Research* **38**, 147–200. Academic Press, London.

Svedersky, L.P., Benton, C.V., Berger, W.H., Rinderknecht, E., Harkins, R.N. and Palladino, M.A. (1984). *J. Exp. Med.* **159**, 812–827.

Sztein, M.B., Steeg, P.S., Johnson, H.M. and Oppenheim, J.J. (1984). *J. Clin. Invest.* **73**, 556–565.

Takiguchi, M., Ting, J.P.-Y., Buessow, S.C., Boyer, C., Gillespie, Y. and Frelinger, J.A. (1985). *Eur. J. Immunol.* **15**, 809–814.

Taylor, P.M., Wraith, D.C. and Askonas, B.A. (1985). *Immunology* **54**, 607–614.

Tovey, M.G., Streuli, M., Gresser, I., Gugenheim, J., Blanchard, B., Guymarho, J., Vignaux, F. and Gigou, M. (1987). *Proc. Natl Acad. Sci. USA* **84**, 5038–5042.

Trent, J.M., Olson, S. and Lawn, R.M. (1982). *Proc. Natl Acad. Sci. USA* **79**, 7809–7813.

Urban, J.L., Shepard, H.M., Rothstein, J.L., Sugarman, B.J. and Schreiber, H. (1986). *Proc. Natl Acad. Sci. USA* **83**, 5233–5237.

Uzé, G., Lutfalla, G. and Gresser, I. (1990). *Cell* **60**, 225–234.

Uzé, G., Lutfalla, G., Bandu, M.T., Proudhon, D. and Mogensen, K.E. (1992). *Proc. Natl Acad. Sci. USA* **89**, 4774–4778.

Veals, S.A., Schindler, C., Leonard, D., Fu, X.Y., Aebersold, R., Darnell, J.E., Jr. and Levy, D.E. (1992). *Mol. Cell Biol.* **12**, 3315–3324.

Velazquez, L., Fellous, M., Stark, G.R. and Pellegrini, S. (1992). *Cell* **70**, 313–322.

Verhaegen-Lewalle, M., Kuwata, T., Zhang, Z.X., De Clercq, E., Cantell, K. and Content, J. (1982). *Virology* **117**, 425–434.

Virelizier, J.L. and Gresser, I. (1978). *J. Immunol.* **120**, 1616–1619.

Virelizier, J.L., Perez, N., Arenzana-Seisdedos, F. and Devos, R. (1984). *Eur. J. Immunol.* **14**, 106–108.

Vogel, S.N., Finbloom, D.S., English, K.E., Rosenstreich, D.L. and Langreth, S.G. (1983). *J. Immunol.* **130**, 1210–1214.

Wallach, D. (1983). *Cell Immunol.* **75**, 390–395.

Wathelet, M., Moutschen, S., Cravador, A., Dewit, L., Defilippi, P., Huez, G. and Content, J. (1986). *FEBS Lett.* **196**, 113–120.

Wathelet, M., De Vries, L., Defilippi, P., Nols, C., Vandenbussche, P., Pohl, V., Huez, G. and Content, J. (1987). In: *The Biology of the Interferon System* (eds K. Cantell and H. Schellekens), Martinus Nijhoff, The Hague, pp. 85–91.

Weissmann, C. and Weber, H. (1986). *Prog. Nucl. Acid Res.* **33**, 251–302.

Williams, B.R.G., Saunders, M.E. and Williard, H.F. (1986). *Somat Cel. Mol. Genet.* **12**, 403–408.

Wong, G.H.W., Clark-Lewis, I., McKimm-Breschkin, J.L., Harris, A.W. and Schrader, J.W. (1983). *J. Immunol.* **131**, 788–793.

Wright, J.R., Jr., Lacy, P.E., Unanue, E.R., Muszynski, C. and Hauptfeld, V. (1986). *Diabetes* **35**, 1174–1177.

Xanthoudakis, S., Cohen, L. and Hiscott, J. (1989). *J. Biol. Chem.* **15**, 1139–1145.

Yamada, Y.K., Meager, A., Yamada, A. and Ennis, F.A. (1986). *J. Gen Virol.* **67**, 2325–2334.

Yoshie, O., Meliman, I.S., Broeze, R.J., Garcia-Blanco, M. and Lengyel P. (1982). *Cell Immunol.* **73**, 128–140.

Zinkernagel, R.M. and Doherty, P.C. (1974). *Nature* **224**, 701–702.

Zinn, K. and Maniatis, T. (1986). *Cell* **45**, 611–618.

Zinn, K., Mellon, P., Ptashne, M. and Maniatis, T. (1982). *Proc. Natl Acad. Sci. USA* **79**, 4897–4901.

Chapter 16

Tumour Necrosis Factor-Alpha

Kevin J. Tracey

Laboratory of Biomedical Science, Department of Surgery, North Shore University Hospital-
Cornell University Medical College, Manhasset, NY, USA

INTRODUCTION

Tumour necrosis factor-α (TNF-α, cachectin), a 17 kDa protein produced by macrophages and other cells, was discovered by separate groups of investigators pursuing mediators of disparate diseases. In one line of research TNF-α was the culmination of years of work directed towards identifying an immunological mediator capable of killing tumour cells. Conversely, TNF-α was also identified (as cachectin) for its potent toxicity, and implicated as a lethal mediator of acute and chronic infection. In part, because these investigative approaches represent two separate avenues to potential therapeutic advance, the convergence of these dual paths into one cytokine created a great deal of interest in both the scientific and lay press. This story evolved over many years, and it continues to evolve, since the final results are pending from clinical trials designed to determine the efficacy of giving exogenous TNF-α to cancer patients, or of inhibiting endogenous TNF-α in infection.

As with other cytokines, the molecular and cellular biology of TNF-α, TNF-α-receptor–ligand interactions, and signal transduction continues to be elaborated. These mechanisms somehow orchestrate the panoply of TNF effects in the mediation of diverse disease states and in health, which is the principal topic of this chapter. Limitations of space prevent citation of all the contributors to this field. In this chapter particular emphasis is placed on the implications of TNF-α to human disease. For additional information the reader is referred to the primary literature as cited, or to one of several recently published volumes devoted entirely to this widely studied cytokine.

TNF-α STRUCTURE

The gene for human TNF-α, located on chromosome 6 near the HLA-B locus, encodes a prohormone of 233 amino acids (Wang et al., 1985; Spies et al., 1986; Davies et al., 1987; Muller et al., 1987). The prohormone is processed by cleavage of a 76-residue peptide that does not have a typical signal sequence. The prohormone may serve to anchor the precursor to the plasma membrane, whereby the mature secreted form of

TNF-α is exposed on the extracellular membrane surface (Kriegler *et al.*, 1988; Jue *et al.*, 1990). The acylation with myristate of lysine residues K19 and K20 (downstream of the hydrophobic membrane-spanning prohormone) appears to contribute to the trafficking to the membrane (Stevenson *et al.*, 1992). The membrane-bound TNF-α exposed to the extracellular environment retains bioactivity, as assayed by cell cytotoxicity (Kriegler *et al.*, 1988; Jue *et al.*, 1990; Perez *et al.*, 1990). This extracellular TNF-α moiety is cleaved during cellular activation to release mature TNF-α, but the proteolytic mechanism, and/or responsible enzyme, remain elusive. Also enigmatic is whether all secreted TNF-α resides initially on the plasma membrane, or whether there is an additional pathway for direct secretion.

Crystallographic studies of the structure of TNF reveal similarity to a 'bell' composed of three monomers associated noncovalently into a compact trimer oriented about a threefold axis of symmetry (Jones *et al.*, 1989). Within this structure each 157-amino-acid monomer is folded back onto itself as a β-pleated sheet; interactions between three adjacent sheets stabilize the trimeric structure (Sprang and Eck, 1992). The N-terminus of each monomer is exposed on the surface, but the C-termini are folded into the complex of β-pleated sheets and are not exposed. Detailed structural analyses suggest that mutations that destabilize the trimeric association of monomers lead to loss of biological activity (Lin, 1992). However, the N-terminus of TNF is not required for binding to the TNF receptor, since mutated forms of TNF missing residues from the N-terminus retain bioactivity (Creasey *et al.*, 1987). Antibodies that neutralize TNF bioactivity presumably interfere sterically to prevent recognition by the receptor. Some antibodies directed against the N-terminus neutralize, but the peptide fragments against which they were raised do not necessarily compete for TNF-α binding to receptor (Socher *et al.*, 1987). Based on the recently published crystallographic structure of lymphotoxin (TNF-β), another cytokine with structural homology to TNF-α, it is thought that the base of the TNF-α trimer binds to three adjacent or clustered receptors (Banner *et al.*, 1993).

TNF-α BIOSYNTHESIS

The biosynthesis of TNF-α is a highly regulated molecular event that has been most rigorously studied in the monocyte/macrophage. The promoter is a TATA box found 20 bp upstream from the transcription site, but other sequences exert regulatory influence (Kruys *et al.*, 1992). These include sequences similar to the nuclear factor κ-B enhancers, to the 'Y'-box promoter, to a cyclic AMP-responsive element, and to the c-*jun*/AP-1 binding site (Brenner *et al.*, 1989; Economou *et al.*, 1989; Kruys *et al.*, 1992). Stimulation of macrophages with bacterial lipopolysaccharide (LPS, endotoxin), a potent inducer of TNF-α secretion, results in a threefold increase of transcription rates (Beutler *et al.*, 1986; Sariban *et al.*, 1988). The TNF-α gene product is regulated at the post-transcriptional level, in part via a conserved consensus octamer present in the 3' untranslated region of the mRNA for TNF-α and other cytokines. The presence of the conserved sequence UUAUUUAU confers a destabilizing influence and shortens the half-life of the mRNA (Shaw and Kamen, 1986). TNF-α mRNA stability is modulated in part by separate degradative pathways, one of which is sensitive to actinomycin D, and another that is insensitive to actinomycin D and accelerated by LPS (Sariban *et al.*, 1988; Han *et al.*, 1991a,b). Another regulatory step linked to the 3' untranslated region is translational derepression, so that following LPS induction the translation rates of TNF-α mRNA are accelerated (Han *et al.*, 1991a,b). The net effect of LPS stimulation is stabilization of the TNF message that accumulates 100-fold (Lindstein *et al.*, 1989; Han *et al.*, 1991).

The release of secreted TNF-α is limited, occurring transiently in tissue culture and *in vivo* systems. Tolerance to LPS develops, so that macrophage production of TNF-α, which is initially upregulated 10 000-fold, becomes refractory to repeat exposure to LPS. A similar form of tolerance occurs *in vivo* with attenuation of serum TNF-α levels after repeat dosing with LPS (Zuckerman *et al.*, 1991; Salkowski and Vogel, 1992; Zuckerman and Evans, 1992). In experimental mammals and man, TNF-α levels peak within 2 h after intravenous administration of LPS, then fall to baseline (undetectable) levels within 4 h (Hesse *et al.*, 1988). Serum TNF-α is usually not detectable in normal healthy volunteers, but high levels are frequently found in disease (see below).

The biosynthesis of TNF-α is suppressed by a number of factors including PGE_2, cAMP, activators of protein kinase C, dexamethasone, pentoxifylline, glucocorticoids, and cyclosporin A. Gamma-interferon is capable of overcoming the glucocorticoid-induced block of TNF-α synthesis, and upregulates the amount of the TNF-α produced in response to LPS (Leudke and Cerami, 1990).

Cell Sources and Stimuli

Although cells from the monocyte/macrophage lineage have been the most extensively studied for TNF-α production, and are believed to be the principal source of TNF-α production *in vivo*, a number of other cells are capable of secreting TNF-α. These other sources include lymphocytes, mast cells, basophils, eosinophils, NK cells, B cells, T cells, astrocytes, Kupffer cells, keratinocytes, and some tumour cells from colon, breast and brain. The most potent stimulus for TNF-α biosynthesis is LPS. The macrophage is exquisitely sensitive to LPS, so that maximal rates of TNF-α production are observed when LPS is present in barely detectable concentrations. Transmembrane signalling of LPS-induced TNF-α release is modulated via interaction of the LPS–LPS-binding protein complex with CD14 (Schumman *et al.*, 1990; Wright *et al.*, 1990). The signalling mechanisms utilized by other microbial products capable of triggering TNF-α biosynthesis (including toxic-shock-syndrome toxin, enterotoxins, and antigenic determinants present on mycobacteria and fungi) are less well understood. An abridged listing of other naturally occurring substances that induce TNF-α includes products of complement activation, TNF-α itself, IL-1, IL-2, GM-CSF, and antibodies that mediate Fc receptor crosslinking.

TNF-α RECEPTORS

There are two forms of the human TNF-α receptor. These differ in size and binding affinity and are present on virtually all cell types except for the red blood cell (Hohmann *et al.*, 1989). The receptors exhibit apparent molecular masses of 55–60 kDa (TNF-α R1 or TNF-α Rp55) and 75–80 kDa (TNF-α R2 or TNF-α Rp75); the dissociation constants (K_d) are $2-5 \times 10^{-10}$ and $3-7 \times 10^{-11}$, respectively. Binding affinity is dependent on the species from which the receptor and ligand are derived; for instance, human TNF-α is bound by both forms of the human receptor but only one form of the murine receptor

(TNF-α R1). Cloning of the cDNAs encoding the two receptors was facilitated by isolation and sequencing of receptor peptide fragments possessing TNF-α-inhibitory activity in urine and serum of patients with fever and other illnesses (Gray *et al.*, 1990; Loetscher *et al.*, 1990; Nophar *et al.*, 1990). These peptides, termed TNF-α-binding proteins (TNF-α BP1, and TNF-α BP2), proved to be degradative products resulting from proteolytic processing of the TNF-α receptors. The enzyme or pathway for receptor processing into TNF-α BPs has not been elucidated. Both receptors are composed of an intracellular region, a transmembrane segment, and an extracellular domain corresponding to the TNF-α BPs. The external domains define the TNF-α receptors as part of a larger receptor family that includes the receptor nerve growth factor and CD40 (Howard *et al.*, 1991).

The two TNF-α receptors mediate the biological effects of TNF-α. As with other potent and conserved hormones, maximal biological activities of TNF-α are induced when 5% or less of the receptors are occupied. After binding, TNF-α is internalized, but signal transduction may occur in the absence of internalization or after binding of agonist anti-receptor antibodies (Engelmann *et al.*, 1990). It has been suggested that signal transduction may be the result of three receptors clustering together to bind a single TNF-α trimer in a mechanism that is analogous to IgE stimulation of mast cells (Banner *et al.*, 1993). A number of postreceptor signal transduction pathways have been implicated in the intracellular effects of TNF-α R1 including phospholipase A_2, phosphatidylcholine-specific phospholipase, guanine-nucleotide-binding proteins, protein kinases A and C, sphingomyelinase, sodium transporters, and nuclear transcription factors. It is unclear if one of these pathways is dominant in modulating the cellular effects of TNF-α. The complex repertoire of postreceptor responses presumably underlies the diversity of biological effects attributable to TNF-α.

Recent studies suggest that differences exist in the biological function of the two TNF-α receptors. The TNF-α R1 function appears to be predominant in mediating cell cytotoxicity (Tartaglia *et al.*, 1991, 1993) and LPS toxicity (Pfeffer *et al.*, 1993). A transgenic mutant-mouse strain made deficient in this receptor is protected against endotoxin- and superantigen-induced shock, and does not activate nuclear factor κ-B in response to TNF-α (Pfeffer *et al.*, 1993). These observations should not be construed as suggesting that the effects stimulated by TNF-α R1 are all bad, because these same mutant animals are severely impaired in their ability to eradicate infection with *Listeria monocytogenes*, which suggests that TNF-α R1 modulates immunological responses that are normally beneficial in this disease (Pfeffer *et al.*, 1993). Less is known about the mechanisms of signal transduction and biological function of TNF-α R2, but it has been implicated in cellular proliferation (Tartaglia *et al.*, 1991).

A number of stimuli have been identified that trigger the cleavage of the TNF-α Rs into TNF-α BPs, thereby causing an increase in the amount of receptor fragments in the circulation. These stimuli include TNF-α and other cytokines, LPS, fever, and other underlying systemic diseases including cancer and HIV infection (Aderka *et al.*, 1991; Digel *et al.*, 1992, Kalinkovich *et al.*, 1992; van Zee *et al.*, 1992; Santos *et al.*, 1993). The function of the TNF-α BPs is dependent upon the quantity available for binding TNF-α. For instance, low levels of TNF-α BPs may stabilize the activity of TNF-α, and provide a reservoir of TNF-α that is available for gradual release (Aderka *et al.*, 1992). By contrast, higher amounts of TNF-αBP antagonize the effects of TNF-α, and act to block cytotoxicity, immunological responses, and organ toxicity (Peppel *et al.*, 1991; van Zee

Table 1. Some biological effects of TNF-α, in health and disease

Central nervous system	Fever
	Anorexia
	Altered pituitary hormone secretion
Cardiovascular	Shock
	ARDS
	Capillary leakage syndrome
Renal	Acute tubular necrosis
	Nephritis
Gastrointestinal	Ischaemia
	Colitis
	Hepatic necrosis
Metabolic	Lipoprotein lipase suppression
	Net protein catabolism
	Net lipid catabolism
	Stress hormone release
	Insulin resistance
Inflammatory	Activation of cell cytotoxicity
	Enhanced NK cell function
	Mediation of IL-2 tumour toxicity

et al., 1992). By virtue of their pleiotropic effects and integral interaction in the cytokine network, the TNF-α BPs are frequently termed cytokines themselves.

BIOLOGICAL EFFECTS OF TNF-α

The biological effects of TNF-α have been studied in isolated tissue culture and organ perfusion systems, laboratory animals, normal human volunteers, and cancer patients. Some of these activities are summarized in Table 1. From these studies has come a general consensus that TNF-α is a key mediator of inflammation and the mammalian host's response to injury or invasion by microbes, parasites, or neoplasia. In the intact organism, and in some isolated organ systems, the net biological effects of TNF-α are influenced by a complex array of factors including the level of tissue exposure to free and unbound TNF-α, the duration of exposure, the production of other cytokines that increase or decrease the effects of TNF-α, the paracrine effects of TNF-α produced locally in different tissues, and the development of tolerance. Unless considered systematically, the influence of these independent factors may confound interpretation of the biological effects of TNF-α in specific tissues or diseases.

Endothelial Cells and Coagulation

Normally the endothelial cell provides a blood vessel lining that reduces the coagulability of blood. TNF-α causes endothelial cells to have procoagulant activity by enhancing the expression of tissue factor and suppressing cofactor activity for the anticoagulant protein C (Belvilacqua *et al.*, 1986; Nawroth and Stern, 1986; Nawroth *et al.*, 1986; Bauer *et al.*, 1989). TNF-α activates endothelial cells to release IL-1 by a mechanism that is dependent upon protein synthesis (Libby *et al.*, 1986; Nawroth *et al.*, 1986). Other TNF-α-induced endothelial factors include major histocompatibility complex antigens HLA-A, -B (Gamble *et al.*, 1985; Collins *et al.*, 1986) and activation antigens that participate in the adherence of leukocytes and platelets to the endothelial surface (Cotran *et al.*, 1986; Pober *et al.*, 1986; Bevilacqua *et al.*, 1989; Lasky, 1992). TNF-α and other cytokines induce rearrangement of actin filaments with structural changes of the endothelial cells and loss of tight junctions that cause capillary leakage syndrome as plasma proteins and water leak into the tissues (Sato *et al.*, 1986; Stolpen *et al.*, 1986; Stephens *et al.*, 1988; Brett *et al.*, 1989; Damle and Doyle, 1989; Kreil *et al.*, 1989). The acute release of large amounts of TNF-α into the circulatory system causes the toxic manifestation of these responses, resulting in diffuse coagulation with necrosis of vital organs and disseminated capillary leakage syndrome leading to dehydration and pulmonary failure (Remick *et al.*, 1987; Tracey *et al.*, 1986, 1987; Natanson *et al.*, 1989; van der Poll *et al.*, 1990).

Central Nervous System

Early studies of TNF-α distribution suggested that only small amounts of TNF-α cross the blood–brain barrier (Beutler *et al.*, 1985). Nonetheless, systemically administered TNF-α causes fever and anorexia because it crosses into the region of the hypo-thalamic centres that regulate body temperature and appetite (areas that are devoid of a blood–brain barrier) (Nawroth *et al.*, 1986; Salaman-Plata, 1988, 1991; Tracey *et al.*, 1988). The anorectic effects of TNF-α are attenuated by insulin and appear to be independent of serotonergic signals (Tracey *et al.*, 1990). The inflammatory effects of TNF-α are pivotal to the development of cerebral inflammation and oedema during meningitis. High levels of TNF-α in cerebrospinal fluid during meningitis are predic-tive of poor outcome (Leist *et al.*, 1988; Mustafa *et al.*, 1989; Waage *et al.*, 1989; Saukkonen *et al.*, 1990). The inflammatory effects of TNF-α have been implicated in the development of the characteristic plaques in patients with multiple sclerosis. Recently antibodies to TNF-α have been used to reduce the severity of brain inflam-mation in an experimental model of MS (Franciotta *et al.*, 1989; Ruddle *et al.*, 1990; Selmaj *et al.*, 1991). It has been hypothesized that TNF-α may participate in the pathogenesis of brain tumour oedema because glial cell lines produce TNF-α in response to LPS, astrocyte proliferation is enhanced by TNF-α, TNF-α is elevated in some patients with brain tumour, and TNF-α induces capillary leakage syndrome in the peritumoral regions (Barna *et al.*, 1990; Tracey *et al.*, 1990; Martin and Tracey, 1991). Recent studies have presented evidence that TNF-α is produced by neurons innervating the regulatory centres of the hypothalamus, where it may function as a neurotransmitter (Breder and Saper, 1990).

Liver

One highly conserved aspect of the mammalian response to injury or invasion is an increased synthesis of acute-phase proteins and triglycerides, and a decreased pro-duction of albumin by hepatocytes. TNF-α upregulates the expression of acute-phase proteins in human hepatocyte-cell lines, induces increases of serum acute-phase protein levels, and suppresses albumin biosynthesis (Perlmutter *et al.*, 1986; Moldawer *et al.*,

1988; Starnes *et al.*, 1988; Delers *et al.*, 1989). TNF-α, a product of Kupffer cells, is capable of mediating these effects directly, but other TNF-α-induced secondary cytokines such as IL-1 and IL-6 may amplify these acute-phase responses (Magilavy and Rothstein, 1988; Guerne *et al.*, 1989). TNF-α acts to stimulate directly the biosynthesis of circulating lipids, and excessive lipogenesis may contribute to hyper-triglyceridaemia frequently observed in the acute-phase response (Feingold and Grunfeld, 1987; Feingold *et al.*, 1989). Other TNF-α-induced cytokines also possess hepatic lipogenesis-promoting activity (Grunfeld *et al.*, 1989). Perhaps to support the increased substrate needs of the anabolic liver, TNF-α enhances hepatic amino acid clearance, and accelerates the rate of glucagon-mediated amino acid transport into hepatocytes (Warren *et al.*, 1988; Charters and Grimble, 1989; Fukushima *et al.*, 1992). These TNF-α-mediated responses promote the transfer of amino acids from the peripheral tissues to liver and may accelerate the nitrogen losses observed in catabolic illness (Tracey, 1992).

Cardiovascular System

The predominant manifestation of the acute release of large amounts of TNF-α into the circulation is hypotension (shock) followed by cardiopulmonary collapse. Shock is caused by several TNF-α-mediated effects including a decrease of peripheral vascular resistance, falling cardiac output, and loss of intravascular volume through capillary leakage (Tracey *et al.*, 1986, 1987; Natanson *et al.*, 1989; Tracey and Lowry, 1990). Infusion of TNF-α derived from different species induces shock in mammals as varied as mouse and man. Species specificity is apparent in toxicity studies, so that lower doses induce shock and tissue injury when the TNF-α is derived from the same animal species. Although a number of other endogenous factors cause hypotension (e.g. IL-1, IL-2, PAF), the toxicity of TNF-α is unique because it is characterized by a constellation of metabolic, humoral, and cardiovascular changes that closely mimic the response to lethal endotoxaemia or infection. Endothelium-derived nitric oxide synthesis is actived by TNF-α; this response has been implicated in both decreases of peripheral vascular tone and cardiac function (Kilbourn *et al.*, 1990; Finkel *et al.*, 1992). IL-1, while less toxic than TNF-α, induces a transient hypotension without extensive tissue injury, but the addition of IL-l to TNF-α synergistically increases the development of shock and tissue injury (Okusawa *et al.*, 1988; Waage and Espevik, 1988). TNF-α is extremely toxic to the lungs and is pivotal in the development of adult respiratory distress syndrome (ARDS), a syndrome characterized by pulmonary oedema, hypoxia, and high mortality. ARDS develops because of TNF-α-induced activation of pulmonary endothelium, margination of leukocytes with degranulation of granulocytes, and capillary leakage, which precipitates the collection of oedematous fluid in alveoli and prevents adequate perfusion and oxygenation (Horvath *et al.*, 1988; Stephens *et al.*, 1988a,b; Zheng *et al.*, 1990).

Muscle

Patients receiving TNF-α injections develop myalgia resembling the symptoms of viral or bacterial infection. Exposure of myocytes to TNF-α leads to a reduction of resting transmembrane potentials and an increase of intracellular sodium (Tracey *et al.*, 1986;

Kagan *et al.*, 1992). These changes have been implicated in the development of sodium sequestration from the intravascular compartment (termed 'third space losses') that occur in shock and critical illness. The metabolic responses of muscle to TNF-α include a depletion of glycogen stores, enhanced amino acid efflux with net protein loss, increased lactate efflux, and initial increases followed by a later suppression of glucose transporters (Lee *et al.*, 1987; Semb *et al.*, 1987; Tracey *et al.*, 1988; Goodman, 1991; Stephens and Pekala, 1991; Zamir *et al.*, 1992). The net muscle proteolytic effects of TNF-α observed *in vivo* do not occur when TNF-α is incubated with isolated myocytes *in vitro*, indicating that this response is mediated via an unknown secondary mediator or pathway (Moldawer *et al.*, 1987; Tracey, 1992).

Adipose

The original bioassay used in the purification of cachectin from activated macrophage supernatants was based on the suppression of lipoprotein lipase in adipocytes (Beutler *et al.*, 1985). Later studies using recombinant cachectin/TNF-α led to the development of an '*in vitro* model of cachexia' because TNF-α stimulates enhanced lipolysis and reduced transcription of several key lipogenic enzymes (Torti *et al.*, 1985). Thus, TNF-α-treated adipocytes are depleted of lipids, exogenous lipid uptake is blocked, and the incorporation of glucose into newly synthesized lipid is prevented. Thus, the combined effects of TNF-α on adipocytes and myocytes promotes the release of amino acids, lactate, and lipids from peripheral tissues which shunts substrates towards the splanchnic bed and liver.

Endocrinological Effects

The endocrinological effects of TNF-α are dependent upon the dose, route of administration, and metabolic or disease state of the host. Within minutes after injection of TNF-α in normal hosts there are increases of ACTH, cortisol, catecholamines, glucagon, and insulin (Tracey *et al.*, 1986, 1987; Evans *et al.*, 1989; Mealey *et al.*, 1990; Lang *et al.*, 1992). An early hyperglycaemia is followed by a profound hypoglycaemia (Tracey *et al.*, 1986; Elias *et al.*, 1987). The molecular basis for these TNF-α-induced hormonal changes is not completely understood. For example, debate continues over whether TNF-α triggers increases in ACTH by a direct effect on the pituicyte, or via stimulation of corticotropin releasing factor (CRF) release by the hypothalamus (reviewed by Martin and Tracey, 1991). A theoretical feedback loop for the regulation of cytokine biosynthesis is mediated through glucocorticoids: as TNF-α and other cytokines accumulate, the rise in glucocorticoids acts to suppress further cytokine biosynthesis (Bertini *et al.*, 1988, 1989; Butler *et al.*, 1989; Zuckerman and Evans, 1992).

Haemopoietic Effects

TNF-α has been implicated in the development of the anaemia of chronic disease (Tracey *et al.*, 1988). Repeated injections of TNF-α cause a decrease of haematocrit and red blood cell mass, because haemopoiesis is suppressed and red blood cell degradation is increased (Tracey *et al.*, 1988; Moldawer *et al.*, 1989). Similar changes are induced by implantation of a genetically engineered tumour that secretes hTNF-α constitutively (Johnson *et al.*, 1989; Tracey *et al.*, 1990). Following an injection of TNF-α there is an initial rise of circulating granulocytes, then a fall as the inflammatory cells are removed from the circulation by margination. Prolonged exposure to IL-1 triggers the appearance of TNF-α which in turn suppresses haemopoiesis (Gasparetto *et al.*, 1989).

Tumour Effects

Early investigators identified TNF-α as the mediator responsible for inducing the haemorrhagic necrosis of certain transplantable tumours *in vivo*, and the cytotoxicity of certain cell lines *in vitro* (Carswell *et al.*, 1975). Later advances in the biology of TNF-α indicated that the initial promise of a broad spectrum anti-neoplastic agent was thwarted by the toxicity of TNF-α against endothelium and normal tissue (Havell *et al.*, 1988; North and Havell, 1988). Moreover, TNF-α is produced by some tumours and cell lines and possesses activity as a growth factor (Sugarman *et al.*, 1985; Gifford and Flick, 1987; Spriggs *et al.*, 1987; Ranges *et al.*, 1988; Beissert *et al.*, 1989). Prolonged TNF-α exposure in animals bearing a TNF-α-secreting tumour may restrict tumour growth, but the animals succumb to the wasting condition (cachexia) caused by chronic TNF-α toxicity (Teng *et al.*, 1991). Clinical trials for TNF-α administration to cancer patients revealed that the metabolic and toxic effects of TNF-α, which were first demonstrated in the early animal studies, were a potential complication (Tracey *et al.*, 1986, 1988; Warren *et al.*, 1987; Spriggs *et al.*, 1988; Starnes *et al.*, 1988). The use of TNF-α in the treatment of cancer is still under investigation in the hope that a better understanding of its toxicity will lead to the development of a treatment strategy that minimizes toxicity but retains anti-tumour activity in some tumours (Frei and Spriggs, 1989).

TOLERANCE TO TNF-α EFFECTS

Early studies of the biology of TNF-α *in vivo* revealed that repeated injections of rhTNF-α in rats was associated with the development of tolerance to the anorectic and weight-losing activities of TNF-α (Tracey *et al.*, 1988). By progressively increasing the daily doses, the anorexia and weight loss returned; these animals were made tolerant to the lethal effects of massive doses of TNF-α (in excess of the normal LD_{100} dose) (Tracey *et al.*, 1988). The molecular basis of this desensitization or tachyphylaxis has been investigated, but remains largely unexplained (Patton *et al.*, 1987; Fraker *et al.*, 1988; Socher *et al.*, 1988; Wallach *et al.*, 1988). Tolerance does not occur in the models employing tumours that secrete TNF-α continuously, but has been observed in animals receiving TNF-α by continuous infusion (Scheringa *et al.*, 1989; Fraker *et al.*, 1990; Tracey *et al.*, 1990; Hoshino *et al.*, 1991). There is some evidence that tolerance is independent of glucocorticoids, and is specific to tissue type (Grunfeld *et al.*, 1989; Mengozzi and Ghezzi, 1991). Since TNF-α is the pivotal mediator of lethal endotoxic shock, this tolerance has been exploited in efforts to prevent the complications of endotoxaemia (Sheppard *et al.*, 1989; Ciancio *et al.*, 1991). The role of receptor expression, function, and release of TNF-α BPs in this development of tolerance has not been defined.

Table 2. TNF-α and the cytokine network (abridged).

Cytokines induced by TNF-α	IL-1
	IL-6
	IL-8
	IFN-γ
	GM-CSF
	NGF
	TGF-β
	PDGF
Cytokines that suppress TNF-α effects	TGF-β
	IL-10
	TNFαBPs
	CNTF
Cytokines that enhance TNF-α effects	IL-1
	IFN-γ
	LPS
	LIF

INTERACTION OF TNF-α WITH OTHER CYTOKINES

The biology of TNF-α *in vivo* is ultimately linked to the biology of the entire cytokine network. Many biological activities overlap, various combinations of cytokines may increase or decrease net biological effects, and these frequently interact in the stimulation or suppression of cytokine biosynthesis. One of the principal biological effects of TNF-α is to trigger the release of a series of other cytokines that amplify and extend the biological activities of TNF-α alone (Table 2). Once initiated, this cascade of factors drives the host response to invasion, injury, or infection, and persists for hours or days, becoming relatively dissociated in time from the inciting event. TNF-α is pivotal in triggering this cytokine cascade in lethal Gram-negative bacteraemia. For example, Gram-negative bacterial products normally stimulate the biosynthesis of IL-1 and IL-6, but when TNF-α is inhibited by passive immunization with anti-TNF-α antibodies, serum IL-1 and IL-6 does not increase, despite overwhelming bacteraemia (Fong *et al.*, 1989). Thus, TNF-α, and not the bacteria themselves, is pivotal to stimulating the injurious cytokine cascade in lethal bacteraemia.

TNF-α IN SEPTIC SHOCK

Septic shock syndrome, a frequently lethal complication of infectious disease, kills 85 000–150 000 people in the USA annually. Early investigators believed that the development of shock and tissue injury in septic shock syndrome was directly attributable to pathogens and their associated toxins. However, studies of TNF-α now suggest that it is the main mediator triggering septic shock and tissue injury. TNF-α is produced in patients with septic shock syndrome and in some cases elevated serum levels predict higher mortality (Girardin *et al.*, 1988; Debets *et al.*, 1989; Marano *et al.*, 1990; Mozes *et al.*, 1991). TNF-α infusions cause shock and tissue injury in normal animals and man (Tracey *et al.*, 1986, 1987; Remick *et al.*, 1987; Evans *et al.*, 1989; Johnson *et al.*, 1989; Hsueh *et al.*, 1990; Ciancio *et al.*, 1991). Passive immunization with inhibitors of TNF-α

prevents the development of shock and tissue injury despite the administration of lethal doses of LPS or bacteria (Beutler *et al.*, 1985; Tracey *et al.*, 1987; Mathison *et al.*, 1988; Hinshaw *et al.*, 1989; Emerson *et al.*, 1992). Clinical trials to assess the efficacy of inhibiting TNF-α with monoclonal antibodies are underway, and preliminary results suggest that this strategy may prove to be of benefit (Exley *et al.*, 1990). The protection conferred by neutralizing TNF-α is believed to result from the combined effect of directly inhibiting TNF-α toxicity to endothelium and other tissues, and of interrupting the cytokine cascade that normally propagates and amplifies the toxicity of TNF-α (for review see Tracey and Lowry, 1990).

TNF-α IN CACHEXIA

Frequently the most dramatic manifestation of cancer or infection (e.g. HIV or tuberculosis) is a loss of body weight. Termed cachexia, this syndrome is characterized by catabolism of protein and lipid stores that ultimately kills the host, sometimes when the total volume of tumour or infected tissue is small. Studies of the biology of TNF-α and other cytokines suggest that cachexia may be caused by chronic exposure to cytokines. The biochemical basis of TNF-α-induced cachexia is in part caused by its catabolic effects on muscle and adipose tissue, with a shunting of energy substrates to the liver for incorporation into acute-phase proteins and lipid (see above). Although there is a large body of evidence confirming that chronic exposure to TNF-α causes cachexia, there is also a general consensus that the molecular basis by which TNF-α increases net protein catabolism is unknown (Oliff *et al.*, 1987; Tracey *et al.*, 1988, 1990). This analysis is confounded by recent studies indicating that the net biological effects of TNF-α are not directly related to the amount of TNF-α in the circulatory system, but are influenced by the paracrine effects of TNF-α produced locally in tissues (e.g. brain versus peripheral tissue) (Tracey *et al.*, 1990). As of this writing there is a general consensus that TNF-α, IL-1, IL-6 and IFN-γ are all capable of causing cachexia, but the underlying mechanisms are unknown, and the role of these factors in causing cachexia in human diseases is also unknown (Gershenwald *et al.*, 1990; Matthys *et al.*, 1991; Strassmann *et al.*, 1992).

TNF-α IN OTHER DISEASES

TNF-α has been implicated in the mediation of a number of other diseases, some of which are summarized in Table 3. The pleiotropic nature of TNF-α prevents generaliz-ation about whether it is beneficial or injurious. It is clear that, in some instances, the local effects of TNF-α improve hose defence mechanisms by mobilizing substrate, increasing immune cell function, and stimulating inflammation. But in other cases the toxicity of TNF-α may cause disease by mediating shock, tissue injury, or catabolic illness. Continued advances in our understanding of the biology of TNF-α and its receptors, the mechanisms of signal transduction, and the pathways that modulate its net biological effects are likely to foster the development of additional therapeutic strategies for a variety of disparate diseases. It is likely that some of these therapies will inhibit the toxicity of TNF-α, whereas others will amplify the immune-enhancing activities of this privotal cytokine.

Table 3.   A list of some of the diseases in which TNF-α has been implicated.

AIDS
Anaemia
Autoimmune disease
Cachexia
Cancer
Cerebral malaria
Diabetes mellitus
Disseminated intravascular coagulopathy
Eurthyroid sick syndrome
Haemorrhagic shock
Hepatitis
Insulin resistance
Leprosy
Leukaemia
Lymphoma
Meningitis
Multiple sclerosis
Myocardial ischaemia
Obesity
Rejection of transplanted organs
Rheumatoid arthritis
Septic shock syndrome
Stroke
Tuberculosis

REFERENCES

Aderka, D., Engelmann, H. and Hornik, V. (1991). *Cancer Res.* **51**, 5602–5607.

Aderka, D., Engelmann, H., Maor, Y., Brakebusch, C. and Wallach, D. (1992). *J. Exp. Med.* **175**, 323–329.

Banner, D.W., D'Arcy, A., Janes, W., Gentz, R., Schoenfeld, H.J., Broger, C., Loetscher, H. and Lesslauer, W. (1993). *Cell* **73**, 431–445.

Barna, B.P., Estes, M.L., Jacobs, B.S., Hudson, S. and Ransohoff, R.M. (1990). *J. Neuroimmunol.* **30**, 239–243.

Bauer, K.A., ten Cate, H., Barzegar, S., Spriggs, D.R., Sherman, M.L. and Rosenberg, R.D. (1989). *Blood* **74**, 165–172.

Beissert, S., Bergholz, M., Maase, I., Lepsien, G., Schauer, A., Pfizenmaier, K. and Kronke, M. (1989). *Proc. Natl Acad. Sci. USA* **86**, 5064–5068.

Bertini, R., Bianchi, M. and Ghezzi, P. (1988). *J. Exp. Med.* **167**, 1708–1712.

Bertini, R., Bianchi, M., Erroi, A., Villa, P. and Ghezzi, P. (1989). *J. Leukoc. Biol.* **46**, 254–262.

Beutler, B., Mahoney, J., Le Trang, N., Pekala, P. and Cerami, A. (1985a). *J. Exp. Med.* **161**, 984–995.

Beutler, B., Milsark, I.W. and Cerami, A. (1985b). *J. Immunol.* **135**, 3972–3977.

Beutler, B., Milsark, I.W. and Cerami, A.C. (1985c) *Science* **229**, 869–871.

Beutler, B., Tkacenko, V., Milsark, I., Krochin, N. and Cerami, A. (1986). *J. Exp. Med.* **164**, 1791–1796.

Bevilacqua, M.P., Pober, J.S., Majeau, G.R., Fiers, W., Cotran, R.S. and Gimbrone, M.A. Jr. (1986). *Proc. Natl Acad. Sci. USA* **83**, 4533–4537.

Bevilacqua, M.P., Stengelin, S., Gimbrone, M.A. Jr. and Seed, B. (1989). *Science* **243**, 1160–1165.

Breder, C.D. and Saper, C.B. (1990). *Soc. Neurosci. Abstr.* **144**, 1280 (Abstr.).

Brenner, D.A., OHara, M., Angel, P., Chojkier, M. and Karin, M. (1989). *Nature* **337**, 661–663.

Brett, J., Gerlach, H., Nawroth, P., Steinberg, S., Godman, G. and Stern, D. (1989). *J. Exp. Med.* **169**, 1977–1991.

Butler, L.D., Layman, N.K., Riedl, P.E., Cain, R.L., Shellhaas, J., Evans, G.F. and Zuckerman, S.H. (1989). *J. Neuroimmunol.* **24**, 143–153.

Carswell, E.A., Old, L.J., Kassel, R.L., Green, S., Fiore, N. and Williamson, B. (1975). *Proc. Natl Acad. Sci. USA* **72**, 3666–3670.

Charters, Y. and Grimble, R.F. (1989). *Biochem. J.* **258**, 493–497.

Ciancio, M.J., Hunt, J., Jones, S.B. and Filkins, J.P. (1991). *Circ. Shock* **33**, 108–120.

Collins, T., Lapierre, L.A., Fiers, W., Strominger, J.L. and Pober, J.S. (1986). *Proc. Natl Acad. Sci. USA* **83**, 446–450.

Cotran, R.S., Gimbrone, M.A. Jr., Bevilacqua, M.P., Mendrick, D.L. and Pober, J.S. (1986). *J. Exp. Med.* **164**, 661–666.

Creasey, A.A., Doyle, L.V., Reynolds, M.T., Jung, T., Lin, L.S. and Vitt, C.R. (1987). *Cancer Res.* **47**, 145–149.

Damle, N.K. and Doyle, L.V. (1989). *J. Immunol.* **142**, 2660–2669.

Davis, J.M., Narachi, M.A., Alton, K. and Arakawa, T. (1987). *Biochem.* **26**, 1322–1326.

Debets, J.M.H., Kampmeijer, R., Van Der Linden, M.P.M.H., Buurman, W.A. and Van Der Linden, C.J. (1989). *Crit. Care Med.* **17**, 489–494.

Delers, F., Mangeney, M., Raffa, D., Vallet Colom, I., Daveau, M., Tran Quang, N., Davrinches, C. and Chambaz, J. (1989). *Biochem. Biophys. Res. Commun.* **161**, 81–88.

Digel, W., Porszolt, F., Schmid, M., Herrmann, F., Lesslauer, W. and Brockhaus, M. (1992). *J. Clin. Invest.* **89**, 1690–1693.

Economou, J.S., Rhoades, K., Essner, R., McBride, W.H., Gasson, J.C. and Morton, D.S. (1989). *J. Exp. Med.* **170**, 321–326.

Elias, J.A., Gustilo, K., Baeder, W. and Freundlich, B. (1987). *J. Immunol.* **138**, 3812–3816.

Emerson, T.E., Lindsey, D.C., Jesmok, G.J., Duerr, M.L. and Fournel, M.A. (1992). *Circ. Shock* **38**, 75–84.

Engelmann, H., Holtmann, H., Brakebusch, C., Avni, Y.S., Sarov, I., Nophar, Y., Hadas, E., Leitner, O. and Wallach, D. (1990). *J. Biol. Chem.* **265**, 14497–14504.

Evans, D.A., Jacobs, D.O., Revhaug, A. and Wilmore, D.W. (1989a). *Ann. Surg.* **209**, 312–321.

Evans, D.A., Jacobs, D.O. and Wilmore, D.W. (1989b). *Am. J. Physiol.* **257**, R1182–R1189.

Exley, A.R., Cohen, J., Buurman, W., Owen, R., Hanson, G., Lumley, J., Aulakh, J.M., Bodmer, M., Riddell, A., Stephens, S. and Perry, M. (1990). *Lancet* i, 1275–1277.

Feingold, K.R. and Grunfeld, C. (1987). *J. Clin. Invest.* **80**, 184–190.

Feingold, K.R., Soued, M., Staprans, I., Gavin, L.A., Donahue, M.E., Huang, B.-J., Moser, A.H., Gulli, R. and Grunfeld, C. (1989). *J. Clin. Invest.* **83**, 1116–1121.

Finkel, M.S., Oddis, C.V., Jacob, T.D., Watkins, S.C., Hattler, B.G. and Simmons, R.L. (1992). *Science* **257**, 387–389.

Fong, Y., Tracey, K.J., Moldawer, L.L., Hesse, D.G., Manogue, K.R., Kenney, J.S., Lee, A.T., Kuo, G.C., Allison, A.C., Lowry, S.F. and Cerami, A. (1989). *J. Exp. Med.* **170**, 1627–1633.

Fraker, D.L., Sheppard, B.C. and Norton, J.A. (1990). *Cancer Res.* **50**, 2261–2267.

Fraker, D.L., Stovroff, M.C., Merino, M.J. and Norton, J.A. (1988). *J. Exp. Med.* **168**, 95–105.

Franciotta, D.M., Grimaldi, L.M.E., Martino, G.V., Piccolo, G., Bergamaschi, R., Citterio, A. and Melzi d'Eril, G.V. (1989). *Ann. Neurol.* **26**, 787–789.

Frei, E. and Spriggs, D. (1989). *J. Clin. Oncol.* **7**, 291–294.

Fukushima, R., Siato, H., Taniwaka, K., Hirmatsu, T., Morioka, Y., Muto, T. and Abumrad, N.N. (1992). *Am. J. Physiol.* **2625**, E275–E181.

Gamble, J.R., Harlan, J.M., Klebanoff, S.J. and Vadas, M.A. (1985). *Proc. Natl Acad. Sci. USA* **82**, 8667–8671.

Gasparetto, C., Laver, J., Abboud, M., Gillio, A., Smith, C., OReilly, R.J. and Moore, M.A. (1989). *Blood* **74**, 547–550.

Gershenwald, J.E., Fong, Y., Fahey, T.J., III, Calvano, S.E., Chizzonite, R., Kilian, P.L., Lowry, S.F. and Moldawer, L.L. (1990). *Proc. Natl Acad. Sci. USA* **87**, 4966–4970.

Gifford, G.E. and Flick, D.A. (1987). *Ciba. Found. Symp.* **131**, 3–20.

Girardin, E., Grau, G.E., Dayer, J.-M., Roux-Lombard, P., The J5 Study Group and Lambert, P.-H. (1988). *N. Engl. J. Med.* **319**, 397–400.

Goodman, M.N. (1991). *Am. J. Physiol.* **260**, E727–E730.

Gray, P.W., Barrett, K., Chantry, D., Turner, M. and Feldman, M. (1990). *Proc. Natl Acad. Sci. USA* **86**, 7380–7384.

Grunfeld, C., Wilking, H., Neese, R., Gavin, L.A., Moser, A.H., Gulli, R., Serio M.K. and Feingold, K.R. (1989). *Cancer Res.* **49**, 2554–2560.

Guerne, P.A., Zuraw, B.L., Vaughan, J.H., Carson, D.A. and Lotz, M. (1989). *J. Clin. Invest.* **83**, 585–592.

Han, J., Beutler, B. and Huez, G. (1991a). *Biochimica et Biophysica Acta* **1090**, 22–28.
Han, J., Heuz, G. and Beutler, B. (1991b). *Journal of Immunology* **146**, 1843–1848.
Havell, E.A., Fiers, W. and North, R.J. (1988). *J. Exp. Med.* **167**, 1067–1085.
Hesse, D.G., Tracey, K.J., Fong, Y., Manogue, K.R., Palladino, M.A. Jr., Cerami, A., Shires, G.T. and Lowry, S.F. (1988). *Surg. Gynecol. Obstet.* **166**, 147–153.
Hinshaw, L., Olson, P. and Kuo, G. (1989). *Circ. Shock,* **27**, 362–369.
Hohmann, H.-P., Remy, R., Brockhaus, M. and van Loon, A.P.G.M. (1989). *J. Biol. Chem.* **264**, 14927–14934.
Horvath, C.J., Ferro, T.J., Josmok, G. and Malik, A.B. (1988). *Proc. Natl Acad. Sci. USA* **85**, 9219–9223.
Hoshino, E., Pichard, C., Greenwood, C.E., Kuo, G.C., Cameron, R.G., Kurian, R., Kearns, J.P., Allard, J.P. and Jeejeebhoy, K.N. (1991). *Am. J. Physiol. Endocrinol. Metab.* **260**, E27–E36.
Howard, S.T., Chan, Y.S. and Smith G.L. (1991). *Virology* **180**, 633–647.
Hsueh, W., Sun, X., Rioja, L.N. and Gonzalez-Crussi, F. (1990). *Immunology,* **70**, 309–314.
Johnson, J., Meyrick, B., Jesmok, G. and Brigham, K.L. (1989). *J. Appl. Physiol.* **66**, 1448–1454.
Johnson, R.A., Waddelow, T.A., Caro, J., Oliff, A. and Roodman, G.D. (1989). *Blood* **74**, 130–138.
Jones, E.Y., Stuart, D.I. and Walker, N.P. (1989). *Nature* **338**, 225–228.
Jue, D.-M., Sherry, B., Leudke, C., Manogue, K.R. and Cerami, A. (1990). *Biochem.* **29**, 8371–8377.
Kagan, B.L., Baldwin, R.L., Munoz, D. and Wisnieski, B.J. (1992). *Science* **255**, 1427–1430.
Kalinkovich, A., Engelmann, H. and Harpaz, N. (1992). *Clin. Exp. Immunol.* **89**, 351–355.
Kilbourn, R.G., Gross, S.S., Jubran, A., Adams, J., Griffith, O.W., Levi, R. and Lodato, R.F. (1990). *Proc. Natl Acad. Sci. USA* **87**, 3629–3632.
Kreil, E.A., Greene, E., Fitzgibbon, C., Robinson, D.R. and Zapol, W.M. (1989). *Circ. Res.* **65**, 502–514.
Kriegler, M., Perez, C., DeFay, K., Albert, I. and Lu, S.D. (1988). *Cell* **53**, 45–53.
Kruys, V., Kemmer, K., Shakhov, A., Jongeneel, V. and Beutler, B. (1992). *Proc. Natl Acad. Sci. USA* **673**, 677.
Lang, C.H., Dobrescu, C. and Bagby, G.J. (1992). *Endo.* **130**, 43–52.
Lasky, L.A. (1992). *Science* **258**, 964–969.
Lee, M.D., Zentella, A., Pekala, P.H. and Cerami, A. (1987). *Proc. Natl Acad. Sci. USA* **84**, 2590–2594.
Leist, T.P., Frei, K., Kam Hansen, S., Zinkernagel, R.M. and Fontana, A. (1988). *J. Exp. Med.* **167**, 1743–1748.
Leudke, C.E. and Cerami, A. (1990). *J. Clin. Invest.* **86**, 1234–1240.
Libby, P., Ordovas, J.M., Auger, K.R., Robbins, A.H., Birinyi, L.K. and Dinarello, C.A. (1986). *Am. J. Path.* **124**, 179–185.
Lin, L.S. (1992). In *Tumor Necrosis Factor: The Molecules and Their Emerging Role in Medicine* (ed. Beutler, B.), Raven Press, New York, pp. 33–48.
Lindstein, T., June, C.H., Ledbetter, J.A., Stella, G. and Thompson, C.B. (1989). *Science* **244**, 339–343.
Loetscher, H., Pan, Y.-C.E., Lahm, H.-W., Gentz, R., Brockhaus, M., Tabuchi, H. and Lesslauer, W. (1990). *Cell* **61**, 351–359.
Magilavy, D.B. and Rothstein, J.L. (1988). *J. Exp. Med.* **168**, 789–794.
Marano, M.A., Fong, Y., Moldawer, L.L., Calvano, S.E., Tracey, K.J., Barie, P.S., Manogue, K.R., Cerami, A., Shires, G.T. and Lowry, S.F. (1990). *Surg. Gynecol. Obstet.* **170**, 32–38.
Martin S.B. and Tracey, K.J. (1991). *Adv. Neuroimmun*
Mathison, J.C., Wolfson, E. and Ulevitch, R.J. (1988). *J. Clin. Invest.* **81**, 1925–1937.
Matthys, P., Dukmans, R., Proost, P., Damme, J.V., Heremans, H., Sobis, H. and Balliau, A. (1991). *Int. J. Cancer.* **49**, 77–82.
Mealy, K., van Lanschot, J.J.B., Robinson, B.G., Rounds, J. and Wilmore, D.W. (1990). *Arch. Surg.* **125**, 42–48.
Mengozzi, M. and Ghezzi, P. (1991). *Endo.* **128**, 1668–1672.
Moldawer, L.L., Svaninger, G., Gelin, J. and Lundholm, K.G. (1987). *Am. J. Physiol.* **253**, C766–C773.
Moldawer, L.L., Andersson, C., Gelin, J., Lonnroth, C. and Lundholm, K. (1988). *Am. J. Physiol.* **254**, G450–G456.
Moldawer, L.L., Marano, M.A., Wei, H., Fong, Y., Silen, M.L., Kuo, G., Manogue, K.R., Vlassara, H., Cohen, H., Cerami, A. *et al.* (1989). *FASEB J.* **3**, 1637–1643.
Mozes, T., Ben-Efraim, S., Tak, C.J.A.M., Heiligers, J.P.C., Saxena, P.R. and Bonta, I.L. (1991). *Immunol. Lett.* **27**, 157–162.
Muller, U., Jongeneel, V., Nedospasov, S.A., Lindahl, K.F. and Steinmetz, M. (1987). *Nature* **335**, 265–267.

Mustafa, M.M., Lebel, M.H., Ramilo, O., Olsen, K.D., Reisch, J.S., Beulter, B. and McCracken, G.H. Jr. (1989). *J. Pediatr.* **115**, 208–213.

Natanson, C., Eichenholz, P.W., Danner, R.L., Eichhacker, P.Q., Hoffman, W.D., Kuo, G.C., Banks, S.M., MacVittie, T.J. and Parrillo, J.E. (1989). *J. Exp. Med.* **169**, 823–832.

Nawroth, P.P. and Stern, D.M. (1986). *J. Exp. Med.* **163**, 740–745.

Nawroth, P.P., Bank, I., Handley, D., Cassimeris, J., Chess, L. and Stern, D. (1986). *J. Exp. Med.* **163**, 1363–1375.

Nophar, Y., Kemper, O., Brakebusch, C., Engelmann, H., Zwang, R., Aderka, D., Holtmann, H. and Wallach, D. (1990). *EMBO J.* **9**, 3269–3278.

North, R.J. and Havell, E.A. (1988). *J. Exp. Med.* **167**, 1086–1099.

Okusawa, S., Gelfand, J.A., Ikejima, T., Connolly, R.J. and Dinarello, C.A. (1988). *J. Clin. Invest.* **81**, 1162–1172.

Oliff, A., Defeo-Jones, D., Boyer, M., Martinez, D., Kiefer, D., Vuocolo, G., Wolfe, A. and Socher, S.H. (1987). *Cell* **50**, 555–563.

Patton, J.S., Peters, P.M., McCabe, J., Crase, D., Hansen, S., Chen, A.B. and Liggit, D. (1987). *J. Clin. Invest.* **80**, 1587–1596.

Peppel, K., Crawford, D. and Beutler, B. (1991). *J. Exp. Med.* **174**, 1483–1489.

Perez, C., Albert, I., DeFay, K., Zachariades, N., Gooding, L. and Kriegler, M. (1990). *Cell* **63**, 251–258.

Perlmutter, D.H., Dinarello, C.A., Punsal, P.I. and Colten, H.R. (1986). *J. Clin. Invest.* **78**, 1349–1354.

Pfeffer, K., Matsuyama, T., Kundig, T.M., Wakeham, A., Kishihara, K., Shahinian, A., Wiegmann, K., Ohashi, P.S., Kronke, M. and Mak, T.W. (1993). *Cell* **73**, 457–467.

Pober, J.S., Bevilacqua, M.P., Mendrick, D.L., Lapierre, L.A., Fiers, W. and Gimbrone, M.A. Jr. (1986). *J. Immunol.* **136**, 1680–1687.

Ranges, G.E., Zlotnik, A., Espevik, T., Dinarello, C.A., Cerami, A. and Palladino, M.A. Jr. (1988). *J. Exp. Med.* **167**, 1472–1478.

Remick, D.G., Kunkel, R.G., Larrick, J.W. and Kunkel, S.L. (1987). *Lab. Invest.* **56**, 583–590.

Ruddle, N.H., Bergman, C.M., McGrath, K.M., Lingenheld, E.G., Grunnet, M.L., Padula, S.J. and Clark, R.B. (1990). *J. Exp. Med.* **172**, 1193–1200.

Salaman-Plata, C.R. (1991). *Neurosci. Biobehav. Rev.* **15**, 185–215.

Salaman-Plata, C.R., Oomura, Y. and Kai, Y. (1988). *Brain Res.* **448**, 106–114.

Salkowski, C.A. and Vogel, S.N. (1992). *J. Immunol.* **149**, 4041–4047.

Santos, A.A., Scheltinga, M.R., Lynch, E., Brown, E.F., Lawton, P., Chambers, E., Browning, J., Dinarello, C.A., Wolff, S.M. and Wilmore, D.W. (1993). *Arch. Surg.* **128**, 138–144.

Sariban, E., Imamura, K., Luebbers, R. and Kufe, D.W. (1988). *J. Clin. Invest.* **81**, 1506–1510.

Sato, N., Goto, T., Haranaka, K., Satomi, N., Nariuchi, H., Mano-Hirano, Y. and Sawasaki, Y. (1986). *JNCI* **76**, 1113–1122.

Saukkonen, K., Sande, S., Cioffe, C., Wolpe, S., Sherry, B., Cerami, A. and Tuomanen, E. (1990). *J. Exp. Med.* **171**, 439–448.

Scheringa, M., Keizer, A., Jeekel, J. and Marquet, R.L. (1989). *Int. J. Cancer* **43**, 905–909.

Schumann, R.R., Leong, S.R., Flaggs, G.W., Gray, P.W., Wright, S.D., Mathison, J.C., Tobias, P.S. and Ulevitch, R.J. (1990). *Science* **249**, 1429–1431.

Selmaj, K., Raine, C.S., Cannella, B. and Brosnan, C.F. (1991). *J. Clin. Invest.* **87**, 949–954.

Semb, H., Peterson, J., Tavernier, J. and Olivecrona, T. (1987). *J. Biol. Chem.* **262**, 8390–8394.

Shaw, G. and Kamen, R. (1986). *Cell* **46**, 659–667.

Sheppard, B.C., Fraker, D.L. and Norton, J.A. (1989). *Surgery* **106**, 156–161; discus.

Socher, S.H., Friedman, A. and Martinez, D. (1988). *J. Exp. Med.* **167**, 1957–1962.

Socher, S.H., Riemen, M.W., Martinez, D., Friedman, A., Tai, J., Quintero, J.C., Garsky, V. and Oliff, A. (1987). *Proc. Natl Acad. Sci. USA* **84**, 8829–8833.

Spies, T., Morton, C.C., Nedospasov, S.A., Fiers, W., Pious, D. and Strominger, J.L. (1986). *Proc. Natl Acad. Sci. USA* **83**, 8699–8702.

Sprang, S.R. and Eck, M.J. (1922). In *Tumor Necrosis Factor: The Molecules and Their Emerging Role in Medicine* (ed. Beutler, B.), Raven Press, New York, pp. 11–32.

Spriggs, D.R., Sherman, M.L., Michie, H.R., Arthur, K.A., Imamura, K., Wilmore, D.W., Frei, W., III, and Kufe, D.W. (1988). *JNCI* **80**, 1039–1044.

Spriggs, D.R., Imamura, K., Rodriguez, C., Horiguchi, J. and Kufe, D.W. (1987). *Proc. Natl Acad. Sci. USA* **84**, 6563–6566.

Starnes, H.R. Jr., Warren, R.S., Jeevanandam, M., Gabrilove, J.L., Larchian, W., Oettgen, H.F. and Brennan, M.F. (1988). *J. Clin. Invest.* **82**, 1321–1325.

Stephens, J.M. and Pekala, P.H. (1991). *J. Biol. Chem.* **266**, 21839–21845.

Stephens, K.E., Ishizaka, A., Larrick, J.W. and Raffin, T.A. (1988a). *Am. Rev. Respir, Dis.* **137**, 1364–1370.

Stephens, K.E., Ishizaka, A., Wu, Z., Larrick, J.W. and Raffin, T.A. (1988b). *Am. Rev. Respir. Dis.* **138**, 1300–1307.

Stevenson, F.T., Burstein, S.L., Locksley, R.M. and Lovett, D.H. (1992). *J. Exp. Med.* **176**, 1053–1062.

Stolpen, A.H., Guinan, E.C., Fiers, W. and Pober, J.S. (1986). *Am. J. Path.* **123**, 16–24.

Strassmann, G., Fong, M., Kenney, J.S. and Jacob, C.O. (1992). *J. Clin. Invest.* **89**, 1681–1684.

Sugarman, B.J., Aggarwal, B.B., Hass, P.E., Figari, I.S., Palladino, M.A. Jr. and Shepard, H.M. (1985). *Science* **230**, 943–945.

Tartaglia, L.A., Weber, R.F., Figari, I.S., Reynolds, C., Palladino, M.A. and Goeddel, D.V. (1991). *Proc. Natl Acad. Sci. USA* **88**, 9292–9296.

Tartaglia, L.A., Rothe, M., Hu, Y.F. and Goeddel. D.W. (1993). *Cell* **73**, 213–216.

Teng, M.N., Park, B.H., Koeppen, H.K.W., Tracey, K.J., Fendly, B.M. and Schreiber, H. (1991). *Proc. Natl Acad. Sci. USA* **88**, 3535–3539.

Torti, F.M., Dieckmann, B., Beutler, B., Cerami, A. and Ringold, G.M. (1985). *Science* **229**, 867–869.

Tracey, K.J. (1992). *Clin. Nutr.* **11**, 1–11.

Tracey, K.J. and Lowry, S.F. (1990). *Adv. Surg.* **23**, 21–56.

Tracey, K.J., Beutler, B., Lowry, S.F., Merryweather, J., Wolpe, S., Milsark, I.W., Hariri, R.J., Fahey, T.J., III, Zentella, A., Albert, J.D., Shires, G.T. and Cerami, A. (1986a). *Science* **234**, 470–474.

Tracey, K.J., Lowry, S.F., Beutler, B., Cerami, A., Albert, J.D. and Shires, G.T. (1986b). *J. Exp. Med.* **164**, 1368–1373.

Tracey, K.J., Fong, Y., Hesse, D.G., Manogue, K.R., Lee, A.T., Kuo, G.C., Lowry, S.F. and Cerami, A. (1987a). *Nature* **330**, 662–664.

Tracey, K.J., Lowry, S.F., Fahey, T.J., III, Albert, J.D., Fong, Y., Hesse, D., Beutler, B., Manogue, K.R., Calvano, S., Wei, H., Cerami, A. and Shires, G.T. (1987b). *Surg. Gynecol. Obstet.* **164**, 415–422.

Tracey, K.J., Wei, H., Manogue, K.R., Fong, Y., Hesse, D.G., Nguyen, H.T., Kuo, G.C., Beutler, B., Cotran, R.S., Cerami, A. and Lowry, S.F. (1988). *J. Exp. Med.* **167**, 1211–1227.

Tracey, K.J., Morgello, S., Koplin, B., Fahey, T.J., III, Fox, J., Aledo, A., Manogue, K.R. and Cerami, A. (1990). *J. Clin. Invest.* **86**, 2014–2024.

van der Poll, T., Buller, H.R., ten Cate, H., Wortel, C.H., Bauer, K.A., van Deventer, S.J.H., Hack, E., Sauerwein, H.P., Rosenberg, R.D. and ten Cate, J.W. (1990). *N. Engl. J. Med.* **322**, 1622–1627.

van Zee, K.J., Kohno, T., Fischer, E., Rock, C.S., Moldawer, L.L. and Lowry, S.F. (1992). *Proc. Natl Acad. Sci. USA* **89**, 4845–4849.

Waage, A. and Espevik, T. (1988). *J. Exp. Med.* **167**, 1987–1992.

Waage, A., Halstensen, A., Shalaby, R., Brandtzaeg, P., Kierulf, P. and Espevik, T. (1989). *J. Exp. Med.* **170**, 1859–1967.

Wallach, D., Holtmann, H., Engelmann, H. and Nophar, Y. (1988). *J. Immunol.* **140**, 2994–2999.

Wang, A.M., Creasey, A.A., Ladner, M.B., Lin, L.S., Strickler, J., van Arsdel, J.N., Yamamoto, R. and Mark, D.F. (1985). *Science* **228**, 149–154.

Warren, R.S., Starnes, J.F. Jr., Gabrilove, J.L., Oettgen, H.F. and Brennan, M.F. (1987). *Arch. Surg.* **122**, 1396–1400.

Warren, R.S., Starnes, H.F. Jr., Alcock, N., Calvano, S. and Brennan, M.F. (1987). *Am. J. Physiol.* **255**, E206–E212.

Wright, S.D., Ramos, R.A., Tobias, P.S., Ulevitch, R.J. and Mathison, J.C. (1990). *Science* **249**, 1431–1433.

Zamir, O., Hasselgren, P.O., Kunkel, S.L., Frederick, J., Higashiguchi, T. and Fischer, J.E. (1992). *Arch. Surg.* **127**, 170–174.

Zheng, H., Crowley, J.J., Chan, J.C., Hoffman, H., Hatherill, J.R., Ishizaka, A. and Raffin, T.A. (1990). *Am. Rev. Respir, Dis.* **142**, 1073–1078.

Zuckerman, S.H. and Evans, G.F. (1992). *Cell Immunol.* **140**, 513–519.

Zuckerman, S.H., Evans, G.F. and Butler, L.D. (1991). *Infect. Immun.* **59**, 2774–2780.

Chapter 17

Tumour Necrosis Factor-Beta/Lymphotoxin-Alpha

Nancy H. Ruddle

Department of Epidemiology and Public Health, Yale University School of Medicine,
New Haven, CT, USA

INTRODUCTION

Tumour necrosis factor-β (TNF-β), also known as lymphotoxin (LT) or LT-α, is a 25 kDa protein produced by activated lymphocytes and was actually the first of the TNFs to be described. At the time of its discovery, Ruddle and Waksman (1968) called it cytotoxic factor and Granger and Williams (1968) coined the term, lymphotoxin (LT). The factor was originally characterized by its toxicity to syngeneic embryo fibroblasts or L929 cells. The realization that LT and tumour necrosis factor (TNF), a protein originally thought to be produced exclusively by activated macrophages, are 35% homologous (Li *et al.*, 1987) and share many activities including killing L929 cells, inducing necrosis of the Meth A sarcoma *in vivo* (Gray *et al.*, 1984), and activating polymorphonuclear leukocytes (Shalaby *et al.*, 1985) prompted a change in the name of lymphotoxin to TNF-β and tumour necrosis factor to TNF-α. It is now clear that TNF-α and TNF-β are members of a gene family that includes yet another member previously termed p33, and now designated LT-β (Browning *et al.*, 1993). The three genes are tightly linked within the MHC and show similar organization. The biologically active forms of secreted TNF-α and TNF-β are homotrimers. To date no heterotrimers of these secreted forms have been described. TNF-α and TNF-β share many biological activities, including competition for the same cell-surface receptors (Aggarwal *et al.*, 1985a). Nevertheless, important differences do exist both with regard to protein sequence and gene regulation. There are also distinct differences in the mode of secretion, in that TNF-α can be displayed as a membrane protein utilizing its long signal sequence (Kriegler *et al.*, 1988) or it can be secreted, whereas TNF-β has a more conventional signal peptide and is secreted. However, TNF-β (LT-α) can be complexed with LT-β as a membrane-associated heterotrimer with two copies of TNF-β and one of LT-β (LT-α_2 LT-β_1). LT-β is anchored to the membrane through its long *N*-terminal leader peptide and has not yet been identified in a secreted form. Differences in target cell sensitivities to the two secreted TNFs exist (Browning and Ribolini, 1989) and there are similarities and differences in the nature of cells producing the members of the family; TNF-α is produced by a wide variety of cells, including fibroblasts, macrophages, and T and B cells, whereas TNF-β and LT-β are predominantly products of lymphocytes (Paul and Ruddle, 1988; Ware *et al.*, 1992).

TNF-β exerts a wide variety of effects in tissue culture ranging from killing tumour cells, to inducing gene expression, to stimulating fibroblast proliferation. To date, no biological activity of the LT-α LT-β complex has been defined. Biological roles of TNF-β include mediation of inflammation and graft rejection. It has been detected in lesions of multiple sclerosis (Selmaj *et al.*, 1991a), and TNF-β, together with TNF-α has been implicated in a mouse model of that disease, experimental allergic encephalomyelitis (Ruddle *et al.*, 1990). Participation in insulin-dependent diabetes mellitus has also been suggested (Picarella *et al.*, 1992). Additional roles in T- and B-cell development and retroviral-associated diseases including AIDS, human T-cell leukaemia virus 1 (HTLV-1) associated myelopathy and hypercalcaemia are under investigation.

CELLS OF ORIGIN

TNF-β is a tightly regulated product of lymphocytes. It is induced from members of some T- and B-cell subsets by any of several different stimuli (Paul and Ruddle, 1988; Turetskaya *et al.*, 1992). TNF-β is released from T cells after activation with antigen, in association with components of the MHC (Conta *et al.*, 1983, 1985), agents that mimic that activation through the T-cell receptor such as anti-CD3 (Ruddle *et al.*, 1990; Steffen *et al.*, 1988; Sung *et al.*, 1988), high levels of IL-2, or nonspecific T cell mitogens such as Con A or phytohaemagglutinin (reviewed in Paul and Ruddle, 1988). It is produced after antigen activation of cytotoxic CD8 T cells and of CD4 T_{H1} or inflammatory cells but not by T_{H2} cells. TNF-β is also produced constitutively at a high level by several HTLV-1-infected cell lines (Ratner *et al.*, 1987; Kronke *et al.*, 1988; Tschachler *et al.*, 1989; Paul *et al.*, 1990). A direct role for that virus is indicated by the observation (Tschachler *et al.*, 1989) that constitutive expression of TNF-β occurs after infection of T-cell clones with HTLV-1. Furthermore, Tax protein induces expression of TNF-β mRNA in B cells (Lindholm *et al.*, 1992) and transfection of the HTLV-1 *tax* gene in T cells activates LT gene promoter activity (Paul *et al.*, 1993). TNF-β is produced from normal human B cells after activation with bacterially derived products such as LPS (Sung *et al.*, 1989). TNF-β mRNA has also been detected in LPS-activated murine B cells (O'Garra *et al.*, 1990). It is produced constitutively by several malignantly transformed murine cell lines that represent early stages of B-cell development (Laskov *et al.*, 1990), human myeloma cells (Garrett *et al.*, 1987), and by human Epstein–Barr virus-transformed B cell lines. It is also induced by the human immunodeficiency virus (HIV) *tat* III gene transfection of B cells (Sastry *et al.*, 1990). Activated cells of the central nervous system, including astrocytes have also been reported to produce TNF-β (Lieberman *et al.*, 1989).

RECEPTORS

Two types of TNF receptors have been characterized and their cDNAs cloned from human and murine tissues. Unfortunately, the nomenclature for the receptors is as confused as that of the ligands. A 55 kDa form has been called p55, Type B, Type II and Type 1; the higher molecular weight form has been called p75, p80, Type A, Type 1 and Type 2. In this document, a molecular mass descriptor will be employed. Both TNF receptors bind TNF-α and TNF-β homotrimers. Their affinity for the LT-α_2 LT-β_1 heterotrimer has not been reported, nor is it known whether LT-β forms homotrimers that bind to any of the previously described TNF receptors. The TNF receptors are members of, and are homologous to, an ever-growing family of proteins characterized by cysteine-rich repeats (Loetscher *et al.*, 1990; Schall *et al.*, 1990; Smith *et al.*, 1990). Other members of this family include the low-affinity nerve growth-factor receptor, OX 40, CD40, CD27, fas, and products of viral open reading frames (Smith *et al.*, 1991). The genes for the ligands for CD40 and CD27 have recently been cloned, and they also show a high degree of homology with TNF-α, TNF-β, and LT-β, indicating the existence of both ligand and receptor families.

The two TNF receptors appear to have different functions, although considerable controversy exists regarding their roles (Heller *et al.*, 1993; Tartaglia *et al.*, 1993). As noted above, both p55 and p75 receptors bind both TNFs and can carry out biological activities after interaction with their ligands. p55 appears to be more ubiquitously expressed, shows no species preference, and is the receptor whose binding induces killing of murine WEHI 164 cells (Barrett *et al.*, 1991). Conversely, p75 is expressed on a rather limited range of cell types, predominantly activated lymphocytes (Ware *et al.*, 1991), and exhibits some degree of species preference, in that murine thymocytes respond to murine but not human TNF (Barrett *et al.*, 1991); it has been identified as a mediator of proliferation and has also been implicated in signalling through NK-κB (Hohmann *et al.*, 1991).

The two types of TNF receptor are regulated differently and their ratio on various cells and response to inductive signals differ. The genes for the receptors are located on different chromosomes; p55 is encoded by a gene on mouse chromosome 6 and on human chromosome 12; p75 is encoded by a gene on mouse chromosome 4 and on human chromosome 1 (summarized by Ruddle, 1992). The signals regulating expression of the two receptors differ. Dibutyric cAMP treatment of HL-60 cells upregulates p75 but not p55 (Hohmann *et al.*, 1991), and IL-2 and anti-CD3 induce expression of p75 but not p55 from resting T cells (Ware *et al.*, 1991). Mice deficient for p55 receptor have been recently produced through genetic engineering (Pfeffer *et al.*, 1993). These p55 knock-out mice appear phenotypically normal, but are highly susceptible to infection by *Listeria monocytogenes* and resistant to endotoxin shock. These data suggest that the p55 receptor plays a crucial role in these two biological activities but shed no information on the role of the p75 receptor. They also provide little insight into the role of the different ligands in these responses. It is most likely that TNF-α, a product of LPS-activated macrophages is the mediator of endotoxin shock. The mediator for *Listeria* resistance could be a macrophage (TNF-α) or a T-cell (TNF-α, TNF-β, LT-β) product.

PROTEIN STRUCTURE

The predominant lymphotoxin species derived from human B-lymphoblastoid cell line RPM1 1788 is a 25 kDa glycoprotein, although a 20 kDa TNF-β species has also been detected in culture supernatants derived from the same cells (Aggarwal *et al.*, 1983, 1985b; Gray *et al.*, 1984). The smaller of the two TNF-β species lacks the 23 *N*-terminal residues and could be a breakdown product. Despite the amino *N*-terminal differences, both forms are cytotoxic for L929 cells. Recombinant human TNF-β and murine TNF-β

kill L929 cells, indicating that glycosylation is not necessary for cytotoxic activity. Recombinant human TNF-β and murine TNF-β translated *in vitro* are usually detected in Western blots as two bands of 18 kDa and 34 kDa (Li *et al.*, 1987); the higher molecular mass form is presumably an oligomer.

TNF-β protein sequences are highly conserved among mammalian species. The sequences depicted in Fig. 1 were derived from human TNF-β protein and human and murine TNF-β cDNA cloning. The rabbit and bovine amino acid sequences were derived only from the genomic sequences. (Gray *et al.*, 1984; Goeddel *et al.*, 1986; Ito *et al.*, 1986; Li *et al.*, 1987; Shakhov *et al.*, 1990b). The cDNAs code for polypeptides of 205 amino acids (human), 204 amino acids (cow), 197 amino acids (rabbit) or 202 amino acids (mouse). There is some divergence in the length and sequences in the *N*-terminal signal of 34 residues (human), 33 residues (cow and mouse) or 26 residues (rabbit).

There have been sporadic reports concerning the existence of additional forms of TNF-β. Descriptions of lymphotoxins with unusual properties included reports of higher molecular weight forms (Aggarwal *et al.*, 1985b) and others of cytotoxic proteins with unusual neutralization properties (Green, 1985; Yamamoto and Karpas, 1989). Yamamoto *et al.* (1986) described a high-molecular-weight cytotoxic factor produced by human lymphoid cells that was only partly neutralized by antibodies to TNF-β but completely neutralized with a mixture of antibodies to TNF-α and TNF-β. Liu *et al.* (1987) also described a high-molecular-weight factor produced by T lymphocytes which was antigenically related to TNF-β and TNF-α and termed leukalexin. Although Northern blot analysis with TNF-α and TNF-β probes did not reveal specific TNF mRNAs, the possibility remains that leukalexin is a combination of previously described cytotoxins coded by the TNF locus.

Several nonmutually exclusive explanations can be invoked to account for the novel TNF-β forms. TNF-β monomers associate into homotrimers and such multimeric forms may be less easily neutralized by antibodies. Many supernants from T- and B-cell cultures undoubtedly also contain TNF-α, and simultaneous addition of both anti-TNF-β and anti-TNF-α antibodies might achieve neutralization. TNF-β/TNF-α oligomers may also exist. It is not yet known whether LT-α_2 LT-β_1 heterotrimers are released or whether they possess biological activity. They could also account for the unusual forms. Post-translational modifications of TNF-β might occur in some cells resulting in changes in antigenicity, or alternatively spliced forms of TNF-β mRNA might occur. A short open reading frame does exist in the 3' untranslated region of the fourth exon of the human, mouse and rabbit TNF-β genes (Shakhov *et al.*, 1990b). The potential 16-residue peptide encoded by this sequence is conserved among the three species analysed and could give rise to a different *C*-terminus. A form that includes this sequence could display antigenic properties different from those of conventional TNF-β. No experimental evidence for such a translated product has been obtained. Another potential form of TNF-β could be derived from an unusual cytoplasmic RNA that includes intron 3 (Weil *et al.*, 1990). This 1.7 kb cytoplasmic RNA has been determined to be associated with polyribosomes (as is the 1.4 kb fully spliced form) and thus could be translated. Again, no protein corresponding to this form has been isolated.

The molecular structure of the biologically active form of TNF-β is a homotrimer (Schoenfeld *et al.*, 1991) which can bind to both TNF (p55 and p75) receptors. TNF-β also crystallizes in the trimeric form (Eck *et al.*, 1992) as does TNF-α (Jones *et al.*, 1989).

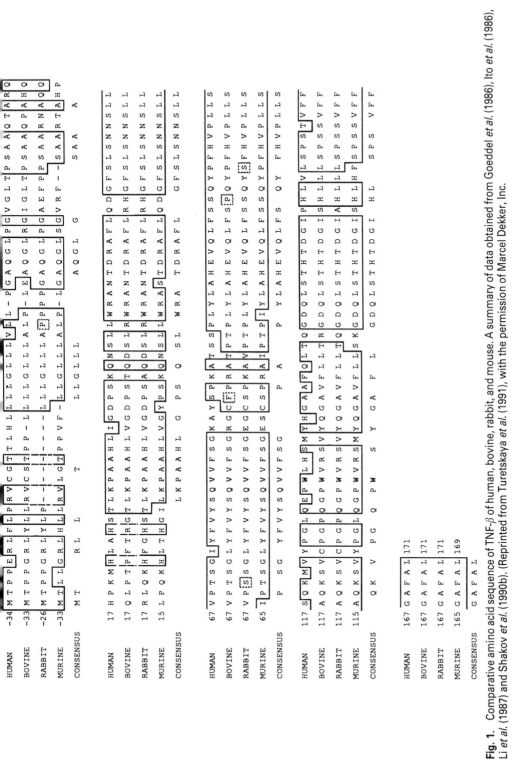

Fig. 1. Comparative amino acid sequence of TNF-β of human, bovine, rabbit, and mouse. A summary of data obtained from Goeddel et al. (1986), Ito et al. (1986), Li et al. (1987) and Shakov et al. (1990b). (Reprinted from Turetskaya et al. (1991), with the permission of Marcel Dekker, Inc.

Analyses of the TNF-β molecule indicate the importance of surface loops near the base of each monomer. Mutation of Asp-50 or Tyr-108 results in loss of L929-killing activity (Goh *et al.*, 1991). These regions of the TNF-β molecule are comparable with regions on the TNF-α molecule which are also crucial for function (Yamagishi *et al.*, 1990; van Ostade *et al.*, 1991). Recently, the TNF-β ligand–receptor complex has been crystallized at 2.85 Å resolution (Banner *et al.*, 1993). This complex is composed of three soluble p55 receptor molecules bound symmetrically to one TNF-β trimer.

ACTIVITIES AND MECHANISM

The tissue culture assay for murine, rat, or human TNF-β is killing of L929 or WEHI 164 cells. Enzyme-linked immunosorbent assays (ELISA) are also available that discriminate between human TNF-α and TNF-β. The ELISA for murine TNF does not discriminate between TNF-α and TNF-β because of the crossreactivity of the monoclonal antibody (Sheehan *et al.*, 1989). As noted above, TNF-β is also active in inducing necrosis in mice of a methylcholanthrene-induced transplanted tumour, which was the original TNF-α assay. TNF-β carries out many activities in tissue culture including killing several different tumour-cell lines, inducing DNA fragmentation, activating fibroblast growth, and activating expression of several genes, including those of MHC and adhesion molecules. TNF-β also acts as an osteoclast activating factor (Bertolini *et al.*, 1986). It is a growth factor for activated B cells (Kehrl *et al.*, 1987) and may act as an autocrine factor for B lymphomas (Seregina *et al.*, 1989) and some Epstein-Barr virus-infected B-cell lines (Estrov *et al.*, 1993). It stimulates replication of HIV (Folks *et al.*, 1989). Its other activities that have been defined *in vitro* are summarized in Paul and Ruddle (1988) where they are also compared with those of TNF-α.

TNF-β and TNF-α carry out many of the same biological activities, although both qualitative and quantitative differences have been noted. The basis for the occasional biological differences is not understood since both receptors bind both ligands with high affinities. Dissociation constants ranging between 10^{-9} M and 10^{-11} M have been reported.

The diversity of the effects of TNF-β on a variety of different targets, from induction of proliferation to killing reflects the variety of ways that target cells can respond to TNF-β and suggests that different signalling mechanisms are used by individual cells in their response to that ligand.

At least one of the two molecular classes of TNF receptors of 55 kDa and 75 kDa have been found on most cell types, with the exception of erythrocytes and resting T cells. The number of receptors found on individual cells range from 2000 to 50 000. Although the presence of a receptor is required for a response to TNF-β, the number of binding molecules expressed by a cell does not necessarily reflect its sensitivity to the ligand, presumably indicating the different biological functions of the receptors.

After TNFs bind to their receptors, they are internalized and degraded (Aggarwal *et al.*, 1985a; Mosselmans *et al.*, 1988). Inhibitors of lysosomal integrity inhibit TNF-α and TNF-β cytotoxicity (Ruff and Gifford, 1981) and manoeuvers that enhance rapid internalization accelerate their cytotoxic effects from 48 to 4 h (Schmid *et al.*, 1985). It is not clear whether these observations indicate that TNFs are active only after internalization or whether receptor internalization and reutilization is necessary for maximal cytotoxicity. The fact that antibodies to the receptor induce killing (Espevik *et al.*, 1990) suggests that a major part of TNF effects occur through signal transduction through the receptor. Several pathways including phosphorylation of a 26 kDa protein (Schutze *et al.*, 1989) and generation of inositol phosphates have been invoked. TNF-α and β enhances expression of many genes at least in part through activation of NF-κB (Folks *et al.*, 1989; Messer *et al.*, 1990).

Both TNF-α and TNF-β induce apoptosis or programmed cell death in some targets, (Schmid *et al.*, 1986, 1987) as do many other members of the TNF family. Although killing by TNF-β requires a fairly long time-course, effects on the structure and integrity of target cell DNA are detectable considerably before actual cell death. This phenomenon, also called 'killing from within', is manifested as degradation of target cell DNA. Radiolabelled DNA is released from the nucleus, to the cytoplasm, to the culture medium from cells after exposure to TNF-β. It is visualized by gel electrophoresis in a laddered pattern, indicating degradation at regular intervals, perhaps at internucleosomal spaces. Whether the effects of TNF-β on DNA are a consequence or a contributor to cell death has not been clearly defined. Several mechanisms have been invoked to explain the effects of TNF on cellular DNA. These include generation of oxygen free radicals and activation or translocation to the nucleus of a cellular endonuclease. TNF-β itself does not degrade DNA, but induces the process. The relationship of apoptosis to TNF-β induction of gene expression is not clear. It is possible that DNA fragmentation is an extreme example of a more subtle effect on chromatin structure. Perhaps TNF-β treatment results in histone release (McGrath *et al.*, 1989) and DNA unfolding and exposure to sites for DNA-binding proteins in those situations in which TNF-β treatment results in increased transcription of certain genes. The conflicting effects of TNF-β on target cells is similar to the effects of several other members of the TNF receptor family when ligand binding may result in proliferation or apoptosis (Rabizadeh *et al.*, 1993).

GENE STRUCTURE AND REGULATION

The complete nucleotide sequence of the TNF-β loci of human, murine, and rabbit genomes has been determined (Ito *et al.*, 1986; Nedospasov *et al.*, 1986a,b; Gardner *et al.*, 1987; Gray *et al.*, 1987; Semon *et al.*, 1987; Shakhov *et al.*, 1990b). A comparison of these gene sequences and organization shows a conserved exon structure and provides information regarding putative regulatory elements. The gene organization and the identification of coding regions were derived from the original sequencing of the human TNF-β protein (Aggarwal *et al.*, 1985b) and the cDNA cloning of human (Gray *et al.*, 1984) and murine TNF-β (Li *et al.*, 1987). The TNF-β gene maps within the MHC in man on chromosome 6 (Nedwin *et al.*, 1985a,b) and in the mouse on chromosome 17 (Nedospasov *et al.*, 1986a; Gardner *et al.*, 1987; Ruddle *et al.*, 1987) between the complement and Class I genes in close proximity to the TNF-α locus (Fig. 2). The 3' end of the TNF-β gene is approximately 1 kbp from the transcription initiation site of the TNF-α gene. The direction of transcription through the TNF complex is from TNF-β to TNF-α and it occurs on the same coding strand. The TNF-β gene organization of four exons and three introns is conserved in mouse, human, rabbit and cow and is similar to that of TNF-α. Its organization and linkage relationships are also conserved between the species. These observations suggest that TNF-β and TNF-α have arisen through a process of gene duplication.

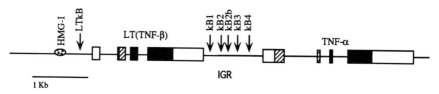

Fig. 2. A schematic comparison of the murine TNF Locus with putative and identified transcriptional elements. Note the presence of five NF-κB sites in the intergenic region (IGR).

Upon alignment of the human, rabbit, and mouse TNF-β genes, extensive similarities are seen. The most complete homology among the three species in the 5′ region is in the 300 bases upstream of the transcription initiation sites (Fashena *et al.*, 1990; Paul *et al.*, 1990; Shakhov *et al.*, 1990a,b). Primer extension and RNase protection analysis of murine TNF-β mRNA derived from anti-CD3-activated T-cell clones and PD and PD31 pre-B cells have revealed two functional cap sites within 15 bases of each other (Fashena *et al.*, 1990). In the three species analysed, within 110 bp upstream of a TATA box, are consensus sites for SP1 transcription factor and near-consensus sites for AP-2. Several NF-κB-like sites are found in the TNF-β genes of human, mouse and rabbit. The human upstream NF-κB-like sequence, which is identical to the murine sequence, forms a complex after incubation with nuclear extracts from a variety of cells (PHA/PMA-activated Jurkat, C81-66-45, MT-2) which are known to contain active NF-κB (Paul *et al.*, 1990). This site has also been determined to be a functional element in TNF-β gene transcription in T cells (Messer *et al.*, 1990; Paul *et al.*, 1990) and to be responsive to activation by HTLV-I *tax* gene product. (Lindholm *et al.*, 1992; Paul *et al.*, 1993).

Additional 5′ regulatory elements in TNF-β regulation were analysed functionally with a nested series of 5′ deletion mutants linked to the bacterial gene encoding chloramphenicol acetyl transferase (CAT). Both positive and negative regulatory elements have been defined that appear to have some tissue specificity (Fashena *et al.*, 1990; Paul *et al.*, 1990). One long poly (dA-dT)-rich region binds a high-mobility group I nonhistone nuclear protein also known as HMGI and is crucial for TNF-β production in pre-B cells (Fashena *et al.*, 1992). This protein does not act as a transcriptional factor *per se*, but rather stabilizes chromatin structure to allow interactions with other transcription factors. HMG-I plays a similar role in IFN-β regulation (Thonos and Maniatis, 1992).

The 3′ region of the TNF-β gene is of considerable interest with regard to transcriptional regulation of both TNF-β and TNF-α. This inter-genic region (IGR) consisting of approximately 1 kb of DNA includes several potential NF-κB sites. In the mouse there are five (Fig. 2). Four of these sites are conserved in the human. Some of these sites have already been demonstrated to bind NF-κB and/or to play some role in LPS induction of TNF-α. (Collart *et al.*, 1990). The possibility that this region contains elements that act as shared enhancers, functioning in those situations in T cells in which both TNF-α and TNF-β are transcribed is under investigation.

TNF-β gene expression is also regulated at the post-transcriptional level. Jongeneel *et al.* (1989) and Ferreri *et al.* (1992) noted that although activation of murine T-cell clones resulted in a 10-fold increase in TNF-β transcription rate, as determined by nuclear run-on analysis, the overall rate of transcription was quite low compared with that of TNF-α. Nevertheless, high levels of TNF-β mRNA accumulate under such activation conditions. This is because TNF-β mRNA has an unusually long half-life, particularly when it is compared to that of TNF-α (English *et al.*, 1991; Millet and Ruddle, 1994). This is probably due, in part, to the fact that TNF-β mRNA is relatively poor in AU-rich sequences compared with TNF-α (Caput *et al.*, 1986). These areas have been implicated in mRNA destabilization (Shaw and Kamen, 1986). Agents that inhibit TNF-β production include prostaglandin E2 which reduces TNF-β mRNA accumulation (Ferreri *et al.*, 1992). TNF-β production is also regulated at the level of mRNA processing. Different activation schemes influence the cytoplasmic accumulation of differently spliced mRNA species. Weil *et al.* (1990) determined that IL-2 induces nuclear accumulation of at least four species of TNF-β mRNA. Two of these, a fully spliced form and an intron-3 retaining form are exported to the cytoplasm with slightly different kinetics. These forms are also induced by anti-CD3 activation of murine T-cell clones (Millet and Ruddle, 1994).

BIOLOGICAL ROLES

TNF-β is, in all likelihood, one of several mediators of killing by cytolytic T cells, 'helper-killer' T cells, NK cells, and LAK cells (Ruddle and Schmid, 1987). It is produced by such cells after stimulation by antigen presented by MHC, their natural targets, or high levels of IL-2, and the cytotoxicity of many CD4 T-cell clones correlates with their production of TNF-β (Tite *et al.*, 1985). Its association with LT-β on the activated T-cell surface (Ware *et al.*, 1992; Browning *et al.*, 1993) suggests that it could also contribute to cell–cell interactions including killing. Other products of cytotoxic cells that also contribute to killing and may synergize with TNF-β to accelerate the process include TNF-α, perforin and serine proteases. The ability of TNF-β to induce DNA fragmentation or apoptosis, a characteristic of cytolytic- but not antibody- and complement-mediated killing, further implicates it in cell-mediated killing (Ruddle and Schmid, 1987). Through its cytotoxic activity, TNF-β probably contributes to graft rejection and to manifestations of graft-versus-host reactions. TNF-β kills virus-infected target cells more effectively than noninfected cells (Aderka *et al.*, 1985). This property suggests that a crucial biological role may include defence against viruses, particularly through TNF-β elimination of virus-infected cells.

Evidence is accumulating that TNF-β and TNF-α are important mediators in the pathogenesis of some autoimmune diseases. Their synergism with IFN and IL-1 in destroying β cells of the islets of Langerhans (Pukel *et al.*, 1988) suggests a role in insulin-dependent diabetes mellitus. Induction by TNF-β of myelin swelling and its cytotoxicity against oligodendrocytes (Selmaj and Raine, 1988; Selmaj *et al.*, 1991b) and its production by cells of the central nervous system (Lieberman *et al.*, 1989), implicate it in certain demyelinating diseases, such as multiple sclerosis. Its presence in the plaques in multiple sclerosis patients also implicates it in the disease (Selmaj *et al.*, 1991a). Its role as an inflammatory mediator also suggests its involvement in such diseases with their prominent mononuclear infiltrates. TNF-β production is positively correlated with the ability of T cells to transfer experimental allergic encephalomyelitis, a murine model of an autoimmune demyelinating disease (Powell *et al.*, 1990). Further evidence implicating TNF-β as an effector molecule of that disease has been derived from studies with a monoclonal antibody that neutralizes both TNF-β and TNF-α and inhibits transfer of symptoms by T-cell clones (Ruddle *et al.*, 1990). This process is due in part to the proinflammatory activities of TNF, particularly induction of adhesion molecules in the central nervous system (Barten and Ruddle, 1994).

The activity of TNF-β *in vivo* as a proinflammatory mediator is apparent from studies in which its production is artifically regulated in transgenic mice. Mice transgenic for a construct consisting of the rat insulin promoter II (RIP) driving TNF-β express high levels of the transgene in β cells in the islets of Langerhans, the kidney, and skin (Picarella *et al.*, 1992). This inappropriate expression has dramatic consequences. The hair has a distinctly ruffled appearance, and there is a marked inflammatory infiltrate in the kidney and around the islets (Picarella *et al.*, 1992, 1993). This infiltrate consists of CD4$^+$ T cells, CD8$^+$ T cells, and B220$^+$ B cells. Presumably this is a response to TNF-β-induced elevated expression of adhesion molecules at these sites. Similar, but not identical patterns of inflammation are seen in the islets of mice transgenic for the RIP–TNF-α construct (Higuchi *et al.*, 1992; Picarella *et al.*, 1993). Despite the high level of TNF expression in such mice, no β-cell destruction is seen, confirming the *in vitro* observations that only a limited range of cells is susceptible to TNF killing, despite their exquisite sensitivity to some of the other activities of the molecule.

Infection with HTLV-I has several sequelae in which TNF-β may play a role. These include hypercalcaemia associated with adult T-cell leukaemia and HTLV-I-associated myelopathy. The presence of TNF-β in the serum of patients with hypercalcaemia (Ishibashi *et al.*, 1991) and the high constitutive TNF-β production by several HTLV-I-infected cell lines (Paul *et al.*, 1990) suggests that TNF-β could contribute to the pathogenesis of clinical manifestations of infection with that virus. Hypercalcaemia could be facilitated through TNF-β's activity as an osteoclast-activating factor, and HTLV-I associated myelopathy through its role as a demyelinating and proinflammatory agent.

Several years ago, I (Ruddle, 1986) suggested that TNF-β contributed to HIV pathogenesis in AIDS. I predicted that HIV could induce cytokines including TNF-β (then known as LT) and that the cytokine would induce T-cell death through T-cell suicide (apoptosis). This hypothesis was made before several facts were known concerning the diverse activities of both TNFs and the variety of pathologies associated with AIDS. The known activities of TNF-β that could contribute to HIV pathogenesis include: cachexia, B-cell activation, T-cell death, oligodendrocyte killing, and inflammation. Its ability to induce HIV activation and replication (Folks *et al.*, 1989) in infected T cells and monocytes has been demonstrated. Presumably, this occurs through the ability of TNF-β to activate NF-κB, an important element in the HIV promoter region. These facts add substantial support to the hypothesis. Experimental evidence has derived from the observation that L929-killing activity is increased in supernatants of HIV-infected cells (Ratner *et al.*, 1987), but discrimination between the TNF-α and TNF-β was not made. The report (Sastry *et al.*, 1990) that transfection of the HIV-1 tat*III* gene results in induction of TNF-β mRNA and protein from Raji cells implicates a specific viral protein and a specific TNF. It is very likely that, as suggested in 1986, cytokines including TNF-β contribute to HIV infection symptoms and disease progression. Advances in treatment can occur through strategies that inhibit induction of TNF and its biological activities.

A complete understanding of the biological role of TNF-β will emerge with the development of agents that specifically inhibit its production or its activity. Treatment of cells with antisense TNF-β mRNA should inhibit its production and render those cells incapable of carrying out functions attributable to TNF-β. Considerations of the role of TNF-β must also take into account the activity of TNF-α, which is frequently produced by the same cells. Analysis with agents that specifically inactivate only one of these two biologically similar factors may be misleading. Disruption of the p55 receptor, as noted above, indicates that all TNF activities are not essential for life. Disruption of the genes for the p75 receptor or TNF-β and/or TNF-α will provide further information on the roles of TNF and the importance (or not) of their redundancy.

NOTE ADDED IN PROOF

Recently it has been demonstrated that TNF-β plays a unique and critical role in lymphoid organ development (De Togni *et al.*, 1994). Mice rendered deficient in TNF-β through the technique of homologous recombination display an absolute absence of lymph nodes and splenic disorganization. These data suggest that TNF-β is expressed by a particular cell in a particular time or place that does not express TNF-α, and indicate that TNF-α and TNF-β are not completely redundant.

ACKNOWLEDGEMENTS

This work was supported by NIH ROI CA-16885 and ROI CA-47874 and National Multiple Sclerosis Society grant RG 2934. I am grateful to Frances Larvey for expert manuscript preparation, to Regina Turetskaya for her contributions to an earlier version of this chapter, and to Nina Paul, Sarah Fashena, Isabelle Millet, Donna Barten, Chang-ben Li, Cheryl Bergman, and Alexander Kratz for helpful discussions.

REFERENCES

Aderka, D., Novick, D., Hahn, T., Rischer, D.G. and Wallach, D. (1985). *Cell Immunol.* **92**, 918–925.
Aggarwal, B.B., Moffat, B. and Harkins, R.N. (1983). In *Interleukins, Lymphokines, and Cytokines* (eds Openheim J.J. and Cohen, S.), Academic Press Inc., New York, pp. 521–525.
Aggarwal, B.B., Eessalu, T.E. and Hass, P.E. (1985a). *Nature* **318**, 665–667.
Aggarwal, B.B., Henzel, W.J., Moffat, B., Kohr, W.J. and Harkins, R.N. (1985b). *J. Biol. Chem.* **260**, 2334–2344.
Banner, D.W., D'Arcy, A., Janes, W., Gentz, R., Schoenfeld, H.-J., Broger, C., Loetscher, H. and Lesslauer, W. (1993). *Cell* **73**, 431–445.
Barten, D.M. and Ruddle, N.H. (1994). *J. Neuroimmunol.* (in press).
Barrett, K., Taylor-Fiswick, D.A., Cope, A.P., Kissonerghis, A.M., Gray, P.W., Feldmann, M. and Foxwell, B.M.J. (1991). *Eur. J. Immunol.* **21**, 1649–1656.
Bertolini, D.R., Nedwin, G.E., Bringman, T.S., Smith, D.D. and Mundy, T.R. (1986). *Nature* **319**, 516–518.
Browning J. and Ribolini, A. (1989). *J. Immunol.* **143**, 1859–1867.
Browning, J.L., Ngam-ek, A., Lawton, P., DeMarinis, J., Tizard, R., Chow, E.P., Hession, C., Greco, B., Foley, S. and Ware, C.F. (1993). *Cell* **72**, 847–856.
Caput, D., Beutler, B., Hartog, K., Thayer, R., Brown-Shimer, S. and Cerami, A. (1986). *Proc. Natl Acad. Sci. USA* **83**, 1670–1674.
Collart, M.A., Baeuerle, P.A. and Vasalli, P. (1990). *Mol. Cell Biol.* **10**, 1498–1506.
Conta, B.S., Powell, M.B. and Ruddle, N.H. (1983). *J. Immunol.* **130**, 2231–2235.
Conta, B.S., Powell, M.B. and Ruddle, N.H. (1985). *J. Immunol.* **134**, 2185–2190.
De Togni, P., Goellner, J., Ruddle, N.H., Streeter, P.R., Fick, A., Mariathasan, S., Smith, S.C., Carlson, R., Shornick, L.P., Strauss-Schoenberger, J., Russell, J.H., Karr, R. and Chaplin, D.D. (1994). *Science*, in press.

Eck, M.J., Ultsch, M. Rinderknech, E., de Vos, A.M. and Sprang, S.R. (1992). *J. Biol. Chem.* **267**, 2119–2122.

English, B.K., Weaver, W.M. and Wilson, C.B. (1991). *J. Biol. Chem.* **266**, 7108–7113.

Espevik, T., Brockhaus, M., Loetscher, H., Nonstad, U. and Shalaby, R. (1990). *J. Exp. Med.* **171**, 415–426.

Estrov, Z., Kurzrock, R., Pocsik, E., Pathak, S., Kantarjiian, H.M., Zipf, T.F., Harris, D., Talpaz, M. and Aggarwal, B.B. (1993). *J. Exp. Med.* **177**, 763–774.

Fashena, S.J., Tang, W.-L., Sarr, T. and Ruddle, N.H. (1990). *J. Immunol.* **45**, 177–183.

Fashena, S.J., Reeves, R. and Ruddle, N.H. (1992). *Mol. Cell Biol.* **12**, 894–903.

Ferreri, N.R., Sarr, T., Askenase, P.W. and Ruddle, N.H. (1992). *J. Biol. Chem.* **267**, 9443–9449.

Folks, T.M., Clouse, K.A., Justement, J., Rabson, A., Duh, E., Kehrl, J.H. and Fauci, A.S. (1989). *Proc. Natl Acad. Sci USA* **86**, 2365–2368.

Gardner, S.M., Mock, B.A., Hilgers, J., Huppi, K.E. and Roeder, W.D. (1987). *J. Immunol.* **139**, 476–483.

Garrett, I.R., Durie, B.G.M., Nedwin, G.E., Gillespie, A., Bringman, T., Sabatini, M., Bertolini, D.R. and Mundy, G.R. (1987). *New Eng. J. Med.* **317**, 526–532.

Goeddel, D.V., Aggarwal, B.B., Gray, P.W., Leung, D.W., Nedwin, G.E., Palladino, M.A., Patton, J.S., Pennica, D., Shepard, H.M., Sugarman, B.J. and Wong, G.H.W. (1986). *Cold Spring Habor Symp. Quant. Biol.* **51**, 597–609.

Goh, C.R., Loh, C.S. and Porter, A.G. (1991). *Protein Eng.* **4**, 785–791.

Granger, G.A. and Williams, T.W. (1968). *Nature* **218**, 1253–1254.

Gray, P.W., Aggarwal, B.B., Benton, C.V., Bringman, T.S., Henzel, W.J., Jarett, J.A., Leung, D.W., Moffat, B., Ng, P., Svedersky, L.P., Palladino, M.A. and Nedwin, G.E. (1984). *Nature* **312**, 721–724.

Gray, P.W., Chen, E., Li, C.-B., Tang, W.-L. and Ruddle, N.H. (1987). *Nucl. Acids Res.* **15**, 3937.

Green, L.M., Stern, M.L., Haviland, D.L., Mills, B.J. and Ware, C.F. (1985). *J. Immunol.* **135**, 4034–4043.

Heller, R.A., Song, K. and Fan, N. (1993). *Cell* **73**, 216.

Higuchi, Y., Herrera, P., Muniesa, P., Huarte, J., Belin, D., Ohashi, A.P., Orci, L., Vassalli, J.-D. and Vassalli, P. (1992). *J. Exp. Med.* **176**, 1719–1731.

Hohmann, H.-P., Brockhaus, M., Baeuerle, P.A., Remy, R., Kolbeck, R. and VanLoon, A.P.G.M. (1991). *J. Biol. Chem.* **265**, 22409–22417.

Ishibashi, K., Ishitsuka, K., Chumon, Y., Otsuka, M., Kwazuru, Y., Iwashi, M., Utsonomiya, A., Handa, S., Sakurami, T. and Arima, T. (1991). *Blood* **77**, 2451–2455.

Ito, H., Shirau, T., Yamamoto, S., Akira, M., Kawahara, S., Todd, C.W. and Wallace, R.B. (1986). *DNA* **5**, 157–165.

Jones, E.Y., Stuart, D.I. and Walker, N.P.C. (1989). *Nature* **338**, 225–228.

Jongeneel, C.V., Shakhov, A.N., Nedospasov, S.A. and Cerottini, J.-C. (1989). *Eur. J. Immunol.* **19**, 549–552.

Kehrl, J.H., Alvarez-Mon, M., Delsing, G.A. and Fauci, A.S. (1987). *Science* **238**, 1144–1146.

Kriegler, M., Perez, C., DeFay, K., Albert, I. and Lu, S.D. (1988). *Cell* **53**, 45–53.

Kronke, M., Hensel, G., Schluter, C., Scheurich, P., Schutze, S. and Pfizenmaier, K. (1988). *Cancer Res.* **48**, 5417–5421.

Laskov, R., Lancz, G., Ruddle, N.H., McGrath, K.M., Specter, S., Klein, T., Djeu, J.Y. and Friedman, H. (1990). *J. Immunol.* **144**, 3424–3430.

Li, C.-B., Gray, P., Lin, P.-F., McGrath, K.M., Ruddle, F.H. and Ruddle, N.H. (1987). *J. Immunol.* **138**, 4496–4501.

Lieberman, A.P., Pitha, P., Shin, H.S. and Shin, M.L. (1989). *Proc. Natl Acad. Sci. USA* **86**, 6348–6352.

Liu, C.-C., Steffen, M., King, F. and Young, J.D.-E. (1987). *Cell* **51**, 393–403.

Loetscher, H., Pan, Y.C.E., Lahm, H.W., Gentz, R., Brockhaus, M., Tabuchi, H. and Lesslauer, W. (1990). *Cell* **61**, 351–359.

Lindholm, P.F., Reid, R.L. and Brady, J.N. (1992). *J. Virol.* **66**, 1294–1302.

McGrath, K.M., Levesque, M.C. and Ruddle, N.H. (1989). In *Cellular Basis of Immune Modulation* (eds Kaplan, J.G., Green D.R. and Bleackley, R.D.), Liss, New York, pp. 299–310.

Messer, G.E., Weiss, H. and Bauerle, P.A. (1990). *Cytokine* **2**, 389.

Millet, I. and Ruddle, N.H. (1994). *J. Immunol.* **152**, 4336–4346.

Mosselmans, R., Hepburn, A., Dumont, J.E., Fiers, W. and Galand, P. (1988). *J. Immunol.* **141**, 3096–3100.

Nedospasov, S.A., Shakhov, A.N., Turetskaya, R.L., Mett, V.A., Hirt, B., Shakhov, A.N., Dobrinin, V.N., Kawashima, E., Accola, R.S. and Jongeneel, C.V. (1986a). *Nucl. Acids Res.* **14**, 7713–7725.

Nedospasov, S.A., Shakov, A.N., Turetskaya, R.L., Mett, V.A., Azizov, M.M., Georgiev, G.P., Korobko, V.G., Dobrinin, V.N., Filippov, S.A., Bystrov, N.S., Boldyreva, E.F., Chuvpilo, S.A., Chumakov, A.M., Shingarova, L.N. and Ovchinnikov, Y.A. (1986b). *Cold Spring Habor Symp. Quant. Biol.* **51**, 611–624.

Nedwin, G.E., Jarett-Nedwin, J., Smith, D.H., Naylor, S.L., Sakaguchi, A.Y., Goeddel, D.V. and Gray, P.W. (1985a). *J. Cell. Biochem.* **29**, 171–181.

Nedwin, G.E., Naylor, S.L., Sakaguchi, A.Y., Smith, D.H., Jarett-Nedwin, J., Pennica, D., Goeddel, D.V. and Gray, P.W. (1985b). *Nucl. Acids Res.* **13**, 6361–6373.

O'Garra, A., Stapleton, G., Dhar, V., Pearce, M., Schumacher, J., Rugo, H., Barbis, D., Stall, A., Cupp, J., Moore, K., Vieira, P., Mosmann, T., Whitmore, A., Arnold, L., Haughton, G. and Howard, M. (1990). *International Immunol.* **2**, 821–832.

Paul, N.L. and Ruddle, N.H. (1988). *Ann. Rev. Immunol.* **6**, 407–438.

Paul, N.L., Lenardo, M.J., Novak, K.D., Sarr, T., Tang, W.-L. and Ruddle, N.H. (1990). *J. Virol.* **64**, 5412–5419.

Paul, N.L., Millet, I. and Ruddle, N.H. (1993). *Cytokine* **5**, 372–378.

Picarella, D.E., Kratz, A., Li, C.-B., Ruddle, N.H. and Flavell, R.A. (1992). *Proc. Natl Acad. Sci. USA* **89**, 10036–10040.

Picarella, D.P., Kratz, A., Li. C.-B., Ruddle, N.H. and Flavell, R.A. (1993). *J. Immunol.* **150**, 4136–4150.

Pfeffer, K., Matsuyama, T., Kundig, T.M., Wakeham, A., Kishihara, K., Shahinian, A., Wiegmann, K., Ohashi, P.S., Kronke, M. and Mak, T.W. (1993). *Cell* **73**, 457–467.

Powell, M.B., Mitchell, D., Lederman, J., Buchmeier, S., Zamvil, S.S., Graham, M., Ruddle, N.H. and Steinman, L. (1990). *Int. Immunol.* **2**, 539–544.

Pukel, C., Baquerizo, H. and Rabinovitch, A. (1988). *Diabetes* **37**, 133–136.

Rabizadeh, S., Oh, J., Zhong, L.-t., Yang, J., Bitter, C.M., Butcher, L.L. and Bredesen, D.E. (1993). *Science* **261**, 345–348.

Ratner, L., Polmar, S.H., Paul, N. and Ruddle, N. (1987). *AIDS Res. Hum. Retroviruses* **3**, 147–154.

Ruddle, N.H. (1986). *Immunol. Today* **7**, 8–9.

Ruddle, N.H. (1992). *Current Op. Immunol.* **4**, 327–332.

Ruddle, N.H. and Schmid, D.S. (1987). *Ann. Inst. Pasteur Immunol.* **138**, 314–320.

Ruddle, N.H. and Waksman, B.H. (1968). *J. Exp. Med.* **128**, 1267–1279.

Ruddle, N.H., Li, C.-B., Tang, W.-L., Gray, P. and McGrath, K.M. (1987). In *Ciba Foundation Symposium* (eds. Block, G. and Marsh, J.), Wiley, Chichester, **131**, pp. 64–82.

Ruddle, N.H., Bergman, C., McGrath, K.M., Lingenheld, E.G., Grunnet, M.L., Padula, S.J. and Clark, R.B. (1990). *J. Exp. Med.* **172**, 1193–1200.

Ruff, M.R. and Gifford, G.E. (1981). In *Lymphokines, Vol. 2* (ed. Rich, E.). Academic Press, New York, pp. 235–240.

Sastry, K.J., Reddy, R.H., Pandito, R., Totpol, K. and Aggarwal, B.B. (1990). *J. Biol. Chem.* **32**, 20091–20093.

Schall, T.J., Lewis, M., Koders, K.J., Lee, A., Rice, G.C., Wong, G.H., Gatanga, T., Granger, G.A., Lentz, R., Raab, H., Kahr, W.J. and Goeddel, D.V. (1990). *Cell* **61**, 361–370.

Schmid, D.S., Powell, M.B., Mahoney, K.A. and Ruddle, N.H. (1985). *Cell. Immunol.* **93**, 68–82.

Schmid, D.S., Tite, J.P. and Ruddle, H.N. (1986). *Proc. Natl Acad. Sci. USA* **83**, 1881–1885.

Schmid, S., Hornung, R., McGrath, K.M., Paul, N. and Ruddle, N.H. (1987). *Lymphokine Res.* **61**, 195–202.

Schoenfeld, H.J., Poeschl, B., Frey, J.R., Loetscher, H., Hunziker, W., Lustig, A. and Zulauf, M. (1991). *J. Biol. Chem.* **266**, 3863–3869.

Schutze, S., Scheurich, P., Pfizenmaier, K. and Kronke, M. (1989). *J. Biol. Chem.* **264**, 3562–3567.

Selmaj, K. and Raine, C.S. (1988). *Ann. Neurol.* **23**, 339–346.

Selmaj, K., Raine, C.S., Cannella, B. and Brosnan, C.S. (1991a). *J. Clin. Invest.* **87**, 949–954.

Selmaj, K., Raine, C.S., Faroog, M., Norton, W.T. and Brosnan, C.F. (1991b). *J. Immunol,* **147**, 1522–1530.

Semon, D., Kwashima, E., Jongeneel, C.V., Shakhov, A.N. and Nedospasov, S.A. (1987). *Nucl. Acids Res.* **15**, 9083–9084.

Seregina, T.M., Mekshenkov, M.I., Turetskaya, R.L. and Nedospasov, S.A. (1989). *Mol. Immunol.* **26**, 339–342.

Shakhov, A.N., Collart, M.A., Vassalli, P., Nedospasov, S.A. and Jongeneel, C.V. (1990a). *J. Exp. Med.* **171**, 35–47.

Shakhov, A.N., Kuprash, D.V., Azizov, M.M., Jongeneel, C.V. and Nedospasov, S.A. (1990b). *Gene* **95**, 215–221.

Shalaby, M.R., Aggarwal, B.B., Rinderknecht, E., Svedersky, L.P., Finkle, B.S. and Palladino, M.A. (1985). *J. Immunol.* **135**, 2069–2073.

Shaw, G. and Kamen, R. (1986). *Cell* **46**, 659–687.

Sheehan, K.C.F., Ruddle, N.H. and Schreiber, R.D. (1989). *J. Immunol.* **142**, 3884–3893.

Smith, C.A., Davis, T., Anderson, D., Solan, L., Bechmann, M.P., Jerzy, R., Dower, S.K., Cosmon, P. and Goodman, R.G. (1990). *Science* **248**, 1019–1023.

Smith, C.A., Davis, T., Wignall, J.M., Din, W.S., Farrah, T., Upton, C., McFadden, G. and Goodwin, R.G. (1991). *Biochem. Biophys. Res. Comm.* **176**, 335–342.

Steffen, M., Ottmann, O.G. and Moore, M.A.S. (1988). *J. Immunol.* **140**, 2621–2624.

Sung, E.-S., Bjorndahl, J., Wang, C.Y., Kao, H.T. and Fu, S.M. (1988). *J. Exp. Med.* **167**, 937–953.

Sung, S.-S.J., Jung, L.K.L., Walters, J.A., Jeffes, E.W.B., Granger, G.A. and Fu, S.M. (1989). *J. Clin. Invest.* **84**, 236–243.

Tartaglia, L.A., Rothe, M., Hu, U.-F. and Goeddel, D.V. (1993). *Cell* **73**, 213–216.

Thonos, D. and Maniatis, T. (1992). *Cell* **71**, 777–789.

Tite, J.P., Powell, M.B. and Ruddle, N.H. (1985). *J. Immunol.* **135**, 23–33.

Tschachler, E., Rober-Gurroff, M., Gallo, R.C. and Reitz, M.S. (1989). *Blood* **73**, 194–201.

Turetskaya, R., Fashena, S.J., Paul, N.L. and Ruddle, N.H. (1992). In *Tumor Necrosis Factors: Structure, Function and Mechanism of Action.* (eds Aggarwal, B. and Vilček, J.). Marcel Dekker Inc., New York, pp. 35–60.

Van Ostade, X., Tavernier, J., Prange, T. and Fiers, W. (1991). *EMBO J.* **10**, 827–836.

Ware, C.F., Crowe, P.D., Vanarsdale, T.L., Andrews, J.L., Grayson, M.H., Jerzy, R., Smith, C.A. and Goodwin, R.G. (1991). *J. Immunol.* **147**, 4229–4238.

Ware, C.F., Crowe, P.D., Grayson, M.H., Andolewicz, M.J. and Browning, J.L. (1992). *J. Immunol.* **149**, 3881–3888.

Weil, D., Brosset, S. and Daubry, F. (1990). *Mol. cell. Biol.* **10**, 5865–5875.

Yamagishi, J., Kawashima, H., Matsuo, N., Ohue, M., Yamayoshi, M., Fukui, T., Kotanim, H., Furuta, R., Nakano, K. and Yamada, M. (1990). *Prot. Eng.* **3**, 713–719.

Yamamoto, R.S., Ware, C.F. and Granger, G.A. (1986). *J. Immunol.* **137**, 1878–1884.

Yamanaka, H.I. and Karpas, A. (1989). *Proc. Natl Acad. Sci. USA* **86**, 1343–1347.

Chapter 18

Transforming Growth Factor-Beta

Rik Derynck

Departments of Growth and Development, and Anatomy, Programs in Cell Biology and
Developmental Biology, University of California at San Francisco, San Francisco, CA, USA

INTRODUCTION

The initial identification of transforming growth factor-β (TGF-β), now more than a decade ago, was based on its ability to reversibly induce phenotypic transformation of select fibroblast cell lines (Moses *et al.*, 1981; Roberts *et al.*, 1981). In some cell lines, this transforming activity was apparent only when both TGF-β and TGF-α were present (Anzano *et al.*, 1982, 1983) or when EGF was added to TGF-β (Roberts *et al.*, 1981). Despite their name, TGF-α and TGF-β are structurally unrelated. However, TGF-α shares structural similarity with EGF and interacts with a common EGF/TGF-α receptor. This chapter will not review the biology of TGF-α (for review, see Derynck, 1992), and will focus only on TGF-β.

The initial detection of TGF-β activity in a transformation assay suggested a role for TGF-β in malignant transformation and tumour development. It is now well established that the activities of TGF-β are by no means restricted to tumour cells, but that TGF-β exerts a multiplicity of biological activities on most cells, both normal or transformed, and regulates many cell physiological processes. The biological response to TGF-β is complex and depends on the cell type (and even on the individual cell line tested) and the physiological conditions. Furthermore, TGF-β also plays an important role in the control of the immune response and wound healing, and in the development of various tissues and organs.

The recent accumulation of knowledge on the biology of TGF-β makes it a daunting task to comprehensively review TGF-β in depth. An excellent review by Roberts and Sporn (1990) makes it unnecessary to extensively elaborate on several areas, such as the spectrum of biological activities of TGF-β. Thus, I will focus mainly on some subject areas that have seen major changes during the last few years. I will first outline our knowledge of the structure of the different TGF-β isoforms and the TGF-β receptors, then elaborate on the role of TGF-β in the control of cell proliferation and the immune response and finally review our knowledge of the involvement of TGF-β in normal and tumour development.

The Cytokine Handbook, 2nd ed.
ISBN 0–12–689661–5

Since the original cDNA cloning of the first TGF-β, i.e. TGF-β_1 (Derynck *et al.*, 1985), extensive protein characterization and cDNA analyses have revealed a large group of structurally related secreted factors. Collectively, these factors are called the TGF-β superfamily, which contains not only the different TGF-β isoforms, but also the activins, bone morphogenetic proteins (BMPs), as well as several other secreted factors. TGF-β-related proteins are found in vertebrate species and the fruitfly *Drosophila*, and are likely also present in *Caenorhabditis elegans*. They are thought to play important roles in cell differentiation and proliferation during development. For an overview of the TGF-β superfamily, which will not be discussed here, I refer the reader to the existing review articles (Massagué, 1990; Hoffmann, 1991; Kingsley, 1994).

THE STRUCTURE OF TGF-β

It was originally assumed that there was only the TGF-β type now known as TGF-β_1, that was purified from platelets (Assoian *et al.*, 1983). Protein purification and cDNA cloning approaches have subsequently revealed three TGF-β isoforms in mammalian cells, each encoded by their own gene. TGF-β_1 (Derynck *et al.*, 1985), TGF-β_2 (de Martin *et al.*, 1987), and TGF-β_3 (Derynck *et al.*, 1988; ten Dijke *et al.*, 1988) are made as larger precursors of 390 amino acids (TGF-β_1) or 412 amino acids (TGF-β_2 and TGF-β_3). Each precursor contains an *N*-terminal signal peptide, a long pro-segment, also called latency-associated polypeptide (LAP), and a 112-amino-acid *C*-terminal poly-peptide that constitutes the mature TGF-β monomer. This monomer is cleaved from the remaining precursor segment following a tetrabasic peptide. The nature of this cleavage site suggests that the protease responsible for this cleavage belongs to the KEX/furin-like proteases, that recognize multibasic sites in secreted proteins (Barr, 1991).

The active form of TGF-β is a hydrophobic, disulphide-linked dimer of the *C*-terminal segment of the pre-pro TGF-β (Assoian *et al.*, 1983; Derynck *et al.*, 1985; Cheifetz *et al.*, 1987). The three TGF-β species with a sequence identity of 70–80% (Derynck *et al.*, 1988; ten Dijke *et al.*, 1988) are thus generated as homodimers of two identical *C*-terminal polypeptides, although heterodimers between TGF-β_1 and -β_2 have also been isolated (Cheifetz *et al.*, 1987). The biological relevance of the heterodimeric species is unclear, especially since they presumably correspond to only minor species. The 112-amino-acid mature TGF-β polypeptide includes nine conserved cysteines, eight of which are paired. All cysteines form intrachain disulphide bonds, with the exception of one intermolecular cysteine bridge responsible for the dimeriza-tion (Daopin *et al.*, 1992; Schlunegger and Grütter, 1992). Three-dimensional structure analysis has revealed an unexpected extended butterfly-like structure of the TGF-β_2 homodimer, rather than the compact globular structure frequently seen in highly stable and temperature- and protease-resistant growth factors (Daopin *et al.*, 1992; Schluneg-ger and Grütter, 1992). Considering the generally conserved sequence features and the number and relative positions of the cysteines among the different TGF-β superfamily members, the three TGF-β isoforms and all members of the TGF-β superfamily are likely to assume similar structural conformations. The sequence between the fifth and sixth cysteine, which has the most sequence divergence among the different TGF-β isoforms and the other members of the TGF-β superfamily, is exposed at the surface of this molecule and may play an important role in the determination of the specificity of the ligand–receptor recognition.

The pro-segments of the three TGF-β precursors show a sequence identity of only 25–35% (Derynck *et al.*, 1988; ten Dijke *et al.*, 1988). Nevertheless, some structural elements are strongly conserved, suggesting critical roles either in the function or in the folding of this pro-segment. Most noteworthy among these conserved features are three cysteine residues and two N-glycosylation sites (Derynck *et al.*, 1988). Two of these three cysteines are involved in intermolecular disulphide bridge formation (Miyazono *et al.*, 1988, 1991). The conserved N-linked carbohydrates are mannose-6-phosphorylated and mediate binding of the pro-segment to the mannose-6-phosphate receptor (Purchio *et al.*, 1988; Kovacina *et al.*, 1989). Finally, a hydrophobic stretch of amino acids closely following the signal peptide is also conserved and may be involved in the folding of the precursor segment (Lopez *et al.*, 1992).

Biochemical characterization has shown that TGF-β is normally secreted as a protein complex, consisting of the mature TGF-β homodimer and two pro-segments which interact noncovalently with the mature dimer. The participation of the mature TGF-β in this complex prevents it from interacting with the TGF-β receptors, thus rendering this complex inactive or 'latent' (Miyazono *et al.*, 1988; Wakefield *et al.*, 1988). Based on antibody recognition studies, it is likely that this interaction of TGF-β with the much larger pro-segments leaves little of the mature TGF-β exposed at the surface of this complex. The TGF-β complex isolated from platelets has revealed the identity of yet another polypeptide that associates with this complex. This polypeptide, named latent TGF-β-binding protein (LTBP), represents a fifth protein in this platelet-derived TGF-β complex (Miyazono *et al.*, 1988, 1991; Wakefield *et al.*, 1988). LTBP is a protein of 125–160 kDa and interacts through at least one disulphide bond with one of the pro-TGF-β segments in the latent complex (Miyazono *et al.*, 1991). Its amino acid sequence reveals 16 EGF-like repeats, the relevance of which is still unknown. In addition, it contains an RGD sequence and an 8-amino-acid sequence identical to the proposed cell-binding domain of the laminin B2 chain (Kanzaki *et al.*, 1990). Northern hybridization suggests that this protein is made by a large variety of cell types, raising the possibility that many cells make the five protein latent complex, rather than the smaller tetrameric complex, and that formation of this type of complex could be subject to regulation as well (Kanzaki *et al.*, 1990; Miyazono *et al.*, 1991; Olofsson *et al.*, 1992).

The expression of the three TGF-β isoforms is differentially regulated. Thus, different inducers or exogenous agents have distinct effects on the secretion of the individual TGF-β species. The complexity of this regulation will not be discussed here, but has been illustrated by Roberts and Sporn (1992). As an example, treatment of cells with TGF-β_1 or TGF-β_2 results in differential changes in the synthesis of the different TGF-β isoforms (Bascom *et al.*, 1989). In addition, retinoic acid treatment results in a strong induction of TGF-β_2 but not TGF-β_1 synthesis (Glick *et al.*, 1989). Finally, interaction of mammary epithelial cells with plastic as substrate induces transcription of TGF-β_1 but not of TGF-β_2 (Streuli *et al.*, 1993). This differential regulation of expression is largely due to a characteristic and independent pattern of transcriptional regulation of the three TGF-β species, which is in turn regulated by distinct control elements in the promoters of the genes (Roberts *et al.*, 1991). In addition, all three TGF-β isoforms have long 5' untranslated sequences (Derynck *et al.*, 1985; Arrick *et al.*, 1991; Kim *et al.*, 1992) which most likely play an isoform-specific role in the regulation of the translation efficiency (Arrick *et al.*, 1991; Kim *et al.*, 1992; Romeo *et al.*, 1993).

THE ROLE OF THE ASSOCIATED PROTEINS IN THE ACTIVATION OF TGF-β

The synthesis of TGF-β as a latent complex raises the questions of how TGF-β is normally activated and what the role is of the associated proteins. The association of the two pro-segments with mature TGF-β may serve several functions: they may be required for secretion of TGF-β, maintenance of TGF-β in an inactive form and targeting of the latent TGF-β. The first of these roles of the pro-segment of TGF-β is suggested by two lines of evidence. Transfection of TGF-β expression plasmids in which the sequence coding for the precursor segment of TGF-β was deleted did not result in the secretion of TGF-β, but synthesis of the pro-segment from a cotransfected plasmid rescued the ability of the cells to secrete TGF-β, albeit at low efficiency (Gray and Mason, 1990). In addition, deletion of some conserved structural elements of the precursor segment, such as the hydrophobic sequence following the signal peptide cleavage site, and the two mannose-6-phosphorylated N-linked carbohydrates, prevents TGF-β secretion (Lopez *et al.*, 1992). Thus, the precursor segment may serve as a chaperone, required for the secretion of TGF-β. Whether this chaperoning function merely facilitates the secretion process or also plays a role in the folding of mature TGF-β is unknown. Once secreted, the pro-segments maintain mature and active TGF-β in the latent complex and prevent its interaction with the TGF-β receptors (Miyazono *et al.*, 1988; Wakefield *et al.*, 1988). Considering the widespread distribution of TGF-β receptors and the potent biological effects of TGF-β, it is indeed strategically most important that TGF-β remains inactive until its required activation at the target site.

The release of active TGF-β from the latent complex occurs, presumably, in a highly regulated manner. The studies of the physiological activation mechanism of latent TGF-β have mainly been carried out in cocultures of smooth muscle cells and endothelial cells (Antonelli-Orlidge *et al.*, 1989; Sato and Rifkin, 1989). Whereas latent TGF-β can be activated by treatment with heat and acid (Miyazono *et al.*, 1990), active TGF-β is under normal physiological conditions and is most likely released following degradation of the pro-segments by proteases such as plasmin and cathepsins (Lyons *et al.*, 1988, 1990; for review see Harpel *et al.*, 1993). In cocultures of endothelial and smooth muscle cells, plasmin is the major protease responsible for the activation of TGF-β_1 (Antonelli-Orlidge *et al.*, 1989; Sato and Rifkin, 1989). Induction of plasminogen activators, e.g. during angiogenesis and invasion, results in conversion of plasminogen into plasmin, which in turn activates latent TGF-β. The activation process presumably occurs at the cell surface, where the pro-segments of the latent TGF-β complexes are retained, at least in part, through interaction of their mannose-6-phosphorylated carbohydrates with the mannose-6-phosphate receptors (Dennis and Rifkin, 1991). The activation can be inhibited by plasmin inhibitors such as antiplasmin (Flaumenhaft *et al.*, 1992a), and by inhibitors of type II transglutaminase (Kojima *et al.*, 1993), suggesting a role for the latter enzyme in the activation mechanism. The role of LTBP in the activation of the latent complex is largely unclear, but antibodies against LTBP and soluble LTBP itself inhibit the activation process. Thus, LTBP may direct the latent complex to the cell surface or the extracellular matrix, as required for activation (Flaumenhaft *et al.*, 1993).

Active TGF-β is also released from other cell sources such as tumour cells, activated macrophages, osteoclasts and osteoblasts (Twardzik *el al.*, 1990; Oursler *et al.*, 1992; Kojima and Rifkin, 1993). Proteases are presumably involved in the activation of TGF-β

by these cells also, although little information is as yet available about the nature of these enzymes and mechanism of activation by these cells. Finally, little is as yet known about how TGF-β_2 and TGF-β_3 are activated. Considering the similar nature of the latent complexes, it is likely that proteolytic mechanisms may be at work, but the extensive sequence differences in the pro-segments suggest mechanistic differences, possibly even the involvement of different proteases.

Once released from the cells, latent and active TGF-β can interact with proteins in the extracellular milieu, especially with various components of the extracellular matrix or basement membrane. These interactions result in yet another type of control mechanism that governs the biological availability and activity of TGF-β. One of the proteins with a high affinity for TGF-β is α-2-macroglobulin, which is present at high levels in the circulation and interacts with various other growth factors and cytokines as well (for a review see James 1990; LaMarre *et al.*, 1991a). Interaction of TGF-β with α-2-macroglobulin sequesters TGF-β into an inactive form that is unable to bind to the TGF-β receptors (O'Connor-McCourt and Wakefield, 1987; Huang *et al.*, 1988). Thus, α-2-macroglobulin may serve as an efficient scavenger that binds all free active TGF-β, especially since almost all TGF-β in plasma is sequestered in this type of complex (O'Connor-McCourt and Wakefield, 1987; Huang *et al.*, 1988). Following transportation to the liver, interaction of the complex with the α-2-macroglobulin receptor may result in the delivery of high concentrations of TGF-β to the liver, where it functions as an active molecule or, perhaps more likely, is degraded (LaMarre *et al.*, 1991b). Other soluble proteins that engage in a high-affinity interaction with TGF-β are decorin and biglycan—two secreted proteoglycans that are part of the extracellular matrix. Interaction of TGF-β with these proteins neutralizes the activity of TGF-β and, thus, could result in a physiological inactivation of TGF-β in the extracellular matrix (Yamaguchi *et al.*, 1990). Finally, thrombospondin (Murphy-Ullrich *et al.*, 1992), fibronectin (Fava and McClure, 1987) and several collagens, including collagen type IV (Paralkar *et al.*, 1991), are also able to bind TGF-β with a high affinity. The interactions of these extracellular matrix components with TGF-β may result in sequestration of active TGF-β into the extracellular matrix, which thus could be considered as a reservoir for TGF-β (and many other growth and differentiation factors). The interactions of TGF-β with thrombospondin and collagen IV keep TGF-β in an active form (Murphy-Ullrich *et al.*, 1992).

THE TGF-β RECEPTORS AND BINDING PROTEINS

Like all secreted growth and differentiation factors, TGF-β interacts with cell-surface receptors to induce its repertoire of biological activities. Various TGF-β-binding polypeptides have been identified at the cell surface following chemical crosslinking using radiolabelled TGF-β. They have been called receptors, even though, for most of them, no evidence has been provided that they are indeed involved in TGF-β-induced signal transduction. At least eight different cell surface polypeptides with an ability to bind TGF-β have been identified to date (for review, see Massagué, 1992; Lin and Lodish, 1993). These receptors have been typified on the basis of the apparent size on gel of the protein crosslinked to ^{125}I-TGF-β. The types I, II, and III receptors are commonly observed on most cells in culture and are best characterized. Although it was originally thought that the biological activities of TGF-β are mediated through the type

III receptors (Cheifetz *et al.*, 1987, 1988), recent studies have revealed that the type I and type II receptors mediate most if not all activities of TGF-β (Laiho *et al.*, 1991a; Geiser *et al.*, 1992; Chen *et al.*, 1993).

The type III receptor, also called betaglycan, is a cell surface proteoglycan, which contains covalently linked heparin sulphate and chondroitin sulphate (Segarini and Seyedin, 1988; Cheifetz and Massagué, 1989), but these side chains may not be required for binding of TGF-β (Cheifetz and Massagué, 1989). Betaglycan can be detected both as a transmembrane and a soluble protein (Andres *et al.*, 1989). It is encoded as an 853-amino-acid protein with a short cytoplasmic domain without known signalling motifs, consistent with the current belief that this receptor does not mediate any signalling activities (Lopez-Casillas *et al.*, 1991; Wang *et al.*, 1991). The type III receptor has sequence homology with endoglin (Gougos and Letarte, 1990), a transmembrane protein expressed by various cells, especially endothelial cells, which has now been shown to bind TGF-β_1 and TGF-β_3 (Cheifetz *et al.*, 1992). Although the overall sequence identity is only about 25%, their intracellular and transmembrane domains are more highly conserved; the biological significance of this homology is unknown. Expression of betaglycan increases binding of TGF-β to the type II receptor, but not the type I receptor, which suggests that the type III receptor may be involved in ligand presentation to that receptor (Lopez-Casillas *et al.*, 1991; Wang *et al.*, 1991). This situation is somewhat reminiscent of the heparin sulphate-enhanced presentation of basic FGF to the FGF receptor (Yayon *et al.*, 1991). Remarkably, the type III receptor can also bind basic FGF and thus could also play a role in the presentation of this growth factor to its receptor (Andres *et al.*, 1991).

The type II TGF-β receptor is a transmembrane serine-threonine kinase encoded as a 567-amino-acid polypeptide (Lin *et al.*, 1992). Its glycosylated extracellular domain is rich in cysteines and its intracellular domain contains all features and consensus sequences characteristic of serine–threonine kinases. Fusion proteins containing the cytoplasmic domain can be autophosphorylated on serines and threonines (Lin *et al.*, 1992). Transfections of cells with a mutated receptor lacking the active kinase site, indicate that the kinase domain is essential for signalling and subsequent biological activities (Wrana *et al.*, 1992). Comparison of the type II receptor sequence with other serine–threonine kinase receptors, such as type II activin receptors (Mathews and Vale, 1991; Attisano *et al.*, 1992) and the *C. elegans* receptor-like protein Daf-1 (Georgi *et al.*, 1990), indicates striking sequence homologies in the extracellular and intracellular domains (Lin *et al.*, 1992). The extracellular domains are short and have an abundance of cysteines, including a characteristic cysteine cluster upstream from the transmembrane region, yet the overall sequence identity is limited. The cytoplasmic domains display all consensus sequences characteristic of serine–threonine kinases. However, the demonstration that purified activin receptor has dual kinase activity *in vitro* for tyrosine and serine–threonine (Nakamura *et al.*, 1992) suggests that other members of this receptor family, including the type II TGF-β receptor may also be dual specificity kinases. It is possible that additional type II TGF-β receptors exist. This is based on the fact that the cloned type II receptor does not bind TGF-β_2 efficiently (Lin *et al.*, 1992; Lawler *et al.*, 1994) and that the *in situ* hybridization pattern of the mouse type II receptor during development localizes the cloned type II receptor at sites of TGF-β_1

expression but not at sites of TGF-β_2 expression (Lawler *et al.*, 1994). More recent cDNA cloning has led to the identification of many other related serine–threonine kinase receptors with as yet unknown specificity. Their sequence identity is largely concentrated in the kinase sequences in the cytoplasmic domains. It is now generally assumed that all TGF-β family members bind to receptors of this transmembrane serine–threonine kinase family.

Finally, the sequence for a type I receptor has recently been determined. This receptor is also a member of the transmembrane serine–threonine kinase receptor family. Its cytoplasmic domain does not have an extension beyond the kinase domain and is of minimal size. The extracellular domain has a defined sequence similarity with the type II TGF-β receptor but is shorter and has only one N-glycosylation site. Although this receptor by itself does not bind TGF-β, cotransfection with the type II receptor results in the expression and TGF-β binding of the type I receptor at the cell surface (Ebner *et al.*, 1993). The required coexpression of the type II receptor for cell surface transport and/or TGF-β binding to the type I receptor is consistent with observations in mutant cell lines that the type II receptor can rescue cell-surface binding to the type I receptor (Wrana *et al.*, 1992). Remarkably, cotransfection of this type I receptor also inhibited the binding of TGF-β to the type II receptor, but the physiological relevance of this dominant negative interference still has to be established (Ebner *et al.*, 1993).

Considering the two types of TGF-β receptors implicated in TGF-β signalling, how are the multiple activities of TGF-β mediated? The conclusions have been rather confusing for some time owing to the lack of specific tools, such as cloned receptor of cDNAs, to dissect the signalling pathways. Analyses of mutated cell lines suggested that the type I receptor was the mediator of biological activities (Boyd and Massagué, 1989), but that the type II receptor may be required also (Laiho *et al.*, 1990b, 1991a). Other observations suggested that the type II receptor was important in the antiproliferative effect of TGF-β (Geiser *et al.*, 1992). Subsequently, it has been proposed that the type II and type I receptor form heterodimers and that this complex signals the variety of biological activities (Wrana *et al.*, 1992). Most recently, abolition of type II receptor signalling by overexpression of a dominant negative mutant of the type II receptor indicated that the type II receptor is required for the inhibition of proliferation by TGF-β. It is not yet known whether this activity of the type II receptor requires a biologically active type I receptor. In contrast, the type I receptor is thought to mediate the induction of several genes by TGF-β, including several effects on the deposition of the extracellular matrix, without requiring a signalling type II receptor (Chen *et al.*, 1993). Thus, two different signalling pathways are associated with the type I and type II receptors. It is unclear whether both pathways are connected with a heterodimeric type I/type II receptor heterodimer or with functional type I and type II homodimer receptors. Finally, the type III receptor may be a component of the signalling receptor complex and may enhance presentation of TGF-β to the type II receptor (Lopez-Casillas *et al.*, 1991, 1993; Wang *et al.*, 1991). It should be stressed that, at this point in time, the nature of the receptor complexes is ill-defined. Whereas there is evidence for complex formation, it is still unclear how the type I, II and III receptors interact physically and physiologically with each other at the cell surface[1].

The Multifunctional Nature of TGF-β

TGF-β exerts a large variety of biological functions in most cells. The wide spectrum of target cells results from the presence of cell-surface TGF-β receptors in nearly all cells in culture. The nature of the biological effects of TGF-β depend critically on several parameters including the cell type, the culture conditions and the cellular environment, the presence and nature of other growth factors and the differentiation state and, thus, on the general physiological context. We will only briefly outline the several classes of activities that have been extensively reviewed by Roberts and Sporn (1990). In the next few sections, we will then focus on the role of TGF-β in some defined contexts.

Many TGF-β-induced effects can be grouped in several categories. One set of activities is related to the potent growth regulatory effect of TGF-β. TGF-β stimulates proliferation or acts as a potent antiproliferative factor depending on the cell type and cell line. We will further elaborate on this activity of TGF-β in the next section. An additional set of activities relates to the interaction of TGF-β with the extracellular matrix (Roberts and Sporn, 1990). In most cells of nonhaemopoietic origin, TGF-β modifies the cellular interaction with the surrounding extracellular matrix and/or basement membrane in several different ways (although, as stressed before, the specific response will depend on the cell type and its physiological environment). First, TGF-β induces the synthesis and secretion of many proteins of the extracellular matrix, including several collagens, fibronectin, thrombospondin, tenascin, osteopontin, osteonectin and proteoglycans. The increased deposition of these proteins should result in an increased formation of extracellular matrix. Second, TGF-β increases the expression of many integrins. These are heterodimeric cell adhesion receptors that, depending on the combination of the α and β transmembrane polypeptide chains, interact with defined structural proteins in the extracellular matrix or basement membrane. These interactions mediate not only cell adhesion but also integrin-mediated intracellular signalling, which affects gene expression and cellular differen-tiation (Damsky and Werb, 1992). The effect of TGF-β on integrin expression again strongly depends on the cell type and on the type of integrin, but frequently results in increased adhesiveness of the cells to the matrix. Third, TGF-β treatment also regulates the synthesis and activity of secreted proteases and protease inhibitors. The generally observed TGF-β-mediated decrease of protease secretion should inhibit degradation of extracellular matrix, whereas increased synthesis of protease inhibitors further accen-tuates the accumulation of extracellular matrix and/or basement membrane. Finally, TGF-β is also a potent chemoattractant for several cell types, especially monocytes (Wahl et al., 1987) and fibroblasts (Postlethwaite et al., 1987). This activity may be very important at sites of wound-healing or other repair processes, where TGF-β is locally activated and may be a major effector of monocyte/macrophage and fibroblast influx.

Effects of TGF-β on Cell Proliferation

TGF-β induces a mitogenic or antiproliferative effect depending on the cell line and cell type (for review see Moses et al., 1990; Arrick and Derynck, 1993). TGF-β promotes cell proliferation in culture in several cell types, predominantly of mesenchymal origin. Example include fibroblasts (Leof et al., 1986), osteoblasts (Centrella et al., 1987), smooth muscle cells (Battegay *et al.*, 1990) and Schwann cells (Ridley *et al.*, 1989). In at least one fibroblast cell line, TGF-β induced an increased number of cell surface receptors for epidermal growth factor (Assoian *et al.*, 1984), suggesting that increased sensitivity to EGF or the related TGF-α in the medium could be the mechanistic basis for the TGF-β-induced increase of proliferation and the synergistic effect with TGF-α or EGF on anchorage-independence (Roberts *et al.*, 1981; Anzano *et al.*, 1983).

The mitogenic effect of TGF-β on some cell types is indirect and due to stimulated production of platelet-derived growth factor (PDGF) that acts in an autocrine manner. TGF-β induces c-*sis* mRNA which encodes the PDGF-B chain, and PDGF (or PDGF-like) protein in the AKR-2B fibroblastic cell line (Leof *et al.*, 1986) whereas, in human foreskin fibroblasts, TGF-β stimulates expression of the A-chain gene of PDGF (Soma and Grotendorst, 1989). In smooth muscle cells, fibroblasts and chondrocytes, TGF-β induces a bimodal response in proliferative behaviour (Battegay *et al.*, 1990). Thus, treatment of these cells with a concentration of TGF-β that is 10-fold higher than that which stimulated DNA synthesis, nearly abolished the mitogenic response. At lower concentrations, TGF-β induced PDGF-A expression, whereas higher concentrations of TGF-β inhibited the expression of the PDGF receptor α subunit. In this manner, a PDGF-based autocrine growth loop stimulated by low concentrations of TBF-β was blocked at the receptor level by higher concentrations of TGF-β (Battegay *et al.*, 1990). Thus, at least in these cells, the effects of TGF-β on cell proliferation reflect the modulation by TGF-β of the autocrine growth regulation by PDGF.

Exogenous TGF-β administration *in vivo* has been shown to result in increased cell density, fibrosis and angiogenesis (Roberts *et al.*, 1986) but, to date, there is little evidence documenting increased cell proliferation in response to TGF-β *in vivo*. Conversely, an increased cell mass in the chicken chorioallantoic membrane system following administration of TGF-β was concomitant with decreased mitogenic activity in the newly formed tissue, which suggests that the increased cell mass was largely the result of cellular influx (Yang and Moses, 1990). Thus, hypercellular lesions at the site of TGF-β injection may be due to an influx of cells as a consequence of the chemotactic activity of TGF-β, rather than a TGF-β-induced increase in cell proliferation.

TGF-β is a potent inhibitor of cell proliferation of many cell types which, in several cases, is achieved by inhibiting the proliferation induced by other growth factors. As an example, TGF-β inhibited the fibroblast growth factor-stimulated proliferation of fibroblast cells without affecting the binding of the growth factor to its receptor or many of the cellular events that occur within the first few hours after mitogen stimulation (Like and Massagué, 1986; Chambard and Pouysségur, 1988). In many cells, TGF-β directly inhibits cellular proliferation. Most studies have been performed on keratinocytes or other epithelial cells, which are arrested by TGF-β in late G1 just prior to the onset of S phase, thus preventing the wave of DNA synthesis (Howe *et al.*, 1990; Laiho *et al.*, 1990a). The mechanistic basis of this inhibition is still largely unclear; however, some interesting functional connections have recently emerged.

A correlation between endogenous c-*myc* expression and TGF-β mediated growth inhibition has become apparent in keratinocytes. Inhibition of murine keratinocyte proliferation by TGF-β was associated with diminished expression of c-*myc*, which is functionally involved in the growth inhibition, but not with a change in expression of c-*fos* or several other proto-oncogenes (Pietenpol *et al.*, 1990a). In addition, TGF-β did not affect the c-*myc* mRNA levels in various tumour-cell lines that are not growth-inhibited by TGF-β (Pietenpol *et al.*, 1990). Whereas early studies attributed the observed reduction in c-*myc* by TGF-β to a post-transcriptional process (Coffey *et al.*, 1988), subsequent analyses have documented an inhibition of transcriptional initiation of c-*myc* by TGF-β. The inhibition of transcription was mapped to a 23-bp sequence in the c-*myc* promoter, termed the TGF-β control element (Pietenpol *et al.*, 1991). This element contains sequences similar to a previously described TGF-β inhibitory element that mediates the TGF-β-induced repression of transcription of the transin/stromelysin gene (Kerr *et al.*, 1990). DNA-binding proteins specific for sequences within the TGF-β control element of the c-*myc* gene have been detected (Pietenpol *et al.*, 1991).

Expression of the transforming proteins from three DNA tumour viruses—E7 from HPV-16, E1A from adenovirus, and large T antigen from SV40—can not only block the TGF-β-induced antiproliferative effect but also the inhibition of c-*myc* transcription by TGF-β (Pietenpol *et al.*, 1990b). These transforming proteins bind to the retinoblastoma gene product, pRB, a tumour suppressor gene known to exert growth inhibitory activities. Thus, pRB and related proteins may serve as mediators of TGF-β growth-inhibitory activity. During the cell cycle, pRB undergoes phosphorylation and dephosphorylation, with the underphosphorylated form predominating in the G1 phase. The growth inhibition of mink lung epithelial cells by TGF-β was associated with decreased phosphorylation of pRB, raising the possibility that TGF-β generates or stabilizes the underphosphorylated form of pRB, which in turn mediates inhibition of cell proliferation (Laiho *et al.*, 1990a,b, 1991). Transforming proteins that associate with, and inactivate or alter the function, of the underphosphorylated form of pRB, would thus effectively block the growth-inhibitory activity of TGF-β. It is not clear whether the effect of TGF-β on the phosphorylation state of pRB is the result of a direct effect of TGF-β or a consequence of the growth arrest in G1. Finally, the finding that pRB can itself modulate expression of the TGF-β_1 gene positively or negatively, depending on cell type, adds yet another level of complexity to this growth regulatory pathway (Kim *et al.*, 1991).

Nuclear factors other than pRB have also been implicated in the antiproliferative activity of TGF-β. Thus, other cellular proteins, perhaps recessive oncogenes themselves, can also be mediators of growth inhibition by TGF-β. Such would also be the conclusion from observations that some breast-cancer cell lines which lack functional pRB retain sensitivity to inhibition of proliferation by TGF-β (Ong *et al.*, 1991). The p53 recessive oncogene product is a candidate alternative mediator of growth inhibition by TGF-β of some cell types. For example, SV40-immortalized human bronchial epithelial cells lose their negative growth responsiveness to TGF-β when transfected with a mutant p53 (Gerwin *et al.*, 1992).

Other late-G1-acting proteins may also be involved in TGF-β growth-inhibitory effects. One such protein is the cyclin-dependent kinase 2 (cdk2), a 34 kDa serine–threonine kinase which fluctuates in activity with the cell cycle and may phosphorylate pRB. Cyclin E–cdk2 complexes may function in controlling progression through G1, whereas cyclin A–cdk2 may play a role in controlling the onset of DNA synthesis (Sherr, 1993). Although TGF-β treatment and subsequent growth arrest did not affect the protein levels of cyclin E and cdk2, the assembly of both protein complexes and the accumulation of the kinase activity were inhibited (Koff *et al.*, 1993). Thus, cyclin-dependent kinases may be direct or indirect targets of TGF-β signalling. It is possible that activation of a specific phosphatase by TGF-β, such as has been reported with protein phosphatase 1 (Gruppuso *et al.*, 1991), may be involved in these changes in the phosphorylation state of cell-cycle regulatory proteins.

TGF-β IN THE IMMUNE SYSTEM

There is considerable evidence for an immunomodulatory role of TGF-β and its function as a potent differentiation modulating and immunosuppressive agent (for reviews see Wahl *et al.*, 1989; Roberts and Sporn, 1990; Kehrl, 1991; Ruscetti *et al.*, 1993). In culture, most cells of the immune system, such as lymphocytes and monocytes synthesize TGF-β which is almost exclusively TGF-β_1 (Kehrl, 1991). The TGF-β released by these cells is mostly latent, suggesting that activation of the latent complex is required before TGF-β can exert its function. The target cells are presumably not only the lymphocytes and monocytes themselves, but also various other cell types in the immediate tissue environment, such as endothelial cells or tumour cells. It is likely that lymphocytes and especially monocytes have the necessary proteases required for TGF-β activation. Stimulation of monocytes induces the secretion of plasmin and cathepsin D, both of which are able to activate TGF-β (Nathan, 1987). These cells also have TGF-β receptors, which suggests that, also in the immune context, TGF-β could function in an autocrine fashion (Wahl *et al.*, 1989; Kehrl, 1991). The receptors are predominantly type II and type I receptors, based on the migration in gel of the ^{125}I-TGF-β crosslinked receptors, although various cells contain only detectable type I receptors. The regulation of the receptor expression and TGF-β responsiveness is still poorly studied, mainly because of the lack, until recently, of the cDNA probes and antibodies. However, it has already been noted that the differentiation of monocytes into macrophages is accompanied by a decrease in TGF-β receptor levels (Wahl *et al.*, 1987, 1990). The expression of TGF-β in lymphocytes and monocytes is also regulated. The low level of TGF-β secretion in unstimulated monocytes and lymphocytes is strongly upregulated in response to mitogenic activation of lymphocytes and lipopolysaccharide activation of monocytes (Kehrl *et al.*, 1986a; Assoian *et al.*, 1987). In addition, TGF-β_1 synthesis by monocytes is strongly induced by TGF-β itself (McCartney-Francis *et al.*, 1990). This auto-induction of TGF-β synthesis, which also occurs in many different cell types, may play a role in amplifying the autocrine response to TGF-β (Wahl *et al.*, 1989).

Treatment of lymphocytes and monocytes with TGF-β results in a large array of biological responses, dependent on the cell type and its differentiation state. One of the most potent activities of TGF-β on lymphocytes is its antiproliferative effect. TGF-β inhibits the proliferation of T lymphocytes, B lymphocytes, thymocytes, large granular lymphocytes, NK cells, and LAK cells (Kehr *et al.*, 1986a,b; Ristow, 1986; Rook *et al.*, 1986; Kuppner *et al.*, 1988; Wahl *et al.*, 1988; Ortaldo *et al.*, 1991). This inhibition is most likely a consequence of a direct inhibition of the progression through the cell cycle (Smeland *et al.*, 1987; Kehrl, 1991), thus resembling the growth inhibitory effect of TGF-β on epithelial cells. The antiproliferative effect of TGF-β strongly contributes to its immunosuppressive effect on these cells. In addition, TGF-β influences a variety of differentiation-associated functions. In B cells, TGF-β suppresses the expression by activated B lymphocytes of membrane immunoglobulin and decreases secretion of immunoglobulin G and M (Kehrl *et al.*, 1986a, 1991). This is likely a result of decreased transcription of the immunoglobulin polypeptide chains (Kehrl *et al.*, 1991). TGF-β

also inhibits the acquisition of the κ light-chain by the murine pre-B cells (Lee *et al.*, 1987). Furthermore, the presence of TGF-β promotes murine B cells stimulated with lipopolysaccharide to undergo isotype switching to IgA, whereas the continued presence of TGF-β inhibits IgA secretion (Coffman *et al.*, 1989). Finally, TGF-β strongly promotes the generation of T_{H1} cells, a subset of helper T cells with a characteristic cytokine secretion pattern (Swain *et al.*, 1991).

The many studies of peripheral blood mononuclear cells, LAK cells and T lymphocytes suggest that TGF-β may function as a strong inhibitor of expression of many cytokines involved in the effector functions of the activated cells (Wahl *et al.*, 1989; Kehrl, 1991; Shull *et al.*, 1992). Thus, TGF-β inhibits the effects and/or the production of IFN-γ, TNF-α and TNF-β and IL-1, IL-2 and IL-3, and the expression of IL-2 receptor (Espevik *et al.*, 1987, 1988; Ohta *et al.*, 1987; Ranges *et al.*, 1987; Roberts and Sporn, 1990; Kehrl, 1991). The endogenous synthesis of TGF-β by most cytokine-producing cells and the increased cytokine production in TGF-β_1-deficient mice (Shull *et al.* 1992) strongly suggest that cytokine production is under autocrine control of TGF-β. The inhibition of cytokine production is presumably a major factor in TGF-β-induced immunosuppression, especially as it relates to the cytolytic activities of the immune system. Indeed, TGF-β has been shown to be a strong inhibitor of the generation and cytolytic activity of cytotoxic T cells, NK cells and LAK cells, and to suppress the natural and lymphokine-activated killing by large granular lymphocytes (Roberts and Sporn, 1990; Kehrl, 1991). Further evidence of the strong immunosuppressive effect of TGF-β on lymphocytes comes from the observation that TGF-β downregulates IFN-γ-induced MHC II antigen expression on both lymphoid and nonlymphoid cells (Czarniecki *et al.*, 1988). The potent inhibition by TGF-β of activities induced by various cytokines is a common theme for the role of TGF-β in the immune system. It is therefore likely that, *in vivo*, TGF-β plays an important role as a negative regulator of various cytokine-induced effects and thus that TGF-β is an important component in the maintenance of the proper balance between the different cytokine-induced effects. The antagonist role of TGF-β and other cytokines is best illustrated by the contrasting activities of TGF-β and TNF-α. TNF-α enhances cytotoxic T-lymphocyte development, IL-2 receptor expression, MHC II antigen expression, IFN-γ production, NK cell activity, thymocyte proliferation and B-cell proliferation, effects that are all potently inhibited and antagonized by TGF-β (Ranges *et al.*, 1987, Espevik *et al.*, 1988).

TGF-β also plays an important role in inflammation, to a large extent because of its potent modulatory effects on monocytes and macrophages (for review see Wahl *et al.*, 1989; Kehrl, 1991). Subcutaneous injection of TGF-β elicits a sequence of inflammatory cell recruitment, fibroblast accumulation and vascular growth that is very similar to the normal inflammatory response to injury (Roberts *et al.*, 1986). At the site of injury, TGF-β may play a key role in the initiation of the inflammatory response by its ability to potently attract monocytes. This chemotactic activity of TGF-β on monocytes is already apparent at femtomolar concentrations (Wahl *et al.*, 1987). It is thus conceivable that TGF-β released by activated degranulating platelets is responsible for the influx of monocytes, that accompanies the initiation of the inflammation. TGF-β is also a chemotactic agent for fibroblasts, which may explain the influx of fibroblasts at the site of injury (Postlethwaite *et al.*, 1987). Following recruitment of monocytes, the TGF-β at the site of inflammation presumably activates monocytes to induce the expression and release of various growth factors and inflammatory mediators, such as IL-1, PDGF,

TNF-α, fibroblast growth factor and also TGF-β_1 (Wahl *et al.*, 1989; McCartney-Francis *et al.*, 1990). These mediators are important in further amplifying the inflammatory response and initiating the repair processes at the site of injury. Besides this strong activating effect on monocytes, TGF-β also exerts a potent deactivating effect, once the monocytes are differentiated into macrophages. TGF-β is a potent inhibitor of the macrophage respiratory burst, as it suppresses H_2O_2 release by the activated macrophages. This inhibition can be reversed by activating agents such as IFN-γ and TNF-α (Tsunawaki *et al.*, 1988). The proinflammatory activity of TGF-β on monocytes and the subsequent deactivating activity on macrophages clearly illustrates the highly coordinated role of TGF-β in the complex response to injury and its modulatory role at the site of repair and inflammation. It is conceivable that, in the absence of TGF-β, exposure of the recruited cells to the uninhibited respiratory-burst capacity of macrophages could be detrimental to the surrounding cells. The anti-inflammatory effect of TGF-β on macrophages is also illustrated by the suppression by TGF-β of TNF-α expression and Ia antigen expression in these cells (Tsunawaki *et al.*, 1988). Finally, TGF-β also inhibits neutrophil and T-lymphocyte adhesion to endothelium and in this way further suppresses the inflammatory response. Thus, also in this context, TGF-α antagonizes the effect of TNF-α which increases the adhesiveness of the endothelial cells (Gamble and Vadas, 1988).

The potent activities of TGF-β on immune cells *in vitro* are also reflected in the various effects of TGF-β in animal model systems (Kehrl, 1991). Exogenous administration of TGF-β *in vivo* markedly depresses inflammatory and immunological responses. For example, TGF-β_1 prolongs the time to rejection of rat islet transplants (Carel *et al.*, 1990, 1993), delays the onset of acute and chronic experimental allergic encephalomyelitis (Kuruvilla *et al.*, 1991) and experimentally induced arthritis (Brandes *et al.*, 1991) and, furthermore, suppresses the generation of the cytotoxic T-cell response (Fontana *et al.*, 1989). The relevance of these findings for the normal immunoregulatory role of TGF-β *in vivo* has to be further evaluated. Endogenous TGF-β may also play a regulatory role in limiting immune function *in vivo* and in some pathological dysfunctions of the immune system, as suggested by several correlative studies. Increased levels of TGF-β in the synovial fluid of joints of patients with rheumatoid arthritis may explain some of the arthritis-associated physiological changes and contribute to the inflammation in this tissue context, and perhaps contribute to the functional changes in synovial lymphocytes (Wahl *et al.*, 1988b; Lotz *et al.*, 1990; Wilder *et al.*, 1990). The suppressed responsiveness of these cells in arthritic patients is similar to the inhibited responsiveness in lymphocytes and macrophages from mice with experimental chronic arthritis (Wahl *et al.*, 1988a,b). Another example of a pathological role of active TGF-β in immune suppression associated with a specific disease is provided by adult T-cell leukaemia (ATL). One of the clinical features of this disease, caused by the HTLV-1 virus, is a suppression of cellular and humoral immunity. ATL mononuclear cells secrete considerably higher levels of TGF-β_1 compared with their normal counterparts, which could be responsible, in part, for their inhibited immune function (Kim *et al.*, 1990). Excessive TGF-β production observed in peripheral blood mononuclear cells from AIDS patients, and in HIV-infected monocytes may similarly play a role in the impairment of the immune response in HIV-infected AIDS-patients (Kekow *et al.*, 1990, 1991; Wahl *et al.*, 1991).

Finally, the best illustration of the endogenous role of TGF-β_1 in normal immune function and infiltration is provided by mice in which the TGF-β_1 gene was functionally inactivated by gene targeting. Shortly after birth, these mice develop a multifocal mixed inflammatory disease with rapid and massive infiltration of lymphocytes and neutrophils in many tissues and subsequent death (Shull et al., 1992; Kulkarni et al., 1993). Thus, TGF-β_1 deficiency results in a severe pathology with dysfunction of the immune and inflammatory systems, which is accompanied by increased production of several cytokine mediators of inflammation, such as IFN-γ, TNF-α and MIP-1α (Shull et al., 1992). In summary, there is ample evidence that TGF-β is a major determinant of the immune and inflammatory response. Among the TGF-β isoforms, TGF-β_1 is most likely the major effector molecule under most conditions, and TGF-β_2 and TGF-β_3 may exert their major normal effects outside the immune system.

TGF-β IN NORMAL MAMMALIAN DEVELOPMENT

To gain insight into the role of TGF-β in normal development, several approaches have been used. They include the study of the effects of TGF-β on cellular differentiation in vitro, the localization of the expression of the three TGF-β isoforms and the receptors in the developing animal, and the transgenic manipulation of the expression of TGF-β and its receptors in mice.

TGF-β has been evaluated for its effects on mesenchymal cell differentiation in vitro. The focus of these studies on mesenchymal differentiation was suggested not only by phenotypic alterations induced by TGF-β, but also by the normal mesenchymal expression of TGF-β during embryonic development. Although the results are sometimes conflicting, they nevertheless indicate the potent ability of TGF-β to influence cell differentiation. Thus, TGF-β has been shown to inhibit myoblast maturation and concomitant myotube formation of several myoblast cell lines in vitro, although the mechanism is unclear (Massagué et al., 1986; Brennan et al., 1991). However, under some culture conditions, TGF-β also stimulates myotube formation (Zentella and Massagué, 1992) and exposure of embryonic stem cells to TGF-β will result in enhanced myogenic differentiation (Slager et al., 1993). Mesenchymal cells also have the ability to differentiate into adipocytes and this line of differentiation is also potently inhibited in vitro by TGF-β (Ignotz and Massagué, 1985). Finally, mesenchymal cells can differentiate into chondrocytes that give rise to cartilage, and osteoblasts that are responsible for bone formation. Cell culture experiments suggest that TGF-β has the ability to guide undifferentiated mesenchymal cells into chondrocyte differentiation. In addition, TGF-β may induce osteoblastic differentiation under some conditions, but also inhibit osteoblast maturation of established osteoblasts (for review see Centrella et al., 1993). These in vitro effects of TGF-β on chondrocyte and osteoblast differentiation are paralleled by in vivo experiments showing that introduction of TGF-β at the site of cartilage- or bone formation results in increased cartilage- and bone synthesis (Joyce et al., 1990). Taken together, these experiments strongly suggest that TGF-β plays an important role in mesenchymal differentiation but they also stress the need to define the role of TGF-β in mesenchymal differentiation in vivo, rather than in cell culture outside the tissue context. Thus, in vivo experiments using transgenic animal models will have to provide better insight into the role of TGF-β in the development of these tissues.

Most studies on the role of TGF-β in normal embryonic development have focused on the localization of the expression of the three TGF-β species during embryonic development in the mouse. The resulting data-base on the temporal and spatial expression patterns (Heine *et al.*, 1987; Lehnert and Akhurst, 1988, Fitzpatrick *et al.*, 1990; Pelton *et al.*, 1990a,b,c; Unsicker *et al.*, 1991), which cannot be discussed comprehensively in this review, is still far from complete but, nevertheless, provides sufficient background to carry out functional studies using transgenic model systems or gene targeting methodology. Some initial immunolocalization studies may not have accurately provided specificity for the individual TGF-β species owing to the lack of isoform-specific antibodies. However, the specificity of *in situ* hybridization studies with isogenic cDNA probes have provided an accurate description of the spatial and temporal expression patterns of the mRNAs for the different TGF-β isoforms. The recent development of reliable isoform-specific antibodies now allows a further definition of the highly regulated expression patterns.

The three TGF-β isoforms have complex but well-defined expression patterns during mouse development, that are often partially overlapping (Pelton *et al.*, 1990c). Most, if not all organs express one or several TGF-β isoforms at defined stages during development, which usually coincide with active tissue differentiation and morphogenesis. Furthermore, the sites of TGF-β synthesis frequently coincide with the deposition of extracellular matrix components, such as collagens, fibronectin and glycosaminoglycans (Heine *et al.*, 1990). Thus, the localization and the activities of TGF-β suggest that TGF-β may play an active role in various differentiation processes and morphogenetic events, which may be closely associated with the activities of TGF-β on extracellular matrix deposition and cell–matrix interactions.

High levels of TGF-β mRNA and protein synthesis are found in tissues of mesodermal origin. Thus, TGF-β synthesis is frequently associated with mesenchyme and especially with cartilage and bone formation (Heine *et al.*, 1987; Lehnert and Akhurst, 1988; Fitzpatrick *et al.*, 1990; Pelton *et al.*, 1990a,b,c). In addition, TGF-β is synthesized in mesenchymal cells at sites of epithelial interactions (Heine *et al.*, 1987; Pelton *et al.*, 1990c). The pattern of TGF-β synthesis frequently depends on the stage of differentiation. Thus, undifferentiated mesenchyme, an abundant source of TGF-β synthesis, makes all three TGF-β isoforms, but differentiation into cartilage and bone coincides with a drastic alteration of the expression pattern of the individual TGF-β isoforms. During mesenchymal condensation preceding cartilage formation, the TGF-β_1 synthesis is strikingly downregulated (Pelton *et al.*, 1990a,b,c). Furthermore, osteoblasts and chondrocytes synthesize all three TGF-β isoforms, whereas periosteal and perichondrial cells make predominantly TGF-β_1 and, to a lesser extent, TGF-β_3 (Pelton *et al.*, 1990a,b,c). Another example of differential expression of the three TGF-β isoforms is the developing tooth. Whereas the pulp cells and the mesodermally derived odontoblasts synthesize high levels of TGF-β_2, the ameloblasts from epithelial origin make primarily TGF-β_1 (Pelton *et al.*, 1990a,b; Heikinheimo *et al.*, 1993). Thus, the embryonic skeletal system is a major site of TGF-β synthesis and differential expression and responsiveness to TGF-β and the structurally related BMPs may play an important role in the successive differentiation steps of cartilage and bone cells (Centrella *et al.*, 1993).

The epithelia and skin are additional major sites of TGF-β synthesis during development (Heine *et al.*, 1987; Lehnert and Akhurst, 1988; Fitzpatrick *et al.*, 1990; Pelton *et al.*, 1990a,b,c). Expression of TGF-β may play an important role in the branching morphogenesis of complex epithelial structures, such as in the developing lung and mammary gland (Robinson *et al.*, 1991). Epithelia of the intestinal tract also synthesize high TGF-β levels, whereas the developing epidermis makes all three different TGF-β types (Pelton *et al.*, 1990a,b,c). The expression pattern of the different TGF-β isoforms may again depend on the stage of development. Furthermore, developing skin makes several BMPs, again suggesting the involvement of multiple TGF-β superfamily members in epidermal differentiation (Pelton *et al.*, 1990c). Another example of highly regulated TGF-β synthesis is the developing brain, which does not make detectable levels of TGF-β_1, but produces high levels of TGF-β_2 and TGF-β_3 (Wilcox and Derynck, 1988; Unsicker *et al.*, 1991). Finally, many striking expression patterns of the different TGF-β species occur during development of many other organs, such as heart, kidney, the vascular system and the developing haemopoietic system. There is some evidence for differential localization of TGF-β mRNA and protein in some organs (Pelton *et al.*, 1990c), but further substantiation of this conclusion is required. For example, some epithelial cell populations synthesize TGF-β mRNA, whereas the protein itself can only be found in the basement membrane or the extracellular matrix of adjacent cell types (Heine *et al.*, 1987; Lehnert and Akhurst, 1988; Fitzpatrick, *et al.*, 1990; Pelton *et al.*, 1990a,b,c). Differential localization of mRNA and protein may also occur in the brain, cartilage and bone.

Little is as yet known about the expression of the TGF-β receptors during development, since only some initial *in situ* hybridization studies have been performed with a type II receptor mRNA probe. The receptor is localized primarily in the undifferentiated mesenchyme and in the developing epidermis in a pattern reminiscent of the TGF-β_1 expression pattern (Lawler *et al.*, 1994). This coincident expression of ligand and receptor confirms that TGF-β exerts an autocrine and paracrine influence during development. No type II receptor mRNA transcripts were detected in condensing mesenchyme that differentiates into cartilage or in the central nervous system, which do not make detectable levels of TGF-β_1, yet clearly synthesize TGF-β_2 and/or TGF-β_3. These localization data together with the low efficiency of binding of TGF-β_2 to the type II receptor suggest the existence of an additional type II receptor species with a high specificity for TGF-β_2 (Lawler *et al.*, 1994).

Few transgenic studies have evaluated the effect of TGF-β on mammalian development. Transgenic expression of TGF-β was not expected to exert any major physiological effects because TGF-β is normally made in a latent form that does not bind to TGF-β receptors. However, the recent finding that expression of a TGF-β precursor, in which two cysteines in the pro-segment are replaced by serines, generates active TGF-β (Brunner *et al.*, 1989) has now allowed the generation of transgenic mice that overexpress active TGF-β. Overexpression of TGF-β in the mammary gland has been shown to inhibit lobuloalveolar development of the mammary gland and inhibit lactation (Jhappan *et al.*, 1993; Pierce *et al.*, 1993). In addition, overexpression of active TGF-β from an epidermal-specific promoter resulted in a hyperkeratotic epidermis with strongly inhibited proliferation and a reduced number of hair follicles, and resulted in early death (Sellheyer *et al.*, 1993). An alternative approach to evaluate the developmental role of TGF-β *in vivo* is to abolish functional gene expression in mice by targeted gene inactivation. Mice lacking a functional TGF-β_1 gene show a massive inflammatory response resulting in early death (Shull *et al.*, 1992; Kulkarni *et al.*, 1993). This effect has been discussed in the context of the effects of TGF-β on the immune response. No developmental defects were apparent, which could be due in part to the fact that the high degree of inflammation and early death has obscured any underlying developmental abnormalities. Alternatively, a partial redundancy in the roles of the three TGF-β isoforms may allow the two other TGF-β isoforms to compensate for the absence of TGF-β_1. Finally, the effects of TGF-β_1 deficiency during development could also have been compensated for by the transplacental transfer of maternal TGF-β *in utero* or by postnatal transfer of TGF-β_1 through the milk, which may have delayed any developmental deficiencies in the absence of TGF-β_1 (Shull *et al.*, 1992).

TGF-β IN TUMOUR DEVELOPMENT

Because of the initial identification of TGF-β in a phenotypic transformation assay (Moses *et al.*, 1981; Roberts *et al.*, 1981), it was originally assumed that TGF-β might play a role in malignant transformation and tumour development. This notion lost considerable enthusiasm as it became clear that TGF-β was made by nearly all cells in culture and that TGF-β inhibited the proliferation of many cell types in culture. Nevertheless, there is now growing evidence that endogenous TGF-β expression may play an important role in tumour development, which is supported by the many instances where TGF-β_1 expression is upregulated in tumours both *in vitro* and *in vivo* (Derynck *et al.*, 1987; Niitsu *et al.*, 1988; Travers *et al.*, 1988; Gomella *et al.*, 1989; Ito *et al.*, 1991). While the TGF-β released by tumour cells into the medium is often mostly in the latent form, the conditioned medium frequently also contains active TGF-β (Knabbe *et al.*, 1987; Liu *et al.*, 1988; Jennings *et al.*, 1991). Whether secreted TGF-β is active or not may not be an accurate reflection of its autocrine and paracrine role, since activation of latent TGF-β presumably occurs in a cell-associated fashion (Dennis and Rifkin, 1991; Arrick *et al.*, 1992; Harpel *et al.*, 1993). It is therefore most likely that the cell-associated TGF-β, and not so much the TGF-β in the conditioned medium, is of physiological importance for the tumour cells. Thus, what advantage if any does increased endogenous TGF-β production provide in tumour formation?

A possible advantage could be that increased TGF-β expression enhances the proliferation rate of the tumour cells. In this scenario, increased TGF-β synthesis in tumour cells that are mitogenically stimulated by TGF-β, such as tumour cells of mesenchymal origin, may result in an autocrine increase of cell proliferation *in vivo*. Conversely, many tumour cells are growth inhibited *in vitro* by TGF-β, which suggests that increased TGF-β synthesis may confer a disadvantage to these tumour cells in an autocrine fashion. At least in one tumour cell line, overexpression of antisense RNA and the resulting inhibition of TGF-β synthesis resulted in increased tumour growth (Wu *et al.*, 1992). This apparent disadvantage of increased TGF-β production may be less important considering the effects of TGF-β overproduction on the tumour environment *in vivo*, which may indirectly stimulate tumour growth (see below). Finally, many tumour cells are not affected in their proliferation by TGF-β (Moses *et al.*, 1990). Thus, many carcinomas are resistant to the antiproliferation effect of TGF-β, in contrast to untransformed epithelial cells. This resistance to the growth-modulatory effects of TGF-β is often considered as a general unresponsiveness of these cells to TGF-β, even though other responses to TGF-β such as the changes in cell–matrix interactions and extracellular matrix production are apparently maintained (Laiho *et al.*, 1991; Arrick *et al.*, 1992). Indeed, inactivation of the growth inhibitory effect of TGF-β either spontaneously or by functional inactivation of pRB or the type II receptor-mediated signalling pathway does not decrease the cellular responses related to cell–matrix interactions and extracellular matrix production (Laiho *et al.*, 1991b; Arrick *et al.*, 1992; Chen *et al.*, 1993). The selective loss of the antiproliferative response of these cells to TGF-β may be considered as a contributory step of the tumour cell in its progression towards autonomous growth and a full malignant phenotype (Hubbs *et al.*, 1989; Wakefield and Sporn, 1990; Haddow *et al.*, 1991; Manning *et al.*, 1991).

The effect of endogenous TGF-β on tumour-cell proliferation may also be of considerable importance in the physiology of hormone-responsive tumours such as breast carcinomas. Treatment of mammary carcinoma cells with oestrogen increases cell proliferation and decreases endogenous TGF-β synthesis, whereas tamoxifen, an oestrogen-based inhibitor of proliferation of hormone-responsive breast cancer cells, increases TGF-β synthesis, which in turn exerts its antiproliferative effect in responsive cells *in vitro* (Knabbe *et al.*, 1987). On the other hand, there is evidence for a marked increase in endogenous TGF-β synthesis when hormone-responsive breast cancers progress to a hormone-unresponsive phenotype (reviewed by Arteaga *et al.*, 1993). Increased TGF-β expression may provide an advantage for the *in vivo* tumour development, especially since overexpression of a transfected TGF-β_1 cDNA in a hormone-responsive mammary carcinoma-cell line has been shown to confer hormone-independence and increased tumour formation (Arteaga *et al.*, 1993).

The direct effects of TGF-β on tumour-cell proliferation may be less important for tumour development than the effects on the direct cellular and tissue environment that promote increased tumour growth. Because of the potent effects of TGF-β on cell–matrix interactions, TGF-β may induce increased matrix formation and integrin synthesis not only in the tumour cells but also in the surrounding cells. Thus, many tumour cells that are no longer responsive to the growth-inhibitory effects of TGF-β, may still increase extracellular matrix production and integrin synthesis in response to TGF-β (Arrick *et al.*, 1993). In addition, TGF-β is chemotactic for fibroblasts and tumour tissue is interspersed with large numbers of fibroblasts, which are responsive to TGF-β. The resulting autocrine and paracrine effects, not only on the tumour cells but also on the fibroblasts, may induce substantial changes in the physiology and growth of the tumour *in vivo*. Indeed, both the tumour cells and fibroblasts in the tumour stroma may, in response to the increased levels of TGF-β, increase their synthesis of extracellular matrix components. In addition, the tumour cells may become more adhesive to the extracellular matrix. As a consequence, increased extracellular matrix deposition and fibroblast infiltration and proliferation will result in extensive stroma formation. Thus, even though TGF-β synthesis by tumour cells would be predicted not to directly influence the proliferation rate or to directly inhibit tumour-cell proliferation, as assessed by *in vitro* proliferation assays, increased tumour-cell growth is likely to occur as a consequence of changes in stroma deposition and increased extracellular matrix formation, which support cell adhesion *in vitro* and proliferation *in vivo*. These effects of TGF-β on the tumour cells and the tumour environment are therefore likely to result in more favourable conditions for tumour growth (Arrick *et al.*, 1992; Steiner and Barrack, 1992; Chang *et al.*, 1993).

Another advantage of increased TGF-β synthesis to the tumour cells is based on the ability of TGF-β to exert a local immunosuppressive effect, as discussed in the previous section. TGF-β suppresses T and B lymphocyte proliferation and function and, perhaps most important in this context, inhibits the generation of cytotoxic T lymphocytes and

NK cells. Thus, increased TGF-β synthesis and activation may result in a localized immunosuppressive environment, that favours tumour growth (Torre-Amione *et al.*, 1990; Chang *et al.*, 1993).

The relative importance of these different effects of TGF-β on the tumour growth *in vivo* is hard to predict and presumably depends on the tumour-cell type and the progression stage of the tumour. Nevertheless, the available data suggest that the effects of TGF-β on the direct tumour environment, due to the combined effect on cell–matrix interaction, stroma formation and localized immunosuppression, may be far more important than any direct effect of TGF-β on cell proliferation. Thus, increased TGF-β synthesis in tumour cells that are growth-inhibited *in vitro* by endogenous TGF-β, may still provide a major advantage *in vivo* and thus result in increased tumour formation (Arrick *et al.*, 1992; Chang *et al.*, 1993).

Based on the different effects of TGF-β on cell–matrix interaction, especially on extracellular matrix synthesis, cell adhesion, and secretion of proteases and protease inhibitors, it is to be expected that TGF-β synthesis will strongly affect the invasive and metastatic behavior of tumour cells *in vivo*. Little is yet known about the importance of TGF-β in tumour metastasis.

CONCLUSION

The role of TGF-β in the different physiological and pathological process *in vivo* is only now starting to be explored. Whereas a multiplicity of biological activities of TGF-β has already been described, the coming years should bring us a better insight into the relevance of these activities *in vivo* and should define the role of TGF-β in the physiology of the cell, tissue and organism and during normal development. Another area of progress will be in the elucidation of how TGF-β induces its activities at the subcellular level and what signalling pathways mediate the biological activities of TGF-β. The recent cloning of some of the complex set of TGF-β receptors is only a first step that should lead to a definition of these molecular mechanisms.

NOTE

Rapid progress has been made in the characterisation of the TGF-β receptors, since the preparation of this chapter. An update of the knowledge of these receptors can be found in Derynck (1994).

REFERENCES

Owing to the very large number of references relevant to the subjects discussed, only a limited set of references could be provided.

Andres, J.L., Stanley, K., Cheifetz, S. and Massagué, J. (1989). *J. Cell Biol.* **109**, 3137–3145.

Andres, J.L., Rönnstrand, L., Cheifetz, S. and Massagué, J. (1991). *J. Biol. Chem.* **266**, 23282–23287.

Antonelli-Orlidge, A., Saunders, K.B., Smith, S.R. and d'Amore, P.A. (1989). *Proc. Natl Acad. Sci. USA* **86**, 4544–4548.

Anzano, M.A., Roberts, A.B., Meyers, C.A., Komoriya, A., Lamb, L.C., Smith J.M. and Sporn, M.B. (1982). *Cancer Res.* **42**, 4776–4778.

338   R. Derynck

Anzano, M.A., Roberts, A.B., Smith, J.M., Sporn, M.B. and DeLarco, J.E. (1983). *Proc. Natl Acad. Sci. USA* **80**, 6264–6268.

Arrick, B.A., Lee, A., Grendell, R.L. and Derynck, R. (1991). *Mol. Cell Biol.* **11**, 4306–4313.

Arrick, B.A., Lopez, A.R., Elfman, F., Ebner, R., Damsky, C.H. and Derynck, R. (1992). *J. Cell Biol.* **118**, 715–726.

Arrick, B.A. and Derynck, R. (1993). In *Oncogenes and Tumor Suppressor Genes in Human Malignancies* (eds Benz, C.and Liu, E.). Kluwer Academic Publishers, Boston, pp. 255–264.

Arteaga, C.L., Cart-Dugger, T., Moses, H.L., Hurd, S.D. and Pietenpol, J.A. (1993). *Cell Growth and Differentiation* **4**, 193–201.

Assoian, R.K., Komoriya, A., Meyers, C.A., Miller, D.M. and Sporn, M.B. (1983). *J. Biol. Chem.* **258**, 7155–7160.

Assoian, R.K., Frolik, C.A., Roberts, A.B., Miller, D.M. and Storn, M.B. (1984). *Cell* **36**, 35–41.

Assoian, R.K., Fleurdelys, B.E., Stevenson, H.C., Miller, P.T., Madtes, D.K., Raines, E.W., Ross, R. and Sporn, M.B. (1987). *Proc. Natl Acad. Sci. USA* **84**, 6020–6023.

Attisano, L., Wrana, J.L., Cheifetz, S. and Massagué, J. (1992). *Cell* **68**, 97–108.

Barr, P.J. (1991). *Cell* **66**, 1–3.

Bascom, C.C., Wolfshohl, J.R., Coffey, R.J., Madisen, L., Webb, N.R., Purchio, A.R., Derynck, R. and Moses, H.L. (1989). *Mol. Cell. Biol.* **9**, 5508–5515.

Battegay, E.J., Raines, E.W., Seifert, R.A., Bowen-Pope, D.F. and Ross, R. (1990). *Cell* **63**, 515–524.

Boyd, F.T. and Massagué, J. (1989). *J. Biol. Chem.* **264**, 2272–2278.

Brandes, M.E., Allen, J.B., Ogawa, Y. and Wahl, S.M. (1991). *J. Clin. Invest.* **87**, 1108–1113.

Brennan, T.J., Edmondson, D.G., Li, L. and Olson, E.N. (1991). *Proc. Natl Acad. Sci. USA* **88**, 3822–3826.

Brunner, A.M., Marquardt, H., Malacko, A.R., Lioubin, M.N. and Purchio, A.F. (1989). *J. Biol. Chem.* **264**, 13660–13664.

Carel, J.C., Schreiber, R.D., Falqui, L. and Lacy, P.E. (1990). *Proc. Natl Acad. Sci. USA* **87**, 1591–1595.

Carel, J.C., Sheehan, K.C., Schreiber, R.D. and Lacy P.E. (1993). *Transplantation* **55**, 456–458.

Centrella, M., McCarthy, T.L. and Canalis, E. (1987). *J. Biol. Chem.* **262**, 2869–2874.

Centrella, M., Horowitz, M.C., Wozney, J.M. and McCarthy, T.L. (1993). *Endocrine Rev.* **15**, 27–39.

Chambard, J.-C. and Pouysségur, J. (1988). *J. Cell Physiol.* **135**, 101–107.

Chang, H.-L., Gillett, N., Figari, I., Lopez, A.R., Palladino, M.A. and Derynck, R. (1993). *Cancer Res.* **53**, 4391–4398.

Cheifetz, S., Weatherbee, J.A., Tsang, M.L.S., Andersen, J.K., Mole, J.E., Lucas, R. and Massagué, J. (1987). *Cell* **48**, 409–415.

Cheifetz, S., Andres, J.L. and Massagué, J. (1988). *J. Biol. Chem.* **263**, 16984–16991.

Cheifetz, S. and Massagué, J. (1989). *J. Biol. Chem.* **264**, 12025–12028.

Cheifetz, S., Bellón, T., Calés, C., Vera, S., Bernabeu, C., Massagué, J. and Letarte, M. (1992). *J. Biol. Chem.* **267**, 19027–19030.

Chen, R.-H., Ebner, R. and Derynck, R. (1993). *Science* **260**, 1335–1338.

Coffey, R.J. Jr., Bascom, C.C., Sipes, N.J., Graves-Deal, R., Weissman, B.E. and Moses, H.L. (1988). *Mol. Cell Biol.* **8**, 3088–3093.

Coffman, R.L., Lebman, D.A. and Schrader, B. (1989). *J. Exp. Med.* **170**, 1039–1044.

Czarniecki, C.W., Chiu, H.H., Wong, G.H.W., McCabe, S.M. and Palladino, M. (1988). *J. Immunol.* **140**, 4217–4223.

Damsky, C.H. and Werb, Z. (1992). *Curr. Opin. Cell Biol.* **4**, 772–781.

Daopin, S., Piez, K.A., Ogawa, Y. and Davies, D.R. (1992). *Science* **257**, 369–373.

de Martin, R., Haendler, B., Hofer-Warbinek, R., Gaugitsch, H., Wrann, M. Schlüsener, H., Seifert, J.M., Bodmer, S., Fontana, A. and Hofer, E. (1987). *EMBO J.* **6**, 3673–3677.

Dennis, P.A. and Rifkin, D.B. (1991). *Proc. Natl Acad. Sci. USA* **88**, 580–584.

Derynck, R., Jarrett, J.A., Chen, E.Y., Eaton, D.H., Bell, J.R., Assoian, R.K., Roberts, A.B., Sporn, M.B. and Goeddel, D.V. (1985). *Nature* **316**, 701–705.

Derynck, R., Goedell, D.V., Ullrich, A., Gutterman, J.U., Williams, R.D., Bringman, T.S. and Berger, W.H. (1987). *Cancer Res.* **47**, 707–712.

Derynck, R., Lindquist, P.B., Lee, A., Wen, D., Tamm, J., Graycar, J.L., Rhee, L., Mason, A.J., Miller, D.A., Coffey, R.J., Moses, H.L. and Chen, E.Y. (1988). *EMBO J.* **7**, 3737–3743.

Derynck, R. (1992). *Adv. Cancer Res.* **58**, 27–52.

Derynck, R. (1994). *Trends Biochem. Sci.* (in press).

Ebner, R., Chen, R.-H., Chum, L., Lawler, S., Zionchek, T.F., Lee, A., Lopez, A.R. and Derynck, R. (1993). *Science* **260**, 1344–1348.

Espevik, T., Figari, I.S., Shalaby, R., Lackides, G.A., Lewis, G., Shepard, H.M. and Palladino, M.A. (1987). *J. Exp. Med.* **166**, 571–576.

Espevik, T., Figari, I., Ranges, G.E. and Palladino, M.A. (1988). *J. Immunol.* **140**, 2312–2316.

Fava, R. and McClure, D.B. (1987). *J. Cell Physiol.* **131**, 184–189.

Fitzpatrick, D.R., Denhez, F., Kondaiah, P. and Akhurst, R. (1990). *Development* **109**, 585–595.

Flaumenhaft, R., Abe, M., Mignatti, P. and Rifkin, D.B. (1992a). *J. Cell Biol.* **118**, 901–909.

Flaumenhaft, R., Kojima, S., Abe, M. and Rifkin, D.B. (1992b). *Adv. Pharmacol.* **24**, 51–76.

Flaumenhaft, R., Abe, M., Sato, Y., Miyazono, K., Harpel, J.G., Heldin, C.-H. and Rifkin, D.B. (1993). *J. Cell Biol.* **120**, 995–1002.

Fontana, A., Frei, K., Bodmer, S., Hofer, E., Schreier, M.H., Palladino, M.A. Jr and Zinkernagel, R.M. (1989). *J. Immunol.* **143**, 3230–3234.

Gamble, J.R. and Vadas, M.A. (1988). *Science* **242**, 97–99.

Geiser, A.G., Burmester, J.K., Webbink, R., Roberts, A.B. and Sporn, M.B. (1992). *J. Biol. Chem.* **267**, 2588–2593.

Georgi, L.L., Albert, P.S. and Riddle, D. (1990). *Cell* **61**, 635–645.

Gerwin, B.I., Spillare, E., Forrester, K., Lehman, T.A., Kispert, J., Welsh, J.A., Pfeifer, A.M.A., Lechner, J.F., Baker, S.J., Vogelstein, B. and Harris, C.C. (1992). *Proc. Natl Acad. Sci. USA* **89**, 2759–2763.

Glick, A.B., Flanders, K.C., Danielpour, D., Yuspa, S.H. and Sporn, M.B. (1989). *Cell Regul.* **1**, 87–97.

Gomella, L.G., Sargent, E.R., Wade, T.P., Anglard, P., Linehan, W.M. and Kasid, A. (1989). *Cancer Res.* **49**, 6972–6975.

Gougos, A. and Letarte, M. (1990). *J. Biol. Chem.* **265**, 8361–8364.

Gray, A.M. and Mason, A.J. (1990). *Science* **247**, 1328–1330.

Gruppuso, P.A., Mikumo, R., Brautigan, D.L. and Braun, L. (1991). *J. Biol. Chem.* **266**, 3444–3448.

Haddow, S., Fowlis, D.J., Parkinson, K., Akhurst, R.J. and Balmain, A. (1991). *Oncogene* **6**, 1465–1470.

Harpel, J.G., Metz, C.N., Kojima, S. and Rifkin, D.B. (1993). *Progress in Growth Factor Research 4*.

Heikinheimo, K., Happonen, R.-P., Miettinen, P.J. and Ritvos, O. (1993). *J. Clin. Invest.* **91**, 1019–1027.

Heine, U.I., Munoz, E.F., Flanders, K.C., Ellingsworth, L.R., Lam, H.-Y.P., Thompson, N.L., Roberts, A.B. and Sporn, M.B. (1987). *J. Cell Biol.* **105**, 2861–2876.

Heine, U.I., Munoz, E.F., Flanders, K.C., Roberts, A.B. and Sporn, M.B. (1990). *Development* **109**, 29–36.

Hoffmann, F.M. (1991). *Curr. Opin. Cell Biol.* **3**, 947–952.

Howe, P.H., Cunningham, M.R. and Leof, E.B. (1990). *Biochem. J.* **266**: 537–543.

Huang, S.S., O'Grady, P. and Huang, J.S. (1988). *J. Biol. Chem.* **263**, 1535–1541.

Hubbs, A.F., Hahn, F.F. and Thomassen, D.G. (1989). *Carcinogenesis* **10**, 1599–1605.

Ignotz, R.A. and Massagué, J. (1985). *Proc. Natl Acad. Sci, USA* **82**, 8530–8534.

Ito, N., Kawata, S., Tamura, S., Takaishi, K., Shirai, Y., Kiso, S., Yabuuchi, I., Matsuda, Y., Nishioka, M. and Tarui, S. (1991). *Cancer Res.* **51**, 4080–4083.

Jennings, M.T., Maciunas, R.J., Carver, R., Bascom, C.C., Juneau, P., Misulis, K. and H.L. Moses, (1991). *Int. J. Cancer* **49**, 129–139.

Jhappan, C., Geiser, A.G., Kordon, E.C., Bagheri, D., Hennighausen, L., Roberts, A.B., Smith, G.H. and Merlino, G. (1993). *EMBO J.* **12**, 1835–1846.

Joyce, M.E., Roberts, A.B., Sporn, M.B. and Bolander, M. (1990). *J. Cell Biol.* **110**, 2195–2207.

Kanzaki, T., Olofsson, A., Morén, A., Wernstedt, C., Hellman, U., Miyazono, K., Claesson-Welsh, L. and Heldin, C.-H. (1990). *Cell* **61**, 1051–1061.

Kehrl, J.H. (1991). *Int. J. Cell Cloning* **9**, 438–450.

Kehrl, J.H., Roberts, A.B., Wakefield, L.M., Jakowlew, S., Sporn, M.B. and Fauci, A.S. (1986a). *J. Immunol.* **137**, 3855–3860.

Kehrl, J.H., Wakefield, L.M., Roberts, A.B., Jakowlew, S., Alvarez-Mon, M., Dernyck, R., Sporn, M.B. and Fauci, A.S. (1986b). *J. Exp. Med.* **163**, 1037–1050.

Kehrl, J.H., Thevenin, C., Rieckmann, R. and Fauci, A.S. (1991). *J. Immunol.* **146**, 4016–4022.

Kekow, J., Wachsman, W., McCutchan, J.A., Cronin, M., Carson, D.A. and Lotz, M. (1990). *Proc. Natl Acad. Sci. USA* **87**, 8321–8325.

Kekow, J., Wachsman, W., McCutchan, J.A., Gross, W.L., Zachariah, M., Carson, D.A. and Lotz, M. (1991). *J. Clin. Invest.* **87**, 1010–1016.

Kerr, L.D., Miller, D.B. and Matrisian, L.M. (1990). *Cell* **61**, 267–278.

Kim, S.-J., Kehrl, J.H., Burton, J., Tendler, C.L., Teang, K.T., Danielpour, D., Thévenin, C., Kim, K.-Y., Sporn, M.B. and Roberts, A.B. (1990). *J. Exp. Med.* **172**, 121–129.

Kim, S.-J., Lee, H.-D., Robbins, P.D., Busam, K., Sporn, M.B. and Roberts, A.B. (1991). *Proc. Natl Acad. Sci. USA* **88**, 3052–3056.

Kim, S.-J., Park, K., Koeller, D., Kim, K.Y., Wakefield, L.M., Sporn, M.B. and Roberts, A.B. (1992). *J. Biol. Chem.* **267**, 13702–13707.

Kingsley, D.M. (1994). *Genes Dev.* **8**, 133–146.

Knabbe, C., Lippman, M.E., Wakefield, L.M., Flanders, K.C., Kasid, A., Derynck, R. and Dickson, R.B. (1987). *Cell* **48**, 417–428.

Koff, A., Ohtsuki, M., Polyak, K., Roberts, J.M. and Massagué, J. (1993). *Science* **260**, 536–539.

Kojima, S. and Rifkin, D.B. (1993). *J. Cell Physiol.* **155**, 323–332.

Kojima, S., Nara, K. and Rifkin, D.B. (1993). *J. Cell Biol.* **12**, 439–448.

Kovacina, K.S., Steele, P.G., Purchio, A.F., Lioubin, M., Miyazona, K., Heldin, C.-H. and Roth, R.A. (1989). *Biochem. Biophys. Res. Commun.* **160**, 393–403.

Kulkarni, A.B., Huh, C.-G., Becker, D., Geiser, A., Light, M., Flanders, K.C., Roberts, A.B., Sporn, M.B., Ward, J.M. and Karlsson, S. (1993). *Proc. Natl Acad. Sci. USA* **90**, 770–774.

Kuppner, M.C., Hamou, M.F., Bodmer, S., Fontana, A. and De Tribolet, N. (1988). *Int. J. Cancer* **42**, 562–567.

Kuruvilla, A.P., Shah, R., Hochwald, G.M., Liggitt, H.D., Palladino, M.A. and Thorbecke, G.J. (1991). *Proc. Natl Acad. Sci. USA* **88**, 2918–2921.

Laiho, M., DeCaprio, J.A., Ludlow, J.W., Livingston, D.M. and Massagué, J. (1990a). *Cell* **62**, 175–185.

Laiho, M., Weis, F.M.B. and Massagué, J. (1990b). *J. Biol. Chem.* **265**, 18518–18524.

Laiho, M., Rönnstrand, L., Heino, J., DeCaprio, J.A., Ludlow, J.W., Livingston, D.M. and Massagué, J. (1991a). *Mol. Cell Biol.* **11**, 972–978.

Laiho, M., Weis, F.M.B., Boyd, F.T., Ignotz, R.A. and Massagué, J. (1991b). *J. Biol. Chem.* **266**, 9108–9112.

LaMarre, J., Hayes, M.A., Wollenberg, G.K., Hussaini, I., Hall, S.W. and Gonias, S.L. (1991a). *J. Clin. Invest.* **87**, 39–44.

LaMarre, J., Wollenberg, G.K., Gonias, S.L. and Hayes, M.A. (1991b). *Lab. Invest.* **65**, 3–14.

Lawler, S., Candia, A.F., Ebner, R., Lopez, A.R., Moses, H.L., Wright, C.V.E. and Derynck, R. (1994). *Development* **120**, 165–175.

Lee, G., Ellingsworth, L.R., Gillis, S., Wall, R. and Kincade, P.K. (1987). *J. Exp. Med.* **166**, 1290–1299.

Lehnert, S.A. and Akhurst, E.J. (1988). *Development* **104**, 263–273.

Leof, E.B., Proper, J.A., Goustin, A.S., Shipley, G.D., DiCorleto, P.E. and Moses, H.L. (1986). *Proc. Natl Acad. Sci. USA* **83**, 2453–2457.

Like, B. and Massagué, J. (1986). *J. Biol. Chem.* **261**, 13426–13429.

Lin, H.Y., Wang, X.-F., Ng-Eaton, E., Weinberg, R.A. and Lodish, H.F. (1992). *Cell* **68**, 775–785.

Lin, H.Y. and Lodish, H.F. (1993). *Trends in Cell Biology* **3**, 14–19.

Liu, C., Tsao, M.S. and Grisham, J.W. (1988). *Cancer Res.* **48**, 850–855.

Lopez, A.R., Cook, J., Deininger, P.L. and Derynck, R. (1992). *Mol. Cell Biol.* **12**, 1674–1679.

Lopez-Casillas, F., Cheifetz, S., Doody, J., Andres, J.L., Lane W.S. and Massagué, J. (1991). *Cell* **67**, 785–795.

Lopez-Casillas, F., Wrana, J.L. and Massagué, J. (1993). *Cell* **73**, 1435–1444.

Lotz, M., Kekow, J. and Carson, D.A. (1990). *J. Immunol.* **144**, 4194–4198.

Lyons, R.M., Keski-Oja, J. and Moses, H.L. (1988). *J. Cell Biol.* **106**, 1659–1665.

Lyons, R.M., Gentry, L.E., Purchio, A.F. and Moses, H.L. (1990). *J. Cell Biol.* **110**, 1361–1367.

Manning, A.M., Williams, A.C., Game, S.M. and Partskeva, C. (1991). *Oncogene* **6**, 1471–1476.

Massagué, J., Cheifetz, S., Endo, T. and Nadal-Ginard, B. (1986). *Proc. Natl Acad. Sci. USA* **83**, 8206–8210.

Massagué, J. (1990). *Annu. Rev. Cell Biol.* **6**, 597–641.

Massagué, J. (1992). *Cell* **69**, 1067–1070.

Mathews, L.S. and Vale, W.W. (1991). *Cell* **65**, 973–982.

McCartney-Francis, N., Mizel, D., Wong, H., Wahl, L.M. and Wahl, S.M. (1990). *Growth Factors* **4**, 27–32.

Miyazono, K., Hellman, U., Wernstedt, C. and Heldin, C.-H. (1988). *J. Biol. Chem.* **263**, 6407–6415.

Miyazono, K., Yuki, K., Takaku, F., Wernstedt, C., Kanzaki, T., Olofsson, A., Hellman, U. and Heldin, C.-H. (1990). *Ann. N.Y. Acad. Sci.* **593**, 51–58.

Miyazono, K., Oloffson, A., Colosetti, P. and Heldin, C.-H. (1991). *EMBO J.* **10**, 1091–1101.

Moses, H.L., Branum, E.L., Proper, J.A. and Robinson, R.A. (1981). *Cancer Res.* **41**, 2842–2848.

Moses, H.L., Yang, E.Y. and Pietenpol, J.A. (1990). *Cell* **63**, 245–247.

Murphy-Ullrich, J.E., Schultz-Cherry, S. and Hook, M. (1992). *Molec Biol. Cell* **3**, 181–188.

Nakamura, T., Sugino, K., Kurosawa, N., Sawai, M., Takio, K., Eto, Y., Iwashita, S., Muramatsu, M., Titani, K., Sugino, H. (1992). *J. Biol. Chem.* **267**, 18924–18928.

Nathan, C.F. (1987). *J. Clin. Invest.* **79**, 319–326.

Niitsu, Y., Urushizaki, Y., Koshida, Y., Terui, K., Mahara, K., Kohgo, Y. and Urushizaki, I. (1988). *Blood* **71**, 263–266.

O'Connor-McCourt, M. and Wakefield, L.M. (1987). *J. Biol. Chem.* **262**, 14090–14099.

Ohta, M., Greenberger, J.S., Anklesaria, P., Bassols, A. and Massagué, J. (1987). *Nature* **329**, 539–541.

Olofsson, A., Miyazono, K., Kanzaki, T., Colosatti, P., Engstrom, U. and Heldin, C.-H. (1992). *J. Biol. Chem.* **267**, 19482–19488.

Ong, G., Sikora, K. and Gullick, W.J. (1991). *Oncogene* **6**, 761–763.

Ortaldo, J.R., Mason, A.T., O'Shea, J.J., Smyth, M.J., Falk, L.A., Kennedy, A.C.S., Longo, D.L. and Ruscetti, F.W. (1991). *J. Immunol.* **146**, 3791–3798.

Oursler, M.J., Cortese, C., Keeting, P., Anderson, M.A., Riggs, B.L. and Spelsberg, T.C. (1991). *Endocrinol.* **129**, 3313–3320.

Paralkar, M.V., Vukicevic, S. and Reddi, A.H. (1991). *Dev. Biol.* **143**, 303–308.

Pelton, R.W., Dickinson, M.E., Moses, H.L. and Hogan, B.L.M. (1990a). *Development* **110**, 609–620.

Pelton, R.W., Hogan, B.L.M., Miller, D.A. and Moses, H.L. (1990b). *Dev. Biol.* **141**, 456–460.

Pelton, R.W., Saxena, B., Jones, M., Moses, H.L. and Gold, L.I. (1990c). *J. Cell Biol.* **115**, 1091–1105.

Pierce, D.F. Jr., Johnson, M.D., Matsui, Y., Robinson, S.D., Gold, L.I., Purchio, A.F., Danid, C.W., Hogan, B.L.M. and Moses, H.L. (1993). *Genes Dev.* **7**, 2308–2317.

Pietenpol, J.A., Holt, J.T., Stein, R.W. and Moses, H.L. (1990a). *Proc. Natl Acad. Sci. USA* **87**, 3758–3762.

Pietenpol, J.A., Stein, R.W., Moran, E., Yaciuk, P., Schlegel, R., Lyons, R.M., Pittelkow, M.R., Münger, K., Howley, P.M. and Moses, H.L. (1990b). *Cell* **61**, 777–785.

Pietenpol, J.A., Münger, K., Howley, P.M., Stein, R.W. and Moses, H.L. (1991). *Proc. Natl Acad. Sci. USA* **88**, 10227–10231.

Postlethwaite, A.E., Keski-Oja, J., Moses, H.L. and Kang, A.H. (1987). *J. Exp. Med.* **165**, 251–256.

Purchio, A.F., Cooper, J.A., Brunner, A.M., Lioubin, M.N., Gentry, L.E., Kovacina, K.S., Roth, R.A. and Marquardt, H. (1988). *J. Biol. Chem.* **263**, 14211–14215.

Ranges, G.E., Figari, I.S., Espevik, T. and Palladino, M.A. (1987). *J. Exp. Med.* **166**, 991–998.

Ridley, A.J., Davis, J.B., Stroobant, P. and Land, H. (1989). *J. Cell Biol.* **109**, 3419–3424.

Ristow, H.J. (1986). *Proc. Natl Acad. Sci. USA* **83**, 5531–5534.

Roberts, A.B., Anzano, M.A., Lamb, L.C., Smith, J.M. and Sporn, M.B. (1981). *Proc. Natl Acad. Sci. USA* **78**, 5339–5343.

Roberts, A.B., Sporn, M.B., Assoian, R.K., Smith, J.M., Roche, N.S., Wakefield, L.M., Heine, U.I., Liotta, L.A., Falanga, V., Kehrl, J.H. and Fauci, A.S. (1986). *Proc. Natl Acad. Sci. USA* **83**, 4167–4171.

Roberts, A.B. and Sporn, M.B. (1990). In *Peptide Growth Factors and their Receptors* (eds Sporn, M.B. and Roberts, A.B.). Springer-Verlag, Heidelberg. pp. 421–472.

Roberts, A.B. and Sporn, M.B. (1992). *Cancer Surveys* **14**, 205–220.

Roberts, A.B., Kim, S.-J., Noma, T., Glick, A.B., Lafyatis, R., Lechleiter, R., Jakowlew, S.B., Geisser, A., O'Reilly, M.A., Danielpour, D. and Sporn, M.B. (1991). *Ciba Found. Symp.* **157**, 7–15.

Robinson, S.D., Silberstein, G.B., Roberts, A.B., Flanders, K.C. and Daniel, C.W. (1991). *Development* **113**, 867–878.

Romeo, D.S., Park, K., Roberts, A.B., Sporn, M.B. and Kim, S.-J. (1993). *Mol. Endocrinol.* **7**, 759–766.

Rook, A.H., Kehrl, J.H., Wakefield, L.M., Roberts, A.B., Sporn, M.B., Burlington, D.B., Lane, H.C. and Fauci, A.S. (1986). *J. Immunol.* **136**, 3916–3920.

Ruscetti, F., Vanesio, L., Ochoa, A. and Ontaldo, J. (1993). *Ann NY Acad. Sci.* **485**, 488–500.

Sato, Y. and Rifkin, D.B. (1989). J. Cell Biol. **109**, 309–315.

Schlunegger, M.P. and Grütter, M.G. (1992). *Nature* **358**, 430–434.

Segarini, P.R. and Seyedin, S.M. (1988). *J. Biol. Chem.* **263**, 8366–8370.

Sellheyer, K., Bickenbach, J.R., Rothnagel, J.A., Bundman, D., Longley, M.A., Krieg, T., Roche, N.S., Roberts, A.B. and Roop, D.R. (1993). *Proc. Natl Acad. Sci. USA* 5237–5241.

Sherr, C.J. (1993). *Cell* **73**, 1059–1065.

Shull, M.M., Ormsby, I., Kier, A.B., Pawlowski, S., Diebold, R.J., Yin, M., Allen, R., Sidman, C., Proetzel, G., Calvin, D., Annunziata, N. and Doetschman, T. (1992). *Nature* **359**, 693–699.

Smeland, E.B., Blonhoff, H.K., Holte, H., Ruud, E., Beiske, K., Funderud, S., Godal, T. and Ohlsson, R. (1987). *Exp. Cell Res.* **171**, 213–222.

Slager, H.G., Van Inzen, W., van den Eijnden-van Raaij, A.J.M. and Mummery, C.L. (1993). *Dev. Gen.* **14**, 212–224.

Soma, Y. and Grotendorst, G.R. (1989). *J. Cell Physiol.* **140**, 246–253.

Steiner, M.S. and Barrack, E.R. (1992). *Mol. Endocrin.* **6**, 15–25.

Swain, S.L., Huston, G., Tonkonogy, S. and Weinberg, A.D. (1991). *J. Immunol.* **147**, 2991–3000.

Streuli, C.H., Schmidhauser, C., Kobrin, M., Bissell, M.J. and Derynck, R. (1993). *J. Cell. Biol.* **120**, 253–260.

ten Dijke, P., Hanson, P., Iwata, K.K., Pieler, C. and Foulkes, J.G. (1988). *Proc. Natl Acad. Sci. USA* **82**, 4715–4719.

Torre-Amione, G., Beauchamp, R.D., Koeppen, H., Park, B.H., Schreiber, H., Moses, H.L. and Rowley, D.A. (1990). *Proc. Natl Acad. Sci. USA* **87**, 1486–1490.

Travers, M.T., Barrett-Lee, P.J., Berger, U., Luqmani, Y.A., Gazet, J.-C., Powers, T.J. and Coombes, R.C. (1988). *Br. Med. J.* **296**, 1621–1624.

Tsunawaki, S., Sporn, M.B., Ding, A. and Nathan, C. (1988). *Nature* **334**, 260–262.

Twardzik, D.R., Mikovits, J.A., Ranchalis, J.E., Purchio, A.F., Ellingsworth, L., Ruscetti, F.W. (1990). *Ann. NY Acad. Sci.* **593**, 276–284.

Unsicker, K., Flanders, K.C., Cissel, D.S., Lafayatis, R. and Sporn, M.B. (1991). *Neuroscience* **44**, 613–625.

Wahl, S.M., Hunt, D.A., Wakefield, L.M., McCartney-Francis, N., Wahl, L.M., Roberts, A.B. and Sporn, M.B. (1987). *Proc. Natl Acad. Sci. USA* **84**, 5788-5792.

Wahl, S.M., Hunt, D.A., Wong, H.L., Dougherty, J., McCartney-Francis, N., Wahl, L.M., Ellingsworth, L., Schmidt, J.A., Hall, G. and Roberts, A.B. (1988a). *J. Immunol.* **140**, 3026–3032.

Wahl, S.M., Hunt, D.A., Bansal, G., McCartney-Francis, N. Ellingsworth, L. and Allen J.B. (1988b). *J. Exp. Med.* **168**, 1403–1417.

Wahl, S.M., McCartney-Francis, N.M. and Mergenhagen, S.E. (1989). *Immunology Today* 258–261.

Wahl, S.M., McCartney-Francis, N., Allen, J.B., Dougherty, E.B. and Dougherty, S.F. (1990). *Ann. NY Acad. Sci.* **593**, 188–196.

Wahl, S.M., Allen, J.B., McCartney-Francis, N., Morganti-Kossman, M.C., Kossman, T., Ellingsworth, L., Mai, U.E., Mergenhagen, S.F. and Orenstein, T.M. (1991). *J. Exp. Med.* **173**, 981–991.

Wakefield, L.M. and Sporn, M.B. (1990). In *Tumor Suppressor Genes* (ed Klein, G.). Marcel Dekker, New York. pp. 216–243.

Wakefield, L.M., Smith, D.M., Flanders, K.C. and Sporn, M.B. (1988). *J. Biol. Chem.* **263**, 7646–7654.

Wang, X.-F., Lin, H.Y., Ng-Eaton, E., Downward, J., Lodish, H.F. and Weinberger, R.A. (1991). *Cell* **67**, 797–805.

Wilder, R., Lafyatis, R., Roberts, A.B., Case, J.P., Kimkumian, G. K., Sano, G., Sporn, M.B. and Remmers, E.F. (1990). *Ann. NY Acad. Sci.* **593**, 197–207.

Wilcox, J.N. and Derynck, R. (1988). *Mol. Cell Biol.* **8**, 3415–3422.

Wrana, J.L., Attisano, L., Carcamo, J., Zentella, A., Doody, J. Laiho, M., Wang, X.-F. and Massagué, J. (1992). *Cell* **71**, 1003–1014.

Wu, S., Theodorescu, D., Kerbel, R.S., Willson, J.K.V., Mulder, K.M., Humphrey, L.E. and Brattain, M.G. (1992). *J. Cell Biol.* **116**, 187–196.

Yamaguchi, Y., Mann, D.M. and Ruoslahti, E. (1990). *Nature* **346**, 281–284.

Yang, E.Y. and Moses, H.L. (1990). *J. Cell Biol.* **111**, 731–741.

Yayon, A., Klagsbrun, M., Esko, J.D., Leder, P. and Ornitz, D. (1991). *Cell* **64**, 841–848.

Zentella, A. and Massagué, J. (1992). *Proc. Natl Acad. Sci. USA* **89**, 5176–5180.

Chapter 19

Granulocyte-Macrophage Colony Stimulating Factor

John E. J. Rasko and Nicholas M. Gough

The Walter and Eliza Hall Institute of Medical Research, and The Cooperative Research
Centre for Cellular Growth Factors, Post Office, Royal Melbourne Hospital, Parkville,
Victoria, 3050, Australia

INTRODUCTION

Granulocyte-macrophage colony stimulating factor (GM-CSF) is one of at least 20 glycoprotein growth factors or cytokines which are able to modulate the growth or differentiation of haemopoietic cells. GM-CSF was one of the first of this large number of factors to be described, purified and cloned. In semi-solid cultures of haemopoietic progenitor cells it is a potent stimulus for the formation of granulocyte and macrophage colonies. GM-CSF was one of the first haemopoietic regulators to be deployed clinically and, along with G-CSF, is now used widely to ameliorate chemotherapy-induced neutropenia and to enhance haemopoietic recovery after bone-marrow transplantation.

It is the purpose of this review to outline our current understanding of the structure of both GM-CSF and its receptor; to summarize its molecular genetics and that of the cell-surface receptor with which it interacts; to examine the biological activities of this cytokine, including its involvement in leukaemia, and discuss its clinical potential.

THE STRUCTURE OF GM-CSF

The structures of murine (Gough et al., 1984, 1985; Sparrow et al., 1985), human (Lee et al., 1985; Wong et al., 1985a), gibbon (Wong et al., 1985b) and bovine (Maliszewski et al., 1988) GM-CSF have been determined by partial amino acid sequence analysis and by deduction from the nucleotide sequence of cDNA clones. In each species the mature protein is preceded by a hydrophobic leader sequence of 25 amino acid residues in length. Mature murine GM-CSF comprises 124 amino acid residues (molecular mass = 14 kDa), whereas human, gibbon and bovine GM-CSF are 3 residues longer. The length difference is due to an insertion of 3 residues between residues 27 and 28 of the murine sequence. Interestingly this is within a region of GM-CSF implicated in binding to the β chain of the receptor, within the first of four α helices (see below). Murine and

The Cytokine Handbook, 2nd ed.
ISBN 0–12–689661–5

Table 1. Cross-species comparison of CSFs and their receptors.

	Mouse: Human amino acid sequence identity (%)	
	Ligand	Receptor (α chain)
Erythropoietin	79	82
M-CSF	75	75
G-CSF	80	63
IL-5	67	71
GM-CSF	56	35
Multi-CSF (IL-3)	29	30

Table 2. Location of α-helices in human GM-CSF.

Helix	Residues
Helix-A	13–28
Helix-B	55–64
Helix-C	74–87
Helix-D	103–116
% α-helix	47

See Diederichs *et al.* (1991)

human GM-CSF, which do not exhibit cross-species biological activity or receptor binding, display only 56% amino acid sequence identity, and thus represent one of the less-well conserved of the myeloid growth factors (see Table 1).

The murine and human GM-CSF polypeptide sequences both contain two potential N-linked glycosylation sites, but interestingly they are at different locations within the respective molecules. GM-CSF isolated from most murine and human sources is glycosylated to approximately 23 000 Da (Nicola *et al.*, 1989). Although native GM-CSF is glycosylated, nonglycosylated *Escherichia coli*-derived recombinant GM-CSF has high biological activity (Libby *et al.*, 1987; Schrimsher *et al.*, 1987; Wingfield *et al.*, 1988). Similarly, yeast-derived (Price *et al.*, 1987) and baculovirus-derived (Chiou and Wu, 1990) recombinant GM-CSF, which exhibit different glycosylation to that of mammalian GM-CSF, are also active. Thus, glycosylation does not appear to be essential for GM-CSF activity, either *in vitro* or *in vivo*, but appears to lead to a decrease in affinity of GM-CSF for its receptor (Kaushansky *et al.*, 1987; Moonen *et al.*, 1987).

The crystal structure of human GM-CSF has been determined (Diederichs *et al.*, 1991) and, in common with a number of other haemopoietic growth factors (Brandhuber *et al.*, 1987; Bazan, 1990a, 1992; Parry *et al.*, 1991; Powers *et al.*, 1992), comprises two pairs of anti-parallel α-helices (see Table 2). The pattern of disulphide bonding has

Table 3. Cell types capable of expressing GM-CSF.

Cell type	Inductive-stimuli
T lymphocytes	Antigen, lectins, IL-2
B lymphocytes	Antigen, LPS, IL-1
Macrophages	LPS, phagocytosis, adherence
Mesothelial cells	
Keratinocytes	
Osteoblasts	Parathyroid hormone, LPS
Uterine epithelial cells	
Synoviocytes	Rheumatoid arthritis
Mast cells	IgE
Fibroblasts	IL-1, TNF-α, NaF, retroviruses
Various solid tumours	
Stromal cells	Mitogens, TNF-α, IL-1
Endothelial cells	IL-1, TNF-α, LPS, oxidized lipoproteins

been determined, with the first and third, and second and fourth residues, respectively, being paired (Schrimsher *et al.*, 1987). The residues on the GM-CSF molecule involved in binding to its cellular receptor are located in four general regions of the molecule: residues 18–22, 34–41, 52–61, and 94–115 (Gough *et al.*, 1987; Clark *et al.*, 1988; Kaushansky *et al.*, 1989; Shanafelt and Kastelein, 1989; LaBranche *et al.*, 1990; Shanafelt *et al.*, 1991a,b). Residues responsible for interaction with the β chain of the receptor to form a high-affinity complex (see below) are located within the first α helix (residues 18–22). In particular, glutamine residue 21 has been implicated as playing an important role in interacting with the β chain: mutation of Gln-21 to an Arg residue gives rise to a mutant in which low-affinity binding to the α chain is unimpaired, but which has essentially lost any ability to interact with the β chain and form a high-affinity complex (Lopez *et al.*, 1992).

EXPRESSION OF GM-CSF

GM-CSF can be produced by a number of different cell types under different circumstances (Metcalf, 1984). Injection of mice with bacterial endotoxin results in a rapid release of GM-CSF into the serum, probably from macrophages and/or endothelial cells. Almost all tissues and organs derived from endotoxin-primed mice which are then cultured *in vitro* release GM-CSF into the culture medium (Nicola *et al.*, 1979). Indeed, the source from which murine GM-CSF was first purified was medium conditioned by lungs from endotoxin-primed mice (Sparrow *et al.*, 1985). Production from organ cultures is continuous over several days and appears to reflect *de novo* synthesis rather than release of preformed protein, since production can be inhibited by protein synthesis inhibitors (Nicola *et al.*, 1979). Studies with purified primary cell cultures and cell lines have identified a number of cell types with the capacity to synthesize GM-CSF, including T lymphocytes, macrophages, endothelial cells, stromal cells, fibroblasts and others (see Table 3). In many cases, GM-CSF production requires stimulation of the producer cell, for example by other cytokines, antigens or inflammatory agents. Potential GM-CSF-producing cells are thus widely dispersed throughout the body and in locations likely to make early contact with products of invading microorganisms. In particular, the location of endothelial cells not only predisposes them to a role in local inflammatory reactions, but also to a role in acute systemic reactions. Thus, the very rapid increase in GM-CSF and other cytokine levels in the serum after intravenous injection of lipopolysaccharide (LPS) may occur through stimulation of a large number of endothelial cells, which would potentially lead to a generalized increase in the number of mature granulocytes and macrophages.

Of the several cell types known to produce GM-CSF, T lymphocytes are perhaps the best studied, due largely to the availability of cloned cell lines (Kelso and Gough, 1987). T lymphocytes can be induced to express a large number of different haemopoietic regulators, including GM-CSF, Multi-CSF (IL-3), IL-2, IL-4, IL-5 and IFN-γ (Kelso et al., 1991). These molecules have diverse, and in some cases opposing, effects within the haemopoietic and lymphoid systems and there has been considerable interest in the possibility that T cells might be subdivided on the basis of profiles of lymphokine production. Many long-term CD4$^+$ T-cell clones could be classified into two subsets on the basis of lymphokine profiles: T_{H1} clones secrete IFN-γ, IL-2, TNF-β, IL-3 and GM-CSF, whereas T_{H2} clones secrete IL-4, IL-5, IL-6, IL-3 and GM-CSF (Mosmann et al., 1986; Bottomly, 1988; Janeway et al., 1988). However, it appears that these two classes do not represent two absolute and mutually exclusive states and that normal T cells are not precommitted to express a restricted lymphokine profile (Kelso and Gough, 1988; Kelso et al., 1991). The major pathway for the activation of GM-CSF synthesis in T cells is induced by ligands of the T-cell antigen receptor, such as lectins, monoclonal antibodies and antigen (for reviews see Imboden et al., 1985). Other stimuli that can induce GM-CSF production in T cells have also been noted, and include IL-1 and the T-cell growth factor, IL-2 (Kelso and Gough, 1987, 1989).

Macrophage populations can also be induced to produce GM-CSF, in conjunction with a different, but overlapping range of cytokines to those coexpressed with GM-CSF in T cells, including G-CSF, TNF-α and IL-1 (Rich, 1986; Thorens et al., 1987; Fibbe et al., 1988). Among the most common signals to induce cytokine production by macrophages is the bacterial cell-wall product LPS (Hamilton and Adams, 1987; Tannenbaum et al., 1988), which, like ligands of the T-cell antigen receptor, appears to generate inositol trisphosphate and diacyl glycerol as second messengers (Prpic et al., 1987). Using short-term cultures of peritoneal exudate cells, substantially enriched for macrophages, a number of different stimuli were demonstrated to induce GM-CSF secretion, including LPS, phagocytosis and adherence (Thorens et al., 1987). Similarly, using longer-term cultures of bone-marrow-derived macrophages (devoid of T lymphocytes, in contrast to the former populations) GM-CSF production by macrophages has also been documented (Rich, 1986).

Endothelial cells are involved in a number of inflammatory reactions, and it has been noted for some time that various factors that act on the growth and differentiation of haemopoietic progenitor cells are produced by stimulated endothelial cells. More recently it has been shown that TNF-α and IL-1, which are released by activated macrophages, induce various phenotypic changes in cultured endothelial cells, including increased adhesiveness for leukocytes (Bevilacqua et al., 1985; Gamble et al., 1985). It is now clear that IL-1, TNF-α, LPS, and oxidized lipoproteins, can induce the expression of not only GM-CSF, but also G-CSF and M-CSF in cultured endothelial cells. Interestingly, TNF-α stimulates production of IL-1 by endothelial cells (Seelentag *et al.*, 1987); thus, autocrine stimulation of endothelial cells by IL-1 at the site of inflammation is a possibility. The stimulation by inflammatory mediators of endothelial cells to produce IL-1 and CSFs may constitute an important step in the inflammatory process. The CSFs could not only functionally activate mature white blood cells at an inflammatory site (and by inhibiting their migration, ensure their retention in the region of inflammation, but could also enhance proliferation and differentiation of progenitor cells. Thus, an initial release of IL-1 and TNF-α from macrophages stimulated by an inflammatory stimulus could mediate an amplification of the local inflammatory response.

Fibroblasts can also be induced to produce GM-CSF by a variety of agents: including TNF-α, IL-1, inflammatory agents and retroviruses. As such, fibroblasts may also contribute to the development of a local inflammatory focus or, in the case of bone-marrow stromal fibroblasts, may also play a role in controlling development of granulocyte-macrophage progenitors.

Although increased transcription of the GM-CSF gene is evident after inductive stimulation of most producer-cell types (Chan *et al.*, 1986; Seelentag *et al.*, 1987; Koeffler *et al.*, 1988; James and Kazenwadel, 1989; Kaushansky, 1989; Brorson *et al.*, 1991), quantitatively the more important mechanism may be post-transcriptional stabilization of the mRNA (Thorens *et al.*, 1987; Ernst *et al.*, 1989; Kaushansky, 1989; Bickel *et al.*, 1990; Akahane *et al.*, 1991; Hahn *et al.*, 1991). Many mRNAs which display short cytoplasmic half-lives, and encode a number of different cytokines and transcription factors, have a 5'-AUUUA-3' motif repeated a variable number of times, generally in the 3' untranslated region (Shaw and Kamen, 1986). The GM-CSF mRNA contains eight tandem copies of this motif, and it appears that this motif mediates, or plays a role in mediating, the instability and degradation of the corresponding mRNA (Shaw and Kamen, 1986). Intriguingly, these sequences and/or sequences closely linked to them in the GM-CSF mRNA, also seem likely to mediate the transient stabilization of the GM-CSF mRNA after cellular stimulation (Akashi *et al.*, 1991; Iwai *et al.*, 1991).

A number of sequences in and around the GM-CSF gene have been implicated as playing a role in its transcription. A family of closely related decanucleotides located 100–300 bp upstream of the transcriptional initiation sites of various cytokine genes, including GM-CSF, have been noted (Kelso and Gough, 1987). These and other sequence elements close to the GM-CSF promoter have been implicated in controlling GM-CSF transcription by the demonstration that their removal or mutation ablates GM-CSF promoter activity (Chan *et al.*, 1986; Miyatake *et al.*, 1988; Nimer *et al.*, 1988, 1990; Nishida *et al.*, 1991). Moreover, specific nuclear proteins have been identified which bind to, or in the vicinity of, these motifs (Schreck and Baeuerle, 1990; Shannon *et al.*, 1990; Sugimoto *et al.*, 1990; Kuczek *et al.*, 1991; Miyatake *et al.*, 1991; Tsuboi *et al.*, 1991). While some of these candidate transcription factors are expressed widely, others display a narrow cellular specificity and, in certain instances, are present only after stimulation of the producer cell. The GM-CSF gene may also be activated by the HTLV-1 viral transcription factor, Tax. Expression of GM-CSF by HTLV-1-infected lymphocytes may be important in the granulocytosis and eosinophilia frequently seen in patients with HTLV-1-induced T-cell leukaemia (Nimer *et al.*, 1989).

Interestingly, a strongly inducible hypersensitive site, whose appearance is inhibited by cyclosporin A (which inhibits GM-CSF and IL-3 expression) is located between the

GM-CSF and IL-3 genes, and has been hypothesized to contain sequences that act as enhancers of both of these closely linked genes (Cockerill *et al.*, 1993).

THE GM-CSF RECEPTOR

Molecular cloning studies have revealed that the GM-CSF receptor is composed of two distinct chains: a primary binding chain (the α chain) which binds GM-CSF with low affinity (K_d = 1–10 nM) and displays rapid dissociation kinetics (Gearing *et al.*, 1989; Park *et al.*, 1992) and a second chain (the β chain (Gorman *et al.*, 1990; Hayashida *et al.*, 1990)) which, despite having no measurable intrinsic binding affinity for GM-CSF alone, is able to interact with and convert the GM-CSF/α-chain complex to a high-affinity state (K_d = 30–100 pMolar) displaying slow dissociation kinetics (Chiba *et al.*, 1990; Hayashida *et al.*, 1990; Park *et al.*, 1992).

While the α chain of the GM-CSF receptor appears to display absolute binding specificity for GM-CSF, the β chain is also a component of the IL-3 and IL-5 receptors (Takaki *et al.*, 1991; Hara and Miyajima, 1992): thus, in each case, the ligand binds with low affinity to an α chain, which has absolute specificity for that particular ligand, and the dimeric complex is then able to interact with, and compete for binding to, the affinity-converting β subunit. Since there is some evidence that the β chain is responsible for cellular signalling, this arrangement may explain some of the shared biological activities of these cytokines. Similarly, this model may also explain the apparent partial crossreactivity for receptor binding displayed by these cytokines (Walker and Burgess, 1985; Nicola, 1987; Lopez *et al.*, 1989). Although the presence of the β chain (as well as the α chain) appears to be required for cellular signalling, signalling *per se* does not apparently require the formation of a high-affinity complex. That is, ligand does not necessarily associate with the β chain to form a high-affinity complex. Rather, the implication is that a direct α–β interaction occurs to precipitate signalling (Metcalf *et al.*, 1990; Lopez *et al.*, 1992; Shanafelt and Kastelein, 1992).

Both components of the GM-CSF receptor are related in structure and are members of the recently defined haemopoietin or cytokine receptor family (Gearing *et al.*, 1989; Bazan, 1990a,b). They each contain a conserved *c*.200 amino acid extracellular domain, the so-called haemopoietin domain, shared with a number of other cytokine receptors, including receptors for growth hormone, prolactin, G-CSF, erythropoietin, IL-2 (β- and γ-chains), IL-3 (α-chain), IL-4, IL-5 (α chain), IL-6 (α chain), LIF (α chain), gp130, CNTF, IL-7, and IL-9. This structural domain is characterized by a number of conserved amino acid residues, including four cysteine residues, which form two internal disulphide loops, a Pro-Pro pair which divides the domain into two subdomains, each of which appears to adopt a seven-stranded β-barrel structure, and the largely conserved sequence Trp–Ser–X–Trp–Ser. Genes encoding a number of haemopoietin receptors appear to give rise to a variety of alternately spliced transcripts, and the GMR-α gene is no exception: two groups have identified an GMR-α mRNA isoform which lacks 97 nucleotides of sequence encompassing the transmembrane region (Crosier *et al.*, 1991). The consequence of this deletion is to remove the transmembrane domain and to introduce a frame-shift and hence a different *C*-terminus to the encoded GM-CSF receptor. Despite the lack of transmembrane region, this mutant appears capable of transducing a proliferative signal in murine FDC-P1 cells, perhaps as a result of interaction with the cell-surface β chain in such cells.

Table 4. Localization of genes for GM-CSF and its receptor chains.

	Mouse	Human
GM-CSF	11A5–B1	5q23–31
GM-CSF Rα	19D2	X/Y PAR
GM-CSF Rβ	15	22q12.3–13.1

SIGNAL TRANSDUCTION

Although many authors currently consider a 'kinase cascade' as a major link between cytokine stimulation and cell response, to date, little is known about the postreceptor signal transduction pathways modulated by GM-CSF (Roberts, 1992). In general, tyrosine phosphorylation of proteins by tryosine kinases (PTKs) have been increasingly implicated as intermediates in the regulation of proliferation, differentiation and leukaemogenesis (Punt, 1992). However, like other members of the haemopoietin receptor superfamily, the GM-CSFR has neither a tyrosine kinase catalytic domain nor any known signalling sequences. In differentiated, but not undifferentiated, WEHI-3B cells, GM-CSF treatment leads to a rapid, transient and concentration-dependent phosphorylation of tyrosine on a number of endogenous proteins (Hallek et al., 1992). Known intermediates phosphorylated and activated consequent to the presence of GM-CSF include pp100 (Quelle et al., 1992), pim-1 kinase (Lilly et al., 1992), Raf-1 kinase (Hallek et al., 1992), p92c-fes kinase and the p42 mitogen-activated (or microtubule-associated) protein serine–threonine kinase family (MAPK) (Gomez et al., 1992; Raines et al., 1992). MAPK appears to transduce a common signalling event elicited by GM-CSF, IL-3, IL-5 and Steel factor (Okuda et al., 1992), but not IL-4 (Welham et al., 1992).

Other molecules implicated in the signal transduction pathway of GM-CSF include priming of neutrophils, possibly by G-protein (Bourgoin et al., 1992) and/or protein kinase Cε (Li et al., 1992) activation of phospholipase D; ras p21 (Satoh et al., 1991); and, inositol lipid metabolism (Nishimura et al., 1992). More controversial is possible involvement of the Na^+/H^+ antiport and Ca^{++}.

GENETICS OF GM-CSF AND ITS RECEPTOR

The GM-CSF gene comprises four exons spread over approximately 2.5 kbp of DNA (Miyatake et al., 1985; Stanley et al., 1985). It is located on murine chromosome 11, at band A5 to B1 (Gough et al., 1984; Barlow et al., 1987; Buchberg et al., 1988; Lee and Young, 1989; Wilson et al., 1990) and on the long arm of human chromosome 5, at 5q23-31 (Huebner et al., 1985, 1990; Le Beau et al., 1986b; van Leeuwen et al., 1989; Frolova et al., 1991) (see Table 4). The most interesting feature to its genetic localization is its close proximity to the gene for Multi-CSF (IL-3): the Multi-CSF gene is located approximately 10 kbp 5′ of the GM-CSF gene in the human genome (Yang et al., 1988; Frolova et al., 1991) and approximately 15 kbp 5′ in the murine genome (Lee and Young, 1989). The reason for such tight and conserved linkage is unclear. Although the two proteins display similar secondary and tertiary structures, in common with a large number of cytokines that interact with receptors of the same family, they display no overt primary sequence homology, suggesting that either the two genes are not the products of divergent evolution from a common ancestral gene or that they are products of quite an ancient duplication event. Either way there is no particular reason to expect tight linkage of the two genes to be conserved in the absence of selective pressure to maintain such linkage. One level at which selective pressure might be exerted is at the control of expression of the two genes: the tight linkage may in some way facilitate or modulate their coexpression in activated T lymphocytes (Gough and Kelso, 1989).

The suggested order of the GM-CSF/IL-3 gene pair on human chromosome 5, based on analysis of the arrangement of the gene pair on a 5q$^-$ chromosome in the HL60 human myeloid leukaemia cell line, is centromere → 5' IL-3 → 5' GM-CSF → qter (Huebner et al., 1990; Nagarajan et al., 1990). However, this assumes that no inversions occurred in the generation of the HL60 5q$^-$ chromosome. If any inversion had occurred during the generation of the 5q$^-$ chromosome, the suggested gene order would be incorrect.

The human GM-CSF gene is located within a region of chromosome 5, which is frequently deleted in certain refractory anaemias (the so-called 5q$^-$ syndrome) and some secondary acute myeloid leukaemias arising after chemo- and radiotherapy (Huebner et al., 1985, 1990; Van den Berghe et al., 1985; Le Beau et al., 1986a,b). In most cases the deletion is interstitial, with the proximal breakpoint between 5q11 and 21 and the distal breakpoint between 5q22 and 34. A survey of a large number of cases of the 5q$^-$ anomaly indicates that although the extent of the deletion is variable, there is a common region involved in all deletions, at or about 5q22–23. The close linkage of various haemopoietic regulator genes to this region of chromosome 5 has raised the suggestion that deletion of the gene(s), for various of these regulators, may be a contributing factor in the genesis of these leukaemias. However, it is hard to see how deletion of one allele of a CSF gene could contribute to neoplasia. Further, although lying close to the minimal critical region common to all 5q$^-$ chromosomes, the CSF gene cluster may not actually lie within it. It is more likely that the relevant gene on 5q is a recessive oncogene linked to, but not identical with, the CSF genes. Indeed, the IFN regulatory factor-1 gene (IRF-1), a gene whose product is a transcriptional activator which manifests anti-oncogenic capacity, has been mapped to 5q31.1, centromeric to GM-CSF and IL-3. Moreover IRF-1 appears to be consistently deleted in all cases of leukaemia and myelodysplasia with aberrations of 5q31 and, in at least one case of acute leukaemia examined, has undergone homozygous inactivation (Willman et al., 1993). In light of the observation that subtle changes in the levels of the IRF-1 transcriptional factor perturb cell growth control (Harada et al., 1993), loss of a single IRF-1 allele may well have profound biological significance, analogous to the loss of other tumour-suppressor genes, such as the MCC gene at 5q21 (Kinzler et al., 1991), the Rb-1 and p53 genes.

In the human genome, the common β-subunit of the GM-CSF, Multi-CSF and IL-5 receptors appears to be encoded by a unique gene, located at 22q12–q13 (Shen et al., 1992). This gene is in the vicinity of the t(1;22)(p13;q13) translocation which occurs frequently and specifically in acute megakaryocytic leukaemia (FAB subtype M7) (Lion et al., 1992), although the relationship, if any, of the GMR-β gene to this translocation has not been determined. In contrast, the murine genome has two closely related genes, Aic2a and Aic2b, which are homologous to the β subunit (see above). These two genes are closely linked to each other (within 250 kbp) in a region of murine chromosome 15 around the *sis* gene, which is known to be syntenic with the q12–13 region of human chromosome 22 (Gorman *et al.*, 1992).

The gene encoding the α chain of the human GM-CSF receptor (CSF2RA) is located in the pseudo-autosomal region (PAR) (Gough *et al.*, 1990), a region of approximately 2.6 Mbp of homologous sequence localized at the tip of the human sex chromosomes which recombines during male meiosis. The CSF2RA gene has been localized to the middle of the PAR, approximately 1200 kbp from the telomere (Rappold *et al.*, 1992). There is a very high frequency of recombination within the PAR and this region is rich in hypervariable repeat sequences and, as a consequence, the CSF2RA gene is highly polymorphic. At the time of its localization, the CSF2RA gene was the first gene of known function to be located within the PAR (one other gene, *MIC2* located close to the boundary of the PAR encodes a cell-surface antigen of unknown function). Since then however, the ANT3 ADP/ATP translocase has been located near to CSF2RA (Slim *et al.*, 1993) and more intriguingly, so has the IL-3 receptor α chain gene (IL3RA) (Kremer *et al.*, 1993). It appears that the gene order of these loci is pter → CSF2RA → IL3RA → ANT3 → cent. The distance between the CSF2RA and IL3RA genes is at most 100 kbp (G. Goodall, personal communication) but the precise distance, and relative orientation of the two genes has yet to be determined. This is particularly intriguing in view of the close physical proximity of the genes encoding the ligands for these two receptors in both the murine and human genomes. The significance of this linkage is, at this point, unclear since in the murine genomes the two corresponding genes are unlinked, and thus the observed linkage of these two genes in the human genome most likely reflects an ancient duplication event in the evolution of these related genes. A similar situation has recently been noted for two genes encoding receptors of the related type II cytokine receptor family, IFNAR and CRF-4 (Lutfalla *et al.*, 1993). In the murine genome the GMR-α chain gene (*Csf2ra*) is autosomal, being located at the distal end of chromosome 19 (Disteche *et al.*, 1992). It has been suggested that repeated sequences at the subtelomeric ends of the sex chromosomes and chromosome 19 may have been responsible for facilitating the rearrangement of the CSF2RA/*Csf2ra* locus (Disteche *et al.*, 1992). By contrast, the *113ra* gene is located at the proximal end of chromosome 14 (Rakar, Gough and Goodall, submitted for publication).

IN VITRO BIOLOGICAL ACTIONS OF GM-CSF

The major actions of GM-CSF involve the regulation of survival, differentiation, proliferative and functional activities in granulocyte-macrophage populations (Metcalf, 1988). However, at least four other glycoproteins are capable of stimulating granulocyte-macrophage progenitors (IL-3, M-CSF, G-CSF and IL-6) and so inherent in the system is a marked apparent subtlety, if not redundancy, owing to numerous combinatorial possibilities.

Survival

Withdrawal of GM-CSF from purified haemopoietic progenitor cells *in vitro*, or from GM-CSF-dependent cell lines, leads to their loss of viability, with a half life from 9 to 24 h (Metcalf and Merchav, 1982; Nicola and Metcalf, 1982). However, if GM-CSF is present then the cells survive and proliferate with extended life spans. Nevertheless, despite the presence of GM-CSF, these differentiated cells eventually die (Begley *et al.*, 1986). Viability of both mature and progenitor cells is maintained *in vitro* by as little as one-hundredth the concentration required to stimulate cell proliferation, implying the priority of survival (Burgess, 1982).

Given their short half-life of several hours, prolonging the survival of myeloid effector cells, for example granulocytes (Colotta *et al.*, 1992), eosinophils (Begley *et al.*, 1986) and basophils (Yamaguchi *et al.*, 1992), may be very important in the facilitation of host inflammatory responses. While the mechanisms by which cytokines prolong survival in haemopoietic cells are far from clear, clues are emerging regarding the means by which GM-CSF protects against apoptotic cell death. Apoptosis, or pro-grammed cell death, is characterized by morphologic changes and oligonucleosomic DNA fragmentation. GM-CSF-treatment of the 7-M12 leukaemic-cell line was able to protect against both TGF-β_1 and chemotherapy-induced apoptosis (Lotem and Sachs, 1992). However, another cell line (M1) was not protected from apoptotic cell death and pIXY321 (a GM-CSF–IL-3 fusion protein) augmented the high dose Ara-C-induced death of human myeloid leukaemic cells (Bhalla *et al.*, 1992). Further, the sequential activation of protein kinase C and the Na^+/H^+ antiport has been implicated in the signal transduction pathway which prevents apoptotic cell death induced by factor withdrawal (Rajotte *et al.*, 1992).

Proliferation

GM-CSF stimulates the formation of a range of myeloid colony types in semi-solid cultures *in vitro* in a dose-dependent manner (Metcalf *et al.*, 1986a). Native and recombinant GM-CSF molecules are both effective stimuli for murine granulocyte (CFU-G) and macrophage (CFU-M) and granulocyte-macrophage (CFU-GM) colony formation at low concentrations of 2–80 pg/ml (Koike *et al.*, 1987). Eosinophil colony formation (CFU-Eo) in semi-solid medium occurs at concentrations of GM-CSF above 80 pg/ml, whereas up to 10-fold greater concentrations are required to stimulate megakaryocyte (CFU-Meg), erythroid (BFU-E) and mixed progenitor colony forma-tion (CFU-GEMM) (Robinson *et al.*, 1987). More recently recognized is the ability of GM-CSF to induce the differentiation of typical dendritic cells in both murine and human systems (as discussed in the following section).

The considerable heterogeneity in the ability of individual progenitor cells to form colonies in semi-solid medium (clonogenicity) in the presence of GM-CSF is demon-strated readily by the sigmoid-shaped dose-response curve (when CSF concentration is plotted on a log scale versus number of colonies developing on a linear scale) (Metcalf, 1987). Although this response may be predicted by a progressive saturation of cell-surface receptors, not only clonogenicity, but the extent and rate of cell division, total number of progeny and entry into cell cycle are all dependent on GM-CSF concen-trations between 1 pM and 100 pM (Metcalf, 1980). The proliferation kinetics may be further complicated by the upregulation of GM-CSFR in the presence of low, but not high, concentrations of rmGM-CSF and rmIL-3 (Fan *et al.*, 1992). By comparison, human bone-marrow cultures reveal a less-marked correlation between GM-CSF concentrations and progenitor cell colony formation for granulocytes, macrophages and eosinophils (Metcalf *et al.*, 1986b), megakaryocytes (Mazur *et al.*, 1987) and erythroid precursors (Migliaccio *et al.*, 1987).

In addition to effects on normal cells, a number of immortalized, growth-factor-dependent cell lines proliferate with minimal differentiation in response to GM-CSF (or often IL-3). The ready availability of such lines has greatly facilitated the study of myeloid cell physiology and transformation. These include the following myeloid lines: FDC-P1, derived from long-term murine bone-marrow culture (Dexter *et al.*, 1980); BAC1, derived from SV40 transformed macrophages (Morgan *et al.*, 1987); and DA1 and NFS-60, derived from leukaemic mice (Hara *et al.*, 1988). T-lymphocyte lines have also been shown to proliferate in the presence of GM-CSF including TALL101, derived from a human leukaemia (Valtieri *et al.*, 1987), and the murine IL-2-dependent HT2 line (Kupper *et al.*, 1987).

The apparent direct proliferative effects of GM-CSF *in vitro* may be less relevant to its *in vivo* actions where combinations of cytokines may lead to a number of additive and synergistic enhancing or even suppressing effects. Moderate superadditive effects on GM-CFCs have been demonstrated when various cytokines have been combined with GM-CSF in several systems (Metcalf, 1984). For example, together with GM-CSF, IL-3 or G-CSF in murine bone marrow (McNeice *et al.*, 1988; Metcalf *et al.*, 1992b) and human progenitor cell cultures (Bot *et al.*, 1990) enhanced GM-CFC formation. Moreover, additive effects of GM-CSF and IL-3 were evident in the stimulation of maximal erythroid, eosinophil and megakaryocyte colony formation (Mazur *et al.*, 1987). SCF dramatically stimulated myeloid and erythroid colony number and size in human bone-marrow culture when combined with GM-CSF, by its direct effect on marrow progenitor cells (McNiece *et al.*, 1991).

In contrast, while GM-CSF plus M-CSF in both murine (Williams *et al.*, 1987) and human (Caracciolo *et al.*, 1987) bone marrow leads to an increase in colony formation, some macrophage colonies are suppressed (Gliniak and Rohrschneider, 1990) owing to loss of clonogenicity and incremental monocyte-macrophage differentiation (Metcalf *et al.*, 1992b). How this phenomenon of synergistic suppression occurs is not resolved, although GM-CSF-induced 'transregulation' of the M-CSFR through induction of a ribonuclease likely contributes (Gliniak *et al.*, 1992). Whatever the mechanism, the existence of suppressive combinations of cytokines *in vitro* demands that the clinical use of 'cocktails' should be tempered with some caution.

Differentiation and Function

Although it may appear somewhat artificial to separate GM-CSF-induced proliferation from differentiation, in that they are typically thought of as coupled, evidence from several sources suggests that they should be studied individually. Certainly GM-CSF is sufficient to generate mature subpopulations of granulocytes, macrophages, eosinophils, megakaryocytes and dendritic cells *in vitro*, as detailed in the previous section. However, the very fact that the various lineages are induced by diverse GM-CSF concentrations suggests heterogeneity in responsiveness of the committed progenitor population. Commitment to differentiation should suggest intrinsic conflict with the processes of proliferation and implied self-renewal (clonal extinction). For example, despite GM-CSF induction of erythroid precursors (BFU-E), complete erythroid differentiation, and consequent loss of clonogenicity, requires the addition of erythropoietin (Erickson and Quesenberry, 1992); other factors may also contribute to the terminal differentiation of eosinophils and megakaryocytes.

Evidence of GM-CSF-concentration-dependent differentiation was provided by paired daughter-cell experiments, each daughter being derived from a single progenitor cell. A high GM-CSF concentration leads to neutrophil lineage commitment whereas a low concentration leads to monocyte commitment (Metcalf, 1980). In similar paired daughter-cell studies in which the initial stimulus of either GM-CSF or M-CSF was then swapped to the other stimulus, GM-CSF was able to irreversibly commit progenitor cells to differentiate toward mature granulocytes (Metcalf and Burgess, 1982). However, precommitment of some daughter cells was still apparent, and selective expansion of such cells could not be ruled out.

Another model system of GM-CSF-induced differentiation is the outgrowth of dendritic, and specifically skin Langerhans cells, from the nonadherent class Ia-negative fraction of murine peripheral blood (Inabe et al., 1992), human CD34[+] progenitor cells (Caux et al., 1992) and lymphocyte-depleted human tonsils (Clark et al., 1992). TNF-α enhances this GM-CSF effect by 10–20-fold (Reid et al., 1992). GM-CSF induces up to 2% of MHC Class II-negative murine bone-marrow precursors to produce typical dendritic cells in mixed colonies in semi-solid medium (Inaba et al., 1993). Hence, GM-CSF is able to induce distinct granulocyte, macrophage and dendritic pathways of development from a common progenitor.

Functional synergy has been demonstrated, for example, in the enhanced complement-dependent phagocytosis of the fungal pathogen, *Cryptococcus neoformans*, seen when GM-CSF and TNF-α were combined (Collins and Bancroft, 1992), and in the GM-CSF-induced potentiation of IL-8 priming of neutrophils (Yuo et al., 1991).

Several cell lines which terminally differentiate in the presence of GM-CSF provide perhaps the most compelling evidence of growth factor-induced lineage commitment. Macrophage commitment and suppression of proliferation was demonstrated in the murine myeloid leukaemia lines, WEHI-3B D[+] (Metcalf, 1979) and a subclone of M1 (Lotem and Sachs, 1988). Similarly, GM-CSF stimulation of HL60, a human promyelocytic cell line, results in initial proliferation and subsequent differentiation with suppression of clonogenicity (Begley et al., 1987b). Of particular interest is UT-7, a recently described factor-dependent pluripotent cell line derived from a human megakaryoblastic leukaemia. UT-7 exhibits erythroid or myeloid lineage commitment in hierarchical response to erythropoietin or GM-CSF at least in part due to 'transmodulation' of cytokine receptors (Hermine et al., 1992).

IN VIVO BIOLOGICAL ACTIONS OF GM-CSF

The *in vivo* effects of native or recombinant purified GM-CSF have been tested by several approaches: administration by various routes in healthy and compromised animal models, particularly mice and primates; haemopoietic reconstitution of mice by cells containing a retrovirally-expressed GM-CSF gene; constitutive expression of GM-CSF in transgenic mice; and human clinical trials. The latter will be discussed in the section entitled Clinical Applications of GM-CSF. As will be seen by much of the evidence cited here, GM-CSF is capable of playing a central role in effecting the rapid cellular responses seen in inflammation (inducible haemopoiesis). Whether GM-CSF acts as a homeostatic regulator under normal conditions (constitutive haemopoiesis) is less clear.

Animal Models

Three normal adult mice strains tested with bacterially synthesized rGM-CSF injected intraperitoneally showed only a twofold rise in peripheral neutrophil counts, as well as a several-fold increase in lung alveolar-sac-wall neutrophils and a 50% rise in spleen weight (Metcalf *et al.*, 1987). This occurred despite the dose of 200 ng being administered three times daily for six days prior to analysis. However, the local peritoneal response was much more impressive, with a dose-related elevation in macrophages (up to 15-fold), neutrophils and eosinophils (up to 100 fold). Whether GM-CSF was administered locally or by the subcutaneous route, peritoneal macrophages exhibited increased phagocytic and mitotic activity (Morrissey *et al.*, 1988). While bone marrow levels of neutrophils and monocytes remained constant, a dose-related fall in total cellularity of 40% and nonerythroid precursors of up to 66% was noted (Metcalf *et al.*, 1987).

In nonhuman primates, the continuous intravenous or intermittent subcutaneous infusion of glycosylated or nonglycosylated human GM-CSF caused a greater than fivefold leukocytosis, typically within 24 h (Mayer *et al.*, 1987). The effect, manifested predominantly as a neutrophilia, eosinophilia, monocytosis, and unexpected lymphocytosis, could be sustained for as long as the infusion continued (1 month) and counts normalized on cessation without evidence of toxicity (Donahue *et al.*, 1986). Of considerable importance was the lack of any effect on platelet or erythrocyte concentrations, despite weeks of GM-CSF administration, particularly since critics had predicted possible 'marrow exhaustion' owing to stem cell over-stimulation toward the myeloid lineage. As had been expected from *in vitro* experiments, the neutrophils were not only numerically increased, but they also manifested enhanced phagocytic and bacterial-killing capacity (Mayer *et al.*, 1987).

Radio- and Chemoprotective Effects

When mice were infused or injected repeatedly with GM-CSF prior to sublethal doses of cytotoxic drugs or irradiation, restoration of haemopoiesis was accelerated (Neta *et al.*, 1988). However, GM-CSF had no radioprotective effect when administered as a single intraperitoneal dose 3 h following lethal irradiation (Neta and Oppenheim, 1988). Nevertheless, GM-CSF was able to synergize with suboptimal doses of rhIL-1α and rhTNF-α to provide optimal radioprotection, perhaps indicating that the interaction of cytokines may be important in the haemopoietic recovery following radiation damage.

Extending the studies involving the direct radioprotective effects of cytokines in animals are murine models of allogeneic bone marrow transplantation using *ex vivo* donor graft incubation with cytokine combinations (Muench and Moore, 1992). Engraftment of T-cell-depleted donor marrow was effectively promoted by GM-CSF, although no effects were seen on post-transplantation mortality, marrow stem-cell capacity or the incidence of graft-versus-host disease (Blazar *et al.*, 1988). Similarly, in sublethally irradiated rhesus monkeys treated with a continuous infusion of rhGM-CSF following autologous bone-marrow transplantation, a sustained and accelerated recovery of neutrophils and platelets was observed (Monroy *et al.*, 1987; Nienhuis *et al.*,

1987). If the infusion was halted prior to recovery, neutrophil counts fell to untreated control values, which suggests that GM-CSF effects haemopoietic reconstitution by stimulating later progenitor cells in the graft, rather than progenitors capable of repopulation (Clark and Kamen, 1987).

Constitutive Over-expression of GM-CSF

One way of analysing the enhanced constitutive expression of GM-CSF has been to transplant lethally irradiated mice with haemopoietic cells expressing a GM-CSF gene introduced by retroviral infection *in vitro* (Johnson *et al.*, 1989). The transplanted animals attain very high circulating GM-CSF levels with a marked concomitant neutrophilia. Within a month after transplantation, the mice had succumbed to neutrophil and macrophage infiltration of spleen, lung, liver, peritoneal cavity, skeletal muscle and heart; the last two also contained increased numbers of eosinophils. Still, notwithstanding the considerable hyperplasia of responsive cells, neither the primary marrow recipients nor secondary recipients developed tumours. No increase in GM-CSFs was seen in bone marrow or spleen, again suggesting that the cytokine stimulation had occurred in later progenitor cells.

An alternate means of obtaining mice with constitutively high GM-CSF levels has been the creation of transgenic lines. Enforced expression was attained by the introduction of retrovirally promoted mGM-CSF into the germ-line of inbred mice (Lang *et al.*, 1987), leading to elevated GM-CSF bioactivity which was detectable in the serum, eye and peritoneal cavity of two separate founder lineages. Although peripheral blood and bone marrow progenitor cell counts were normal, marked accumulation of up to 100-fold were seen in pleural and peritoneal cavity macrophage numbers owing to increased local proliferation (Metcalf *et al.*, 1992a). These increased peritoneal macrophages in transgenic animals exhibited higher rates of phagocytosis and bacteriolysis when compared to macrophages from their normal littermates (Tran *et al.*, 1990). Elevations in macrophage numbers were also seen in the retina, resulting in eventual blindness, and striated muscle, leading to muscle weakness, progressive weight loss and premature death from 'wasting' (Lang *et al.*, 1987). Another feature of the GM-CSF transgenic mice was the occurrence of spontaneous intraperitoneal bleeding associated with increased local urokinase-type plasminogen activator activity (Elliott *et al.*, 1992).

The phenotype seen in both the transgenic and retrovirally over-expressed GM-CSF animals may not be due solely to GM-CSF itself. It is known that GM-CSF induces the *in vitro* production of TNF-α and IL-1α and IL-1β in monocytes (Cannistra *et al.*, 1987), and IL-1 in neutrophils (Lindemann *et al.*, 1988). Since the granulocytes and macrophages in the GM-CSF transgenic mice display GM-CSF receptors (Nicola, 1987), if they express GM-CSF then they may well be self-stimulating (autocrine). Hybridization histochemistry analysis of affected tissues in the GM-CSF transgenics and their normal littermates has demonstrated increased expression of TNF-α, IL-1α and IL-1β and bFGF in the former, produced directly or indirectly as a consequence of probable autocrine stimulation of granulocytes and macrophages by GM-CSF (Lang *et al.*, 1992). In summary, the common pathological effects of increased endogenous GM-CSF are primarily related to the functional activation of mature inflammatory effector cells, rather than haemopoietic progenitor cell derangement or leukaemic transformation.

Role of GM-CSF in the Pathogenesis of Leukaemia

The restraints imposed on normal myeloid cells are abrogated in leukaemic cells: in particular, the neoplastic clone escapes from the otherwise essential balance between self-renewal and differentiation. That is, any normally proliferating population of cells should not exceed 50% self-regenerative divisions if homeostasis is to be maintained. However, cells that have extremely high rates of self-regeneration (or conversely low rates of differentiation) may not necessarily be leukaemogenic—for example, the immortalized but nonleukaemogenic, factor-dependent myeloid cell lines FDC-P1 and 32D (Metcalf, 1989). The mechanisms by which neoplastic clones may achieve freedom from the above restraints have included models of autocrine growth factor production or abnormal responses to proliferative stimuli, since studies by Furth and collaborators in the 1950s. In its simplest form the autocrine hypothesis of leukaemogenesis requires the neoplastic clone to secrete a growth factor to which it may respond and thereby lead to a self-sustained proliferative loop (Sporn and Roberts, 1985).

A number of problems face the simple autocrine model, not the least of which is the fact that mice overproducing GM-CSF (see previous section Constitutive Over-expression of GM-CSF) are not ostensibly preleukaemic. Hence GM-CSF overproduc-tion is not sufficient for the development of leukaemia, but it could perhaps be a necessary step along the pathway to neoplasia. Support for this possibility comes from experiments in which immortalized, but nontransformed, FDC-P1 murine cells were infected with a retrovirus expressing GM-CSF. The cells were rendered not only factor-independent, but leukaemogenic in syngeneic recipients (Lang et al., 1985). Similarly, nine out of eleven factor-independent mutants of the IL-3 or GM-CSF-dependent D35 murine cell line have been shown to secrete either IL-3 or GM-CSF, the genes of which had been activated by retroviral insertion (Stocking et al., 1988). All of the factor-independent mutants were rendered leukaemogenic compared with the nonleukaemo-genic parent cell. In this way, then, GM-CSF behaves as a transforming gene (proto-oncogene?) at the least facilitating leukaemogenesis.

The autocrine hypothesis also predicts that 'spontaneous' myeloid leukaemias be factor-independent. However, in vitro analysis of most human myeloid leukaemias at diagnosis reveals that they remain factor-dependent and responsive to a number of cytokines at typical concentrations (Begley et al., 1987a; Kelleher et al., 1987; Vellenga et al., 1987). Nevertheless, genuine cases of autocrine leukaemias have been docu-mented (Young and Griffin, 1986), a few with unusually large transcripts from rearranged GM-CSF loci (Cheng et al., 1988). In general, since most leukaemias remain factor-dependent, it is clear that GM-CSF and other cytokines are essential cofactors facilitating the in vivo expansion of the transformed myeloid clone into manifest leukaemia.

Perhaps the most intriguing model of leukaemic transformation comes from the analysis of tumorigenic mutants arising in vivo following the injection of non-tumorigenic, factor-dependent FDC-P1 cells. Transplantable leukaemia of donor karyotype developed in all irradiated syngeneic mice receiving intravenous FDC-P1 cells (Duhrsen, 1988; Duhrsen and Metcalf, 1988). The leukaemogenic variants exhibited a range of in vitro growth characteristics from absolute factor-dependency to autonomy; this was remarkably similar to the pattern seen in human leukaemia where, as described above, cells commonly remain factor-dependent (Moore et al., 1974b). A similar pattern of transformation is seen when FDC-P1 cells are injected into GM-CSF transgenic mice (Metcalf and Rasko, 1993). All GM-CSF transgenic recipients, but no normal littermates, developed transplantable leukaemias, many with rearranged GM-CSF or IL-3 loci possibly occurring as secondary events. Analysis of the mechanism(s) by which FDC-P1 cell transformation occurs may provide further insights into human leukaemogenesis.

Role of GM-CSF in Other Clinical Disorders

A number of studies using marrow bioassays have, in the past, attempted to correlate CSF levels in serum, urine or other body fluids with clinical disorders (see Table 2 in review by Morstyn and Burgess, 1988). In retrospect, it was not possible to clearly distinguish which of the four CSFs were being detected. To date, no definite GM-CSF deficiency state or syndrome of cell resistance/nonresponsiveness or hyper-responsiveness has been identified. Nevertheless, the following examples demand further investigation.

The congenital cytopenias have provided investigators with a number of hetero-geneous natural experiments in which to examine pathogenetic mechanisms involving CSFs (Moore, 1991). For example, cyclic neutropenia in humans is characterized by a fluctuation in peripheral blood cells and bone-marrow progenitor cells with a 21-day periodicity. Although serum or urine levels of CSFs have been shown to cycle in these patients (Moore et al., 1974a), current evidence suggests that the defect may lie in G-CSF or GM-CSF signal transduction. This conclusion is based on the reduced responsiveness of GM progenitor cells in these patients, despite normal G-CSF binding affinity, as well as the cure achieved by bone-marrow transplantation (Kyas et al., 1992). In severe congenital neutropenia of the Kostmann Syndrome, a G-CSF-related defect was suggested because serum levels were raised in all 10 patients examined, which implies a state of reduced responsiveness (Mempel et al., 1991).

In the myelodysplastic syndromes (MDS), patients often succumb to the conse-quences of cytopenias. In a recent study, 25% of MDS patients had elevated GM-CSF serum levels compared with normal controls (Zwierzina et al., 1992). In the same groups no abnormality was detected in serum IL-3 levels or in the expression of GM-CSF or IL-3 receptor levels. The suggested conclusion is that pathways down-stream of the receptor may be implicated in the pathogenesis of MDS-related cytope-nias. Conversely, in the chronic myeloproliferative syndrome polycythemia vera, haemopoietic progenitor cells have been shown to be hyper-responsive to IL-3 and GM-CSF—an effect unlikely to be mediated by enhanced binding (Dai et al., 1992). In patients with tumour-related thrombocytosis, a GM-CSF megakaryocyte colony stimu-lating activity was detected (Suzuki et al., 1992).

Abnormal cytokine levels may contribute to the pathogenesis of a number of other diseases of nonhaemopoietic organs. In the plasma and synovial fluid of patients with rheumatoid arthritis (and plasma of patients with systemic lupus erythematosus), GM-CSF concentrations were significantly raised compared with control specimens from patients with noninflammatory arthritis (Agro et al., 1992; Fiehn et al., 1992). Altered GM-CSF expression has been implicated in the development of the interstitial lung disease (Agostini et al., 1992) and impaired immunity (Re et al., 1992) seen in patients with AIDS, as well as contributing to the granulomata of pulmonary sarcoidosis

(Itoh, 1992). In bronchial epithelial cells and bronchoalveolar lavage fluid from patients with asthma, elevated GM-CSF and other cytokine levels may contribute to the persistence of inflammation (Marini *et al.*, 1992) by eosinophil priming (Warringa *et al.*, 1992).

CLINICAL APPLICATIONS OF GM-CSF

There are at least three major areas in which sargramostim (the generic drug name for rhGM-CSF) has been considered for clinical use: amelioration of acute and chronic states of neutropenia, including facilitation of bone marrow and peripheral blood stem-cell transplantation; adjunctive therapy with anti-microbials in nonneutropenic states; and anti-neoplastic effects via differentiation of the malignant phenotype, recruitment of leukaemic cells to enhance the efficacy of chemotherapy or enhancement of anti-tumour immunity. From early 1993 in the USA, rhGM-CSF has been approved only for use as a means of accelerating engraftment following autologous bone marrow transplantation (ABMT) in patients with lymphoid malignancies.

The pharmacokinetics and pharmacodynamics of rhGM-CSF have been studied using various measures of efficacy and toxicity. While dosing schedules will probably be optimized for each individual indication, current clinical protocols have favoured the subcutaneous route (at approximately 5 μg/kg.day as a single dose (Edmondson *et al.*, 1991)) above bolus or continuous intravenous injection, due to an improved therapeutic index (Cebon *et al.*, 1992). Using typical therapeutic doses, patients may experience flushing, fever, bone and muscle pain, tiredness and generalized, as well as local, skin eruptions (Lieschke *et al.*, 1989b; Mehregan *et al.*, 1992). In general, these side effects are well tolerated and may be treated symptomatically. Of greater concern is the 'first-dose' effect occurring within several hours of GM-CSF administration, the main features of which are hypoxaemia and hypotension (Lieschke *et al.*, 1989a).

The major relative contraindications for GM-CSF relate to possible exacerbation/ reactivation of chronic inflammatory or autoimmune diseases, such as rheumatoid arthritis (Hazenberg *et al.*, 1989), thyroiditis (Hoekman *et al.*, 1991), haemolytic anaemia (Logothetis *et al.*, 1990; Berney *et al.*, 1992), and idiopathic thrombocytopenic purpura (Lieschke *et al.*, 1989b).

Following each injection of GM-CSF, a rapid onset neutropenia, eosinophilopenia and monocytopenia lasting from 1 to 3 h occur (Devereux *et al.*, 1987). It is thought that margination of leucocytes owing to increased endothelial adherence in the lung (Hovgaard *et al.*, 1992; Yong *et al.*, 1992) and perhaps liver (Spolarics *et al.*, 1992) account for the drop in peripheral white cells. A minor thrombocytopenia associated with an increase in platelet volume has also been noted within days of GM-CSF therapy (Antman *et al.*, 1988). After the transient leukopenia, the peripheral concentration of neutrophils, eosinophils, monocytes and progenitor cells rises. A sixfold increase in the circulating half-life of neutrophils, allied with a 1.5 fold increase in neutrophil production rate, probably accounts for most of the neutrophilia (Lord *et al.*, 1992), although the leftward shift in peripheral neutrophils has possibly led to overestimates in the past.

The effects of GM-CSF administration on bone-marrow morphology include increases in cellularity owing to an expansion of the myeloid compartment as well as a shift toward more primitive myeloid cells. There is, however, no change in the content of progenitor cells in bone marrow. Biochemical effects include increases in amino-transferases, cobalamin, lactate dehydrogenase and alkaline phosphatase; and decreases in albumin and cholesterol (Nimer *et al.*, 1988a; Lieschke *et al.*, 1989b). Functional effects of GM-CSF include increases in stimulatable superoxide production in neutrophils (Sullivan *et al.*, 1989), possible impairment of neutrophil motility at sites of inflammation (Addison *et al.*, 1989), regulation of neutrophil anti-tumour activity by increased CD11/CD18 and FcRII expression (Kushner and Cheung, 1992) and increased monocyte cytotoxicity.

At least 12 heterogeneous congenital cytopenias act on the myeloid compartment (Table 2 in Moore, 1991). While G-CSF has been quite successful in ameliorating the neutropenias of patients with congenital, idiopathic chronic and cyclic neutropenia (Hammond *et al.*, 1989; Migliaccio *et al.*, 1990) for up to 2 years without evidence of stem-cell depletion, GM-CSF has generally been inferior. However, in aplastic anaemia (and possibly agranulocytosis or neutropenia associated with large granular lymphocyte proliferation) (Mulder *et al.*, 1992) preliminary results for patients receiving GM-CSF have been encouraging (Nissen *et al.*, 1988; Vadhan *et al.*, 1988a,b; Champlin *et al.*, 1989). Clear guidelines are not available and the results of well-controlled studies are awaited (Schuster *et al.*, 1990).

In attempting to ameliorate chemotherapy-induced myelotoxicity, GM-CSF has been tested as part of many different protocols in a variety of solid and haematological malignancies (reviewed by Demetri and Antman, 1992; Lieschke and Burgess, 1992). As mentioned above, to date, only in supporting recovery from ABMT for lymphoid neoplasms has GM-CSF been proven to offer a clinical benefit. The improvement is achieved by accelerating neutrophil recovery (Khwaja *et al.*, 1992), and by reducing hospital stay (Gorin *et al.*, 1992) and the number of bacterial infections (Nemunaitis *et al.*, 1991; Link *et al.*, 1992). Despite these cost-effective benefits (Gulati and Bennett, 1992), no improvement in survival has been demonstrated. Facilitation of dose intensification with (Table 4 in Lieschke and Burgess, 1992) or without (Neidhart *et al.*, 1992; Vadhan *et al.*, 1992) progenitor cell transplantation has not been an unqualified success either, insofar as profound neutropenia and consequent infections still occur.

Nevertheless, the use of GM-CSF to treat patients suffering from graft failure after bone marrow transplantation offers some hope in this often fatal situation (Nemunaitis *et al.*, 1990), and combinations of cytokines as well as *ex vivo* expansion of stem cells may improve efficacy. For example, GM-CSF (and/or G-CSF) administered to enrich for circulating haemopoietic progenitor cells (Siena *et al.*, 1989; Villeval *et al.*, 1990) which may then be harvested by leukapheresis (Gianni *et al.*, 1989) accelerates haemopoietic recovery (Elias *et al.*, 1992), even in paediatric populations (Takaue *et al.*, 1992). The *in vitro* preincubation of bone marrow cells with various CSFs for patients receiving allogeneic bone marrow transplants also promises to enhance haemopoietic recovery (Haylock *et al.*, 1992; Naparstek *et al.*, 1992) as well as possibly facilitate novel gene delivery systems (Hughes *et al.*, 1989; Bregni *et al.*, 1992).

By increasing sensitivity to cell-cycle-active drugs such as cytarabine, GM-CSF has also been considered for improving the efficacy of chemotherapeutic regimes (Bhalla *et al.*, 1988; Miyauchi *et al.*, 1989; Andreeff *et al.*, 1990). Although a significant amount of *in vitro* data support the kinetic rationale for using GM-CSF (Griffin *et al.*, 1986; Tafuri and Andreeff, 1990), or combined IL-3 and GM-CSF (Bhalla *et al.*, 1991, 1992;

Hiddemann *et al.*, 1992) in patients the results have been somewhat disappointing (Preisler *et al.*, 1992; Archimbaud *et al.*, 1993).

GM-CSF has been administered in a number of other disparate disease states. In AIDS, GM-CSF stimulated HIV replication in monocyte macrophages and increased p24 antigen levels (Perno *et al.*, 1992), whereas neutrophil function and the anti-viral effects of AZT were enhanced (Baldwin *et al.*, 1988; Pluda *et al.*, 1990). Haemopoietic failure owing to retroviral/antimicrobial therapy or AIDS itself has been treated with GM-CSF with favourable results (Groopman *et al.*, 1987).

Understandably, concern has been raised regarding the use of cytokines in the myelodysplastic syndromes and myeloid leukaemia, for fear of increasing further the malignant clone's growth advantage. In practice, progression towards, or exacerbation of, acute leukaemia has not been clearly evident, although most authors still advise caution (Buchner *et al.*, 1991; Ganzer *et al.*, 1992; Willemze *et al.*, 1992). In particular, increasingly abnormal karyotypes have been noted in some patients with myelodysplasia who received GM-CSF (Gradishar *et al.*, 1992; Verhoef *et al.*, 1992;).

Nonetheless, there are novel developments involving GM-CSF which may be of considerable clinical importance. In a B16 melanoma model in which 10 different molecules were assessed for their ability to enhance tumour immunogenicity, GM-CSF was the most potent stimulator of sustained, specific anti-tumour immunity (Dranoff *et al.*, 1993). Since the effect requires $CD4^+$ and $CD8^+$ cells, it is tempting to speculate on the mechanism which may involve localized enhancement of host tumour–antigen presenting cell activity as outlined in the section Differentiation and Function.

REFERENCES

Addison, I.E., Johnson, B., Devereux, S., Goldstone, A.H. and Linch, D.C. (1989). *Clin. Exp. Immunol.* **76**, 149–153.
Agostini, C., Trentin, L., Zambello, R., Bulian, P., Caenazzo, C., Cipriani, A., Cadrobbi, P., Garbisa, S. and Semenzato, G. (1992). *J. Immunol.* **149**, 3379–3385.
Agro, A., Jordana, M., Chan, K.H., Cox, G., Richards, C., Stepien, H. and Stanisz, A.M. (1992). *J. Rheumatol.* **19**, 1065–1069.
Akahane, K., Cohen, R.B., Bickel, M. and Pluznik, D.H. (1991). *J. Immunol.* **146**, 4190–4196.
Akashi, M., Shaw, G., Gross, M., Saito, M. and Koeffler, H.P. (1991). *Blood* **78**, 2005–2012.
Andreeff, M., Tafuri, A. and Hegewisch, B.S. (1990). *Hamatol. Bluttransfus.* **33**, 747–762.
Antman, K.S., Griffin, J.D., Elias, A., Socinski, M.A., Ryan, L., Cannistra, S.A., Oette, D., Whitley, M., Frei, E. and Schnipper, L.E. (1988). *N. Engl. J. Med.* **319**, 593–598.
Archimbaud, E., Fenaux, P., Reiffers, J., Cordonnier, C., Leblond, V., Travade, P., Troussard, X., Tilly, H., Auzanneau, G., Marie, J.-P., Ffrench, M. and Berger, E. (1993). *Leukemia* **7**, 372–377.
Baldwin, G.C., Gasson, J.C., Quan, S.G., Fleischmann, J., Weisbart, R., Oette, D., Mitsuyasu, R.T. and Golde, D.W. (1988). *Proc. Natl Acad. Sci. USA* **85**, 2763–2766.
Barlow, D.P., Bucan, M., Lehrach, H., Hogan, B.L. and Gough, N.M. (1987). *EMBO J.* **6**, 617–623.
Bazan, J.F. (1990a). *Immunol. Today* **11**, 350–354.
Bazan, J.F. (1990b). *Proc. Natl Acad. Sci. USA* **87**, 6934–6938.
Bazan, J.F. (1992). *Science* **257**, 410–413.
Begley, C.G., Lopez, A.F., Nicola, N.A., Warren, D.J., Vadas, M.A., Sanderson, C.J. and Metcalf, D. (1986). *Blood* **68**, 162–166.
Begley, C.G., Metcalf, D. and Nicola, N.A. (1987a). *Leukemia* **1**, 1–8.
Begley, C.G., Metcalf, D. and Nicola, N.A. (1987b). *Int. J. Cancer* **39**, 99–105.
Berney, T., Shibata, T., Merino, R., Chicheportiche, Y., Kindler, V., Vassalli, P. and Izui, S. (1992). *Blood* **79**, 2960–2964.

Bevilacqua, M.P., Pober, J.S., Wheeler, M.E., Cotran, R.S. and Gimbrone, M.J. (1985). *J. Clin. Invest.* **76**, 2003–2011.

Bhalla, K., Birkhofer, M., Arlin, Z., Grant, S., Lutzky, J. and Graham, G. (1988). *Leukemia* **2**, 810–813.

Bhalla, K., Holladay, C., Arlin, Z., Grant, S., Ibrado, A.M. and Jasiok, M. (1991). *Blood* **78**, 2674–2679.

Bhalla, K., Tang, C., Ibrado, A.M., Grant, S., Tourkina, E., Holladay, C., Hughes, M., Mahoney, M.E. and Huang, Y. (1992). *Blood* **80**, 2883–2890.

Bickel, M., Cohen, R.B. and Pluznik, D.H. (1990). *J. Immunol.* **145**, 840–845.

Blazar, B.R., Widmer, M.B., Soderling, C.C., Urdal, D.L., Gillis, S., Robison, L.L. and Vallera, D.A. (1988). *Blood* **71**, 320–328.

Bot, F.J., van, E.L., Schipper, P., Backx, B. and Lowenberg, B. (1990). *Leukemia* **4**, 325–328.

Bottomly, K. (1988). *Immunol. Today* **9**, 268–274.

Bourgoin, S., Poubelle, P.E., Liao, N.W., Umezawa, K., Borgeat, P. and Naccache, P.H. (1992). *Cell Signal* **4**, 487–500.

Brandhuber, B.J., Boone, T., Kenney, W.C. and McKay, D.B. (1987). *Science* **238**, 1707–1709.

Bregni, M., Magni, M., Siena, S., Di, N.M., Bonadonna, G. and Gianni, A.M. (1992). *Blood* **80**, 1418–1422.

Brorson, K.A., Beverly, B., Kang, S.M., Lenardo, M. and Schwartz, R.H. (1991). *J. Immunol.* **147**, 3601–3609.

Buchberg, A.M., Bedigian, H.G., Taylor, B.A., Brownell, E., Ihle, J.N., Nagata, S., Jenkins, N.A. and Copeland, N.G. (1988). *Oncogene Res.* **2**, 149–165.

Buchner, T., Hiddemann, W., Koenigsmann, M., Zuhlsdorf, M., Wormann, B., Boeckmann, A., Freire, E.A., Innig, G., Maschmeyer, G., Ludwig, W.D. *et al.* (1991). *Blood* **78**, 1190–1197.

Burgess, A.W., Nicola, N.A., Johnson, G.R. and Nice, E.C. (1982). *Blood* **60**, 1219–1223.

Cannistra, S.A., Rambaldi, A., Spriggs, D.R., Herrmann, F., Kufe, D. and Griffin, J.D. (1987). *J. Clin. Invest.* **79**, 1720–1728.

Caracciolo, D., Shirsat, N., Wong, G.G., Lange, B., Clark, S. and Rovera, G. (1987). *J. Exp. Med.* **166**, 1851–1860.

Caux, C., Dezutter, D.C., Schmitt, D. and Banchereau, J. (1992). *Nature* **360**, 258–261.

Cebon, J., Lieschke, G.J., Bury, R.W. and Morstyn, G. (1992). *Br. J. Haematol.* **80**, 144–150.

Champlin, R.E., Nimer, S.D., Ireland, P., Oette, D.H. and Golde, D.W. (1989). *Blood* **73**, 694–699.

Chan, J.Y., Slamon, D.J., Nimer, S.D., Golde, D.W. and Gasson, J.C. (1986). *Proc. Natl Acad. Sci. USA* **83**, 8669–8673.

Cheng, G.Y., Kelleher, C.A., Miyauchi, J., Wang, C., Wong, G., Clark, S.C., McCulloch, E.A. and Minden, M.D. (1988). *Blood* **71**, 204–208.

Chiba, S., Shibuya, K., Piao, Y.F., Tojo, A., Sasaki, N., Matsuki, S., Miyagawa, K., Miyazono, K. and Takaku, F. (1990). *Cell. Regul.* **1**, 327–335.

Chiou, C.J. and Wu, M.C. (1990). *FEBS Lett.* **259**, 249–253.

Clark, E.A., Grabstein, K.H. and Shu, G.L. (1992). *J. Immunol.* **148**, 3327–3335.

Clark, L.I., Lopez, A.F., To, L.B., Vadas, M.A., Schrader, J.W., Hood, L.E. and Kent, S.B. (1988). *J. Immunol.* **141**, 881–889.

Clark, S.C. and Kamen, R. (1987). *Science* **236**, 1229–1237.

Cockerill, P.N., Shannon, M.F., Bert, A.G., Ryan, G.R. and Vadas, M.A. (1993). *Proc. Natl Acad. Sci. USA* **90**, 2466–2470.

Collins, H.L. and Bancroft, C.J. (1992). *Eur. J. Immunol.* **22**, 1447–1454.

Colotta, F., Re, F., Polentarutti, N., Sozzani, S. and Mantovani, A. (1992). *Blood* **80**, 2012–2020.

Crosier, K.E., Wong, G.G., Mathey, P.B., Nathan, D.G. and Sieff, C.A. (1991). *Proc. Natl Acad. Sci. USA* **88**, 7744–7748.

Dai, C.H., Krantz, S.B., Dessypris, E.N., Means, R.J., Horn, S.T. and Gilbert, H.S. (1992). *Blood* **80**, 891–899.

Demetri, G.D. and Antman, K.H. (1992). *Semin. Oncol.* **19**, 362–385.

Devereux, S., Linch, D.C., Campos, C.D., Spittle, M.F. and Jelliffe, A.M. (1987). *Lancet* **ii**, 1523–1524.

Dexter, T.M., Garland, J., Scott, D., Scolnick, E. and Metcalf, D. (1980). *J. Exp. Med.* **152**, 1036–1047.

Diederichs, K., Boone, T. and Karplus, P.A. (1991). *Science* **254**, 1779–1782.

Disteche, C.M., Brannan, C.I., Larsen, A., Adler, D.A., Schorderet, D.G., Gearing, D., Copeland, N.G., Jenkins, N.A. and Parks, L.S. (1992). *Nature Genetics* **1**, 333–336.

Donahue, R.E., Wang, E.A., Stone, D.K., Kamen, R., Wong, G.G., Sehgal, P.K., Nathan, D.G. and Clark, S.C. (1986). *Nature* **321**, 872–875.

Dranoff, G., Jaffee, E., Lazenby, A., Columbek, P., Levitsky, H., Brose, K., Jackson, V., Hamada, H., Pardoll, D. and Muligan, R.C. (1993). *Proc. Natl Acad. Sci. USA* **90**, 3539–3543.

Duhrsen, U. (1988) *Leukemia* **2**, 334–342.

Duhrsen, U. and Metcalf, D. (1988). *Leukemia* **2**, 329–333.

Edmonson, J.H., Hartmann, L.C., Long, H.J., Colon, O.G., Fitch, T.R., Jefferies, J.A., Braich, T.A. and Maples, W.J. (1991). *Cancer* **70**, 2529–2539.

Elias, A.D., Ayash, L., Anderson, K.C., Hunt, M., Wheeler, C., Schwartz, G., Tepler, I., Mazanet, R., Lynch, C., Pap, S., Pelaez, J., Reich, E., Critchlow, J., Demetri, G., Bibbo, J., Schnipper, L., Griffin, J.D., Frei III, E. and Antman, K.H. (1992). *Blood* **79**, 3036–3044.

Elliott, M.J., Faulkner, J.B., Stanton, H., Hamilton, J.A. and Metcalf, D. (1992). *J. Immunol.* **149**, 3678–3681.

Erickson, N. and Quesenberry, P.J. (1992). *Med. Clin. North Am.* **76**, 745–755.

Ernst, T.J., Ritchie, A.R., O'Rourke, R. and Griffin, J.D. (1989). *Leukemia* **3**, 620–625.

Fan, K., Ruan, Q., Sensenbrenner, L. and Chen, B.D. (1992). *J. Immunol.* **149**, 96–102.

Fibbe, W.E., Kluck, P.M., Duinkerken, N., Voogt, P.J. Willemze, R. and Falkenburg, J.H. (1988). *Eur. J. Haematol.* **41**, 352–358.

Fiehn, C., Wermann, M., Pezzutto, A., Hufner, M. and Heilig, B. (1992). *Z. Rheumatol.* **51**, 121–126.

Frolova, E.I., Dolganov, G.M., Mazo, I.A., Smirnov, D.V., Copeland, P., Stewart, C., O'Brien, S.J. and Dean, M. (1991). *Proc. Natl Acad. Sci. USA* **88**, 4821–4824.

Gamble, J.R., Harlan, J.M., Klebanoff, S.J. and Vadas, M.A. (1985). *Proc. Natl Acad. Sci. USA* **82**, 8667–8671.

Ganser, A., Seipelt, G., Eder, M., Geissler, G., Ottmann, O.G., Hess, U. and Hoelzer, D. (1992). *Semin. Oncol.* **19**, 95–101.

Gearing, D.P., King, J.A., Gough, N.M. and Nicola, N.A. (1989). *EMBO J.* **8**, 3667–3676.

Gianni, A.M., Siena, S., Bregni, M., Tarella, C., Stern, A.C., Pileri, A. and Bonadonna, G. (1989). *Lancet* **ii**, 580–585.

Gliniak, B.C. and Rohrschneider, L.R. (1990). *Cell* **63**, 1073–1083.

Gliniak, B.C., Park, L.S. and Rohrschneider, L.R. (1992). *Mol. Biol. Cell* **3**, 535–544.

Gomez, C.J., Huang, C.K., Gomez, C.T., Waterman, W.H., Becker, E.L. and Sha'afi, R.I. (1992). *Proc. Natl Acad. Sci. USA* **89**, 7551–7555.

Gorin, N.C., Coiffier, B., Hayat, M., Fouillard, L., Kuentz, M., Flesch, M., Colombat, P., Boivin, P., Slavin, S. and Philip, T. (1992). *Blood* **80**, 1149–1157.

Gorman, D.M., Itoh, N., Kitamura, T., Schreurs, J., Yonehara, S., Yahara, I., Arai, K. and Miyajima, A. (1990). *Proc. Natl Acad. Sci. USA* **87**, 5459–5463.

Gorman, D.M., Itoh, N., Jenkins, N.A., Gilbert, D.J., Copeland, N.G. and Miyajima, A. (1992). *J. Biol. Chem.* **267**, 15842–15848.

Gough, N.M. and Kelso, A. (1989). *Growth Factors* **1**, 287–298.

Gough, N.M., Gough, J., Metcalf, D., Kelson, A., Grail, D., Nicola, N.A., Burgess, A.W. and Dunn, A.R. (1984). *Nature* **309**, 763–767.

Gough, N.M., Metcalf, D., Gough, J., Grail, D. and Dunn, A.R. (1985). *EMBO J* **4**, 645–653.

Gough, N.M., Grail, D., Gearing, D.P. and Metcalf, D. (1987). *Eur. J. Biochem.* **169**, 353–358.

Gough, N.M., Gearing, D.P., Nicola, N.A., Baker, E., Pritchard, M., Callen, D.F. and Sutherland, G.R. (1990). *Nature* **345**, 734–736.

Gradishar, W.J., Le, B.M., O'Laughlin, R., Vardiman, J.W. and Larson, R.A. (1992). *Blood* **80**, 2463–2470.

Griffin, J.D., Young, D., Herrmann, F., Wiper, D., Wagner, K. and Sabbath, K.D. (1986). *Blood* **67**, 1448–1453.

Groopman, J.E., Mitsuyasu, R.T., DeLeo, M.J., Oette, D.H. and Golde, D.W. (1987). *N. Engl. J. Med.* **317**, 593–598.

Gulati, S.C. and Bennett, C.L. (1992). *Ann. Intern. Med.* **116**, 177–182.

Hahn, S., Woodnar, F.A., Nair, A.P. and Moroni, C. (1991). *Oncogene* **6**, 2327–2332.

Hallek, M., Druker, B., Lepisto, E.M., Wood, K.W., Ernst, T.J. and Griffin, J.D. (1992). *J. Cell. Physiol.* **153**, 176–186.

Hamilton, T.A. and Adams, D.O. (1987). *Immunol. Today* **8**, 151–158.

Hammond, W., Price, T.H., Souza, L.M. and Dale, D.C. (1989). *N. Engl. J. Med.* **320**, 1306–1311.

Hara, K., Suda, T., Suda, J., Eguchi, M., Ihle, J.N., Nagata, S., Miura, Y. and Saito, M. (1988). *Exp. Hematol.* **16**, 256–261.

Hara, T. and Miyajima, A. (1992). *EMBO J.* **11**, 1875–1884.

Harada, H., Kitagawa, M., Tanaka, N., Yamamoto, H., Harada, K., Ishihara, M. and Taniguchi, T. (1993). *Science* **259**, 971–974.

Hayashida, K., Kitamura, T., Gorman, D.M., Arai, K., Yokota, T. and Miyajima, A. (1990). *Proc. Natl Acad. Sci. USA* **87**, 9655–9659.

Haylock, D.N., To, L.B., Dowse, T.L., Juttner, C.A. and Simmons, P.J. (1992). *Blood* **80**, 1405–1412.

Hazenberg, B.P., Van, L.M., Van, R.M., Stern, A.C. and Vellenga, E. (1989). *Blood* **74**, 2769–2770.

Hermine, O., Mayeux, P., Titeux, M., Mitjavila, M.T., Casadevall, N., Guichard, J., Komatsu, N., Suda, T., Miura, Y., Vainchenker, W. *et al.* (1992). *Blood* **80**, 3060–3069.

Hiddemann, W., Kiehl, M., Zuhlsdorf, M., Busemann, C., Schleyer, E., Wormann, B. and Buchner, T. (1992). *Semin. Oncol.* **19**, 31–37.

Hoekman, K., von, B.v.d.F.B., Wagstaff, J., Drexhage, H.A. and Pinedo, H.M. (1991). *Lancet* **338**, 541–542.

Hovgaard, D., Schifter, S., Rabol, A., Mortensen, B.T. and Nissen, N.I. (1992). *Eur. J. Haematol.* **48**, 202–207.

Huebner, K., Isobe, M., Croce, C.M., Golde, D.W., Kaufman, S.E. and Gasson, J.C. (1985). *Science* **230**, 1282–1285.

Huebner, K., Nagarajan, L., Besa, E., Angert, E., Lange, B.J., Cannizzaro, L.A., van den Berghe, H., Santoli, D., Finan, J., Croce, C.M. and Nowell, P.C. (1990). *Am. .J Hum. Genet.* **46**, 26–36.

Hughes, P.F., Eaves, C.J., Hogge, D.E. and Humphries, R.K. (1989). *Blood* **74**, 1915–1922.

Imboden, J.B., Weiss, A. and Stobo, J.B. (1985). *Immunol. Today* **6**, 328–331.

Inaba, K., Inaba, M., Deguchi, M., Hagi, K., Yasumizu, R., Ikehara, S., Maramatsu, S., and Steinman, R.M. (1993). *Proc. Natl Acad. Sci.* **90**, 3038–3042.

Inaba, K., Steinman, R.M., Pack, M.W., Aya, H., Inaba, M., Sudo, T., Wolpe, S. and Schuler, G. (1992). *J. Exp. Med* **175**, 1157–1167.

Itoh, A. (1992). *Hokkaido Igaku Zasshi* **67**, 365–375.

Iwai, Y., Bickel, M., Pluznik, D.H. and Cohen, R.B. (1991). *J. Biol. Chem.* **266**, 17959–17965.

James, R. and Kazenwadel, J. (1989). *Proc. Natl Acad. Sci. USA* **86**, 7392–7396.

Janeway, C.J., Carding, S., Jones, B., Murray, J., Portoles, P., Rasmussen, R., Rojo, J., Saizawa, K., West, J. and Bottomly, K. (1988). *Immunol. Rev.* **101**, 39–80.

Johnson, G.R., Gonda, T.J., Metcalf, D., Hariharan, I.K. and Cory, S. (1989). *EMBO J.* **8**, 441–448.

Kaushansky, K. (1989). *J. Immunol.* **143**, 2525–2529.

Kaushansky, K., O'Hara, P.J., Hart, C.E., Forstrom, J.W. and Hagen, F.S. (1987). *Biochemistry* **26**, 4861–4867.

Kaushansky, K., Shoemaker, S.G., Alfaro, S. and Brown, C. (1989). *Proc. Natl Acad. Sci. USA* **86**, 1213–1217.

Kelleher, C., Miyauchi, J., Wong, G., Clark, S., Minden, M.D. and McCulloch, E.A. (1987). *Blood* **69**, 1498–1503.

Kelso, A. and Gough, N. (1987). In *The Lymphokines* (ed D.R. Webb and D.V. Goeddel), Academic Press, New York, pp. 209–238.

Kelso, A. and Gough, N.M. (1988). *Proc. Natl Acad. Sci. USA* **85**, 9189–9193.

Kelso, A. and Gough, N.M. (1989). *Growth Factors* **1**, 165–177.

Kelso, A., Troutt, A.B., Maraskovsky, E., Gough, N.M., Morris, L., Pech, M.H. and Thomson, J.A. (1991). *Immunol. Rev.* **123**, 85–114.

Khwaja, A., Linch, D.C., Goldstone, A.H., Chopra, R., Marcus, R.E., Wimperis, J.Z., Russell, N.H., Haynes, A.P., Milligan, D.W., Leyland, M.J. *et al.* (1992). *Br. J. Haematol.* **82**, 317–323.

Kinzler, K.W., Nilbert, M.C., Vogelstein, B., Bryan, T.M., Levy, D.B., Smith, K.J., Preisinger, A.C., Hamilton, S.R., Hedge, P., Markham, A. *et al.* (1991). *Science* **251**, 1366–1370.

Koeffler, H.P., Gasson, J. and Tobler, A. (1988). *Mol. Cell Biol.* **8**, 3432–3438.

Koike, K., Ogawa, M., Ihle, J.N., Miyake, T., Shimizu, T., Miyajima, A., Yokota, T. and Arai, K. (1987). *J. Cell Physiol.* **131**, 458–464.

Kremer, E., Baker, E., D'Andrea, R.J., Slim, R., Phillips, H., Moretti, P.A.B., Lopez, A., Petit, C., Vadas, M.A., Sutherland, G.R. and Goodall, G.J. (1993). *Blood* **82**.

Kuczek, E.S., Shannon, M.F., Pell, L.M. and Vadas, M.A. (1991). *J. Immunol.* **146**, 2426–2433.

Kupper, T., Flood, P., Coleman, D. and Horowitz, M. (1987). *J. Immunol.* **138**, 4288–4292.

Kushner, B.H. and Cheung, N.K. (1992). *Blood* **79**, 1484–1490.

Kyas, U., Pietsch, T. and Welte, K. (1992). *Blood* **79**, 1144–1147.

LaBranche, C.C., Clark, S.C., Johnson, G.D., Ornstein, D., Sabath, D.E., Tushinskio, R., Paetkau, V. and Prystowsky, M.B. (1990). *Arch. Biochem. Biophys.* **276**, 153–159.

Lang, R.A., Metcalf, D., Gough, N.M., Dunn, A.R. and Gonda, T.J. (1985). *Cell* **43**, 531–542.

Lang, R.A., Metcalf, D., Cuthbertson, R.A., Lyons, I., Stanley, E., Kelso, A., Kannourakis, G., Williamson, D.J., Klintworth, G.K., Gonda, T.J. and Dunn, A.R. (1987). *Cell* **51**, 675–686.

Lang, R.A., Cuthbertson, R.A. and Dunn, A.R. (1992). *Growth Factors* **6**, 131–138.

Le Beau, M.M., Pettenati, M.J., Lemons, R.S., Diaz, M.O., Westbrook, C.A., Larson, R.A., Sherr, C.J. and Rowley, J.D. (1986a). *Cold Spring Harb. Symp. Quant. Biol.* **2**, 899–909.

Le Beau, M.M., Westbrook, C.A., Diaz, M.O., Larson, R.A., Rowley, J.D., Gasson, J.C., Golde, D.W. and Sherr, C.J. (1986b). *Science* **231**, 984–987.

Lee, F., Yokota, T., Otsuka, T., Gemmell, L., Larson, N., Luh, J., Arai, K. and Rennick, D. (1985). *Proc. Natl Acad. Sci. USA* **82**, 4360–4364.

Lee, J.S. and Young, I.G. (1989). *Genomics* **5**, 359–362.

Li, F., Grant, S., Pettit, G.R. and McCrady, C.W. (1992). *Blood* **80**, 2495–2502.

Libby, R.T., Braedt, G., Kronheim, S.R., March, C.J., Urdal, D.L., Chiaverotti, T.A., Tushinski, R.J., Mochizuki, D.Y., Hopp, T.P. and Cosman, D. (1987). *DNA* **6**, 221–229.

Lieschke, G.J. and Burgess, A.W. (1992). *N. Engl. J. Med.* **327**, 99–106.

Lieschke, G.J., Cebon, J. and Morstyn, G. (1989a). *Blood* **74**, 2634–2643.

Leischke, G.J., Maher, D., Cebon, J., O'Connor, M., Green, M., Sheridan, W., Boyd, A., Rallings, M., Bonnem, E., Metcalf, D., Burgess, A.W., McGrath, K., Fox, R.M. and Montyn, G. (1989b). *Ann. Intern. Med.* **110**, 357–364.

Lilly, M., Le, T., Holland, P. and Hendrickson, S.L. (1992). *Oncogene* **7**, 727–732.

Lindemann, A., Riedel, D., Oster, W., Meuer, S.C., Blohm, D., Mertelsmann, R.H. and Herrmann, F. (1988). *J. Immunol.* **140**, 837–839.

Link, H., Boogaerts, M.A., Carella, A.M., Ferrant, A., Gadner, H., Gorin, N.C., Harabacz, I., Harousseau, J.L., Herve, P., Holldack, J., Kolb, H.-J., Krieger, O., Labar, B., Linkesch, W., Mandelli, F., Margninchi, D. Naparstek, E. Nicola, N., Niederweiser, D., Reiffers, J., Rizzoli, V., Siegert, W., Vernant, J.-P. and de Witte, T. (1992). *Blood* **80**, 2188–2195.

Lion, T., Haas, O.A., Harbott, J., Bannier, E., Ritterbach, J., Jankovic, M., Fink, F.M., Stojimirovic, A., Herrmann, J., Riehm, H.J., Lampert, F., Ritter, J., Koch, H. and Gadner, H. (1992). *Blood* **79**, 3325–3330.

Logothetis, C.J., Dexeus, F.H., Sella, A., Amato, R.J., Kilbourn, R.G., Finn, L. and Gutterman, J.U. (1990). *J. Natl Cancer Inst.* **82**, 667–672.

Lopez, A.F., Eglinton, J.M., Gillis, D., Park, L.S., Clark, S. and Vadas, M.A. (1989). *Proc. Natl Acad. Sci. USA* **86**, 7022–7026.

Lopez, A.F., Shannon, M.F., Hercus, T., Nicola, N.A., Cambareri, B., Dottore, M., Layton, M.J. Eglinton, L. and Vadas, M.A. (1992). *EMBO J* **11**, 909–916.

Lord, B.I., Gurney, H., Chang, J., Thatcher, N., Crowther, D. and Dexter, T.M. (1992). *Int. J. Cancer* **50**, 26–31.

Lotem, J. and Sachs, L. (1988). *Blood* **71**, 375–382.

Lotem, J. and Sachs, L. (1992). *Blood* **80**, 1750–1757.

Lutfalla, G., Gardiner, K. and Uze, G. (1993). *Genomics* **16**, 366–373.

McNiece, I.K., Stewart, F.M., Deacon, D.M. and Quesenberry, P.J. (1988). *Exp. Hematol.* **16**, 383–388.

McNiece, I.K., Langley, K.E. and Zsebo, K.M. (1991). *Exp. Hematol.* **19**, 226–231.

Maliszewski, C.R., Schoenborn, M.A., Cerretti, D.P., Wignall, J.M., Picha, K.S., Cosman, D., Tushinski, R.J., Gillis, S. and Baker, P.E. (1988). *Mol. Immunol.* **25**, 843–850.

Marini, M., Avoni, E., Hollemborg, J. and Mattoli, S. (1992). *Chest* **102**, 661–669.

Mayer, P., Lam, C., Obenaus, H., Liehl, E. and Besemer, J. (1987). *Blood* **70**, 206–213.

Mazur, E.M., Cohen, J.L., Wong, G.G. and Clark, S.C. (1987). *Exp. Hematol.* **15**, 1128–1133.

Mehregan, D.R., Fransway, A.F., Edmonson, J.H. and Leiferman, K.M. (1992). *Arch. Dermatol.* **128**, 1055–1059.

Mempel, K., Pietsch, T., Menzel, T., Zeidler, C. and Welte, K. (1991). *Blood* **77**, 1919–1922.

Metcalf, D. (1979). *Int. J. Cancer* **24**, 616–623.

Metcalf, D. (1980). *Proc. Natl Acad. Sci. USA* **77**, 5327–5330.

Metcalf, D. (1984). *The Colony Stimulating Factors.* Elsevier, Amsterdam.

Metcalf, D. (1987). *Proc. R. Soc. Lond. Biol.* **230**, 389–423.

Metcalf, D. (1988). *The Molecular Control of Blood Cells.* Harvard University Press, Cambridge. MA.

Metcalf, D. (1989). *Cancer Res.* **49**, 2305–2311.

Metcalf, D. and Burgess, A.W. (1982). *J. Cell Physiol.* **111**, 275–283.

Metcalf, D. and Merchav, S. (1982). *J. Cell Physiol.* **112**, 411–418.

Metcalf, D. and Rasko, J.E.J. (1993) *Leukaemia* **7**, 878–886.

Metcalf, D., Begley, C.G, Johnson, G.R., Nicola, N.A., Vadas, M.A., Lopez, A.F., Williamson, D.J., Wong, G.G., Clark, S.C. and Wang, E.A. (1986a). *Blood* **67**, 37–45.

Metcalf, D., Burgess, A.W., Johnson, G.R., Nicola, N.A., Nice, E.C., DeLamarter, J., Thatcher, D.R. and Mermod, J.J. (1986b). *J. Cell Physiol.* **128**, 421–431.

Metcalf, D., Begley, C.G., Williamson, D.J., Nice, E.C., De, L.J., Mermod, J.J., Thatcher, D. and Schmidt, A. (1987). *Exp. Hematol.* **15**, 1–9.

Metcalf, D., Nicola, N.A., Gearing, D.P. and Gough, N.M. (1990). *Proc. Natl Acad. Sci. USA* **87**, 4670–4674.

Metcalf, D., Elliott, M.J. and Nicola, N.A. (1992a). *J. Exp. Med.* **175**, 877–884.

Metcalf, D., Nicola, N.A., Gough, N.M., Elliott, M., McArthur, G. and Li, M. (1992b). *Proc. Natl Acad. Sci. USA* **89**, 2819–2823.

Migliaccio, A.R., Bruno, M. and Migliaccio, G. (1987). *Blood* **70**, 1867–1871.

Migliaccio, A.R., Migliaccio, G., Dale, D.C. and Hammond, W.P. (1990). *Blood*, **75**, 1951–1959.

Miyatake, S., Otsuka, T., Yokota, T., Lee, F. and Arai, K. (1985). *EMBO J.* **4**, 2561–2568.

Miyatake, S., Seiki, M., Yoshida, M. and Arai, K. (1988). *Mol. Cell Biol.* **8**, 5581–5587.

Miyatake, S., Shlomai, J., Arai, K. and Arai, N. (1991). *Mol. Cell Biol.* **11**, 5894–5901.

Miyauchi, J., Kelleher, C.A., Wang, C., Minkin, S. and McCulloch, E.A. (1989). *Blood* **73**, 1272–1278.

Monroy, R.L., Skelly, R.R., MacVittie, T.J., Davis, T.A., Sauber, J.J., Clark, S.C. and Donahue, R.E. (1987). *Blood* **70**, 1696–1699.

Moonen, P., Mermod, J.J., Ernst, J.F., Hirschi, M. and DeLamarter, J.F. (1987). *Proc. Natl Acad. Sci. USA* **84**, 4428–4431.

Moore, M.A. (1991). *Blood* **78**, 1–19.

Moore, M.A., Spitzer, G., Metcalf, D. and Penington, D.G. (1974a). *Br. J. Haematol.* **27**, 47–55.

Moore, M.A., Sptizer, G., Williams, N., Metcalf, D. and Buckley, J. (1974b). *Blood* **44**, 1–18.

Morgan, C., Pollard, J.W. and Stanley, E.R. (1987). *J. Cell Physiol.* **130**, 420–427.

Morrissey, P.J., Bressler, L., Charrier, K. and Alpert, A. (1988). *J. Immunol.* **140**, 1910–1915.

Morstyn, G. and Burgess, A.W. (1988). *Cancer Res.* **48**, 5624–5637.

Mosmann, T.R., Cherwinski, H., Bond, M.W., Giedlin, M.A. and Coffman, R.L. (1986). *J. Immunol.* **136**, 2348–2357.

Muench, M.O. and Moore, M.A. (1992). *Exp. Hematol.* **20**, 611–618.

Mulder, A.B., de, W.J., Smit, J.W., van, O.J. and Vellenga, E. (1992). *Ann Hematol* **65**, 91–95.

Nagarajan, L., Lange, B., Cannizzaro, L., Finan, J., Nowell, P.C. and Huebner, K. (1990). *Blood* **75**, 82–87.

Naparstek, E., Hardan, Y., Ben, S.M., Nagler, A., Or, R., Mumcuoglu, M., Weiss, L., Samuel, S. and Slavin, S. (1992). *Blood* **80**, 1673–1678.

Neidhart, J.A., Mangalik, A., Stidley, C.A., Tebich, S.L., Sarmiento, L.E., Pfile, J.E., Oette, D.H. and Oldham, F.B. (1992). *J. Clin. Oncol.* **10**, 1460–1469.

Nemunaitis, J., Singer, J.W., Buckner, C.D., Durnam, D., Epstein, C., Hill, R., Strob, R., Thomas, E.D. and Appelbaum, F.R. (1990). *Blood* **76**, 245–253.

Nemunaitis, J., Rabinowe, S.N., Singer, J.W., Bierman, P.J., Vose, J.M., Freedman, A.S., Onetto, N., Gillis, S., Oette, D., Gold, M., Buckner, C.D., Hansen, J.A., Ritz, J., Appelbaum, F.R. and Armitage, J.O. (1991). *N. Engl. J. Med.* **324**, 1773–1778.

Neta, R. and Oppenheim, J.J. (1988). *Blood* **72**, 1093–1095.

Neta, R., Oppenheim, J.J. and Douches, S.D. (1988). *J. Immunol.* **140**, 108–111.

Nicola, N.A. (1987). *Immunol. Today* **8**, 134–140.

Nicola, N.A., Burgess, A.W. and Metcalf, D. (1979). *J. Biol. Chem.* **254**, 5290–5299.

Nicola, N.A. and Metcalf, D. (1982). *J. Cell Physiol.* **112**, 257–264.

Nienhuis, A.W., Donahue, R.E., Karlsson, S., Clark, S.C., Agricola, B., Antinoff, N., Pierce, J.E., Turner, P., Anderson, W.F. and Nathan, D.G. (1987). *J. Clin. Invest.* **80**, 573–577.

Nimer, S.D., Champlin, R.E. and Golde, D.W. (1988a). *JAMA* **260**, 3297–3300.

Nimer, S.D., Morita, E.A., Martis, M.J., Wachsman, W. and Gasson, J.C. (1988b). *Mol. Cell Biol.* **8**, 1979–1984.

Nimer, S.D., Gasson, J.C., Hu, K., Smalberg, I., Williams, J.L., Chen, I.S. and Rosenblatt, J.D. (1989). *Oncogene* **4**, 671–676.

Nimer, S., Fraser, J., Richards, J., Lynch, M. and Gasson, J. (1990). *Mol. Cell Biol.* **10**, 6084–6088.

Nishida, J., Yoshida, M., Arai, K. and Yokota, T. (1991). *Int. Immunol.* **3**, 245–254.

Nishimura, M., Kaku, K., Azuno, Y., Okafuji, K., Inoue, Y. and Kaneko, T. (1992). *Blood* **80**, 1045–1051.

Nissen, C., Tichelli, A., Gratwohl, A., Speck, B., Milne, A., Gordon, S.E. and Schaedelin, J. (1988). *Blood* **72**, 2045–2047.

Okuda, K., Sanghera, J.S., Pelech, S.L., Kanakura, Y., Hallek, M., Griffin, J.D. and Druker, B.J. (1992). *Blood* **79**, 2880–2887.

Park, L.S., Martin, U., Sorensen, R., Luhr, S., Morrissey, P.J., Cosman, D. and Larsen, A. (1992). *Proc. Natl Acad. Sci. USA* **89**, 4295–4299.

Parry, D.A., Minasian, E. and Leach, S.J. (1991). *J. Mol. Recog.* **4**, 63–75.

Perno, C.F., Cooney, D.A., Gao, W.Y., Hao, Z., Johns, D.G., Foli, A., Hartman, N.R., Calio, R., Broder, S. and Yarchoan, R. (1992). *Blood,* **80**, 995–1003.

Pluda, J.M., Yarchoan, R., Smith, P.D., McAtee, N., Shay, L.E., Oette, D., Maha, M., Wahl, S.M., Myers, C.E. and Broder, S. (1990). *Blood* **76**, 463–472.

Powers, R., Garrett, D.S., March, C.J., Frieden, E.A., Gronenborn, A.M. and Clore, G.M. (1992). *Science* **256**, 1673–1677.

Preisler, H.D., Raza, A. and Larson, R.A. (1992). *Blood* **80**, 2600–2603.

Price, V., Mochizuki, D., March, C.J., Cosman, D., Deeley, M.C., Klinke, R., Clevenger, W., Gillis, S., Baker, P. and Urdal, D. (1987). *Gene* **55**, 287–293.

Prpic, V., Weiel, J.E., Somers, S.D., DiGuiseppi, J., Gonias, S.L., Pizzo, S.V., Hamilton, T.A., Herman, B. and Adams, D.O. (1987). *J. Immunol.* **139**, 526–533.

Punt, C.J. (1992). *Leuk. Res.* **16**, 551–559.

Quelle, F.W., Quelle, D.E. and Wojchowski, D.M. (1992). *J. Biol. Chem.* **267**, 17055–17060.

Raines, M.A., Golde, D.W., Daeipour, M. and Nel, A.E. (1992). *Blood* **79**, 3350–3354.

Rajotte, D., Haddad, P., Haman, A., Cragoe, E.J. and Hoang, T. (1992). *J. Biol. Chem.* **267**, 9980–9987.

Rappold, G., Willson, T.A., Henke, A. and Gough, N.M. (1992). *Genomics* **14**, 455–461.

Rakar, S.J., Goodall, E.J., Maretti, P.A.B., D'Andrea, R.J. and Gough, N.M. (1994) (Submitted).

Razanajaona, D., Maroc, C., Lopez, M., Mannoni, P. and Gabert, J. (1992). *Cell Growth Differ.* **3**, 299–305.

Re, M.C., Zauli, G., Furlini, G., Giovannini, M., Ranieri, S., Ramazzotti, E., Vignoli, M. and La, P.M. (1992). *Microbiologica* **15**, 265–270.

Reid, C.D., Stackpoole, A., Meager, A. and Tikerpae, J. (1992). *J. Immunol.* **149**, 2681–2688.

Rich, I.N. (1986). *Exp. Hematol.* **14**, 738–745.

Roberts, T.M. (1992). *Nature* **360**, 534–535.

Robinson, B.E., McGrath, H.E. and Quesenberry, P.J. (1987). *J. Clin. Invest.* **79**, 1648–1652.

Satoh, T., Nakafuku, M., Miyajima, A. and Kaziro, Y. (1991). *Proc. Natl Acad. Sci. USA* **88**, 3314–3318.

Schreck, R. and Baeuerle, P.A. (1990). *Mol. Cell Biol.* **10**, 1281–1286.

Schrimsher, J.L., Rose, K., Simona, M.G. and Wingfield, P. (1987). *Biochem. J.* **247**, 195–199.

Schuster, M.W., Liu, E.T., Solberg, L.A. *et al.* (1990). *Blood* **76**, 47.

Seelentag, W.K., Mermod, J.J., Montesano, R. and Vassalli, P. (1987). *EMBO J.* **6**, 2261–2265.

Shanafelt, A.B. and Kastelein, R.A. (1989). *Proc. Natl Acad. Sci. USA* **86**, 4872–4876.

Shanafelt, A.B., Johnson, K.E. and Kastelein, R.A. (1991a). *J. Biol. Chem.* **266**, 13804–13810.

Shanafelt, A.B., Miyajima, A., Kitamura, T. and Kastelein, R.A. (1991b). *EMBO J.* **10**, 4105–4112.

Shanafelt, A.B. and Kastelein, R.A. (1992). *J. Biol. Chem.* **267**, 25466–25472.

Shannon, M.F., Pell, L.M., Lenardo, M.J., Kuczek, E.S., Occhiodoro, F.S., Dunn, S.M. and Vadas, M.A. (1990). *Mol. Cell Biol.* **10**, 2950–2959.

Shaw, G. and Kamen, R. (1986). *Cell* **46**, 659–667.

Shen, Y., Baker, E., Callen, D.F., Sutherland, G.R., Willson, T.A., Rakar, S. and Cough, N.M. (1992). *Cytogenet. Cell Genet.* **61**, 175–177.

Siena, S., Bregni, M., Brando, B., Ravagnani, F., Bonadonna, G. and Gianni, A.M. (1989). *Blood* **74**, 1905–1914.

Slim, R., Levilliers, J., Ludecke, H.-J., Claussen, U., Nguyen, V.-C., Gough, N.M., Horsthemke, B. and Petit, C. (1993). *Genomics* **16**, 26–33.

Sparrow, L.G., Metcalf, D., Hunkapiller, M.W., Hool, L.E. and Burgess, A.W. (1985). *Proc. Natl Acad. Sci. USA* **82**, 292–296.

Spolarics, Z., Schuler, A., Bagby, C.J., Lang, C.H., Nelson, S. and Spitzer, J.J. (1992). *J. Leukoc. Biol.* **51**, 360–365.

Sporn, M.B. and Roberts, A.B. (1985). *Nature* **313**, 745–747.

Stanley, E., Metcalf, D., Sobieszczuk, P., Gough, N.M. and Dunn, A.R. (1985). *EMBO J.* **4**, 2569–2573.

Stocking, C., Loliger, C., Kawai, M., Suciu, S., Gough, N. and Ostertag, W. (1988). *Cell* **53**, 869–879.

Sugimoto, K., Tsuboi, A., Miyatake, S., Arai, K. and Arai, N. (1990). *Int. Immunol.* **2**, 787–794.

Sullivan, R., Fredette, J.P., Socinski, M., Elias, A., Antman, K., Schnipper, L. and Griffin, J.D. (1989). *Br. J. Haematol.* **71**, 475–479.

Suzuki, A., Takahashi, T., Nakamura, K., Tsuyuoka, R., Okuno, Y., Enomoto, T., Fukumoto, M. and Imura, H. (1992). *Blood* **80**, 2052–2059.

Tafuri, A. and Andreeff, M. (1990). *Leukemia* **4**, 826–834.

Takaki, S., Mita, S., Kitamura, T., Yonehara, S., Yamaguchi, N., Tominaga, A., Miyajima, A. and Takatsu, K. (1991). *EMBO J.* **10**, 2833–2838.

Takaue, Y., Watanabe, T., Abe, T., Okamoto, Y., Saito, S., Shimizu, T., Sato, J., Hirao, A., Suzue, T., Koyama, T., Kawano, Y., Ninomiya, T., Shimokawa, T., Yokobayashi, A., Takehara, H. and Kuroda, Y. . (1992). *Bone Marrow Transplant* **10**, 241–248.

Tannenbaum, C.S., Koerner, T.J., Jansen, M.M. and Hamilton, T.A. (1988). *J. Immunol.* **140**, 3640–3645.

Thorens, B., Mermod, J.J. and Vassalli, P. (1987). *Cell* **48**, 671–679.

Tran, H.T., Metcalf, D. and Cheers, C. (1990). *Immunology* **71**, 377–382.

Tsuboi, A., Sugimoto, K., Yodoi, J., Miyatake, S., Arai, K. and Arai, N. (1991). *Int. Immunol.* **3**, 807–817.

Vadhan, R.S., Buescher, S., Broxmeyer, H.E., LeMaistre, A., Lepe, Z.J., Ventura, G., Jeha, S., Horwitz, L.J., Trujillo, J.M., Gillis, S., Hittelman, W.M. and Gutterman, J.U. . (1988a). *N. Engl. J. Med.* **319**, 1628–1634.

Vadhan, R.S., Buescher, S., LeMaistre, A., Keating, M., Walters, R., Ventura, C., Hittelman, W., Broxmeyer, H.E. and Gutterman, J.U. (1988b). *Blood* **72**, 134–141.

Vadhan, R.S., Broxmeyer, H.E., Hittelman, W.N., Papadopoulos, N.E., Chawla, S.P., Fenoglio, C., Cooper, S., Buescher, E.S., Frenck, R.J., Holian, A., Perkins, R.C., Schuele, R.K., Gutterman, J.U., Salem, P. and Benjamin, R.S. (1992). *J. Clin. Oncol.* **10**, 1266–1277.

Valtieri, M., Santoli, D., Caracciolo, D., Kreider, B.L., Altmann, S.W., Tweardy, D.J., Gemperlein, I., Mavilio, F., Lange, B. and Rovera, G. (1987). *J. Immunol.* **138**, 4042–4050.

Van den Berghe, H., Vermaelen, K., Mecucci, C., Barbieri, D. and Tricot, G. (1985). *Cancer Genet. Cytogenet.* **17**, 189–255.

van Leeuwen, B.H., Martinson, M.E., Webb, G.C. and Young, I.G. (1989). *Blood* **73**, 1142–1148.

Vellenga, E., Young, D.C., Wagner, K., Wiper, D., Ostapovicz, D. and Griffin, J.D. (1987). *Blood* **69**, 1771–1776.

Verhoef, G., Van, d.B.H. and Boogaerts, M. (1992). *Leukemia* **6**, 766–769.

Villeval, J.L., Duhrsen, U., Morstyn, G. and Metcalf, D. (1990). *Br. J. Haematol.* **74**, 36–44.

Walker, F. and Burgess, A.W. (1985). *EMBO J.* **4**, 933–939.

Warringa, R.A., Mengelers, H.J., Kuijper, P.H., Raaijmakers, J.A., Bruijnzeel, P.L. and Koenderman, L. (1992). *Blood* **79**, 1836–1841.

Welham, M.J., Duronio, V., Sanghera, J.S., Pelech, S.L. and Schrader, J.W. (1992). *J. Immunol.* **149**, 1683–1693.

Willemze, R., van, d.L.N., Zwierzina, H., Suciu, S., Solbu, G., Gerhartz, H., Labar, B., Visani, G., Peetermans, M.E., Jacobs, A., Stryckmans, P., Fenaux, P., Haak, H.L., Ribeiro, M.M., Baumelou, E., Baccarani, M., Mandelli, F., Jaksic, B., Louwagie, A., Thyss, A., Hayat, M., de Cataldo, F., Stern, A.C. and Zittoun, R. (1992). *Ann. Hematol.* **64**, 173–180.

Williams, D.E., Straneva, J.E., Cooper, S., Shadduck, R.K., Waheed, A., Gillis, S., Urdal, D. and Broxmeyer, H.E. (1987). *Exp. Hematol.* **15**, 1007–1012.

Willman, C.L., Sever, C.E., Pallavicini, M.G., Harada, H., Tanaka, N., Slovak, M.L., Yamamoto, H., Harada, K., Meeker, T.C., List, A.F. and Taniguchi, T. (1993). *Science* **259**, 968–971.

Wilson, S.D., Billings, P.R., D'Eustachio, P., Fournier, R.E., Geissler, E., Lalley, P.A., Burd, P.R., Housman, D.E., Taylor, B.A. and Dorf, M.E. (1990). *J. Exp. Med.* **171**, 1301–1314.

Wingfield, P., Graber, P., Moonen, P., Craig, S. and Pain, R.H. (1988). *Eur. J. Biochem.* **173**, 65–72.

Wong, G.G., Witek, J.S., Temple, P.A., Wilkens, K.M., Leary, A.C., Luxenberg, D.P., Jones, S.S., Brown, E.L., Kay, R.M., Orr, E.C., Shoemaker, C., Golde, D.W., Kaufman, R.J., Hewick, R.M., Wang, E.A. and Clark, S.C. (1985a) *Science* **228**, 810–815.

Wong, G.G., Witek, J.S., Temple, P.A., Wilkens, K.M., Leary, A.G., Luxenberg, D.P., Jones, S.S., Brown, E.L., Kay, R.M. and Orr, E.C. (1985b). In *Cancer Cells* (eds J. Feramisco, B. Ozanne, and C. Stiles), Cold Spring Harbor Laboratory Press, New York, pp. 235–242.

Yamaguchi, M., Hirai, K., Morita, Y., Takaishi, T., Ohta, K., Suzuki, S., Motoyoshi, K., Kawanami, O. and Ito, K. (1992). *Int. Arch. Allergy Appl. Immunol.* **97**, 322–329.

Yang, Y.C., Kovacic, S., Kriz, R., Wolf, S., Clark, S.C., Wellems, T.E., Nienhuis, A. and Epstein, N. (1988). *Blood* **71**, 958–961.

Yong, K.L., Rowles, P.M., Patterson, K.G. and Linch, D.C. (1992). *Blood* **80**, 1565–1575.

Young, D.C. and Griffin, J.D. (1986). *Blood* **68**, 1178–1181.

Yuo, A., Kitagawa, S., Kasahara, T., Matsushima, K., Saito, M. and Takaku, F. (1991). *Blood* **78**, 2708–2714.

Zwierzina, H., Schollenberger, S., Herold, M., Schmalzl, F. and Besemer, J. (1992). *Leuk. Res.* **16**, 1181–1186.

Chapter 20

Granulocyte Colony Stimulating Factor and its Receptor

Shigekazu Nagata

Osaka Bioscience Institute, Osaka 565, Japan

INTRODUCTION

More than 70% of white blood cells are neutrophilic granulocytes (neutrophils), which play important roles in protecting mammals from bacterial infection. Neutrophils have a short half-life, and need to be constantly replenished from pluripotent stem cells in the bone marrow. Granulocyte colony stimulating factor (G-CSF) is a glycoprotein of M_r about 20 000, which regulates the production of neutrophils and enhances their maturation. It is produced by activated macrophages, endothelial cells and fibroblasts. Using recombinant DNA technology, G-CSF can be produced in large quantity in *Escherichia coli* and mammalian cells, and it is widely used clinically to treat patients suffering from neutropenia after cancer chemotherapy.

The activity of G-CSF to stimulate proliferation and differentiation of cells is mediated by its receptor. The G-CSF receptor is specifically expressed in the neutrophilic progenitors and mature neutrophils. The G-CSF receptor has been biochemically and genetically characterized. It carries a single transmembrane domain which divides the molecule into extracellular and cytoplasmic domains, and it is a member of the haemopoietic growth factor receptor family. The G-CSF receptor binds G-CSF with high affinity as a homodimer, and can transduce proliferation and differentiation signals into cells. The detailed mechanism of the signal transduction is unknown. However, since the G-CSF receptor does not contain apparent signalling elements, the receptor presumably couples to the signalling components such as tyrosine kinases. Here, the biochemical and genetic properties of G-CSF and the G-CSF receptor are summarized.

GRANULOCYTE COLONY STIMULATING FACTOR

Biochemical Properties of G-CSF

G-CSF was initially identified by the pioneering works of D. Metcalf and his colleagues as a factor that induced the terminal differentiation of murine myelomonocytic leukaemia WEHI-3BD$^+$ cells into granulocytes and monocytes. This factor was

The Cytokine Handbook, 2nd ed.
ISBN 0–12–689661–5

designated granulocyte-macrophage differentiation factor (GM-DF), and purified from medium conditioned by the lungs from mice previously injected with endotoxin (Nicola *et al.*, 1983). Using ordinary column chromatography and high-performance liquid chromatography (HPLC), GM-DF was purified about 500 000-fold with a yield of 30%, and about 5 μg of protein was obtained from 800 mice. Since the purified GM-DF stimulated colony formation of neutrophilic granulocytes in semi-solid culture of bone-marrow cells, the factor was redesignated as granulocyte colony-stimulating factor (G-CSF). Murine G-CSF is an acidic glycoprotein of M_r 24 000–25 000 (pI 4.5–5.8). It is relatively stable to extreme pH levels (pH 2–10), temperature (50% loss of the activity at 70°C for 30 min), and strong denaturation agents (6 M guanidine hydrochloride, 8 M urea, 0.1% SDS).

Malignant tumours in patients are often accompanied by marked granulopoiesis without apparent bacterial infection (Asano *et al.*, 1980). Cell lines established from these tumours indicate that they constitutively produce large amounts of colony stimulating factor. The colony stimulating factor produced by human squamous carcinoma CHU-2 and bladder carcinoma 5637 cell lines was purified from their conditioned medium. The factor purified from CHU-2 cells was designated G-CSF since it specifically stimulated colony formation of neutrophilic granulocytes (Nomura *et al.*, 1986). Conversely, the factor purified from 5637 cells was initially named pluripoetin because it stimulated colony formation of not only neutrophilic granulo-cytes but also erythroid cells, megakaryocytes, and macrophages (Welte *et al.*, 1985). However, it was later renamed G-CSF because when bone-marrow cells depleted of mature myeloid and lymphoid cells were used as targets, the factor exclusively stimulated colony formation of neutrophilic granulocytes (Strife *et al.*, 1987). Human G-CSF is a glycoprotein with an apparent M_r of 19 000 and a pI of 5.5–6.1 depending on the degree of sialylation (Nomura *et al.*, 1986).

Using the amino acid sequence of the purified human G-CSF, its cDNA was independently isolated from human CHU-2 and 5637 cell lines (Nagata *et al.*, 1986a, b; Souza *et al.*, 1986). Human G-CSF is composed of 174 amino acids with a 30-amino-acid signal sequence. The calculated molecular mass of the core protein is 18 671 Da. Human G-CSF does not carry the consensus sequence for N-glycosylation (Asn–X–Thr/Ser), but it is O-glycosylated at Thr-133, which explains the difference between the calculated M_r and that of the native protein. The structure of the sugar moiety attached to the human G-CSF is N-acetyl-neuramic acid α(2-6)[galactose β(1-3)] N-acetylgalactosamine (Souza *et al.*, 1986; Oheda *et al.*, 1988). The sugar moiety is not essential for biological activity as the recombinant G-CSF produced in *E. coli* is as active as native glycosylated G-CSF. However, it contributes to the stability of the molecule by preventing its aggregation, especially under neutral and alkaline con-ditions (Oheda *et al.*, 1990). Human G-CSF contains five cysteine residues, four of which are connected by disulphide bonds (Cys-36–Cys-42 and Cys-64–Cys-74). Muta-tional analysis of the cysteine residues indicated that these disulphide bonds are essential for proper folding of the molecule and biological activity (Lu *et al.*, 1989).

Based upon homology with human G-CSF, murine G-CSF cDNA was isolated from a mouse carcinoma-cell line which constitutively produces G-CSF (Tsuchiya *et al.*, 1986). Mouse G-CSF consists of 178 amino acids with a 30-amino-acid leader sequence, and does not contain an N-glycosylation site. The difference between the M_r calculated from the amino acid sequence (19 061) and that of the native protein (25 000) seems to be due to O-glycosylation. As shown in Fig. 1, human and mouse G-CSFs are 73.6% identical at the amino acid sequence level, and fully crossreact both biologically and at the receptor-binding level (Nicola *et al.*, 1985). The positions of the cysteine residues connected by disulphide bonds are conserved between human and mouse G-CSFs.

G-CSF has a significant sequence homology with other cytokines such as IL-6, LIF and oncostatin M (OSM), which have a variety of activities upon several target cells including myeloid cells, hepatocytes, adipocytes, embryonic cells and neurons (Kishimoto *et al.*, 1989; Malik *et al.*, 1989; Hilton, 1992). X-ray diffraction analysis of human G-CSF indicates that it has a four α-helical bundle structure as found in other cytokines, such as IFN, IL-2, growth hormone and GM-CSF. Mutational analysis of human G-CSF and epitope mapping of neutralizing antibodies indicated that the amino acid residues from 20–46 as well as the *C* terminus are important for binding to the receptor (Kuga *et al.*, 1989; Layton *et al.*, 1991).

Genetic Properties of G-CSF and its Expression

There is only one G-CSF chromosomal gene per haploid genome in the human and murine systems. The G-CSF gene is localized on human chromosome 17q21–q22 (Kanda *et al.*, 1987) and on mouse chromosome 11 (Buchberg *et al.*, 1988). The human and mouse G-CSF genes are about 2.5 kb in length and contain five exons (Nagata *et al.*, 1986b; Tsuchiya *et al.*, 1987a). The G-CSF mRNA is about 1.5 kb, and the human, but not the mouse G-CSF gene produces alternatively spliced mRNAs (Nagata *et al.*, 1986b). The alternatively spliced form of the human G-CSF mRNA, which constitutes a minor population of human G-CSF mRNA, codes for 177 amino acids (Nagata *et al.*, 1986a). The human G-CSF consisting of 177 amino acids has at least 10 times less specific activity than authentic human G-CSF consisting of 174 amino acids. Like other cytokine mRNAs, the G-CSF mRNA carries several AUUUA sequences in the 3' noncoding region, which confers instability (Shaw and Kamen, 1986).

G-CSF activity is detected in the serum of mice injected with endotoxins or infected with bacteria (Burgess and Metcalf, 1980; Cheers *et al.*, 1988). Accordingly, peritoneal macrophages or macrophage cell lines can be induced *in vitro* to produce G-CSF in response to bacterial endotoxins such as *E. coli* LPS, TNF-α and IL-1 (Metcalf and Nicola, 1985; Lu *et al.*, 1988; Vellenga *et al.*, 1988; Nishizawa and Nagata, 1990). In addition, fibroblasts and endothelial cells can be stimulated to produce G-CSF using IL-1 or TNF-α (Broudy *et al.*, 1987; Koeffler *et al.*, 1987; Seelentag *et al.*, 1987; Kaushansky *et al.*, 1988). These results suggest that during the inflammatory process, endotoxins stimulate macrophages to produce not only G-CSF but also several monokines, including IL-1 and TNF-α, which then induce the release of G-CSF from fibroblasts and endothelial cells. The G-CSF accumulated in the serum appears to be responsible for the granulopoiesis that accompanies inflammation. In addition to the inducible expression of G-CSF in macrophages, endothelial cells and fibroblasts, some carcinoma cells constitutively produce large quantities of G-CSF. These include squamous carcinoma CHU-2, bladder carcinoma 5637, melanoma LD-1, glioblastoma U87MG and hepatoma SK-HEP-1 cell lines (Nagata, 1990; Tweardy *et al.*, 1987).

G-CSF gene expression is transcriptionally and post-transcriptionally regulated, and is insensitive to cycloheximide (Koeffler *et al.*, 1988; Ernst *et al.*, 1989; Nishizawa and Nagata, 1990). Stabilization of the mRNA by binding of proteins to the AUUUA

```
                 -30                                     -20                                 -10
Human:  Met Ala Gly Pro Ala Thr Gln Ser Pro Met Lys Leu Met Ala Leu Gln Leu Leu Leu Trp His Ser Ala Leu Trp Thr Val
Mouse:  Met Ala Gln Leu Ser Ala Gln Arg Arg Met Lys Leu Met Ala Leu Gln Leu Leu Leu Trp Gln Ser Ala Leu Trp Ser Gly
                 -30                                     -20                                 -10

                 -1  1                                              10
Human:  Gln Glu Ala Thr Pro Leu --- --- --- Gly Pro Ala Ser Ser Leu Pro Gln Ser Phe Leu Leu Lys Cys Leu
Mouse:  Arg Glu Ala Val Pro Leu Val Thr Val Ser Ala Leu Pro Pro Ser Leu Pro Leu Pro Arg Ser Phe Leu Leu Lys Ser Leu
                 -1  1                              10                        20

                                                                   40
Human:  Glu Gln Val Arg Lys Ile Gln Gly Asp Gly Ala Ala Leu Gln Glu Lys Leu Cys Ala Thr Tyr Lys Leu Cys His Pro Glu
Mouse:  Glu Gln Val Arg Lys Ile Gln Gly Ala Ser Val Leu Leu Gln Gln Leu Cys Ala Thr Tyr Lys Leu Cys His Pro Glu
             30                          50                        60                70

Human:  Glu Leu Val Leu Leu Gly His Ser Leu Gly Ile Pro Trp Ala Pro Leu Ser Ser Cys Pro Ser Gln Ala Leu Gln Leu Ala
Mouse:  Glu Leu Val Leu Leu Gly His Ser Leu Gly Ile Pro Lys Ala Ser Leu Ser Gly Cys Ser Ser Gln Ala Leu Gln Leu Ala
                              80                                   90

                                                         100                               110                        120
Human:  Gly Cys Leu Ser Gln Leu His Ser Gly Leu Phe Leu Tyr Gln Gly Leu Leu Gln Ala Leu Glu Gly Ile Ser Pro Glu Leu
Mouse:  Gln Leu Ser Gln Leu His Ser Gly Leu Cys Leu Tyr Gln Gly Leu Leu Gln Ala Leu Ser Gly Ile Ser Pro Ala Leu

                                             130                                 140                        150
Human:  Gly Pro Thr Leu Asp Thr Leu Gln Leu Asp Val Ala Asp Phe Ala Thr Thr Ile Trp Gln Gln Met Glu Glu Leu Gly Met
Mouse:  Ala Pro Thr Leu Asp Thr Leu Gln Leu Asp Val Ala Asn Phe Ala Thr Thr Ile Trp Gln Gln Met Glu Gln Leu Gly Met

                                 160                                 170
Human:  Ala Pro Ala Met Pro Ala Phe Ala Ser Ala Phe Gln Arg Arg Ala Gly Gly Val Leu Val
Mouse:  Ala Pro Ala Met Pro Ala Phe Ala Ser Ala Phe Gln Arg Arg Ala Gly Gly Val Leu Ala

Human:  Ala Ser His Leu Gln Ser Phe Leu Glu Val Ser Tyr Arg Val Leu Arg His Leu Ala Gln Pro
Mouse:  Ile Ser Tyr Leu Gln Ser Phe Leu Glu Val Ser Tyr Arg Val Leu Arg His Leu Ala Leu Ala
```

Fig. 1. Primary structure of human and murine G-CSF. The amino acids that are identical between human and murine G-CSF are shown in bold characters, and the cysteine residues connected by disulphide bonds are underlined.

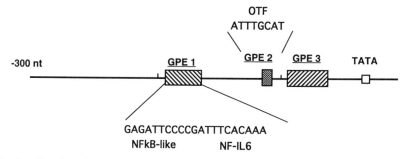

Fig. 2. Functional regulatory elements in the promoter of the G-CSF gene.

sequences in the 3' noncoding sequence may be responsible for the post-transcriptional regulation. The transcriptional activation of the G-CSF gene is mediated by a promoter sequence located at the 5' flanking region of the G-CSF gene. About 300 nucleotides upstream of the ATG initiation codon are well conserved (about 80% homology) between human and mouse G-CSF genes (Tsuchiya *et al.*, 1987a). This region is sufficient for the inducible expression of the G-CSF gene in macrophages and its constitutive expression in carcinoma cells (Nishizawa and Nagata, 1990; Nishizawa *et al.*, 1990). At least three regulatory elements (G-CSF promoter elements, GPE1, GPE2 and GPE3) have been identified in this region by mutational analyses (Fig. 2). GPE1 is composed of an NF-κB-like CSF box (PuGAGPuTTCCACPu) which can be found in the promoter of IL-3 and GM-SCF genes, and an NF-IL6 binding site (TT/GNNNGNAAT/G). GPE2 is the octamer transcription factor (OTF) binding site (ATTTGCAT). GPE3 is an unique element for the G-CSF gene, and it can be divided into two subregions (Asano and Nagata, 1992). During activation of macrophages by endotoxins, all three GPEs and their cognate transcription factors seem to be activated in a concerted fashion (Asano *et al.*, 1991). A transcription factor cDNA (GPEI-BP or Ig/EBP) which binds to the GPE1 has been isolated (Nishizawa *et al.*, 1991). GPE1-BP carries a basic domain and a leucine zipper motif, and is a member of the C/EBP family (Landschulz *et al.*, 1989). GPE1-BP does not carry a transcription activation domain, and cannot activate the GPE1-mediated transcription. Heterodimerization of GPE1-BP with other C/EBP or ATF (activation transcription factor) family members may be responsible for activation of the G-CSF gene through GPE1 (Nishizawa and Nagata, 1992).

In Vitro Biological Activities of G-CSF

G-CSF specifically stimulates the colony formation of neutrophilic granulocytes in semi-solid cultures of bone-marrow cells. In this assay, G-CSF has a specific activity of about 2×10^8 units/mg protein (where 50 units/ml is the concentration required for half-maximal stimulation) (Nomura *et al.*, 1986; Tsuchiya *et al.*, 1987b). Other types of colonies are occasionally observed in G-CSF-supported cultures but these seem to be indirect effects mediated by accessory cells (Strife *et al.*, 1987). In addition to its ability to stimulate proliferation and differentiation of the neutrophilic progenitors, G-CSF can prolong the survival of the mature neutrophils and enhance their functional capacity (Kitagawa *et al.*, 1987; Yuo *et al.*, 1989, 1990; Williams *et al.*, 1990). Several mouse and human myeloid leukaemia-cell lines also respond to G-CSF. For example, G-CSF can induce differentiation of mouse myeloid leukaemia WEHI-3B D$^+$ (Nicola *et al.*, 1983), 32D C13 (Valtieri *et al.*, 1987) and L-G cells (Lee *et al.*, 1991) into neutrophils. In accord with normal differentiation of neutrophilic granulocytes (Bainton, 1990), G-CSF induces the expression of various neutrophil-specific genes such as myeloperoxidase, lactoferrin and chloroacetate esterase in 32DC13 cells during differentiation (Valtieri *et al.*, 1987). Furthermore, downregulation of c-*myc* and c-*myb* gene expression and upregulation of the c-*fos* gene was observed during the late stage of the differentiation of WEH1-3BD$^+$ cells by G-CSF (Gonda and Metcalf, 1984). Conversely, mouse myeloid leukaemia NFS60 cells only proliferate in response to G-CSF (Weinstein *et al.*, 1986) and do not differentiate, probably owing to integration of the retrovirus and rearrangement of the c-*myb* and c-*evi*-1 genes (Morishita *et al.*, 1988).

In Vivo Activities of G-CSF and its Clinical Use

Using recombinant G-CSF produced in *E. coli* and mammalian cells, many groups have studied the *in vivo* effects of G-CSF (Cohen *et al.*, 1987; Tsuchiya *et al.*, 1987b; Welte *et al.*, 1987). When G-CSF was administered to mice, hamsters and monkeys, the number of neutrophils in the blood increased immediately after injection in a dose-dependent manner, and reached 5–10 times the basal level within 24 h. This effect of G-CSF is specific for neutrophilic granulocytes, and no significant changes were observed in other blood cell numbers such as erythrocytes, monocytes, lymphocytes and platelets. The injected G-CSF was cleared in a biexponential manner with a distribution half-life of 30 min and an elimination half-life of 3.8 h (Cohen *et al.*, 1987). When the administration of the G-CSF ceased, the number of neutrophils in the blood returned to the basal level within 48 h. The effect of G-CSF was then studied in animals with neutropenia induced by chemical drugs such as 5-fluorouracil or cyclophosphamide (Cohen *et al.*, 1987; Tamura *et al.*, 1987; Welte *et al.*, 1987). In every case, G-CSF remarkably accelerated the recovery from granulopenia. Furthermore, when G-CSF was administered to mice pretreated with a cytotoxic drug, it protected them from lethal infections by *E. coli*, *Staphylococcus aureus*, and *Candida albicans* (Matsumoto *et al.*, 1987).

Mice were chronically exposed to high circulating levels of G-CSF by infecting mouse bone-marrow cells with a G-CSF expression vector (Chang *et al.*, 1989) or by implanting fibroblasts transfected with a similar expression vector (Tani *et al.*, 1989). Under both conditions, the mice showed sustained neutrophilia and infiltration of neutrophilic granulocytes into various organs, such as liver and lungs. However, in contrast to the tissue damage associated with chronic overexpression of either GM-CSF or IL-3 (Lang *et al.*, 1987; Wong *et al.*, 1989), no significant tissue damage was observed in mice exposed to high dosages of G-CSF (Chang, *et al.*, 1989).

Encouraged by the data obtained from the animal model system, G-CSF is now widely used clinically in patients with granulopenia (Davis and Morstyn, 1991; Gabrilove, 1992). G-CSF is administered to cancer patients receiving chemotherapy with or without bone-marrow transplantation and to patients receiving immunosuppressive agents after organ transplantation. In both types of patients, G-CSF accelerates the recovery of neutrophilic granulocytes, and diminishes the risk of severe bacterial and fungal infections after chemotherapy. G-CSF has almost no adverse side effects; at most, there may be slight bone pain, which is tolerated well by patients. These results suggest that higher dosage of anti-cancer chemical drugs can be used for treatment. However, some myeloid leukaemia or endothelial tumour cells respond to G-CSF by proliferation *in vitro* (Pebusque *et al.*, 1988; Bussolino *et al.*, 1989). Although such acute myeloid leukaemia cells may not respond to G-CSF *in vivo* (Ohno *et al.*, 1990), the clinical application of G-CSF in these patients should be carefully controlled. In this regard, G-CSF therapy may become more effective if the ability of tumour cells to respond to G-CSF is examined *in vitro* by G-CSF binding or proliferation assay before its administration *in vivo*. G-CSF is also being used successfully to treat patients with congenital cyclic neutropenia (Hammond *et al.*, 1989). Unfortunately, when G-CSF was administered to patients with congenital agranulocytosis (Kostman's disease) some did not respond, and defects in G-CSF signal transduction were suggested in these patients (Welte *et al.*, 1990).

RECEPTOR FOR G-CSF

Biochemical Properties of the G-CSF Receptor

The function of G-CSF is triggered by binding of G-CSF to its receptor. Except for the placenta (Uzumaki *et al.*, 1989), the G-CSF receptor can be found only in neutrophilic progenitors, mature neutrophils and in various myeloid leukaemia cells such as NFS-60, WEHI-3B D^+ and HL-60 cells which respond to G-CSF (Nicola and Peterson, 1986; Park *et al.*, 1989; Fukunaga *et al.*, 1990a). This agrees with the fact that G-CSF specifically regulates the production of neutrophilic granulocytes. The number of the receptor is relatively low, being around 300–1000 molecules per cell, and G-CSF binds to the receptor with a dissociation constant (K_d) of about 100 pM. This value is much higher than the concentration (10 pM) required for the half-maximal biological response, indicating that the biological responses to G-CSF occur at low levels of receptor occupancy.

   The G-CSF receptor has been purified from a mouse myeloid NFS-60 cell line which expresses the receptor at a relatively high level (2000 molecules per cell) (Fukunaga *et al.*, 1990a). The membrane fraction from 3×10^{11} cells was solubilized by CHAPS, and the G-CSF receptor was purified by G-CSF affinity column chromatography and gel filtration on Superose 12. The purified G-CSF receptor had a M_r of 100 000–130 000, which agreed with the value obtained by chemically crosslinking the cell-surface receptor with ^{125}I-labelled G-CSF (Fukunaga *et al.*, 1990a). Scatchard analysis of the G-CSF binding to the purified receptor suggested two forms of the receptor, one with high affinity (K_d = 120–360 pM) and the other with low affinity for G-CSF (K_d= 2.6–4.2 nM). Analysis of the purified receptor by sucrose density gradient centrifugation indicated that the dimeric and monomeric forms of the receptor bind G-CSF with high and low affinity, respectively. Furthermore, when the purified receptor was analysed by the polyacrylamide gel electrophoresis under nonreducing conditions in the presence of SDS, most proteins migrated as the monomeric form, and a minor fraction behaved like oligomers. Ligand blotting with ^{125}I-G-CSF showed that the oligomeric form has much higher affinity for G-CSF than the monomeric form.

Structure of the G-CSF Receptor

Murine G-CSF receptor cDNA has been isolated from a NFS-60 cDNA library by expression cloning (Fukunaga et al., 1990b). When the cDNA was expressed in heterologous mammalian cells such as COS, the cells specifically bound G-CSF with high affinity (about 100 pM), indicating that the single polypeptide coded by the cloned cDNA is sufficient to constitute a high-affinity binding site. Since the dimer of the purified receptor binds G-CSF with high affinity, as described above, these results suggest that the G-CSF receptor on the cell surface functions as a homodimer to bind G-CSF with high affinity.

The murine G-CSF receptor mRNA of about 3.7 kb codes for a protein consisting of 837 amino acids, including a 25-amino-acid signal sequence at the N-terminus. The polypeptide contains a single transmembrane region of 24 amino acids which divides the molecule into extracellular and cytoplasmic regions of 601 and 187 amino acids, respectively. There are 11 predicted N-glycosylation sites (Asn–X–Thr/Ser) in the extracellular region. Glycosylation of the protein seems to explain the difference between the M_r predicted from the amino acid sequence (90 814) and that of the native protein (100 000–130 000). The extracellular region of the G-CSF receptor has a composite structure. The N-terminal domain of 100 amino acids has an Ig-like sequence. The following 200-amino-acid domain (CRH domain) is related to the domain of the extracellular region of various haemopoietic growth factor receptors, as described below. This region contains four conserved cysteine residues at the N-terminal half, and the consensus Trp–Ser–X–Trp–Ser element at the C-terminus. Between the CRH and the transmembrane domains, the G-CSF receptor contains three fibronectin type III domains (FNIII). The cytoplasmic region of the G-CSF receptor carries no motif for enzymatic activities such as tyrosine kinase and phosphatase, but does have a proline-rich region called Box 1, proximal to the transmembrane domain (Fukunaga et al., 1991).

Based upon homology with the murine G-CSF receptor, human G-CSF receptor cDNA was isolated from human myeloid leukaemia U937 cells and human placenta (Fukunaga et al., 1990c; Larsen et al., 1990). At least four alternative transcripts for human G-CSF were isolated. Major human G-CSF receptor mRNA codes for a protein consisting of 813 amino acids with a calculated M_r of 89 743. The overall structure of the human G-CSF receptor is similar to that of the mouse, and it has an amino acid sequence similarity of 62.5%. A small percentage of the G-CSF receptor mRNAs expressed in U937 cells code for a soluble receptor in which an 88 bp internal deletion removes the transmembrane domain and changes the reading frame, resulting in 149 different amino acids at the C-terminus. The third and fourth types of G-CSF receptor mRNA are found in the placenta. They contain an insertion coding for an extra 27 amino acids in the cytoplasmic region or carry a sequence for 34 amino acids at the C-terminus that are different from those of the authentic G-CSF receptor. The functional significance of these aberrant forms of the G-CSF receptor is unknown. The human G-CSF receptor gene is located on chromosome 1p35–34.3 (Inazawa et al., 1991), and is composed of 17 exons spanning about 17 kb (Seto et al., 1992). Exons 3–17 code for the G-CSF receptor protein, and the subdomains of the receptor are coded by a set of exons. This gene organization is similar to that of the chromosomal genes for other haemopoietic growth-factor receptors (Godowski et al., 1989; Shibuya et al., 1990;

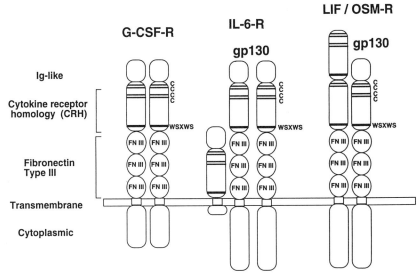

Fig. 3. The G-CSF receptor subfamily. The G-CSF, IL-6 and LIF/OSM receptors are shown schematically. The conserved cysteine residues and the WSXWS motif in the CRH domain are indicated by thin and thick bars, respectively.

Youssoufian *et al.*, 1990; Gorman *et al.*, 1992; Wrighton *et al.*, 1992). The regulatory elements in the promoter of the G-CSF receptor gene have not yet been characterized. However, an element of 18 nucleotides located 100 bp upstream of the transcriptional initiation site of the G-CSF receptor gene can be found at the corresponding position of the myeloperoxidase and neutrophil elastase genes, which are also expressed only in neutrophilic granulocytes (Seto *et al.*, 1992).

The G-CSF receptor is a member of the haemopoietic growth-factor receptor family which includes the IL-2 receptor β and γ chains and receptors for IL-3-7, GM-CSF, LIF, growth hormone and prolactin, as well as the gp130, IL-6 receptor β-chain (Bazan, 1990). A domain of about 200 amino acids (CRH domain) in the extracellular region is conserved among the members of this family. Mutational analyses of the growth hormone and G-CSF receptors indicate that this region is the ligand-binding domain (Cunningham and Wells, 1989; Fukunaga *et al.*, 1991). The LIF receptor and gp130 have an overall structure similar to the G-CSF receptor, and their amino acid sequences show significant homology to the G-CSF receptor (Fig. 3). These results suggest that the G-CSF receptor, the LIF receptor and gp130 constitute a cytokine receptor subfamily (Nagata and Fukunaga, 1991, 1993). On the other hand, except for the CRH domain, there is little homology among the members of this haemopoietic growth factor receptor family.

The Function of the G-CSF Receptor

G-CSF stimulates the proliferation and differentiation of the progenitor cells of neutrophilic granulocytes. The cloned G-CSF receptor can mediate these signals into cells. G-CSF receptor cDNA has been expressed in IL-3-dependent cell lines such as the myeloid precursor FDC-P1, the pro-B-cell line BAF-B03, and the IL-2-dependent

T-cell line CTLL2 (Fukunaga *et al.*, 1991), which normally do not express the G-CSF receptor. The transformants acquired the ability to bind G-CSF with high affinity. The FDC-P1 and BAF-B03 transformants, but not those of CTLL2 expressing the G-CSF receptor, also proliferated in response to G-CSF. This indicates that the cloned G-CSF receptor can not only bind G-CSF but can also transduce the growth signal. Furthermore, it also suggests that the signal transducing system used by the G-CSF receptor is similar or common to that for the IL-3 receptor system, but it may differ from that used for the IL-2 receptor system.

In addition to growth-promoting activity, G-CSF can induce the terminal differentiation of neutrophilic granulocytes. When FDC-P1 transformants expressing the G-CSF receptor are cultured in the presence of IL-3, they express Thy-1 and F4/80 antigens on their cell surface. Conversely, when they were shifted to culture medium containing G-CSF, the expression of these cell surface antigens was highly suppressed within 7 days (Fukunaga *et al.*, 1993). Since Thy-1 and F4/80 antigens are normally expressed in premature cells and not in mature neutrophils, these results suggest that G-CSF receptor can mediate the differentiation signal. G-CSF powerfully induced the expression of neutrophil-specific genes, such as myeloperoxidase and leukocyte elastase in FDC-P1 transformants expressing the G-CSF receptor. This differentiation-inducing activity was specific for G-CSF, and neither GM-SCF nor IL-3 could induce the expression of the myeloperoxidase gene. Rather, GM-CSF and IL-3 worked as inhibitors of the G-CSF receptor-mediated differentiation signal. Furthermore, this signal was specific for myeloid cells; that is, myeloperoxidase gene induction by G-CSF was observed only in myeloid precursor FDC-P1 cells but not in the pro-B-cell line.

The functional domain of the G-CSF receptor was determined by expressing various deletion mutants of the G-CSF receptor in FDC-P1 cells (Fukunaga *et al.*, 1991). This analysis indicated that the CRH domain of the G-CSF receptor was indispensable for binding G-CSF, whereas the Ig-like domain, the FNIII domains and the entire cytoplasmic region were not required. A 76-amino-acid stretch proximal to the transmembrane domain in the cytoplasmic region is essential for transducing the growth signal (Fukunaga *et al.*, 1993; Ziegler *et al.*, 1993), while both *N*-terminal and *C*-terminal domains of the cytoplasmic region are indispensable for transducing the differentiation signal (Fukunaga *et al.*, 1993). These results indicate that different domains of the G-CSF receptor, and thus different signal transducing systems are utilized for the G-CSF-induced proliferation and differentiation of neutrophilic progenitor cells (Fig. 4). It will be of interest to determine what kinds of signalling molecules are involved in proliferation and differentiation signalling pathways evoked by G-CSF. Various cytokines activate tyrosine kinase although their receptors do not carry kinase domains. Recently, we also observed activation of tyrosine kinase(s) by G-CSF (Pan *et al.*, 1993). In the IL-2 receptor system, the IL-2 receptor β-chain associates with a *src* family kinase, *lck*, and activates it (Hatakeyama *et al.*, 1991). Various kinases may also be involved in the signal transduction system through the G-CSF receptor.

Dimerization of the G-CSF Receptor

Most haemopoietic growth factor receptors such as IL-2, IL-3, GM-CSF and IL-6 receptors are composed of two or three subunits, and function as a heterodimer or

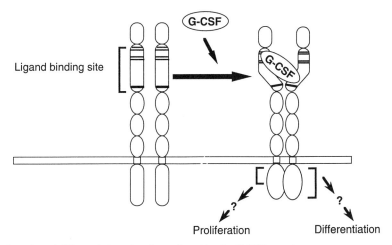

Fig. 4. Growth and differentiation signals mediated by the G-CSF receptor.

heterotrimer to bind their respective ligands with high affinity (Nicola and Metcalf, 1991; Miyajima *et al.*, 1992). The growth hormone, prolactin and G-CSF receptors, however, seem to function as a homodimer form. Mutational analyses of the growth hormone and its receptor indicate that the growth hormone interacts with the CRH domain of the extracellular region of the growth hormone receptor at two sites (site 1 and site 2) (Cunningham *et al.*, 1991). Accordingly, the X-ray diffraction analysis revealed a complex composed of a single growth hormone and two receptor molecules (de Vos *et al.*, 1992).

To examine the dimerization of the G-CSF receptor, a series of chimaeric receptors between the growth hormone and G-CSF receptors were constructed (Ishizaka-Ikeda *et al.*, 1993). In these chimaeric receptors, the extracellular region of the G-CSF receptor was replaced with that of the growth hormone receptor by exon swapping. All chimaeric receptors, including the growth hormone receptor itself, could transduce the proliferation signal in FDC-P1 cells upon growth hormone stimulation (Fuh *et al.*, 1992; Ishizaka-Ikeda *et al.*, 1993). However, the growth response occurred only at growth hormone concentrations from 10 pM to 100 nM. At higher concentrations, growth hormone could not stimulate the proliferation of the transformants expressing the chimaeric receptor or the authentic growth hormone receptor. This result can be explained as follows (Fuh *et al.*, 1992). At the optimal concentration, the growth hormone binds the receptor through site 1. The growth hormone then binds a second receptor at site 2, which results in dimerization of the receptor and signal transduction. At a higher concentration of growth hormone, all the growth hormone receptor would be occupied by a single growth hormone, which would inhibit dimerization of the receptor. Since the chimaeric receptor carries the cytoplasmic region of the G-CSF receptor, this indicates that dimerization of the G-CSF receptor is essential for the signal transduction mediated by the G-CSF receptor (Fig. 4). Recently, a similar result, that is, dimerization of gp130, was reported (Murakami *et al.*, 1993). As postulated for the growth hormone receptor system, it is conceivable that a single G-CSF molecule induces dimerization of the receptor, which is an active form that transduces the signal.

CONCLUSION

About 10 years have elapsed since G-CSF was identified as a factor which stimulates proliferation and differentiation of neutrophilic progenitors. Extensive biochemical and biological characterization of this factor, and clinical trials have shown that G-CSF is one of the best cytokines that can be used to treat patients. This is because G-CSF has a rather strict target-cell-specificity, and it specifically regulates the production of neutrophils. Because of this, G-CSF has proved to be very beneficial in treating patients suffering from neutropenia. Furthermore, this ability of G-CSF provides an ideal model system with which to examine the molecular mechanism of cell growth and differentiation in general.

ACKNOWLEDGEMENTS

I thank Drs O. Hayaishi and C. Weissmann for their encouragement and discussion. The work in our laboratory was carried out in collaboration with Drs R. Fukunaga, E. Ishizaka-Ikeda, Y. Seto, C.-X. Pan and Y. Itoh, and supported in part by Grants-in-Aid from the Ministry of Education, Science and Culture of Japan. I also thank Ms K. Mimura for secretarial assistance.

REFERENCES

Asano, M. and Nagata, S. (1992). *Gene* **121**, 371–375.
Asano, M., Nishizawa, M. and Nagata, S. (1991). *Gene* **107**, 241–246.
Asano, S., Sato, N., Mori, M., Ohsawa, N., Kosaka, N. and Ueyama, Y. (1980). *Br. J. Cancer* **41**, 689–694.
Bainton, D.F. (1990). In *Hematology* 4th edn (eds W.J. Williams, E. Beutler, A.J. Erslev, and M.A. Lichtman) McGraw-Hill Publishing Co., New York, pp. 761–769.
Bazan, J.F. (1990). *Proc. Natl Acad. Sci. USA* **87**, 6934–6938.
Broudy, V.C., Kaushansky, K., Harlan, J.M. and Adamson, J.W. (1987). *J. Immunol.* **139**, 464–468.
Buchberg, A.M., Bedigian, H.G., Taylor, B.A., Brownell, E., Ihle, J.N., Nagata, S., Jenkins, N.A. and Copeland, N.G. (1988). *Oncogene Res.* **2**, 149–166.
Burgess, A.W. and Metcalf, D. (1980). *Int. J. Cancer* **26**, 647–654.
Bussolino, F., Wang., J.M., Defilippi, P., Turrini, F., Sanavio, F., Edgell, C.-J.S., Aglietta, M., Arese, P. and Mantovani, A. (1989). *Nature* **337**, 471–473.
Chang, J.M., Metcalf, D., Gonda., T.J. and Johnson, G.R. (1989). *J. Clin. Invest.* **84**, 1488–1496.
Cheers, C., Haigh, A.M., Kelso, A., Metcalf, D., Stanley, E.R. and Young, A.M. (1988). *Infect. Immun.* **56**, 247–251.
Cohen, A.M., Zsebo, K.M., Inoue, H., Hines, D., Boone, T.C., Chazin, V.R., Tsai, L., Ritch, T. and Souza, L.M. (1987). *Proc. Natl Acad. Sci. USA* **84**, 2848–2488.
Cunningham, B.C. and Wells, J.A. (1989). *Science* **244**, 1081–1085.
Cunningham, B.C., Ultsch, M., de Vos, A.M., Mulkerrin, M.G., Clauser, K.R. and Wells, J.A. (1991). *Science* **254**, 821–825.
Davis, I. and Morstyn, G. (1991). *Semi. Hematol.* **28**, 25–33.
de Vos, A.M., Ultsch, M. and Kossiakoff, A.A. (1992). *Science* **255**, 306–312.
Ernst, T.J., Ritchie, A.R., Demetri, G.D. and Griffin, J.D. (1989). *J. Biol. Chem.* **264**, 5700–5702.
Fuh, G., Cunningham, B.C., Fukunaga, R., Nagata, S., Goeddel, D.V. and Wells, J.A. (1992). *Science* **256**, 1677–1680.
Fukunaga, R., Ishizaka-Ikeda, E. and Nagata, S. (1990a). *J. Biol. Chem.* **265**, 14008–14015.
Fukunaga, R., Ishizaka-Ikeda, E., Seto, Y. and Nagata, S. (1990b). *Cell* **61**, 341–350.
Fukunaga, R., Seto, Y., Mizushima, S. and Natata, S. (1990c). *Proc. Natl Acad. Sci. USA* **87**, 8702–8706.
Fukunaga, R., Ishizaka-Ikeda, E., Pan, C.-X., Seto, Y. and Nagata, S. (1991). *EMBO J.* **10**, 2855–2865.
Fukunaga, R., Ishizaka-Ikeda, E. and Nagata, S. (1993). *Cell* **74**, 1079–1087.

Gabrilove, J.L. (1992). *Growth Factors* **6**, 187–191.

Godowski, P.J., Leung, D.W., Meachan, L.R., Galgani, J.P., Hellmiss, R., Keret, R., Rotwein, P.S., Park, J.S., Laron, Z. and Wood, W.I. (1989). *Proc. Natl Acad. Sci. USA* **86**, 8083–8087.

Gonda, T.J. and Metcalf, D. (1984). *Nature* **310**, 249–251.

Gorman, D.M., Itoh, N., Jenkins, N.A., Gilbert, D.J., Copeland, N.G. and Miyajima, A. (1992). *J. Biol. Chem.* **267**, 15842–15848.

Hammond, W.P., Price, T.H., Souza, L.M. and Dale, D.C. (1989). *N. Engl. J. Med.* **320**, 1306–1311.

Hatekeyama, M., Kono, T., Kobayashi, N., Kawahara, A., Levin, S.D., Perlmutter, R.M. and Taniguchi, T. (1991). *Science* **252**, 1523–1528.

Hilton, D.J. (1992). *TIBS* **17**, 72–76.

Inazawa, J., Fukunaga, R., Seto, Y., Nakagawa, H., Misawa, S., Abe, T. and Nagata, S. (1991). *Genomics* **10**, 1075–1078.

Ishizaka-Ikeda, E., Fukunaga, R., Wood, W.I., Goeddel, D.V. and Nagata, S. (1993). *Proc. Natl Acad. Sci. USA* **90**, 123–127.

Kanda, N., Fukushige, S.-I., Murotsu, T., Yoshida, M.C., Tsuchiya, M., Asano, S., Kaziro, Y. and Nagata, S. (1987). *Somat. Cell Mol. Genet.* **13**, 679–684.

Kaushansky, K., Lin, N. and Adamson, J.W. (1988). *J. Clin. Invest.* **81**, 92–97.

Kishimoto, T., Akira, S. and Taga, T. (1992). *Science* **258**, 593–597.

Kitagawa, S., Yuo, A., Souza, L.M., Saito, M., Miura, Y. and Takaku, F. (1987). *Biochem. Biophys. Res. Commun.* **144**, 1143–1146.

Koeffler, H.P., Gasson, J., Ranyard, J., Souza, L., Shepard, M. and Munker, R. (1987). *Blood* **70**, 55–59.

Koeffler, H.P., Gasson, J. and Tobler, A. (1988). *Mol. Cell. Biol.* **8**, 3432–3438.

Kuga, T., Komatsu, Y., Yamasaki, M., Sekine, S., Miyaji, H., Nishi, T., Sato, M., Yokoo, Y., Asano, M., Okabe, M., Morimoto, M. and Itoh, S. (1989). *Biochem. Biophys. Res. Commun.* **159**, 103–111.

Landschulz, W.H., Johnson, P.F., Adashi, E.Y., Graves, B.J. and McKnight, S.L. (1988). *Genes Devel.* **2**, 786–800.

Lang, R.A., Metcalf, D., Cuthbertson, R.A., Lyons, I., Stanley, E., Kelso, A., Kannourakis, G., Williamson, D.J., Klintworth, G.K., Gonda, T.J. and Dunn, A.R. (1987). *Cell* **51**, 675–686.

Larsen, A., Davis, T., Curtis, B.M., Gimpel, S., Sims, J.E., Cosman, D., Park, L., Sorensen, E., March, C.J. and Smith, C.A. (1990). *J. Exp. Med.* **172**, 1559–1570.

Layton, J.E., Morstyn, G., Febri, L.J., Reid, G.E., Burgess, A.W., Simpson, R.J. and Nice, E.C. (1991). *J. Biol. Chem.* **266**, 23815–23823.

Lee, K.H., Kinashi, T., Tohyama, K., Tashiro, K., Funato, N., Hama, K. and Honjo, T. (1991). *J. Exp. Med.* **173**, 1257–1266.

Lu, H.S., Boone, T.C., Souza, L.M. and Lai, P.H. (1989). *Arch. Biochem. Biophys.* **268**, 81–92.

Lu, L., Walker, D., Graham, C.D., Waheed, A., Shadduck, R.K. and Broxmeyer, H.E. (1988). *Blood* **72**, 34–41.

Malik, N., Kallestad, J.C., Gundereson, N.L., Austin, S.D., Neubauer, M.G., Ochs, V., Marquardt, H., Zarling, J.M., Shoyab, M., Wei, C., Linsley, P.S. and Rose, T.M. (1989). *Mol. Cell. Biol.* **9**, 2847–2853.

Matsumoto, M., Matsubara, S., Matsuno, T., Tamura, M., Hattori, K., Nomura, H., Ono, M. and Yokota, T. (1987). *Infect. Immun.* **55**, 2715–2720.

Metcalf, D. and Nicola, N.A. (1985). *Leukemia Res.* **1**, 35–50.

Miyajima, A., Kitamura, T., Harada, N., Yokota, T. and Arai, K. (1992). *Annu. Rev. Immunol.* **10**, 295–331.

Morishita, K., Parker, D.S., Mucenski, M.L., Jenkins, N.A., Copeland, N.G. and Ihle, J.N. (1988). *Cell* **54**, 831–840.

Murakami, M., Hibi, M., Nakagawa, N., Nakagawa, T., Yasukawa, K., Yamanishi, K., Taga, T. and Kishimoto, T. (1993). *Science* **260**, 1808–1810.

Nagata, S. (1990). In *Handbook of Experimental Pharmacology* Vol. 95, (eds M.B. Sporn and A. B. Roberts), Springer-Verlag, Berlin, pp. 699–722.

Nagata, S. and Fukunaga, R. (1991). *Prog. Growth Factor Receptor* **3**, 131–141.

Nagata, S. and Fukunaga, R. (1993). *Growth Factor* **8**, 99–107.

Nagata, S., Tsuchiya, M., Asano, S., Kaziro, Y., Yamazaki, T., Yamamoto, O., Hirata, Y., Kubota, N., Oheda, M., Nomura, H. and Ono, M. (1986a). *Nature* **319**, 415–418.

Nagata, S., Tsuchiya, M., Asano, S., Yamamoto, O., Hirata, Y., Kubota, N., Oheda, M., Nomura, H. and Yamazaki, T. (1986b). *EMBO J.* **5**, 575–581.

Nicola, N.A. and Metcalf, D. (1991). *Cell* **67**, 1–4.

Nicola, N.A. and Peterson, L. (1986). *J. Biol. Chem.* **261**, 12384–12389.

Nicola, N.A., Metcalf, D., Matsumoto, M. and Johnson, G.R. (1983). *J. Biol. Chem.* **258**, 9017–9023.
Nicola, N.A., Begley, C.G. and Metcalf, D. (1985). *Nature* 314, 625–628.
Nishizawa, M. and Nagata, S. (1990). *Mol. Cell Biol.* **10**, 2002–2011.
Nishizawa, M. and Nagata, S. (1992). *FEBS Lett.* **299**, 36–38.
Nishizawa, M., Tsuchiya, M., Watanabe-Fukunaga, R. and Nagata, S. (1990). *J. Biol. Chem.* **265**, 5897–5902.
Nishizawa, M., Wakabayashi-Ito, N. and Nagata, S. (1991). *FEBS Lett.* **282**, 95–97.
Nomura, H., Imazeki, I., Oheda, M., Kubota, N., Tamura, M., Ono, M., Ueyama, Y. and Asano, S. (1986). *EMBO J.* **5**, 871–876.
Oheda, M., Hase, S., Ono, M. and Ikenaka, T. (1988). *J. Biochem.* **103**, 544–546.
Oheda, M., Hasegawa, M., Hattori, K., Kuboniwa, H., Kojima, T., Orita, T., Tomonou, K., Yamazaki, T. and Ochi, N. (1990). *J. Biol. Chem.* **265**, 11432–11435.
Ohno, R., Tomonaga, M., Kobayashi, T., Kanamaru, A., Shirakawa, S., Masaoka, T., Omine, M., Oh, H., Nomura, T., Sakai, Y., Hirano, M., Yokomaku, S., Nakayama, S., Yoshida, Y., Miura, A.B., Morishima, Y., Dohy, H., Niho, Y., Hamajima, N. and Takaku, F. (1990). *N. Engl. J. Med.* **323**, 871–877.
Pan, C.-X., Fukunaga, R., Yonehara, S. and Nagata, S. (1993). *J. Biol. Chem.* **268**, 25818–25823.
Park, L.S., Waldron, P.E., Friend, D., Sassenfeld, H.M., Price, V., Anderson, D., Cosman, D., Andrews, R.G., Bernstein, I.D. and Urdal, D.L. (1989). *Blood* 74, 56–65.
Pebusque, M.-J., Lafage, M., Lopez, M. and Mannoni, P. (1988). *Blood* 72, 257–265.
Seelentag, W.K., Mermod, J.-J., Montesano, R. and Vassalli, P. (1987). *EMBO J.* **6**, 2261–2265.
Seto, Y., Fukunaga, R. and Nagata, S. (1992). *J. Immunol.* **148**, 259–266.
Shaw, G. and Kamen, R. (1986). *Cell* **46**, 659–667.
Shibuya, H., Yoneyama, M., Nakamura, Y., Harada, H., Hatakeyama, M., Minamoto, S., Kono, T., Doi, T., White, R. and Taniguchi, T. (1990). *Nucl. Acids Res.* **18**, 3697–3703.
Souza, L.M., Boone, T.C., Gabrilove, J., Lai, P.H., Zsebo, K.M., Murdock, D.C., Chazin, V.R., Bruszewski, J., Lu, H., Chen, K.K., Barendt, J., Platzer, E., Moore, M.A.S., Mertelsmann, R. and Welte, K. (1986). *Science* **232**, 61–65.
Strife, A., Lambeck, C., Wisniewski, D., Gulati, S., Gasson, J.C., Golde, D.W., Welte, K., Gabrilove, J.L. and Clarkson, B. (1987). *Blood* **69**, 1508–1523.
Tamura, M., Hattori, K., Nomura, H., Oheda, M., Kubota, N., Imazeki, I., Ono, M., Ueyama, Y., Nagata, S., Shirafuji, N. and Asano, S. (1987). *Biochem. Biophys., Res. Commun.* **142**, 454–460.
Tani, K., Ozawa, K., Ogura, H., Takahashi, T., Okano, A., Watari, K., Matsudaira, T., Tajika, K., Karasuyama, H., Nagata, S., Asano, S. and Takaku, F. (1989). *Blood* **174**, 1274–1280.
Tsuchiya, M., Asano, S., Kaziro, Y. and Nagata, S. (1986). *Proc. Natl Acad. Sci. USA* **83**, 7663–7637.
Tsuchiya, M., Kaziro, Y. and Nagata, S. (1987a). *Eur. J. Biochem.* **165**, 7–12.
Tsuchiya, M., Nomura, H., Asano, S., Kaziro, Y. and Nagata, S. (1987b). *EMBO J.* **6**, 611–616.
Tweardy, D.J., Caracciolo, D., Valtieri, M. and Rovera, G. (1987). *Ann. NY Acad. Sci.* **511**, 30–38.
Uzumaki, H., Okabe, T., Sakaki, N., Hagiwara, K., Takaku, F., Tobita, M., Yasukawa, K., Ito, S. and Umezawa, Y. (1989). *Proc. Natl Acad. Sci. USA.* **86**, 9323–9326.
Valtieri, M., Tweardy, D.J., Carraci, D., Johnson, K., Mavilio, F., Altman, S., Santoli, D. and Rovela, G. (1987). *J. Immunol.* **138**, 3829–3835.
Vellenga, E., Rambaldi, A., Ernst, T.J., Ostapovicz, D. and Griffin, J.D. (1988). *Blood* 71, 1529–1532.
Weinstein, Y., Ihle, J.N., Lavu, S. and Reddy, E.P. (1986). *Proc. Natl Acad. Sci. USA* 83, 5010–5014.
Welte, K., Platzer, E., Lu, L., Gabrilove, J.L., Levi, E., Mertelsmann, R. and Moore, M.A.S. (1985). *Proc. Natl Acad. Sci. USA* **82**, 1526–1530.
Welte, K., Bonilla, M.A., Gillio, A.P., Boone, T.C., Potter, G.K., Gabrilove, J.L., Moore, M.A.S., O'Reilly, R.J. and Souza, L.M. (1987). *J. Exp. Med.* **165**, 941–948.
Welte, K., Zeidler, C., Reiter, A., Müller, W., Odenwald, E., Souza, L. and Riehm, H. (1990). *Blood* **175**, 1056–1063.
Williams, G.T., Smith, C.A., Spooncer, E., Dexter, T.M. and Taylor, D.R. (1990). *Nature* 343, 76–79.
Wong, P.M.C., Chung, S.-W., Dunbar, C.E., Bodine, D.M., Ruscetti, S. and Nienhuis, A.W. (1989). *Mol. Cell. Biol.* **9**, 798–808.
Wrighton, N., Campbell, L.A., Harada, N., Miyajima, A. and Lee, F. (1992). *Growth Factors* **6**, 103–118.
Youssoufian, H., Zon, L.I., Orkin, S.H., D'Andrea, A.D. and Lodish, H.F. (1990). *Mol. Cell. Biol.* **10**, 3675–3682.

Yuo, A., Kitagawa, S., Ohsaka, A., Ohta, M., Miyazono, K., Okabe, T., Urabe, A., Saito, M. and Takaku, F. (1989). *Blood* **74**, 2144–2149.
Yuo, A., Kitagawa, S., Ohsaka, A., Saito, M. and Takaku, F. (1990). *Biochem. Biophys. Res. Commun.* **171**, 491–497.
Ziegler, S.F., Bird, T.A., Morella, K.K., Mosley, B., Gearing, D.P. and Baumann, H. (1993). *Mol. Cell. Biol.* **13**, 2384–2390.

Chapter 21

Colony Stimulating Factor-1 (Macrophage Colony Stimulating Factor)

E. Richard Stanley

Department of Developmental and Molecular Biology, Albert Einstein College of Medicine,
Bronx, NY, USA

INTRODUCTION

Colony stimulating factor-1 (CSF-1) is one of a group of growth factors termed colony stimulating factors because of their ability to stimulate the formation of colonies of mature myeloid cells from single immature hemopoietic precursor cells plated in semi-solid medium (Pluznik and Sachs, 1965; Bradley and Metcalf, 1966). The homodimeric glycoprotein CSF-1 was the first of these factors to be purified (Stanley and Heard, 1977) and was shown to stimulate the formation of colonies of macrophages (Stanley *et al.*, 1978; Stanley and Guilbert, 1980). CSF-1 was formally demonstrated to be distinct from the other colony stimulating factors by antibody neutralization and its detection in specific radioimmuno- and radioceptor assays (Stanley, 1979; Das *et al.*, 1980, 1981). It was shown to be identical to macrophage growth factor (MGF) (Stanley *et al.*, 1976), which stimulates the proliferation of activated peritoneal macrophages (Virolainen and Defendi, 1967) and had been partially purified (Mauel and Defendi, 1971). CSF-1 is also known as macrophage colony stimulating factor (M-CSF) and has been formerly referred to as colony stimulating factor (CSF) or macrophage and granulocyte inducer IM (MGI-IM). It is synthesized by a variety of different cell types. Secreted glyco-protein and proteoglycan forms of CSF-1 are found at biologically active concentrations in the circulation, the latter form probably being sequestered from the circulation to particular sites. In addition, a membrane-spanning, cell-surface glycoprotein form plays an important role in local regulation by this growth factor. Our understanding of the biology of CSF-1 has been greatly increased by the recent discovery that an inactivating mutation in the CSF-1 gene is the basis of the defect in the CSF-1-less osteopetrotic (op/op) mouse (Wiktor-Jedrzejczak *et al.*, 1990; Yoshida *et al.*, 1990). CSF-1 has been shown to regulate a variety of cell types other than macrophages and their precursors, including decidual cells, trophoblastic cells, microglia and osteoclasts (reviewed in Stanley, 1990; Roth and Stanley, 1992). Its target cells generally have trophic and scavenger function and, as such, have important roles in organogenesis and tissue remodelling. The biological effects of CSF-1 are mediated by the CSF-1 receptor

The Cytokine Handbook, 2nd ed.
ISBN 0–12–689661–5

(CSF-1R) (Guilbert and Stanley, 1980), a protein tyrosine-kinase receptor that is identical to the c-*fms* proto-oncogene product (Sherr *et al.*, 1985). The responses mediated by the CSF-1 receptor depend on the responding cell type but, in general, are pleiotropic, including survival, proliferation and differentiation (Stanley *et al.*, 1983). A detailed understanding of the post CSF-1R signal transduction pathways in the macrophage has not yet been attained. However, fibroblasts transfected with the CSF-1 receptor gene are dependent on CSF-1 for their proliferation in semi-solid medium (Roussel and Sherr, 1989) and have been studied in detail. Many components in the signal transduction pathways regulating macrophage proliferation are shared with those identified in the fibroblasts. This chapter describes the structure, function and biology of CSF-1 and its receptor. For aspects of earlier work on CSF-1 not covered here, readers are referred to previous review articles (Stanley and Guilbert, 1981; Stanley *et al.*, 1983; Stanley, 1985, 1990; Sherr, 1990; Sherr and Stanley, 1990; Roth and Stanley, 1992).

THE BIOSYNTHESIS AND STRUCTURE OF CSF-1

The CSF-1 gene is localized to human chromosome 1p13–p21 (Morris *et al.*, 1991; Saltman *et al.*, 1992) and to mouse chromosome 3 at the *op* locus (Buchberg *et al.*, 1989; Gisselbrecht *et al.*, 1989). The human gene is approximately 21 kb in length, comprising 10 exons (Ladner *et al.*, 1987; Kawasaki and Ladner, 1990) (Fig. 1). Alternative mRNA splicing in exon 6 can result in shortened coding regions in CSF-1 mRNAs that affect the processing of the CSF-1 protein precursors they encode (Kawasaki *et al.*, 1985; Ladner *et al.*, 1987; Wong *et al.*, 1987; Cerretti *et al.*, 1988). Alternative use of different 3′ untranslated regions encoded by exon 9 (0.68 kb) and 10 (2 kb) results in further CSF-1 mRNA heterogeneity (Ladner *et al.*, 1987; Wong *et al.*, 1987) (Fig. 1). The exon 10-encoded 3′ untranslated region contains AU-rich sequences, which may confer mRNA instability (Shaw and Kamen, 1986). The 5′ promoter regions of both the human (Ladner *et al.*, 1987) and mouse (Harrington *et al.*, 1991) CSF-1 genes have been cloned and exhibit 80% sequence similarity in the region 450 bp upstream of the transcription start site. Several elements, presumably involved in the regulation of CSF-1 gene expression, are located within this region.

Several human (Fig. 1) and murine cDNAs have been isolated and sequenced (Kawasaki *et al.*, 1985; DeLamarter *et al.*, 1987; Ladner *et al.*, 1987, 1988; Rajavashisth *et al.*, 1987; Wong *et al.*, 1987; Cerretti *et al.*, 1988; Pampfer *et al.*, 1991b). The predicted full-length coding region of the human CSF-1 mRNA (Fig. 2) comprises a 32-amino-acid signal sequence, followed by 522 additional residues which contain four potential N-linked glycosylation sites, a single consensus sequence for glycosaminogly-can addition (acidic residues–Ser–Gly–X–Gly/Ala) at Ser-277 and a hydrophobic stretch of 23 amino acids at residues 464–486 that encodes the transmembrane domain and is followed by a sequence of charged amino acids (Arg–Trp–Arg–Arg–Arg) that apparently functions as a stop transfer (Sabatini *et al.*, 1982) sequence (Kawasaki *et al.*, 1985; Ladner *et al.*, 1987; Wong *et al.*, 1987). Excluding its 32-amino-acid signal sequence, the full-length coding region of the mouse transcript predicts a precursor of 520 amino acids with 59.6% sequence similarity to human CSF-1 and all of the aforementioned features of human CSF-1 (Lander *et al.*, 1988) (Fig. 2). The highest degree of sequence similarity (80.5%) occurs for the *N* terminal residues 1–149, which have been shown to be required for *in vitro* biological activity (Kawasaki and Ladner, 1990). As expected, the cysteine residues involved in intrachain (Cys-7–Cys-90, Cys-48–Cys-139, Cys-102–Cys-146) and interchain, (Cys-31–Cys-31, Cys-157–Cys-157, Cys-159–Cys-159) disulphide bonding in human CSF-1 (Glocker *et al.*, 1993; Wilkins *et al.*, 1993) are highly conserved.

Recent studies of the biosynthesis and secretion of mouse CSF-1 indicate that the secreted forms are homodimeric glycoprotein and proteoglycan molecules (Price *et al.*, 1992). Reinterpretation of earlier data (Heard *et al.*, 1987b; Rettenmier *et al.*, 1987; Manos, 1988; Manos *et al.*, 1988; Rettenmier and Roussel, 1988) on the biosynthesis and secretion of human CSF-1 (Price *et al.*, 1992), as well as more recent work on human CSF-1 (Suzu *et al.*, 1992b), indicates that a significant proportion of the secreted form of human CSF-1, previously thought to be exclusively glycoprotein, is proteoglycan. As shown in Fig. 1, CSF-1 encoded by an mRNA containing a full-length coding region is cotranslationally N-glycosylated in the endoplasmic reticulum. The resulting membrane-spanning precursor rapidly undergoes a dimerization that involves the formation of interchain disulphide bonds (Manos, 1988; Rettenmier and Roussel, 1988). The homodimeric precursor moves to the Golgi, where the N-linked oligosaccharides are converted from high mannose to complex type and O-linked oligosaccharides are added. Among these O-linked oligosaccharides is an 18 000 kDa chondroitin sulphate chain that is added to Ser-277 (human) or Ser-276 (mouse) within the consensus sequence for glycosaminoglycan addition (Price *et al.*, 1992). The secreted forms of the mature CSF-1 are cleaved from the precursor in the secretory vesicle. Depending on whether the proteolytic cleavage takes place on the *N* terminal side or the *C* terminal side of the glycosaminoglycan addition site, they are secreted as either the glycoprotein (80–100 kDa) or proteoglycan (130–160 kDa) forms. These forms rapidly accumulate in the extracellular medium with a half-life of 40 min (Price *et al.*, 1992).

At least three sequenced human CSF-1 cDNAs possess shorter than full-length coding regions due to alternative splicing in exon 6 (Kawasaki *et al.*, 1985; Cerretti *et al.*, 1988; Pampfer *et al.*, 1991b). These clones encode precursor monomers of 224 (CSF-1^{224}) (Kawasaki *et al.*, 1985; Pampfer *et al.*, 1991b) or 406 (CSF-1^{406}) (Cerretti *et al.*, 1988) amino acids in which the amino acids 150–447 and 332–447 have been spliced out (Fig. 1). The expression of CSF-1^{224} differs significantly from the expression and processing of the full-length precursor CSF-1^{522}. CSF-1^{224} encodes a precursor in which the region encoding the proteolytic cleavage sites, the sites for O-linked oligosaccharide addition, including the glycosaminoglycan site, and half the potential N-linked glycosylation sites has been deleted. This molecule, like CSF-1^{522}, is cotranslationally glycosylated in the endoplasmic reticulum, rapidly dimerizes there and then moves to the Golgi, where its N-linked oligosaccharides are converted to complex type. In the secretory vesicle, however, it is not proteolytically cleaved, but instead is expressed as a membrane-spanning protein on the cell surface (Rettenmier *et al.*, 1987). In contrast to the cells expressing CSF-1^{522}, fixed-cell layers expressing CSF-1^{224} stimulate the proliferation of overlayered macrophages, indicating that the membrane-spanning form is biologically active (Stein *et al.*, 1990). Studies in mouse L cells indicate that this form of CSF-1 is stably expressed at the cell surface ($t_{1/2} = 11$ h) (Price *et al.*, 1992) although release of CSF-1 by proteolysis from CSF-1^{224} at the cell surface is greatly stimulated by activation of protein kinase C (Stein and Rettenmier, 1991), a response in which the *C*-terminal Val is likely to be an important determinant (Bosenberg *et al.*, 1992).

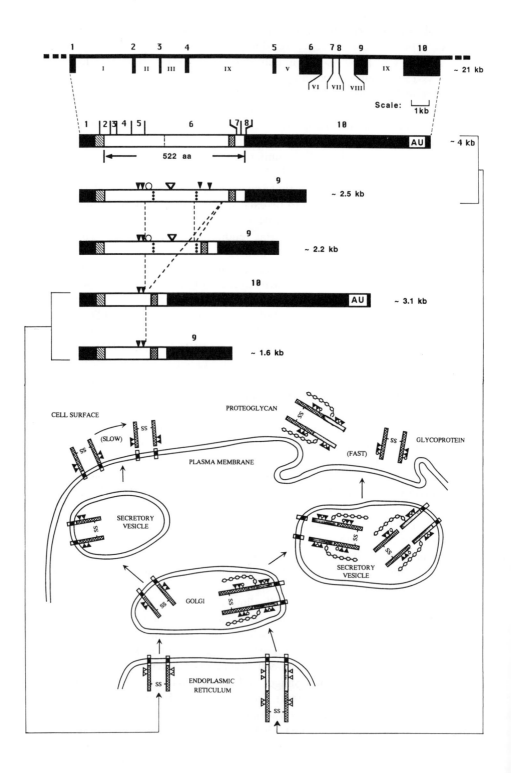

It is not clear how the processing of CSF-1[406] occurs, although it is possible that it encodes the cell-surface form and the secreted glycoprotein form.

A comparison of the extracellular domains of CSF-1[224] with the extracellular domain of stem cell factor reveals a ≈16% identity and a ≈32% sequence similarity, indicating that these dimeric cytokines are related (Bazan, 1991). This region is conserved in all biologically active forms of CSF-1 and is required for *in vitro* biological activity (Heard *et al.*, 1987b; Kawasaki and Ladner, 1990). Its crystal structure (amino acids 4–158) has recently been determined (Pandit *et al.*, 1992) and the structure predicted by Bazan (Bazan, 1991) was confirmed. Despite its lack of sequence similarity with members of the cytokine family, it also possesses a similar four α-helical bundle/anti-parallel β-ribbon structure. The CSF-1 monomer is an antiparallel four α-helical bundle in which the helices run up–up–down–down, similar to the connectivity observed in GM-CSF and growth hormone, yet differing from the more common up–down–up–down connectivity of other four helical bundles (Presnell and Cohen, 1989). The similarity in secondary and tertiary structure between this *N* terminal region of CSF-1 and these two other cytokines is quite remarkable. Differences are in the relative lengths of the helices and the connecting loops and the differences in the disulphide bonds in all three proteins (Pandit *et al.*, 1992). Interestingly, the exon–intron junctions occur at nearly the same positions in the three-dimensional structure of all three, at the end of helix A, at the beginning of helix B, at the end of helix C and the end of helix D (Fig. 2). The CSF-1 dimer is formed by linking two monomers end-to-end, yielding a very flat, elongated structure with dimensions of approximately 80 by 30 by 20 Å (Pandit *et al.*, 1992). As indicated above, there are three intrachain disulphide bonds per monomer and three interchain disulphide bonds that maintain the dimeric state (Glocker *et al.*, 1993; Wilkins *et al.*, 1993). Recent studies indicate that the interchain disulphide bonds are not necessary for activity and that monomeric CSF-1 is biologically active provided the intrachain disulphide bonds remain intact (Krantwald and Baccarini, 1993).

THE BIOSYNTHESIS AND STRUCTURE OF THE CSF-1R

The CSF-1R is encoded by the c-*fms* proto-oncogene product (Sherr *et al.*, 1985; Coussens *et al.*, 1986) and belongs to a family of protein tyrosine kinases that includes the α and β platelet-derived growth factor receptors (PDGFRs) (Yarden *et al.*, 1986) and the c-*kit* proto-oncogene product or SCF receptor (Besmer *et al.*, 1986; Yarden *et al.*, 1987). The human CSF-1R gene is located on chromosome 5q33.3 (Groffen *et al.*, 1983; Roussel *et al.*, 1983; Gimbrone *et al.*, 1989) and is the 3′ neighbour of the gene for

---

Fig. 1. Human CSF-1 genomic organization, transcripts and expression. The top half of the diagram depicts the intron–exon relationships and the five cDNA clones that have been sequenced. Exons (1–10), 5′ and 3′ untranslated regions (filled) and coding region (open), including signal peptide (hatched) and transmembrane domain (crosshatched), are indicated, together with the N-linked (filled arrowheads) and O-linked (open circles) glycosylation sites, the site of glycosaminoglycan addition (open arrowhead) and the approximate intracellular proteolytic cleavage sites (dotted lines). The bottom half of the figure shows the processing of CSF-1 homodimers encoded by both the short and long coding regions. Hatched regions are those present in the mature secreted or released glycoprotein forms while both hatched and open regions are present in the major secreted proteoglycan form. The symbols for glycosylation are as described above except that the glycosaminoglycan chain is shown as linked, open hexagons and the filled region represents the transmembrane domain.

Human CSF-1 [522]
Murine CSF-1 [520]

	Human CSF-1	Murine CSF-1	
-32	Met Thr Ala Pro Gly Ala Ala	* * Arg * * Thr Ala	-26
-25	Gly Arg Cys Pro Pro Thr Thr Trp Leu Gly Ser Leu Leu Leu Leu Val Cys Leu Leu Ala Ser Arg Ser Ile Thr	* * * * Ser Ser His * * * * Arg Asn * * * * * * Met Gln * * Ala Met	-1
1	Glu Glu Val Ser Glu Tyr Cys Ser His Met Ile Gly Ser Gly His Leu Gln Ser Leu Gln Arg Leu Ile Asp Ser	Lys * * * His * * * Ala * * Asn * Arg * * Lys Val * Gln * Asp *	25
26	Gln Met Glu Thr Ser Cys Gln Ile Thr Phe Glu Phe Val Asp Gln Glu Gln Leu Lys Asp Pro Val Cys Tyr Leu	* * Phe * * * * * Ala * Asp * * Glu * * * * Asp *	50
51	Lys Lys Ala Phe Leu Leu Val Gln Asp Ile Met Glu Asp Thr Met Arg Phe Arg Asp Asn Thr Pro Asn Ala Ile	* * * Phe * * * Lys * * * * * * * * Glu His Asp Lys	75
76	Ala Ile Val Gln Leu Gln Glu Leu Ser Leu Arg Leu Lys Ser Cys Phe Thr Lys Asp Tyr Glu Glu His Asp Lys	Thr Glu Arg * Asn * Asn * * Gln Asn	100
101	Ala Cys Val Arg Thr Phe Tyr Glu Thr Pro Leu Gln Leu Leu Glu Lys Val Lys Asn Val Phe Asn Glu Thr Lys	Thr * * * His * * * * * * Ile * Phe *	125
126	Asn Leu Leu Asp Lys Asp Trp Asn Ile Phe Ser Lys Asn Cys Asn Asn Ser Phe Ala Glu Cys Ser Ser Gln Asp	* * Glu * Glu * * Thr * * Thr * Lys Arg	150
151	Val Val Thr Lys Pro Asp Cys Asn Cys Leu Tyr Pro Lys Ala Ile Pro Ser Ser Asp Pro Ala Ser Val Ser Pro	* * * * * * Thr * * * *	175
176	His Gln Pro Leu Ala Pro Ser Met Ala Pro Val Ala Gly Leu Thr Trp Glu Asp Ser Glu Gly Thr Glu Gly Ser	* * Pro Pro * * Leu * Asp Ala Gln Arg	200
201	Ser Leu Leu Pro Gly Glu Gln Pro Leu His Thr Val Asp Pro Gly Ser Ala Lys Gln Arg Pro Pro Arg Ser Thr	Ser * * * Leu Arg Ile Glu Ala	225

Helix A   Helix B   Helix C   Helix D   β1   β2

226	Cys	Gln	Ser	Phe	Glu	Pro	Pro	Glu	Thr	Pro	Val	Val	Lys	Asp	Ser	Thr	Ile	Gly	Gly	Ser	Pro	Gln	Pro	Arg	Pro	250
226	*	*	Thr	Leu	*	Ser	Thr	*	Gln	*	Asn	His	Gly	*	Arg	Leu	Thr	Glu	Asp	*	-	*	*	His	*	249
251	Ser	Val	Gly	Ala	Phe	Asn	Pro	Gly	Met	Glu	Asp	Ile	Leu	Asp	Ser	Ala	Met	Gly	Thr	Asn	Trp	Val	Pro	Glu	Glu	275
250	*	Ala	*	Gly	Pro	Val	*	*	Val	*	*	*	*	Glu	*	Ser	Leu	*	*	*	*	*	Leu	*	*	274
276	Ala	Ser	Gly	Glu	Ala	Ser	Glu	Ile	Pro	Val	Pro	Gln	Gly	Thr	Glu	Leu	Ser	Pro	Ser	Arg	Pro	Gly	Gly	Gly	Ser	300
275	*	*	*	*	*	*	*	Gly	Phe	Leu	Thr	*	Glu	Ala	Lys	Phe	*	*	*	Thr	*	Val	*	*	*	299
301	Met	Gln	Thr	Glu	Pro	Ala	Arg	Pro	Ser	Asn	Phe	Leu	Ser	Ala	Ser	Ser	Pro	Leu	Pro	Ala	Ser	Ala	Lys	Gly	Gln	325
300	Ile	*	Ala	*	Thr	Asp	*	*	-	Arg	Ala	*	*	*	*	-	*	Phe	*	Lys	*	Thr	Glu	Asp	*	322
326	Gln	Pro	Ala	Asp	Val	Thr	Gly	Thr	Ala	Leu	Pro	Arg	Val	Gly	Pro	Val	Arg	Pro	Thr	Gly	Gln	Asp	Trp	Asn	His	350
323	Lys	*	Val	*	Ile	*	Asp ↳2	Arg	Pro	*	Thr	Glu	*	Asn	*	Met	*	*	Ile	*	*	Thr	Gln	*	Asn	347
351	Thr	Pro	Gln	Lys	Thr	Asp	His	Pro	Ser	Ala	Leu	Leu	Arg	Asp	Pro	Pro	Glu	Pro	Gly	Ser	Pro	Arg	Ile	Ser	Ser	375
348	*	*	Glu	*	*	*	Gly	Thr	*	Thr	*	Arg	Glu	*	His	Gln	*	*	*	*	*	His	*	Ala	Thr	372
376	Leu	Arg	Pro	Gln	Gly	Leu	Ser	Asn	Pro	Ser	Thr	Leu	Ser	Ala	Gln	Pro	Gln	Leu	Ser	Arg	Ser	His	Ser	Ser	Gly	400
373	Pro	Asn	*	*	Arg	Val	*	*	Ser	Ala	*	Pro	Val	*	*	Leu	Leu	*	Pro	Lys	*	*	*	Trp	*	397
401	Ser	Val	Leu	Pro	Leu	Gly	Glu	Leu	Glu	Gly	Arg	Arg	Ser	Thr	Arg	Asp	Arg	Arg	Ser	Pro	Ala	Glu	Pro	Glu	Gly	425
398	Ile	*	*	*	*	*	*	*	*	*	Lys	*	*	*	*	*	*	*	*	*	*	*	Leu	*	*	422
426	Gly	Pro	Ala	Ser	Glu	Gly	Ala	Ala	Arg	Pro	Leu	Pro	Arg	Phe	Asn	Ser	Val	Pro	Leu	Thr	Asp	Thr	Gly	His	Glu	450
423	*	Ser	*	*	*	*	*	*	*	*	Val	Ala	*	*	*	*	Ile	*	*	*	*	* 1,2	*	*	Val	447
451	Arg	Gln	Ser	Glu	Gly	Ser	Ser	Ser	Pro	Gln	Leu	Gln	Glu	Ser	Val	Phe	His	Leu	Leu	Val	Pro	Ser	Val	Ile	Leu	475
448	Glu	*	His	*	*	*	*	Asp	*	*	Ile	Pro	*	*	*	*	*	*	*	*	*	Gly	Ile	*	*	472
476	Val	Leu	Leu	Ala	Val	Gly	Gly	Leu	Leu	Phe	Tyr	Arg	Trp	Arg	Arg	Arg	Ser	His	Gln	Glu	Pro	Gln	Arg	Ala	Asp	500
473	*	*	*	Thr	*	*	*	*	*	*	*	Lys	*	Lys	Trp	*	*	*	Arg	Asp	*	*	Thr	Leu	*	497
501	Ser	Pro	Leu	Glu	Gln	Pro	Glu	Gly	Ser	Pro	Leu	Thr	Gln	Asp	-	Asp	Arg	Gln	Val	Glu	Leu	Pro	Val			522
498	*	Ser	Val	Gly	Arg	*	*	Asp	*	Ser	*	*	*	*	Glu	*	*	*	*	*	*	*	*			520

Fig. 2. The primary structure of CSF-1. Predicted amino acid sequences of the human CSF-1^{522} and mouse CSF-1^{520} precursors. In mouse CSF-1^{520}, amino acid identity with the human sequence is indicated by an asterisk. Maximal alignment of sequences was achieved by introducing four gaps, each indicated by a dash. Signal peptide and transmembrane domains are indicated by filled boxes, N-linked glycosylation sites by the open boxes and cysteines involved in the disulphide bonds by dashed open boxes. The consensus sequence for glycosaminoglycan addition (heavy underline) and the four α-helical and two β-pleated regions (overlined) are also shown. Amino acids 150–447 (between arrows numbered 1) and 332–447 (between arrows numbered 2) are deleted in truncated forms that are derived from alternatively spliced mRNAs.

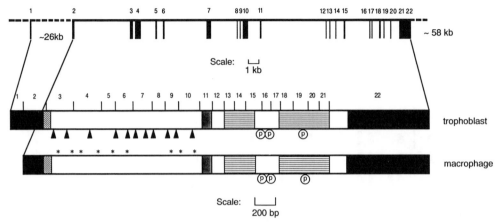

Fig. 3. The human CSF-1R genomic organization and transcripts. The intron–exon relationships of the CSF-1R gene are shown, together with a schematic representation of the mRNAs expressed in placental trophoblasts and macrophages. The untranslated regions (filled), signal sequence (hatched), transmembrane domain (shaded) and interrupted tyrosine kinase catalytic domain (striped) are shown, together with the potential N-linked glycosylation sites (arrowheads), positions of the extracellular cysteine residues (asterisks) and tyrosine phosphorylation sites (P). (Based on Hampe *et al.*, 1989), from Roth and Stanley, 1992.

PDGFR-β (Yarden *et al.*, 1986; Roberts *et al.*, 1988). These genes are juxtaposed head-to-tail, with the CSF-1R promoter located within 0.5 kb of the PDGFR-β polyadenylation signal, raising the possibility that transcription of the former is influenced by transcription of the latter (Roberts *et al.*, 1988). The CSF-1R gene is 58 kb in length and comprises 21 introns and 22 exons (Hampe *et al.*, 1989; reviewed in Sherr, 1990) (Fig. 3). Exon 1 encodes non-translated sequences and is 26 kb upstream of the signal peptide encoding exon 2. CSF-1R gene transcription occurs in a tissue-specific fashion from two distinct promoters. Transcription is initiated upstream of exon 1 in placental trophoblasts. However, in macrophages it is initiated immediately upstream of exon 2 (Visvader and Verma, 1989; Roberts *et al.*, 1992). The receptor possesses a highly glycosylated extracellular ligand-binding domain (493 amino acids) a hydrophobic transmembrane domain (25 amino acids) and an intracellular tyrosine kinase domain (436 amino acids) (Coussens *et al.*, 1986; Rothwell and Rohrschneider, 1987; Hampe *et al.*, 1989; Borycki *et al.*, 1992) (Fig. 4). In line with the other members of this receptor family, the extracellular domain of the CSF-1R is characteristic of members of the immunoglobulin gene superfamily and the tyrosine kinase domain is interrupted by an interkinase domain of 73 amino acids. The *C*-terminal tail of the CSF-1R has been shown to negatively regulate signal transduction in that both human and feline CSF-1Rs mutated in this region exhibit increased transforming activity (Roussel *et al.*, 1987; Woolford *et al.*, 1988) while exchange of this sequence in the v-*fms* viral oncogene product with the c-*fms* encoded sequence decreases transforming activity (Browning *et al.*, 1986).

CSF-1 SIGNAL TRANSDUCTION

Studies of the interaction of [125]-labelled CSF-1 with macrophages at both 4°C and at 37°C (Guilbert and Stanley, 1980, 1986; Guilbert *et al.*, 1986), together with

Sequence alignment of Human CSF-1R and Murine CSF-1R (amino acid residues 1–325). In the Murine row, an asterisk (*) indicates a residue identical to the Human sequence; where a residue is shown, it differs from the Human sequence. Boxed residues denote conserved cysteines (Cys) and potential N-linked glycosylation sites (Asn). Residue numbers for each line are shown at left (start) and right (end).

Line (Human / Murine start)	Sequence	End
Human CSF-1R	Met Gly Pro Gly Val Leu Leu Leu Leu Leu Val Ala Thr Ala Trp His Gly Gln Gly Ile Pro Val Ile Glu Pro	25
Murine CSF-1R	Glu Leu * Pro * * * * * Val * Val * * * * * * * * Ala * * * *	25
26 Human	Ser Val Pro Glu Leu Val Val Lys Pro Gly Ala Thr Val Thr Leu Arg Cys Val Gly Asn Gly Ser Val Glu Trp	50
26 Murine	* Gly * Ala * * * * * * Ser * * Thr * * * * Ile * Ser * * Arg Thr	50
51 Human	Asp Gly Pro Pro Ser Pro His Trp Thr Leu Tyr Ser Asp Gly Ser Ser Ser Ile Leu Ser Thr Asn Asn Ala Thr	75
51 Murine	* * Ala * * Ala * * * * * Thr Thr * * * Gly * * * * * Thr Thr *	75
76 Human	Phe Gln Asn Thr Gly Thr Tyr Arg Cys Thr Glu Pro Gly Asp Pro Leu Gly Gly Ser Ala Ala Ile His Leu Tyr	100
76 Murine	* Lys * * * * * * * * * Met * Glu Glu * * * * Thr Thr Ala Thr Leu Val	100
101 Human	Val Lys Asp Pro Ala Arg Pro Trp Asn Val Leu Ala Gln Glu Val Val Val Phe Glu Asp Gln Asp Ala Leu Leu	125
101 Murine	* * * * * * * * * * Met * * * * * Gln Gln Gly Gly Ala Glu Asp Gln Val	125
126 Human	Pro Cys Leu Leu Thr Asp Pro Val Leu Glu Ala Gly Val Ser Leu Val Arg Val Arg Gly Arg Pro Leu Met Arg	150
126 Murine	* * Leu Ile * * * Ala * Lys Asp * Ser * * * Met * Gly Gly Arg Gln Val Leu *	150
151 Human	His Thr Asn Tyr Ser Phe Ser Pro Trp His Gly Phe Thr Ile His Arg Ala Lys Phe Ile Gln Ser Gln Asp Tyr	175
151 Murine	Lys Val Asn Val Phe * * * Arg Arg * Val Ser * * * Lys * Val Leu * Asn Asp Thr Thr	175
176 Human	Gln Cys Ser Ala Leu Met Gly Gly Arg Lys Val Met Ser Ile Ser Ile Arg Leu Lys Val Gln Lys Val Ile Pro	200
176 Murine	Val Val Lys Thr Met Thr Thr Trp * Arg * Ile * * Gly * * Glu Thr * * Asn Lys Arg His	200
201 Human	Gly Pro Pro Ala Leu Thr Leu Val Pro Ala Glu Leu Val Arg Ile Arg Gly Glu Ala Ala Gln Ile Val Cys Ser	225
201 Murine	* Glu Gln * * * Lys * Glu * * Ser * Arg Arg * * * * * * Pro Gln Val Ser	225
226 Human	Ala Ser Ser Val Asp Val Asn Phe Asp Val Phe Leu Gln His Asn Asn Thr Lys Leu Ala Ile Pro Gln Gln Ser	250
226 Murine	* Thr Asn Ala Glu * * * * Ile Lys * * * Asn Asn Asp Arg Gly * * Glu Leu Asn *	250
251 Human	Asp Phe His Asn Asn Arg Tyr Gln Lys Val Leu Thr Leu Asn Leu Asp Gln Val Asp Phe Gln His Ala Gly Asn	275
251 Murine	* Phe His Gln Asp * Tyr Gln Lys Lys Arg Tyr * * Ser Thr Ala * Asn Ala * Met Phe Arg Gln	275
276 Human	Tyr Ser Cys Val Ala Ser Asn Val Gln Gly Lys His Ser Thr Ser Met Phe Phe Arg Val Val Glu Ser Ala Tyr	300
276 Murine	* Ser Cys Val Ala Ala * * Asp Gln Gln Gly Ser Gln Gln * * Phe Arg Asn Gly Glu Val Ala Tyr	300
301 Human	Leu Asn Leu Ser Glu Gln Gly Leu Leu Asn Leu Asp Gly Val Lys Leu Asn Ile Ser Gly Val Val Lys Met Val	325
301 Murine	* Asn Ser Thr Thr * Ser Asn Asn Asn Ser Tyr Ala Glu * * Ala Asp Gly * * Thr Lys His Ala	325

Protein sequence alignment (two sequences). Three-letter amino acid codes; "*" marks identical residues; boxed/shaded regions highlight conserved motifs. Left numbers = block start, right numbers = block end for each sequence pair.

Start	Sequence (top / bottom, * = identity)	End
326 / 326	Glu Ala Tyr Pro Gly Leu Gln Gly Phe Asn Trp Thr Tyr Leu Pro Phe Ser Asp His Gln Pro Glu Pro Lys / Asp · · · Ser Ile · His Tyr (boxed Asn Trp Thr) · · · · Phe Glu Asp · – · Arg ·	350 / 348
351 / 349	Leu Ala Asn Ala Thr Thr Lys Asp Tyr Arg Thr Phe Leu Ser Phe / · Glu Phe Ile · Gln Arg Ala · · Lys Phe · Ala ·	375 / 373
376 / 374	Ala Gly Arg Tyr Ser Phe Leu Arg Asn Pro Gly Ala Leu Thr Phe / · · Gln · Phe Leu Met · Gln Lys Ala · · · Asn	400 / 398
401 / 399	Pro Pro Glu Glu Val Val Ser Val Ile Trp Phe Thr Gly Asn Gly Thr Gly Leu Leu Val Ala Ala Ser Cys / · · · · · · · Thr Met Pro · Asp Val Asp · Phe	425 / 423
426 / 424	Gln Pro Asn Val Thr Trp Leu Cys Ser Gly His Thr Asp Arg Cys Gly Ala Gln Val Gln Leu Ala / · · Ser · · Met Glu · Arg · · · His Asp · ·	450 / 448
451 / 449	Asp Asp Pro Tyr Pro Glu Gln Leu Ser Val Thr His Lys Val Thr Val Leu Ser Leu Leu Thr Val Glu / Asn · Thr His · · · Asp · Ile Ile · · Gln Pro · Ile Gly	475 / 473
476 / 474	Thr Leu Glu His Thr Gln Tyr Glu Cys Arg Asn His Pro Pro Asp Gly Ser Asn Ser Val Val Ala Trp Ala Phe Ile Pro	500 / 498
	· Lys · · · Met Phe · · Lys · · · · · · Asn Ser · · Gln Tyr · Arg	
501 / 499	Ile Ser Ala Gly Ala His Thr His Pro Pro Asp Glu Phe Leu Ser Phe Thr Pro Val Val Ala Cys Met Ser Ile / Val · · · Gln Ser Lys · Leu · Ser · · ·	525 / 523
526 / 524	Met Ala Leu Leu Leu Leu Leu Leu Leu Leu Tyr Lys Tyr Gln Lys Pro Lys Tyr Asn Pro Thr Gln Val Arg Trp / · Ser · · Val · · · · · · · · · · ·	550 / 548
551 / 549	Lys Ile Glu Tyr Ser Gly Asn Ser Tyr Thr Phe Ile Asp Pro Thr Gln Leu Pro Tyr Asn Glu Lys Trp / · · · · · · · · · · · · ·	575 / 573
576 / 574	Glu Phe Pro Arg Asn Leu Gln Phe Gly Lys Thr Leu Gly Ala Phe Ala Gly Phe Lys Val Val Glu Ala Thr / · · · · · · · · · · · · · ·	600 / 598
601 / 599	Ala Phe Gly Glu Leu Asp Ala Val Lys Val Ala Val (616) Lys Met Leu Lys Ser Thr Ala His Ala Asp / · · · · · · · · · Ile · · ·	625 / 623
626 / 624	Glu Lys Ala Leu Met Ser Glu Lys Leu Lys Ile Met Ser His His Gly Leu Gln His Val Asn Ile Leu / · · · · · · · · · · · ·	650 / 648

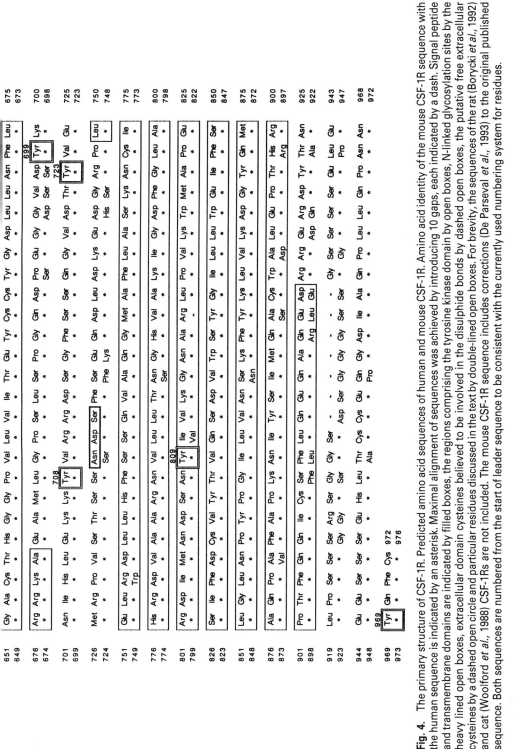

Fig. 4. The primary structure of CSF-1R. Predicted amino acid sequences of human and mouse CSF-1R. Amino acid identity of the mouse CSF-1R sequence with the human sequence is indicated by an asterisk. Maximal alignment of sequences was achieved by introducing 10 gaps, each indicated by a dash. Signal peptide and transmembrane domains are indicated by filled boxes, the regions comprising the tyrosine kinase domain by open boxes, N-linked glycosylation sites by the heavy lined open boxes, extracellular domain cysteines believed to be involved in the disulphide bonds by dashed open boxes, the putative free extracellular cysteines by a dashed open circle and particular residues discussed in the text by double-lined open boxes. For brevity, the sequences of the rat (Borycki *et al.*, 1992) and cat (Woolford *et al.*, 1988) CSF-1Rs are not included. The mouse CSF-1R sequence includes corrections (De Parseval *et al.*, 1993) to the original published sequence. Both sequences are numbered from the start of leader sequence to be consistent with the currently used numbering system for residues.

crosslinking studies (Morgan and Stanley, 1984), demonstrated that there is a single class of high-affinity receptor sites through which all the biological effects of CSF-1 are mediated. Early studies had also shown that CSF-1 exerts pleiotropic effects, e.g. survival, proliferation, differentiation, on mononuclear phagocytes (reviewed in Stanley *et al.*, 1983). Rapid, visible responses of macrophages to CSF-1 include plasma membrane ruffling, filopodia formation, the appearance of vesicles, reorganization of the actin cytoskeleton, cell spreading (1 min) and vacuole formation (5 min) (Tushinski *et al.*, 1982; Boocock *et al.*, 1989). The stimulation of ruffling and vesicle formation is associated with the rapid stimulation of pinocytosis and solute flow through the endocytic compartment (Tushinski *et al.*, 1982; Racoosin and Swanson, 1989, 1992; Knight *et al.*, 1992). CSF-1 stimulation causes other rapid changes, including increased protein tyrosine phosphorylation (Downing *et al.*, 1988; Sengupta *et al.*, 1988), enhanced Na^+/H^+ antiport and Na^+/K-ATPase activities (Vairo and Hamilton, 1985; Hartmann *et al.*, 1990; Vairo *et al.*, 1990), an increased rate of glucose uptake (Hamilton *et al.*, 1986, 1988; Rist *et al.*, 1990), an increased rate of protein synthesis (Tushinski and Stanley, 1983) and an inhibition of the rate of protein degradation (Tushinski and Stanley, 1983; Morgan *et al.*, 1987). Early reports with impure cell and/or growth factor preparations suggested that CSF-1-induced cyclooxygenase activity resulted in an observed increase in prostaglandin E_2 production (Kurland *et al.*, 1979; Orlandi *et al.*, 1989). However, subsequent experiments have indicated that CSF-1 inhibits prostaglandin E_2 production (Jackowski *et al.*, 1990; Puri *et al.*, 1992). Other responses are the increased expression of the mRNAs for c-*myc*, c-*fos*, (Müller *et al.*, 1985; Orlofsky and Stanley, 1987) and c-*fgr* (Willman *et al.*, 1987), proto-oncogenes, and for the KC and JE genes (Orlofsky and Stanley, 1987). CSF-1 has been shown to increase the urokinase-type plasminogen activator mRNA and enzyme activity of macrophages (Lin and Gordon, 1979; Hamilton *et al.*, 1980, 1991), an effect which could be mediated by protein kinase C and phospholipase C (Hamilton *et al.*, 1991). CSF-1-induced monocyte and macrophage proliferation has been shown to be a pertussis toxin-sensitive event (Imamura and Kufe, 1988; Ball *et al.*, 1990; Imamura *et al.*, 1990). Pertussis-sensitive G-proteins have been implicated as mediators of the CSF-1-induced Na^+ influx (Imamura and Kufe, 1988) which, although apparently not involved in early responses (increases in protein synthetic rate, *fos* and *myc* mRNAs), appears to be required in late G1 for entry of mouse macrophages into S-phase (Vairo *et al.*, 1990).

CSF-1 stimulation of macrophages is not associated with hydrolysis of inositol lipids (Whetton *et al.*, 1986; Hamilton *et al.*, 1989; Imamura *et al.*, 1990) and the failure of CSF-1 to alter intracellular Ca^{++} (Whetton *et al.*, 1986; Cook *et al.*, 1989) is consistent with its failure to stimulate inositol phosphate turnover and the failure of Ca^{++} ionophores to mimic many CSF-1 responses of the macrophage (Hamilton *et al.*, 1989, 1991). However, elevated 1,2-diacylglycerol (DAG) turnover, possibly mediated via phospholipase C (PLC) phosphatidyl-choline (PC) hydrolysis and/or the combined activities of phospholipase D and phosphatidate phosphohydrolase has been reported for CSF-1-stimulated human monocytes (Imamura *et al.*, 1990) and mouse bone-marrow derived macrophages but not for resident peritoneal macrophages, which exhibit a poor proliferative response (Veis and Hamilton, 1991). Within 15 min of stimulation of the mouse macrophage cell line, BAC1.2F5, CSF-1 causes a four-fold elevation in the levels of CTP:phosphocholine cytidylyltransferase, the rate-controlling enzyme for PC biosynthesis in these cells (Tessner *et al.*, 1991); related studies indicate that PC hydrolysis and c-*myc* expression are in collaborating mitogenic pathways activated by CSF-1 (Xu *et al.*, 1993). CSF-1 also activates protein kinase C (PKC) in monocytes (Imamura *et al.*, 1990) and recent studies indicate that CSF-1 stimulates PC hydrolysis in human monocytes by inducing cytoplasmic phospholipase A_2 activity (Nakamura *et al.*, 1992). Additional evidence for a role of PKC in CSF-1 signal transduction is supported by studies in which phorbol esters acutely elicit similar responses, chronically inhibit such responses and are themselves weakly mitogenic (Vairo and Hamilton, 1991).

Several of the early events discussed above, such as the induction of Na^+/H^+ exchange and activation of PKC, appear to be necessary for the proliferative response since their inhibition leads to inhibition of cell entry into S-phase. However, none of the early events appear to be sufficient for mitogenesis, consistent with the requirement for CSF-1 to be present throughout the entire G1 period for the entry of macrophages into S phase (Tushinski and Stanley, 1985).

Kinetic studies of the very early CSF-1-induced changes in the CSF-1R and of protein tyrosine phosphorylation have been carried out utilizing the CSF-1-dependent mouse macrophage cell line BAC1.2F5 (Morgan *et al.*, 1987). BAC1-2F5 cells possess ≈120 000 CSF-1R per cell, exhibit a strong proliferative responsive to CSF-1 and a weaker proliferative response to GM-CSF (Morgan and Stanley, 1984; Morgan *et al.*, 1987). Like bone marrow-derived macrophages, BAC1.2F5 cells exhibit rapid morphological changes that are apparent within 60 s of stimulation (Tushinski *et al.*, 1982; Boocock *et al.*, 1989). However, they have the additional advantage that somatic cell genetic approaches can be used in studies of CSF-1 signal transduction (Dello Sbarba *et al.*, 1991; Pollard *et al.*, 1991). Within 60 s of its addition to BAC1.2F5 macrophages at 37°C, CSF-1 causes changes in the CSF-1R and stimulates the tyrosine phosphorylation of several proteins (Downing *et al.*, 1988; Sengupta *et al.*, 1988). Since these changes are also observed over a longer time-interval (≈180 min) at 4°C (Sengupta *et al.*, 1988), lower temperature studies utilizing high ligand concentrations have been carried out in order to establish the kinetic relationships between these early events. In contrast to the situation at 37°C, at 4°C the binding of CSF-1 to the receptor is irreversible and the receptor–ligand complex fails to be internalized (Stanley and Guilbert, 1981; Guilbert *et al.*, 1986; Guilbert and Stanley, 1986). As shown in Fig. 5, prior to exposure to CSF-1 the receptors are apparently either aggregated or undergoing rapid dimer–monomer interconversion. Addition of CSF-1 at concentrations that saturate binding sites within 1 min causes either noncovalent dimerization of monomeric receptors or stabilizes noncovalent dimeric forms and leads, presumably by the transphosphorylation of one kinase domain by another (Lee and Nienhuis, 1990; Otsuka *et al.*, 1990; Roussel *et al.*, 1990c), to an initial wave of CSF-1R tyrosine phosphorylation, which is complete by 2–5 min at 4°C (Baccarini *et al.*, 1991; Li and Stanley, 1991). This is followed by the tyrosine phosphorylation of a group of primarily cytoplasmic proteins, which appear in a particular order (Sengupta *et al.*, 1988; Li and Stanley, 1991; Li *et al.*, 1991). The concentration of these phosphoproteins is maximal by 45 min, but significantly earlier, as their rate of appearance slows, extracellular covalent linkage of monomeric units of the 380-kDa CSF-1R homodimers occurs via disulphide bonds. This covalent linkage of the 380-kDa CSF-1R homodimer leads to the formation, by 90 min at 4°C, of a 450 kDa heterodimer comprising the 165-kDa CSF-1R monomer and a modified 215 kDa or

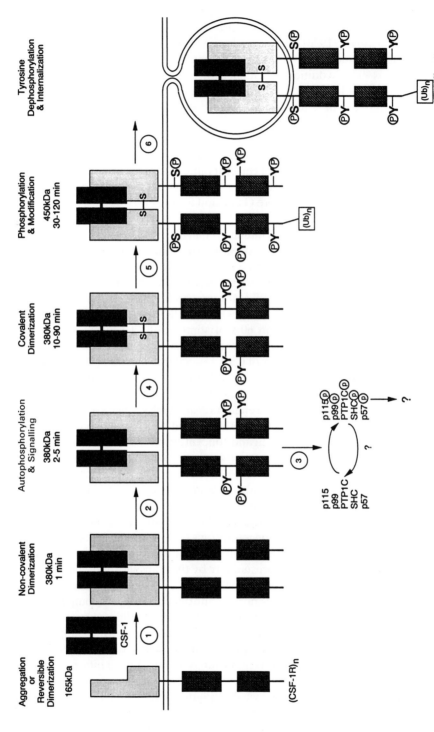

Fig. 5. Schematic representation of the ligand-induced changes in CSF-1R prior to internalization of the receptor–ligand complex. Six steps and the times of their duration at 4°C are depicted. The exact locations of the phosphorylation (encircled P) and polyubiquitination ((Ub)$_n$) sites associated with the various steps are unknown. The noncovalently associated 450 kDa heterodimer is not shown but its appearance is coincident with the appearance of the covalently associated 450 kDa heterodimer.

250 kDa form which remains either cthe ovalently or noncovalently associated (Li and Stanley, 1991). Experiments in this and the PDGF system indicate that this modification is the result of polyubiquitination of the cytoplasmic domain (Mori *et al.*, 1992), which is apparently required for its degradation following internalization of the receptor–ligand complex. At the time of the conversion of the 380-kDa CSF-1 homodimer to the 450-kDa heterodimer, there is a further increase in CSF-1R tyrosine and serine phosphorylation (Baccarini *et al.*, 1991; Li and Stanley, 1991). Thus, the transient existence of the noncovalent 380 kDa homodimeric form of the receptor is temporally correlated with the period of active receptor signalling (cytoplasmic protein tyrosine phosphorylation). Furthermore, studies at 37°C indicate that the subsequently modified heterodimeric form of the receptor is selectively internalized. Consistent with these observations, pretreatment of the cells with the alkylating agent iodoacetic acid prevents formation of the disulphide-bonded 380 kDa homodimer, causing an eight fold increase in the cellular protein tyrosine phosphorylation and inhibiting internalization (Li and Stanley, 1991). These studies suggest that ligand–induced noncovalent CSF-1 receptor-kinase is the active signalling form, whereas the extracellular disulphide bond formation and subsequent modifications lead to kinase inactivation, phosphotyrosine dephosphorylation (and internalization) and internalization and destruction of the receptor–ligand complex.

Mouse 3T3 cells expressing the human CSF-1R exhibit CSF-1-dependent anchorage-independent growth (Roussel *et al.*, 1987). This system, and others in which the mouse or feline CSF-1Rs are expressed in rat fibroblasts (Roussel *et al.*, 1988; Woolford *et al.*, 1988; Van der Geer and Hunter, 1991), have been used to study CSF-1-regulated cell proliferation. Fibroblasts produce CSF-1, but high concentrations of mouse and cat CSF-1 are unable to bind the human CSF-1R and binding to the feline CSF-1R is only observed at very high concentrations of mouse CSF-1. The disadvantage of these systems is that although many of the components of the pathways regulating proliferation in the macrophage and the fibroblast are shared, there may well be differences in how cell proliferation is regulated in these two cell types. In addition, the heterologous nature of these systems (human/mouse, cat/rat or mouse/rat) may significantly alter the complicated processes involved. Finally, these systems obviously provide no information on the CSF-1 regulation of macrophage-specific pathways and the interaction of receptors with macrophage-specific cell components. However, the advantage of being able to examine the action of genetically engineered CSF-1R in fibroblasts has provided valuable information about CSF-1R structure–function relationships. Furthermore, by expressing the mouse CSF-1R in CSF-1R-less mouse haemopoietic cell lines homologous systems have been created in which CSF-1-regulated proliferation and differentiation can be studied (Rohrschneider and Metcalf, 1989; Kato and Sherr, 1990).

Extracellular domain mutations of the CSF-1R, in some cases in the context of a C-terminal truncation (Woolford *et al.*, 1988) constitutively activate the kinase, resulting in ligand-independent transformation (Roussel *et al.*, 1988; Van Daalen Wetters *et al.*, 1992). In at least one case, the substitution of serine for leucine at codon 301 in the human CSF-1R, the mutation did not affect ligand affinity, but altered enzyme activity, suggesting that mutations may result in changes in the extracellular domain that somehow mimic the ligand-induced changes in wild-type receptors. Consistent with the induction of a conformational change(s), only certain amino acid substitutions at codon 301 are transforming (Roussel *et al.*, 1990a) and novel activating mutations have been identified within sequences separating the third and fourth immunoglobulin-like loops (Van Daalen Wetters *et al.*, 1992).

Analysis of cells coexpressing kinase negative and active forms of the receptor (Ohtsuka *et al.*, 1990), together with evidence for ligand-induced dimerization (Li and Stanley, 1991), suggest that the initial ligand-induced tyrosine phosphorylation of the CSF-1R is due to autophosphorylation involving the phosphorylation of one kinase domain by the other within the ligand-induced homodimer. Although it appears that not all of the CSF-1R tyrosine phosphorylation sites have been discovered (Downing *et al.*, 1991), several have been identified and their requirement for signal transduction has been investigated using site-directed mutagenesis. Those mapped include Tyr-697 and Tyr-706 in the kinase insert domain and Tyr-807 in the kinase domain of the mouse CSF-1R (Tapley *et al.*, 1990; Van der Geer and Hunter, 1990). These correspond to Tyr-699, Tyr-708 and Tyr-809 in the human CSF-1R. It seems likely that Tyr-721 (mouse) is also a site (Downing *et al.*, 1991; Carlberg *et al.*, 1991). In contrast to other receptor kinases, in which the binding of proteins containing *src* homology region 2 (SH2) is believed to be important for intracellular signalling (Pawson and Gish, 1992), the tyrosine-phosphorylated CSF-1R does not appear to physically associate with many other intracellular signalling molecules. In macrophages, the activated CSF-1R has been shown to bind phosphatidylinositol 3'-kinase (PI3K) (Varticovski *et al.*, 1989) and it has also recently been claimed to associate with *src* family kinases (Courtneidge *et al.*, 1993), but it does not stably associate with phospholipase C-γ (Downing *et al.*, 1989a), RAF-1 (Baccarini *et al.*, 1990), rasGAP (Reedijk *et al.*, 1990), protein tyrosine phosphatase 1C (Yeung *et al.*, 1992) or other proteins that can be labelled with ^{35}S-methionine or ^{32}P-phosphate (Baccarini and Stanley, unpublished observations). The association of PI3K appears to be mediated via tyrosine phosphorylation site(s) in the kinase insert domain (Reedijk *et al.*, 1990; Shurtleff *et al.*, 1990). Studies indicate that the region defined by residues 701–721 at least partly overlap the PI3K binding site (Downing *et al.*, 1991), that phosphorylation of the putative Tyr-723 site (human CSF-1R) is necessary (Downing *et al.*, 1991; Sherr, 1991; Van der Geer and Hunter, 1991; Reedijk *et al.*, 1992), that a minority of the tyrosine-phosphorylated receptors stably associate with PI3K (Downing *et al.*, 1991) and that association is mediated by the SH2 domains of the noncatalytic p85α subunit of PI3K (McGlade *et al.*, 1992; Reedijk *et al.*, 1992). Since CSF-1R mutants lacking the entire kinase insert domain can still induce cell proliferation (Taylor *et al.*, 1989; Reedijk *et al.*, 1990; Shurtleff *et al.*, 1990), it seems unlikely that association of PI3K with the activated CSF-1R is necessary for mitogenicity.

In contrast, phosphorylation of Tyr-809 (human) or Tyr-807 (mouse) is important for the mitogenic response (Roussel *et al.*, 1990b; Van der Geer and Hunter, 1991). The Phe-809 mutant exhibited only partially impaired tyrosine kinase activity, CSF-1-dependent association with PI3K and induction of c-*fos* and *jun*B mRNAs, but was unable to mediate a mitogenic response (Roussel *et al.*, 1990b) or induction of c-*myc* mRNA (Roussel *et al.*, 1991). The Phe-807 mutant exhibited a 40–60% decrease in kinase activity, and two- to threefold decrease in CSF-1R phosphorylation, whereas CSF-1R association with PI3K and induction of the mRNAs for c-*fos*, c-*jun* and *egr*-1 were indistinguishable from those mediated by wild-type receptors (Van der Geer and Hunter, 1991). However, both the growth rate in response to CSF-1 and the CSF-1-induced morphological responses were also significantly reduced in cells expressing this mutant receptor. Interestingly, in cells expressing the Phe-809 mutation, which were unable to maximally induce expression of c-*myc* mRNA in response to CSF-1, CSF-1-induced mitogenesis is rescued by constitutive expression of the c-*myc* (Roussel *et al.*, 1991) or c-*ets*-2 genes (Langer *et al.*, 1992). On the basis of these results, it has been suggested that there is a bifurcation of CSF-1-induced effector signals at the immediate postreceptor level, with one arm targeting c-*fos/jun* B in the other c-*ets*/c-*myc* (Roussel *et al.*, 1991; Langer *et al.*, 1992). Studies with the Phe-706 and Gly-706 mutations in the mouse CSF-1R support this concept since the induction of c-fos, c-jun and egr-1 were differentially decreased in cells expressing these mutant receptors (Van der Geer and Hunter, 1991), while other aspects of the response were essentially wild type. One caveat concerning this interpretation is that there is some loss of receptor kinase activity and a decrease in the degree of protein tyrosine phosphorylation in cells expressing both the Phe-809 and the Phe-807 mutations, and various arms of the response might be differentially sensitive to quantitative changes in receptor kinase activity.

The 40 C-terminal amino acids in the normal CSF-1R are replaced by 11 unrelated amino acids in the feline v-*fms* gene product, deleting a region containing a C-terminal tyrosine, Tyr-969 (Coussens *et al.*, 1986). Coexpression of human CSF-1R bearing Phe-969 with human CSF-1 in mouse NIH 3T3 cells significantly increases the transforming potential of the CSF-1R (Roussel *et al.*, 1987), raising the possibility that phosphorylation at Tyr-969 negatively regulates receptor kinase activity in a manner analogous to the phosphorylation of Tyr-527 in the c-*src* gene product (Cooper *et al.*, 1986). However, there is no evidence that the equivalent tyrosine in the mouse CSF-1R (Tyr-973) is phosphorylated following CSF-1 stimulation (Van der Geer and Hunter, 1990), which suggests that Tyr-973 might simply be conformationally important for negative regulation by the CSF-1R tail.

In the absence of CSF-1, the CSF-1R turns over with a half-life of 3–4 h (Rettenmier *et al.*, 1987), whereas the ligand-induced internalization and intracellular degradation of both ligand and receptor leads to a dramatically shorter half-life (Guilbert and Stanley, 1986; Rettenmier *et al.*, 1987; Downing *et al.*, 1988). Studies with mutated receptors indicate that neither the kinase activity of the CSF-1R nor the interkinase domain appear to be necessary for its ligand-induced internalization, but that both are required for ligand-induced degradation (Downing *et al.*, 1989b; Carlberg *et al.*, 1991). Since mutation of the major sites of tyrosine autophosphorylation in the kinase insert region failed to affect CSF-1R degradation (Carlberg *et al.*, 1991), with the exception of Tyr-721 (mouse) which was not tested, one possible interpretation is that ligand-induced degradation of the CSF-1R requires tyrosine phosphorylation of a non CSF-1R protein and the kinase insert region may be necessary for recognition of this substrate.

The macrophage proteins that are rapidly phosphorylated on tyrosine in response to CSF-1 are primarily cytoplasmic (Sengupta *et al.*, 1988), as a group represent only 0.1% of the total cytosolic fraction and are tyrosine phosphorylated in a particular order (Li *et al.*, 1991). One of them, p120 (Downing and Reynolds, 1991), is also tyrosine phosphorylated in pp60^{src}-transformed cells and is related to the cadherin-binding factors, b-catenin, plakoglobin and *armadillo* (Reynolds *et al.*, 1992). Efficient purification procedures for mouse macrophage phospho-tyrosyl proteins of 70 000 kDa or less have been developed (Yeung *et al.*, 1992) and two SH2-domain-containing proteins, protein tyrosine phosphatase-1C (PTP-1C) (Shen *et al.*, 1991) and a protein with a collagen-related sequence, SHC (Pelicci *et al.*, 1992), were identified by direct sequencing (Yeung *et al.*, 1992; Yeung, Lee and Stanley, unpublished observations). PTP-1C, which is selectively expressed in epithelial and haemopoietic cells (Yi *et al.*, 1992), is of particular interest because the specific activity of the tyrosine phosphorylated enzyme is several-fold higher than that of the unphosphorylated enzyme (Berg, Einstein and Stanley, in preparation) and because an inactivating mutation in the PTP-1C gene is responsible for the recessive mouse mutation, motheaten (*me*) (Tsui *et al.*, 1993; Shultz *et al.*, 1993). An important aspect of the phenotype of the *me/me* mouse is the accumulation of macrophages in the periphery (Shultz, 1988). Thus, this observation coupled with the tyrosine phosphorylation and increased activity of PTP-1C in macrophages in response to CSF-1 is consistent with PTP-1C playing an important negative regulatory role in CSF-1-mediated macrophage survival, proliferation or differentiation. The identification of SHC and PTP-1C, proteins with important roles in signal transduction, demonstrates that direct sequencing of tyrosine phosphorylated macrophage proteins will be useful in the future identification of proteins involved early in CSF-1 signal transduction.

In macrophages, RAF-1, which is phosphorylated on serine and activated in response to CSF-1 (Baccarini *et al.*, 1990), is important for the proliferative response. Interestingly, however, the phosphorylation and activation of MAP kinase is not regulated by RAF-1 and is, kinetically, an earlier event than the phosphorylation of RAF-1 (Büscher *et al.*, 1993). Studies in CSF-1R-expressing NIH 3T3 cells indicate that the CSF-1-induced cell transformation requires activation of the c-*ras* protein (Bortner *et al.*, 1991), which leads to induction of the *ets* transcription factors and the *myc* gene product (Langer *et al.*, 1992). Further downstream are two cyclin genes originally termed cyclin-like genes 1 (CYL1) and 2 (CYL2) (Matsushime *et al.*, 1991) and now referred to as the D cyclins, that are regulated by CSF-1 in macrophages during G1 and whose expression may be necessary for entry of cells into S phase. Cyclin D1 and protein are maximally expressed at 6 h after stimulation and remain elevated throughout the remainder of the cell cycle, despite the fact that Cyclin D1 is apparently not required for late S, G2 or M phase. Cyclin D2 mRNA is increased during mid-G1, is maximally expressed at the G1–S interface and is degraded during early S-phase. During G1, both Cyclin D gene products form complexes with $p34^{cdc2}$-like polypeptides, suggesting that they function as regulatory subunits of serine kinases that are involved in growth-factor regulated cell-cycle progression (Matsushime *et al.*, 1991).

THE BIOLOGY OF CSF-1 AND ITS RECEPTOR

Cellular Sources of CSF-1

CSF-1 is synthesized by a variety of different types of normal cell, including endothelial cells (Seelentag *et al.*, 1987), fibroblasts (Tushinski *et al.*, 1982), bone-marrow stromal cells (Lanotte *et al.*, 1982; Fibbe *et al.*, 1988), osteoblasts (Elford *et al.*, 1987), thymic epithelial cells (Le *et al.*, 1988), keratinocytes (Chodakewitz *et al.*, 1990), astrocytes (Théry *et al.*, 1990), myoblasts (Leibovitch *et al.*, 1989), mesothelial cells (Demetri *et al.*, 1989), liver parenchymal cells (Tsukui *et al.*, 1992) and by uterine epithelial cells (Pollard *et al.*, 1987) during pregnancy. Its synthesis is stimulated following the activation of several other cell types including monocytes (Haskill *et al.*, 1987;

Horiguchi *et al.*, 1987; Rambaldi *et al.*, 1987; Horiguchi *et al.*, 1988; Lu *et al.*, 1988; Oster *et al.*, 1988), endothelial cells (Seelentag *et al.*, 1987), T lymphocytes (Cerdan *et al.*, 1990), B lymphocytes (Reisbach *et al.*, 1989), fibroblasts (Henschler *et al.*, 1990) and mesangial cells (Mori *et al.*, 1990). It is synthesized by several leukaemic and lymphoma-cell lines and by adenocarcinomas of the lung, pancreas, breast, ovary and endometrium (reviewed in Roth and Stanley, 1992).

Regulation of Mononuclear Phagocytes by CSF-1

CSF-1 was initially defined as a macrophage colony stimulating factor (Stanley, 1979; Das *et al.*, 1980; Das *et al.*, 1981) or macrophage growth factor (Stanley *et al.*, 1976). While its action is now clearly not limited to mononuclear phagocytes, these cells, including osteoclast precursors, represent the major target population. In haemopoietic and lymphoid tissues, the CSF-1R is exclusively expressed on mononuclear phagocytic cells (Guilbert and Stanley, 1980; Byrne *et al.*, 1981). In cultures of primary bone-marrow-derived macrophages that have been incubated overnight in the absence of CSF-1, each macrophage possesses $\approx 5 \times 10^4$ cell-surface receptors (Guilbert and Stanley, 1986). By comparison, more primitive cells express fewer cell surface CSF-1R (Byrne *et al.*, 1981; Bartelmez *et al.*, 1985) and very primitive haemopoietic cells, that are precursors of the determined but undifferentiated mononuclear phagocyte precursors possess only 2×10^3 cell surface receptors per cell (Bartelmez and Stanley, 1985) (Fig. 1). *In vivo*, circulating monocytes are noncycling cells. However, in the mouse, monocytes and their precursors, macrophage precursor cells, monoblast and promonocytes are all capable of forming macrophage colonies in the presence of CSF-1 with very high plating efficiency. Macrophages that are recently derived from monocytes possess a slightly reduced plating efficiency, while resident tissue macrophage populations have relatively poor plating efficiencies, containing many macrophages that are incapable of proliferating in response to CSF-1 (Stanley *et al.*, 1978, 1983; Chen *et al.*, 1979). In contrast to mouse mononuclear phagocytes, human mononuclear phagocytes generally exhibit a poorer proliferative response to CSF-1 (Das *et al.*, 1981) and the proliferative response of monocytes and macrophages is virtually nonexistent (Bennett *et al.*, 1992).

The primary role of CSF-1 in regulating mononuclear phagocyte production *in vivo* has been shown in experiments with mice (Hume *et al.*, 1988) and with nonhuman primates (Munn *et al.*, 1990), in which administration of recombinant human CSF-1 results in an increase of up to 10-fold in the circulating monocyte concentration, and increases in macrophage numbers in certain areas of the periphery. Conversely, the absence of CSF-1 in the *op/op* mouse is associated with a large decrease in the concentration of circulating monocytes, some tissue macrophages and osteoclasts (Marks and Lane, 1976; Wiktor-Jedrzejczak *et al.*, 1982, 1991; Naito *et al.*, 1991; Cecchini *et al.*, 1994). In humans, elevated peripheral blood monocyte counts in the newborn are associated with a threefold increase in circulating CSF-1 (Roth, 1991).

Experiments involving the intravenous administration of CSF-1 in normal (Hume *et al.*, 1988) and in *op/op* (Wiktor-Jedrzejczak *et al.*, 1991; Cecchini *et al.*, 1994) mice, suggest that circulating CSF-1 has a major regulatory role in the production of blood monocytes and in the development and maintenance of mononuclear phagocytes in the liver, kidney, spleen and dermis. In normal mice, 94% of circulating CSF-1 (half-life, 10 min) is cleared by CSF-1R-mediated endocytosis and intracellular degradation by

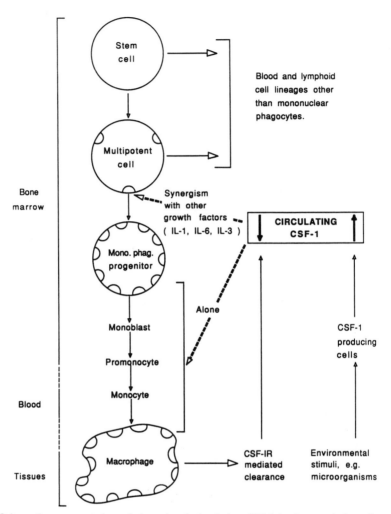

Fig. 6. Schematic representation of the role of circulating CSF-1 in the regulation of mononuclear phagocyte production and the role of sinusoidally located macrophages and environmental stimuli in the regulation of circulating CSF-1. CSF-1R expression is represented by small semicircles. (From Stanley, 1990).

sinusoidally located macrophages in the liver and spleen; only 5% is filtered through the kidney. This clearance by macrophages of the growth factor that is responsible for their generation represents a negative-feedback loop and is the basic coarse control for macrophage production regulated by circulating CSF-1 (Bartocci *et al.*, 1987). Superimposed upon this coarse control, rapid increases in circulating CSF-1 in response to stimuli and infections are mediated by the increased synthesis and release of the growth factor by endothelial cells of several organs (Roth, Bartocci and Stanley, unpublished observations) (Fig. 6).

CSF-1 does not appear to have a significant role in regulating the normal development and maintenance of the majority of macrophages in the thymus, lymph nodes or epidermis (Takahashi *et al.*, 1992, 1993; Cecchini *et al.*, 1994; Witmer-Pack *et al.*,

1993). These observations are consistent with immunological studies in which it has been shown that *op/op* mice possess normal *in vivo* phagocytic function, normal delayed-type hypersensitivity and normal humoral and cellular immune responses to sheep red blood cells (Wiktor-Jedrzejczak *et al.*, 1992a). Except for its capacity to enhance the killing of *Candida albicans* (Karbassi *et al.*, 1987; Cenci *et al.*, 1991) and *Listeria monocytogenes* (Kayashima *et al.*, 1991), its production in inflammatory exudates (Stanley *et al.*, 1976) and the impaired ability of *op/op* mice to release TNF-α and G-CSF into the circulation in response to bacterial endotoxin (Wiktor-Jedrzejczak *et al.*, 1992b), all of which might be explained by its chemotactic role or its role of stimulating macrophage production, CSF-1 does not appear to have a very significant immunological role (reviewed in Roth and Stanley, 1992).

CSF-1 is either synthesized locally, or the proteoglycan form is specifically sequestered (Price *et al.*, 1992; Suzu *et al.*, 1992a), in the regulation of macrophages of muscle, tendon, periosteum, synovium, bladder, salivary gland, gut, adrenals and bone marrow (Cecchini *et al.*, 1994).

Irrespective of whether the tissue macrophage requirement is for circulating or locally produced CSF-1, the requirement is, in many cases, prenatal as well as postnatal. In general, it appears that macrophages requiring either locally produced or circulating CSF-1 for their establishment or maintenance appear to have trophic or scavenger roles important in organogenesis and tissue remodelling (physiological processes), whereas CSF-1-independent macrophages are primarily involved in immune and inflammatory responses (pathological processes). Many aspects of the *op/op* phenotype, including reduced weight, hypoplastic and hypertrophic dermis, poor fertility and synovial membrane and neuromuscular disfunction appear to be a direct consequence of the lack of the physiologically active macrophage populations whose development and maintenance are regulated by CSF-1 (Cecchini *et al.*, 1994).

In vitro CSF-1 stimulates the spreading of cultured macrophages (Boocock *et al.*, 1989) and the morphology of macrophages grown in the presence of GM-CSF is more rounded (Akagawa *et al.*, 1988; Falk and Vogel, 1988). Consistent with these observations, macrophages in the CSF-1-dependent tissue macrophage populations of the *op/op* mouse are more round and possess less developed organelles than macrophages from normal mice (Naito *et al.*, 1991; Pollard *et al.*, 1991b; Cecchini *et al.*, 1994). The functional significance of their more rounded morphology is not clear.

The development of osteoclasts during the prenatal period is also CSF-1 dependent and they appear to be derived from mononuclear phagocyte precursors (Hofstetter *et al.*, 1992; Suda *et al.*, 1992). In *op/op* mice, the osteopetrosis is radiologically recognizable at birth (Felix *et al.*, 1990). The effect of CSF-1 on osteoclasts appears to be primarily to stimulate the differentiation of osteoclast precursor cells to osteoclasts rather than to stimulate proliferation of osteoclasts themselves. As in the case of certain macrophage populations (Cecchini *et al.*, 1994), osteoclast precursors require an additional factor(s) besides CSF-1 to develop appropriately (Suda *et al.*, 1992).

CSF-1 administration to hyperliperdemic rabbits or cynomolgus monkeys rapidly lowers blood cholesterol levels (Shimano *et al.*, 1990; Stoudemire and Garnick, 1991). CSF-1 has been shown to enhance the uptake and degradation of acetylated low density lipoproteins and cholesterol esterification by macrophages *in vitro* (Ishibashi *et al.*, 1990) and its expression in atherosclerotic lesions (Rosenfeld *et al.*, 1992) indicates that it may have a role in the pathogenesis of atherosclerosis (reviewed by Ross, 1993).

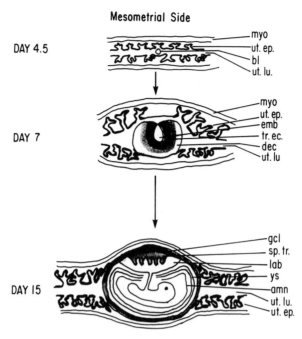

Fig. 7. CSF-1 and CSF-1R mRNA expression during placental development in the mouse. CSF-1 (filled) and CSF-1R (stippled; density of stippling proportional to intensity) mRNA expression is shown at days 4.5, 7 and 15 of pregnancy. Implantation takes place at day 5. myo, myometrium; ut. ep., uterine epithelium; bl, blastocyst; ut. lu., uterine lumen; emb, embryo; tr. ec., trophectoderm; dec, decidua; gcl, giant cell layer; sp. tr., spongiotrophoblast cells; lab, labyrinthine trophoblast cells; ys, yolk sac; amn, amnion. (From Stanley, 1990).

Action of CSF-1 in the Female Reproductive Tract

Mouse CSF-1 is synthesized by the lumenal and glandular secretory epithelium of the uterus during pregnancy (Pollard *et al.*, 1987) and, at least in the early stages of pregnancy, its synthesis is regulated synergistically by a combination of oestradiol-17β and progesterone (Pollard *et al.*, 1987; Wood *et al.*, 1992). Increased uterine expression of CSF-1 mRNA can be detected as early as 2 days after mating and increases throughout both the pre- and postimplantation periods (Arceci *et al.*, 1989). In the postimplantation period, the decidual stimulus apparently enhances CSF-1 synthesis (Pollard *et al.*, 1987) and the concentration of CSF-1 at term is approximately 1000 times higher than in nonpregnant uterus (Bartocci *et al.*, 1986). There is a constant, high, but less elevated concentration of CSF-1 in the placenta (Bartocci *et al.*, 1986) with elevated concentration in the amniotic fluid and comparatively little CSF-1 in the fetus (Bartocci *et al.*, 1986). *In situ* and other evidence indicate that the ultimate source of the elevated CSF-1 in the extra-embryonic tissues is apparently the uterine epithelium (Bartocci *et al.*, 1986; Pollard *et al.*, 1987; Arceci *et al.*, 1989, 1992; Pollard *et al.*, 1991a) (Fig. 7). In contrast to the 1000-fold increase in CSF-1 concentration in the uterus during pregnancy, the circulating concentration of CSF-1 is only increased 1.4-fold and its concentration in tissues other than placenta is increased only slightly (Bartocci *et al.*, 1986), indicating that the large elevation in CSF-1 concentration is

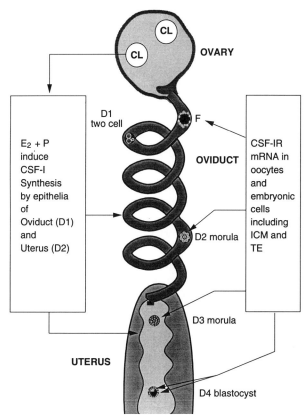

Fig. 8. Schematic representation of pre-implantation development within the female reproductive system of the mouse, indicating the expression of CSF-1 and CSF-1R mRNAs. Cl, corpus luteum; D, day; E$_2$, oestradiol; P, progesterone; ICM, inner cell mass; TE, trophectoderm.

restricted to the female reproductive tract. Interestingly, CSF-1 is not only synthesized by the uterus during pregnancy, as CSF-1 mRNA has been shown to also be present in cumulus cells and in the oviduct during the entire preimplantation period (Arceci *et al.*, 1992) (Fig. 8). The CSF-1 mRNA in the pregnant mouse uterus is predominantly the 2.3 kb species containing the full coding region and the 3' untranslated region encoded by exon 9 (Pollard *et al.*, 1987; Arceci *et al.*, 1989; Regenstreif and Rossant, 1989; Pollard *et al.*, 1991b). *In situ* hybridization and RP-PCR studies indicate that CSF-1 mRNA is not detected in oocytes or embryos during the preimplantation period up until the blastocyst stage (Arceci *et al.*, 1992). However, experiments with pregnant *op/op* mice bearing both +/*op* and *op/op* fetuses indicate that postimplantation embryos do synthesize the growth factor (Pollard *et al.*, 1991b).

In the mouse, the level of CSF-1R mRNA increases during the maturation of oocytes and is abundant in the unfertilized oocyte. Following fertilization, its concentration drops off rapidly and it cannot be detected at the early two-cell stage. However, by the late two-cell stage low levels, presumably of embryonic CSF-1 mRNA, are again detectable and this low level of expression is maintained throughout the preimplantation period (Arceci *et al.*, 1992) (Fig. 8). Both fetally and maternally derived cells express the CSF-1R in postimplantation embryos. Predominant expression is by trophectodermal cells, cells of the ectoplacental cone and secondary giant trophoblasts. In the mature placenta, the expression is greatest on cells of the giant cell layer, followed by cells of the spongiotrophoblast and labyrinthine layers (Arceci *et al.*, 1989; Regenstreif and Rossant, 1989). The cells of the yolk sac express low levels of CSF-1R mRNA (Arceci *et al.*, 1989). Maternal CSF-1 mRNA expression is found in the primary decidual zone, especially in the maternal tissue surrounding the ectoplacental cone (Arceci *et al.*, 1989; Regenstreif and Rossant, 1989) (Fig. 7). Maternal macrophages, expressing the CSF-1R also accumulate in the uterus during the pregnancy. Macrophage numbers are increased at days 1 and 2 and then increase further in the postimplantation period (Pollard *et al.*, 1991b; De *et al.*, 1993). During these periods, they are often concentrated around epithelia known to synthesize CSF-1 (De *et al.*, 1993), possibly as a result of the known chemotactic activity of CSF-1 (Wang *et al.*, 1988; Pierce *et al.*, 1990).

The action of CSF-1 on these various CSF-1R-bearing cell types of the female reproductive tract is under investigation. The possibility that a direct effect of CSF-1 on early embryos may be important for preimplantation development is suggested by the observed enhancement by CSF-1 of the *in vitro* growth of two-cell embryos to the blastocyst stage (Pampfer *et al.*, 1991a). Since macrophages are greatly decreased in the uteri of pregnant *op/op* mice (Pollard *et al.*, 1991b), it seems likely that CSF-1 increases the recruitment and/or local proliferation of maternal macrophages. However, despite the poorer fertility of *op/op* females and the reduced postimplantation survival of their fetuses, the placental weights of pregnant *op/op* mice are normal (Pollard *et al.*, 1991b), which suggests that CSF-1 is not the sole regulator of the proliferation and differentiation of decidual and trophoblastic cells. While CSF-1 has been shown to be mitogenic for primary placental cell types (Athanassakis *et al.*, 1987) and for some placental-cell lines (Pollard *et al.*, 1991d), these cells have not been unequivocally identified as trophoblastic cells. It is possible that CSF-1 regulates the endocrine functions of trophoblastic cells, such as the stimulation of gonadotrophin production.

Breeding experiments with *op/op* mice indicate that *op/op* × *op/op* crosses have very low fertility. The fertility of *op/op* females mated with *op/+* males is reduced by 60% and only 10% of *op/op* mothers can nurture their young (Pollard *et al.*, 1991b). Their infertility is contributed to by pre- and postimplantation problems. In pregnant *op/op* mice, in which circulating CSF-1 has been restored, the postimplantation problem remains (Wiktor-Jedrzejczak *et al.*, 1991), consistent with an important role for locally produced CSF-1 in pregnancy.

Experiments in humans suggest that CSF-1 has a similar role. During pregnancy, CSF-1 is elevated three- to fourfold in the endometrium, twofold in the circulation and also increases in the amniotic fluid (Ringler *et al.*, 1989; Daiter *et al.*, 1992). Both the uterus and placenta express elevated CSF-1 mRNA (Azuma *et al.*, 1990; Daiter *et al.*, 1992; Pampfer *et al.*, 1992) and CSF-1 has been immunohistochemically localized to the maternal glandular and lumenal epithelia and to cells lining the endometrial blood vessels (Daiter *et al.*, 1992). In placenta, CSF-1 is localized to the cytotrophoblast and extravillous cytotrophoblast in the first and second trimesters and various stromal cells in the villous mesenchyme at the second trimester and thereafter. By the third trimester, CSF-1 is localized to cells lining the fetal vessels in villi (Daiter *et al.*, 1992) and may contribute to the observed elevation of CSF-1 in fetal cord blood at term

(Roth, 1991). The CSF-1 mRNA expressed in uterus and placenta is primarily a 4.0 kb species with the full-length coding region and a 3' untranslated region encoded by exon 10 (Daiter *et al.*, 1992) (Fig. 1). However, a 3.0 kb species, possessing a short exon 6 and exon 10 (Fig. 1) is also expressed in significant amounts (Pampfer *et al.*, 1991b; Daiter *et al.*, 1992), representing ≈40% of the total CSF-1 mRNA in the glandular epithelium (Pampfer *et al.*, 1991b). This mRNA, encoding a cell-surface form of CSF-1 is differentially expressed throughout the menstrual cycle in a pattern reflecting female sex steroid regulation (Pampfer *et al.*, 1991b).

Human CSF-1R and CSF-1R mRNA are present in both placenta and uterus (Müller *et al.*, 1983; Hoshina *et al.*, 1985; Azuma *et al.*, 1990; Pampfer *et al.*, 1992). Transcription in placenta and chorion, which contains extravillous trophoblasts is initiated upstream of exon 1, while the exon 2 promoter is used in nonpregnant endometrium and gland epithelium (Pampfer *et al.*, 1992), suggesting a mechanism for differentially regulated maternal and fetal CSF-1R mRNA expression. The maternal cells expressing the CSF-1R during pregnancy are the glandular and lumenal epithelium and decidual cells (Pampfer *et al.*, 1992). However, CSF-1R has also been localized to placental cytotrophoblasts and extravillous cytotrophoblasts (Pampfer *et al.*, 1992).

Thus, in contrast to the mouse, CSF-1 and CSF-1R are both expressed in maternal epithelia and in cytotrophoblasts, raising the possibility of autocrine as well as paracrine roles for the growth factor. However, in both mouse and man, the elevated expression of CSF-1 and the CSF-1R-bearing cells in the female reproductive tract during pregnancy is consistent with observations in the mouse which suggest that CSF-1 plays an important role in regulation that goes beyond its action on mononuclear phagocytic cells.

Role in Neoplasia

The role of CSF-1 and the CSF-1R in neoplasia has been reviewed in detail elsewhere (Sherr, 1990; Sherr and Stanley, 1990; Stanley, 1990; Roth and Stanley, 1992). The v-*fms* gene is capable of inducing the formation of tumours derived from haemopoietic cells (Heard *et al.*, 1987a) and the c-*fms* gene has been shown to be expressed in a number of different human neoplasms. In v-*fms*, several point-mutations in the extracellular domain, besides the initially reported point-mutation at residue 301, appear to cause transformation (Van Daalen Wetters *et al.*, 1992). Thus further analysis of such neoplasms, especially those that do not express CSF-1, for the presence of subtly altered and autonomously transforming forms of the CSF-1R is warranted.

The normal CSF-1 or c-*fms* gene can cause transformation in situations where either is inappropriately expressed (reviewed in Stanley, 1990). This may be as a secondary event in tumour development that leads to inappropriate coexpression of both CSF-1 and the CSF-1R in the same cell type and consequent autocrine regulation by the growth factor (Baumbach *et al.*, 1987). Coexpression of both CSF-1 and CSF-1R has been described for human adenocarcinomas of the endometrium, ovary and breast, as well as leukaemias (Rambaldi *et al.*, 1988; Kacinski *et al.*, 1989a, b, 1991). In addition, many patients with neoplasms of these types possess significantly elevated concentrations of circulating CSF-1 (Gilbert *et al.*, 1989; Kacinski *et al.*, 1989a, 1990; Janowska-Wieczorek *et al.*, 1991).

Potential Clinical Applications

CSF-1 has a number of potential clinical applications, many of which have been reviewed elsewhere (Roth and Stanley, 1992). They include its therapeutic use as an adjunct in the treatment of infection and malignancies, as well as in the acceleration of haemopoietic recovery following chemotherapy or bone-marrow transplantation. In addition, elevated levels of circulating CSF-1 may be useful as a tumour marker for certain neoplastic diseases, particularly those of the female reproductive and lympho-haemopoietic systems. The development of effective antagonists is another potential area of application, because of the elevation of circulating CSF-1 in specific chronic diseases.

CONCLUSIONS

Several exciting developments over the last few years have contributed to the large increase in our knowledge of CSF-1, its receptor and biology. In addition to the identification of the proteoglycan form of CSF-1, the determination of the CSF-1 crystal structure and a further understanding of CSF-1 signal transduction, the utilization of the CSF-1-less *op/op* mouse has provided us with much new information about the nature of the various CSF-1 target populations and their regulation by CSF-1. The many questions that remain concerning the nature of the regulation by the various forms of CSF-1 can be conveniently studied utilizing this mutant. Other discoveries, both molecular and biological, have provided specific information concerning CSF-1 and CSF-1R that will be useful in understanding their involvement in neoplastic and other disorders.

ACKNOWLEDGEMENTS

I thank Dr Fiona Pixley for help in preparation of the Figures. This work was supported by NIH grants CA 26504, CA32551, a grant from the Lucille P. Markey Charitable Trust and the Albert Einstein Core Cancer Grant P30-CA 13330.

REFERENCES

Akagawa, K.S., Kamoshita, K. and Tokunaga, T. (1988). *J. Immunol.* **141**, 3383–3390.
Arceci, R.J., Shanahan, F., Stanley, E.R. and Pollard, J.W. (1989). *Proc. Natl Acad. Sci. USA* **86**, 8818–8822.
Arceci, R.J., Pampfer, S. and Pollard, J.W. (1992). *Dev. Biol.* **151**, 1–8.
Athanassakis, I., Bleackley, R.C., Paetkau, V., Guilbert, L.J., Barr, P.J. and Wegmann, T.G. (1987). *J. Immunol.* **138**, 37–44.
Azuma, C., Saji, F., Kimura, T., Tokugawa, Y., Takemura, M., Samejima, Y. and Tanizawa, O. (1990). *J. Mol. Endocrinol.* **5**, 103–108.
Baccarini, M., Sabatini, D.M., App, H., Rapp, U.R. and Stanley, E.R. (1990). *EMBO J.* **9**, 3649–3657.
Baccarini, M., Li, W., Dello Sbarba, P. and Stanley, E.R. (1991). *Receptor* **1**, 243–259.
Ball, R.L., Tanner, K.D. and Carpenter, G. (1990). *J. Biol. Chem.* **265**, 12836–12845.
Bartelmez, S.H. and Stanley, E.R. (1985). *J. Cell. Physiol.* **122**, 370–378.
Bartelmez, S.H., Sacca, R. and Stanley, E.R. (1985). *J. Cell. Physiol.* **122**, 362–369.
Bartocci, A., Pollard, J.W. and Stanley, E.R. (1986). *J. Exp. Med.* **164**, 956–961.

Bartocci, A., Mastrogiannis, D.S., Migliorati, G., Stockert, R.J., Wolkoff, A.W. and Stanley, E.R. (1987). *Proc. Natl Acad. Sci. USA* **84**, 6179–6183.

Baumbach, W.R., Stanley, E.R. and Cole, M.D. (1987). *Mol. Cell. Biol.* **7**, 664–671.

Bazan, J.F. (1991). *Cell* **65**, 9–10.

Bennett, S., Por, S.B., Stanley, E.R. and Breit, S.N. (1992). *J. Immunol. Methods* **153**, 201–212.

Besmer, P., Murphy, J.E., George, P.C., Qiu, F., Bergold, P.J., Lederman, L., Snyder, H.W., Jr, Brodeur, D., Zuckerman, E.E. and Hardy, W.D. (1986). *Nature* **320**, 415–421.

Boocock, C.A., Jones, G.E., Stanley, E.R. and Pollard, J.W. (1989). *J. Cell Sci.* **93**, 447–456.

Bortner, D.M., Ulivi, M., Roussel, M.F. and Ostrowski, M.C. (1991). *Genes Dev.* **5**, 1777–1785.

Borycki, A-G., Guillier, M., Leibovitch, M-P. and Leibovitch, S.A. (1992). *Growth Factors* **6**, 209–218.

Bosenberg, M.W., Pandiella, A. and Massagué, J. (1992). *Cell* **71**, 1157–1165.

Bradley, T.R. and Metcalf, D. (1966). *Aust. J. Exp. Biol. Med. Sci.* **44**, 287–299.

Browning, P.J., Bunn, H.F., Cline, A., Shuman, M. and Nienhuis, A.W. (1986). *Proc. Natl Acad. Sci. USA* **83**, 7800–7804.

Buchberg, A.M., Jenkins, N.A. and Copeland, N.G. (1989). *Genomics* **5**, 363–367.

Byrne, P.V., Guilbert, L.J. and Stanley, E.R. (1981). *J. Cell Biol.* **91**, 848–853.

Büscher, D., Dello Sbarba, P., Hipskind, R.A., Rapp, U.R., Stanley, E.R. and Baccarini, M. (1993). *Oncogene* **8**, 3323–3332.

Carlberg, K., Tapley, P., Haystead, C. and Rohrschneider, L. (1991). *EMBO J.* **10**, 877–883.

Cecchini, M.G., Dominguez, M.G., Mocci, S., Wetterwald, A., Felix, R., Fleisch, H., Chisholm, O.T., Pollard, J.W., Hofstetter, W. and Stanley, E.R. (1994). *Development* (in press).

Cenci, E., Bartocci, A., Puccetti, P., Mocci, S., Stanley, E.R. and Bistoni, F. (1991). *Infect. Immun.* **59**, 868–872.

Cerdan, C., Courcoul, M., Razanajaona, D., Pierrès, A., Maroc, N., Lopez, M., Mannoni, P., Mawas, C., Olive, D. and Birg, F. (1990). *Eur. J. Immunol.* **20**, 331–335.

Cerretti, D.P., Wignall, J., Anderson, D., Tushinski, R.J., Gallis, B.M., Stya, M., Gillis, S., Urdal, D.L. and Cosman, D. (1988). *Mol. Immunol.* **25**, 761–770.

Chen, D.M., Lin, J.S., Stahl, P. and Stanley, E.R. (1979). *Exp. Cell Res.* **121**, 103–109.

Chodakewitz, J.A., Lacy, J., Edwards, S.E., Birchall, N. and Coleman, D.L. (1990). *J. Immunol.* **144**, 2190–2196.

Cook, N., Dexter, T.M., Lord, B.I., Cragoe, E.J., Jr. and Whetton, A.D. (1989). *EMBO J.* **8**, 2967–2974.

Cooper, J.A., Gould, K.L., Cartwright, C.A. and Hunter, T. (1986). *Science* **231**, 1431–1434.

Courtneidge, S.A., Dhand, R., Pilat, D., Twamley, G.M., Waterfield, M.D. and Roussel, M.F. (1993). *EMBO J.* **12**, 943–950.

Coussens, L., Van Beveren, C., Smith, D., Chen, E., Mitchell, R.L., Isacke, C.M., Verma, I.M. and Ullrich, A. (1986). *Nature* **32**, 277–280.

Daiter, E., Pampfer, S., Yeung, Y.G., Barad, D., Stanley, E.R. and Pollard, J.W. (1992). *J. Clin. Endocrinol. Metab.* **74**, 850–858.

Das, S.K., Stanley, E.R., Guilbert, L.J. and Forman, L.W. (1980). *J. Cell. Physiol.* **104**, 359–366.

Das, S.K., Stanley, E.R., Guilbert, L.J. and Forman, L.W. (1981). *Blood* **58**, 630–641.

De, M., Sanford, T. and Wood, G.W. (1993). *J. Leukocyte Biol.* **53**, 240–248.

De Parseval, N., Bordereaux, D., Gisselbrecht, S. and Sola, B. (1993). *Nucl. Acids Res.* **21**, 750.

DeLamarter, J.F., Hession, C., Semon, D., Gough, N.M., Rothenbuhler, R. and Mermod, J-J. (1987). *Nucl. Acids Res.* **15**, 2389–2390.

Dello Sbarba, P., Pollard, J.W. and Stanley, E.R. (1991). *Growth Factors* **5**, 75–85.

Demetri, G.D., Zenzie, B.W., Rheinwald, J.G. and Griffin, J.D. (1989). *Blood* **74**, 940–946.

Downing, J.R. and Reynolds, A.B. (1991). *Oncogene* **6**, 607–613.

Downing, J.R., Rettenmier, C.W. and Sherr, C.J. (1988). *Mol. Cell. Biol.* **8**, 1795–1799.

Downing, J.R., Margolis, B.L., Zilberstein, A., Ashmun, R.A., Ullrich, A., Sherr, C.J. and Schlessinger, J. (1989a). *EMBO J.* **8**, 3345–3350.

Downing, J.R., Roussel, M.F. and Sherr, C.J. (1989b). *Mol. Cell. Biol.* **9**, 2890–2896.

Downing, J.R., Shurtleff, S.A. and Sherr, C.J. (1991). *Mol. Cell. Biol.* **11**, 2489–2495.

Elford, P.R., Felix, R., Cecchini, M., Trechsel, U. and Fleisch, H. (1987). *Calcif. Tissue Int.* **41**, 151–156.

Falk, L.A. and Vogel, S.N. (1988). *J. Leukocyte Biol.* **43**, 148–157.

Felix, R., Cecchini, M.G. and Fleisch, H. (1990). *Endocrinology* **127**, 2592–2594.

Fibbe, W.E., Van Damme, J., Billiau, A., Goselink, H.M., Voogt, P.J., van Eeden, G., Ralph, P., Altrock, B.W. and Falkenburg, J.H. (1988). *Blood* **71**, 430–435.

Gilbert, H.S., Praloran, V. and Stanley, E.R. (1989). *Blood* **74**, 1231–1234.

Gimbrone, M.A., Jr., Obin, M.S., Brock, A.F., Luis, E.A., Hass, P.E., Hébert, C.A., Yip, Y.K., Leung, D.W., Lowe, D.G., Kohr, W.J., Darbonne, W.C., Bechtol, K.B. and Baker, J.B. (1989). *Science* **246**, 1601–1603.

Gisselbrecht, S., Sola, B., Fichelson, S., Bordereaux, D., Tambourin, P., Mattei, M.G., Simon, D. and Guenet, J.L. (1989). *Blood* **73**, 1742–1745.

Glocker, M.O., Arbogast, B., Schreurs, J. and Deinzer, M.L. (1993). *Biochemistry* **32**, 482–488.

Groffen, J., Heisterkamp, N., Spurr, N., Dana, S., Wasmuth, J.J. and Stephenson, J.R. (1983). *Nucl. Acids Res.* **11**, 6331–6399.

Guilbert, L.J. and Stanley, E.R. (1980). *J. Cell Biol.* **85** 153–159.

Guilbert, L.J. and Stanley, E.R. (1986). *J. Biol. Chem.* **261**, 4024–4032.

Guilbert, L.J., Tynan, P.W. and Stanley, E.R. (1986). *J. Cell. Biochem.* **31**, 203–216.

Hamilton, J.A., Stanley, E.R., Burgess, A.W. and Shadduck, R.K. (1980). *J. Cell. Physiol.* **103**, 435–445.

Hamilton, J.A., Vairo, G. and Lingelbach, S.R. (1986). *Biochem. Biophys. Res. Commun.* **138**, 445–454.

Hamilton, J.A., Vairo, G. and Lingelbach, S.R. (1988). *J. Cell. Physiol.* **134**, 405–412.

Hamilton, J.A., Veis, N., Bordun, A.-M., Vairo, G., Gonda, T.J. and Phillips, W.A. (1989). *J. Cell. Physiol.* **141**, 618–626.

Hamilton, J.A., Vairo, G., Knight, K.R. and Cocks, B.G. (1991). *Blood* **77**, 616–627.

Hampe, A., Shamoon, B.M., Gobet, M., Sherr, C.J. and Galibert, F. (1989). *Oncogene Res.* **4**, 9–17.

Harrington, M.A., Edenberg, H.J., Saxman, S., Pedigo, L.M., Daub, R. and Broxmeyer, H.E. (1991). *Gene* **102**, 165–170.

Hartmann, T., Seuwen, K., Roussel, M.F., Sherr, C.J. and Pouysségur, J. (1990). *Growth Factors* **2**, 289–300.

Haskill, S., Warren, M.K., Becker, S., Ladner, M.B., Johnson, C., Eierman, D., Ralph, P. and Mark, D.F. (1987). *J. Leukocyte Biol.* **42**, 359.

Heard, J.M., Roussel, M.F., Rettenmier, C.W. and Sherr, C.J. (1987a). *Cell* **51**, 663–673.

Heard, J.M., Roussel, M.F., Rettenmier, C.W. and Sherr, C.J. (1987b). *Oncogene Res.* **1**, 423–440.

Henschler, R., Mantovani, L., Oster, W., Lübbert, M., Lindemann, A., Mertelsmann, R. and Herrmann, F. (1990). *Br. J. Haematol.* **76**, 7–11.

Hofstetter, W., Wetterwald, A., Checchini, M.C., Felix, R., Fleisch, H. and Mueller, C. (1992). Proc. Natl Acad. Sci. USA **89**, 9637–9641.

Horiguchi, J., Warren, M.K. and Kufe, D. (1987). *Blood* **69**, 1259–1261.

Horiguchi, J., Sariban, E. and Kufe, D. (1988). *Mol. Cell. Biol.* **8**, 3951–3954.

Hoshina, M., Nishio, A., Bo, M., Boime, I. and Mochizuki, M. (1985). *Acta Obsta Gynaec. JPN* **37**, 2791–2798.

Hume, D.A., Pavli, P., Donahue, R.E. and Fidler, I.J. (1988). *J. Immunol.* **141**, 3405–3409.

Imamura, K. and Kufe, D. (1988). *J. Biol. Chem.* **263**, 14093–14098.

Imamura, K., Dianoux, A., Nakamura, T. and Kufe, D. (1990). *EMBO J.* **9**, 2423–2429.

Ishibashi, S., Inaba, T., Shimano, H., Harada, K., Inoue, I., Mokuno, H., Mori, N., Gotoda, T., Takaku, F. and Yamada, N. (1990). *J. Biol. Chem.* **265**, 14109–14117.

Jackowski, S., Rettenmier, C.W. and Rock, C.O. (1990). *J. Biol. Chem.* **265**, 6611–6616.

Janowska-Wieczorek, A., Belch, A.R., Jacobs, A., Bowen, D., Paietta, E. and Stanley, E.R. (1991). *Blood* **77**, 1796–1803.

Kacinski, B.M., Bloodgood, R.S., Schwartz, P.E., Carter, D. and Stanley, E.R. (1989a). *Cancer Cells* **7**, 333–337.

Kacinski, B.M., Stanley, E.R., Carter, D., Chambers, J.T., Chambers, S.K., Kohorn, E.I. and Schwartz, P.E. (1989b). *Int. J. Radiat. Oncol. Biol. Phys.* **17**, 159–164.

Kacinski, B.M., Chambers, S.K., Stanley, E.R., Carter, D., Tseng, P., Scata, K.A., Chang, D.H.-Y., Pirro, M.H., Nguyen, J.T., Ariza, A., Rohrschneider, L.R. and Rothwell, V.M. (1990). *Int. J. Radiat. Oncol. Biol. Phys.* **19**, 619–626.

Kacinski, B.M., Scata, K.A., Carter, D., Yee, L.D., Sapi, E., King, B.L., Chambers, S.K., Jones, M.A., Pirro, M.H., Stanley E.R. and Rohrschneider, L.R. (1991). *Oncogene* **6**, 941–952.

Karbassi, A., Becker, J.M., Foster, J.S. and Moore, R.N. (1987). *J. Immunol.* **139**, 417–421.

Kato, J-Y. and Sherr, C.J. (1990). *Blood* **75**, 1780–1787.

Kawasaki, E.S., Ladner, M.B., Wang, A.M., Van Arsdell, J., Warren, M.K., Coyne, M.Y., Schweickart, V.L., Lee, M.T., Wilson, K.J., Boosman, A. *et al.* (1985). *Science* **230**, 291–296.

Kawasaki, E.S. and Ladner, M.B. (1990). In *Colony-Stimulating Factors. Molecular and Cellular Biology* (eds T.M. Dexter, J.M. Garland and N.G. Testa), Marcel Dekker Inc., New York pp. 155–176.

Kayashima, S., Tsuru, S., Shinomiya, N., Katsura, Y., Motoyoshi, K., Rokutanda, M. and Nagata, N. (1991). *Infect. Immun.* **59**, 4677–4680.
Knight, K.R., Vairo, G. and Hamilton, J.A. (1992). *J. Leukocyte Biol.* **51**, 350–359.
Krantwald, S. and Baccarini, M. (1993). *Biochem. Biophys. Res. Commun.* **192**, 720–727.
Kurland, J.I., Pelus, L.M., Ralph, P., Bockman, R.S. and Moore, M.A.S. (1979). *Proc. Natl Acad. Sci. USA* **76**, 2326–2330.
Ladner, M.B., Martin, G.A., Noble, J.A., Nikoloff, D.M., Tal, R., Kawasaki, E.S. and White, T.J. (1987). *EMBO J.* **6**, 2693–2698.
Ladner, M.B., Martin, G.A., Noble, J.A., Wittman, V.P., Warren, M.P., McGrogan, M. and Stanley, E.R. (1988). *Proc. Natl Acad. Sci. USA* **85**, 6706–6710.
Langer, S.J., Bortner, D.M., Roussel, M.F., Sherr, C.J. and Ostrowski, M.C. (1992). *Mol. Cell. Biol.* **12**, 5355–5362.
Lanotte, M., Metcalf, D. and Dexter, T.M. (1982). *J. Cell. Physiol.* **112**, 123–127.
Le, P.T., Kurtzberg, J., Brandt, S.J., Niedel, J.E., Haynes, B.F. and Singer, K.H. (1988). *J. Immunol.* **141**, 1211–1217.
Lee, A.W. and Nienhuis, A.W. (1990). *Proc. Natl Acad. Sci. USA* **87**, 7270–7274.
Leibovitch, S.A., Leibovitch, M-P., Borycki, A-G. and Harel, J. (1989). *Oncogene Res.* **4**, 157–162.
Li, W. and Stanley, E.R. (1991). *EMBO J.* **10**, 277–288.
Li, W., Yeung, Y.G. and Stanley, E.R. (1991). *J. Biol. Chem.* **266**, 6808–6814.
Lin, H-S. and Gordon, S. (1979). *J. Exp. Med.* **150**, 231–245.
Lu, L., Walker, D., Graham, C.D., Waheed, A., Shadduck, R.K. and Broxmeyer, H.E. (1988). *Blood* **72**, 34–41.
McGlade, C.J., Ellis, C., Reedijk, M., Anderson, D., Mbamalu, G., Reith, A.D., Panayotou, G., End, P., Bernstein, A., Kazlauskas, A., Waterfield, M.D. and Pawson, T. (1992). *Mol. Cell. Biol.* **12**, 991–997.
Manos, M.M. (1988). *Mol. Cell. Biol.* **8**, 5035–5039.
Manos, M.M., Shadle, P.J. and Ting, Y. (1988). In *Viral Vectors* (eds Y. Gluzman and S.H. Hughes), Cold Spring Harbor Laboratory Press, New York, pp. 45–50.
Marks, S.C., Jr. and Lane, P.W. (1976). *J. Hered.* **67**, 11–18.
Matsushime, H., Roussel, M.F., Ashmun, R.A. and Sherr, C.J. (1991). *Cell* **65**, 701–713.
Mauel, J. and Defendi, V. (1971). *Exp. Cell Res.* **65**, 33–42.
Morgan, C.J. and Stanley, E.R. (1984). *Biochem. Biophys. Res. Commun.* **119**, 35–41.
Morgan, C.J., Pollard, J.W. and Stanley, E.R. (1987). *J. Cell. Physiol.* **130**, 420–427.
Mori, S., Heldin, C.H. and Claesson-Welsh, L. (1992). *J. Biol. Chem.* **267**, 6429–6434.
Mori, T., Bartocci, A., Satriano, J., Zuckerman, A., Stanley, R., Santiago, A. and Schlondorff, D. (1990). *J. Immunol.* **144**, 4697–4702.
Morris, S.W., Valentine, M.B., Shapiro, D.N., Sublett, J.E., Deaven, L.L., Foust, J.T., Roberts, W.M., Cerretti, D.P. and Look, A.T. (1991). *Blood* **78**, 2013–2020.
Munn, D.H., Garnick, M.B. and Cheung, N.-K.V. (1990). *Blood* **75**, 2042–2048.
Müller, R., Slamon, D.J., Adamson, E.D., Tremblay, J.M., Müller, D., Cline, M.J. and Verma, I.M. (1983). *Mol. Cell. Biol.* **3**, 1062–1069.
Müller, R., Curran, T., Müller, D. and Guilbert, L. (1985). *Nature* **314**, 546–548.
Naito, M., Hayashi, S., Yoshida, H., Nishikawa, S., Shultz, L.D. and Takahashi, K. (1991). *Am. J. Pathol.* **139**, 657–667.
Nakamura, T., Lin, L.-L., Kharbanda, S., Knopf, J. and Kufe, D. (1992). *EMBO J.* **11**, 4917–4922.
Ohtsuka, M., Roussel, M.F., Sherr, C.J. and Downing, J.R. (1990). *Mol. Cell. Biol.* **10**, 1664–1671.
Orlandi, M., Bartolini, G., Minghetti, L., Luchetti, S., Giuliucci, B., Chiricolo, M. and Tomasi, V. (1989). *Prostaglandins Leukot. Essent. Fatty Acids* **36**, 101–106.
Orlofsky, A. and Stanley, E.R. (1987). *EMBO J.* **6**, 2947–2952.
Oster, W., Lindemann, A., Mertelsmann, R. and Herrmann, F. (1988). *Blood Cells* **14**, 443–462.
Pampfer, S., Arceci, R.J. and Pollard, J.W. (1991a). *BioEssays* **13**, 535–540.
Pampfer, S., Tabibzadeh, S., Chuan, F.-C. and Pollard, J.W. (1991b). *Mol. Endocrinol.* **5**, 1931–1938.
Pampfer, S., Daiter, E., Barad, D. and Pollard, J.W. (1992). *Biol. Reprod.* **46**, 48–57.
Pandit, J., Bohm, A., Jancarik, J., Halenbeck, R., Koths, K. and Kim, S.-H. (1992). *Science* **258**, 1358–1362.
Pawson, T. and Gish, G.D. (1992). *Cell* **71**, 359–362.
Pelicci, G., Lanfrancone, L., Grignani, F., McGlade, J., Cavallo, F., Forni, G., Nicoletti, I., Pawson, T. and Pelicci, P.G. (1992). *Cell* **70**, 93–104.

Pierce, J.H., Di Marco, E., Cox, G.W., Lombardi, D., Ruggiero, M., Varesio, L., Wang, L.M., Choudhury, G.G., Sakaguchi, A.Y., Di Fiore, P.P. and Aaronson, S.A. (1990). *Proc. Natl Acad. Sci. USA* **87**, 5613–5617.
Pluznik, D.H. and Sachs, L. (1965). *J. Cell. Comp. Physiol.* **66**, 319–324.
Pollard, J.W., Bartocci, A., Arceci, R., Orlofsky, A., Ladner, M.B. and Stanley, E.R. (1987). *Nature* **330**, 484–486.
Pollard, J.W., Arceci, R.J., Bartocci, A. and Stanley, E.R. (1991a). In *Molecular and Cellular Immunobiology of the Maternal-fetal Interface* (eds T.G. Wegmann, T. Gill and E. Nisbet-Brown), Oxford University Press, Oxford, pp. 243–260.
Pollard, J.W., Hunt, J.W., Wiktor-Jedrzejczak, W. and Stanley, E.R. (1991b). *Dev. Biol.* **148**, 273–283.
Pollard, J.W., Morgan, C.J., Dello Sbarba, P., Cheers, C. and Stanley, E.R. (1991c). *Proc. Natl Acad. Sci. USA* **88**, 1474–1478.
Pollard, J.W., Pampfer, S., Daiter, E., Barad, D. and Arceci, R.J. (1991d). In *Growth Factors in Reproduction* (ed D.W. Schomberg), Plenum Press, New York, pp. 219–229.
Presnell, S.R. and Cohen, F.E. (1989). *Proc. Natl Acad. Sci. USA* **86**, 6592–6596.
Price, L.K.H., Choi, H.U., Rosenberg, L. and Stanley, E.R. (1992). *J. Biol. Chem.* **267**, 2190–2199.
Puri, J., Pierce, J.H. and Hoffman, T. (1992). *Prostaglandins Leukot. Essent. Fatty Acids* **45**, 43–48.
Racoosin, E.L. and Swanson, J.A. (1989). *J. Exp. Med.* **170**, 1635–1648.
Racoosin, E.L. and Swanson, J.A. (1992). *J. Cell Sci.* **102**, 867–880.
Rajavashisth, T.B., Eng, R., Shadduck, R.K., Waheed, A., Ben-Avram, C.M., Shively, J.E. and Lusis, A.J. (1987). *Proc. Natl Acad. Sci. USA* **84**, 1157–1161.
Rambaldi, A., Young, D.C. and Griffin, J.D. (1987). *Blood* **69**, 1409–1413.
Rambaldi, A., Wakamiya, N., Vellenga, E., Horiguchi, J., Warren, M.K., Kufe, D. and Griffin, J.D. (1988). *J. Clin. Invest.* **81**, 1030–1035.
Reedijk, M., Liu, X. and Pawson, T. (1990). *Mol. Cell. Biol.* **10**, 5601–5608.
Reedijk, M., Liu, X., Van der Geer, P., Letwin, K., Waterfield, M.D., Hunter, T. and Pawson, T. (1992). *EMBO J.* **11**, 1365–1372.
Regenstreif, L.J. and Rossant, J. (1989). *Dev. Biol.* **133**, 284–294.
Reisbach, G., Sindermann, J., Kremer, J.P., Hültner, L., Wolf, H. and Dörmer, P. (1989). *Blood* **74**, 959–964.
Rettenmier, C.W., Roussel, M.F., Ashmun, R.A., Ralph, P., Price, K. and Sherr, C.J. (1987). *Mol. Cell. Biol.* **7**, 2378–2387.
Rettenmier, C.W. and Roussel, M.F. (1988). *Mol. Cell. Biol.* **8**, 5026–5034.
Reynolds, A.B., Herbert, L., Cleveland, J.L., Berg, S.T. and Gaut, J.R. (1992). *Oncogene* **7**, 2439–2445.
Ringler, G.E., Coutifaris, C., Strauss III, J.F., Allen, J.I. and Geier, M.D. (1989). *Am. J. Obstet. Gynecol.* **160**, 655–656.
Rist, R.J., Jones, G.E. and Naftalin, R.J. (1990). *Biochem. J.* **265**, 243–249.
Roberts, W.M., Look, A.T., Roussel, M.F. and Sherr, C.J. (1988). *Cell* **55**, 655–661.
Roberts, W.M., Shapiro, L.H., Ashmun, R.A. and Look, A.T. (1992). *Blood* **79**, 586–593.
Rohrschneider, L.R. and Metcalf, D. (1989). *Mol. Cell. Biol.* **9**, 5081–5092.
Rosenfeld, M.E., Ylä-Herttuala, S., Lipton, B.A., Ord, V.A., Witztum, J.L. and Steinberg, D. (1992). *Am. J. Pathol.* **140**, 291–300.
Ross, R. (1993). *Nature* **362**, 801–809.
Roth, P. (1991). *J. Pediatr.* **119**, 113–116.
Roth, P. and Stanley, E.R. (1992). *Curr. Top. Microbiol. Immunol.* **181**, 141–167.
Rothwell, V.M. and Rohrschneider, L.R. (1987). *Oncogene Res.* **1**, 311–324.
Roussel, M.F. and Sherr, C.J. (1989). *Proc. Natl Acad. Sci. USA* **86**, 7924–7927.
Roussel, M.F., Sherr, C.J., Barker, P.E. and Ruddle, F.H. (1983). *J. Virol.* **48**, 770–773.
Roussel, M.F., Dull, T.J., Rettenmier, C.W., Ralph, P., Ullrich, A. and Sherr, C.J. (1987). *Nature* **325**, 549–552.
Roussel, M.F., Downing, J.R., Rettenmier, C.W. and Sherr, C.J. (1988). *Cell* **55**, 979–988.
Roussel, M.F., Downing, J.R. and Sherr, C.J. (1990a). *Oncogene* **5**, 25–30.
Roussel, M.F., Shurtleff, S.A., Downing, J.R. and Sherr, C.J. (1990b). *Proc. Natl Acad. Sci. USA* **87**, 6738–6742.
Roussel, M.F., Transy, C., Kato, J.-Y., Reinherz, E.L. and Sherr, C.J. (1990c). *Mol. Cell. Biol.* **10**, 2407–2412.
Roussel, M.F., Cleveland, J.L., Shurtleff, S.A. and Sherr, C.J. (1991). *Nature* **353**, 361–363.
Sabatini, D.D., Kreibich, G., Morimoto, T. and Adesnik, M. (1982). *J. Cell Biol.* **92**, 1–22.

Saltman, D.L., Dolganov, G.M., Hinton, L.M. and Lovett, M. (1992). *Biochem. Biophys. Res. Commun.* **182**, 1139–1143.

Seelentag, W.K., Mermod, J.J., Montesano, R. and Vassalli, P. (1987). *EMBO J.* **6**, 2261–2265.

Sengupta, A., Liu, W-K., Yeung, Y.-G., Yeung, D.C-Y., Frackelton, A.R. and Stanley, E.R. (1988). *Proc. Natl Acad. Sci. USA* **85**, 8062–8066.

Shaw, G. and Kamen, R. (1986). *Cell* **46**, 659–667.

Shen, S.-H., Bastien, L., Posner, B.I. and Chrétien, P. (1991). *Nature* **352**, 736–739.

Sherr, C.J. (1990). *Blood* **75**, 1–12.

Sherr, C.J. (1991). *Trends Genet.* **7**, 398–402.

Sherr, C.J. and Stanley, E.R. (1990). In *Handbook of Experimental Pharmacology, Vol. 95/I, Peptide Growth Factors and Their Receptors* (eds M.B. Sporn and A.B. Roberts), Springer-Verlag, Berlin, pp. 667–698.

Sherr, C.J., Rettenmier, C.W., Sacca, R., Roussel, M.F., Look, A.T. and Stanley, E.R. (1985). *Cell* **41**, 665–676.

Shimano, H., Yamada, N., Motoyoshi, K., Matsumoto, A., Ishibashi, S., Mori, N. and Takaku, F. (1990). *Ann. NY Acad. Sci.* **587**, 362–370.

Shultz, L.D. (1988). *Curr. Top. Microbiol. Immunol.* **137**, 216–222.

Shultz, L.D., Schweitzer, P.A., Rajan, T.V., Yi, T., Ihle, J.N., Matthews, R.J., Thomas, M.L. and Beier, D.R. (1993). *Cell* **73**, 1445–1454.

Shurtleff, S.A., Downing, J.R., Rock, C.O., Hawkins, S.A., Roussel, M.F. and Sherr, C.J. (1990). *EMBO J.* **9**, 2415–2421.

Stanley, E.R. (1979). *Proc. Natl Acad. Sci. USA* **76**, 2969–2973.

Stanley, E.R. (1985). *Methods Enzymol.* **116**, 564–587.

Stanley, E.R. (1990). In *Genetics of Pattern Formation and Growth Control* (ed. A.P. Mahowald), Wiley-Liss, New York, pp. 165–180.

Stanley, E.R. and Guilbert, L.J. (1980). In *Mononuclear Phagocytes—Functional Aspects* (ed. R. van Furth), Martinus Nijhoff, Boston, pp. 417–433.

Stanley, E.R. and Guilbert, L.J. (1981). *J. Immunol. Methods* **42**, 253–284.

Stanley, E.R. and Heard, P.M. (1977). *J. Biol. Chem.* **252**, 4305–4312.

Stanley, E.R., Cifone, M., Heard, P.M., and Defendi, V. (1976). *J. Exp. Med.* **143**, 631–647.

Stanley, E.R., Chen, D.M. and Lin, H-S. (1978). *Nature* **274**, 168–170.

Stanley, E.R., Guilbert, L.J., Tushinski, R.J. and Bartelmez, S.H. (1983). *J. Cell. Biochem.* **21**, 151–159.

Stein, J. and Rettenmier, C.W. (1991). *Oncogene* **6**, 601–605.

Stein, J., Borzillo, G.V. and Rettenmier, C.W. (1990). *Blood* **76**, 1308–1314.

Stoudemire, J.B. and Garnick, M.B. (1991). *Blood* **77**, 750–755.

Suda, T., Takahashi, N. and Martin, T.J. (1992). *Endocr. Rev.* **13**, 66–80.

Suzu, S., Ohtsuki, T., Makishima, M., Yanai, N., Kawashima, T., Nagata, N. and Motoyoshi, K. (1992a). *J. Biol. Chem.* **267**, 16812–16815.

Suzu, S., Ohtsuki, T., Yanai, N., Takatsu, Z., Kawashima, T., Takaku, F., Nagata, N. and Motoyoshi, K. (1992b). *J. Biol. Chem.* **267**, 4345–4348.

Takahashi, K., Naito, M. and Shultz, L.D. (1992). *J. Invest. Dermatol.* **99**, 46S–47S.

Takahashi, K., Naito, M., Shultz, L.D., Hayashi, S. and Nishikawa, S. (1993). *J. Leukocyte Biol.* **53**, 19–28.

Tapley, P., Kazlauskas, A., Cooper, J.A. and Rohrschneider, L.R. (1990). *Mol. Cell. Biol.* **10**, 2528–2538.

Taylor, G.R., Reedijk, M., Rothwell, V., Rohrschneider, L. and Pawson, T. (1989). *EMBO J.* **8**, 2029–2037.

Tessner, T.G., Rock, C.O., Kalmar, G.B., Cornell, R.B. and Jackowski, S. (1991). *J. Biol. Chem.* **266**, 16261–1624.

Théry, C., Hétier, E., Evrard, C. and Mallat, M. (1990). *J. Neurosci. Res.* **26**, 129–133.

Tsui, H.W., Siminovitch, K.A., de Souza, L. and Tsui, F.W.L. (1993). *Nature Genetics* **4**, 124–129.

Tsukui, T., Kikuchi, K., Mabuchi, A., Sudo, T., Sakamoto, T., Sato, N., Tsuneoka, K., Shikita, M., Aida, T., Asano, G., Watari, E. and Yokomuro, K. (1992). *J. Leukocyte Biol.* **52**, 383–389.

Tushinski, R.J. and Stanley, E.R. (1983). *J. Cell Physiol.* **116**, 67–75.

Tushinski, R.J. and Stanley, E.R. (1985). *J. Cell. Physiol.* **122**, 211–228.

Tushinski, R.J., Oliver, I.T., Guilbert, L.J., Tynan, P.W., Warner, J.R. and Stanley, E.R. (1982). *Cell* **28**, 71–81.

Vairo, G. and Hamilton, J.A. (1991). *Immunol. Today* **12**, 362–369.

Vairo, G. and Hamilton, J.A. (1985). *Biochem. Biophys. Res. Commun.* **132**, 430–437.

Vairo, G., Argyriou, S., Bordun, A.-M., Gonda, T.J., Cragoe, E.J., Jr. and Hamilton, J.A. (1980). *J. Biol. Chem.* **265**, 16929–16939.

Van Daalen Wetters, T., Hawkins, S.A., Roussel, M.F. and Sherr, C.J. (1992). *EMBO J.* **11**, 551–557.

Van der Geer, P. and Hunter, T. (1990). *Mol. Cell. Biol.* **10**, 2991–3002.

Van der Geer, P. and Hunter, T. (1991). *Mol. Cell. Biol.* **11**, 4698–4709.

Varticovski, L., Druker, B., Morrison, D., Cantley, L. and Roberts, T. (1989). *Nature* **343**, 699–702.

Veis, N. and Hamilton, J.A. (1991). *J. Cell. Physiol.* **147**, 298–305.

Virolainen, M. and Defendi, V. (1967). *Wistar Inst. Symp. Monogr.* **7**, 67–85.

Visvader, J. and Verma, I.M. (1989). *Mol. Cell. Biol.* **9**, 1336–1341.

Wang, J.M., Chen, Z.G., Colella, S., Bonilla, M.A., Welte, K., Bordignon, C. and Mantovani, A. (1988). *Blood* **72**, 1456–1460.

Whetton, A.D., Monk, P.N., Consalvey, S.D. and Downes, C.P. (1986). *EMBO J.* **5**, 3281–3286.

Wiktor-Jedrzejczak, W., Ahmed, A., Szczylik, C, and Skelly, R.R. (1982). *J. Exp. Med.* **156**, 1516–1527.

Wiktor-Jedrzejczak, W., Bartocci, A., Ferrante, A.W., Jr., Ahmed-Ansari, A., Sell, K.W., Pollard, J.W. and Stanley, E.R. (1990). *Proc. Natl Acad. Sci. USA* **87**, 4828–4832.

Wiktor-Jedrzejczak, W., Urbanowska, E., Aukerman, S.L., Pollard, J.W., Stanley, E.R., Ralph, P., Ansari, A.A., Sell, K.W. and Szperl, M. (1991). *Exp. Hematol.* **19**, 1049–1054.

Wiktor-Jedrzejczak, W., Ansari, A.A., Szperl, M. and Urbanowska, E. (1992a). *Eur. J. Immunol.* **22**, 1951–1954.

Wiktor-Jedrzejczak, W., Ratajczak, M.Z., Ptasznik, A., Sell, K.W., Ahmed-Ansari, A. and Ostertag, W. (1992b). *Exp. Hematol.* **20**, 1004–1010.

Wilkins, J.A., Cone, J., Randhawa, Z.I., Wood, D., Warren, M.K. and Witkowska, H.E. (1993). *Protein Science* **2**, 244–254.

Willman, C.L., Stewart, C.C., Griffith, J.K., Stewart, S.J. and Tomasi, T.B. (1987). *Proc. Natl Acad. Sci. USA* **84**, 4480–4484.

Witmer-Pack, M.D., Hughes, D.A., Schuler, G., Lawson, L., McWilliam, A., Inaba, K., Steinman, R.M. and Gordon, S. (1993). *J. Cell Sci.* **104**, 1021–1029.

Wong, G.G., Temple, P.A., Leary, A.C., Witek Giannotti, J.S., Yang, Y.C., Ciarletta, A.B., Chung, M., Murtha, P., Kriz, R., Kaufman, R.J. *et al.* (1987). *Science* **235**, 1504–1508.

Wood, G.W., De, M., Sanford, T. and Choudhuri, R. (1992). *Dev. Biol.* **152**, 336–343.

Woolford, J., McAuliffe, A. and Rohrschneider, L.R. (1988). *Cell* **55**, 965–977.

Xu, X.X., Tessner, T.G., Rock, C.O. and Jackowski, S. (1993). *Mol. Cell. Biol.* **13**, 1522–1533.

Yarden, Y., Escobedo, J.A., Kuang, W.J., Yang-Fang, T.L., Daniel, T.O., Tremble, P.M., Chen, E.Y., Ando, M.E., Harkins, R.N., Francke, U., Fried, V.A., Ullrich, A. and Williams, L.T. (1986). *Nature* **323**, 226–232.

Yarden, Y., Kuang, W.J., Yang-Feng, T., Coussens, L., Munemitsu, T.J., Dull, T.J., Chen, E., Schlessinger, J., Francke, U. and Ullrich, A. (1987). *EMBO J.* **6**, 3341–3351.

Yeung, Y.-G., Berg, K.L., Pixley, F.J., Angeletti, R.H. and Stanley, E.R. (1992). *J. Biol. Chem.* **267**, 23447–23450.

Yi, T., Cleveland, J.L. and Ihle, J.N. (1992). *Mol. Cell. Biol.* **12**, 836–846.

Yoshida, H., Hayashi, S.-I., Kunisada, T., Ogawa, M., Nishikawa, S., Okamura, H., Sudo, T., Shultz, L.D. and Nishikawa, S.-I. (1990). *Nature* **345**, 442–444.

Chapter 22

The Chemokines

Thomas J. Schall

DNAX Research Institute, CA 94304, USA

INTRODUCTION

How is leukocyte trafficking accomplished? This question has occupied immunologists for over a century. Metchnikov predicted the necessity of cell-specific attractant signals late in the 19th century, a direct result of his penchant for placing rose thorns in starfish larvae. His observations surrounding amoebocyte attacks on the foreign body and his peculiar yet appealing concept of organismal harmony and disharmony led him to postulate that 'physiological inflammation' was a necessary condition of living systems. But like many of his ideas, debate over the nature of the attracting signals for phagocytes, which are necessary for physiological inflammation and, hence, for the functioning of an active, adaptive, and dynamic host defence, was sidetracked for over 50 years. Metchnikov's vision gave way to the humoral immunologists and their decades-long quest to decipher the mechanisms of antibody recognition.

Recent immunological history has witnessed the appreciation of what seem on the surface to be entirely new areas of immunobiology, but whose roots can be traced to Metchnikov's time. Nowhere is this better exemplified than in the explosion of two fields over the last decade: (1) the leukocyte adhesion molecules and (2) the recently discovered superfamily of immune cytokines we have come to call the chemokines.

This chapter concerns itself with the biology of the chemokines. Although the properties of these molecules have only recently begun to be elucidated, the bulk of the evidence to date suggests that the chemokines function as regulators of inflammatory and immunoregulatory processes, particularly through their specific leukocyte chemo-attractant effects. This chapter will investigate what these effects are and how they may be involved in what Metchnikov might have described as physiologic inflammation, as well as in processes of pathologic inflammation.

The structure of this chapter is designed to help the reader make sense of a rapidly expanding field that touches upon various biomedical disciplines. In it the attempt is made first to organize the complicated history of the discovery of the chemokine proteins. Accordingly, a brief overview of the history of the identification of each molecule in the superfamily is given. A more detailed description of the bioactivities is given in subsequent sections, with a particular emphasis placed on their potential roles in leukocyte biology in general and leukocyte trafficking in particular. The chapter will then examine the complex receptor–ligand interactions in the chemokine superfamily, as we seek to understand through what mechanisms the overlapping and distinct bioactivities of the chemokine proteins are mediated. These concepts yield naturally to a review of the current ideas of the involvement of chemokines in various diseases. Because more information is available from the human than murine studies (and for reasons of simplicity) there is an admitted bias towards using the human chemokine nomenclature throughout this report. Nevertheless, every attempt is made to discuss and refer to chemokines in other species.

A BRIEF HISTORY OF THE CHEMOKINES

Like the physicists' *dark matter*, the existence of chemokines had been suspected, but their nature in the immunological cosmos was undefined until relatively recently. Once appreciated as molecular entities, however, the roles of these small secreted proteins are beginning to be thought of as central to a cohesive model of immune function.

The chemokines have been called a 'bewildering, burgeoning family' of proteins (see Shaw, first edition of this volume, 1991). This is a fair comment since nowhere else in the field of cytokine research is one exposed to such a large family of structurally and functionally related proteins. It is interesting to note that in this volume of *The Cytokine Handbook* there are more chemokines alone (~20 distinct proteins) to be covered in this one chapter than there are in all the other chapters, each covering predominantly one cytokine combined. Thus, to adequately cover the subject in detail is beyond the scope of this work. Fortunately, at least one other chemokine, IL-8, is the subject of its own chapter in this volume. Additionally several reviews have been written in the past few years which may be of interest (Stoeckle and Barker, 1990; Oppenheim *et al.*, 1991; Schall, 1991; Miller and Krangel 1992a).

Part of the difficulty in coming to grips with the chemokines is their sheer number. A great many were identified in rapid succession in the period 1986–89, but even now new members of this superfamily are ghosting themselves into the literature. A roster of the human chemokine superfamily, current as of this writing, is given in Fig. 1. Structurally these proteins form a superfamily of proteins that are related by a four-cysteine motif. The superfamily is subdivided into two branches based upon whether the first two cysteines in the motif are either adjacent (termed the C–C branch) or spaced by an intervening residue (the C–X–C chemokines; Fig. 1). The term chemokine has only recently been decided on by an international committee (see Lindley *et al.*, 1993). Other terms used in the past have included the intercrines, the scy (small cytokine) family, and SIS (small inducible, secreted) cytokines. Chemokine is now the sanctioned usage. This term, a contraction of chemoattractant cytokine, is used to describe molecules which share this four-cysteine motif. The other key presumption implicit in the name is that the proteins that comprise the chemokine superfamily will all display some chemoattractant activity but, as discussed below, this has by no means been shown in all cases. It should also be noted that not all cytokines possessing chemo-attractant activity (TGF-β, for example) are considered chemokines since the name is based as much on structural as functional considerations.

In number, degree of relatedness, and complexity, the chemokines are quite unlike anything that has previously been seen in the study of cytokines. The route to the

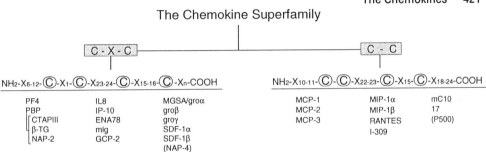

Fig. 1. Organization of the chemokine superfamily. Diagrammatic representation showing the relationship of the mature protein structures of C–X–C and C–C chemokines in the superfamily. Cysteine residues are encircled and the number of intervening amino acids between them (X) in a typical human chemokine is denoted by the subscript. C terminal residues for the C–X–C branch (X_n) range from 15–53 amino acids. The designations for the molecules listed are those for the human chemokines except in the case of murine C10 and 17 where no human molecule has yet been identified. The line connecting CTAP III, β-TG, and NAP-2 to PBP indicates that these proteins are thought to be derived from a common precursor. Molecules listed in parentheses (NAP-4 and P500) are chemokine variants that lack some of the cysteines in the canonical four-cysteine motif.

discovery of most of the chemokines has also been unusual. For example, traditionally studied cytokines (virtually all of the early interleukins, interferons, and TNF, to name a few) were discovered first by observations of soluble bioactivities, followed by rigorous biochemical analysis and purification of protein entities responsible for those activities. Although some of the early chemokines were identified by such methods, most of the members of the superfamily were, by contrast, discovered as a result of molecular cloning techniques. Typically, investigators were attempting to identify novel genes that were characteristically expressed in a cell-type-specific (e.g. by T cells or monocytes) or activation-state-specific (e.g. after mitogen or antigen exposure) fashion. Thus, the chemokine superfamily was originally little more than a collection of cDNAs encoding small, secreted, structurally related proteins of unknown function which resulted from such experiments.

It is impossible to embark on a discussion of the functions of the chemokines without a review of the discovery of each of the members of the superfamily. Accordingly, this section will briefly consider the history of members of the two subgroups C–C and C–X–C individually.

The C–X–C Chemokines

The Platelet α Granule Proteins: PF4, PBP, β-TG, CTAP-III and NAP-2

Long before a chemokine superfamily was identified, there was platelet factor 4 (PF4). Thirty years before the discovery of the next chemokines PF4 and the related protein β-thromboglobulin (β-TG, discussed below) were investigated because of their presence in blood platelets and because of PF4's ability to bind strongly to heparin, thereby promoting blood coagulation (Deutsch *et al.*, 1955, Deutsch and Kain, 1961). PF4 is stored in the α granules of blood platelets, and is thought to be released along with PDGF, TGF-β, and β-TG from these granules upon platelet stimulation. This platelet release response has long been thought to play a role in inflammation and wound healing.

PF4 is probably the most extensively studied of all the chemokines. However, it is a little appreciated fact among modern chemokine biologists that the number of publications, abstracts and patent applications concerning PF4 almost certainly surpasses all of those concerning the other chemokines combined. Ironically, PF4 is not a topic of mainstream research within the chemokine community. The Third International Symposium on Chemotactic Cytokines (Baden bei Wien, Austria, 1992), the forum which has come to concern itself almost exclusively with chemokine research, contained few presentations on PF4 biology.

The amino acid sequence of PF4 was fully determined in 1977 (Deuel *et al.*), setting it as the archetype of chemokine structure: a relatively small mature protein (70 amino acids) containing four cysteines. The cDNAs for rat and human PF4 were cloned 10 years later (Doi *et al.*, 1987; Poncz *et al.*, 1987). The crystal and NMR structures of PF4 have been solved and the molecule appears to exist as a homotetramer which adopts a shape reminiscent of that of MHC Class I molecules (Bjorkman *et al.*, 1987; Mayo and Chen, 1989; St. Charles *et al.*, 1989). The overall structure of PF4 is shared with another C–X–C chemokine, IL-8, the subject of another chapter of this volume.

PF4 also proved to be the archetypal chemokine in terms of some of its biological activities. Although these activities, and those of the other chemokines, will be examined in greater detail in the following sections, it is instructive to note some of the properties of this prototype chemokine here. Deuel and colleagues (1981) showed PF4 to be chemotactic protein which induced the migration of neutrophils and monocytes. In this respect PF4 sets the stage for chemokines as chemoattractant molecules while, at the same time, excepting itself from what has subsequently developed as a rule of thumb for chemokine activities. As discussed in detail below, C–X–C chemokines generally attract neutrophils but not monocytes, while C–C chemokines act conversely: attracting monocytes but not neutrophils. PF4 is one of the few chemokines that does not follow this guideline, at least *in vitro*, the others being IP-10 and possibly murine TCA3 (see below).

The lessons of PF4 biology were not readily recognized by modern chemokinologists when we first characterized new cDNAs encoding molecules of undefined functions in the mid- to late 1980s. First, the existence of the conserved four-cysteine motif was only just becoming apparent, and it was not clear at the time that this motif would exist in two variations. Second, the amount of primary structural identity between PF4 and, say, C–C chemokines such as MIP-1α and RANTES, is only around 20%, so to many workers the idea that the proteins encoded by the new cDNA clones would have chemotactic activities was not obvious. Had this been recognized earlier, many of the chemokines that existed for a time as orphan cDNA clones might have had biological functions assigned to them earlier. The lessons of PF4 biology have still probably not been fully appreciated. Whereas, for example, PF4 is known to stimulate the chemotaxis of fibroblasts (Senior *et al.*, 1983) most of the other chemokines have not been tested for fibroblast attractant activity.

As has been noted by other authors (Zucker and Katz, 1991; Miller and Krangel, 1992a), the biology of PF4 also provides a model for a link between thrombosis, inflammation, and wound healing—processes which are known to be physiologically coordinated. Thrombogenic stimulation, including aggregation of platelets, results in the release of the contents of α granules including PF4. PF4 then could recruit phagocytic leukocytes (neutrophils and monocytes) to the affected site to wall-off the tissue injury and to clear any introduced pathogens. Some products of the recruited monocytes, macrophages, and activated neutrophils could then amplify the inflammatory response, while others could mediate the healing response. Furthermore, PF4 would directly participate in wound healing via its fibroblast attractant effects.

PF4 is a more potent chemoattractant for fibroblasts than for monocytes or neutrophils (Senior *et al.*, 1983). It is not yet known whether the different potencies of PF4 for leukocytes and fibroblasts are of physiological relevance, but concentration-dependent specificity for various cell types responding to a given chemokine is a theme replayed with other chemokines. In addition, different chemokines have different potencies for the attraction of the same cell types.

β-TG, CTAP-III and NAP-2 are Proteolytically Derived from PBP

It is now clear that several other C–X–C chemokines can be found in the α granules of platelets, but they all derive from the proteolytic processing of a single protein. Differential processing of Platelet Basic Protein (PBP) at its *N*-terminus yields at least three distinct molecules with differing bioactivities: β-thrombogulin (TG), Connective Tissue Activating Protein III (CTAP-III) and Neutrophil Activating peptide 2 (NAP-2). β-TG was the original PBP derivative identified when it was found along with PF4 in platelet α granules, as described above. Begg *et al.* (1978) showed β-TG to be an 81 amino acid, highly basic protein containing the same four-cysteine motif as PF4. Also, like PF4, β-TG was shown to be a chemoattractant for fibroblast, and was more potent than PF4 in this activity (Senior *et al.*, 1983). Unlike PF4, β-TG has not been shown to be a neutrophil or monocyte attractant.

The role of CTAP-III is somewhat unclear. Also localized to the α granules of platelets, CTAP-III was originally thought to be mitogenic for synovial cells and fibroblasts (Castor *et al.*, 1979, 1983). However, these activities have not been found in highly purified CTAP-III (Holt *et al.*, 1986). The sequence of CTAP-III determined it to be identical to β-TG, except that CTAP-III was *N*-terminally extended by four amino acids (Rucinski *et al.*, 1979). This observation was followed by the purification and characterization of PBP (Holt *et al.*, 1986), which revealed two things: PBP was the precursor of both CTAP-III and β-TG, and PBP did not itself possess the bioactivities of the processed molecules. The cDNA for PBP/CTAP-III has been isolated (Wegner *et al.*, 1989).

The latest variation on the PBP theme was discovered when Walz and colleagues (1989) isolated a novel, potent neutrophil attractant and activator from platelets. This protein, NAP-2, was discovered to be yet another cleavage product of PBP. NAP-2 appears to affect neutrophils but not monocytes (note that neither CTAP-III on β-TG has been reported to have this activity). In this fashion, NAP-2 is similar to the C–X–C chemokines IL-8 and MGSA/gro (see below).

Thus, PBP can be processed to yield CTAP-III, β-TG, or NAP-2; each resulting molecule having its own bioactivity. There is reason to believe that CTAP-III is the primary species within α granules (Holt *et al.*, 1986), but further processing after degranulation is suspected. The processing steps responsible for the generation of these distinct molecules is yet unclear. There is no evidence to suggest that the processing of PBP to the smaller molecules occurs sequentially, and distinct proteolytic mechanisms are thought to be in place. Perhaps the most interesting feature of the PBP derivatives is how proteolytic processing of the N-terminus unmasks new activities. Much remains to be discovered how this specificity is imparted at the level of receptor–ligand interactions for these molecules.

There is one twist in the chemokines-derived-from-platelets story that should be mentioned here. A molecule designated neutrophil activating protein-4 (NAP-4, where under the NAP nomenclature, NAP-1 is identical to IL-8, NAP-2 has been described above, and NAP-3 has been used to describe MGSA/gro-α, discussed below) has been isolated by Schröder and colleagues (1990b) from platelet lysates. NAP-4 is mildly chemotactic for neutrophils ($ED_{50} \approx 400$ ng/ml), and will crossreact with an anti-IL-8 monoclonal antibody (Schröder et al., 1990b). The N-terminal sequence of NAP-4 revealed it to be a novel protein with a high degree of similarity to PF4. However, NAP-4 lacks the first two canonical cysteines in the C–X–C motif that would place it clearly in the chemokine family. Since the name chemokine by definition refers to structure as well as function (see Lindley et al., 1993), NAP-4 is destined to reside in a nether region of chemokine biology. There it may be joined by other ill-defined 'quasi-chemokines', including molecules such as P500 discussed below.

The Nonplatelet C–X–C Chemokines: IL-8, IP-10, MGSA/gro Proteins, ENA78, mig, and GCP-2

The C–X–C chemokines not found in platelets are a collection of molecules derived from a variety of tissue sources. Probably the most extensively studied of these is IL-8 NAP-1 which is the subject of another chapter in this volume. The interaction of IL-8 with its receptors, however, will be examined briefly in the receptor–ligand section below. Here we will review the other nonplatelet-derived C–X–C chemokines in the order of their first characterizations.

IFN-γ-inducible protein 10 (IP-10) was identified by molecular cloning as a cDNA encoding a 10 kDa protein of undefined function (Luster et al., 1985). IP-10 mRNA was found in monocytes, fibroblasts and endothelial cells. In addition, IP-10 secretion has been detected in monocytes, keratinocytes and activated T cells. IP-10 has been localized to sites of delayed-type hypersensitivity (DTH) reactions, such as the skin of leprosy patients injected with purified protein derivative of mycobacteria (Kaplan et al., 1987). The murine homologue of human IP-10 is encoded by the mouse cDNAs crg-2 or C7 (Ohmori and Hamilton, 1990; Vanguri and Farber, 1990). A biological activity of IP-10 has only recently been demonstrated in vitro. The chemotactic and proadhesive effects of IP-10 for blood leukocytes are discussed in detail in the next section.

Melanocyte growth stimulatory activity (MGSA) was purified as an approximately 15 kDa protein by Richmond and colleagues (1988) as an autocrine growth factor for a human melanoma cell line. MGSA cDNA was identical to one representing the gro gene, cloned a year previously by Anisowicz et al. (1987). Hamster gro was cloned by subtractive hybridization as a transcript represented much more abundantly in a tumorigenic chinese hamster embryo fibroblast (CHEF) cell line than in nontumorigenic CHEF cells. The human homologue was obtained from fibroblasts, where its transcription was apparently growth related, hence its designation as the gro gene. Generally speaking the cDNAs from both hamster and human studies and the proteins they encode are referred to as MGSA or MGSA/gro-α. The α designation was necessitated by the discovery of three distinct, nonallelic forms of gro; gro-β and gro-γ are 90% and 86% identical to the original gro (Haskill et al., 1990; Iida and Grotendorst, 1990). These three distinct human *gro* genes are thought to be the homologues of the murine KC, MIP-2α, and MIP-2β (Oquendo *et al.*, 1989; Wolpe *et al.*, 1989; Tekamp-Olson *et al.*, 1990).

Most recent published reports using recombinant or purified MGSA/*gro* protein do not concern themselves primarily with either growth or tumorigenic properties. MGSA/*gro* is now widely regarded as neutrophil attractant and activator (Balentien *et al.*, 1990; Derynck *et al.*, 1990; Moser *et al.*, 1990; Schröder *et al.*, 1990a). MGSA/*gro* biology is puzzling in several aspects. It is not clear why at least three distinct isoforms of *gro* exist. It is also not yet clear whether a specific *gro* receptor exists, or whether it utilizes only a common IL-8 receptor (Type B) as described below. It is also speculated, although not yet proven, that KC, MIP-2α, and MIP-2β (the murine *gro* homologues) perform the functions of IL-8 in mice, since there are no reports of a defined molecular homologue of IL-8 in mice (despite many attempts to identify one). Interestingly, an IL-8 receptor homologue is clearly present in mice (Wood, W., Gerard, C., Ceretti, D., personal communication, and in Dayhoff protein database as *MUSIL8GROA-1*).

Monokine induced by IFN-γ (mig-γ) was obtained first as a cDNA representing a transcript induced by IFN-γ in murine macrophages (Farber, 1990). The mig cDNA encodes a C–X–C protein predicted to be larger than most other proteins in the superfamily. The predicted mig protein is to be 127 amino acids including the signal peptide, and 104 amino acids in the mature form, and is extremely basic (pI > 11.0). The *C*-terminal extension which makes mig larger than other chemokines contains fully 50% basic residues. The human homologue has recently been found (Farber, 1993), but no functional information about the role of the mig protein has been reported.

Conversely, more is known about the function of epithelial-derived neutrophil attractant-78 (ENA-78). Walz *et al.* (1991) purified ENA-78 from the supernatants of IL-1- or TNF-stimulated A549 cells, a lung type II alveolar epithelial cell line. The known properties of ENA-78 are much like those of other C–X–C chemokines in that it functions as a neutrophil attractant and activator *in vitro*, probably by acting via a common C–X–C chemokine receptor on that cell type. The murine homologue of ENA-78 has not yet been reported.

The last C–X–C chemokines to be reported are two cDNAs designated stromal cell-derived Factors-1α and -1β (SDF-1α, 1β). These were isolated as orphan clones by Honjo and colleagues (Tashiro *et al.*, 1993) as part of a cloning strategy designed to isolate cDNAs encoding secreted molecules and Type I membrane proteins. Granulocyte chemotactic protein-2 (GCP-2, where GCP-1 has been used as a designation for IL-8/NAP-1) is an approximately 6 kDa protein isolated from the supernatants of stimulated MG63 cells, an osteosarcoma cell type (Proost *et al.*, 1993). In these cells GCP-2 exists, like gro-α, gro-γ, and IP-10, in different *N*-terminally truncated forms. Like IL-8, MGSA, NAP-2, and ENA-78, GCP-2 attracts and activates neutrophils *in vitro*, and causes granulocyte accumulation after *in vivo* injection (Proost *et al.*, 1993).

An amino acid alignment of 13 of the known distinct human C–X–C chemokines is shown in Fig. 2. The questions presented by these molecules are extremely interesting. Why has nature been so generous with the number of C–X–C chemokines? Why has it seen fit to dispense with what many have considered to be the most important one, IL-8, in mice and rats? If so many C–X–C chemokines can compensate for each other (i.e., if the actions are redundant) then why is there emerging evidence for the primacy of the role of IL-8 in neutrophil-mediated damage in animal models of inflammation and lung

```
PBP    1  S S T K G Q T K R N L A K G K E E S L D S D L Y A E L R C M C I K T   T S G I H P K N I Q S L E V I
CTAP   1          N L A K G K E E S L D S D L Y A E L R C L C I K T   T S G I H P K N I Q S L E V I
BTG    1              G K E E S L D S D L Y A E L R C M C I K T   T S G I H P K N I Q S L E V I
NAP.2  1                            A E L R C M C I K T   T S G I H P K N I Q S L E V I
PF4    1                E A E E D G D L Q C L C V K T   T S Q V R P R H I T S L E V I
groa   1                 A S V A T E L R C Q C L Q T   L Q G I H P K N I Q S V N V K
grob   1                 A P L A T E L R C Q C L Q T   L Q G I H L K N I Q S V K V K
grog   1                 A S V V T E L R C Q C L Q T   L Q G I H L K N I Q S V N V R
IL8    1              A V L P R S A K E L R C Q C I K T Y S K P F H P K F I K E L R V I
IP10   1                 V P L S R T V R C T C I S I S N Q P V N P R S L E K L E I I
ENA78  1            A G P A A A V L R E L R C V C L Q T   T Q G V H P K M I S N L Q V F
mig    1                  T P V V R K G R C S C I S T N Q G T I H L Q S L K D L K Q F
GCP-2  1                 G P V S A V L T E L R C T C L R V   T L R

PBP    50 G K G T H C N Q V E V I A T L   K D G R K I C L D P D A P R I K K I V Q K K L A G D E S A D
CTAP   41 G K G T H C N Q E N E I A T L   K D G R K I C L D P D A P R I K R I V Q K K L A G D E S A D
BTG    37 G K G T H C N Q V E V I A T L   K D G R K I C L D P D A P R I K K I V Q K K L A G D E S A D
NAP.2  26 G K G T H C N Q V E V I A T L   K D G R K I C L D P D A P R I K K I V Q K K L A G D E S A D
PF4    31 K A G P H C P T A Q L I A T L   K N G R K I C L D L Q A P L Y K K I I K K L L E S
groa   30 S P G P H C A Q T E V I A T L   K N G R K A C L N P A S P I V K K I I E K M L N S D K S N
grob   30 S P G P H C A Q T E V I A T L   K N G Q K A C L N P A S P M V K K I I E K M L K N G K S N
grog   30 S P G P H C A Q T E V I A T L   K N G K K A C L N P A S P M V Q K I I E K I L N K G S T N
IL8    34 E S G P H C A N T E I I V K L   S D G R E L C L D P K E N W V Q R V V E K F L K R A E N S
IP10   31 P A S Q F C P R V E I I A T M K K K G E K R C L N P E S K A I K N L L K A V S K E M S K R S P
ENA78  34 A I G P Q C S K V E V V A S L   K N G K E I C L D P E A P F L K K V I Q K I L D G G N K E N
mig    31 A P S P S C E K I E I I A T L   K N G V Q T C L N P D S A D V K E L I K K W E K Q V S Q K K

mig    76 K Q K N G K K H Q K K K V L K V R K S Q R S R Q K K T T
```

Fig. 2.   Primary structure of the human C–X–C chemokines. Alignment of predicted amino acid sequences of the mature proteins (devoid of signal peptides) is shown. Conserved four-cysteine motif and other residues conserved in all the proteins are boxed.

injury? If nature has already provided us with an IL-8 'knock-out' mouse (all of them), then why is there an 'IL-8 receptor' in mice? What will happen when this is knocked out?

The C–C Chemokines

Whereas many of the C–X–C chemokines were identified first by protein chemistry, most of the C–C chemokines were identified by molecular cloning. An amino acid alignment of the currently known C–C chemokines is given in Fig. 3. There are fewer C–C chemokines than C–X–C chemokines to examine in this report but this is partly because less *N*-terminal processing of the C–C chemokines (leading to molecules of distinct bioactivities, as in the case of PBP) has been reported. However, more bioactivities for C–C chemokines as a class have been reported. These bioactivities are leading to the view that C–C chemokines act as links between monocytes, lymphocytes, basophils and eosinophils during immune and inflammatory processes. In contrast, the C–X–C chemokines have been reported to act primarily on neutrophils.

Reasonably detailed treatments of the individual C–C chemokines have been given in at least two recent review articles (Schall, 1991; Miller and Krangel, 1992a). Accordingly, the early discovery and characterization of the C–C chemokines is only briefly sketched here; the reader is referred to the earlier reports for details. The biological

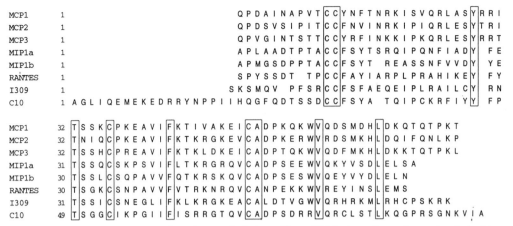

Fig. 3. Amino acid alignment of the human C–C chemokines. C10 is the only murine molecule in this alignment.

activities of the C–C chemokines are only beginning to be appreciated, however, and these are covered in more detail in the following sections.

There are seven distinct human C–C chemokines reported in the literature, and perhaps two more reported from mice for which no human homologue has yet been found (Figs 1 and 3). The macrophage inflammatory proteins (MIP)-1α and MIP-1β were characterized in the mouse as a single small (c. ~8–12 kDa) protein species (MIP-1) purified from a stimulated mouse macrophage cell line (Wolpe et al., 1988). The name derives from the cell source and from the fact that this protein preparation elicited an inflammatory response upon injection into mice footpads. Subsequent cloning of cDNA for murine MIP-1α (Davatelis et al., 1988) showed it to be the probable homologue to a human cDNA obtained three years earlier, designated LD78, which was isolated from human tonsillar lymphocytes stimulated with phorbol ester (Obaru et al., 1986). LD78 was the first reported C–C chemokine cDNA sequence, but other human MIP-1α (hMIP-1α) cDNAs have been subsequently reported cloned: PAT464 (Zipfel et al., 1989), and GOS-19 (Blum et al., 1990). In addition, other murine MIP-1α cDNAs have been called TY-5 (Brown et al., 1989), stem cell inhibitor (SCI, Graham et al., 1990), and the usefully named L2G25B (Kwon and Weissman, 1989). Modern usage, however, typically refers to all of these as either murine or human MIP-1α (MIP-1α, hMIP-1α). There is evidence to suggest that there are at least three distinct and nonallelic genes that encode hMIP-1α proteins (Irving et al., 1989; Nakao et al., 1990; Hirashima et al., 1992) but the significance of this is not yet clear. The cloning of murine MIP-1β (Sherry et al., 1988), was followed by a flurry of cloning reports identifying the human homologue variously as Act-2 (Lipes et al., 1988), H400 (Brown et al., 1989), HC21 (Chang and Reinherz, 1989), PAT744 (Zipfel et al.,1989), G26 (Miller et al., 1989), MAD-5 (Sporn et al., 1990), and LAG-1 (Baixeras et al., 1990). The predicted protein products of these cDNAs differ by a few amino acids, likely to be the result of different nonallelic MIP-1β genes. A detailed analysis of these variations can be found in the two recent reviews (Schall, 1991; Miller and Krangel, 1992a).

MIP-1α and MIP-1β in mouse and man are both about 70% identical to each other in their mature secreted forms (68–69 amino acids). Unlike nearly all of the other chemokines, MIP-1α and MIP-1β are both acidic in nature (pI ≈ 4.5), although they both have been reported to bind to heparin, which is also acidic. Despite a great deal of structural homology, MIP-1α and MIP-1β appear to have distinct specificities for their cellular targets, as detailed below.

Data from a number of laboratories suggest that both MIP-1α and MIP-1β are expressed primarily in T cells, B cells, and monocytes after stimulation with antigen or mitogen. In these cases, stimulation of mRNA accumulation for the MIP-1s is swift and massive (Schall, 1991; Miller and Krangel, 1992a). MIP-1β transcription has also been reported to occur after monocyte adherence to different substrates (Sporn et al., 1990). MIP-1α has been shown to be transcribed and produced by activated neutrophils (Kasama et al., 1993; S. McColl, personal communication), and to be regulated upon the induction of anergy in T cell clones (Schall et al., 1992a). The biological effects of the MIP-1 proteins are detailed below. In addition, some of the properties of both the MIP-1 and MIP-2 proteins have been reviewed (Wolpe and Cerami, 1989; Sherry et al., 1992).

T-cell activation gene 3 (TCA3) was identified using subtractive hybridization as a murine T-cell transcript induced upon activation of those cells by antigen or Con A (Burd et al., 1987). TCA3 is encoded, like MIP-1α and MIP-1β, as a 92-amino-acid precursor protein (68 amino acids in the mature form). TCA3 protein expressed in CHO cells is secreted as a basic 16 kDa glycoprotein (Wilson et al., 1990). The expression of TCA3 mRNA has been detected in activated T cells and mast cells (Burd et al., 1988), and the production of TCA3 protein as a function of T-cell activation has been confirmed using monoclonal antibodies (Luo et al., 1993). No biological activities have been described for purified TCA3 from in vitro studies, but its proinflammatory properties from injections into mice and rabbits are described in the next section.

The murine cDNA clone P500 (Brown et al., 1989) probably represents a splice variant of TCA3 (see Miller et al., 1990). P500 is identical to TCA3 except that it contains an insert of 99 bp in the C-terminal coding region. This insert results in an altered C terminus of the predicted P500 protein relative to TCA3, and leads to a presumed mature P500 protein 62 amino acids in length rather than 69 for TCA3. Importantly, P500 would also lack the last of the canonical four cysteines in the conserved family motif as well as the site for N-glycosylation thought to be functionally linked to a glycan in TCA3. This loss of conservation of the four-cysteine motif technically excludes P500, like NAP-4 described above, from the chemokine designation. The P500 protein, if translated in nature, would clearly not share the typical two-disulphide-bridged structure proposed for all other members of the chemokine super-family. Some molecular genetic evidence described below suggests that P500 is an active transcript. In addition, recombinant P500 has been produced in unpurified form and may indeed be biologically active in vitro (Dorf, M., personal communication).

Human I-309 was identified by Miller and colleagues (1989) as a transcript present in a γ/δ T-cell line but not in EBV-transformed B cells. Recombinant I-309 protein has been prepared (Miller and Krangel, 1992b), and its effects on monocytes, as described in a later section, makes it similar to other C–C chemokines. Judging by sequence homology alone, there is little to suggest that the human molecule I-309 and TCA3 are species counterparts. However, although the amount of amino acid identity is only 42% between the two proteins, they share an extra pair of cysteine residues not found in other chemokines. Moreover, the genomic loci for I-309 and TCA3 has been characterized, and the two genes share marked nucleotide sequence homology in their 5' flanking regions (Miller *et al.*, 1990). These similarities have led to the conclusion that I-309 and TCA3 are species homologues, although they have diverged considerably in sequence and possibly in function.

Genomic sequencing of the I-309 and TCA3 genes may also shed some light on the status of P500. The TCA3 gene carries two distinct splice acceptor sites in the second intron. The utilization of the alternative sites could result in different transcripts with distinct third exons. The 99 bp insert present in P500 described above represents an insertion immediately 5' to the start of exon 3 of the TCA3 transcript (Miller *et al.*, 1990). The isolation of P500 by Brown *et al.* (1989) from a cDNA library suggests that this splicing does occur. While alternative splicing of the human I-309 transcript has not been described, I-309 and TCA3 exhibit a perfectly conserved stretch of 14 nucleotides that span the P500 alternative splice site in the second intron. The overall nucleotide homology elsewhere in that intron is only 36%. Thus, alternative mature mRNA transcripts may exist for both TCA3 and I-309, and encode translated chemokine variants.

RANTES was also originally identified by molecular cloning as a transcript expressed in T cells but not in B cells (Schall *et al.*, 1988). The name, which has been acronymized to make it editorially palatable, is actually derived from the space alien/asylum inmate protagonist in an Argentinian film (*Man Facing Southeast,* Filmdallas Productions 1986, in Spanish with English subtitles). The mature protein encoded by RANTES is a basic 8 kDa protein (Schall *et al.*, 1990) with no N-linked glycosylation, though it may be O-glycosylated at two serine residues in the *N*-terminal portion of the protein (Kameyoshi *et al.*, 1992). It is fascinating that 35 years after the isolation of PF4 from platelet granules, RANTES has been purified from this source (Kameyoshi *et al.*, 1992), and is the only C–C chemokine known to be in platelets.

RANTES production has been detected not only in T cells and platelets, but in selected tumour-cell lines (Schall, 1991) and stimulated rheumatoid synovial fibroblasts (Rathanaswami *et al.*, 1993), where it is subjected to a fascinating regulation by IL-1, TNF, IFN-γ, and IL-4. Preliminary data suggest that the list of the types of cells and tissues capable of producing RANTES will grow (to include perhaps epithelial and endothelial cells), but RANTES does not appear to be as widely expressed nor as readily inducible as the C–C chemokine MCP-1 (see below). RANTES is becoming one of the most interesting and versatile of the chemokines in its ability to affect lymphocytes, monocytes, basophils and eosinophils. These activities are discussed by cell type in the next section.

Murine RANTES has been identified (Schall *et al.*, 1992b), and though the mRNA in the mouse is clearly shorter in the 3' UT region than its human counterpart, the proteins encoded by the two species are 85% identical. This is the highest degree of identity yet described between mouse and human chemokines.

There is a vast literature concerning the discovery, characterization, and biological activities of monocyte chemotactic protein (MCP-1) and its presumed murine counterpart, JE. However, it is probably fair to summarize most of the accumulated knowledge regarding MCP-1 at the time of writing as quite simply: almost all cells or tissues examined will make MCP-1 upon stimulation by a variety of agents, but the targets of MCP-1 appear to be limited to monocytes and basophils.

The history of MCP-1 can be traced to the discovery of murine JE in 1983 (Cochran *et al.*) and its subsequent cloning and characterization by Rollins and colleagues (1988). Like most C–C chemokines the path to the discovery of JE was a molecular one: it was a transcript induced rapidly in fibroblasts by PDGF. (The murine C–X–C chemokine KC was identified in the same way). The biological role of JE was a mystery until the discovery and purification of a human monocyte chemoattractant protein by at least two groups in 1989. This protein, variously known as lymphocyte-derived chemotactic factor (LDCF), glioma-derived chemotactic factor (GDCF), or monocyte chemotactic and activating factor (MCAF), was purified from the supernatants of stimulated human PBMC, glioma cells, or from a monocytic cell line (Matsushima *et al.*, 1989; Yoshimura *et al.*, 1989a, b). Amino acid sequencing of these proteins, as well as cDNA cloning, led to the realization that all groups were working with the same molecule, and it was likely to be the human homologue of murine JE (Chang *et al.*, 1989; Furutani *et al.*, 1989; Robinson *et al.*, 1989; Rollins *et al.*, 1989; Yoshimura *et al.*, 1989c). Oddly, the murine and human molecules are distinct in that the JE protein is *C*-terminally extended by 53 amino acids, making it considerably larger than MCP-1. Human MCP-1 is secreted from mammalian cells in perhaps three forms, each resulting from different post-translational carbohydrate modifications (Jiang *et al.*, 1990, 1991; Leonard and Yoshimura, 1990; Yoshimura and Leonard, 1990a). The biological differences, if any, between these forms is not clear.

The general use of the term MCP-1 (and MCP-2, below) is perhaps unfortunate. Care should be taken to avoid confusion with the defensin molecules designated macrophage cationic proteins 1 and 2 (MCP-1, 2) which are abundant antimicrobial peptides found in rabbit alveolar macrophages. It is surprising that more confusion has not occurred, given that the defensins are also small, cysteine-containing macrophage proteins which possess some chemoattractant activities (Selsted *et al.*, 1983, 1985; Ganz *et al.*, 1989; Linzheimer *et al.*, 1993).

The literature concerning the various types of tissues that produce MCP-1 is too vast for an adequate treatment in this chapter. More thorough reviews can be obtained by reading Miller and Krangel (1992a), Schall (1991), Leonard and Yoshimura (1990) and Yoshimura and Leonard (1991).

Recent reports have revealed the existence of monocyte chemotactic protein-2, and monocyte chemotactic protein-3 (MCP-2 and MCP-3). Van Damme and colleagues (1992) purified novel monocyte chemotactic activities from the human osteosarcoma cell line MG63. The resulting proteins were sequenced and found to be C–C chemokines with 62% (MCP-2) and 73% (MCP-3) amino acid identity to MCP-1. MCP-2 is the same molecule as the previously mentioned, though never fully described HC14 (Chang *et al.*, 1989). MCP-2 and MCP-3 share the chemoattractant specificity of MCP-1 for monocytes *in vivo* (Van Damme *et al.*, 1992). Our preliminary data with MCP-2 cDNA indicate that MCP-2 is not as widely expressed as MCP-2 (Rathanaswami *et al.*, 1994). The cDNA for MCP-3 has also been isolated (Opendakker *et al.*, 1993), and a murine cDNA designated MARC is likely to be the murine homologue of either MCP-2 or MCP-3 (Kulmburg *et al.*, 1992). Interestingly, murine MARC protein is about the same size as human MCP-2 or MCP-3, and is not *C*-terminally extended like the presumed MCP-1 homologue JE.

The MCPs comprise a distinct subgroup within the C–C family. It is now difficult to assign specific species homologues between these molecules, particularly when one considers the peculiar size difference of murine JE relative to all the other known MCP molecules. The significance of the existence of this MCP group within the chemokine family is not yet clear.

Murine chemokines have been identified for which no human homologue are yet known. C10 is a mouse cDNA identified by Orlofsky *et al.* (1991) as a transcript induced in bone-marrow cells after stimulation with GM-CSF. The deduced amino acid sequence derived from the C10 cDNA predicts a C–C chemokine that is longer than most other C–C chemokines. C10 protein would be 116 amino acids long, including the signal peptide (compared with 92 amino acids for RANTES) and the extra amino acids in C10 would make it likely to have an extended *N*-terminus relative to other chemokines. The protein also contains an extra pair of cysteine residues not found in other chemokines. The expression of C10 mRNA has been detected in some murine myeloid lineage cells, where its expression is induced by GM-CSF. In addition, C10 mRNA has been detected in an IL-2-dependent murine T-cell line, where expression of the mRNA is substantially reduced following stimulation of the cells. The only other chemokine known to exhibit such a reduction in mRNA accumulation after T-cell stimulation is RANTES. No reports of C10 protein have been published and its biological activities are still unknown.

It is known that T-helper cells can be made unresponsive, or anergic, when they are stimulated only through their T-cell receptor in the absence of costimulation through the CD28 molecule. These anergic T cells produce little or no IL-2, suboptimal amounts of IFN-γ, and are unresponsive to subsequent stimulation by antigen. The search for T-cell molecules that may be associated with the anergic phenotype has recently yielded a new member of the murine C–C chemokine family. A cDNA designated clone 17, which is more highly expressed in mouse T cells stimulated solely with an anti-CD3 antibody than in T cells stimulated both with anti-CD3 and anti-CD28, has been isolated (Jenkins, M. personal communication). Clone 17 mRNA is well expressed not only under anergy-inducing conditions but it appears to be maintained in the anergic state, and is unperturbed by subsequent stimulation of the cells with conditions that mimic antigen stimulation. It is not yet known whether the protein product of clone 17 is involved in the induction or maintenance of anergic phenotype.

Chemokine Gene Organization

The genomic configurations of the C–X–C chemokines PF4, IP-10, MGSA/gro, and IL-8 have been reported. All of these genes have been localized in man to chromosome 4 between q12 and q21 (Griffin *et al.*, 1987; Luster *et al.*, 1987; Richmond *et al.*, 1988; Modi *et al.*, 1990). The C–C chemokines genes studied to date appear to be similarly clustered but on a different chromosome. The genes for hMIP-1α, hMIP-1β, I-309, MCP-1, and RANTES have been localized to chromosome 17 (q11–q21) (Irving *et al.*, 1989; Donlon *et al.*, 1990; Miller *et al.*, 1990; Modi *et al.*, 1991; Rollins *et al.*, 1991b; Hirashima *et al.*, 1992). The characterized murine C–C chemokine genes are similarly clustered on a syntenic region of mouse chromosome 11. With the exception of PF4, all C–X–C chemokines genes have a four exon, three intron structure, with the intron/exon junctions highly conserved. The C–C chemokine genes all appear to be configured in a three exon, two intron arrangement. PF4 is the only C–X–C reported, to date, to share this C–C gene motif. A more thorough analysis of the molecular genetics of the chemokines can be found in Miller and Krangel (1992a), Schall (1991), and Miller *et al*. (1990).

THE EFFECTS OF CHEMOKINES ON BLOOD LEUKOCYTES: AN ANALYSIS BY CELL TYPE

The chemokines have been so named mainly because of their ability to induce the migration of various white blood cell populations. The establishment of chemoattractant activity can be made from either *in vivo* or *in vitro* experiments. Both approaches contain pitfalls of interpretation. IL-1 or TNF injected into mouse footpads clearly induces an inflammatory response characterized by the profound infiltration of various leukocyte populations. However, neither of these two molecules seems to profoundly and directly induce the migration of leukocytes. Therefore, to assign chemoattractant activity to a molecule based solely on *in vivo* experiments is to risk ascribing a direct effect to the injected molecule when the infiltration of cells may be an indirect consequence of its presence. However, *in vitro* assignments of chemotactic activity are also fraught with difficulties.

The Boyden chamber is the preferred microchemotaxis assay system used for the *in vitro* investigation of chemoattractant substances. This type of assay is arguably crude, certainly flawed, but also undeniably effective. In this assay, a series of wells is drilled into a plexiglass block. Each well consists of two chambers, upper and lower, which are separated by any one of several types of porous filters, nitrocellulose and polycarbonate being two common examples. Into the top chamber of each well is added the cell of interest, for example, neutrophils or peripheral blood mononuclear cells (PBMC). To the bottom chamber is added the test substance, or chemoattractant of interest. Simply stated, if the cells in the top chamber are attracted to the substance in the bottom chamber, they will migrate along the theoretical concentration gradient which exists in solution, crawl through the pores of the filter, and adhere for a while to the bottom side of that filter. After a suitable incubation period the filters can be removed from the wells and cells on the underside of the filters (those that have migrated) can be stained and counted by eye or by semi-automated processes.

Now consider the limitations of this sort of assay, and contrast this with what is likely to be happening *in vivo*. First, the *in vitro* assay depends partially on the ability of the tested cells to adhere to plastic and other nonphysiological substrates. Second, the assay is dependent on the cells' innate chemotactic ability, that is, the ability to recognize, and migrate along, a gradient in the fluid phase. It may be more physiologically relevant, however, to consider normal cells as responding in a haptotactic fashion, that is, migrating in response to proteins bound to a substratum, rather than in free solution. The evidence for the relevance of such a situation for the chemokines is discussed in more detail in the following section.

Thus, the use of the standard *in vitro* assays to accurately predict physiologically relevant chemoattractant activities is undeniably limited, and more sophisticated systems are being developed. Nevertheless, the current experimental models are providing evidence for a fascinating spectrum of chemokine activities for each of the

Table 1. Chemoattraction *in vitro* of monocytes and neutrophils.

Neutrophils		Monocytes	
PF4	(C–X–C)	MCP-1	(C–C)
IL-8	(C–X–C)	MCP-2	(C–C)
NAP-2	(C–X–C)	MCP-3	(C–C)
MGSA/gro-α	(C–X–C)	RANTES	(C–C)
GCP-2	(C–X–C)	MIP-1α	(C–C)
ENA.78		MIP-1β	(C–C)
NAP-4		I-309	(C–C)
		IP-10	(C–X–C)
		PF4	(C–X–C)

Based on purified recombinant or natural material.

five major classes of blood leukocytes: neutrophils, monocytes, lymphocytes, basophils, and eosinophils.

Monocytes and Neutrophils

If one examines the effects of the chemokines on monocytes and neutrophils *in vitro* a simple (though not absolute) pattern emerges. Generally speaking, C–X–C chemokines affect neutrophils but not monocytes, while C–C chemokines affect monocytes but not neutrophils. This general trend is shown in Table 1. The biological activities most actively investigated *in vitro* with these two cell types include chemoattraction and activation. MGSA/gro-α, IL-8, ENA-78, GCP-2, NAP-2 (and NAP-4) have all been reported to preferentially attract neutrophils *in vitro* and to induce activation, as measured by shape change, transient increases in cytoplasmic calcium concentration, degranulation, respiratory burst, increased adhesive properties, and enhanced ability to kill pathogens (reviewed by Oppenheim *et al.*, 1991, and Van Damme, Chapter 10 in this volume). The situation with the C–X–C chemokines is also relatively simple *in vivo*. Injection studies using rats, mice, and rabbits commonly show an influx of neutrophils in response to the C–X–C chemokines which are known to be active *in vitro*.

The monocyte activities of the C–C chemokines, when tested *in vitro*, are also fairly straightforward: RANTES, MCP-1, MCP-2, MCP-3, hMIP-1α, hMIP-1β, and I-309 have all been reported to induce the migration of monocytes, but not neutrophils in microchemotaxis assays. MCP-1 has also been reported to elicit degranulation and respiratory burst in monocytes (Zachariae *et al.*, 1990; Rollins *et al.*, 1991a), and regulate adhesion molecule expression and cytokine production in these cells (Jiang *et al.*, 1992). The designation of MCP-1 as a monocyte chemotactic and *activating* factor (MCAF) was given after the chemokine was observed to enhance the ability of monocytes to inhibit the growth of certain tumour cells *in vitro* (Matsushima *et al.*, 1989). Little has been reported on the monocyte activating capabilities of other C–C chemokines. One study does report that murine MIP-1α will enhance macrophage cytotoxicity for tumour targets and cause the induction of IL-1, TNF and IL-6 in elicited mouse peritoneal macrophages (Fahey *et al.*, 1992). This is significant since chemokines have been typically thought of as end-stage cytokines. The finding that a chemokine can induce the production of primary regulatory cytokines such as IL-1 and TNF runs counter to this notion.

Where does the C–C/monocyte and C–X–C/neutrophil paradigm not hold true? With *in vitro* studies there are only two obvious exceptions. PF4 has been reported to attract both neutrophils and monocytes (Deuel *et al.*, 1981), although its effects on neutrophil functions *in vitro* have been more thoroughly studied (Bebawy *et al.*, 1986). IP-10, another C–X–C chemokine, has never been shown to attract neutrophils, but it has recently been reported to behave like a C–C chemokine—attracting monocytes but not neutrophils (Taub *et al.*, 1993b).

It is primarily with *in vivo* studies that the distinction has not been rigorously tested, and some studies call the paradigm's validity into question. One example is the case of the murine protein preparation MIP-1 (a combination of MIP-1α and MIP-1β). Originally MIP-1 was shown to elaborate an inflammatory response characterized by a neutrophil influx when injected into mouse footpads (Wolpe *et al.*, 1988). In the same study, mild attraction of neutrophils *in vitro* was reported. However, subsequent *in vitro* studies using purified recombinant material have failed to detect any neutrophil migration (McColl *et al.*, 1993; Wang *et al.*, 1993b). One detailed report showed clearly that while the recombinant hMIP-1 proteins induced a modest transient Ca^{++} flux in neutrophils, this signal was not linked to other standard measures of neutrophil function including actin polymerization, chemotaxis, degranulation, respiratory burst, or activation of the Na/H^+ antiport (McColl *et al.*, 1993). *In vivo* studies with the same material results in a large monocyte influx, but also a modest neutrophil infiltration (own unpublished data).

The murine C–C chemokine TCA3 has been reported to cause neutrophil influx upon injection into mouse footpads. This response has been shown to be rapid, and has been observed with both partially and highly purified recombinant material (Wilson *et al.*, 1990; Dorf, M. personal communication). As stated above, TCA3 is thought to be the homologue of human I-309; but I-309 has clearly been shown to be a monocyte, not neutrophil, chemoattractant *in vitro* (Miller and Krangel, 1992b). Preliminary indications suggest that recombinant P500 protein (the TCA3 variant which may represent the product of alternative splicing) also appears to attract neutrophils *in vitro* (Dorf, M. personal communication). Obviously, direct comparison of the molecules both *in vitro* and in animals is required to determine their similarities and differences in modes of action.

It is probably fair to say that, on the balance, the data *in vitro* and *in vivo* support the hypothesis that C–X–C chemokines act primarily on neutrophils while C–C chemokines act preferentially on monocytes. This has clear implications for the roles of the two chemokine subgroups in acute and chronic inflammatory processes. This is also relevant in light of the actions of chemokines on another class of cells known to be involved in chronic inflammatory processes: the lymphocyte.

Lymphocytes

At the time of writing three C–C and two C–X–C chemokines have been reported to have differential chemoattractant and adhesive effects on lymphocytes: RANTES, hMIP-1α, hMIP-1β, IL-8, and IP-10. In the C–C branch RANTES was first shown to be an attractant of memory (CD45 RO$^+$) cells in 1990 (Schall *et al.*). Preliminary data on the chemoattractant effects of MIP-1α and MIP-1β were presented in 1991 (Schall), and two recent reports have detailed that MIP-1α and MIP-1β preferentially attract CD8$^+$ and CD4$^+$T cells, respectively (Schall *et al.*, 1993a; Taub *et al.*, 1993a). Additionally, MIP-1α is the only chemokine which has been shown to be an attractant for B cells (Schall *et al.*, 1993a). While the C–X–C chemokine IP-10 has been reported to be a mild chemoattractant of stimulated (αCD3 treated) CD4$^+$/CD29$^+$ T cells, (Taub *et al.*, 1993b), the chemotactic response of T cells to IL-8 has become contentious. The interleukin designation for what had been previously known as NAP-1 (among other terms) was conferred as a result of its attractant effects on T cells both *in vitro* and *in vivo* (Larsen *et al.*, 1989). However, Taub *et al.* (1993a) show no *in vitro* chemoattractant effects for IL-8, even though RANTES, MIP-1α, and MIP-1β are active in the same assays. Clearly, further examination of the role of IL-8 in T-cell migration is needed.

Of the two groups who have reported lymphocyte chemoattraction in response to chemokines, some minor differences in experimental results are seen, but there are also clear similarities. Both groups agree that MIP-1α and MIP-1β preferentially attract CD8$^+$ and CD4$^+$ T cells, respectively, though one report (Schall *et al.*, 1993a) detects a concentration dependency in the chemoattractant specificity of MIP-1α. In addition, while Taub *et al.* suggest that MIP-1α, MIP-1β (1993a), and IP-10 (1993b) will attract T cells only after αCD3 stimulation of those cells, the other study shows no such requirement for chemokine-mediated attraction of T lymphocytes (Schall *et al.*, 1993a). These discrepancies are likely a result of differences in the methods used for T cell isolation, as well as in details concerning the microchemotaxis assays as employed by the different investigators. (Compare Bacon *et al.*, 1988; Schall *et al.*, 1990, 1993a; Taub *et al.*, 1993a, b). One should not let these relatively minor differences obscure what might be considered the important message obtained from these experiments: different chemokines, when tested together in the same assays (making direct comparisons possible) appear to attract distinct subsets of lymphocytes.

In addition to the lymphocyte attractant activities of the chemokines, three reports have defined the lymphocyte adhesion-inducing properties of some of the chemokines. The first report showed that MIP-1β increased the adhesiveness of CD8$^+$ T lymphocytes when proteoglycan-immobilized chemokine was presented to the cells (Tanaka *et al.*, 1993). The same report demonstrated that this chemokine could be localized by immunostaining to lymph node endothelium, supporting the idea that immobilization by charged glycosoaminoglycans on molecules such as CD44 could be a means by which chemokines establish solid-phase gradients *in vivo*. The adhesive effects of MIP-1β and MIP-1α have also been examined by Taub *et al.* (1993a). In that report, however, MIP-1β appeared to enhance the adhesion of CD4$^+$ T cells, the same population that it preferentially attracts. Similarly, MIP-1α induced the adhesion of CD8$^+$ T cells. The reason for the differences between the Tanaka and the Taub reports with respect to the proadhesive specificities of the hMIP-1 proteins are not yet clear. IP-10 and RANTES have also been reported to increase the adhesion of CD3-activated T cells for IL-1-stimulated HUVEC (Taub *et al.*, 1993b).

B-cell function appears to be affected by at least two chemokines. Not only does MIP-1α attract B cells, as mentioned above, but IL-8 has been reported to selectively inhibit IgE production in IL-4-stimulated B cells (Kimata *et al.*, 1992).

Basophils

Blood basophils can be induced to degranulate and release histamine in the absence of IgE. Histamine release factors (HRF) have been postulated to effect this action via an IgE-independent pathway, and extracts of stimulated monocyte supernatants have been shown to contain potent HRF activity (Thueson et al., 1979; Baeza et al., 1989). Several groups over the last few years have been dissecting the defined protein components that comprise HRF. Notable success has been achieved recently; it has been shown that the C–C chemokine MCP-1 is a potent histamine releasing agent, and is probably the major histamine inducer in crude HRF (Alam et al., 1992c; Bischoff et al., 1992; Kuna et al., 1992a). In addition, RANTES has been also shown to be effective at histamine release and, to a lesser extent, so has hMIP-1α (Alam et al., 1992b; Kuna et al., 1992b; Bischoff et al., 1993). Finally, the related C–X–C chemokines CTAP-III and NAP-2 appear to be weak inducers of histamine release (Reddigari et al., 1992), as does PF4 and its C-terminal amino acids 59–70 (Brindley et al., 1983). Interestingly, pretreatment of basophils with heterologous chemokines has been shown to desensitize the histamine-releasing capacity of MCP-1 (Kuna et al., 1991, 1992b; Alam et al., 1992a). As is true for crude HRF, chemokine activation of basophils appears to be independent of IgE induced activation pathways (Kuna et al., 1992a, b, 1993). Basophils can also be induced to migrate in response to C–C chemokines. RANTES and MCP-1 have been shown to potent basophil chemoattractants in vitro (Leonard et al., 1991; Bischoff et al., 1993).

Eosinophils

Excessive activation of eosinophils (and basophils/mast cells) is thought to be central to asthma and other allergic diseases. The role of eosinophils in inflammatory processes, lung disorders, and in host defence against parasitic infection has been well documented (see, for example, Gleich, 1990). The existence of defined eosinophil chemotactic proteins has been postulated for some time, but except for the complement fragment C5a, few proteins tested appeared to be genuinely potent eosinophil attractants. Possible cytokine eosinophil attractants include lymphocyte chemotactic factor (LCF; Rand et al., 1991), and IL-5 (Wang et al., 1989), although the latter appears to be a rather weak attractant in many assays. Three recent reports provide strong evidence that C–C chemokines are potent eosinophil chemoattractants. Schröder and colleagues purified an eosinophil chemoattractant from thrombin-stimulated blood platelets. N-terminal sequencing of this protein revealed it to be identical to RANTES (Kameyoshi et al., 1992). The chemoattraction of eosinophils to RANTES was independently observed by Rot et al. (1992) using purified recombinant material; the report also showed MIP-1α to possess eosinophil attractant activity, although its potency was less than RANTES. No activity was detected in response to MIP-1β or MCP-1. Rot and colleagues also showed that RANTES and MIP-1α would induce a modest activation of eosinophils, as measured by the release of eosinophil cationic proteins (ECP), and superoxide production. In addition, Alam et al. (1993) have shown ECP release, a modest upregulation of the CD11/CD18 adhesion markers, and the induction of hypodensity (the state most often observed in asthma and rhinitis) in eosinophils after RANTES stimulation.

Table 2. Chemoattractant effects *in vitro* of chemokines for cells other than monocytes and neutrophils.

	T Cells	B cells	Eosinophils	Basophils	Fibroblasts
PF4					+
β-TG					+
IL-8	±			−	
IP-10	+				
RANTES	+	−	+	+	
MCP-1				+	
MIP-1α	+	+	+	±	
MIP-1β	+	−	−	−	

Taken together these results show that C–C chemokines can be potent regulators of eosinophil function. These activities, especially in combination with their basophil attractant and activating functions, suggest that the chemokines may be key regulators of allergic rhinitis, asthma, and other respiratory pathologies.

A MODEL OF CHEMOKINE INVOLVEMENT IN LEUKOCYTE TRAFFICKING

What is the biological role and significance of the selective chemoattractant (as summarized in Tables 1 and 2) and proadhesive effects of the chemokines for leukocytes? The adhesion of white blood cells to endothelial cells is a necessary component for the development of immune and inflammatory responses. But the problem of leukocyte trafficking is to get the right cell to the right location at the right time. The selective activities of the chemokines for lymphocyte subsets as described primarily in the five reports discussed (Schall *et al.*, 1990, 1993a; Tanaka *et al.*, 1993; Taub *et al.*, 1993a, b), make them ideal candidates to play a key role in a solution of the trafficking problem for lymphocytes. If this one small family of factors possesses the dual properties of promoting both cell subtype-specific chemoattraction and adhesion, then their elaboration at an inflammatory site could provide an economical way of directing lymphocyte trafficking.

However, one must contrast the typical *in vitro* microchemotaxis and adhesion assay systems by which the chemokine data were obtained to what is likely to be happening *in vivo*. Although on the simplest level leukocyte trafficking can be thought to contain two main components: sticking and crawling, the *in vivo* requirements for a trafficking cell include circulation, adhesion, diapedesis, and migration, and is likely to be an immensely complicated process. Leukocytes must overcome haemodynamic forces to adhere to the endothelial cell surface lining the typical vessel wall. Having done this, they must crawl their way along and migrate through junctions between endothelial cells and penetrate the basement membrane before gaining entry into, and migrating through, the tissue spaces. How is this done? The coordinate expression of adhesion receptors on the surface of the leukocytes and their countereceptors on the surface of endothelial cells is thought to be the key link in the process.

Let us first consider the initial step of the trafficking process, cellular adhesion. Models of cellular adhesion have been refined by Springer (1990), Butcher (1991), and Lasky (1992; see also Springer and Lasky 1991). The current view espouses a three-step process where rolling of leukocyte along the vasculature is followed by an activation step, resulting in firm adhesion, which leads ultimately to extravasation.

The selectins, which bind carbohydrate ligands, probably provide the first step in the recognition cascade. Selectin–carbohydrate interactions are thought to be somewhat transient, allowing for the rolling of the leukocyte along the vessel wall under physiological flow conditions. Selectins are undoubtedly induced in situations of thrombosis or inflammation. Lawrence and Springer (1991) and others have elegantly shown that the transition from rolling to firm adhesion requires an activation step which can be induced by chemoattractants such as the bacterial tripeptide chemoattractant fMLP (see also Smith *et al.*, 1991). After activation, firm adhesion is thought to be mediated through integrin molecules.

Butcher (1991) suggests that the activation step for lymphocytes is generally mediated through pertussis-toxin (PT) sensitive pathways. This is perfectly consistent with Lawrence and Springer's observations, as fMLP acts through a seven-transmembrane-spanning (7TM), G-protein linked, PT-sensitive receptor system (Boulay *et al.*, 1990, 1991). There is much speculation that IL-8 and other chemokines will confer the same sort of activation and firm adhesion to various populations of leukocytes. This is an appealing concept since, as discussed below, all chemokine receptors identified to date appear to share the same general 7TM architecture, and many chemokine-mediated effects are accordingly PT sensitive. Thus, although it has not been proven, chemokine mediation of the activation step of adhesion is an attractive hypothesis. Once adhered, cells could then migrate along a concentration gradient of chemokine to accomplish diapedesis and extravasation into the tissues.

In addition to potentially playing a large role in the first steps of leukocyte diapedesis, chemokines are likely to be required for the subsequent migration into, and invasion of, the interstitial spaces. Huber and colleagues (1991) have shown that IL-8 is required not only for binding of neutrophils in an *in vitro* vessel-wall model, but that the cells extravasated as a function of the presence of IL-8 on the basolateral, but not apical, side of the chamber. Moreover, IL-8 was shown to be made by the endothelium and sequestered in the subendothelial matrix produced by those same cells. This situation would obviously allow for the maintenance of a stable gradient of chemokine to direct migration of, in this case, neutrophils (Huber *et al.*, 1991). The creation of solid-phase chemotactic gradients is a physiologically sound approach. Under normal conditions of blood flow, a gradient present only in solution is apt to be washed away and would require constant replenishment by the cell producing the chemoattractant. By contrast, if the chemoattractant could be sequestered and maintained by stable components of, say, the extracellular matrix, then a single release of chemokine (as might happen during platelet degranulation) might be sufficient to initiate the inflammatory cascade. The inflammatory response could then be fine-tuned as each cell which trafficked through could leave its own signals bound in solid phase.

Is there any support for a model of sequestration of chemokines in a solid phase? Evidence has accumulated that chemokines are likely to form chemical gradients in an immobilized phase via electrostatic interactions with negatively charged proteoglycans. The work of Rot (1992) provides support for a model of IL-8 binding to endothelial cell surfaces, thus facilitating neutrophil emigration. Tanaka *et al.* (1993) provide good evidence for an association of MIP-1β with glycososaminoglycans

(GAGs) on the proteoglycan CD44, the complex then provides a scaffolding for the stimulation of T cells, resulting in a upregulation of T-cell adhesion to endothelial cells.

Many of the elements of the model discussed in this section are summarized in Fig. 4 which shows the central role chemokines may play in leukocyte trafficking.

CHEMOKINES IN TUMOUR BIOLOGY

Chemokines in Tumour Transduction Models In Vivo

The leukocyte attractant effects of chemokines have been tested (and exploited) *in vivo* in murine tumour-transduction models. The premise of the experiments is simple: can the growth of murine tumours be affected if those tumours are engineered to produce chemokines? It has been shown that chemokine secretion by tumours inhibits tumour growth. Rollins and Sunday (1991) engineered mouse CHO cells, which are normally tumorigenic in nude mice, to produce MCP-1. CHO cells so engineered failed to grow in recipient nude mice, while the parent cells formed large tumours in each case (Rollins and Sunday, 1991). Although the mechanism of inhibition was not established, a large number of monocytes and macrophages were associated with the injection site, leaving the modified CHO cells. Walter *et al.* (1991) also report that the growth of sarcoma clones expressing MCP-1 was negatively affected as a function of the amount of MCP-1 secreted. Another model has been examined in immunocompetent mice by Mulé and colleagues (1994). In that study various weakly immunogenic and nonimmunogenic murine tumours were engineered to secrete RANTES. In all cases, RANTES abolished the tumorigenicity of the transformed cells: RANTES-bearing tumour cells always failed to grow, while the unmodified cells formed large tumours in every case. The mechanism of the inhibition of tumour growth was also examined. Coadministration of antibodies which inhibited T-cell function or macrophage migration rescued the growth of the tumours. These results confirmed that the inhibition of tumour growth was an immune-mediated phenomenon dependent on monocytes/macrophages and T cells, confirming that migration phenomena observed *in vitro* are likely to occur *in vivo*.

These studies suggest that chemokines could be used in anti-tumour strategies, but at the same time they raise an interesting paradox. This paradox arises from the fact that many tumour cells, and even some primary tumours, appear to be making chemokines.

Expression of Chemokines by Tumour Cells

It has long been appreciated that macrophages and lymphocytes infiltrate the regions surrounding growing tumour cells and can comprise the majority of the mass of certain solid tumour types (Botazzi *et al.*, 1983; Mantovani, 1990). Many chemokines including MCP-1, 2, 3, GCP-2, MGSA/gro were first isolated from tumour-cell lines. In addition, Graves and colleagues have shown MCP-1 expression by a variety of malignant cells (Graves *et al.*, 1989; Graves and Valente, 1991) and in primary human melanoma (Graves *et al.*, 1992). It is not at all clear what advantage tumour cells would derive from chemokine production *in vivo*, but some compelling ideas can be raised. The normal physiological process of leukocyte diapedesis mirrors, in some ways, the pathologic

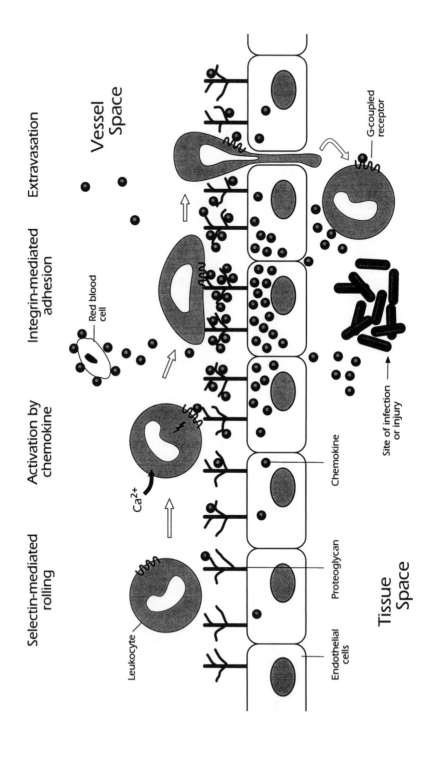

Selectin-mediated rolling | Activation by chemokine | Integrin-mediated adhesion | Extravasation

Vessel Space

G-coupled receptor

Red blood cell

Ca²⁺

Leukocyte

Site of infection or injury

Chemokine

Proteoglycan

Endothelial cells

Tissue Space

process of tumour-cell metastasis. Both the normally trafficking leukocyte and the metastasizing tumour cell must bind to endothelial cells, penetrate their junctions, and invade the basement membrane to reach the interstitial spaces. To begin the metastatic process, tumour cells must first go through this process in reverse in order to leave their initial tissue location and gain access to the circulation. Bevilaqua and colleagues have shown that certain tumour-cell types adhere to endothelial cell surfaces in the same way as normal leukocytes (Rice *et al.*, 1988; Rice and Bevilaqua, 1989). The intriguing possibility is therefore raised that chemokines somehow play a role in the invasive and metastatic potentials of certain types of tumour cells. Why then is tumour growth profoundly inhibited in experimental models of tumour transduction with chemokines? There are a few possibilities. First, the production of chemokines by native tumour cells may be stage-specific. Production of the chemokine at too early a stage (as modelled in the tumour-transduction experiments) could stop the growth of the nascent tumour via immune-mediated mechanisms. At later stages the immune cells may be ineffective against either the sheer number of transformed cells or by inactivating agents released by the mature tumour mass. Second dosage effects may be in play. The *in vivo* tumour may secrete either too much or too little chemokine to trigger an effective immune response. In the first case, too much chemokine could actually prevent leukocyte migration. It is known from *in vitro* studies that cells migrate only within a 'window' of chemokine concentration and above or below that concentration no migration is observed. High localized concentrations could also be employed by tumours to desensitize immune cells, causing them to be inadequate effector cells. Finally, small amounts of chemokine production by tumours might not trigger immune intervention, but may be sufficient to accomplish the migratory aims of the tumour.

OTHER CHEMOKINE ACTIVITIES

Haemopoiesis

The MIP proteins have been reported to have some interesting effects on haemopoietic precursor cells. Both MIP-1 and murine MIP-2, in synergy with GM-CSF and M-CSF, will enhance the formation of granulocyte-macrophage colonies by murine CFU-GM

Fig. 4.   Schematic representation of a model for chemokine involvement in leukocyte trafficking. In this multistep model, specific leukocyte populations circulating near the site of injury or infection (represented by the rods), could be signalled to adhere and extravasate by the presence of specific chemokines (small spheres) in the tissue spaces and bound to extracellular matrix components. Cytokines produced in response to the pathogen (e.g. IL-1 or TNF) induce changes in the endothelium including the upregulation of adhesion molecules and the production of certain chemokines. Chemokine production by tissue fibroblasts and platelets is known to occur, and could contribute to the initiation of the cascade. The establishment of a solid-phase chemotactic or haptotactic gradient could occur as a result of the association of chemokines with glycosoaminoglycan determinants on such molecules as CD44 (represented by the branched structures). Free chemokines escaping into the circulation are scavenged by binding to red blood cells for clearance and to maintain the gradient. The formation of the gradient leads to activation of the rolling leukocytes to form firmly adhered cells which migrate along the endothelial cell surface and eventually through endothelial cell junctions into the tissue space. Selectivity for the leukocyte migration could be supplied by the different chemokines, based on their *in vitro* activities. The adhesion molecules involved are not shown, and the proteoglycans themselves are not thought to be adhesive during the inflammatory process. Adapted from Lasky (1993).

(Broxmeyer *et al.*, 1989). However, None of the MIP preparations contains any enhancing activities in themselves. MIP-1α has also been reoported to enhance osteoclast differentiation (Kukita *et al.*, 1992). At the earliest stages of the haemopoiesis MIP-1α may actually have inhibitory effects. It has been identified as stem cell inhibitor (SCI), a protein which can reversibly inhibit the proliferation of haemopoietic stem cells (Graham *et al.*, 1990). One report indicates that the closely related MIP-β does not appear to share this activity, and may antagonize the inhibitory effect of MIP-1α (Broxmeyer *et al.*, 1991), but this is not wholly consistent with the findings of Graham *et al.* (1993). The *in vitro* observations have been supported by *in vivo* studies. Recombinant MIP-1α confers protection to the CFU-S compartment from the cell-cycle-specific toxins arabinoside (ARA-C) or hydroxyurea (HU) (Dunlop *et al.*, 1992; Lord *et al.*, 1992). In addition, exogenously administered recombinant MIP-1α, but not MIP-1β, decreased the cycling rates and numbers of myeloid progenitor cells in mouse bone-marrow and spleen, and induced a 50% decrease in the number of circulating neutrophils (Maze *et al.*, 1992). MIP-1α has also been reported to inhibit the cycling of normally quiescent long-term reconstituting stem cells *in vivo* (Quesniaux *et al.*, 1993). In two other studies, Mantel *et al.* (1993) and Graham *et al.* (1994) showed that MIP-1α, which has a tendency to polymerize and aggregate (Wolpe *et al.*, 1988), is inactive and unable to effect myelosuppression in the larger molecular-mass form; the active moiety is the MIP-1α monomer. It seems likely, although it has not been proven, that this will be true also for the other bioactivities of MIP-1α.

Are the inhibitory activities of the MIP-1α chemokine restricted to haemopoietic stem cells? There are some preliminary indications which suggest not. Heufler *et al.* (1992a, b) report that Langerhans-cell-derived MIP-1α inhibits the proliferation of keratinocyte stem cells, and Matsue and colleagues (1992) have noted Langerhans-cell production of MIP-1α. Graham and Pragnell (1992) also discuss the inhibitory effects of MIP-1α on clonogenic epidermal cells. Moreover, the antiproliferative effects of MIP-1α have not been observed solely on very early progenitor cells. One group suggests that MIP-1α can inhibit the proliferation of mature T cells (Oh *et al.*, 1991; Kwon *et al.*, 1992).

In addition to MIP-1α, Broxmeyer *et al.* (1993) report that MIP-2α, PF-4, IL-8, and MCP-1 all have some ability to suppress the colony formation of immature myeloid progenitors that have been stimulated by GM-CSF plus kit ligand. This effect is not observed when RANTES, MIP-1β, MIP-2β, gro-α, NAP-2 are tested in parallel. Although not yet tested *in vivo*, the suggestion is that multiple chemokines may have a role in the regulation of blood-cell development.

Pyrogenic Effects

Pyrogenic activities have also been ascribed to the MIP-1 proteins. Davatelis and colleagues (1989) first showed that the murine MIP-1 protein preparation induced an increase in basal temperature upon injection into rabbits. This action was unique in that it appeared to occur in a prostaglandin-independent fashion. That is, unlike IL-1 and TNF, whose fever-inducing properties can be blocked by agents such as aspirin or ibuprofen (which block the cyclooxygenase pathway), the activity of MIP-1 was unaffected by these agents. The pharmacological aspects of the pyrogenic activity of MIP-1 have been detailed in several reports by Myers and colleagues (Minano and

Meyers 1991; Minano *et al.*, 1991a, b, 1992). The evidence from these studies suggests that MIP-1 exerts its febrile effects by some direct interaction with the hypothalamus in the brain.

PF4 in the Inhibition of Tumour Growth and Megakaryopoiesis, the Alleviation of Immunosuppression, and Bactericidal Activities

On the C–X–C side of the chemokine superfamily, PF4 has been reported to have many interesting activities. It appears to be a growth inhibitor of various transformed tumour-cell lines including human erythroid leukaemia (HEL) and osteosarcoma cell lines (Han *et al.*, 1992; Tatakis, 1992). Both growth inhibition and even anti-tumour effects of PF4 have been seen *in vivo*. For example, the growth of melanoma and human colon carcinoma in mouse models has been shown to be inhibited by administration of PF4 and PF4 analogues (Sharpe *et al.*, 1990; Maione *et al.*, 1991). The anti-tumour effects of PF4 appear to be largely a function of the chemokine's anti-angiogenesis properties. As such, recombinant human PF4 inhibits angiogenesis in a chicken chorioallantoic membrane system in a dose-dependent fashion (Maione *et al.*, 1990). In that model PF4 appears to inhibit endothelial cell (EC) proliferation, as well as EC migration. The migration-blocking effects of PF4 may be due to the ability of this chemokine to block the binding of basic fibroblast growth factor to its receptors on EC (Sato *et al.*, 1990). The anti-tumour effects of PF4 have led to its current clinical trials as an anti-cancer therapeutic in humans.

Growth inhibition is also seen in the ability of PF4 to inhibit megakaryopoiesis (Gerwitz *et al.*, 1989; Han *et al.*, 1990). Interestingly, both the anti-angiogenic effects and the megakaryopoietic-inhibitory activity of PF4 appear to be a property of the *C*-terminal portion of the protein. For megakaryopoietic inhibition, the 24 amino acids at the *C*-terminals are active, while the *C*-terminal tridecapeptide (AA 58–70) is not. The anti-angiogenic effects of PF4 have been also observed with a peptide consisting of the 12 *C*-terminal residues (Maione *et al.*, 1990).

Native PF4 and its *C*-terminal peptide derivatives have also been reported to alleviate con-A-induced immunosuppression in mice (Katz *et al.*, 1985, 1986a, b, 1991; Barone *et al.*, 1988; Yin *et al.*, 1988, Zucker *et al.*, 1989; Gregg *et al.*, 1990). This activity is as fascinating as its mechanism is mysterious. In these experiments, the murine immune response to sheep red blood cells can be suppressed by injection of syngeneic mouse lymphoma cells or Con A. The suppression is measured by a decrease in the number of plaque-forming cells in the spleens of challenged mice, as measured by the technique of Jerne and Nordin (1963) and Mishell and Dutton (1967). The suppression can be overcome by the administration of PF4 (references above), and to a far lesser extent by β-TG (Katz *et al.*, 1986a, b; Zucker *et al.*, 1989). IL-8, however, is inactive in the assay (Katz *et al.*, 1991). Again the *C*-terminal peptides of PF4 seem to retain the ability to reverse the immunosuppression.

Antibacterial activity has been attributed to the last 13 amino acids of the *C*-terminus of PF4 (Darveau *et al.*, 1992). Amino acid substitutions predicted to disrupt the α-helical or amphipathic properties of this peptide abolish the activity. Other activities assigned to PF4 during its long history include stimulation of leukocyte elastase (Lonky and Wohl 1981), and an inhibition of collagenase (Hiti-Harper *et al.*, 1978). MGSA/gro-α has been examined by Unemori *et al.* (1993) and found to decrease collagen expression by human fibroblasts. Other chemokines tested (both C–C and C–X–C) did not show this activity within the narrow concentration ranges in which they were tested.

Thus, the spectrum of chemokine activities is broad, encompassing a range of shared and specific activities on all the major classes of blood leukocytes (and their subsets), as well as a much more diverse constellation of nonhaemopoietic cells and tissues. The central questions of chemokine biology are these: how are these various biologic activities accomplished at the level of cell surface interactions; how many chemokine receptors are there to accomplish the varied actions of the chemokines; what is the molecular nature of these receptors?

CHEMOKINE RECEPTOR–LIGAND INTERACTIONS

As we have seen, there are over 20 different chemokines known in two separate subfamilies. For blood leukocytes, the molecules share activities (the C–X–C for neutrophils, the C–C for monocytes, for example), as well as having distinct activities; for example, RANTES attracts eosinophils while MCP-1 does not; NAP-2 attracts neutrophils, while β-TG (which is the same protein with a few more N-terminal amino acids) does not. How is this redundancy and specificity of action imparted at the level of cell surface receptors? How many chemokine receptors are there?

A number of studies have attempted to characterize chemokine receptor–ligand interactions. These studies have generally been done on various leukocyte populations and fall into four basic categories: (1) direct binding and displacement studies with radiolabelled ligands and unlabelled competitors; (2) signal transduction studies attempting to predict the number of distinct receptors based upon Ca^{++} signal desensitization profiles in response to various chemokines; (3) molecular cloning of chemokine receptors; and (4) structure function studies employing mutagenesis techniques. Here we will examine the evidence provided by these various types of studies that the chemokines are likely to bind to an array of shared and specific receptors to accomplish their varied immunoregulatory tasks.

Direct Binding Studies

Most early direct binding studies have been done with IL-8 and MCP-1. The binding of these radiolabelled chemokines and displacement with themselves or each other led to the early observations that: (1) IL-8 would bind mostly to neutrophils; (2) MCP-1 would bind to monocytes; and (3) these two chemokines did not bind to the same receptors. The various studies of IL-8- and MCP-1 binding are typified by such reports as Yoshimura and Leonard (1990b; see also Leonard and Yoshimura, 1990) showing that MCP-1 bound monocytes with a $K_d \approx 2$ nM and this binding could not be displaced by IL-8. No MCP-1 binding to lymphocytes was detected. These data were not dissimilar to those obtained by Valente et al. (1991). For IL-8, Samanta et al. (1989) define a $K_d \approx 5$ nM on human neutrophils, with no displacement by C–C chemokines.

A fair number of reports have concerned themselves with the binding properties of MIP-1α and MIP-1β. The K_d for MIP-1α has been variously assigned at between c. 400 pM and 5 nM on monocytes, monocyte-cell lines, and T cells (Oh et al., 1991; Yamamura et al., 1992; Graham et al., 1993; McColl et al., 1993; Wang et al., 1993b). MIP-1β has been reported to bind peripheral blood mononuclear cells with an affinity of ≈ 10 nM (Napolitano *et al.*, 1990) and THP-1 monocytic cells of ≈ 400 pM (Wang *et al.*, 1993b). The Wang report also provides some binding and displacement data that support the model that there are at least three types of chemokine receptors on monocytes: (1) a MIP-1α/MIP-1β shared receptor; (2) a MCP-1-specific receptor; and (3) a MCP-1/MIP-1α/MIP-1β common receptor. Two recent papers have also examined the binding properties of RANTES, assigning its K_d on THP-1 cells and monocytes at between *c.* 450 pM and 960 pM (Van Riper *et al.*, 1993; Wang *et al.*, 1993a). Both reports suggest that MCP-1 can displace RANTES, and that MCP-1 binds to the presumed RANTES receptor with a lower relative affinity. The Wang report also shows competition for the RANTES binding site by MIP-1α.

It should also be noted that many investigators have observed anomalous binding properties with some of the chemokines. Several groups have reported difficulty in performing successful binding displacement experiments. With RANTES, for example, studies in this author's laboratory have consistently found a puzzling phenomenon of positive association, instead of displacement, of the radiolabelled RANTES protein in the presence of increasing concentrations of unlabelled competitor chemokine (Neote *et al.*, 1993b; own unpublished data). We have been able to rule out the possibility that the anomalous RANTES binding is an artifact of the reagents employed in the binding assay because in one special case the direct binding of RANTES can be readily assessed. This special case involves binding of chemokines to red blood cells and is discussed in detail below.

The reasons for the binding anomalies are not yet clear, but it should be kept in mind that binding to specific, signal-transducing cell-surface receptors is probably not the only type of binding relationship that chemokines are likely to engage in. Most of the chemokines are highly basic molecules and all seem to have positively charged domains that are likely to be capable of interacting with immobilized carbohydrates such as heparin sulphate or with proteoglycan carbohydrate moieties. Saturable PF4 binding to umbilical vein endothelium, glomerular microvascular matrix, bovine aorta, and cultured endothelial cells can be variously abolished by heparinase from platelets, or *Flavobacterium* heparinase, but not by chondroitin-ABCase or hyaluronidase (for review see Zucker and Katz, 1991). This suggests that these binding interactions are not with a specific cell-surface receptor but rather with cell-surface-associated heparin sulphates. Note also that evidence has accumulated that other chemokines such as IL-8 (Rot, 1992) and MIP-1β (Tanaka *et al.*, 1993) are likely to form chemical gradients in an immobilized phase via electrostatic interactions with negatively charged proteoglycans. Thus, the difficulty of characterizing chemokine binding to specific cell-surface receptors may be a function of the interference resulting from less-specific interactions of the ligands with extracellular matrix components.

Signal Transduction Studies: How Many Chemokine Receptors?

The measurement of the mobilization of intracellular Ca^{++} can provide a straightforward indication of early signal transduction in leukocytes. In addition, it has been shown to have a predictive value in ascertaining whether various ligands signal through the same or different cell-surface receptors. Rapid, successive exposure to the same ligand is known to desensitize the signalling capacity of G-protein-linked receptors

(Schild, 1973), and desensitization can also occur when the two different agonists signal through the same receptor.

Ca^{++} flux assays have been used in several published reports to address whether the C–C chemokines use the same or distinct receptors on panels of target cells. These reports are not all consistent with one another but, nevertheless, they reveal an emerging unusual pattern of Ca^{++} signalling desensitization in chemokine-challenged cells. Sozzani *et al.* (1991, 1993) used human monocytes freshly isolated from peripheral blood. These monocytes were loaded with calcium indicator (Fura-2 or INDO-1AM are typically used) and challenged with different combinations of MCP-1, RANTES, and MIP-1α in succession. When MCP-1 was used as the first agonist, a clear rise in intracellular calcium ion concentration (measured in a spectrofluorimeter) was observed, but no subsequent rise in calcium occurred if another dose of MCP-1 was added, or if RANTES or MIP-1α was added after MCP-1. Thus, MCP-1 has desensitized the cell to itself and to the other chemokines. The simplest explanation is that the chemokines are occupying the same receptor and the engagement of this receptor's associated G-protein complex upon MCP-1 binding triggers the Ca^{++} flux and renders the signalling complex insensitive to subsequent rapid engagement through the same receptor. However, Sozzani *et al.* (1991, 1993) report that if either RANTES or MIP-1α is added before MCP-1, two distinct calcium fluxes are observed: one in response to the first chemokine challenge (either RANTES or hMIP-1α) and one in response to the subsequent MCP-1 challenge. Finally, RANTES and hMIP-1α desensitize each other regardless of the order in which they are added. This asymmetrical pattern of signal desensitization suggests an array of shared and specific receptors. The phenomena observed by Sozzani *et al.* (1991, 1993) can be explained in terms of a two-receptor model. In fresh monocytes one can envision a receptor shared by RANTES, MIP-1α, and MCP-1, as well as a MCP-1-specific receptor. If RANTES or MIP-1α are presented first to the cells, Ca^{++} flux occurs via the shared receptor. Subsequent exposure to MCP-1 results in a second Ca^{++} flux via the specific receptor. To reverse the order of ligand challenge, however, results in only a single flux as MCP-1 occupies all of the available binding sites.

Interestingly, this pattern of desensitization is dependent on what type of target cell is being challenged with the chemokines. Bischoff and colleagues (1993) show that the pattern of calcium signal desensitization seen on basophils and eosinophils in response to RANTES, MCP-1, and MIP-1α is distinct from the pattern seen on fresh blood monocytes. However, the model presented for fresh blood monocytes can be extended to basophils and eosinophils by postulating the existence of: (1) in basophils, a RANTES-specific receptor, a MCP-1-specific receptor, and a RANTES/MIP-1α shared receptor; and (2) in eosinophils, no MCP-1 receptor, a RANTES-specific receptor, and a RANTES/MIP-1α shared receptor.

The picture becomes even more complex when four C–C chemokines are used in various combinations to challenge cultured monocytes (Schall *et al.*, 1993b). If MIP-1α is the first chemokine added to the cells, it will induce an appreciable transient Ca^{++} increase, but no other chemokine added after MIP-1α is capable of Ca^{++} mobilization in these cells. This indicates that MIP-1α desensitizes the cell to all other chemokines tested. In contrast, if MCP-1 is added first, followed by MIP-1β, then RANTES, then MIP-1α, four Ca^{++} fluxes are clearly induced. In fact, depending solely on the order in which the same ligands are added to the cells, all combinations of 1, 2, 3 and 4 fluxes are observed. In this case, one would need to invoke the rather baroque arrangement of four distinct chemokine receptors, all of which can bind hMIP-1α and each of which will bind its own combination of chemokines in the following fashion: receptor 1 binds MIP-1α/RANTES/MIP-1β/MCP-1; receptor 2 binds MIP-1α/RANTES/MIP-1β; receptor 3 binds MIP-1α/RANTES; receptor 4 binds MIP-1α alone.

One cautionary note has been sounded recently regarding this kind of model building. The cloned receptor isolated by Neote *et al.* (1993b), the C–C CKR-1, behaves as if it were two receptors. MIP-1α challenge of C–C CKR-1-transfected cells will desensitize those cells to a subsequent challenge with RANTES, but the reverse is not true: RANTES added first, followed by MIP-1α, results in two calcium signals (Neote *et al.*, 1993b). This raises the possibility that some unusual signalling mechanisms are linked to this single receptor.

Molecular Characterization of Chemokine Receptors

Four types of chemokine receptors have been cloned at the time of writing. These receptors, whose amino acid sequences are aligned in Fig. 5, share a seven transmembrane (7TM) domain architecture whose archetype is bacterial rhodopsin, are thought to be linked to heterotrimeric G-protein complexes. Two C–X–C receptors have been identified, designated the IL-8RA (sometimes called IL-8 receptor type I; Holmes *et al.*, 1991) and IL-8RB (sometimes called IL-8R type II; Murphy and Tiffany, 1991). The designation of the IL-8RB receptor is something of a misnomer: this clone is likely to bind to many C–X–C chemokines, such as—IL-8, MGSA/gro, NAP-2, and ENA78 with high affinity (Cerreti *et al.*, 1992; Lee *et al.*, 1992; Schumacher *et al.*, 1992; Gayle *et al.*, 1993). For the other branch of the superfamily, a receptor designated the C–C chemokine receptor-1 (C–C CKR-1) has been isolated. The C–C CKR-1 binds MIP-1α, RANTES, MIP-1β and MCP-1 with varying affinities, but it transduces a signal in transfected kidney cells primarily in response to MIP-1α and RANTES (Neote *et al.*, 1993b). An independent report (Gao *et al.*, 1993) calls this same receptor the MIP-1α/RANTES receptor, possibly because the experimental system used in that study was *Xenopus* oocytes and direct binding experiments using multiple ligands were not performed.

A second C–C chemokine receptor was identified at the molecular level in the report by Neote *et al.* (1993b). Interestingly, this receptor is encoded by a cytomegalovirus (CMV) open reading frame designated US28, whose function was previously undefined. The CMV chemokine receptor binds all of the C–C chemokines tested, but not the C–X–C chemokine IL-8. In addition, the viral receptor binds MIP-1α with a higher affinity ($K_d \approx 1$ nM) than does the human receptor ($K_d \approx 6$ nM) in the same system. This suggests C–C chemokines play a role in antiviral immunity or in immune evasion by CMV. Table 3 summarizes what ligands have been shown to bind to the cloned receptors.

Receptor–Ligand Structure Function Studies

Several studies have shown that the *N*-terminal portion of IL-8 is important in receptor binding and possibly neutrophil activation. The sequence Glu–Leu–Arg (ELR) at positions 4–5–6 preceding the cysteine residues in the *N*-terminal portion of the 72

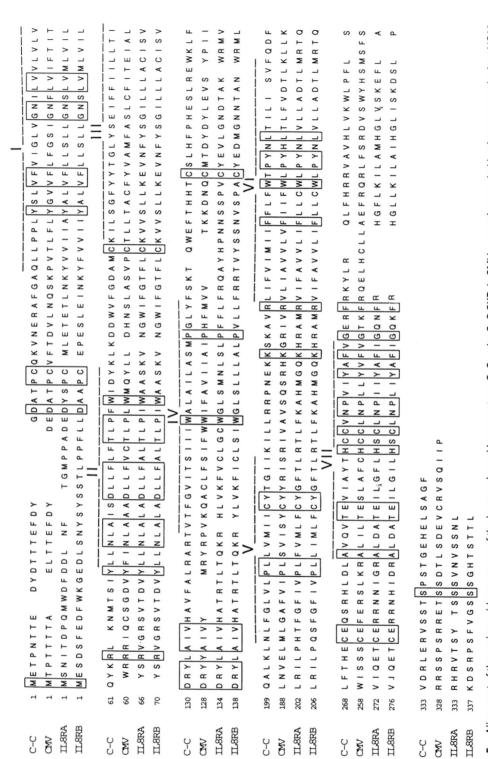

Fig. 5. Alignment of the amino acid sequences of the known chemokine receptors. C–C = the C–C CKR-1; CMV = protein encoded by the cytomegalovirus US28 open reading frame; IL-8RA, IL-8RB = IL-8 receptors. Dotted overlines numbered with roman numerals depict each of the predicted seven transmembrane-spanning domains. Amino acids conserved identically throughout are boxed.

Table 3. Chemokine binding to cloned receptors.

C–X–C		C–C	
Receptor	Ligand	Receptor	Ligand
IL-8RA	IL-8	C–C CKR-1	MIP-1α MCP-1β
IL-8RB	IL-8		MCP-1
	MGSA/gro		RANTES
	NAP 2		
	ENA 78	CMV US28	MIP-1α
			MIP-1β
			MCP-1
			RANTES

amino acid form of IL-8 is thought to be essential, but perhaps not solely responsible, for IL-8 binding (Clark-Lewis *et al.*, 1991; Hébert *et al.*, 1991). Moser *et al.* (1993) have gone on to make IL-8 antagonists which are synthesized IL-8 peptides that are either truncated or substituted at the ELR positions. Paradoxically, PF4, which has been shown to contain most of its bioactivities in its *C* terminus, can be made to bind to IL-8 receptors when its *N*-terminus is modified to contain ELR (Clark-Lewis *et al.*, 1993). Modification of the *N*-terminal regions of the C–X–C chemokine IP-10 or the C–C chemokine MCP-1 failed to result in IL-8R binding, suggesting a role for other regions in receptor binding. Curiously, one report suggests that changing two amino acids in MCP-1 to the corresponding amino acids present in IL-8 can cause the loss of MCP-1 activities and the concomitant gain of IL-8-like activities. Substitutions in MCP-1, Y28 to L and R30 to V respectively, resulted in a substantial decrease in monocyte chemoattractant activity, and the acquisition of neutrophil attractant activity in the mutant molecule (Beall *et al.*, 1992). No detailed binding studies using this interesting mutant on any of the cloned receptors have yet been reported.

The *N*-terminal regions of the chemokine receptors are also likely to be important in chemokine binding interactions. Substitution of the *N*-terminal domains of the two IL-8R proved that these regions are responsible for the differences in binding specificity between the A and B receptors. Placing of a type B *N* terminus on the A receptor results in a chimaeric receptor binding with a normal B specificity and vice versa (Gayle *et al.*, 1993).

Chemokine Interactions with Red Blood Cells

Red blood cells possess a promiscuous chemokine receptor on their surface, and may therefore act as regulators of chemokines in circulation. The red blood cell chemokine receptor (RBC CKR), originally postulated to be a sink for IL-8 (Darbonne *et al.*, 1991), binds chemokines of both C–C and C–X–C classes with a K_d of about 5 nM, and is present at about 5000 sites per cell (Neote *et al.*, 1993a). To our knowledge, the RBC CKR is the only binding structure that will accommodate both C–C and C–X–C chemokines, and is therefore distinct from chemokine receptors on neutrophils, monocytes, or lymphocytes. The existence of the RBC CKR suggests that, unlike previously studied immune cytokines, the chemokines are likely to interact with a complex array of receptors *in vivo*.

Further studies by Horuk and colleagues (1993) have revealed that the RBC CKR has a fascinating dual identity. It appears to be the same molecule as the Duffy antigen (Cutbush *et al.*, 1950; Nichols *et al.*, 1987), which acts as the receptor for the malarial parasite *Plasmodium vivax* (Miller *et al.*, 1976). The first clue to the dual identity of the RBC CKR was that it was not present on the surface of erythrocytes from black donors. The Duffy antigen is also known to be absent in this population (Miller *et al.*, 1976). This distribution, as well as the size and biochemical properties of the RBC CKR (Neote *et al.*, 1993a), suggests that there may be a relationship between the RBC CKR and the Duffy antigen. In addition, an anti-Duffy antibody was shown to inhibit chemokine binding to red blood cells, and chemokines were shown to inhibit the infection of red cells by *P. vivax* (Horuk *et al.*, 1993). Thus, the red blood cell may have evolved a chemokine receptor to control the levels of proinflammatory peptides in circulation. This regulatory function could be complemented by the existence of naturally occurring anti-chemokine antibodies, as reported by Leonard and colleagues (Sylvester *et al.*, 1992). The RBC CKR could have been subsumed by the malarial parasite, and this evolutionary pressure could have led to the loss of the RBC CKR in black populations, thus rendering them resistant to *P. vivax* infection.

CHEMOKINES IN DISEASE

The leukocyte attractant and activating properties of the chemokines make them logical candidates for involvement in a variety of disease processes possessing an inflammatory component. For example, could some of the C–C chemokines, with their ability to preferentially attract monocytes and T lymphocytes, be involved in the pathogenesis of chronic inflammatory or autoimmune process where these cells are thought to play a central role? The hypothesis is an attractive one, and one that has been investigated at least at the first level. High levels of chemokines can be found in many chronic inflammatory disease states, but the correlation of the presence of chemokines in pathologies by no means shows a causal relationship of chemokines in the disease process. This connection is largely unproven, though a few reports are beginning to test this notion more thoroughly.

MCP-1 mRNA expression or protein production has been detected in a variety of conditions where monocytes predominate in the pathology. In a sense, this is not surprising, since MCP-1 can be induced easily in many cells and tissues by a variety of agents including IL-1 and TNF-α. In experimental models of EAE (Hulkower *et al.*, 1993) MCP-1 mRNA expression levels correlate with the onset of disease and disappear at its resolution. Rat models of lung injury have also shown induction of MCP-1 (Brieland *et al.*, 1992), and one model of immune-complex-induced alveolitis revealed that anti-MCP-1 antibody administration lessened the severity of the disease (Jones *et al.*, 1992). MCP-1 production has also been well scrutinized in rheumatoid arthritis, human idiopathic pulmonary fibrosis, and in atherosclerosis. Hachicha *et al.* (1993) examined the production of MCP-1 in type B human rheumatoid synoviocytes, and Koch and colleagues (1992) thoroughly analysed MCP-1 production in both RA synovial fibroblasts and RA synovial macrophages. The latter study showed that while MCP-1 expression could be induced in the synovial fibroblasts (this is probably not dissimilar to normal fibroblasts), synovial macrophages constitutively express the chemokine. The authors also showed MCP-1 immunostaining in rheumatoid synovial tissues. Similar findings have been reported by Villiger *et al.* (1992a), who also showed that articular cartilage can be induced to produce MCP-1 (Villiger *et al.*, 1992b). Two groups have examined the expression of MCP-1 in human idiopathic pulmonary fibrosis (Antoniades *et al.*, 1992; Standiford *et al.*, 1993), and one has noted an increase in MCP-1 (JE) and KC in a rat model of renal ischemia (Safirstein *et al.*, 1991). MIP-2 and KC mRNAs have also been observed to be increased in pulmonary inflammation models (Driscoll *et al.*, 1992; Huang *et al.*, 1992).

A role for chemokines in atherosclerosis has been widely postulated, since leukocyte infiltration is a hallmark of human atheromatous plaques. One of the earliest detectable lesions in atherosclerosis is the fatty-streak—a deposition of lipid-laden macrophages known as foam cells. These cells are derived from blood monocytes that have migrated to the site of the nascent atherosclerotic lesion.

Hints that chemokines in general, and MCP-1 in particular, may play a role in this process date to at least 1988 when Valente and coworkers purified what was later identified as MCP-1 from baboon vascular smooth muscle cells. Shortly after that it became clear that minimally modified low-density lipoprotein (MM-LDL) would induce MCP-1 expression in both human endothelial cells and in smooth muscle cells (Cushing *et al.*, 1990). This, coupled with the fact the MM-LDL appeared to be biologically active *in vivo* (Liao *et al.*, 1991), led to the hypothesis that MCP-1 would be a key mediator of monocyte attraction in atherogenesis. Correlative support for this hypothesis comes from studies showing that primates undergoing diet-induced hyper-cholesterolaemia exhibit increased levels of presumably smooth-muscle-derived MCP-1 *in vivo* (Yu *et al.*, 1992). MCP-1 expression has been localized to atheromatous plaques in animal models and in humans (Nelken *et al.*, 1991; Yla-Herttuala *et al.*, 1991). Preliminary data reveal other C–C chemokines are expressed also in these lesions (Schall, 1991).

Monocyte transmigration into the subendothelial space of cocultures of human aortic endothelial and smooth-muscle cells has been investigated *in vitro* (Navab *et al.*, 1991). This transmigration was shown to correlate with an increase in MCP-1 production by the cocultures upon serum stimulation, and migration was substantially inhibited in the presence of an anti-MCP-1 antibody. Interestingly, monocyte transmigration was also profoundly inhibited by high-density lipoprotein (HDL). The same coculture system has since been used to show the efficacy of the anti-inflammatory compound leumedin to reduce the MCP-1 in the cocultures and subsequently to abrogate the transmigration of monocytes (Navab *et al.*, 1993). This inhibition has been postulated to occur as a result of the formation of a stable complex between leumedin and LDL, thus preventing LDL-induced MCP-1 production. In another model, aortic injury induced by balloon angioplasty was shown to induce MCP-1/JE production *in vivo* (Taubman *et al.*, 1992).

The potential role of chemokines in cardiovascular diseases has been reviewed in several recent reports (Schwartz *et al.*, 1991, 1993; Clinton and Libby, 1992; Valente *et al.*, 1992; Ross, 1993; Edgington, 1993). What is currently lacking is a definitive proof of a causal connection between any chemokines and the pathogenesis of atheroma. No study has yet shown, for example, that the progression of atheroma is blocked by the absence or inhibition of any chemokine.

A causal connection for MIP-1α might be conjectured for MIP-1α in the formation of granulomatous lesions in a schistosoma model. Not only was MIP-1α found to be present in, and secreted from, schistosoma egg pulmonary granuloma, but adminis-

Table 4. Summary of chemokine source and target cells and tissues.

Chemokine	Sources	Targets
C–X–C		
PF4	Platelets	Neutrophils
		Monocytes
		Fibroblasts
		Endothelial cells
		Megakaryocytes
PBP	Platelets	unknown
CTAPIII	Platelets/PBP	Fibroblasts?
β-TG	Platelets/PBP	Fibroblasts
NAP2	Platelets/PBP	Neutrophils
IL-8	Many tissues	Neutrophils
		B cells
		T cells
MGSA/gro-α	Fibroblasts	Neutrophils
	Melanoma cell line	Melanoma cell line
	Monocytes	
gro-β	Monocyte/macrophages	same as gro-α?
gro-γ	Monocyte/macrophages	same as gro-α?
ENA78	Type II alveolar lung epithelial cell line	Neutrophils
GCP-2	Osteosarcoma cell line	Neutrophils
IP-10	Monocytes	Monocytes
	Fibroblasts	T cells
	Endothelial cells	
	Keratinocytes	
mig	Macrophages	unknown
C–C		
MCP-1	Many tissues	Monocytes
		Basophils
MCP-2	Monocyte/macrophages	Monocytes
	Fibroblasts	
	Osteosarcoma cell line	
MCP-3	Osteosarcoma cell line	Monocytes
RANTES	T cells	Monocytes
	Monocytes	T cells
	Fibroblasts	Basophils
	Platelets	Eosinophils
	Endothelial cells	
	Epithelial cells?	
I-309	T cells	Monocytes
MIP-1α	T cells	Monocytes
	B cells	T cells
	Monocytes/macrophages	B cells
	Neutrophils	Eosinophils
	Langerhans cells	Basophils
	Astrocytes	Stem cells
		CFU-GM
		CFU-B
		Osteoclasts
		Hypothalamus
MIP-1β	T cells	Monocytes
	B cells	T cells
	Monocytes/macrophages	
C10[a]	Bone-marrow cells	unknown
	T cells	
17[a]	T cells	unknown

a: Murine cDNA; human homologue unidentified.

tration of an anti-MIP-1α antiserum decreased granuloma formation in the model (Lukacs *et al.*, 1993). Thus, the inhibition of MIP-1α may decrease monocyte attraction and lessen granuloma formation. A report by Appelberg (1992) provides evidence for the involvement of both MIP-1 and MIP-2 in chronic, T-cell-dependent neutrophilia in mycobacterium-infected mice.

Clearly, further definitive proof of causal connections between chemokines and pathologic conditions await the development of better inhibitory antibodies or other chemokine-specific antagonists. Some progress towards such proof appears to be at hand. For example, Matsushima and colleagues present preliminary findings which show inhibition of neutrophil migration to sites of LPS injection into skin by an anti-IL-8 antibody (Harada *et al.*, 1993). One conclusion from such a finding is that IL-8 is essential for the induction of inflammation in this model. An additional and, perhaps fundamentally important, conclusion is that IL-8 is the most important chemokine involved in the inflammatory cascade involving neutrophils, since an anti-IL-8 antibody alone blocks the inflammatory response, while a number of C–X–C chemokines are known to attract neutrophils. Clearly, the substantiation of such models awaits further testing, including the demonstration that anti-IL-8 antibodies used in such experiments are definitively IL-8-specific, and not crossreacting with other chemokines. This is particularly relevant in light of a recent study by Mulligan *et al.* (1993). Here it was shown that an anti-human IL-8 antibody inhibited lung inflammation in a glycogen induced injury model in the rat. The noteworthy feature here is that mice and rats do not appear to have a molecular homologue of IL-8. Thus, either such a homologue exists, and it shares antigenic but not nucleic acid similarity with human IL-8, or the antibody is crossreacting with another protein or proteins, probably chemokines, with neutrophil-attractant activity. The use of chemokine and chemokine receptor knockout mice could also be of considerable utility. The potential scientific, clinical, and therapeutic benefits which may be derived from the establishment of such proofs of concept are enormous (Table 4).

ACKNOWLEDGEMENTS

This chapter was written while the author was at Genentech, Inc. Accordingly, I wish to thank the Genentech staff including Evelyn Berry for data management and word processing, Louis Tamayo and Kerry Andow for artwork, and Barb Gilmore and Rueben Diaz for literature searches. Thanks also to Drs D. Taub, D. Cerretti, C. Gerard, L. Lasky, and K. Neote for useful discussions.

REFERENCES

Alam, R., Forsythe, P.A., Lett-Brown, M.A. and Grant, J.A. (1992a). *Am. J. Respir. Cell Mol. Biol.* **7**, 427–433.
Alam, R., Forsythe, P.A., Stafford, S., Lett-Brown, M.A. and Grant, J.A. (1992b). *J. Exp. Med.* **176**, 781–786.
Alam, R., Lett-Brown, M.A., Forsythe, P.A., Anderson-Walters, D.J., Kenamore, C., Kormos, C. and Grant, J.A. (1992c). *J. Clin. Invest.* **89**, 723–728.
Alam, R., Stafford, S., Forsythe, P., Harrison, R., Faubion, D., Lett-Brown, M.A. and Grant, J.A. (1993). *J. Immunol.* **150**, 3442–3447.
Anisowicz, A., Bardwell, L. and Sager, R. (1987). *Proc. Natl Acad. Sci. USA* **84**, 7188.
Antoniades, H.N., Neville-Golden, J. Galanopoulos, T., Kradin, R.L., Valente, A.J. and Graves, D.T. (1992). *Proc. Natl Acad. Sci. USA* **89**, 5371–5375.

Appelberg, R. (1992). *Clin. Exp. Immunol.* **89**, 269–273.

Bacon, K.B., Camp, R.D.R., Cunningham, F.M. and Woollard, P.M. (1988). *Br. J. Pharmacol.* **95**, 966–974.

Baeza, M.L., Reddigari, S.R., Haak-Frendscho, M. and Kaplan, A.P. (1989). *J. Clin. Invest.* **83**, 1204–1210.

Baixeras, E., Roman-Roman, S., Jitsukawa, S., Genevee, C., Mechiche, S., Viegas-Pequignot, E., Hercend, T. and Triebel, F. (1990). *Mol. Immunol.* **27**, 1091–1102.

Balentien, E., Han, J.H., Thomas, H.G., Wen, D., Samantha, A.K., Zachariae, C.O., Griffin, P.R., Brachmann, R., Wong, W.L., Matsushima, K.,*et al.* (1990). *Biochemistry* **29**, 10225–10233.

Barone, A.D., Ghrayeb, J., Hammerling, U., Zucker, M.B. and Thorbecke, G.J. (1988). *J. Biol. Chem.* **265**, 8710–8715.

Beall, C.J., Mahajan, S., Kolattukudy, P.E. (1992). *J. Biol. Chem.* **267**, 3455–3459.

Bebawy, S.T., Gorka, J., Hyers, T.M. and Webster, R.O. (1986). *J. Leukocyte Biol.* **39**, 423–434.

Begg, C.S., Pepper, D.S., Chesterman, C.N. and Morgan, F.J. (1978). *Biochemistry* **17**, 1739–1744.

Bischoff, S.C., Krieger, M., Brunner, T. and Dahinden, C.A. (1992). *J. Exp. Med.* **175**, 1271–1275.

Bischoff, S.C., Krieger, M., Brunner, T., Rot, A., Tscharner, V., Baggiolini, M. and Dahinden, C.A. (1993). *Eur. J. Immunol.* **23**, 761–767.

Bjorkman, P.J., Saper, M.A., Samraoui, B., Bennett, W.S., Strominger, J.L. and Wiley, D.C. (1987). *Nature* **329**, 506–512.

Blum, S., Forsdyke, R.E. and Forsdyke, D.R. (1990). *DNA Cell Biol.* **9**, 589–602.

Bottazzi, B., Polentarutti, N. and Acero, R. (1983). *Science* **220**, 210–212.

Boulay, F., Mery, L., Tardif, M., Brouchon, L. and Vignais, P. (1991). *Biochemistry* **30**, 2993–2999.

Boulay, F., Tardif, M., Brouchon, L. and Vignais, P. (1990). *Biochemistry* **29**, 11123–11133.

Brieland, J.K., Jones, M.L., Clarke, S.J., Baker, J.B., Warren, J.S. and Fantone, J.C. (1992). *Am. J. Respir. Cell. Mol. Biol.* **7**, 134–139.

Brindley, L.L., Sweet, J.M., Goetzl, E.J. (1983). *J. Clin. Invest.* **72**, 1218–1223.

Brown, K.D., Zurawski, S.M., Mosmann, T.R. and Zurawaski, G. (1989). *J. Immunol.* **142**, 679–687.

Broxmeyer, H.E., Sherry, B., Lu, L., Cooper, S., Carrow, C., Wolpe, S.D. and Cerami, A. (1989). *J. Exp. Med.* **170**, 1583–1594.

Broxmeyer, H.E., Sherry, B., Cooper, F.W., Ruscetti, F.W., Williams, D.E., Arosio, P., Kwon, B.S. and Cerami, A. (1991). *J. Immunol.* **147**, 2586–2594.

Broxmeyer, H.E., Sherry, B., Cooper, S., Lu, L., Maze, R., Beckmann, M.P., Cerami, A. and Ralph, P. (1993). *J. Immunol.* **150**, 3448–3458.

Burd, P.R., Freeman, G.J., Wilson, S.D., Berman, M., DeKruyff, R., Billings, P.R. and Dorf, M.E. (1987). *J. Immunol.* **139**, 3126–3131.

Burd, P.R., Rogers, H.W., Gordon, J.R., Martin, C.A., Jay, S., Wilson, S.D., Dvork, A.M., Galli, S.J. and Dorf, M.E. (1989). *J. Exp. Med.* **170**, 245–257.

Butcher, E.C. (1991). *Cell* **67**, 1033–1036.

Castor, C.W., Ritchie, J.C., Williams, C.H., Jr., Scott, M.E., Whitney, S.L., Myers, S.L., Sloan, T.B. and Anderson, B.E. (1979). *Arth. Rheum.* **22**, 260–272.

Castor, C.W., Miller, J.W. and Walz, D.A. (1983). *Proc. Natl Acad. Sci. USA* **80**, 765–769.

Cerretti, D.P., Kozlosky, C.J., Vanden Bos, T., Nelson, N., Gearing, D. and Beckmann, M.P. (1992). *Mol. Immunol.* 359–367.

Chang, H.C., Hsu, F., Freeman, G.J., Griffin, J.D. and Reinherz, E.L. (1989). *Int. Immunol.* **1**, 388–397.

Chang, H.C. and Reinherz, E.L. (1989). *Eur. J. Immunol.* **19**, 1045–1051.

Clark-Lewis, I., Schumacher, C., Baggiolini, M. and Moser, B. (1991). *J. Biol. Chem.* **266**, 23128–23132.

Clark-Lewis, I., Dewald, B., Geiser, T., Moser, B. and Baggiolini, M. (1993). *Proc. Natl Acad. Sci. USA* **90**, 3574–3577.

Clinton, S.K. and Libby, P. (1992). *Arc. Pathol. Lab. Med.* **116**, 1292–1300.

Cochran, B.H., Reffel, A.C. and Stiles, C.D. (1983). *Cell* **33**, 939–947.

Cushing, S.D., Berliner, J.A., Valente, A.J., Territo, M.C., Navab, M., Parhami, F., Gerrity, R., Schwartz, C.J. and Fogelman, A.M. (1990). *Proc. Natl Acad. Sci. USA* **87**, 5134–5138.

Cutbush, M., Mollison, P.L. and Parkin, D.M. (1950). *Nature* **165**, 188–189.

Darbonne, W.C., Rice, G.C., Mohler, M.A., Apple, T., Hebert, C.A. Valente, A.J. and Baker, J. (1991). *J. Clin. Invest.* **88**, 1362–1369.

Darveau, R.P., Balek, J., Seachord, C.L., Cosand, W.L., Cunningham, M.D., Cassiano-Clough, L. and Maloney, G. (1992). *J. Clin. Invest.* **90**, 447–455.

Davatelis, G., Tekamp-Olson, P., Wolpe, S.D., Hermsen, K., Luedke, C., Gallegos, C., Coit, D., Merryweather, J. and Cerami, A. (1988). *J. Exp. Med.* **167**, 1939–1944.

Davatelis, G., Wolpe, S.D., Sherry, B., Dayer, J.M., Chicheportiche, R. and Cerami, A. (1989). *Science* **243**, 1066–1068.

Derynck, R., Balentien, E., Han, J.H., Thomas, H.G., Wen, D., Samantha, A.K., Zachariae, C.O., Griffin, P.R., Brachmann, R., Wong, W.L., *et al.* (1990). *Biochemistry* **29**, 10225.

Deuel, T.F., Keim, P.S., Farmer, M. and Heinrikson, R.L. (1977). *Proc. Natl Acad. Sci. USA* **74**, 2256–2258.

Deuel, T.F., Senior, R.M., Chang, D., Griffin, G.L., Heinrikson, R.L. and Kaiser, E.T. (1981). *PNAS USA* **78**, 4584–4587.

Deutsch, E., Johnson, S.A. and Seegers, W.H. (1955). *Circ. Res.* **3**, 110–115.

Deutsch, E. and Kain, W. (1961). In *Blood Platelets*, (ed. S.A. Johnson) Little Brown, Boston, pp. 337.

Doi, T., Greenberg, S.M. and Rosenberg, R.D. (1987). *Mol. Cell. Biol.* **7**, 898–904.

Donlon, T.A., Krensky, A.M., Wallace, M.R., Collins, F.S., Lovett, M. and Clayberger, C. (1990). *Genomics* **6**, 548–553.

Driscoll, K.E., Hassenbein, D.H., Asquith, T., Takigiku, R., Purdon, M., Whitten, J.J, Grant, R.A. and Poynter, J. (1992). *Fed. Am. Sci. Exp. Biol.* **6**, A2048.

Dunlop, D.J., Wright, E.G., Lorimore, S., Graham, G.J., Holyoake, T., Kerr, D.J., Wolpe, S.D. and Pragnell, I.B. (1992). *Blood* **79**, 2221–2225.

Edgington, S.M. (1993). *Biotechnology* **11**, 676–681.

Fahey, T.J., Tracey, K.J., Tekamp-Olson, P., Cousens, L.S., Jones, W.G., Shires, G.T., Cerami, A. and Sherry, B. (1992). *J. Immunol.* **148**, 2764–2769.

Farber, J.M. (1990). *Proc. Natl Acad. Sci. USA* **87**, 5238–5242.

Farber, J.M. (1993). *Biochem. Biophys. Res. Commun.* **192**, 223–230.

Furutani, Y., Nomura, H., Notake, M., Oyamada, Y., Fukui, T., Yamada, M., Larsen, C.G., Oppenheim, J.J. and Matsushima, K. (1989). *Biochem. Biophys. Res. Commun.* **159**, 249–255.

Ganz, T., Rayner, J.R., Valore, E.V., Tumolo, A., Talmadge, K. and Fuller, F. (1989). *J. Immunol.* **143**, 1358–1365.

Gao, J.-L., Kuhns, D.B., Tiffany, H.L., McDermott, D., Li, X., Francke, U. and Murphy, P.M. (1993). *J. Exp. Med.* **177**, 1421–1427.

Gayle, R.B.I., Sleath, P.R., Srinivason, S., Birks, C.W., Weerawarna, K.S., Cerretti, D.P., Kozlosky, C.J., Nelson, N., Vanden Bos, T. and Beckmann, M.P. (1993). *J. Biol. Chem.* **268**, 7283–7289.

Gewirtz, A.M., Calabretta, B., Rucinski, B., Niewiarowski, S. and Xu, W.Y. (1989). *J. Clin. Invest.* **83**, 1477–1486.

Gleich, G.J. (1980). *J. Allergy Clin. Immunol.* **85**, 422–436.

Graham, C.J., Zhou, L., Weatherbee, J.A., Tsang, M.L., Napolitano, M., Leonard, W.J. and Pragnell, I.B. (1993). *Gell Growth Differ.* **4**, 137–146.

Graham, G.J. and Pragnell, I.B. (1992). *Dev. Biol.* **151**, 377–381.

Graham, G.J., Wright, E.G., Hewick, R., Wolpe, S.D., Wilkie, N.M., Donaldson, D., Lorimore, S. and Pragnell, I.B. (1990). *Nature* **344**, 442–444.

Graham, G.J., MacKenzie, J., Lowe, S., Tsang, M.L.-S., Weatherbee, J.A., Issacson, A., Medicherla, J., Fang, F., Wilkinson, P.C. and Pragnell, I.B. (1994). *J. Biol. Chem.* **269**, 4974–4978.

Graves, D.T. and Valente, A.J. (1991). *Biochem. Pharm.* **41**, 333–337.

Graves, D.T., Jiang, Y.L., Williamson, M.J. and Valente, A.J. (1989). *Science* **245**, 1490–1493.

Graves, D.T. Barnhill, R., Galanopoulos, T. and Antoniades, H.N. (1992). *Am. J. Pathol.* **140**, 9–14.

Gregg, E.O., Yarnood, L., Wagstaffe, M.J., Pepper, D.S. and Macdonald, M.C. (1990). *Immunology* **70**, 230–234.

Griffin, C.A., Emanuel, B.S., LaRocco, P., Schwartz, E. and Poncz, M. (1987). *Cytogenet. Cell Genet.* **45**, 67–69.

Hachicha, M., Rathanaswami, P., Schall, T.J. and McColl, S.R. (1993). *Arth. Rheum.* **36**, 26–34.

Han, Z.C., Bellucci, S., Tenza, D. and Caen, J.P. (1990). *Br. J. Haematol.* **74**, 395–401.

Han, Z.C., Maurer, A.M., Bellucci, S., Wan, H.Y., Y, K., Bertrand, O. and Caen, J.P. (1992). *J. Lab. Clin. Med.* **120**, 645–660.

Harada, A., Skido, N., Kuno, K., Akiyama, M., Kasahara, T., Nakanishi, I., Mukaida, N. and Matsushima, K. (1993). *J. Immunol.* **150**, 125A.

Haskill, S., Peace, A., Morris, J., Sporn, S.A., Anisowicz, A., Lee, S.W., Smith, T., Martin, G., Ralph, P. and Sager, R. (1990). *Proc. Natl Acad. Sci. USA* **87**, 7732–7736.

Hébert, C.A., Vitangcol, R.V. and Baker, J.B. (1991). *J. Biol. Chem.* **266**, 18989.

Heufler, C., Parkinson, E.K., Graham, G.J., Koch, F., Topar, G., Kampgen, E., Romani, N., Pragnell, I.B. and Schuler, G. (1992a). *J. Invest. Dermatol.* **98**, 515.

Heufler, C., Topar, G., Koch, F., Trockenbacher, B., Kampgen, E., Romani, N. and Schuler, G. (1992b). *J. Exp. Med.* **176**, 1221–1226.

Hirashima, M., Ono, T., Nakao, M., Nishi, H., Kimura, A., Nomiyama, H., Hamada, F., Yoshida, M.C. and Shimada, K. (1992). *DNA Seq.* **3**, 203–212.

Hiti-Harper, J., Wohl, H. and Harper, E. (1978). *Science* **248**, 1408–1410.

Holmes, W.E., Lee, J., Kuang, W.-J., Rice, G.C. and Wood, W.I. (1991). *Science* **253**, 1278–1280.

Holt, J.C., Harris, M.E., Holt, A.M., Lange, E., Henschen, A. and Niewiarowski, S. (1986). *Biochemistry* **25**, 1988–1996.

Horuk, R., Chitnis, C., Darbonne, W.R., Colby, T., Rybicki, A. and Miller, L. (1993). *Science* **261**, 1182–1184.

Huang, S., Paulauskis, J.D., Godleski, J.J. and Kobzik, L. (1992). *Am. J. Pathol.* **141**, 981–988.

Huber, A.R., Kunkel, S.L., Todd, R.F.I. and Weiss, S.J. (1991). *Science* **254**, 99–102.

Hulkower, K., Brosnan, C.F., Aquino, D.A., Cammer, W., Kulshrestha, S., Guida, M.P., Rapoport, D.A. and Berman, J.W. (1993). *J. Immunol.* **150**, 2525–2533.

Iida, N. and Grotendorst, G.R. (1990). *Mol. Cell. Biol.* **10**, 5596–5599.

Irving, S.G., Zipfel, P.F., Balke, J., McBride, O.W., Morton, C.C., Burd, P.R., Siebenlist, U. and Kelly, K. (1989). *Nucl. Acids. Res.* **18**, 3261–3270.

Jerne, N.K. and Nordin, A.A. (1963). *Science* **140**, 405.

Jiang, Y., Valente, A.J., Williamson, M.J., Zhang, L. and Graves, D.T. (1990). *J. Biol. Chem.* **265**, 18318–18321.

Jiang, Y., Tabak, L.A., Valente, A.J. and Graves, D.T. (1991). *Biochem. Biophys. Res. Commun.* **178**, 1400–1404.

Jiang, Y., Beller, D.I., Frendl, G. and Graves, D.T. (1992). *J. Immunol.* **148**, 2423–2428.

Jones, M.L., Mulligan, M.S., Flory, C.M., Ward, P.A. and Warren, J.S. (1992). *J. Immunol.* **149**, 2147–2154.

Kameyoshi, Y., Dörschner, A., Mallet, A.I., Christophers, E. and Schröder, J.-M. (1992). *J. Exp. Med.* **176**, 587–592.

Kaplan, G., Luster, A.D., Hancock, G. and Cohn, Z.A. (1987). *J. Exp. Med.* **166**, 1098–1108.

Kasama, T., Strieter, R.M., Standiford, T.J., Burdick, M.D. and Kunkel, S.L. (1993). *J. Exp. Med.* **178**, 63–72.

Katz, I.R., Hoffmann, M.K., Zucker, M.B., Bell, M.K. and Thorbecke, G.J. (1985). *J. Immunol.* **134**, 3199–3203.

Katz, I.R., Bell, M.K., Hoffmann, M.K. and Thorbecke, G.J. (1986a). *Cell. Immunol.* **100**, 57–65.

Katz, I.R., Thorbecke, G.J., Bell, M.K., Yin, J.-Z. and Zucker, M.B. (1986b). *PNAS* **83**, 3491–3495.

Katz, I.R., Zucker, M.B. and Thorbecke, G.J. (1991). *Immunoregulatory Effects of Platelet Factor 4.* (eds M. Meltzer and A. Mantovani) *Cellular and Cytokine Networks in Tissue Immunity. Progress in Leukocyte Biology,* Vol. 11. Wiley-Liss, New York.

Kimata, H., Yoshida, A., Ishioka, C., Lindley, I. and Mikawa, H. (1992). *J. Exp. Med.* **176**, 1227–1231.

Koch, A.E., S.L., K., Harlow, L.A., Johnson, B., Evanoff, H.L., Haines, G.K., Burdick, M.D., Pope, R.M. and Strieter, R.M. (1992). *J. Clin. Invest.* **90**, 772–779.

Kukita, T., Nakao, J., Hamada, F., Kukita, A., Inai, T., Kurisu, K. and Nomiyama, H. (1992). *Bone and Mineral* **19**, 215–223.

Kulmburg, P.A., Huber, N.E., Scheer, B.J., Wrann, M. and Baumruker, T. (1992). *J. Exp. Med.* **176**, 1773–1778.

Kuna, P., Reddigari, S.R., Kornfeld, D. and Kaplan, A.P. (1991). *J. Immunol.* **147**, 1920–1924.

Kuna, P., Reddigari, S.R., Rucinski, D., Oppenheim, J.J. and Kaplan, A.P. (1992a). *J. Exp. Med.* **175**, 489–493.

Kuna, P., Reddigari, S.R., Schall, T.J., Rucinski, D., Viksman, M.Y. and Kaplan, A.P. (1992b). *J. Immunol.* **149**, 636–642.

Kuna, P., Reddigari, S.R., Schall, T.J., Rucinski, D., Sadick, M. and Kaplan, A.P. (1993). *J. Immunol.* **150**, 1932–1943.

Kwon, B.S. and Weissman, S.M. (1989). *Proc. Natl Acad. Sci. USA* **86**, 1963–1967.

Kwon, B.S., Zhou, Z., Pollok, K. and Kim, Y. (1992). *Fed. Am. Soc. Exp. Biol.* **6**, A1147.

Larsen, C.G., Anderson, A.O., Appella, E., Oppenheim, J.J. and Matsushima, K. (1989). *Science* **243**, 1464–1466.

Lasky, L.A. (1992). *Science* **258**, 964–969.

Lasky, L.A. (1993). *Curr. Biology* **6**, 366–368.

Lawrence, M.B. and Springer, T.A. (1991). *Cell* **65**, 859–873.

Lee, J., Kuang, W.J., Rice, G.C. and Wood, W.I. (1992). *J. Immunol.* **148**, 1261–1264.

Leonard, E.J. and Yoshimura, T. (1990). *Immunol. Today* **11**, 97–101.

Leonard, E.J., Skeel, A. and Yoshimura, T. (1991). *Adv. Exp. Med. Biol.* **305**, 57–64.

Liao, F., Berliner, J.A., Mehrabian, M., Navab, M., Demer, L.L., Lusis, A.J. and Fogelman, A.M. (1991). *J. Clin. Invest.* **87**, 2253–2257.

Lindley, I.J.D., Westwick, J. and Kunkel, S.L. (1993). *Immunol. Today* **14**, 24.

Linzmeier, R., Michaelson, D., Liu, L. and Ganz, T. (1993). *FEBS Lett.* **321** 267–273.

Lipes, M.A., Napolitano, M., Jeang, K.-T., Chang, N.T. and Leonard, W.J. (1988). *Proc. Natl Acad. Sci. USA* **85**, 9704–9708.

Lonky, S.A. and Wohl, H. (1981). *J. Clin. Invest.* **67**, 817–826.

Lord, B.I., Dexter, T.M., Clements, J.M., Hunter, M.A. and Gearing, A.J.H. (1992). *Blood* **79**, 2605–2609.

Lukacs, N.W., Kunkel, S.L., Strieter, R.M., Warmington, K. and Chensue, S.W. (1993). *J. Exp. Med.* **177**, 1551–1559.

Luo, Y., Laning, J. and Dorf, M.E. (1993). *J. Immunol.* **150**, 971–979.

Luster, A.D., Unkeless, J.C. and Ravetch, J.V. (1985). *Nature* **315**, 672–676.

Luster, A.D., Jhanwar, S.C., Chaganti, R.S.K., Kersey, J.H. and Ravetch, J.V. (1987). *Proc. Natl Acad. Sci. USA* **84**, 2868–2871.

McColl, S.R., Hachicha, M., Levasseur, S., Neote, K. and Schall, T.J. (1993). *J. Immunol.* **150**, 4550–4560.

Maione, T.E., Gray, G.S., Hunt, A.J. and Sharpe, R.J. (1991). *Cancer Res.* **51**, 2077–2083.

Maione, T.E., Gray, G.S., Petro, J., Hunt, A.J., Donner, A.L., Bauer, S.I., Carson, H.F. and Sharpe, R.J. (1990). *Science* **247**, 77–79.

Mantel, C., Kim, Y.J., Cooper, S., Kwon, B. and Broxmeyer, H.E. (1993). *Proc. Natl Acad. Sci. USA* **90**, 2232–2236.

Mantovani, A. (1990). *Curr. Opin. Immunol.* **2**, 689–692.

Matsue, H., Cruz, P.D.J., Bergstresser, P.R. and Takashima, A. (1992). *J. Invest. Dermatol.* **99**, 537–541.

Matsushima, K., Larsen, C.G., DuBois, G.C. and Oppenheim, J.J. (1989). *J. Exp. Med.* **169**, 1485–1490.

Mayo, K.H. and Chen, M.-J. (1989). *Biochemistry* **28**, 9469–9478.

Maze, R., Sherry, B., Kwon, B.S., Cerami, A. and Broxmeyer, H.E. (1992). *J. Immunol.* **149**, 1004–1009.

Miller, L.H., Mason, S.J., Clyde, D.F. and McGinniss, M.H. (1976). *N. Engl. J. Med.* **295**, 302–304.

Miller, M.D. and Krangel, M.S. (1992a). *Crit. Rev. Immunol.* **12**, 17–46.

Miller, M.D. and Krangel, M.S. (1992b). *PNAS USA* **89**, 2950–2954.

Miller, M.D., Hata, S., de Waal Malefyt, R. and Krangel, M.S. (1989). *J. Immunol.* **143**, 2907.

Miller, M.D., Wilson, S.D., Dorf, M.E., Seuanez, H.N., O'Brien, S.J. and Krangel, M.S. (1990). *J. Immunol.* **145**, 2737–2744.

Minano, E.J., Vizcaino, M. and Myers, R.D. (1991a). *Pharmacol. Biochem. Behav.* **39**, 535–539.

Minano, F.J. and Myers, R.D. (1991). *Brain Res. Bull.* **27**, 273–278.

Minano, F.J., Sancibrian, M. and Myers, R.D. (1991b). *Brain Res. Bull.* **27**, 701–706.

Minano, F.J., Vizcaino, M. and Myers, R.D. (1992). *Neuropharmacology* **31**, 193–199.

Mishell, T.I. and Dutton, R.W. (1967). *J. Exp. Med.* **126**, 423–442.

Modi, W.S., Dean, M., Seuanez, H.N., Mukaida, N., Matsushima, K. and O'Brien, S.J. (1990). *Hum. Genet.* **84**, 185–187.

Modi, W.S., Napolitano, M., Cevario, S.J., Gnarra, J.R., Seuanez, H.N. and Leonard, W.J. (1991). *Cytogenet. Cell Genet.* **58**, 2008.

Moser, B., Clark-Lewis, I., Zwahlen, R. and Baggiolini, M. (1990). *J. Exp. Med.* **171**, 1797–1802.

Moser, B., Dewald, B., Barella, L., Schumacher, C., Baggiolini, M. and Clark-Lewis, I. (1993). *J. Biol. Chem.* **268**, 7125–7128.

Mulé, J.T., Custer, M., Averbook, B., Weber, J.S., Goeddel, D.V., Rosenberg, S.A. and Schall, T.J. (1994). *J. Exp. Med.* submitted.

Mulligan, M.S., Jones, M.L., Bolanowski, M.A., Baganoff, M.P., Deppeler, C.L., Meyers, D.M., Ryan, U.S. and Ward, P.A. (1993). *J. Immunol.* **150**, 5585–5595.

Murphy, P.M. and Tiffany, H.L. (1991). *Science* **253**, 1280–1283.

Nakao, M., Nomiyama, H. and Shimada, K. (1990). *Mol. Cell. Biol.* **10**, 3646–3658.

458   T. J. Schall

Napolitano, M., Seamon, K.B. and Leonard, W.J. (1990). *J. Exp. Med.* **172**, 285–289.
Navab, M., Imes, S.S., Hama, S.Y., Hough, G.P., Ross, L.A., Bork, R.W., Valente, A.J., Berliner, J.A., Drinkwater, D.C., Laks, H., *et al.* (1991). *J. Clin. Invest.* **88**, 2039–2046.
Navab, M., Hama, S.Y., Van Lenten, B.J., Drinkwater, D.C. Laks, H. and Fogelman, A.M. (1993). *J. Clin. Invest.* **91**, 1225–1230.
Nelken, N.A., Coughlin, S.R., Gordon, D. and Wilcox, J.N. (1991). *J. Clin. Invest.* **88**, 1121–1127.
Neote, K., Darbonne, W., Ogez, J., Horuk, R. and Schall, T.J. (1993a). *J. Biol. Chem.* **268**, 12247–12249.
Neote, K., DiGregorio, D., Mak, J.Y., Horuk, R. and Schall, T.J. (1993b). *Cell* **72**, 415–425.
Nichols, M.E., Rubinstein, P., Barnwell, J., Rodriguez de Cordoba, S. and Rosenfield, R.E. (1987). *J. Exp. Med.* **166**, 776–785.
Obaru, K., Fukuda, M., Maeda, S. and Shimada, K. (1986). *J. Biochem.* **99**, 885–894.
Oh, K.O., Zhou, Z., Kim, K.K., Samanta, H., Fraser, M., Kim, Y.J., Broxmeyer, H.E. and Kwon, B.S. (1991). *J. Immunol.* **147**, 2978–2983.
Ohmori, Y. and Hamilton, T.A. (1990). *Biochem. Biophys. Res. Commun.* **168**, 1261–1267.
Opdenakker, G., Froyen, G., Fiten, P., Proost, P. and Van Damme, J. (1993). *Biochem. Biophys. Res. Commun.* **191**, 535–542.
Oppenheim, J.J., Zachariae, C.O., Mukaida, N. and Matsushima, K. (1991). *Ann. Rev. Immunol.* **9**, 617–648.
Oquendo, P., Alberta, J., Wen, D., Graycar, J.L., Derynch, R. and Stiles, C.D. (1989). *J. Biol. Chem.* **264**, 4133–4137.
Orlofsky, A., Berger, M.S. and Prystowsky, M.B. (1991). *Cell Reg.* **2**, 403–413.
Poncz, M., Surrey, S., LaRocco, P., Weiss, M.J., Rappaport, E.F., Conway, T.M. and Schwartz, E. (1987). *Blood* **69**, 219–223.
Proost, P., De Wolf-Peeters, C., Conings, R., Opdenakker, G., Billiau, A. and Van Damme, J. (1993). *J. Immunol.* **150**, 1000–1010.
Quesniaux, V.F.J., Graham, G.J., Pragnell, I., Donaldson, D., Wople, S.D., Iscove, N.N. and Fagg, B. (1993). *Blood* **81**, 1497–1504.
Rand, T.H., Cruikshank, W.W., Center, D.M. and Weller, P.E. (1991). *J. Exp. Med.* **173**, 1521–1528.
Rathanaswami, P., Hachicha, M., Neote, K., Schall, T.J. and McColl, S.R. (1994). *J. Biol. Chem.* Submitted.
Rathanaswami, P., Hachicha, M., Sadick, M., Schall, T.J. and McColl, S.R. (1993). *J. Biol. Chem.* **268**, 5834–5839.
Reddigari, S.R., Kuna, P., Miragliotta, G.F., Kornfield, D., Baeza, M.L., Castor, C.W. and Kaplan, A.P. (1992). *J. Allergy Clin. Immunol.* **89**, 666–672.
Rice, G.E. and Bevilacqua, M.P. (1989). *Science* **246**, 1303–1306.
Rice, G.E., Gimbrone, M.A.J. and Bevilacqua, M.P. (1988). *Am. J. Pathol.* **133**, 204–210.
Richmond, A., Balentien, E., Thomas, H.G., Flaggs, G., Barton, D.E., Spiess, J., Bordoni, R., Francke, U. and Derynck, R. (1988). *EMBO J.* **7**, 2025–2033.
Robinson, E.A., Yoshimura, T., Leonard, E.J., Tanaka, S., Griffin, P.R., Shabanowitz, J., Hunt, D.F. and Appella, E. (1989). *Proc. Natl Acad. Sci. USA* **86**, 1850–1854.
Rollins, B.J. and Sunday, M.E. (1991). *Mol. Cell. Biol.* **11**, 3125–3131.
Rollins, B.J., Morrison, E.D. and Stiles, C.D. (1988). *Proc. Natl Acad. Sci. USA* **85**, 3738–3742.
Rollins, B.J., Stier, P., Ernst, T. and Wong, G.G. (1989). *Mol. Cell. Biol.* **9**, 4687–4695.
Rollins, B.J., Walz, A. and Baggiolini, M. (1991a). *Blood* **78**, 1112–1116.
Rollins, B.J., Morton, C.C., Ledbetter, D.H., Eddy, R.L.J. and Shows, T.B. (1991b). *Genomics* **10**, 489–492.
Ross, R. (1993). *Nature* **362**, 801–809.
Rot, A. (1992). *Immunol. Today* **13**, 291–294.
Rot, A., Krieger, M., Brunner, T., Bischoff, S.C., Schall, T.J. and Dahinden, C.A. (1992). *J. Exp. Med.* **176**, 1489–1495.
Rucinski, B., Niewiarowski, S., James, P., Walz, D.A. and Budzynski, A.Z. (1979). *Blood* **53**, 47–62.
Safirstein, R., Megyesi, J., Saggi, S.J., Price, P.M., Poon, M., Rollins, B.J. and Taubman, M.B. (1991). *Am. J. Physiol.* **261**, 1095–1101.
Samanta, A.K., Oppenheim, J.J. and Matsushima, K. (1989). *J. Exp. Med.* **169**, 1185–1189.
Sato, Y., Abe, M. and Takaki, R. (1990). *Biochem. Biophys. Res. Commun.* **172**, 595–600.
Schall, T.J. (1991). *Cytokine* **3**, 165–183.
Schall, T.J., Jongstra, J., Byer, B.J., Jorgensen, J., Clayberger, C., Davis, M.M. and Krensky, A.M. (1988). *J. Immunol.* **141**, 1018–1025.

Schall, T.J., Bacon, K., Toy, K.J., and Goeddel, D.V. (1990). *Nature* **347**, 669–671.

Schall, T.J., O'Hehir, R.E., Goeddel, D.V. and Lamb, J.R. (1992a). *J. Immunol.* **148**, 381–387.

Schall, T.J., Simpson, N.J. and Mak, J.Y. (1992b). *Eur. J. Immunol.* **22**, 1477–1481.

Schall, T.J., Bacon, K., Camp, R.D.R., Kaspari, J.W. and Goeddel, D.V. (1993a). *J. Exp. Med.* **177**, 1821–1825.

Schall, T.J., Mak, J.Y., DiGregorio, D. and Neote, K. (1993b). In (ed. I. Lindley) *Chemotactic Cytokines 2*, Plenum, New York.

Schild, H.O., *Receptor classification with special reference to β-adrenergic receptors*. H.P. Rang, Eds., Drug Receptors (University Park Press, Baltimore, MD, 1973).

Schröder, J.-M., Persoon, N.L.M. and Christophers, E. (1990a). *J. Exp. Med.* **171**, 1091–1100.

Schröder, J.-M., Sticherling, M., Persoon, N.L. and Christophers, E. (1990b). *Biochem. Biophys. Res. Commun.* **172**, 898–904.

Schumacher, C., Clark-Lewis, I., Baggiolini, M. and Moser, B. (1992). *Proc. Natl Acad. Sci. USA* **89**, 10542–10546.

Schwartz, C.J., Valente, A.J., Sprague, E.A., Kelley, J.L. and Nerem, R.M. (1991). *Clin. Cardiol.* **14**, 11–16.

Schwartz, C.J., Valente, A.J. and Sprague, E.A. (1993). *Am. J. Cardiol.* **71**, 9B–14B.

Selsted, M.E., Brown, D.M., DeLange, R.J. and Lehrer, R.I. (1983). *J. Biol. Chem.* **258**, 14485–14489.

Selsted, M.E., Brown, D.M., DeLange, R.J., Harwig, S.S. and Lehrer, R.I. (1985). *J. Biol. Chem.* **260**, 4579–4584.

Senior, R.M., Griffin, G.L., Huang, J.S., Walz, D.A. and Deuel, T.F. (1983). *J. Cell. Biol.* **96**, 382–385.

Sharpe, R.J., Byers, H.R., Scott, C.F., Bauer, S.I. and Maione, T.E. (1990). *JNCI* **82**, 848–853.

Sherry, B., Tekamp-Olson, P., Gallegos, C., Bauer, D., Davatelis G., Wolpe, S.D., Masiarz, F., Coit, D. and Cerami, A. (1988). *J. Exp. Med.* **168**, 2251–2259.

Sherry, B., Horii, Y., Manogue, K.R., Widmer, U. and Cerami, A. (1992). *Cytokines* **4**, 117–130.

Smith, C.W., Kishimoto, T.K., Abbass, O., Hughes, B., Rothlein, R., McIntire, L.V., Butcher, E. and Anderson, D.C. (1991). *J. Clin. Invest.* **87**, 609–618.

Sozzani, S., Luini, W., Molino, M., JiLek, P., Bottazzi, B., Cerletti, C., Matsushima, K. and Mantovani, A. (1991). *J. Immunol.* **147**, 2215–2221.

Sozzani, S., Molino, M., Locati, M., Luini, W., Cerletti, C., Vecchi, A. and Mantovani, A. (1993). *J. Immunol.* **150**, 1544–1553.

Sporn, S.A., Eierman, D.F., Johnson, C.E., Morris, J., Martin, G., Ladner, M. and Haskill, S. (1990). *J. Immunol.* **144**, 4434–4441.

Springer, T.A. (1990). *Nature* **346**, 425–434.

Springer, T.A. and Lasky, L.A. (1991). *Nature* **349**, 196–197.

St. Charles, R., Walz, D.A. and Edwards, B.F.P. (1989). *J. Biol. Chem.* **264**, 2092–2099.

Standiford, T.J., Rolfe, M.R., Kunkel, S.L., Lynch, J.P., Becker, F.S., Orringer, M.B., Phan, S. and Strieter, R.M. (1993). *Chest* **103**, 121S.

Stoeckle, M.Y. and Barker, K.A. (1990). *New Biol.* **2**, 313–323.

Sylvester, I., Yoshimura, T., Sticherling, M., Schröder, J.-M., Ceska, M., Peichl, P. and Leonard, E.J. (1992). *J. Clin. Invest.* **90**, 471–481.

Tanaka, Y., Adams, D.H., Hubscher, S., Hirano, H., Siebenlist, U. and Shaw, S. (1993). *Nature* **361**, 79–82.

Tashiro, K., Tada, H., Heilker, R., Shirozu, M., Nakano, T. and Honjo, T. (1993). *Science* **261**, 600–603.

Tatakis, D.N. (1992). *Biochem. Biophys. Res. Commun.* **187**, 287–293.

Taub, D., Conlon, K., Lloyd, A., Oppenheim, J. and Kelvin, D. (1993a). *Science* **260**, 355–358.

Taub, D.D., Lloyd, A.R., Conlon, K., Wang, J.M., Ortaldo, J.R., Harada, A., Matsushima, K., Kelvin, D.J. and Oppenheim, J.J. (1993b). *J. Exp. Med.* **177**, 1809–1814.

Taubman, M.B., Rollins, B.J., Poon, M., Marmur, J., Green, R.S., Berk, B.C. and Nadal-Ginard, B. (1992). *Circ. Res.* **70**, 314–325.

Tekamp-Olson, P. Gallegos, C., Bauer, D., McClain, J., Sherry, B., Fabre, M., van Deventer, S. and Cerami, A. (1990). *J. Exp. Med.* **172**, 911–919.

Thueson, D.O., Speck, L.S., Lett-Brown, M.A. and Grant, J.A. (1979). *J. Immunol.* **123**, 626–632.

Unemori, E., Amento, E.P., Bauer, E. and Horuk, R. (1993). *J. Biol. Chem.* **268**, 1338–1342.

Valente, A.J., Graves, D.T., Vialle-Valentin, C., Delgado, R. and Schwartz, C.J. (1988). *Biochemistry* **27**, 4162–4168.

Valente, A.J., Rozek, M.M., Schwartz, C.J. and Graves, D.T. (1991). *Biochem. Biophys. Res. Commun.* **176**, 309–314.

Valente., A.J., Rozek, M.M., Sprague, E.A. and Schwartz, C.J. (1992). *Circulation* **86**, 11120–11125.

Van Damme, J., Proost, P., Lenaerts, J.-P. and Opdenakker, G. (1992). *J. Exp. Med.* **176**, 59–65.

Van Riper, G., Siciliano, S., Fischer, P.A., Meurer, R., Springer, M.S. and Rosen, H. (1993). *J. Exp. Med.* **177**, 851–856.

Vanguri, P. and Farber, J.M. (1990). *J. Biol. Chem.* **265**, 15049–15057.

Villiger, P.M., Terkeltaub, R. and Lotz, M. (1992a). *J. Immunol.* **149**, 722–727.

Villiger, P.M., Terkeltaub, R. and Lotz, M. (1992b). *J. Clin. Invest.* **90**, 488–496.

Walter, S., Bottazzi, B., Govoni, D., Colotta, F. and Mantovani, A. (1991). *Int. J. Cancer* **49**, 431–435.

Walz, A., Burgener, R., Car, B., Baggiolini, M., Kunkel, S.L. and Strieter, R.M. (1991). *J. Exp. Med.* **174**, 1355–1362.

Walz, A., Dewald, B., von Tscharner, V. and Baggiolini, M. (1989). *J. Exp. Med.* **170**, 1745–1750.

Wang, J.M., McVicar, D.W., Oppenheim, J.J. and Kelvin, D.J. (1993a). *J. Exp. Med.* **177**, 699–705.

Wang, J.M., Rambaldi, A., Biondi, A., Chen, Z.G., Sanderson, C.J. and Mantovani, A. (1989). *Eur. J. Immunol.* **19**, 701–705.

Wang, J.M., Sherry, B., Fivash, M.J. Kelvin, D.J. and Oppenheim, J.J. (1993b). *J. Immunol.* **150**, 3022–3029.

Wegner, R.H., Wicki, A.N., Walz, A., Kieffer, N. and Clemetson, K.J. (1989). *Blood* **73**, 1498–1503.

Wilson, S.D., Kuchroo, V.K., Israel, D.I. and Dorf, M.E. (1990). *J. Immunol.* **145**, 2745–2750.

Wolpe, S.D. and Cerami, A. (1989). *FASEB J.* **3**, 2565–2573.

Wolpe, S.D., Davatelis, G., Sherry, B., Beutler, B., Hesse, D.G., Nguyen, H.T., Moldawer, L.L., Nathan, C.F., Lowry, S.F. and Cerami. A. (1988). *J. Exp. Med.* **167**, 570–581.

Wolpe, S.D., Sherry, B., Juers, D., Davatelis, G., Yurt, R.W. and Cerami, A. (1989). *Proc. Natl Acad. Sci. USA* **86**, 612–616.

Yamamura, Y., Hattori, T., Ohmoto, Y. and Takatsuki, K. (1992). *Int. J. Hematol.* **55**, 131–137.

Yin, J.-Z., Zucker, M.B., Clarke, D., Bell, M.K. and Thorbecke, G.J. (1988). *Cell. Immunol.* **115**, 221–227.

Yla-Herttuala, S., Lipton, B.A., Rosenfeld, M.E., Sarkioja, T., Yoshimura, T., Leonard, E.J., Witztum, J.L. and Steinberg, D. (1991). *Proc. Natl Acad. Sci. USA* **88**, 5252–5256.

Yoshimura, T. and Leonard, E.J. (1990a). *J. Immunol.* **144**, 2377–2383.

Yoshimura, T. and Leonard, E.J. (1990b). *J. Immunol.* **145**, 292–297.

Yoshimura, T. and Leonard, E.J. (1991). *Adv. Exp. Med. Biol.* **305**, 47–56.

Yoshimura, T., Robinson, E.A. Tanaka, S., Appella, E., Kuratsu, J.I. and Leonard E.J. (1989a). *J. Exp. Med.* **169**, 1449–1459.

Yoshimura, T., Robinson, E.A., Tanaka, S., Appella, E. and Leonard, E.J. (1989b). *J. Immunol.* **142**, 1956–1962.

Yoshimura, T., Yuhki, N., Moore, S.K., Appella, E., Lerman, M.I. and Leonard, E.J. (1989c). *FEB* **244**, 487–493.

Yu, X., Dluz, S. and Graves, D.T. (1992). *Proc. Natl Acad. Sci. USA* **89**, 6953–6957.

Zachariae, C.O.C., Anderson, A.O., Thompson, H.L., Appella, E., Mantovani, A., Oppenheim, J.J. and Matsushima, K. (1990). *J. Exp. Med.* **171**, 2177–2182.

Zipfel, P.F., Balke, J., Irving, S.G., K., K. and Siebenlist, U. (1989). *J. Immunol.* **142**, 1582–1590.

Zucker, M.B. and Katz, I.R. (1991). *Proc. Soc. Exp. Biol. Med.* **198**, 693–702.

Zucker, M.B., Katz, I.R., Thorbecke, G.J. and Milot, D.C. (1989). *Proc. Natl Acad. Sci. USA* **86**, 7571–7574.

Chapter 23

Prospects for Cytokines in Human Immunotherapy

Catherine Haworth[1], Ravindir Nath Maini and Marc Feldmann

Kennedy Institute for Rheumatology, Lurgan Avenue, Hammersmith, London W6 8LW, and
[1]Leicester Royal Infirmary, Child Health Unit, Leicester, LE1 5WW, UK

INTRODUCTION

In the broadcast terminology cytokines include all those peptides involved in growth regulation, differentiation and function. It was anticipated that there would be a wide variety of diseases in which these aspects of cell biology are disturbed, and which would hence provide opportunities for cytokine therapy. In practice, successful clinical application has been slow to materialize and has been limited to relatively few cytokines. In this chapter we will discuss potential benefits of cytokines in disorders of immunity, in infections, and in malignancy and also the difficulties in realizing this potential, and discuss the steps that are being taken to overcome some of these problems. We highlight the difficulties of using models, both *in vitro* and animal, to assess future developments, for example the use of combinations of cytokines in order to obtain synergistic effects on the disease process whilst diluting the undesired effects of the cytokines. The problems of attempting to obtain prolonged therapeutic benefit from agents that under normal circumstances have extremely short half-lives and marked local effects are discussed.

Since the cloning of the genes for growth regulatory molecules and the expression of pure and abundant cytokines, initially IFN-γ in 1982 (Gray *et al.*, 1982), it has become apparent that the majority of the cytokines have multiple biological effects. At present some cytokines appear to have a relatively limited spectrum of activity: these include the haemopoietic growth factors GM-CSF, M-CSF and G-CSF, although even these cytokines have been found to have effects outside the haemopoietic system. For example M-CSF plays a major role in trophoblast growth (Pollard *et al.*, 1987) and GM-CSF receptors are expressed on normal endothelial cells and some malignant cell lines (Dedhar *et al.*, 1988). In these examples the clinical applications are limited to the haemopoietic system. The relative specificity reduces (but does not completely eliminate) the problem of toxicity, and therapeutic applications and limitations are now well on the way to being understood. Other cytokines, especially those involved in the acute inflammatory response (e.g. the proinflammatory molecules TNF and IL-1, IFNs, IL-4 and IL-6) have a wider variety of effects in a number of cell systems. In general, at present, the greater the numbers of biological effects and hence the number of potential side-effects shown by an individual molecule, the less clear are its indications for clinical use. Greater clinical use no doubt will eventually result from finer targeting of effects.

Activation at the site of inflammation of both resident cells (e.g. endothelial cells, macrophages and fibroblasts) and migratory cells (e.g. T cells, B cells, neutrophils and monocytes) leads to cytokine production. The final result under optimal circumstances is limitation of the cause of the inflammation and the repair of any damaged tissue, which is mediated by the action of cytokines on target cells. Activation of target cells results in the production of a cascade of cytokines acting on neighbouring cells which includes positive and negative feedback loops. This results in induction of a 'repertoire' of cytokines; however, the cytokine profile may vary depending on the method of initiating the inflammatory response. Within the inflammatory response cytokines do not act in isolation. Their effect depends on:

(1) the other cytokines they induce: although some cytokines (e.g. TNF-α and IL-1 are more powerful inducers of cytokines than others, most if not all cytokines are inducers of other cytokines under some circumstances, and there are probably no truly 'end-stage' cytokines;

(2) coexisting cytokines, that may be synergistic or inhibitory;

(3) the target cells present, whether or not they express receptors, their physiological state (i.e. active or quiescent; Gerlach *et al.*, 1989) possibly the orientation of the target cells to the cytokine (Poo and Janeway, 1988) and their mode of activation (e.g. IFN-γ inhibits mouse B-cell proliferation induced by soluble but not by bound anti-immunoglobulin antibodies (Mond *et al.*, 1985);

(4) individual variation: examples of interspecies variation and, in laboratory animals, interstrain variation suggest that in outbred species individual variation may be important (Jacob and McDevitt, 1988);

(5) interaction with noncytokine mediators (e.g. neuropeptides and eicosanoids) which may also induce, and be induced by, cytokines (Lotz *et al.*, 1988);

(6) the concentrations of cytokine inhibitors: within the past few years, it has become apparent that there are many cytokine inhibitors present in biological fluids such as serum and urine. The majority of these are the shed extracellular domains of cytokine receptors, among which the best studied are the TNF inhibitors (Seckinger *et al.*, 1988; Engleman *et al.*, 1989). There is a single receptor antagonist, a member of the IL-1 family termed IL-1 receptor antagonist (IL-1Ra) (Seckinger *et al.*, 1987). Clearly the relative abundance of the inhibitors will greatly modify the cytokine response. It is noteworthy that cytokines regulate cytokine inhibitors, both the soluble receptors and the IL-1Ra are regulated via cytokines.

Before there is greater application of cytokines for therapy it will be necessary to add to our understanding of the cytokine network and the properties of individual cytokines. This includes the effects of unphysiological doses of cytokines *in vivo* on cells normally expressing low levels of receptor: as cells differentiate within the hierarchy of the haemopoietic system, they both acquire and lose receptors. In the presence of physiological concentrations of ligand some cells may not have sufficient numbers of occupied receptors to generate a response, but they may respond with unpredictable effects to high concentrations of ligand associated with almost 100% receptor occupancy.

Animal models solve some of the above problems but the interspecies variability of

Table 1. Immunotherapy with IL-1.

Property	Therapeutic potential	Pathological potential
Induction of haemopoietic growth factors	Protection from infections	
Neutrophil adhesion		
Neutrophil and monocyte/ macrophage activation		
Induction of IL-6		
Endogenous pyrogen		
Bone and cartilage lysis		Malignant bone destruction Rheumatoid arthritis
Radioprotection	Radioprotection	
Induction of MnSOD		
T-cell activation	May enchance IL-2 therapy	
Activation of NK cells		
Stimulation of fibroblast proliferation		Implicated in fibrosis (?)
Stimulation of division of haemopoietic precursors		(Autocrine) leukaemic cell growth factor
Basophil degranulation		Histamine release

the properties of some cytokines makes direct extrapolation difficult. For example, IL-5 (Eo-CSF) is a growth factor for mouse B cells but activity has been difficult to demonstrate for human B cells (Kinashi *et al.*, 1986), although recent work suggests that it may stimulate EBV and lymphoma cells (Baumann and Paul, 1992) while IL-4 enhances IL-2-generated LAK cell activity in the mouse but inhibits it in humans (Brooks and Rees, 1988; Gallagher *et al.*, 1988). In addition to the differences in cytokine properties, the models of disease being tested may not be strictly analogous to the human disease: there are differences between transplanted tumours in the mouse and their naturally occurring human counterparts, as there are between animal models of autoimmunity and the human diseases.

We now discuss the cytokines which may be of therapeutic benefit in disorders of immunity, cancer and infection: IL-1, IL-2, IL-4, IL-6, IL-7, IL-10, IL-12, TNF, TGF-β, and the type 1 and type 2 interferons. We consider how downregulation of cytokines may be important in some conditions, and refer to work that has been carried out in our laboratory on the importance of understanding the cytokine network in one inflammatory disease, rheumatoid arthritis.

IL-1

IL-1 is a proinflammatory molecule, the major source of which is activated macrophages (see Dinarello, 1988). Its wide spectrum of activities is summarized in Table 1. It acts on target cells both directly and via the induction of further cytokines, such as IL-6, TNF, GM-CSF, M-CSF and G-CSF, and may even also induce further IL-1 production (Selentaag *et al.*,1987; Howells *et al.*, 1988; Sironi *et al.*, 1989). In addition, it synergizes with TNF in a wide variety of effects. IL-1 has a short half-life, which localizes the effects of the molecule adjacent to the site of production, and the use of IL-1 in systemic therapy is limited by its systemic toxicity.

The properties of IL-1 which suggest therapeutic potential are radioprotection, enhancement of haemopoiesis and stimulation of T cells and NK cells. Mice given IL-1, 20 h prior to lethal doses of radiation show enhanced survival compared to untreated mice (Neta *et al.*, 1986). The mechanism of survival is related partly to the ability of IL-1 (shared also with TNF) to induce MnSOD in target cells, which are therefore able to detoxify the radiation-induced superoxides (Wong and Goeddel, 1988), and possibly to the induction of CSFs and IL-6. As a nonspecific radioprotectant a therapeutic application would be in the anticipation of massive whole-body irradiation to normal individuals (e.g. in nuclear disasters). Much more frequent could be its use as an adjuvant to therapeutic radiation, thus allowing increased radiation dose to the tumour.

The effect of IL-1 on haemopoiesis is complex and is mediated by the direct effect on progenitor cells, where it has been shown to induce cell cycling *in vivo*, by its effect in synergizing with some haemopoietic growth factors (e.g. G-CSF; Neta *et al.*, 1987; Moore and Warren, 1987) and by its inducing haemopoietic growth factors in fibroblasts and endothelial cells. It is therefore possible that nontoxic doses of IL-1 will be used in combination with other haemopoietic growth factors to enhance haemopoietic recovery following intensive chemotherapy or radiotherapy. A further therapeutic option is that of using IL-1 in synergy with IL-2 in immunotherapy for cancer, as it has been shown to be synergistic with IL-2 in the induction of tumour cytotoxicity in mouse.

Because IL-1 is a growth factor for some malignant cells (e.g. human myeloid leukaemias; Cozzolino *et al.*, 1989) and because it induces a further series of cytokines that also may act as growth factors for malignancies, such as IL-6 (myeloma), TNF (some lymphoid leukaemias) there are theoretical limits to its widespread use. It is difficult to assess whether these will be practical problems on the basis of experiments performed *in vitro* or in animal models.

IL-1 is itself implicated in many pathologies and thus it is appropriate to downregulate the molecule. This may be achieved in three ways, by the soluble receptor (Sims *et al.*, 1988), by the natural inhibitor, IL-1Ra (Arend *et al.*, 1989) or by antibodies (Köck *et al.*, 1986). Thus, inhibitors of IL-1 are likely to be of therapeutic potential for example in downregulating the immune response in graft rejection, in autoimmunity, in overwhelming sepsis, and possibly as an adjuvant in therapy for IL-1-dependent tumours (e.g. some examples of acute myeloblastic leukaemia).

To date there are limited data available in man using the soluble IL-1R and IL-1Ra. A pilot trial of soluble IL-1R (type II) has been reported in patients with cutaneous allergy. This receptor does not appear to be involved in signalling and may be only important as a source of inhibitor (Sims *et al.*, 1993). Prior injection of 1–100 μg of recombinant human IL-1 type II receptor has led to diminution of the allergic response, at low doses only in the same arm, but in higher doses in both. No toxicity was seen (Mullarkey *et al.*, 1993). Trials are planned in other conditions, such as rheumatoid arthritis.

IL-1Ra binds to receptors but does not activate them. Since IL-1 activates target cells at low receptor occupancy, a large excess of IL-1Ra is needed to inhibit IL-1 action. Despite this theoretical disadvantage, experiments in animal models have led to clinical trials in sepsis and in rheumatoid arthritis. In sepsis a preliminary study was most

Table 2. Immunotherapy with IL-2.

Property	Therapeutic potential	Pathological potential
Activates proliferation and cytokine production in cells bearing high-affinity IL-2 receptors: T cells, NK cells, activated monocytes	Induces nonMHC-restricted cell-killing (LAK) cells Vaccine adjuvant	Induces further cytokines with toxic effects Growth factor for malignant cells expressing IL-2R Autoimmune disease

encouraging, with a dose-dependent amelioration of mortality (Catalono *et al.*, 1993). However, a large randomized study failed to show significant benefit, in a trial with much lower mortality. There is still a probability that clinical benefit will be shown in the most severe subset. In rheumatoid arthritis, preliminary data on patients injected with 300 mg/day has been reported, with a degree of benefit in some patients. Larger studies are currently in progress (Catalono *et al.*, 1993).

IL-2

IL-2 acts on cells that express high-affinity IL-2 receptors. The latter comprise the α (p70) and β (p55, Tac) chains, and a third chain, the γ chain, has been shown to be necessary for response (Saragovic and Malek, 1990). Until recently it was believed that this confined the effect of IL-2 to T cells and NK cells, which are stimulated to undergo proliferation and activation (see Table 2). The recognition of high-affinity IL-2 receptors on activated B cells and monocytes has broadened the spectrum of IL-2 target cells (Malkovsky *et al.*, 1987). Because of its role as a major activator of T- and NK-cell function, IL-2 has received much attention with regard to its therapeutic potential in conditions where enhancement of T- and NK-responses may be advantageous. These include malignancy, immunodeficiency and chronic infections.

The use of IL-2 in trials in refractory malignancy stems from the observations that prolonged stimulation of peripheral lymphocytes by high doses of IL-2 results in the production of a population of cytotoxic cells where cell killing is restricted neither by MHC specificity, as is the case with conventional cytotoxic T cells, nor to conventional NK-cell targets (Burns *et al.*, 1984). These LAK cells are heterogeneous both phenotypically (CD3$^+$ CD16$^-$ and CD3$^-$ CD16$^+$ cells) and functionally, but among them are populations which will kill tumour targets. IL-2 induces the target cell population to produce a variety of cytokines including TNF and IFN-γ which may be the agents responsible for tumour-cell killing (Chong *et al.*, 1989). Various therapeutic regimes have been studied, such as administration of LAK cells alone, cytokine alone, the two in combination and intrasplenic cytokine. It is possible that the differing routes of therapy may generate differing populations of effector cells. The precise mechanism of the IL-2 response is not well understood (Parmiani, 1990). The main responses have been seen with tumours which have previously been recognized as susceptible to immunomodulation, e.g. melanomas and renal carcinomas. In pilot studies of IL-2 and LAK cells in a variety of tumours (mainly melanomas, renal carcinomas and colorectal tumours) eight out of 106 patients had complete remission, the average duration of which was 10 months. A further 25 patients showed some improvement. In the same study, when IL-2 was used alone (49 patients), there was one complete remission and a further six patients showed some evidence of response (Rosenberg et al., 1987). The IL-2/LAK cell therapy schedule, as originally studied, comprised 5 days of 8-hourly pulses of IL-2, followed by 5 days of leukophoresis to generate LAK cells in vitro and, immediately following the last leukophoresis, the daily infusion of the LAK cells generated in vitro together with further IL-2. The therapy is therefore, of necessity, expensive. It is also toxic, with an overall mortality of about 4%.

Several strategies have been developed to improve the ratio of toxicity to benefit. One development has been to define a more effective subpopulation of IL-2 target cells, by isolating the T cells from the tumour (tumour-infiltrating lymphocytes, or TILs) and expanding them in vitro. Another approach has been to use IL-2 in combination with other cytokines. In the mouse, IL-4 acts in synergy with IL-2 to induce LAK cells. However, in man IL-4 inhibits IL-2-induced LAK-cell activity, possibly through TGF-β. Other adjuvant cytokines have been considered and the most popular is IFN-α. IFN-α in combination with IL-2 might at least have an additive effect, based on the cytostatic effect of interferons. It might also be able to enhance cytotoxic cell killing because of the induction of MHC class I antigens and the IFN-mediated induction of TNF receptors. However, NK activity is reported to be reduced against cells that express higher levels of MHC antigens, and LAK-cell killing is MHC independent. Combination of IL-2 with noncytokines such as flavanoids (e.g. flavone acetic acid) has been studied (Haworth et al., 1993).

Other possibilities are:

(1) to define better the target cell population which responds to IL-2: for example, it has been suggested that melanoma cells expressing high levels of the product of the myc oncogene are more susceptible to LAK-cell killing (Versteeg et al., 1989);
(2) to target the LAK cells to the tumour site(s);
(3) to isolate from the cells incubated with IL-2 those with the highest tumour killing activity (e.g. by immunophenotyping);
(4) genetic modification of tumour-infiltrating lymphocytes, for example with TNF-α is currently being attempted (Yanelli et al., 1993).

Experiments in the mouse suggest that LAK cells may also be able to kill the cells responsible for GVHD and to enhance the engraftment of incompatible donor marrow (Azuma et al., 1989; Sykes et al., 1990). However, it has also been shown that LAK cells themselves are capable of causing GVHD and so it is difficult to ensure the outcome. Trials of IL-2 therapy as an adjuvant to bone-marrow transplantation have been carried out (Brenner et al., 1990) but the potential for IL-2 to act as a growth factor for malignant monocytes, T cells and B cells must also be taken into consideration when selecting suitable patients for study.

IL-2 stimulates T cells to produce not only IL-2, which acts as an autocrine T-cell growth factor but also other cytokines (IL-4 and IL-6, which act as B-cell growth factors), TNF and IFN-γ. It therefore plays a critical role in generating a successful immune response. Thus, it has been a candidate for enhancing the immune response in a variety of situations. In immunocompromised patients it has been used to increase the success of immunization under circumstances when success is usually low: for example, it has been given with hepatitis vaccine in patients with renal failure (Meuer et al.,

Table 3. Immunotherapy with IL-4.

Property	Therapeutic potential	Pathological potential
Stimulates helper T cells		
Generates cytotoxic T cells	TIL generation	
Costimulates haemopoietic progenitor cells		? Growth factor for leukaemic cells
Stimulates B-cell IgE production		Allergy
Inhibits cytokine production and superoxide production in monocytes		Immunosuppression
Induces B-cell IL-6 production		
Mast-cell growth factor (with IL-3)		Systemic mastocytosis (?)

1989). Refractory patients were first given vaccine which was followed 4 h later by IL-2. This schedule resulted in seroconversion in seven of 10 previously unresponsive patients. IL-2 has also been studied as an adjuvant to rabies vaccine (Nunberg *et al.*, 1989). It has been shown to have an effect on the cutaneous lesions of lepromatous leprosy (Kaplan *et al.*, 1989, 1990) and the development of topical preparations may make this a feasible option. In one patient with SCID, whose T cells failed to produce IL-2 on stimulation *in vitro*, IL-2 given in low doses at home three times per week was associated with clinical improvement (Pahwa *et al.*, 1989).

The critical role of IL-2 has also made it a target for downregulation of the immune response in allograft rejection and autoimmune disorders. Possible methods of downregulating the effects of IL-2 include the administration of soluble IL-2 receptor, or of IL-2 conjugated to a toxic module, for example diphtheria toxin (Bacha *et al.*, 1988) or *Pseudomonas* enterotoxin (IL-2 PE40). By deleting activated T cells the latter has been used to improve the survival of cardiac allografts in mouse (Lorberboum-Galski *et al.*, 1989) and to improve collagen arthritis in the rat (Case *et al.*, 1989). Collagen arthritis has been used as a model of rheumatoid arthritis in the human, but in our studies it has been difficult to demonstrate that IL-2 has an important role in rheumatoid arthritis, even though activated T cells expressing high-affinity IL-2R are present. Human adult T-cell leukaemia (ATLL) is characterized by the expression of high-affinity IL-2 receptors and in the early stage of the disease the cells are dependent on IL-2 for growth. It is therefore possible that downregulation of IL-2 may have a role in the management of this disease; preliminary studies have shown responses in some patients and anti-Tac has shown responses in 11/17 patients in one series.

IL-4

As can be seen from Table 3, IL-4 shares some features with IL-2. It is an autocrine growth factor for T cells (Kupper *et al.*, 1987) and appears to play a critical role during thymic ontogeny. IL-4 has been investigated for therapeutic activity in similar situations to IL-2. In the mouse IL-4 is an adjuvant to IL-2 in the induction of LAK cells. Tumours carrying a high expression vector with IL-4 when transplanted into congenic mice are less lethal than tumours not expressing IL-4. However, similar results were obtained when the tumours were transplanted into nude mice, which suggests that the IL-4 effect is not mediated entirely through T-cells (Tepper *et al.*, 1989). IL-4 is a cytotoxic T-cell growth factor and, when used with IL-2 to generate TIL, is found to enhance the anti-tumour effect. However, in man, it reduces the anti-tumour effect of nonspecific LAK cells.

Unlike IL-2, IL-4 has anti-inflammatory effects. It antagonizes many of the effects of IFN-γ, and in the mouse IL-4-producing T-cell (T$_{H2}$) clones inhibit IFN-γ production by T$_{H1}$ cells (Wagner *et al.*, 1989; Fiorentino *et al.*, 1989). This anti-inflammatory effect extends to monocytes, where IL-4 inhibits TNF, IL-1, IL-6 and prostaglandin production in LPS-stimulated human monocytes (Hart *et al.*, 1989). It has been suggested that induction of higher levels of MHC class II may make cells more susceptible to IL-4-induced cytotoxic T-cell killing. In human B cells, however, it has been shown that IFN-γ inhibits IL-4 induced class II expression and therefore this combination may be less effective in B-cell tumours (Mond *et al.*, 1986).

IL-4 receptors are also expressed on nonlymphoid cells. IL-4 is a growth factor for haemopoietic progenitor cells (Peschel *et al.*, 1987) and we have shown that it stimulates the proliferation of some leukaemic cell lines and also fresh leukaemic cells (our unpublished data). It is a growth and differentiation factor for mast cells and therefore therapy may lead to undesirable allergic responses (Hamaguchi *et al.*, 1987). Endothelial cells also express IL-4 receptors, although the effect of IL-4 on this target cell population has still to be assessed fully.

IL-4 is a growth and differentiation factor for B cells and is involved in the control of class switching to IgG$_1$ and IgE. It also induces further cytokine production and, in particular induces B cells to produce IL-6 (Smeland *et al.*, 1989), which again may be a contraindication to its use in the therapy of B-cell tumours for which IL-4 and/or IL-6 may be growth factors, such as multiple myeloma.

It has been suggested from work in the mouse that some pathogens are more susceptible to killing via an IFN-γ-dependent pathway and some more sensitive to an IL-4-dependent pathway. The many mechanisms whereby IL-4 and IFN-γ inhibit each other would support a hypothesis that only one of the two cytokines is effective against an infectious agent. Excess IL-4 may be lethal in some infections such as leishmaniasis (Lehn *et al.*, 1989), and this may be due to the fact that, in contrast to IFN-γ, IL-4 inhibits superoxide production in some phagocytic cells (Abramson and Gallin, 1990). Because of its role in stimulating IgE production (Finkelman *et al.*, 1988) it is important in the response to parasitic infections, as has been demonstrated in the mouse against *Nippostrongylus brasiliensis*. The imbalance between T$_{H1}$ and T$_{H2}$ cells may be important, for example, in insulin-dependent diabetes mellitus and other autoimmune diseases, and resetting the balance using a combination of IL-4 and IL-10 may be beneficial.

Because of the role of IL-4 in the allergic response, that is stimulating IgE production and the activation of mast cells, it is likely that downregulation of the IL-4 response (e.g. via soluble IL-4 receptor) is likely to receive as much attention as a therapeutic modality as IL-4 itself (Mosley *et al.*, 1989).

Table 4. Immunotherapy with IL-6.

Property	Therapeutic potential	Pathological potential
Synergizes with other haemopoietic growth factors for differentiation	Induces differentiation of some leukaemic cells	
Endogenous pyrogen		
Stimulates acute-phase response	Septic shock	
Induces IgG production in activated B cells		Hyperimmunoglobulinaemia in HIV (?) Associated with autoimmunity Growth factor for myeloma
Induces IL-2R in T cells	Anti-tumour in combination with IL-2	
Induces cytotoxic T cells		

IL-6

The properties of IL-6 are summarized in Table 4. Many cells are capable of both producing and responding to IL-6, and therefore it is capable of being an autocrine regulator of growth and/or differentiation in many systems. Within the immune system it has been shown to be an (autocrine) activator of peripheral T and NK cells, an effect which is mediated, in part, via IL-2 (Garman et al., 1987). In thymic ontogeny it may be important alongside IL-2, IL-4 and IL-7 in thymic development. It also stimulates function (but not growth) in normal activated B cells, inducing IgG secretion and is an important mediator of the acute-phase response, inducing the liver to produce acute-phase proteins and inhibiting the production of albumin (Morrone et al., 1988). Increased production of IL-6 secondary to some tumours (e.g. cardiac myxomas and cervical carcinomas) has been implicated in causing autoimmune phenomena in these diseases, for example, production of rheumatoid factor and anti-nuclear factor (Hirano et al., 1988). High levels have also been observed in other autoimmune conditions, for example in synovial fluid of rheumatoid arthritis. As an important mediator of the acute inflammatory response IL-6 has been sought in other conditions and has been demonstrated, for example, in high levels in psoriatic skin (Grossman et al., 1989).

Because IL-6 has been implicated in many cell–cell interactions, it is natural that it should be considered either as the pathological agent or the therapeutic modality of many disease states. At present, studies aimed at testing the therapeutic potential of IL-6 have been associated with its effect on the immune system. The increased activation of NK cells by IL-2 if the cells are treated with IL-6 has led to the suggestion that IL-6 may improve the efficacy of LAK therapy (Luger et al., 1989). IL-6 has a variety of effects on the haemopoietic system: for example, it has been shown to have a direct effect on haemopoietic progenitor cells in increasing their response to other haemopoietic growth factors and with IL-3, has been shown to enhance the growth of megakaryocytes (Ishibashi et al., 1989). Thus, IL-6 may have a beneficial effect in stimulating haemopoietic reconstitution. At later stages of haemopoiesis IL-6 has been shown to be associated with growth arrest during differentiation (Resnitzky et al., 1986) and it has also been implicated in the differentiation of leukaemic cell lines both in man (U937) and mouse (M1 and WEHI 3B) (Chiu and Lee, 1989). In this context it is interesting to note that IL-6 is distantly related genetically to the specific haemopoietic growth factor G-CSF and to the chicken myelomonocytic growth factor (cMGF). It therefore appears that IL-6 is a candidate for adjuvant therapy in myeloid leukaemias. Prior to this, however, it is necessary that rigorous *in vitro* studies be carried out on a variety of fresh leukaemic cells to assess the potential of IL-6 as a growth stimulator in these diseases. In the B-cell system IL-6 stimulates function but not growth of mature B cells, whereas it is widely accepted that IL-6 is a growth factor for myeloma both in man and mouse (Kawano *et al.*, 1988). In myeloma it is unclear whether IL-6 is an autocrine growth factor or whether it is derived from the macrophages in the bone marrow.

As IL-6 appears to be an important growth regulator in many systems it may therefore be effective as an adjuvant therapy in malignancies other than those within the haemopoietic system. It has been shown to inhibit colony formation by breast cancer-cell lines but this is also associated with increased cell motility (Tamm *et al.*, 1989) which, in theory, could enhance metastasis formation. However, together with its effect on T-cell killing, IL-6 may be an effective anti-tumour agent although as some tumours produce IL-6 in large amounts it would be expected that IL-6 would not be beneficial in all cases.

IL-6 therapy would be expected to be associated with pathological states that are associated with IL-6 activity, such as pyrexia, fall in serum albumen, autoimmune phenomena and possibly plasma cell proliferation. Because of its implication in pathological states, downregulation of IL-6 is important in many situations, for example in multiple myeloma. Unlike many soluble receptors (IL-1, IL-2, IL-4, IL-7), the soluble IL-6 receptor (IL-6R) appears to be able to mediate signalling, as it can complex with the second membrane-bound protein (gp130), and hence soluble IL-6R does not block IL-6 response (Taga *et al.*, 1989). Downregulation of IL-6 activity would appear to be limited to the use of monoclonal antibodies and IL-6 PE40 (Morrissey *et al.*, 1989), as studied in endotoxic shock and myeloma.

There have been reports of injecting antibodies to IL-6 in man. The largest study has been in myeloma patients, in which a murine antibody to IL-6 has been injected with clear but short-term benefit (Klein *et al.*, 1990). As this is a murine monoclonal, duration of benefit would be rapidly limited by development of an antibody response. An interesting feature of this study was that the antibody trapped IL-6 in the serum. From the rise in serum IL-6 levels it was calculated that $10\,\mu g$ of IL-6 was produced per day (Lu *et al.*, 1992). A small study of monoclonal anti-IL-6 in rheumatoid arthritis (5 patients) has also been reported at a conference (D. Wendling, 4th French Congress Rheumatology). Benefit was noted in some patients, which lasted 2–3 months. There was a rapid onset of improvement, with a 50% reduction of ESR and normalization of CRP.

IL-7

Originally identified as a pre-B-cell growth factor, IL-7 has been found to have growth stimulatory properties for thymocytes and peripheral T cells which are, at least in part, independent of IL-2 (Okazaki *et al.*, 1989). It is particularly important in stimulating $CD4^-$ $CD8^-$T cells expressing either α/β or γ/δ T-cell receptors (Londei *et al.*, 1990). At present, the only recognized source of IL-7 protein is bone-marrow stroma,

Table 5. Immunotherapy with TNF-α

Property	Therapeutic potential	Pathological potential
Induces bone and cartilage resorption		Rheumatoid arthritis Bone lysis in malignancy
Induces inflammatory cytokines (IL-1, IL-6, GM-CSF) in many target cells	Protection from lethal infection	Critical to the maintenance of a chronic inflammatory response
Enhances HLA class I and II responses		
Alters lipid and carbohydrate metabolism		Cachexia
Stimulates neutrophil activation/migration	Protection from lethal infection	
Stimulates macrophage activation		Activates decidua causing premature labour (?)
Activates endothelial cells: Adherence molecules (ICAM-1, VCAM-1) Coagulation factors		Lowering peripheral WBC Ischaemic graft necrosis, DIC
Direct cytotoxicity Fibroblast proliferation	Anti-cancer Wound healing	Pulmonary fibrosis (various aetiologies) Chronic GVHD

WBC = White Blood Cells
GVHD = Graft versus Host Disease
DIC = disseminated intravascular coagulation

although large amounts of mRNA have been detected in thymic stroma in mice. It is therefore not known if IL-7 plays any role in the immune response. However, its ability to stimulate CD4$^-$ CD8$^-$ T cells, both subtypes of which are effective NK cells, suggests that IL-7 may be useful adjuvant therapy in malignancy. Again, however, IL-7 is likely to be a growth factor for some haemopoietic malignancies, particularly of pre-B cells (e.g. common ALL (cALL)), and also of early T cells, particularly those that express the double-negative phenotype. At present there are insufficient data concerning the physiology of IL-7 and its pathology to predict its therapeutic role. IL-7 has the capacity to induce proinflammatory cytokines such as IL-1 and TNF, and this may lead to side-effects if administered.

IL-10

Mosmann and colleagues reported that a 35 kDa protein, produced by T_{H2} CD4$^+$ T cells, had the ability to inhibit IFN-γ synthesis by T_{H1} CD4$^+$ T cells, and termed the molecule cytokine synthesis inhibitory factor (Fiorentino et al., 1989). Since then it has been shown to be produced by monocytes, CD5$^+$ B cells and keratinocytes; like many cytokines, its list of properties has expanded greatly, and it is now known to act on many cells. It is a costimulator of thymocyte growth, mast cells and B cells and suppresses

T-cell growth both by effects on APC (monocytes and B cells) and directly. One of its major effects is inhibition of monokine production (IL-1, TNF-α, IL-6, IL-8 and GM-CSF). Nitric oxide production by human monocytes and murine peritoneal macrophages is inhibited. The production of IL-1Ra is upregulated (reviewed by Howard and O'Garra, 1992).

These properties *in vitro* suggest that IL-10 would have profound anti-inflammatory properties *in vivo*. To some extent, this prediction has been substantiated, with protective effects of IL-10 against lethal endotoxaemia (Howard *et al.*, 1993). However, some of its effects *in vivo* were not anticipated. In transgenic mice IL-10 led to the upregulation of endothelial adhesion molecules and lymphocyte diapedesis (Wogensen *et al.*, 1993). Whether these effects are direct or indirect is not yet clear, but they may limit the immunosuppressive effectiveness of IL-10 if used in isolation.

Based on the available data, trials of the use of IL-10 in sepsis would seem to be warranted, and the results are eagerly awaited, as other forms of new therapy for this condition, e.g. anti TNFα, and IL-1Ra, have not lived up to their promise.

IL-12

IL-12, previously termed natural killer cell stimulatory factor, and cytotoxic lymphocyte maturation factor is a heterodimeric protein, consisting of subunits of 40 kDa and 35 kDa, covalently linked. The p40 chain has homology to the cytokine receptor family, in particular with IL-6 receptor.

IL-12 is produced by monocytes and B cells. p40 is produced in excess. IL-12 has a wide range of biological effects. Among the most important are the induction of IFN-γ in T and NK cells, and synergy with IL-2 and other activation events. It exerts a comitogenic effect on resting T cells, with other activating signals, but is directly mitogenic on activated T cells and NK cell blasts. It enhances the cytotoxic activity of NK and T cells, and synergizes with IL-2 to generate LAK cells (reviewed Chehimi *et al.*, 1993).

Recently, it has been shown that IL-12 can influence the cytokine profile of human T cells, reducing the capacity to produce IL-4, but augmenting capacity to produce *in vitro* IFN-γ (Manetti *et al.*, 1993). This capacity to deviate the cytokine profile into the T_{H1} pathway has been tested *in vivo* also, and resolution of cutaneous leishmaniasis in mice is augmented in suceptible BALB/c mice, concomitantly with augmented IFN-γ and diminished IL-4 production (Sypek *et al.*, 1993).

These results suggest that IL-12 may have a role in diminishing allergic-type immune responses and augmenting the delayed-type hypersensitivity response. This may be useful in diseases such as tuberculosis, leprosy and leishmaniasis, as an adjunct to other therapy.

TNF-α/β

Although closely associated at the genetic level (they are 1.2 kb apart in the HLA cluster), TNF-α and TNF-β (lymphotoxin, LT) have a low degree of homology (26%) at the protein level, but act on the same receptor molecules and therefore have similar actions (Table 5). There is evidence for heterogeneity of TNF receptors with the identification and cloning of two TNF receptors (p55 and p75) (Gray *et al.*, 1990;

Loetscher *et al.*, 1990; Schall *et al.*, 1990). TNF-α is produced by a wider variety of cells (e.g. T lymphocytes, NK cells and macrophages) and has been demonstrated to play important roles in many physiological and pathological states. TNF-α is the only one of the two which has been available in large amounts for experimental and therapeutic assessment. Therefore most of this section will be devoted to the potential use of TNF-α.

TNF-α is one of the major proinflammatory cytokines having major direct and indirect effects through further cytokine induction, especially of IL-1 and IL-6, in many systems (Dinarello *et al.*, 1986). TNF-α has many effects on cell growth and differentiation. Tumour necrosis, the property by which the cytokine was identified and named, may be related to underlying basic properties of TNF-α; it is probably not caused by the direct cytotoxic action but by the activation of procoagulant activity in endothelial cells. The preliminary observations led to numerous experimental and clinical studies of the effect of TNF-α on tumours, with a view to developing it as a therapeutic option. TNF-α has growth-inhibiting effects and growth stimulatory effects on a variety of cell types: in normal cells, it is directly growth inhibitory on haemopoietic precursors (Broxmeyer *et al.*, 1986) but is stimulatory for a variety of lymphoid cells (Ranges *et al.*, 1988). In addition, it induces a wide variety of target cells, including fibroblasts, endothelial cells and macrophages, to produce further cytokines which may have properties that oppose its direct effect. For example, it induces the synthesis of many of the haemopoietic growth factors that are stimulatory for those target cells on which TNF-α itself is directly inhibitory (Koeffler *et al.*, 1987). The picture is made more complicated in that TNF-α may stimulate growth in malignant cells but be inhibitory in their normal counterpart: myeloid leukaemic cells may be stimulated by TNF-α, whereas the normal counterparts are inhibited (Hoang *et al.*, 1989). TNF-α resistance of tumours emerges rapidly both *in vitro* and *in vivo* (Lattime and Stutman, 1989). Some tumours produce TNF-α and it may be an autocrine growth factor, for example in B-cell malignancies (Cordingley *et al.*, 1988). In addition, the effect of TNF-α on some target cells may vary depending on the state of the targets. It has been shown to have greater effect on endothelium that is actively growing than on confluent endothelium (Gerlach *et al.*, 1989). With these difficulties in predicting cell growth in response to TNF-α it is not surprising that initial trials of TNF-α in cancer therapy have had disappointing results. In one study (Selby *et al.*, 1987) three out of 18 patients had short-lived responses. Toxicity problems included rigors and hypotension. TNF-α resistance and *erb* B2 (HER 2/*neu*) expression have been found to be related (Hudziak *et al.*, 1988). It may thus be possible to use TNF-α together with therapies directed against markers of TNF-α resistance as a combined modality, for example in the treatment of breast cancer.

At present, the only successful reports of TNF-α for human cancer come from the work of F. Lejeune in peripheral sarcomas or melanomas. Limbs were perfused with IFN-γ, and melphalan prior to infusion of TNF-α, using isolation–perfusion and extra-corporal circulation to obviate potential toxicity (see Lejeune *et al.*, 1993). Endothelial activation, (upregulation of ELAM-1, ICAM-1, VCAM-1) thrombosis and tumour necrosis were all noted, and 90% of patients had a complete remission in melanoma, and 44% in sarcoma.

TNF-α plays a pivotal role in the acute inflammatory response both by inducing further cytokines and by its direct action on cells: it stimulates HLA class II expression, activates neutrophils and macrophages and can kill virally infected cells. Inhibition of its production leads to inadequate resolution of the acute response, which may be fatal. In mice, differential abilities to produce TNF-α in different strains of mice have led to pathologies which may be ameliorated by TNF-α therapy, for example cutaneous leishmaniasis in Balb/c mice (Titus *et al.*, 1989). However, high levels of TNF-α are important in the aetiology of Gram negative and toxic-shock syndromes (Tracey *et al.*, 1987). TNF-α has been shown to be important in resistance to nonbacterial infections such as schistosomiasis and *Candida albicans* infection. However, excess TNF-α has been associated with severe cerebral malaria (Grau *et al.*, 1988). The difficulty in predicting the role of TNF-α, and hence its therapeutic potential, in bacterial infections extends to viral infections; although TNF-α is cytotoxic for most virally infected cells, it stimulates the transcription of the HIV genome via the 5' promoter region through NF-κB (Poli *et al.*, 1990).

The role of TNF-α in disorders of the immunoregulatory system is equally difficult to assess. We have demonstrated that it plays a pivotal role in maintaining the chronic inflammatory response in rheumatoid arthritis, where it may be implicated not only in direct joint destruction but also in the induction of further proinflammatory cytokines such as IL-1 and GM-CSF (Brennan *et al.*, 1989). We have therefore proposed that downregulation of TNF-α may be an effective therapeutic strategy. In contrast, in some strains of mouse which can produce only suboptimal TNF-α responses, autoimmune disorders may be improved by TNF-α administration, as in systemic lupus erythematosus (SLE) in NZB/W mice (Jacob and McDevitt, 1988; Jacob *et al.*, 1990). In non-obese diabetic (NOD) mice the situation is more complex, as treatment of young NOD mice, from birth precipitates early disease, whereas therapy with TNF later is protective (Jacob *et al.*, 1990; Yang and McDevitt, unpublished data).

Anti-TNF monoclonal antibody therapy has been used in 16 long-standing active rheumatoid arthritis patients. The antibody used was chimaeric (human IgG$_1$/mouseFv) high-affinity anti-TNF-α, cA2, produced by Centocor. The dose used was based on that which was effective in ameliorating collagen-induced arthritis in the DBA/1 mouse, if injected after onset of arthritis (a total of 20mg/kg, divided doses) and has resulted in marked (>70%) improvement of all the patients for a prolonged period, with a median duration of benefit of 17 weeks. Benefit was noted in all parameters—subjective (pain and morning stiffness), semi-objective ones (joint swelling and tenderness) and objective e.g. ESR and CRP. The last normalized in most patients (Elliott *et al.*, 1993).

TNF-α has also been implicated in pathologies associated with its ability to induce fibroblast proliferation and collagen deposition. It has been implicated in pulmonary fibrosis, especially in relation to bleomycin and silica (Piguet *et al.*, 1989). Chronic therapy may therefore have similar pathological implications. The pulmonary capillary-leak syndrome secondary to high-dose IL-2 therapy is believed by some authors to be associated with TNF-α (Goldstein *et al.*, 1989). The side-effects of OKT3 therapy are caused by TNF, as they are ameliorated by anti-TNF therapy (Ferrar *et al.*, 1991).

The activities of TNF-α may be modulated by a variety of other cytokines: for example, its actions are often similar to those of IL-1 and the two may be synergistic both *in vitro* and *in vivo* at low doses possibly giving beneficial effects with lower toxicity than associated with either cytokine alone (Cross *et al.*, 1989). The overlapping properties of the two cytokines include MnSOD induction and radioprotection (Wong

Table 6. Immunotherapy with TGF-β

Property	Therapeutic potential*	Pathological potential
Inhibits activation of T cells	Inhibits graft rejection	
Stimulates fibroblast proliferation and collagen deposition		Pulmonary and retinal fibrosis
Inhibits cell division in some target cells		Loss of responsiveness may accompany malignant change
Induces bone resorption		Implicated in rheumatoid arthritis (?)
Induces integrins		

*All theoretical therapeutic applications are limited by toxicity.

et al., 1988). IFN-γ also enhances the effect of TNF-α in a variety of situations, such as growth inhibition, induction of haemopoietic cytokines, viral toxicity, activation of neutrophil and macrophage function, and therefore combinations of these two cytokines are likely to be studied in a variety of situations.

THE TGF-β FAMILY

Despite their name, the transforming growth factors (TGF-β_1, TGF-β_2 and TGF-β_3) are also growth-inhibitory cytokines and have multiple actions. Their clinical application is potentially limited by the degree of toxicity they may induce, especially on early haemopoietic progenitor cells, and also by the fact that some malignancies are associated with escape from inhibitory control by TGF-β (Ohta *et al.*, 1987). In addition to its more usual growth-inhibitory properties, TGF-β has growth stimulatory properties (see Table 6) (for fibroblasts, possibly via induction of PDGFR) and its increased production has been associated with pulmonary fibrosis. It may induce further cytokine production: it has been demonstrated to stimulate IL-6 synthesis in monocytes and chondrocytes (Guerne *et al.*, 1990) and, as with IL-6, it inhibits the translation of those genes that are downregulated in the acute response (e.g. albumin). TGF-β is associated with inhibition of cytokine effects; it inhibits thymocyte proliferation in response to IL-1 and also, but to a lesser degree, in response to IL-4 and IL-7 (Chantry *et al.*, 1989).

TGF-β has antiproliferative effects on epithelial and other cells, and is capable of inhibiting immune responses, especially if given prior to immunization. Thus, it has potential for therapy in inflammatory diseases, such as arthritis and psoriasis. However, *in vitro*, TGF-β has no effect on rheumatoid arthritis joint-cell cultures, and it is conceivable that the maximum degree of immune suppression has already been observed. However in combination with anti-inflammatory therapy, such as anti-TNF antibody, TGF-β may be effective, especially as it promotes repair of connective tissues, bone and cartilage. In psoriasis its antiproliferative effect on epithelium may be helpful.

The TGF-β super family of genes includes hormones involved in the pituitary-gonadal axis, namely, activin and inhibin. Both are dimers: activin is a homodimer of B

Table 7. Immunotherapy with IFN-α/β.

Property	Therapeutic potential	Pathological potential
Antiviral	Hepatitis B Human papilloma virus	
Pyrogen		
Antimitotic	Inhibits some malignant cells (e.g. HCL, CGL, MM)	Bone-marrow depression
Enhances MHC response	Enhances cytotoxic T-cell killing (may reduce LAK killing)	

HCL = Hairy cell leukaemia
CGL = Chronic myeloid-leukaemia
MM = Multiple myeloma

chains which are related to TGF-β, while inhibin is a heterodimer of this B chain and a second chain, the A chain. These two proteins have indirect effects on erythropoiesis. Activin stimulates erythropoiesis by a mechanism which is dependent on accessory cells (Murata *et al.*, 1988). Inhibin inhibits this effect but does not inhibit erythropoiesis induced by any other mechanism. Activin is a less effective stimulator of erythropoiesis than erythropoietin and it has effects outside the haemopoietic system not shared by erythropoietin. For clinical use other properties will need to be demonstrated. In some studies it appears to induce higher levels of haemoglobin F and so may have potential benefits in disorders of defective β-chain production such as sickle-cell anaemia or thalassaemia. However, clinical studies have not supported the initial *in vitro* studies.

IFN

Both type 1 (IFN-α and IFN-β) and type 2 (IFN-γ) interferons were originally recognized for their antiviral activity, but are now regarded as cytokines with growth-regulating and differentiation-inducing properties in a wide variety of target cells (see Tables 7 and 8). The properties include the stimulation of cytotoxic T cells and NK cells. The type 1 IFNs act through a common receptor and have growth-inhibitory effects on a wide variety of target cells, including normal haemopoietic cells and numerous malignant cell lines. In addition, they are associated with the induction of higher levels of MHC class I antigens on some target cells. IFN-γ acts through its own specific receptor. It has weaker anti-viral properties than IFN-α and IFN-β. Its growth-inhibitory properties are less on many target cells, with the exception of haemopoietic precursors. It differs in several properties, including the ability to induce MHC Class II antigens on some target cells and the fact that it is a major activator of macrophage function (Boraschi *et al.*, 1984; Groenewegen *et al.*, 1986).

The IFNs were the first cytokines to be produced in pharmacological amounts, both by bulk culture of naturally producing cell lines and by recombinant DNA technology. It is to be expected, therefore, that IFN therapy accounts for the major experience of cytokines in the two fields anti-cancer therapy and anti-viral therapy. This is enhanced by the relative lack of toxicity compared with other proinflammatory cytokines. The

Table 8. Immunotherapy with IFN-γ

Property	Therapeutic potential	Pathological potential
Antiviral		
Antimitotic	Cancer therapy	Bone-marrow suppression
Synergizes with TNF	Adjuvant for TNF therapy	
Stimulates HLA class II response	May enhance TIL therapy	May be associated with (exacerbation of) autoimmune disease
Activates macrophages and neutrophils	Chronic granulomatous disease	
Inhibits fibroblast collagen production	In disease with excess fibrosis (?)	
Downregulates transferrin receptors on monocytes	Inhibiton of intracellular pathogens, e.g. *Legionella*	
Stimulates monocyte expression of MSH receptors	Inhibits melanoma growth	Postinflammatory skin pigmentation
Stimulates IL-2R	May stimulate LAK	

anti-cancer effects of the IFNs may be mediated by one or more of the above known properties.

The clinically responsive tumours in man are not those predicted from animal studies. IFN-α is now recognized as an effective therapy for hairy-cell leukaemia (overall response rate 80%, with 10–15% complete recovery (Quesada *et al.*, 1986) and has a significant role in the management of Philadelphia chromosome positive chronic myeloid leukaemia (Talpaz *et al.*, 1986) and myeloma (Castanzi *et al.*, 1985). In chronic myeloid leukaemia up to 75% of patients have been reported to show some response, with 5% losing karyotypic evidence of Ph$^+$, although analysis by PCR has shown that this is not always associated with complete eradication of the abnormal clone. It is interesting to note that in patients treated with IFN-α, blast transformation to acute disease is associated with a higher incidence of lymphoid blast crises, suggesting that the IFN therapy may inhibit myeloid cells more than lymphoid cells. In multiple myeloma, IFN was used initially in the plateau phase of the disease, and was shown to prolong this period. IFN is now being assessed in induction and maintenance schedules. Data are accruing concerning its effect in other low-grade lymphoid malignancies but the very nature of these diseases means that long follow-up periods will be necessary before the effect on survival can be evaluated. IFN has been evaluated in solid tumours and some positive responses noted in those found to be sensitive to immunomodulation (e.g. renal carcinoma and melanoma).

Recently results of a trial of IFN-β in multiple sclerosis have been reported. Low doses (1.6×10^6 units) self-injected subcutaneously every second day had a slight effect, whereas 8×10^6 units every second day had a more dramatic effect over a 3-year trial period. There was a 33% reduction in annual exacerbation rate, and more patients were exacerbation free in the treated than placebo group. However disability scores changed little in both treated and placebo groups. Serial magnetic resonance imaging showed less activity in the high dose group (IFN-β Multiple Sclerosis Study Group, 1993). These encouraging results could make IFN-β the drug of choice for a period of time.

IFN-γ has not been demonstrated to have a role in common malignant diseases, but this does not exclude a potentially important role in some less common malignancies. Its properties as an inducer of haemopoietic differentiation have led to ongoing studies in haemopoietic disorders in which failure of normal differentiation is a feature, such as myelodysplastic syndromes. It is now the treatment of choice in a rare group of genetically variable inherited disorders of neutrophil function associated with defective intracellular bacterial killing, termed chronic granulomatous disease (Sechler et al., 1988). IFN-γ therapy is associated with induction of oxidative enzymes within the neutrophils and cells of the monocyte/macrophage system. A dose of 0.01–0.05 mg/m^2 subcutaneously has been shown to be effective in the management of all the genetic variants of this disease and reconstitutes defective bactericidal activity in monocytes and neutrophils, although within each group some patients have failed to respond (Esekowitz, 1991).

The antiviral properties of the interferons have also been exploited therapeutically. They have no role in acute viral infections but are effective in the management of persistent viral infections such as hepatitis B and hepatitis C, which may lead to long-term organ damage (e.g. cirrhosis) or where there is an association with malignant transformation, for example hepatitis B and human papilloma virus in condylomata acuminata and laryngeal papillomas. In chronic hepatitis B infections, a 12-week course of lymphoblastoid interferon three times weekly provides a response in 48% of patients, as assessed by conversion to core antibody positivity (Scully et al., 1987). This is associated with improvement of liver function and histology. It is interesting to note that the patients who respond are those who appear to have had a suboptimal immune response to the primary infection. Patients who have acquired hepatitis B neonatally do not appear to respond to IFN therapy. Treatment of condylomata acuminata by local injection three times per week led to higher incidence of complete clearance of the lesion and smaller average lesion size than in untreated controls (Eron et al., 1986). Laryngeal papillomas show an initial marked response to intravenous IFN-α, but this is only short-term and the papillomas progress even though treatment is continued (Healy et al., 1988). Kaposi's sarcoma, which is suspected to be induced virally may occur sporadically or be associated with HIV infection: in the latter group, six of 20 patients were reported to respond to IFN (Groopman et al., 1984). IFN-γ has been shown to be a successful adjuvant to malaria vaccination in the mouse, an observation which may have considerable benefit if extended to man (Playfair and De Souza, 1986).

The limitations of IFN use are the lack of efficacy in the majority of malignant disorders, the haemopoietic toxicity, and the theoretical problem that IFN may induce autoimmune disorders by stimulating MHC expression. There is evidence of transient thyroiditis occurring during therapy for breast carcinoma (Buurman et al., 1985). IFN-γ especially has been implicated in the aetiology of immune disease via induction of MHC class II and its use has been found to exacerbate multiple sclerosis (Patitch et al., 1987). Excess production of IFN-γ has been implicated in pathology of cerebral malaria via the induction of TNF-α (Grau et al., 1989).

Studying the properties of the IFNs shows that there are many theoretical interactions between IFN and other cytokines which may enhance therapeutic effectiveness. The following combinations have theoretical advantages.

(1) Interferons activate cytotoxic T cells and NK cells and therefore may enhance IL-2-induced LAK therapy and IL-2/IL-4-induced TIL therapy. IFN-γ downregulates IL-4-induced MHC class II expression in B cells, and therefore may be contraindicated in clinical situations where B cell class II expression may be advantageous.

(2) IFN-γ and TNF-α share many properties in which they synergize and could therefore be used to give therapeutic responses (in part, the enhancement of TNF response may occur through the IFN induction of TNF receptors, therefore dose scheduling may be important in this combination). A phase I trial studied 200 $\mu g/m^2$ of IFN-γ in combination with variable doses of TNF-α, both as 24-h infusions overlapping by 12 h. The maximum tolerated dose of TNF-α was 205 $\mu g/m^2$ with indomethacin cover. Of 36 patients with a variety of tumours only two out of six sarcoma patients showed evidence of response (Demetri *et al.*, 1989).

It is possible that IFN may inhibit therapy with other cytokines: although enhanced MHC expression may help CTL killing, it may reduce NK cell and LAK cell-mediated killing.

FUTURE DEVELOPMENTS

To enhance the use of immunoregulatory cytokines certain objectives should be achieved and these are set out in the following sections.

Prediction of Patient Responses to Individual Cytokines

Full Documentation of In Vitro *Effects of Cytokines*

The properties of the cytokines have become known by a variety of techniques. One approach has been the addition of cytokine to single cell types and examination for effects. The disadvantage of this technique is that it presupposes a knowledge of the likely effects, for which evidence is then sought. It leaves the possibility that induction of properties occurs for which positive search has not been made and this therefore remains undetected. This point has been highlighted now that cytokine receptors are detectable by a variety of techniques, and effects must be sought to hitherto unsuspected target cell populations, for example it has been difficult to attribute any physiological importance to the fact that endothelial cells express IL-4 (Howells *et al.*, 1991) and GM-CSF receptors (Dedhar *et al.*, 1988).

The Unphysiological Nature of Pure Cell Populations

Cells in culture are in an unnatural environment. We have already stressed that the state of the target cells is important in defining the response and therefore it is difficult to extrapolate directly from the *in vitro* to the *in vivo* situation.

Study of Physiologically More Appropriate Mixtures of Cells

Mixtures of cells have been studied successfully using short-term cultures isolated from synovial membranes or fluids in order to document cytokine production. By using neutralizing antibodies to cytokines (e.g. anti-IL-1, GM-CSF, IFN-γ and its receptor) we have been able to assess the contribution of individual cytokines to the maintenance of the chronic inflammatory response in rheumatoid arthritis and have demonstrated a critical role for TNF-α (Brennan *et al.*, 1989). However, longer-term studies are frustrated by the overgrowth of certain cell populations, especially fibroblasts, which limits the usefulness of this approach.

Physiological Importance of Cytokine Cascades

Under varying circumstances the great majority of cytokines will induce the production of other cytokines in target cells. In theory, it is then easy to build up cytokine cascades in which positive- and negative-feedback loops influence the primary target cells. It is difficult *in vitro* to test the biological relevance of these theoretical loops—such work needs to be investigated *in vivo*.

As can be inferred from the preceding paragraphs and tables, cytokines may exhibit properties that, in various situations, are theoretically both beneficial and harmful. It is therefore important to have better models in which to test cytokines under more physiological circumstances and preferably for longer periods of study, in order to reproduce the clinical situation more closely. Long-term high levels of cytokine are mimicked by transgenic animals which may therefore give some idea of the effect of high levels experienced for long periods, and hence indicate the potential chronic toxicities. Although levels of cytokine expressed in transgenic mice may be too high and therefore toxicity will be overstated as in the case of IL-2R and GM-CSF transgenic animals (Lang *et al.*, 1987; Gearing *et al.*, 1989; Ishida *et al.*, 1989), these models may provide pointers for potential toxicities. In addition, some cytokines (e.g. IL-1, TNF-α) are too toxic for high-expression transgenic mice and therefore need to be expressed under the control of less-active promoters to give more appropriate models. Diseases can then be introduced against the transgenic background, but again it is necessary to interpret the results in the knowledge that the models do not truly reflect human disease.

Extension of Studies to Combination Therapy

With greater knowledge of the effects of single cytokines it will be possible to study the effects of combinations of cytokines:

(1) with other cytokines: as shown in Table 9 cytokine combinations can be chosen in which the desired properties are shared but the undesired effects (side-effects) are not; in addition, cytokines may be used sequentially to maximize their effect (e.g. by induction of receptor molecules or adhesion molecules);
(2) with chemotherapy;
(3) with inhibition of unwanted coinduced cytokines, for example through the use of soluble receptors, inhibitors, or monoclonal antibodies.

The logistics of evaluating these combinations are formidable. It will require many studies to optimize doses and scheduling and to decide which of many similar combinations (e.g. IL-1 plus GM-CSF/G-CSF/IL-3) is optimal.

New Cytotoxic Cell Populations

The role of all cells in the inflammatory response is not fully understood. Activated NK cells and CTLs are currently being studied for immunotherapy. Other cell populations may also be amenable, for example, the use of CD4$^-$ CD8$^-$ T cells which grow in

Table 9. Combination immunotherapy using cytokines.

Cytokine combination	Desirable effects	Undesirable effects
IL-1/TNF	Radioprotection	Tumour cell growth Toxicity
IL-1/IL-2	CTL production	
IL-1/G-CSF IL-1/GM-CSF IL-1/IL-3	} Haemopoietic reconstitution	Leukaemic cell growth
TNF/INF	Tumour cell killing due to CTLs ↓ TNF-induced bone resorption and collagen deposition	NK killing (?)
IL-2/IL-4	LAK production (in mouse)	↓ LAK production (in man) Lymphohaemopoietic tumour cell growth
IL-4/INF-γ	CTL production	INF-γ inhibits IL-4-induced MHC class II response
IL-6/INF-γ	Anti-leukaemia	
IL-6/IL-4	TIL generation	
IL-6/IL-2	LAK generation	
IL-6/(G)M-CSF	ADCC	
IL-7/IL-2	NK activity	T-cell tumour growth
IL-7/IL-4	CTL production	T-cell tumour growth

ADCC = Antibody Dependent Cell-mediated Cytotoxity

response to IL-3 and IL-7. In addition, it may be possible to target cells specifically toward tumours by introducing genes to cause specific adhesion.

Drug Delivery

As has been stated previously, the majority of potentially useful cytokines have multisystemic effects, whereas in the therapeutic context, one may wish to influence only a limited cell population. It may therefore be advantageous to target cytokine therapy by one of the following means.

(1) Physical localization, for example: (1) to the skin to improve wound healing, for therapy for infectious diseases, and for tumour therapy: studies along these lines are already in progress, with the use of IFN locally for papilloma virus infections; (b) possible local delivery to the lung and gastrointestinal tract; or (c) intra-arterially to localized disease: pilot studies of IL-2 administered either via the hepatic or splenic artery to 28 patients with liver metastases showed significant tumour regression in two patients.

(2) Functional localization. Receptor molecules may vary on different target cell populations: there is evidence for this with both TNF (Locksley *et al.*, 1987) and IL-1 (Bomsztyk *et al.*, 1989). It may therefore be possible to inhibit the response in certain

cell populations by specific receptor blockade (e.g. the IL-1 inhibitor blocks T cell/ fibroblast receptor but not the bone-marrow receptor) or by using cytokine combinations that inhibit the undesired effects of the primary therapeutic agent (e.g. IFN-γ inhibits the bone resorption and collagen deposition induced by TNF-α).

(3) Improvement of dose schedules. Currently most cytokines are administered intravenously in pulse doses or subcutaneously: experimenting with the scheduling may improve therapeutic effect and reduce toxicity. In addition, for those agents for which long-term therapy is required and which are relatively nontoxic (e.g. IFN in leukaemias or hepatitis, or G-CSF in congenital neutropenias), depot preparations may become available.

Cytokines as Adjuvants

The use of IL-2 as an adjuvant to vaccination and the suggestion of action of IL-2 and IL-4 in anti-tumour therapy leads to the speculation that cytokines may be used as adjuvant to cancer therapy and possibly immunization, as antigenic determinants of tumour are better understood (Pardoll, 1993). Candidate antigens include tumour specific proteins e.g. bcr-abl; specific lymphoma-related surface immunoglobulin (Tao and Levy, 1993) or T-cell receptor and possibly modulation by cytokine-transfected tumour cells.

Better Disease Models

Most anti-tumour studies are performed on transferable syngeneic tumours, which may differ biologically from naturally occurring tumours. Further, the mechanism of seeding from large intravenous or peritoneal injections may differ in cytokine control compared with spontaneous disease. Human tumours may be assessed by clonogenicity *in vitro* in semi-solid culture or by growing tumour spheroids, but both these systems lack the appropriate microenvironment and select subpopulations of the tumour cells. We have already stressed that animal models are far from ideal but a compromise situation may be developed using human tissue inoculated into SCID mice.

AIDS

As AIDS is one of the major health problems of the late twentieth century it is perhaps important to address separately the question of the use of cytokine in its management. AIDS is a viral disease associated with immune dysfunction and therefore it might have been thought to be suitable for cytokine therapy which, in theory, could stimulate T-cell function and viral killing. In practice, this has proved to be problematic, in part because the HIV 5' region contains an NF-κB site which results in enhanced transcription of the virus in response to those agents which mediate their effect at the DNA level through NF-κB, and TNF (Poli *et al.*, 1990). Enhancing monocyte/macrophage function with GM-CSF is also associated with the release of increased amounts of HIV *in vitro*, though the *in vivo* effect is not certain. Thus, it is important to understand fully the interactions between HIV and cytokines. It is possible that downregulation of cytokines (e.g. TNF blocking) may have an application in the management of AIDS. This can be achieved with antibodies, or drugs such as pentoxyfilline or thalidomide. There are planned clinical trials with N-acetyl cysteine which may act by interfering with TNF-mediated HIV activation. IL-2, however, does not appear to activate HIV and trials of low dose IL-2 therapy currently are being undertaken to improve the immune responses in HIV$^+$ individuals.

CONCLUSION

It has been shown that, in theory at least, cytokine therapy may be effective in malignancy, infection and immune disorders. Preliminary studies in man have, to date, been limited to a few cytokines in which toxicity, either direct or mediated via the induction of further cytokines, is less problematic. Even so, many of the cytokines used commonly induce rigors and hypotension, which may be blocked partly by nonsteroidal anti-inflammatory drugs, but still prove to be dose limiting. In malignant disease, this means that the widespread use of large doses of cytokines (e.g. IL-2 and TNF) is not likely to be adopted. However, individual diseases may be sensitive to acceptable doses of single cytokines. It is a formidable task to investigate all these potential disease/cytokine combinations. Vaccine adjuvant therapy does, however, provide a potentially large population who may benefit from single doses of cytokine given with the vaccine, and it is practically feasible. Again, rare inherited diseases may respond to single cytokine therapies (e.g. chronic granulomatous disease to IFN-γ).

The next step is to investigate whether in common malignancies the toxic side-effects may be overcome by using synergistic therapeutic combinations with differing side-effects. Again, the task of studying the vast numbers of combinations is formidable and success is likely to take time.

Cytokines themselves may play pivotal roles in malignant and inflammatory states and because of the greater specificity which is intrinsic to such systems, it is likely that the future for therapy with cytokine-inhibiting agents in malignancy, autoimmunity and allergy is as bright as that for the cytokines themselves, if not brighter.

REFERENCES

Abramson, S.L. and Gallin, J.I. (1990). *J. Immunol.* **144**, 625–630.

Arend, W.P., Joslin, F.G., Thompson, R.C. and Hannum, C.H. (1989). *J. Immunol.* **143**, 1851–1858.

Azuma, E., Yamamoto, H. and Kaplan, J. (1989). *J. Immunol.* **143**, 1524–1529.

Bacha, P., Williams, D.P., Waters, C., Williams, J.M., Murphy, J.R. and Strom, T.B. (1988). *J. Exp. Med.* **167**, 612–622.

Baumann, M.A. and Paul, C.C. (1992). *Blood* **79**, 1763–1767.

Bomsztyk, K., Sims, J.E., Stanton, T.H., Slack, J., McMahan, C.J., Valentine, M.A. and Dower, S.K. (1989). *Proc. Natl Acad. Sci. USA* **86**, 8034–8038.

Boraschi, D., Censini, S. and Tagliabue, A. (1984). *J. Immunol.* **133**, 764–768.

Brennan, F., Chantry, D., Jackson, A., Maini, R.N. and Feldmann, M. (1989). *Lancet* **ii**, 244–247.

Brenner, M.K., Gottlieb, D.J., Heslop, H.E., Bello-Fernandez, C., Reittie, J.E., Hoffbrand, A.V., Mehta, A.B. and Prentice, H.G. (1990). *J. Cell. Biochem.* **14A**, 260.

Brooks, B. and Rees, R.C. (1988). *Clin. Exp. Immunol.* **74**, 162–165.

Broxmeyer, H.E., Williams, D.E., Lu, L., Cooper, S., Anderson, S.L., Beyer, G.S., Hoffman, R. and Rubin, B.Y. (1986). *J. Immunol.* **136**, 4487–4495.

Buurman, P., Karlsson, F.A., Oberg, K. and Alm, G. (1985). *Lancet* **ii**, 100–101.

Burns, G.F., Triglia, T. and Werkmeister, J.A. (1984). *J. Immunol.* **133**, 1656–1663.

Case, J.P., Lorberboum-Galski, H., Lafyatis, R., Fitzgerald, D., Wilder, R.L. and Pastan, I. (1989). *Proc. Natl Acad. Sci. USA* **86**, 287–291.

Castanzi, J.J., Cooper, M.R., Scarffe, J.H., Ozer, H., Grubbs, S.S., Ferraresi, R.W., Pollard, R.B. and Spiegel, R.J. (1985). *J. Clin. Oncol.* **3**, 654–659.

Catalono, M. (1993). *J. Cell. Biochem. Suppl.* **178**, 55.

Chantry, D., Turner, M., Abney, E. and Feldmann, M. (1989). *J. Immunol.* **142**, 4295–4300.

Chehimi, J., Starr, S.E., Frank, I., Rengaraju, M., Jackson, S.J., Llanes, C., Kobayashi, M., Perussia, B., Young, D., Nickbarg, E., Wolf, S.F. and Trinchieri, G. (1992). *J. Exp. Med.* **175**, 789–796.

Chiu, C.-P. and Lee, F. (1989). *J. Immunol.* **142**, 1909–1915.

Chong, A.S.-F., Scuderi, P., Grimes, W.J. and Hersh, E.M. (1989). *J. Immunol.* **142**, 2133–2139.

Cordingley, F.T., Bianchi, A., Hoffbrand, A.V., Reittie, J.E., Heslop, H.E., Vyakarnam, A., Turner, N., Meager, A. and Brenner, M.K. (1988). *Lancet* **i**, 969–971.

Cozzolino, F., Rubartelli, A., Aldinucci, D., Sitia, R., Torcia, M., Shaw, A. and Di Guglielmo, R. (1989). *Proc. Natl Acad. Sci. USA* **86**, 2369–2373.

Cross, A.S., Sadoff, J.C., Kelly, N., Bernton, E. and Gemski, P. (1989). *J. Exp. Med.* **169**, 2021–2027.

Dedhar, S., Gaboury, L., Galloway, P. and Eaves, C. (1988). *Proc. Natl Acad. Sci. USA* **85**, 9253–9257.

Demetri, G.D., Spriggs, D.R., Sherman, M.L., Arthur, K.A., Kimamura, K. and Kufe, D.W. (1989). *J. Clin. Oncol.* **7**, 1545–1553.

Dinarello, C.A. (1988). *FASEB J.* **2**, 108–115.

Dinarello, C.A., Cannon, J.G., Wolff, S.M., Bernheim, H.A., Beutler, B., Cerami, A., Figari, I.S., Palladino, M.A., Jr. and O'Connor, J.V. (1986). *J. Exp. Med.* **163**, 1433–1450.

Elliott, M.J., Maini, R.N., Feldmann, M., Long-Fox, A., Charles, P., Katsikis, P., Brennan, F.M., Walker, J., Bijl, H., Ghrayeb, J. and Woody, J. (1993). *Arthr. Rheum.* **36**, 1681–1690.

Engelmann, H., Aderka, D., Rubinstein, M., Rotman, D. and Wallach, D. (1989). *J. Biol. Chem.* **274**, 11974–11980.

Eron, L.J., Judson, F., Tucker, S., Prawer, S., Mills, J., Murphy, K., Hickey, M., Rogers, M., Flannigan, S., Hien, N., Katz, H.I., Goldman, S., Gottlieb, A., Adams, K., Burton, P., Tanner, D., Taylor, E. and Peets, E. (1986). *N. Engl. J. Med.* **315**, 1059–1064.

Esekowitz, R.A.B. (1991). *N. Engl. J. Med.* **325**, 1516–1517.

Ferrar, C., Dy, M., Sheehan, K., Schreiber, R., Gran, G., Bluestone, J., Bach, J.-F. and Chatenaud, L. (1991). *Eur. J. Immunol.* **21**, 2349–2353.

Finkelman, F.D., Katona, I.M., Urban, J.F., Holmes, J., Ohara, J., Tung, A.S., Sample, J.G. and Paul, W.E. (1988). *J. Immunol.* **141**, 2335–2341.

Fiorentino, D.F., Bond, M.W. and Mosmann, T.R. (1989), *J. Exp. Med.* **170**, 2081–2096.

Gallagher, G., Wilcox, F. and Al-Azzawi, F. (1988). *Clin. Exp. Immunol.* **74**, 166–170.

Garman, R.D., Jacobs, K.A., Clark, S.C. and Raulet, D.H. (1987). *Proc. Natl Acad. Sci. USA* **84**, 7629–7633.

Gearing, A.J., Metcalf, D., Moore, J.G. and Nicola, N.A. (1989). *Immunology* **67**, 216–220.

Gerlach, H., Liebermann, H., Bach, R., Godman, G., Brett, J. and Stern, D. (1989). *J. Exp. Med.* **170**, 655–663.

Goldstein, D., Sosman, J., Hank, J., Weil-Hillman, G., Moore, K.H., Borchert, A., Bechhofer, R., Storer, B., Kohler, P.C., Levitt, D. and Sondel, P. (1989). *Am. Soc. Clin. Oncology Proc.* **8**, 193.

Grau, G.E., Kindler, V., Piguet, P.-F., Lambert, P.-H. and Vassalli, P. (1988). *J. Exp. Med.* **168**, 1499–1504.

Grau, G.E., Heremans, H., Piguet, P.-F., Pointaire, P., Lambert, P.-H., Billiau, A. and Vassilli, P. (1989). *Proc. Natl Acad. Sci. USA* **86**, 5572–5574.

Gray, P.W., Leung, D.W., Pennica, D., Yelverton, E., Najarian, R., Simonsen, C.C., Derynck, R., Sherwood, P.J., Wallace, D.M., Berger, S.L., Levinson, A.D. and Goeddel, D.V. (1982). *Nature* **295**, 503–508.

Gray, P.W., Barrett, K., Chantry, D., Turner, M. and Feldmann, M. (1990). *Proc. Natl Acad. Sci. USA* **88**, 7380–7384.

Groenewegen, G., de Ley, M., Jeunhomme, G.M.A.A. and Buurman, W.A. (1986). *J. Exp. Med.* **164**, 131–143.

Groopman, J.E., Gottlieb, M.S., Goodman, J., Mitsuyasu, R.T., Conant, M.A., Prince, H., Fahey, J.L., Derezin, M., Weinstein, W.M., Casavante, C., Rothman, J., Rudnick, S.A. and Voberding, P.A. (1984). *Ann. Intern. Med.* **100**, 671–676.

Grossman, R.M., Krueger, J., Yourish, D., Granelli-Piperno, A., Murphy, D.P., May, L.T., Kupper, T.S., Sehgal, P.B. and Gottlieb, A.B. (1989). *Proc. Natl Acad. Sci. USA* **86**, 6367–6371.

Guerne, P.-A., Carson, D.A. and Lotz, M. (1990). *J. Immunol.* **144**, 499–505.

Hamaguchi, Y., Kanakura, Y., Fujita, J., Takeda, S.-I., Nakano, T., Tarui, S., Honjo, T. and Kitamura, Y. (1985). *J. Exp. Med.* **165**, 268–273.

Hart, P.H., Vitti, G.F., Burgess, D.R., Whitty, G.A., Piccoli, D.S. and Hamilton, J.A. (1989). *Proc. Natl Acad. Sci. USA* **86**, 3803–3807.

Haworth, C., O'Reilly, S.M., Chu, E., Rustin, G.J.S. and Feldmann, M. (1993). *Br. J. Cancer* **67**, 1346–1350.

Healy, G.B., Gelber, R.D., Trowbridge, A.L., Grundfast, K.M., Ruben, R.J. and Price, K.N. (1988). *N. Engl. J. Med.* **319**, 401–407.

Hirano, T., Matsuda, T., Turner, M., Miyasaka, N., Buchan, G., Tang, B., Sato, K., Shimizu, M., Maini, R.N., Feldmann, M. and Kishimoto, T. (1988). *Eur. J. Immunol.* **18**, 1797–1801.

Hoang, T., Levy, B., Onetto, N., Haman, A. and Rodriguiz-Cimadevilla, J.C. (1989). *J. Exp. Med.* **170**, 15–26.

Howard, M. and O'Garra, A. (1992). *Immunol. Today* **12**, 198.

Howard, M., Muchamuel, A., Andrade, S. and Menon, S. (1993). *J. Exp. Med.* **177**, 1205–1208.

Howells, G.L., Chantry, D. and Feldmann, M. (1988). *Immunol. Lett.* **19**, 169–174.

Howells, G., Pham, P., Taylor, D., Foxwell, B. and Feldmann, M. (1991). *Eur. J. Immunol.* **21**, 97–101.

Hudziak, R.M., Lewis, G.D., Shalaby, M.R., Eessalu, T.E., Aggarwal, B.B., Ullrich, A. and Shepard, H.M. (1988). *Proc. Natl Acad. Sci. USA* **85**, 5102–5106.

IFNB Multiple Sclerosis Study Group (1993). *Neurology* **43**, 655–661.

Ishibashi, T., Kimura, H., Uchida, T., Kariyone, S., Friese, P. and Burstein, S.A. (1989). *Proc. Natl Acad. Sci. USA* **86**, 5953–5957.

Ishida, Y., Nishi, M., Taguchi, O., Inaba, K., Hattori, M., Minato, N., Kawaichi, M. and Honjo, T. (1989). *J. Exp. Med.* **170**, 1103–1115.

Jacob, C.O. and McDevitt, H.O. (1988). *Nature* **331**, 356–358.

Jacob, C.O., Aiso, S., Michie, S.A., McDevitt, H.O. and Acha-Orba, H. (1990). *Proc. Natl Acad. Sci. USA* **87**, 968–972.

Kaplan, G., Pereira Sampaio, E., Walsh, G.P., Burkhardt, R.A., Fajardo, T.T., Guido, L.S., Machado, A. de M., Cellona, R.V., Abalos, R.M., Sarno, E.N. and Cohn, Z.A. (1989). *Proc. Natl Acad. Sci. USA* **86**, 6269–6273.

Kaplan, G., Kiessling, R., Teklemariam, S., Hancock, G., Sheftel, G., Job, C.K., Converse, P., Ottenhoff, T.H.M., Becx-Bleumink, M., Dietz, M. and Cohn, Z.A. (1990) *J. Exp. Med.* **169**, 893–907.

Kawano, M., Hirano, T., Matsuda, T., Taga, T., Horii, Y., Iwato, K., Asaoku, T., Tang, B., Tanabe, O., Tanaka, H., Kuramoto, A. and Kishimoto, T. (1988). *Nature* **332**, 83–85.

Kinashi, J., Harada, N., Severinson, E., Tanabe, T., Sideras, P., Konishi, M., Athma, C., Tominaga, A., Bergnledt-Lindquist, S., Takahashi, M. and Matsuda, F. (1986). *Nature* **324**, 70–73.

Klein, B., Wijdenes, J., Jourdan, M., Boiron, J.M., Sany, J. and Bataille, R. (1990). *Blood* **76**, 1418.

Köck, A., Danner, M., Stadler, B.M. and Luger, T.A. (1986). *J. Exp. Med.* **163**, 463–468.

Koeffler, H.P., Gasson, J., Ranyard, J., Souza, L., Shepard, M. and Munker, R. (1987). *Blood* **70**, 55–59.

Kupper, T., Horowitz, N., Lee, F., Robb, R. and Flood, P.M. (1987). *J. Immunol.* **138**, 4280–4287.

Lang, R.A., Metcalf, D., Cuthbertson, R.A., Lyons, I., Stanley, E., Kelso, A., Kannourakis, G., Williamson, D.J., Klintworth, G., Gonda, T.J. and Dunn, A.R. (1987). *Cell* **51**, 675–686.

Lattime, E.C. and Stutman, O. (1989). *J. Immunol.* **143**, 4317–4323.

Lehn, M., Weishu, W.Y., Engelhorn, S., Gillis, S. and Remold, H.G. (1989). *J. Immunol.* **143**, 3020–3024.

Lejeune, F., Lenard, D., Eggermont, A.M.M. and Géran, J. (1993). In: *Tumour Necrosis Factor: Molecular and Cellular Biology and Clinical Relevance* (eds W. Fiers and W.A. Buurman), Karger, Basel.

Locksley, R.M., Heinzel, F.P., Shepard, H.M., Agosti, J., Eessalu, T.E., Aggarwal, B.B. and Harlan, J.M. (1987). *J. Immunol.* **139**, 189.

Loetscher, H., Pan, Y-C.E., Lahm, H.-W., Gentz, R., Brockhaus, M., Tabuchi, H. and Lesslauer, W. (1990) *Cell* **61**, 351–359.

Londei, M., Verhoef, A., Hawrylowicz, C., Groves, J., De Berardinis, P. and Feldmann, M. (1990). *Eur. J. Immunol.* **20**, 425–428.

Lorberboum-Galski, H., Barrett, L.V., Kirkman, R.L., Ogata, M., Willingham, M.C., Fitzgerald, D.J. and Pastan, I. (1989). *Proc. Natl Acad. Sci. USA* **86**, 1008–1012.

Lotz, M., Vaughan, J.H. and Carson, D.A. (1988). *Science* **241**, 1218–1221.

Lu, Z.Y., Brochier, J., Wijdenes, J., Brailly, H., Bataille, R. and Klein, B. (1992). *Eur. J. Immunol.* **22**, 2819–2824.

Luger, T.A., Krutman, J., Kimbauer, R., Urbanski, A., Schwarz, T., Klappacher, G., Köck, A., Micksche, M., Malejczyk, J., Schauer, E., May, L.T. and Sehgal, P.B. (1989). *J. Immunol.* **143**, 1206–1209.

Malkovsky, M., Loveland, B., North, M., Asherson, G.L., Gao, L., Ward, P. and Fiers, W. (1987). *Nature* **325**, 262–265.

Manetti, R., Parronchi, P., Giudizi, M.G., Piccini, M-P., Maggi, E., Trinchieri, G. and Romagnani, S. (1993) *J. Exp. Med.* **177**, 1199–1204.

Meuer, S.C., Duman, H., Meyer zum Buschenfelde, K.H. and Koher, H. (1989). *Lancet* **i**, 15–18.

Mond, J.J., Finkelman, F.D., Sarma, C., Ohara, J. and Serrate, S. (1985). *J. Immunol.* **135**, 2513–2517.

Mond, J.J., Carman, J., Sarma, C., Ohara, J. and Finkelman, F.D. (1986). *J. Immunol.* **137**, 3534–3540.

Moore, M.A.S. and Warren, D.J. (1987). *Proc. Natl Acad. Sci. USA* **84**, 7134–7138.

Morrissey, P.J., Goodwin, R.G., Nordan, R.P., Anderson, D., Grabstein, K.H., Cosman, D., Sims, J., Lupton, S., Acres, B., Reed, S.G., Mochizuki, D., Eisenman, J., Conlon, P.J. and Namen, A.E. (1989). *J. Exp. Med.* **169**, 707–716.

Morrone, G., Ciliberto, G., Oliviero, S., Arcone, R., Dente, L., Content, J. and Cortese, R. (1988). *J. Biol. Chem.* **263**, 12554–12558.

Mosley, B., Beckmann, M.P., March, C.J., Idzerda, R.L., Gimpel, S.D., VandenBos, T., Friend, D., Albert, A., Anderson, D., Jackson, J., Wignall, J.M., Smith, C., Gallis, B., Sims, J.E., Urdal, D., Widmer, M.B., Cosman, D. and Park, L.S. (1989). *Cell* **59**, 335–348.

Mullarkey, M.F., Rubin, A.S., Roux, E.R., Hanna, R.K. and Jacob, C.A. (1993). *J. Cell. Biochem, Suppl.* **17B**, 55.

Murata, M., Eto, Y., Shibai, H., Sakai, M. and Muramatsu, M. (1988). *Proc. Natl Acad. Sci. USA* **85**, 2434–2438.

Neta, R., Douches, S.D. and Oppenheim, J.J. (1986). *J. Immunol.* **136**, 2483.

Neta, R., Sztein, M.B., Oppenheim, J.J., Gillis, S. and Douches, S.D. (1987). *J. Immunol.* **139**, 1861–1866.

Nunberg, J.H., Doyle, M.V., York, S.M. and York, C.J. (1989). *Proc. Natl Acad. Sci. USA* **86**, 4240–4243.

Ohta, M., Greenberger, J.S., Ankelsaria, R.K., Bassols, A. and Massagué, J. (1987). *Nature* **329**, 539–541.

Okazaki, H., Ito, M., Sudo, T., Hattori, M., Kano, S., Katsura, Y. and Minato, N. (1989). *J. Immunol.* **143**, 2917–2922.

Pahwa, R., Chatila, T., Pahwa, S., Paradise, C., Day, N.K., Geha, R., Schwartz, S.A., Slade, H., Oyaizu, N. and Good, R.A. (1989). *Proc. Natl Acad. Sci. USA* **86**, 5069–5073.

Pardoll, D.M. (1993). *Trends in Pharm. Sci.* **14**, 202–207.

Parmiani, G. (1990). *Immunol. Today* **11**, 113–115.

Patitch, H.S., Hirsch, R.L., Haley, A.S. and Johnson, K.P. (1987). *Lancet* **i**, 893–894.

Peschel, C., Paul, W.E., Ohara, J. and Green, I. (1987). *Blood,* **70**, 254–263.

Piguet, P.F., Collart, M.A., Grau, G.E., Kapanci, Y. and Vassalli, P. (1989). *J. Exp. Med.* **170**, 913–931.

Playfair, J.H.L. and De Souza, J.B. (1986). *Clin. Exp. Immunol.* **67**, 5–10.

Poli, G., Kinter, A., Justement, J.S., Kehrl, J.H., Bressler, P., Stanley, S. and Fauci, A. (1990). *Proc. Natl Acad. Sci. USA* **87**, 782–787.

Pollard, J.W., Bartocci, A., Arceci, R., Orlofsky, A., Ladner, M.B. and Stanley, E.R. (1987). *Nature* **330**, 484–487.

Poo, W.J. and Janeway, C.A. (1988). *Nature* **332**, 378–380.

Quesada, J.R., Reuben, J., Manning, J.T., Hersh, E.M. and Gutterman, J.U. (1986). *N. Engl. J. Med.* **310**, 15–18.

Ranges, G.E., Zlotnik, A., Espevik, T., Dinarello, C.A., Cerami, A. and Palladino, M.A. (1988). *J. Exp. Med.* **167**, 1472–1478.

Resnitzky, D., Yarden, A., Zipori, D. and Kimchi, A. (1986). *Cell* **46**, 31–40.

Rosenberg, S.A., Lotze, M.T., Muul, L.M., Chang, A.E., Avis, F.P., Leitman, S., Linehan, W.M., Robertson, C.N., Lee, R.E., Rubin, J.T., Seipp, C.A., Simpson, C.G. and White, D.E. (1987). *N. Engl. J. Med.* **316**, 889–897.

Saragovic, H. and Malek, T.R. (1990). *Proc. Natl Acad. Sci. USA* **87**, 11–15.

Schall, T.J., Lewis, M., Koller, K.J., Lee, A., Rice, G.C., Wong, G.H.W., Gatanaga, T., Granger, G.A., Lentz, R., Raab, H., Kohr, W.J. and Goeddel, D.V. (1990). *Cell* **61**, 361–370.

Scully, L.J., Shen, R., Karayiannis, P., McDonald, J.D. and Thomas, H.C. (1987). *J. Hepatol.* **5**, 51–58.

Sechler, J.M.G., Malech, H.L., White, C.J. and Gallin, J.I. (1988). *Proc. Natl Acad. Sci. USA* **85**, 4874–4878.

Seckinger, P., Isaaz, S. and Dayer, J-M. (1988). *J. Exp. Med.* **167**, 1511–1516.

Seckinger, P., Williamson, K., Balauoine, J.F., Mach, B., Mazzoi, G., Shaw, A., Dayer, J-M. (1987). *J. Immunol.* **139**, 1541–1545.

Selby, P., Hobbs, S., Viner, C., Jackson, E., Jones, A., Newell, D., Calvert, A.H., McElwain, T., Fearon, K., Humphreys, J. and Shiga, T. (1987). *Br. J. Cancer* **56**, 803–808.

Selentaag, W.K., Mermod, J.J., Montesano, R. and Vassali, P. (1987). *EMBO J* **6**, 2261–2265.

Sims, J., March, C.J., Cosman, D., Widmer, M.R., MacDonald, H.R., MacMahon, C.J., Grubin, C.K., Wignall, J.M., Jackson, J.L., Call, S.M., Friend, D., Alpert, A.R., Green, S., Urdal, D.L. and Dower, S.K. (1988). *Science* **241**, 585–589.

Sims, J., Gayle, M.A., Slack, J.L., Alderson, M.R., Bird, T.A., Giri, J.G., Colotta, F., Re, F., Mantovani, A., Shanebeck, K., Grabstein, K.H. and Dower, S.K. (1993). *Proc. Natl Acad. Sci. USA* **90**, 6155–6159.

Sironi, M., Breviario, F., Proserpio, P., Biondi, A., Vecchi, A., Van Damme, J., Dejania, E. and Mantovani, A. (1989). *J. Immunol.* **142**, 549–553.

Smeland, E.B., Blomhoff, H.K., Funderud, S., Shalaby, M.R. and Espevik, T. (1989). *J. Exp. Med.* **170**, 1463–1468.

Sykes, M., Romick, M.L., Hoyles, K.A. and Sachs, D.H. (1990). *J. Exp. Med.* **171**, 645–658.

Sypek, J.P., Chung, C.L., Mayer, S.E.H., Subramanyam, J.M., Goldman, S.J., Sieburth, D.S., Wolf, S.F. and Schaub, R.G. (1993). *J. Exp. Med.* **177**, 1797–1802.

Taga, T., Hibi, M., Hirata, Y., Yamasaki, K., Yasukawa, K., Matsuda, T., Hirano, T. and Kishimoto, T. (1989). *Cell* **58**, 573–581.

Talpaz, M., Kantarjian, H.M., McCredie, K., Trujillo, J.M., Keating, M.J. and Gutterman, J.U. (1986). *N. Engl. J. Med.* **314**, 1065–1069.

Tamm, I., Cardinale, I., Krueger, J., Murphy, J.S., May, L.T. and Sehgal, P.B. (1989). *J. Exp. Med.* **170**, 1649–1669.

Tepper, R.I., Pattengale, P.K. and Leder, P. (1989). *Cell* **57**, 503–512.

Titus, R.G., Sherry, B. and Cerami, A. (1989). *J. Exp. Med.* **170**, 2097–2104.

Tracey, K.J., Fong, Y., Hesse, D.G., Manogue, K.R., Lee, A.T., Kuo, G.C., Lowry, S.F. and Cerami, A. (1987). *Nature* **330**, 662–664.

Versteeg, R., Peltenburg, L.T.C., Plomp, A.C. and Schrier, P.E. (1989). *J. Immunol.* **143**, 4331–4337.

Wagner, F., Fischer, N., Lersch, C., Hart, R. and Dancygier, H. (1989). *Immunol. Lett.* **21**, 237–242.

Wogensen, L., Huang, X. and Sarvetnick, N. (1993). *J. Exp. Med.* **178**, 175–185.

Wong, G.H.W. and Goeddell, D.W. (1988). *Science* **242**, 941–943.

Yanelli, J.R., Hyatt, C., Johnson, S., Hwu, P. and Rosenberg, S.A. (1993). *J. Immunol. Methods* **161**, 77–90.

Chapter 24

Future Prospects of Therapy with Haemopoietic Growth Factors

Peter G. Bardy, Angel F. Lopez, M. Frances Shannon and
Mathew A. Vadas

Hanson Centre for Cancer Research,
Institute of Medical and Veterinary Science,
Adelaide, South Australia, 5000

INTRODUCTION

The purpose of this chapter is to extrapolate from our current knowledge to the future uses of cytokines as therapeutic agents. The therapeutic uses of cytokines to date have been based on our understanding of their *in vitro* effects (Table 1) (Vadas *et al.*, 1981; Dessein *et al.*, 1982; Lopez *et al.*, 1983; Vadas and Lopez, 1984; Morstyn and Burgess, 1988; Nicola, 1989). However, as our knowledge of *in vivo* actions expands so too will the list of potential therapeutic indications.

It is clear that in any biologically complex system novel therapeutic agents can be designed. Whether the clinically useful ones will come from alterations of cytokine structure, alternative modes of administration, combinations of treatment or interventions at the gene level is as yet not known. Our aim has been to survey a large number of possibilities and attempt to indicate the relative likelihood of the success of different approaches.

Table 1. Major *in vitro* effects of haemopoietic growth factors.*

1. Survival of progenitor and mature cells
2. Proliferation
3. Differentiation
4. Functional activation of mature cells

*Vadas *et al.* (1981); Dessein *et al.* (1982); Lopez *et al.* (1983, 1986); Vadas and Lopez (1984); Nicola (1989); Morstyn and Burgess (1988).

The Cytokine Handbook, 2nd ed.
ISBN 0–12–689661–5

CURRENT AND PROJECTED THERAPEUTIC USAGE

Single-agent Therapy

The early clinical trials, principally with G-CSF and GM-CSF, used single agents and made use predominantly of their proliferative and differentiative effects; phase 1, phase 2 and, more recently, phase 3 studies with these single recombinant agents have provided clear indications of optimal dosages and routes of administration (Bronchud *et al.*, 1987; Groopman *et al.*, 1987; Vandhan-Raj *et al.*, 1987, 1988a; Antin *et al.*, 1988; Antman *et al.*, 1988; Brandt *et al.*, 1988; Gabrilove *et al.*, 1988; Morstyn *et al.*, 1988; Lieschke *et al.*, 1989a, 1990; Sheridan *et al.*, 1989; Nemunaitis *et al.*, 1991). Increasing experience of *in vivo* effects has confirmed predictions from *in vitro* studies that certain cytokines will be suited to particular clinical conditions. For example, G-CSF is now the treatment of choice for cyclic neutropenia, an isolated neutrophil disorder (Hammond *et al.*, 1989). It also has an established role in the amelioration of postchemotherapy and BMT neutropenia (Sheridan *et al.*, 1989). Other *in vivo* findings have not been predicted by *in vitro* studies. The finding that stem cells mobilized by G-CSF and infused following high doses of chemotherapy speeds both platelet and neutrophil recovery was unexpected (Sheridan *et al.*, 1992; Chao *et al.*, 1993). Similarly, the multilineage *in vitro* effects of IL-3 and GM-CSF have not translated into their ability to speed platelet recovery after cytotoxic therapy (Leung *et al.*, 1987; Sieff *et al.*, 1987; Lopez *et al.*, 1988; Nemunaitis *et al.*, 1991; Biesma *et al.*, 1992; Stahl *et al.*, 1992).

Combination Therapy

Successful *in vivo* combinations of cytokines are anticipated from *in vitro* experiments (Donahue *et al.*, 1988; Paquette *et al.*, 1988; Warren and Moore, 1988; Ulich *et al.*, 1990; Haylock *et al.*, 1992; Brugger *et al.*, 1993). For example, IL-3 treatment allows 10–20-fold lower doses of GM-CSF for the same biological effect *in vitro* (Paquette *et al.*, 1988). A similar degree of synergism has been confirmed *in vivo* in nonhuman primates (Donahue *et al.*, 1988; Warren and Moore, 1988).

It should be noted, however, that the IL-3/GM-CSF combination worked optimally when IL-3 was administered before GM-CSF (Donahue *et al.*, 1988; Mayer *et al.*, 1989, Stahl *et al.*, 1992). This is likely to be due to the fact that IL-3 acts on a more primitive progenitor which it allows to mature into a GM-CSF-responsive state (Donahue *et al.*, 1988). These observations suggest that the timing of administration of combinations may be critical to the choice of cytokines.

It is not unreasonable to anticipate that unique combinations of cytokines will be prescribed for a particular clinical indication. For example, *in vivo* administrations of G-CSF and of GM-CSF are characterized by lack of consistent thrombopoietic effect (Antin *et al.*, 1988; Gabrilove *et al.*, 1988; Nemunaitis *et al.*, 1988; Vandhan-Raj *et al.*, 1988a; Ishibashi *et al.*, 1990). It has recently been shown that IL-6, SCF and IL-11 have such effects *in vivo* (Asarro *et al.*, 1990; Hill *et al.*, 1990; Patchen *et al.*, 1991, 1993; Du *et al.*, 1993; Schuening *et al.*, 1993). In order to achieve a better thrombopoietic response, combinations of these cytokines could be envisaged in therapy.

A number of groups have recently described the use of cytokine combinations to expand stem-cell populations *ex vivo* (Haylock *et al.*, 1992; Brugger *et al.*, 1993). Such an approach has the potential to allow multiple reinfusions of stem cells and/or differentiated cells with multilineage potential following chemotherapy. Such therapy may facilitate faster recovery.

Newer Therapeutic Targets

There are a number of effects of cytokines that have not yet been explored clinically. For example, much attention is being paid to therapeutic strategies that could inhibit atherogenesis. A suitable target of therapy might be the first recognizable event in the generation of atherosclerosis, namely, the adhesion of cholesterol-loaded monocytes to endothelium (Ross, 1986).

Recently, two observations have suggested that cytokines may be used to modulate the process of atherosclerosis. First, IL-4 has been shown to inhibit the adhesion of monocytes to endothelial cells (Elliott *et al.*, 1991), an observation that might also anticipate usefulness in the prevention of vascular diseases. It is important that potential use is put into context: should IL-4 be useful in this regard, it would have to be administered chronically and its other potentially deleterious effects, for example, that of enhanced production of IgE (Coffman *et al.*, 1989), would need to be countered. Second, clinical trials with GM-CSF have reported a totally unanticipated effect of lowering blood cholesterol (Lieschke *et al.*, 1990). This raises the possibility of lipid-lowering effects in chronic use. However, should the hypocholesterolaemic effect be due to enhanced uptake by monocytes or endothelial cells, an accelerated atherogenic process can be anticipated.

MODES OF ADMINISTRATION

Pharmacology

The pharmacology of the cytokines is in its infancy. Extensive *in vivo* studies in humans have been performed only for G-CSF and GM-CSF (Gabrilove *et al.*, 1988; Morstyn *et al.*, 1988, 1989b; Leischke *et al.*, 1990; Cebon *et al.*, 1992; Petros *et al.*, 1992). It is clear from these studies that subcutaneous administration is more efficacious than intravenous infusion when production of neutrophils is used as an end-point. This effect may be secondary to slow release from a subcutaneous reservoir. The phenomenon suggests that there may be a role for slow-release formulations. A number of depot delivery systems have recently been described that allow the slow release of molecules of variable size (e.g. drugs complexed to polymers (Laurenin *et al.*, 1982)) encapsulated together with liposomes in microspheres (Kibat *et al.*, 1990) or complexed to polyethylene glycol, as recently described for GM-CSF (Malik *et al.*, 1992).

Side-effects

The toxicity profiles of cytokines vary. Some (e.g. G-CSF) have minimal *in vivo* toxicity (Bronchud *et al.*, 1987; Morstyn *et al.*, 1988; Lieschke *et al.*, 1989a; Sheridan *et al.*, 1989). GM-CSF, however, has significant dose-related toxicity (Antman *et al.*, 1988; Leischke *et al.*, 1990). In addition, it has a number of side-effects that are not dose-limiting and are variable in incidence (e.g. first-dose syndrome, rash, fever) (Lieschke *et al.*, 1989b). The mechanism of toxicity is unclear but it may relate to activation of mature blood cells with the release of pharmacological mediators (*ibid.*). It can therefore be predicted that the toxicity of a cytokine will relate to the types of cells activated. SCF may be expected to exhibit toxicity mediated by mast-cell activation. Activation of monocytes may be particularly relevant, given their capacity to produce other cytokines. It might also be expected that a cytokine which activates a broad spectrum of cells, such as IL-6, will have considerable toxicity that will be very difficult to minimize (Nemunaitis *et al.*, 1988; Kishimoto, 1989; Weber *et al.*, 1993). The response of mature cells to some cytokines *in vitro* has been shown to vary markedly between individuals (Vadas *et al.*, 1985; Gamble *et al.*, 1990). Whether this heterogenicity can be explored to predict those individuals at particular risk of toxicity awaits further study.

The long-term effects of chronic administration of cytokines will become evident with time. At present there is little evidence to support concerns regarding exhaustion of progenitors or the development of *de novo* leukaemia (*ibid.*). One group has, however, reported that progenitor numbers were depleted in mice following sequential cyclophosphamide and GM-CSF or G-CSF treatment, an effect that could be ameliorated by IL-1 administration (Hornung and Longo, 1992).

The clinical significance of the toxicity manifested in experimental animals chronically expressing very high levels of circulating cytokines is at present unclear (Lang *et al.*, 1987; Chang *et al.*, 1989; Johnson *et al.*, 1989). Such experimental models may be of value in defining the potential spectrum of toxicity in humans. However, it is likely that most of these effects may be avoided by minimizing circulating cytokine levels.

Very Low-Dose Therapy

The affinity of receptors for cytokines in very high (10^{-11}M) and for many *in vitro* biological effects 10–20% occupancy appears to be sufficient (Nicola and Metcalf, 1988; Elliott *et al.*, 1989). For GM-CSF the extension of mature cell survival in particular appears to require the lowest doses *in vitro* (Elliott *et al.*, 1989). The mechanism of this effect is unclear but it may be secondary to the inhibition of programmed cell death or apoptosis (Williams *et al.*, 1990).

The therapeutic effects of the administration of very low doses of cytokines, sufficient to occupy only high-affinity receptors, are not known. The efficacy of *in vivo* administration has, until now, been measured predominantly by increases in circulation levels of mature cells, an effect that is clearly dose-related with G-CSF and GM-CSF. We do not at present know what component of this effect is mediated by high-affinity receptors. It is also unclear whether *in vitro* effects such as prolonged cell survival will extrapolate to the *in vivo* setting. It is tempting to suggest that this effect may be manifest as a heightened resistance to cytotoxic agents. Such an action would raise the possibility of very low-dose infusions being used in a chemoprotective role.

Local Therapy

Local administration of cytokines may provide a mechanism for maximizing local effect while limiting systemic toxicity. Loco-regional administration has been suggested particularly for cytokines with major *in vivo* toxicities such as IL-2 (Margolin *et al.*, 1989; Ishihara *et al.*, 1989). GM-CSF or G-CSF could be used similarly at sites of localized resistant infection (e.g. osteomyelitis) to maximize neutrophil activation and thus perhaps healing.

ENDOGENOUS PRODUCTION OF CYTOKINES

Control of Cellular Production of Cytokines

Modulating the production of cytokines *in vivo* could obviate the need for their systemic administration. While some of the stimuli that lead to cellular production of cytokines *in vitro* are well characterized (Guba *et al.*, 1989; Kishimoto, 1989; Sieff *et al.*, 1989), the control mechanisms operating *in vivo* are unknown. The mechanisms that control the basal level of production of the normal spectrum of haemopoietic cells are not understood. It is also unclear how changes such as the selective neutrophilia seen in response to pyogenic infection are produced. In both situations there is likely to be a tightly controlled balance between positive and negative regulators of cytokine production. At present this latter group, the negative regulators, is the least well defined.

TNF, TGF-β and IFN-α have some negative effects on haemopoiesis and may be involved in some circumstances (Broxmeyer *et al.*, 1986; Kishi *et al.*, 1989). However, it is likely that additional specialized and perhaps new cytokines will be discovered that will fulfil the role of selective negative regulators. Cytokines may also play a role in the autocrine and paracrine stimulation of transformed haemopoietic cells. Examples include the production of IL-6 by malignant plasma cells (Kwano *et al.*, 1988) and the production of a number of cytokines by leukaemic cells in acute myeloid leukaemia (Young *et al.*, 1987; Oster *et al.*, 1989; Reilly *et al.*, 1989; Van der Schoot *et al.*, 1989; Russell, 1992). Determining the mechanisms of altered cytokine production in transformed cells may lead to specific therapies aimed at modifying potential autocrine stimulation.

Control of Cytokine Gene Expression

Cytokine genes are expressed in a tissue-specific and inducible manner. The control points are likely to be complex, with some shared and some gene-specific controlling agents. For example, although the GM-CSF and IL-3 genes are closely associated on chromosome 5 at 5q 21-31 (Le Beau *et al.*, 1987; Yang *et al.*, 1988) have significant homologies in both their 5' promoter and 3' noncoding regions (Fig. 1) and have a similar, although not identical spectrum of activities *in vitro* (Lopez *et al.*, 1986; Morstyn and Burgess, 1988; Nicola, 1989), the IL-3 gene is expressed only in T cells while GM-CSF is much more widely expressed (on monocytes, T cells, endothelial cells, etc.) (Guba *et al.*, 1989; Sieff *et al.*, 1989; Gasson, 1991). Understanding the nature of this difference may suggest ways of altering the expression of these two genes.

One reason for the difference in expression may relate to differences in transcriptional control of the two genes. Distinct transcription factors appear to interact with the IL-3 and GM-CSF proximal promoter regions. A protein termed NF-GMa interacts with a conserved region (CK-1) in both promoters (Shannon *et al.*, 1990). The GM-CSF

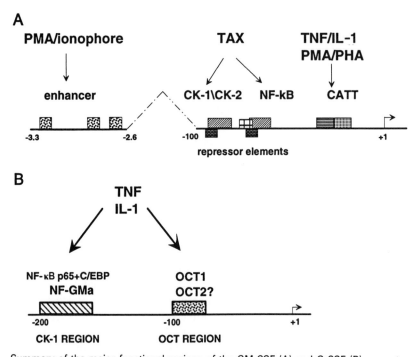

Fig. 1. Summary of the major functional regions of the GM-CSF (A) and G-CSF (B) promoters. A. The regions of the GM-CSF proximal promoter (−100 to +1) that are involved in the response to PMA/PHA in Jurkat T cells, TNF and IL-1 in endothelial cells and fibroblasts and to the HTLV-1 transactivator, *tax* in T cells are shown. Repressor elements that inhibit the TNF/IL-1 response of the CATT repeat regions are also shown. An enhancer located between −3.3 and −2.6 upstream of the GM-CSF promoter is also indicated. The three boxes represent NFAT sites (Cockerill *et al.*, 1993). B. The G-CSF proximal promoter (−200 to +1) is shown with the two TNF/IL-1 responsive regions (CK-1 and Oct) indicated. The transcription factors that bind to these sequences are also shown.

promoter has a functional NF-κB site (Schreck and Baeurle, 1990; M.F. Shannon, L.S. Coles and S.R. Himes, unpublished) as well as CATT repeat sequences which also appear to be required for function (Fig. 1) (Nimer *et al.*, 1989). The IL-3 promoter does not have identifiable NF-κB or CATT repeat sequences but has a functional API site and an octamer/OAP type site similar to that described for the T-cell specific IL-2 promoter (Davies *et al.*, 1993). The OAP/OCT site may be involved in restricting expression of the IL-3 gene to T cells, whereas the NF-κB site of GM-CSF may function in many cell types.

Recently, an enhancer region has been identified 3kb upstream from the GM-CSF gene (Fig. 1) (Cockerill *et al.*, 1993). This enhancer functions when linked to either the GM-CSF or IL-3 promoter following T-cell activation and its activity can be blocked by cyclosporin (Cockerill *et al.*, 1993). It is not known if this enhancer functions in other cell types but if it is T-cell specific it may provide a target to modulate the expression of these genes in a cell-specific manner.

The ability to regulate G-CSF expression may be important for treatment following high-dose chemotherapy and bone-marrow transplantation where administration of G-CSF is currently used (see above). The ability to block G-CSF expression may be important in inflammatory diseases, such as rheumatoid arthritis and psoriasis (Gabrilove, 1992). At least three families of transcription factors appear to be involved in G-CSF promoter function (Fig. 1). They are the octamer, C/EBP and NF-κB families of proteins (Shannon *et al.*, 1992; Dunn and Shannon, submitted). The inflammatory cytokines, TNF-α and IL-1β, mediate activity of NF-κB and some C/EBP proteins such as NF-IL6 and C/EBP (Akira and Kishimoto, 1992; Kinoshita *et al.*, 1992). The TNF response region of G-CSF binds the NF-κB p65 protein and NF-IL6 in a cooperative manner (Dunn *et al.*, 1994). It is likely that direct protein–protein interaction is required for this activity. The gene for IL-8 is also activated by inflammatory cytokines (Mukaida *et al.*, 1990). It is intriguing that the IL-8 gene promoter also contains adjacent binding sites for NF-κB p65 and NF-IL6 which behave as a functional unit (C. Kunsch, R.K. Lang, C.A. Rosen and M.F. Shannon, personal communication). The ability to downregulate G-CSF and IL-8 transcription by blocking NF-κB/C/EBP interactions may be useful in decreasing adverse inflammatory reactions.

Post-transcriptional control mechanisms, mediated at least in part by the 3′ AU-rich sequences, may also vary between the genes. The AU-rich region is common to a number of transiently expressed genes and has been shown to decrease the half-life of a normally stable mRNA when added to its 3′ untranslated region (Shaw and Kamen, 1986). At present, the relative importance of transcriptional and post-transcriptional control mechanisms for IL-3 is unclear. Both mechanisms, however, appear to be operating for both G-CSF and GM-CSF gene expression (Thorens *et al.*, 1987; Koeffler *et al.*, 1988; Ernst *et al.*, 1989).

Modifying Endogenous Production of Cytokines

Our ability to modify the production of cytokines awaits an improved understanding of the mechanisms that control gene expression *in vivo*. It is, however, challenging to postulate the use of specific transcription factors or their derivatives as therapeutic agents. It may be possible to develop dominant negative derivatives of transcription factors that can bind DNA but lack the ability to activate transcription. Such dominant negative factors exist in nature. Examples are the Id protein which interacts with, and blocks the function of, the Myo-D-related proteins by preventing DNA binding (Benezra *et al.*, 1990). An alternative translation product of the *LAP* (NF-IL6) gene called LIP can heterodimerize with other C/EBP proteins and bind DNA, but lacks a transactivation domain and therefore lacks function (Descombes and Schibler, 1991). Since the activation of transcription often depends not only on protein–DNA but also protein–protein interaction it may be possible to prevent protein–protein interactions through the use of modified proteins or drugs.

Drugs that interact with specific promoter regions or with specific transcription factors to block correct protein–DNA interactions may be developed. An example of such an agent is the chemotherapeutic drug, cisplatin. It is known to bind to DNA and covalently modify G/C dinocleotides (Evans and Gralla, 1988). There is come evidence that it can preferentially inhibit transcription from genes containing CC-rich promoter regions (*ibid.*). The steroid hormones exert their effects by promoting interaction between their receptor and promoter sequences in target genes (Evans, 1988). The expression of many cytokine genes is downregulated by glucocorticoids (e.g. Ray *et al.*, 1990). How steroids negatively regulate gene transcription is not clearly understood.

Steroid hormone receptors can interact with and sequester other transcription factors such as AP1, thus preventing activation by these proteins (Schule *et al.*, 1990). They also bind to composite DNA sequences with other transcription factors, having a negative or positive effect depending on the DNA-sequence context (Gaub *et al.*, 1990). The IL-6 promoter contains several glucocorticoid-responsive elements that overlap known transcription activator regions, which suggests that glucocorticoids may alter IL-6 gene transcription through an occlusion mechanism (Kishimoto, 1989). It may be possible, with an increased knowledge of the precise mechanism of action of these agents, to use steroid hormone treatment to target defined genes.

The immunosuppressant drug, cyclosporin, functions by blocking the activation of a component of the T-cell specific transcription factor, NFAT (reviewed in Schreiber, 1992). Cyclosporin, once bound to its receptor (cyclophilin) interacts with calcineurin, a calmodulin-dependent phosphatase, and prevents its action on a cytoplasmic factor, thus preventing its nuclear translocation (Schreiber, 1992). (For further details see Chapter 26 of this volume.) Thus, it can be envisaged that drugs with similar properties may be designed to inactivate or activate other transcription factors.

NEW CYTOKINES

Deglycosylated Molecules

The initial clinical trials used unmodified recombinant molecules. The recombinant products do vary, however, in their degree of glycosylation (Cebon *et al.*, 1990). GM-CSF glycosylation has been shown to have a powerful effect on *in vitro* potency, with the deglycosylated molecule having a six-fold increased potency when compared with the glycosylated form. The *in vivo* half-life of deglycosylated recombinant human GM-CSF injected into rats, however, was lower than the glycosylated forms (Cebon *et al.*, 1990). The overall impact of these conflicting effects has not been determined.

New Variants

Variant or 'second-generation' cytokines are an attractive area for development. The rational design of second-generation cytokines depends on an understanding of the three-dimensional structure of the cytokine, the residues involved in binding to its receptor, the properties of the receptor and an understanding of the pharmacodynamics of the agent.

Structure–Function Analysis
In the light of the above remarks, structure–function studies of cytokines appear to be a fertile ground for investigation. An example of this approach was described recently for the mouse IL-2 receptor (Zurawski and Zurawski, 1989). The functional receptor for IL-2 contains three noncovalently linked binding polypeptides: the low-affinity p55 chain and the intermediate-affinity p70 chain and a non-binding γ chain (Smith, 1988; Takeshita *et al.*, 1990). These chains act together to bind IL-2 with high affinity. The three-dimensional structure of human IL-2 reveals a backbone of six α-helices (*ibid.*). Amino acid substitutions in the first α helix resulted in specific inhibition of p70 receptor binding while substitution in the fifth helix specifically inactivated binding to the p55

Table 2. Desired properties of second generation haemopoietic cytokines.

Desired property	Intermediate aim	Likelihood of achievement
Absorption through skin	Severely truncated forms; probably less than 1–6 kDa	±
Prolonged half-life	Reduced clearance	±
Decreased toxicity	Definition of target cells	±
Enhanced potency	Increased binding affinity	++
Antagonism	Partial agonist/antagonists	±
Selective function	Selective binding to low- and high-affinity receptors	++
Broadened function	Coupled cytokines, chimaeras	±

± Not very likely; ++ likely to happen.

chain of the receptor. Thus, two distinct parts of the IL-2 molecule are required for binding to two distinct parts of the IL-2 receptor. A similar approach utilizing chemical synthesis of truncated GM-CSF proteins has defined a region between residues −14 and −24 critical for activity (Clark-Lewis *et al.*, 1988). Further studies in this region, performed using site-directed mutagenesis, showed that Glu-21 was a crucial residue for biological activity (Lopez *et al.*, 1992a). Significantly expression of a mutant in CHO cells with Arg substituted for Glu-21 led to a GM-CSF analogue still able to recognize fully the low-affinity GM-CSF receptor α chain but defective at binding to the high-affinity (α and β) receptor (Lopez *et al.*, 1992a). The selective loss of interaction with the β chain shows that GM-CSF has two distinct domains that can recognize the α or β chain of its receptor (Lopez *et al.*, 1992a). Analysis of mutated human IL-1α molecules has also revealed 15 residues in the *N* terminal important for *in vitro* activity (Yonofsky and Zurawski, 1990).

Human IL-3 has been subjected to mutagenesis and Leu-111 in the predicted helix D of the molecule was shown to be crucial for activity (Lokker *et al.*, 1991). However, the hydrophobic and conserved (among other cytokines) nature of this residue suggests that rather than being involved in receptor binding, it may be important for the structural integrity of IL-3. Conversely, mutation of residues 101 and 116 led to the production of an IL-3 analogue with increased biological activity (Lopez *et al.*, 1992b).

Second-generation Cytokines
Having used the above techniques to determine which residues are critical for receptor binding and function, the potential exists to manufacture clinically useful mutant molecules. Table 2 lists some desired properties of potential clinically useful second-generation cytokines. Some of these ideal properties are unlikely to be achievable in the short term for the reasons outlined below.

Defining the minimal size necessary for activity may allow manufacture of truncated molecules that are sufficiently small to be absorbed percutaneously. The clear limitation here is that of size: only molecules less than approximately 1 kDa in size can be efficiently absorbed through the skin (Ridaut *et al.*, 1988). Whether it will be feasible to mutate a cytokine to alter clearance will depend on mechanisms of clearance. If it is mediated by binding and internalization by haemopoietic cells, impairing clearance may require impairing receptor binding and thus function. The development of competitive antagonists will require a molecule that binds to a receptor but has minimal or no agonist activity. As discussed below, selective function may be achieved by mutating individual binding sites in a cytokine where multiple sites mediate binding to different receptors. Cytokine function may be broadened by coupling cytokines or forming chimaeras containing active sites of a number of cytokines. It may be anticipated, however, that such molecules will reflect properties not of the mutant ligand but of the receptor they occupy. The recent report of the mutagenesis of human prolactin to allow binding to a human growth-hormone receptor (Cunningham *et al.*, 1990) suggests that the production of such 'designer cytokines' will be possible. The *in vivo* effects of such molecules clearly await further studies.

CYTOKINE RECEPTOR INTERACTIONS

Cytokine Receptors in Normal Haemopoiesis

As our understanding of cytokine receptor–ligand interactions expands, so too does our appreciation of their complexity. The GM-CSF receptor, which is a member of a recently recognized new family of cytokine receptors, will be used as an example (Gearing *et al.*, 1989; Goodwin *et al.*, 1990). The use of ^{125}I-labelled GM-CSF has indicated that in both human and murine systems there are small numbers of GM-CSF receptors on both normal and leukaemic haemopoietic cells (Gasson *et al.*, 1986; Park *et al.*, 1986, 1989), as well as on some nonhaemopoietic tumour cells (Baldwin *et al.*, 1989). These receptors appear to be heterogenous (Table 3), in that in some cells they bind GM-CSF with high affinity while in others they do so with much lower affinity. Furthermore, some cell types express both high- and low-affinity forms. To add to the complexity some high-affinity receptors crossreact IL-3 (Elliott *et al.*, 1989).

The structural basis for the different receptor affinities and for the cross-competition have recently been elucidated with the molecular cloning of several receptor chains (reviewed in Lopez *et al.*, 1992c). The GM-CSF receptor (R) as well as the IL-3R and IL-5R are heterodimeric receptors that comprise an α chain and a β chain. While the α chain is of low affinity and specific for each cytokine, the β chain does not detectably bind GM-CSF, IL-3 or IL-5 but confers high-affinity binding. The fact that the β chain is common to all three receptors explains the cross-competition between GM-CSF, IL-3 and IL-5. These data, together with the observation that cells concomitantly expressing two or three receptors are stimulated to perform the same functions and to the same degree by the corresponding ligand, suggest that the β chain may be the common signal transducer in this receptor complex.

Cytokine Receptors in Transformed Cells

The presence of cytokine receptors on leukaemic cells and some solid tumour-cell lines raises the possibility of transformed cells proliferating in response to *in vivo* cytokine administration. This effect may be used therapeutically in, for instance, acute myeloid leukaemia, in an attempt to drive resting cells into the cell cycle thus making them more chemosensitive (Cannistra *et al*, 1989). Equally, however, the effect could be deleterious should unwanted proliferation be induced in transformed cells, as in patients with myelodysplastic syndromes or solid tumours (Gasser *et al.*, 1989; Herrmann *et al.*, 1989). A potential mechanism for avoiding this would be to tailor cytokines that bind

Table 3. Complexity of GM-CSF interaction with its receptor.

Cell type	Class of receptor	Affinity (K_d)	Cross-competition with IL-3	Biological responses		Reference
				Activation	Proliferation	
Neutrophil	High affinity	10^{-11} M	–	+	–	Di Persio et al. (1988)
Eosinophil	High affinity	10^{-11} M	+	+	–	Lopez et al. (1989)
Monocytes	High + low affinity	10^{-9}, 10^{-11} M	+ (High)	+	+	Elliott et al. (1989)
Endothelial cells	Low affinity	10^{-9} M	?	Migration	+	Bussolino et al. (1989)

only to receptors on normal haemopoietic cells. Such an approach will rely on the definition of clear differences in receptors between normal and transformed cells.

Abnormal receptors may play an aetiological role in the process of transformation of haemopoietic cells. The M-CSF receptor is hypothesized to do so in some cases of acute myeloid leukaemia. As discussed elsewhere, this receptor is a proto-oncogene, c-*fms*, the human cellular homologue of the v-*fms* oncogene. Specific point mutations in the receptor's extracellular domain act as potent activating mutations, enabling transformation of cells in the absence of the ligand M-CSF. This ligand-independent activation is not associated with alteration of the ligand-binding site and therefore the presence of M-CSF could lead potentially to further proliferation of the transformed cells (Sherr, 1989). Although only a minority of cases of myelodysplastic syndrome and acute myeloid leukaemia examined to date have shown evidence of these specific point-mutations (Ridge *et al.*, 1990), other, as yet undefined mutations may be relevant in human haemopoietic neoplasms expressing this receptor. There is, however, no evidence for gross rearrangement of the GM-CSF Rα chain in patients with acute myeloid leukaemia (Bardy *et al.*, 1992; Brown *et al.*, 1993).

The recent localization of a low affinity GM-CSF receptor gene to a site nonrandomly deleted in a significant proportion of FAB subtype M2 acute myeloid leukaemia raises the possibility that abnormality in this receptor may also play a role in leukemogenesis (Gough *et al.*, 1990). If one allele is truly deleted the other may be mutated, potentially leading to abnormal phenotypes. Mutations in the region encoding the GM-CSF binding domain could therefore lead to a phenotype with decreased GM-CSF responsiveness and therefore arrested differentiation. Alterations in the signal transduction domain may lead to a similar phenotype or alternatively to one characterized by constitutive activation of the receptor.

Given that altered receptors may be expressed on the surface of transformed cells, the potential exists to target them therapeutically. An example may be the use of specific ligands labelled with toxin. However, such approaches suffer first, from a lack of discrimination between normal and transformed cells and second, from the problem of clearance of the toxin. These difficulties may be minimized in a system where either the number of receptors expressed on the target cells is greater than on normal cells, or the receptors are altered in some way which allows the production of a tumour-specific ligand.

As stated above, cytokine receptors may also play a role in malignant-cell proliferation through participation in autocrine loops, as is the case for IL-6 in multiple myeloma (Kwano *et al.*, 1988). Such autocrine loops may be interrupted by the introduction of solubilized receptors. Circulating forms of cytokine receptor may have a role in the normal clearance of the ligand and have been described in IL-4, IL-6, and IL-7 (Goodwin *et al.*, 1990). Increasing the circulation levels may interrupt autocrine stimulation of transformed cells by the removal of the ligand.

CONCLUSIONS

The advent of recombinant cytokines will have a profound effect on haemopoietic therapeutics. Some agents will soon enter our therapeutic armamentarium as the first phase-3 clinical trials reach completion. Other agents can be anticipated to follow in the near future as they enter phase 1 and phase 2 studies.

In this chapter we have gone beyond a review of the current status of preclinical and clinical trials, which has recently been done by others (Morstyn, 1990). Rather, we have attempted to survey how our ever-expanding knowledge of the biology of haemopoietic cytokines is likely to lead to the development of new therapeutic agents.

In the immediate future we are likely to see an expansion of trials using an array of new cytokines (IL-3, IL-6, IL-4, M-CSF). The most exciting advances, however, are likely to come in the longer term with the development of second-generation cytokines. It is likely that the designer cytokine—tailored to specific indications with toxicity minimized—will become a reality. Where improved understanding of the mechanisms that control cytokine production in both normal and abnormal haemopoiesis will lead us is, as discussed, unclear and will depend on the successful identification of mechanisms that alter gene expression.

ACKNOWLEDGEMENTS

This work was supported by the National Health and Medical Research Council (Australia), the Anti-Cancer Foundation of the Universities of South Australia and the National Cancer Institute of the National Institutes of Health.

REFERENCES

Akira, S. and Kishimoto, T. (1992). *Immunol. Rev.* **127**, 25–50.

Antin, J.H., Smith, B.R., Holmes, W. and Rosenthal, D.S. (1988). *Blood* **72**, 705–713.

Antman, J.H., Griffin, J.D., Elias, A., Socinski, M.A., Ryan, L., Cannistra, S.A., Oette, D., Whiteley, M., Frei, E. and Schnipper, E. (1988). *N. Eng. J. Med.* **319**, 543–598.

Asarro, S., Okuno, A., Ozawa, K., Nakahata, T., Ishibashi, T., Koike, K., Kimura, H., Tanioku, Y., Shibuya, A., Hirano, T., Kishimoto, T., Takaku, F. and Akiyama, Y. (1990). *Blood* **75**, 1602–1605.

Baldwin, G.C., Gasson, J.C., Kauffman, S.E., Quan, S.G., Williams, R.E., Avalos, B.R., Garder, A.F., Golde, D.W. and Dispersio, J.F. (1989). *Blood* **73**, 1033.

Bardy, P.G., Lopez, A.F., Moore, S., Park, L.S., Vadas, M.A. and Shannon, M.F. (1992). *Leukemia* **6**, 893–897.

Benezra, R., Davis, R.L., Lockshon, D., Turner, D.L. and Weintraub, H. (1990). *Cell* **61**, 49–59.

Biesma, B., Willemse, P.H., Mulder, N.H., Sleijfer, D.T., Gietema, J.A., Mull, R., Limburg, P.C., Bouma, J., Vellenga, E. and de Vries, E.G. (1992). *Blood* **80**, 1141–1148.

Brandt, S.J., Peters, W.P., Atwater, S.K., Kurtzerg, J., Borowitz, M.J., Jones, R.B., Shpull, E.J., Bast, R.C., Gilbert, C.J. and Oette, D.M. (1988). *N. Engl. J. Med.* **318**, 869–876.

Bronchud, M.H., Scarffe, J.H., Thatcher, N., Crowther, D., Souza, L.M., Alton, N.K., Testa, N.G. and Dexter, T.M. (1987). *Br. J. Cancer* **56**, 809–813.

Brown, M.A., Gough, N.M., Willson, T.A., Rockman, S. and Begley, C.G. (1993). *Leukaemia* **7**, 63–74.

Broxmeyer, H., Williams, D., Lu, L., Cooper, S., Anderson, S., Beyer, G., Hoffman, R. and Rubin, B. (1986). *J. Immunol.* **136**, 4487–4495.

Brugger, W., Mocklin, W., Heimfeld, S., Berenson, R.J., Mertelsmann, R. and Kanz, L. (1993). *Blood* **81**, 2579–2584.

Bussolino, F., Wang, J., DeFilipii, D., Turrini, F., Sanavio, F., Edgell, C.-J., Aglietta, M., Anese, P. and Mantovani, A. (1989). *Nature* **337**, 471–473.

Cannistra, S., Groshek, P. and Griffin, J. (1989). *Leukaemia* **3**, 328–334.

Cebon, J., Nicola, N., Ward, M., Gardner, I., Dempsey, P., Layton, J., Duhrsen, U., Burgess, A., Nice, E. and Morstyn, G. (1990). *J. Biol. Chem.* **265**, 4483–4491.

Cebon, J., Lieschke, G.J., Bury, R.W. and Morstyn, G. (1992). *Brit. J. Haemat.* **80**, 144–150.

Chang, J.M., Metcalf, D., Gonda, T.J. and Johnson, G.R. (1989). *J. Clin. Invest.* **84**, 1488–1496.

Chao, N.J., Schriber, J.R., Grimes, K., Long, G.D., Negrin, R.S., Raimondi, C.M., Homing, S.J., Brown, S.L., Miller, L. and Blume, K.G. (1993). *Blood* **81**, 2031–2035.

Clark-Lewis, I., Lopez, A.F., L. Bik To, Vadas, M., Schrader, J., Hood, L. and Kent, S. (1988). *J. Immunol.* **141**, 881–889.

Cockerill, P.N., Shannon, M.F., Bert, A.G., Ryan, G.R. and Vadas, M.A. (1993). *Proc. Natl Acad. Sci. USA* **90**, 2466–2470.

Coffman, R., Seymour, B., Hudak, S., Jackson, J. and Rennick, D. (1989). *Science* **245**, 308–310.

Cunningham, B., Henner, D. and Wells, J. (1990). *Science* **247**, 1461–1465.

Davies, K., TePas, E.C., Nathan, D.G. and Mathey-Prevot, B. (1993). *Blood* **81**, 928–934.

Descombes, P. and Schibler, U. (1991). *Cell* **67**, 569–579.

Dessein, A., Vadas, M.A., Nicola, N., Metcalf, D. and David, J.R. (1982). *J. Exp. Med.* **156**, 90–103.

Di Persio, J., Billing, P., Kaufman, S., Eghtesady, P., Williams, R. and Gasson, J. (1988). *J. Biol. Chem.* **263**, 1834–1841.

Donahue, R.E., Seehra, J., Metzger, M., Letebve, D., Rock, B., Carbone, S., Nathan, D.G., Carnick, M., Sehgal, P.K., Laston, D., La Vallie, E., McCoy, J., Schendel, P.F., Norton, C., Turner, K., Yang, Y.-C. and Clark, S.C. (1988). *Science* **241**, 1820–1822.

Du, X.X., Neben, T., Goldman, S. and Williams, D.A. (1993). *Blood* **81**, 27–34.

Dunn, S.M., Coles, L.S., Lang, R.K., Gerondakis, S., Vadas, M.A. and Shannon, M.F. (1994). *Blood* (in press).

Elliott, M.J., Vadas, M.A., Eglinton, J., Park, L., L. Bik To, Cleland, L., Clark, S. and Lopez, A. (1989). *Blood* **74**, 2349–2359.

Elliott, M.J., Gamble, J.R., Park, L.S., Vadas, M.A. and Lopez, A.F. (1991). *Blood* **77**, 2739–2745.

Ernst, T., Ritchie, A. and Griffin, J.D. (1989). *J. Biol. Chem.* **264**, 5700–5703.

Evans, G.-L. and Gralla, J.D. (1988). *J. Cell. Biochem.* (Suppl 12D), 184 (Abstr.).

Evans, R. (1988). *Science* **240**, 884–895.

Gabrilove, J. (1992). *Blood* **80**, 1382–1385.

Gabrilove, J.L., Jakubowski, A., Fain, K., Grous, J., Scher, H., Sternberg, C., Wong, G., Graus, J., Fuin, K., Moore, M., Clarkson, B., Oettgen, H., Alton, K., Welte, K. and Souza, L. (1988). *N. Eng. J. Med.* **318**, 1414–1422.

Gamble, J., Rand, T., Lopez, A., Clark-Lewis, I. and Vadas, M.A. (1990). *Exp. Haematol.* **18**, 897–902.

Gasser, A., Volkers, B., Greher, J., Ottman, O.G., Wolther, F., Becher, R., Bergman, L., Schulz, G. and Hoelzer, D. (1989). *Blood* **73**, 31–37.

Gasson, J.C. (1991). *Blood* **6**, 1131–1145.

Gasson, J.C., Kauffman, S.E., Weisbart, R.H., Tomonaga, M. and Golde, D.W. (1986). *Proc. Natl Acad. Sci. USA* **83**, 669–673.

Gaub, M.-P., Bellard, M., Scheuer, I., Chambon, P. and Sassone-Corsi, P. (1990). *Cell* **63**, 1267–1276.

Gearing, D., King, J., Gough, N. and Nicola, N. (1989). *EMBO J.* **8**, 3667–3676.

Gewirtz, A. and Calabretta, B. (1988). *Science* **242**, 1303.

Goodwin, R., Friend, D., Ziegler, S., Jerzy, R., Falk, B., Gimpel, S., Cosman, D., Dower, S., March, C., Namen, A. and Park, L.S. (1990) *Cell* **60**, 941–951.

Gough, N., Gearing, D., Nicola, N., Baker, E., Pritchard, M., Callen, D. and Sutherland, G.R. (1990). *Nature* **345**, 734–736.

Groopman, J.E., Mitsuyasu, R.T., DeLeo, M.J., Oette, D.M. and Golde, D.W. (1987). *N. Eng. J. Med.* **317**, 593–598.

Guba, S., Stella, G., Turku, L., June, C., Thompson, C. and Emerson, G. (1989). *J. Clin. Invest.* **84**, 1701–1706.

Hammond, W.P., Price, T.H., Souza, L.M. and Dale, D.C. (1989). *N. Eng. J. Med.* **320**, 1306–1311.

Haylock, D.N., To, L.B., Dose, T.L., Juttner, C.A. and Simmons, P.J. (1992). *Blood* **80**, 1405.

Herrmann, F., Lindemann, A., Klein, H., Labbert, M., Schultz, G. and Mertelsman, R. (1989). *Leukaemia* **3**, 335–338.

Hill, R., Warren, K. and Levin, J. (1990). *J. Clin. Invest* **85**, 1242–1247.

Hornung, R.L. and Longo, D.L. (1992). *Blood* **80**, 77–83.

Ishibashi, T., Kimura, H., Shikama, Y., Uchida, T., Karyone, S. and Muruyama, Y. (1990). *Blood* **75**, 1433–1438.

Ishihara, K., Hayasaka, K. and Yamazaki, H. (1989). *J. Invest. Dermatol.* **92**, 3265–3285.

Johnson, G.R., Gonda, T.J., Metcalf, D., Hariharan, I. and Cory, S. (1989). *EMBO J.* **8**, 441–448.

Kibat, P.G., Igari, Y., Wheatley, M.A., Eisen, H.M. and Langer, R. (1990). *FASEB J.* **4**, 2533–2539.

Kinoshita, S., Akira, S and Kishimoto, T. (1992). *Proc. Natl Acad. Sci. USA* **89**, 1473–1476.

Kishi, K., Ellingsworth, L. and Ogawa, M. (1989). *Leukaemia* **3**, 687–691.

Kishimoto, T. (1989). *Blood* **74**, 1–10.

Koeffler, H.P., Gasson, J. and Tobler, A. (1988). *Mol. Cell. Biol.* **8**, 3432–3438.

Kwano, M., Hirano, T., Matsuda, T., Toya, T., Horii, Y., Iwato, K., Asaobu, H., Targ, B., Tanabe, O., Tanake, H., Kuramoto, A. and Kishimoto, T. (1988). *Nature* **332**, 83–84.

Lang, R.A., Metcalf, D., Cuthbertson, R.A., Lyons, I., Stanley, E., Kelso, A., Kannourakis, G., Williamson, D.J., Klintworth, G.K., Gonda, T.J. and Dunn, A.R. (1987). *Cell* **51**, 675–686.

Laurenin, C.T., Koh, M.J., Nunan, T., Allcock, H.R. and Lanyer, R. (1982). *J. Biomed. Mater. Res.* **21**, 1231–1246.

Le Beau, M.M., Epstein, N.D., O'Brien, S.J., Nienhuis, A.W., Yang, Y.-C., Clark, S.C. and Rowley, J.D. (1987). *Proc. Natl Acad. Sci. USA* **84**, 5913.

Leung, A., Yu-Chung Yang, Clark, S., Gasson, J., Golde, D. and Ogawa, M. (1987). *Blood* **70**, 1343–1348.

Lieschke, G., Cebon, J. and Morstyn, G. (1989a). *Blood* **74**, 2634–2643.

Lieschke, G.J., Maher, D., Cebon, J., O'Connor, M., Green, M., Sheridan, W., Boyd, A., Rallings, M., Bomen, E., Metcalf, D. *et al.* (1989b). *Ann. Int. Med.* **110**, 357–364.

Lieschke, G., Mayer, D., Oconnon, M., Green, M., Sheridan, W., Rallings, M., Bonnem, E., Burgess, W., McGrath, K., Fox, R. and Morsytn, G. (1990). *Cancer Res.* **50**, 606–614.

Lokker, N.A., Zenke, G., Stritmatter, U., Fagg, B. and Movva, R. (1991). *EMBO J.* **10**, 2125–2131.

Lopez, A.F., Nicola, N., Burgess, A., Metcalf, D., Battye, F., Sewell, W. and Vadas, M.A. (1983). *J. Immunol.* **131**, 2983–2988.

Lopez, A.F., Williamson, D.J., Gamble, J.R, Begley, C.G., Harlan, J.M., Klebanoff, S.J., Waltersdorph, A., Wong, G., Clark, S.C. and Vadas, M.A. (1986). *J. Clin. Invest.* **78**, 1220–1228.

Lopez, A.F., Dyson, P., Bik-To, L., Elliott, M.J. *et al.* (1988). *Blood* **72**, 1797–1805.

Lopez, A., Eglinton, J., Gillis, D., Park, L.S. and Vadas, M.A. (1989). *Proc. Natl Acad. Sci. USA* **86**, 7022–7026.

Lopez, A.F., Elliott, M.J., Woodcock, J.M. and Vadas, M.A. (1992a). *Immunol Today* **13**, 495–500.

Lopez, A.F., Shannon, M.F., Barry, S., Phillips, J.A., Cambareri, B., Dottore, M., Simmons, P. and Vadas, M.A. (1992b). *Proc. Natl Acad. Sci. USA* **89**, 11842–11846.

Lopez, A.F., Shannon, M.F., Hercus, T., Nicola, N.A., Cambareri, B., Dottore, M., Layton, M., Eglinton, J. and Vadas, M.A. (1992c). *EMBO J.* **11**, 909–916.

Malik, F., Delgado, C., Knusli, C., Irvine, A.E., Fisher, D. and Francis, G.E. (1992). *Exp. Haematol.* **20**, 1028–1035.

Malter, J.S. (1990). *Science* **246**, 664–666.

Margolin, K.A., Rayner, A.A., Hawkins, M.J., Atkins, M.B., Dutcher, J.P., Fisher, R.I., Weiss, G.R., Doroshow, J.H., Jaffe, H.S., Roper, M., Parkinson, D.R., Wjernik, P.H., Creekmore, S.P. and Boldt, D.H. (1989). *J. Clin. Oncol.* **7**, 486–488.

Mayer, P., Valent, P., Schmidt, G., Liehl, E. and Bettelheim, P. (1989). *Blood* **74**, 613–621.

Morstyn, G. (1990). *Br. J. of Haematol.* **75**, 303–307.

Morstyn, G. and Burgess, A. (1988). *Cancer Res.* **48**, 5624–5637.

Morstyn, G., Campbell, L., Souza, L.M., Alton, N.K., Keech, J., Green, M., Sheridan, W., Metcalf, D. and Fox, R. (1988). *Lancet* **i**, 667–672.

Morstyn, G., Campbell, L., Lieschke, G., Layton, J.E., Maher, D., O'Connor, M., Green, M., Sheridan, W., Vincent, M., Alton, K., Souza, L., McGrath, K. and Fox, R.M. (1989a). *J. Clin. Oncol.* **7**, 1554–1562.

Morstyn, G., Lieschke, G., Sheridan, W., Layton, J. and Cebon, J. (1989b). *Trends Pharmacol. Sci.* **10**, 154–159.

Mukaida, N., Mahe, Y. and Matsushima, K. (1990). *J. Biol. Chem.* **265**, 21128–21133.

Nemunaitis, J., Singer, J.W., Buckner, C.D., Mill, R., Storb, R., Thomas, E.D. and Appelbaum, F. (1988). *Blood* **72**, 834–836.

Nemunaitis, J., Rabinowe, S.N., Singer, J.W., Bierman, P.J., Vose, J.M., Freedman, A.S., Onetto, N., Gillis, S., Oette, D., Gold, M., Buckner, C.D., Hansen, J.A., Ritz, J., Appelbaum, F.R., Armitage, J.O. and Nadler, L.M. (1991). *N. Engl. J. Med.* **324**, 1773–1778.

Nicola, N.A. (1989). *Annu. Rev. Biochem.* **58**, 45–77.

Nicola, N. and Metcalf, D. (1988). *Growth Factors* **1**, 29–39.

Oster, W., Nicola, C., Klein, M., Hirano, T., Kishimoto, T., Albrecht, L., Mertelsmann, R. and Herrmann, F. (1989). *J. Clin. Invest.* **84**, 451–457.

Paquette, R.L., Zhou, J.Y., Yang, Y.-C., Clark, S.C. and Koeffler, H.P. (1988). *Blood* **71**, 1596–1600.

Park, L.S., Friend, D., Gillis, S. and Urdal, D.L. (1986). *J. Exp. Med.* **164**, 251–262.

Park, L.S., Waldron, P., Friend, D., Sassenfeld, H., Price, V., Anderson, D., Cosman, D., Andrews, R.G., Bernstein, I.D. and Urdal, D.L. (1989). *Blood* **74**, 56–65.

Patchen, M.L., Fischer, R. and MacVittie, T.J. (1993). *Exp. Hematol.* **21**, 338–344.

Patchen, M.L., MacVittie, T.J., Williams, J.L., Schwartz, G.N. and Souza, L.M. (1991). *Blood* **77**, 472–480.

Petros, W.P., Rabinowitz, J., Stuart, A.R., Gilbert, C.J., Kanakura, Y., Griffin, D. and Peters, W.P. (1992). *Blood* **70**, 1134–1140.

Ray, A., LaForge, K.S. and Sehgal, P.B. (1990). *Mol. Cell Biol.* **10**, 5736–5746.

Reilly, Kozlowski, R. and Russell, N.H. (1989). *Leukemia* **3**, 145–150.

Ridaut, G., Santus, G. and Guy, R. (1988). *Clin. Pharmacokinetics* **15**, 114–131.

Ridge, S., Worwood, M., Oscier, D., Jacobs, A. and Padua, R. (1990). *Proc. Natl Acad. Sci. USA* **87**, 1377–1380.

Ross, R. (1986). *N. Engl. J. Med.* **314**, 488–500.

Russell, N.H. (1992). *Blood Reviews* **6**, 149–156.

Schreck, R. and Baeuerle, P.A. (1990). *Mol. Cell Biol.* **10**, 1281–1286.

Schreiber, S.L. (1992). *Cell* **70**, 365–368.

Schule, R., Rangarajan, P., Kllewer, S., Ransome, L.J., Bolado, J., Yang, N., Verma, I.M. and Evans, R.M. (1990). *Cell* **62**, 1217–1226.

Shannon, M.F., Pell, L.M., Lenardo, M.J., Kuczek, E.S., Occhiodoro, F.S., Dunn, S.M. and Vadas, M.A. (1990). *Mol. Cell Biol.* **10**, 2950–2959.

Shannon, M.F., Coles, L.S., Fielke, R.K., Goodall, G.J., Lagnado, C.A. and Vadas, M.A. (1992). *Growth Factors* **7**, 181–193.

Shaw, G. and Kamen, R. (1986). *Cell* **46**, 659–667.

Sheridan, W., Morstyn, G., Wolt, M., Dodds, A., Lusk, J., Maher, D., Layton, J., Green, M., Souza, L. and Fox, R. (1989). *Lancet* **ii**, 891–895.

Sheridan, W.P., Begley, C.G., Juttner, C.A., Szer, J., To, L.B., Maher, D., McGrath, K.M., Morstyn, G. and Fox, R.M. (1992). *Lancet* **339**, 640–644.

Sherr, C. (1989). *Blood* **75**, 1–12.

Schuening, F.G., Appelbaum, F.R., Deeg, H.J., Sullivan-Pepe, M., Graham, T.C., Hackman, R., Zsebo, K.M. and Storb, R. (1993). *Blood* **81**, 20–26.

Sieff, C.A., Niemeyer, C.M., Nathan, D.G., Ebern, S.C., Bieber, F., Yang, Y.-C., Wong, G. and Stark, S. (1987). *J. Clin. Invest.* **80**, 818–823.

Sieff, C., Niemeyer, C., Mentzers, and Fallen, D. (1989). *Blood* **73**, 945–951.

Smith, K.A. (1988). *Science* **240**, 1169–1176.

Stahl, C.P., Winton, E.F., Monroe, M.C., Haff, E., Holman, R.C., Myers, L., Liehl, E. and Evatt, B.L. (1992). *Blood* **80**, 2479–2485.

Takeshita, T., Asa, H., Ohtani, olshii, N., Kumaki, S., Tanaka, N., Munakata, O., Nakamura M. and Sugamura, K. (1990). *Science* **257**, 379–382.

Thorens, B., Mermod, J.-J. and Vassalli, P. (1987). *Cell* **48**, 671–679.

Ulich, T., Castillo, J., McNeice, I., Yin, S., Irwin, B., Busser, K. and Guo, K. (1990). *Blood* **75**, 48–53.

Vadas, M.A. and Lopez, A.F. (1984). *Lymphokine Res.* **3**, 45–50.

Vadas, M.A., Dessein, A., Nicola, N. and David, J. (1981). *Aust. J. Exp. Biol. Med. Sci.* **59**, 739–741.

Vadas, M.A, Clarke, S.C., Nicola, N.A. and Lopez, A.F. (1985). *Blood* **66**, 738–741.

Van der Schoot, C., Jansen, P., Poorten, M., Wester, M., von dem Borne, A., Aarden, L and van Oers, R. (1989). *Blood* **74**, 2081–2087.

Vandhan-Raj, S., Keating, M., Lemaistre, A., Hittelman, W.N,. McCredie, K., Trujillo, J.M., Broxmeyer, H.E., Henney, C. and Gutterman, J.H. (1987). *N. Eng. J. Med.* **317**, 1545–1552.

Vandhan-Raj, S., Buescher, S., Broxmeyer, H.E., LeMaistre, A., Lepe Zuninga, J.L., Ventura, G., Jeha, S., Horowitz, L., Trujillo, J., Gillis, S., Hittelman, W. and Gutterman, J. (1988). *N. Eng. J. Med.* **319**, 1628–1634.

Warren, D.J. and Moore, M.A.S. (1988). *J. Immunol.* **140**, 94–99.

Weber, J., Yang, Y.-C., Topalian, S.L., Parkinson, D.R., Schwartzentruber, D.S., Ettinghausen, S.E. *et al.* (1993). *J. Clin. Onc.* **11**, 499–506.

Williams, G., Smith, C.A., Spoonier, E, Dexter, T.M. and Taylor, D. (1990). *Nature* **343**, 76–79.

Yang, Y.-C., Kovacic, S., Kriz, R., Wolf, S., Clark, S.C., Wellems, T.E., Nienhuis, A. and Epstein, N. (1988). *Blood* **71**, 958–961.

Yang, Y.-C. and Clark, S.C. (1988). *Lymphokines* **15**, 375–391.

Yanofsky, S. and Zurawski, G. (1990). *J. Biol. Chem.* **265**, 1300–1306.

Young, D., Wagner, K. and Griffin, J.D. (1987). *J. Clin. Invest.* **79**, 100–106.

Zurawski, M. and Zurawski, G. (1989). *EMBO J.* **8**, 2583–2590.

Biological and Immunological Assays for Cytokines

Andrew J.H. Gearing[1], Judith E. Cartwright[1] and Meenu Wadhwa[2]

[1]British Biotechnology Ltd, Watlington Road, Cowley, Oxford, UK
[2]NIBSC, Blanche Lane, South Mimms, Herts., UK

INTRODUCTION

Many other chapters in this book have described the huge range of biological activities that cytokines can elicit. At some stage most of these activities have formed the basis of cytokine bioassays. No bioassays fulfil the criteria of an ideal assay system: specificity, sensitivity, simplicity, speed and reliability. This has stimulated the development of immunological or receptor-based assays. In this chapter we will first review the general techniques for biological, immunological and receptor assays, and subsequently describe specific bioassay details for individual cytokines.

BIOLOGICAL ASSAY READOUTS

Cytokine assays fall into six basic categories with readouts of: proliferation, cytotoxicity, changes in intracellular, cell membrane or secreted proteins, cell motility and in some cases *in vivo* responses.

Proliferation

Proliferation or enhanced cell survival assays are first choice for many cytokines. Measurement techniques include direct counting of cells by eye as in colony assays (Metcalf, 1984), enzyme-based colour changes as in the MTT assay (Mosmann, 1983), in which yellow MTT is converted to a purple derivative by mitochondria, the colour change being proportional to the number of mitochondria and hence to cell number, and tritiated thymidine incorporation assays in which the amount of new DNA synthesis and hence proliferative activity is estimated by the amount of radiolabelled thymidine incorporated into DNA.

Cytotoxicity

Cytotoxicity assays can use similar readouts to proliferation assays, although in the most common systems the target cells are normally not highly proliferative and hence tritiated thymidine is not useful. In these situations simple vital stains such as crystal violet or amido blue-black give adequate results.

Intracellular Changes
Some cytokines cause intracellular changes in cells resulting in, for example, enhanced killing of ingested bacteria.

Membrane Protein Changes
Changes in membrane protein expression can be monitored by binding of specific antibodies, or when the protein is a receptor by binding of its ligand. Quantification can be by microscope with fluorescent or enzyme labels, by fluorescence-activated cell analyser, PANDEX formats, or in ELISA or IRMAs.

Protein Secretion
Secreted protein levels can be measured by ELISA, IRMA or by specific bioassays.

Motility
Cell movements can be monitored using either Boyden chamber-type systems where cells are allowed to migrate through filters of defined pore size, or out of drops of gelled agar. Directional movement can be assessed by monitoring polarization of individual cells in a gradient of cytokine or by following bulk cell movements.

In vivo *Responses*
In vivo assays have been used for some cytokines, for example the pyrogen response for IL-1 (reviewed by Dinarello, 1990). These are unreliable, costly, nonspecific and insensitive and should be avoided.

IMMUNOASSAYS

Immunoassays for most cytokines have been published and many are now commercially available from a number of companies. The delay between initial publication of a cytokine cDNA sequence and the sale of immunoassays is becoming relatively short. Most investigators would not therefore need to develop their own assays, although there are numerous straightforward methods to develop these (Wadhwa *et al.*, 1990; Meager A., 1991; Poole, S., 1991). Most commercial cytokine immunoassays are either two-site ELISAs or radioimmunoassays with sensitivities of tens to hundreds of pg/ml. All immunoassays suffer from the same potential advantages and disadvantages. They are reliable, rapid, specific, do not require cell culture and can be sensitive, but are expensive, are usually species specific and, depending on the component antibodies, can also detect biologically inactive precursors of cytokines; they may have differential sensitivity for the particular cytokine preparation to which their component antibodies were raised, or may not detect partially cleaved but active forms (Bird *et al.*, 1991). Careful selection of antibodies based on knowledge of the behaviour of particular cytokines should prevent these problems. The specificity of immunoassays may have some disadvantages when the biological activity of a cytokine is due to more than one closely related molecule. Interleukin-1 activity is the result of a balance between IL-1α, IL-1β and IL-1 receptor antagonist which are antigenically distinct and yet bind to shared receptors. Estimation of total IL-1 activity would therefore require three different immunoassays.

RECEPTOR-BASED ASSAYS

An alternative approach to measuring cytokine levels that does not require the production of antibodies is to use the cytokine receptors on cells as capture for labelled cytokine (Park *et al.*, 1987). Displacement of the labelled cytokine by cytokine in a sample can be used to quantify levels. Fluorescent or radiolabelled derivatives of most cytokines are commercially available. The use of purified soluble receptors in assay formats is still experimental but must be a promising approach.

ASSAYS FOR CYTOKINE RECEPTORS

The measurement of soluble forms of cytokine receptors is a topic of increasing interest. A great deal of information has been obtained using ELISAs for the p55 IL-2 receptor, suggesting a correlation between blood levels and disease activity (Eastgate *et al.*, 1988). Many other receptors, particularly for the hemopoietic cytokines are now known to be shed by cells (Cosman, 1993). ELISAs for many of these receptors are available. For some cytokines, TNF for example, the soluble receptors are known to act as natural antagonists (Gatanaga *et al.*, 1990), measurement of both receptor and cytokine levels is therefore of interest in estimating the overall activity of a particular cytokine.

EX VIVO ASSAYS

Many groups have measured the capacity of blood cells or tissues to release cytokines *in vitro* as a reflection of cytokine production *in vivo*. Such assays are useful when access to tissue fluids or blood is limited, or when a particular cytokine is rapidly inactivated or inhibited *in vivo*. The results from such studies should be backed up by immunohistology or *in situ* hybridization studies.

DETECTION OF CYTOKINES IN CELLS AND TISSUES

Specific immunohistochemical techniques can be used to provide semi-quantitative information on tissue distribution of cytokines (Sander *et al.*, 1991). The limiting features of these techniques are the quality of the antibody and amplification system used, and the nature of the tissue; these govern the extent of artefactual staining and the ability to detect the low levels of cytokine found in many tissues. There are also a number of commonly used immunocytochemical procedures for the detection or quantification of cells producing cytokines. These include cytofluorography (Labalette-Houache *et al.*, 1991; Sander *et al.*, 1991); reverse haemolytic plaque assays (Lewis *et al.*, 1990) and ELISPOT (Lewis, 1991). Many of these approaches are also being complemented by the use of *in situ* hybridization techniques for detection of cytokine mRNA in tissue sections or cell smears (Baldino and Lewis, 1989; Naylor and Balkwill, 1991; Zheng *et al.*, 1991).

CHOICE OF ASSAY

Choice of assay system depends on the type of sample being studied and the purpose of the measurement. Commercial producers of cytokines from recombinant DNA expression systems are working with cytokines in isolation and for them any bioassay system is normally adequate to assess potency of the product. Potential problems arise when microbial expression systems also release other substances, for example endotoxin, which can give positive results in some bioassays, or with some mammalian expression systems, for example cho cells, which can themselves secrete cytokines such as IL-6 which can interfere in bioassays (Gearing *et al.*, 1989).

For most workers, cytokine levels are being measured in culture samples or blood and other tissue fluids. These measurements are complicated by the fact that cytokines are never produced in isolation but as a mixture of cytokines which may have similar or opposing actions on particular bioassays. Other biologically active proteins or lipids may also be coproduced and interfere. In these circumstances the most specific bioassay available should be used; high sensitivity is also helpful where inhibitors can be diluted out. When the identity of interfering cytokines is known these can be blocked with specific antibodies (Mosmann and Fong, 1989). With tissue fluids or blood samples a frequent problem is the presence of soluble receptors, cytokine autoantibodies or other binding proteins which can mask activity. Several protocols have been published for sample extraction prior to assay which can overcome this (Cannon *et al.*, 1988; Thorpe *et al.*, 1992). The optimal method for quantifying cytokine levels should involve using a specific bioassay in conjunction with two-site immunoassays for the cytokine and known inhibitors. Correlation of results between the two should inspire confidence in the value obtained. In real life such correlations may not always occur (Gearing *et al.*, 1990), normally the bioassay fails to detect material because of inhibitors that are not detected in the immunoassays.

STANDARDIZATION OF ASSAYS

The inherent variability of immunoassays and particularly biological assays means that every assay must include a standard of reference preparation. Each laboratory should have an aliquoted preparation of solution containing the cytokine to be measured. The aliquots should be kept under conditions ensuring maximum stability, normally frozen or freeze dried. Each assay should include at least one standard curve of the laboratory standard. The laboratory standard can be assigned an arbitrary potency of x units/ml which can then be compared with the activity of unknown samples by probit analysis (Finney, 1978). For most human cytokines and some murine cytokines, an official WHO standard or reference reagent is available from NIBSC, Blanche Lane, South Mimms, Potters Bar, Herts, UK or in the USA from BRMP, National Cancer Institutes, Frederick, Maryland 21701 (Table 1). The official standards can be used to calibrate laboratory standards and hence ensure comparability of results between labs even in different continents. The use of International Units (IU) is to be preferred even when using recombinant cytokines. This is because the standard defines a biological potency. Different preparations of recombinant cytokine may have different biological potencies owing to incorrect folding, partial degradation or glycosylation differences (Mire-Sluis, 1993).

INTERLEUKIN-1

The interleukin-1 gene family has three members, IL-1α, IL-1β and IL-1 receptor antagonist. The most productive source of IL-1 is endotoxin-stimulated monocytes or

Table 1. Availability of cytokine standards and reference reagents.

Cytokine	Abbreviation	Cytokine standards			
		Availability	Status	Source	Cat. No.
Interleukin-1 alpha, rDNA	IL-1α	+	IS	NIBSC*	86/632
Interleukin-1 beta, rDNA	IL-1β	+	IS	NIBSC*	86/680
Interleukin-2, cell line derived	IL-2	+	IS	NIBSC*	86/504
Interleukin-2, rDNA	IL-2	+	RR	NIBSC	86/654
Interleukin-3, rDNA	IL-3	+	RR	NIBSC*	88/780
Interleukin-4, rDNA	IL-4	+	RR	NIBSC*	88/656
Interleukin-5, rDNA	IL-5	+	RR	NIBSC*	90/586
Interleukin-6, rDNA	IL-6	+	IS	NIBSC*	89/548
Interleukin-7, rDNA	IL-7	+	RR	NIBSC*	90/530
Interleukin-8, rDNA	IL-8	+	RR	NIBSC*	89/520
Rantes, rDNA	Rantes	+	RR	NIBCS	92/520
Macrophage inflammatory protein-1 alpha, rDNA	MIP-1α	+	RR	NIBSC	92/518
Interleukin-9, rDNA	IL-9	+	RR	NIBSC	91/678
Interleukin-10, rDNA	IL-10	+	RR	NIBSC	92/516
Interleukin-11, rDNA	IL-11	+	RR	NIBSC	92/788
Interleukin-12	IL-12	–	–	–	–
Interleukin-13	IL-13	–	–	–	–
Macrophage colony stimulating factor, rDNA	M-CSF	+	IS	NIBSC*	89/512
Granulocyte colony stimulating factor, rDNA	G-CSF	+	IS	NIBSC*	88/502
Granulocyte macrophage colony stimulating factor, rDNA	GM-CSF	+	IS	NIBSC*	88/646
Leukaemia inhibitory factor, rDNA	LIF	+	RR	NIBSC*	91/602
Stem cell factor, rDNA	SCF	+	RR	NIBSC	91/682
Transforming growth factor $\beta1$, rDNA	TGF-$\beta1$	+	RR	NIBSC*	89/514
Transforming growth factor $\beta2$, rDNA	TGF-$\beta2$	+	RR	NIBSC	90/696
Tumour necrosis factor alpha	TNF-α	+	IS	NIBSC*	87/650
Tumour necrosis factor beta	TNF-β	+	RR	NIBSC	87/640
Interferon alpha, leukocyte derived	IFN-α_{Le}	+	IS	NIBSC	69/19
Interferon alpha-1, rDNA	IFN-$\alpha1$	+	IS	NIBSC	83/514
Interferon alpha-2a, rDNA	IFN-$\alpha2a$	+	IS	NIAID	Gxa01-901-535
Interferon alpha-2b, rDNA	INF-$\alpha2b$	+	IS	NIBSC	82/576
Interferon beta, fibroblast derived	IFN-β	+	2nd IS	NIAID	Gb23-902-531
Interferon beta [Ser^{17}], rDNA	IFN-β [Ser^{17}]	+	IS	NIAID	Gg23-901-530
Interferon gamma, leukocyte derived	IFN-γ	+	IS	NIAID	Gg23-901-530

rDNA, recombinant DNA; IS, international standard; RR, reference reagent; NIBSC, National Institute for Biological Standards and Control, South Mimms, Herts EN6 3QG, UK; NIAID, National Institute of Allergy and Infectious Diseases, National Institutes of Health, Bethesda, Maryland 20205, USA.
*Indicates availability from BRMP, Biological Response Modifiers Program, National Cancer Institute, Frederick, Maryland 21701, USA.

monocytic cell lines. There are two murine T-cell assay systems which are most commonly used to measure IL-1 biological activity: the D10 proliferation assay, and conversion assays typified by EL4/CTLL systems (reviewed in Symons *et al.*, 1987 and Gearing and Thorpe, 1989). These assays are responsive to IL-1 from most vertebrate species.

D10 cells and various subclones proliferate in a dose-dependent fashion in response to IL-1 (Orencole and Dinarello, 1989). The D10S subclone can be maintained in 5% dilution of a Concanavalin-A-stimulated rat spleen cell conditioned medium (as a source of growth factors). Other subclones require regular mitogen or antigen stimulation. Proliferation of the D10 cells can be measured using ^{3}H-thymidine incorporation after a 3-day culture period, or by MTT after 2 days. Published results using D10S indicate a 50% maximal response to 10 fg/ml of IL-1 with a useful range between 100 fg/ml to 100 ag/ml. Other subclones give 50% response at 5–10 pg/ml with a range of 1–100 pg/ml. D10 cells are responsive to lectins, IL-2, mIL-4, IL-7 and to very high concentrations of IL-6 (Suda *et al.*, 1989). The IL-2 and IL-4 response can be abrogated by performing assays in saturating concentrations of IL-2 and IL-4 (Hopkins and Humphreys, 1989).

Conversion assays involve stimulation by IL-1 of T-cell lines, such as LBRM 33 or EL4 subclones, to produce IL-2 which is then detected by proliferation of a second cell line, usually CTLL. Maintenance is straightforward for EL4 and LBRM33, the CTLL require 5% Concanavalin A supernatant as a source of IL-2. Several assay formats have been described, the most simple involves co-culture of CTLL with a thymidine kinase deficient EL4 clone, for example EL4 6.1, ^{3}H-thymidine incorporation in such cultures is limited to the CTLL cells. Using the NOB-1 subclone of EL4 6.1, we routinely achieve 50% response at 2–5 pg/ml with a range of 500 fg/ml–50 pg/ml. CTLL responses to IL-2 and mIL-4 can be overcome by introducing a sample preincubation (Gearing *et al.*, 1987). EL4 cells show some IL-2 production in response to high levels of mTNF (10 ng/ml) and hTNF (100 ng/ml).

Bell-shaped dose response curves are normally seen when measuring IL-1 levels in tissue culture supernatants and particularly in body fluids, indicating the presence of inhibitors. These inhibitors include IL-1 receptor antagonist, transforming growth factor β, prostaglandin E, or nonspecific binding proteins such as α2 macroglobulin. Chloroform extraction or polyethylene glycol (PEG) precipitation have been used as simple alternatives to chromatography to separate IL-1 from inhibitory substances (Cannon *et al.*, 1988).

Alternative assay systems include the thymocyte assay (LAF assay), in which lectin stimulated murine thymocytes proliferate in response to IL-1 (Gery *et al.*, 1972). This assay is slow, unreliable and nonspecific. Several fibroblast based systems have also been used, measuring proliferation or secretion of prostaglandins. These assays are slow, insensitive and nonspecific.

INTERLEUKIN-2

Interleukin-2 is produced by lectin stimulated T cells or T cell lines. Human IL-2 is active on murine cells but not vice versa. The most common assay for IL-2 uses clones of the murine CTLL line first described in 1978 by Gillis *et al.*, and used as a component of the IL-1 assay above. Other lines which are used include HT-2, FDCP-2 or MT-1.

CTLL cells proliferate in the presence of IL-2 and to a lesser extent to mIL-4. Proliferation can be measured using ^{3}H-thymidine or MTT; MTT however, requires more CTLL cells per assay well (2×10^4 compared with 5×10^3 cells/well) to give an adequate signal. Typical experiments give 50% response to 7 ng/ml IL-2 (1 IU/ml, Gearing and Thorpe, 1988) with a range of 50 pg/ml–50 ng/ml. The murine CT-6 line has been reported to proliferate in response to IL-2 but not to IL-4.

Most biological fluids contain inhibitors of CTLL proliferation. A possible inhibitor is the secreted form of the 55 kDa IL-2 receptor which is found in culture supernatants of activated T cells and even in serum from patients with rheumatoid arthritis (Eastgate *et al.*, 1988).

INTERLEUKIN-3

Interleukin-3 is produced by activated T cells. Human and murine IL-3 sharing only 30% amino acid sequence homology do not act across species and therefore require separate assay systems (rat IL-3 has even been reported not to act on murine cells). The original defining assays for IL-3 (and also G, M, and GM-CSF) were colony assays in which bone marrow cells are cultured as single-cell suspensions in soft agar (Metcalf, 1984; Testa *et al.*, 1991). Stimulation with IL-3 leads to formation of colonies of cells derived from individual precursors. These colonies contain mixed cell lineages the hallmark of IL-3 or multi-CSF as it is also known. Quantification requires counting the number of colonies with greater than 40 cells by eye using a binocular microscope, as automated methods are not yet reliable. Colony number can be directly related to IL-3 concentration. Staining of dried and fixed gels allows identification of cell types in colonies. These assays are not easy to master and involve some subjectivity and regular checking of results. Standard protocols are also slow, taking from 7–14 days for completion. Being mixed populations of cells these assays are also prone to interference by many other cytokines giving potentiation or inhibition of responses. Cell lines that proliferate in response to IL-3 are available for more rapid measurement of either human or murine factor. None of the murine IL-3-dependent lines are specific: DA1 cells also respond to IL-4, GM-CSF and LIF; NFS60 cells to IL-4, IL-6, GM-CSF and G-CSF; Ea3.17 cells to IL-2 and IL-4; FDCP cells to IL-2 and IL-4; and 32DC1 cells to IL-2, IL-4 and G-CSF (Gascan *et al.*, 1989). None of the human IL-3-dependent cells are specific. AML 193 cells also respond to GM-CSF and G-CSF, MO-7 cells to IL-4, GM-CSF and G-CSF, and TF-1 cells respond to GM-SCF, IL-5 and erythropoietin, with cell survival enhanced by IL-1, IL-4 and IL-6 (Fig. 1).

INTERLEUKIN-4

Interleukin-4 is produced by activated T cells. IL-4 is highly species restricted. The classical assay for hIL-4 is B cell costimulation (Callard *et al.*, 1987). B cells are purified from tonsil or blood by T-cell depletion using nylon wool or AET-SRBC rosetting, followed by adherence to remove monocytes. The B cells are then stimulated with anti-IgG, *Staphylococcus aureus* Cowan or phorbol ester. Proliferation assessed by ^{3}H-thymidine incorporation after 3-day culture is enhanced by IL-4. Alternatively, the T-cell growth-promoting properties of IL-4 can be measured using PHA-induced

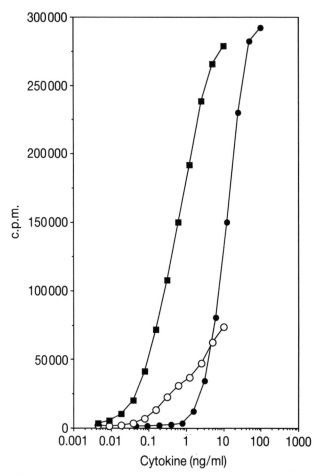

Fig. 1. Differential effects of IL-3 (■), IL-9 (○), and stem-cell factor (●) on the proliferation of the megakaryoblastic leukaemic cell line MO-7e.

lymphoblasts. PBLs are stimulated for 2 days with PHA, IL-2 is added to maintain proliferation, cells are left for a further 3 days, washed, and IL-4 added. Proliferation is determined after 2 days using [³H]thymidine or MTT. These assays give 50% maximal responses at about 1 ng/ml IL-4 with a range of 200 pg/ml–20 ng/ml. Specificity of these assays is poor (any lymphocytic growth factor would be expected to give a response, e.g. IL-2, IL-6, IL-7); they are also slow.

Some human cell lines are available which respond to IL-4 with, for example, induction of CD23 (FceR2) on a range of B-cell lines such as RAMOS. CD23 is measured either by flow cytometer or more conveniently using a fluorescence immunoassay with a Pandex FCA machine (Custer and Lotze, 1990). This assay gives 50% maximal expression at about 2 ng/ml with a range of 500 pg/ml–10 ng/ml IL-4.

Cell lines that proliferate in response to IL-4 include MO-7 and TF-1. These lines respond to many other factors including CSFs and IL-3, with TF-1 also responding to IL-5, IL-13 and even Epo. Sensitivity of TF-1 is about 1 ng/ml, giving 50% maximal response with a range of 10 pg/ml–100 ng/ml, MO-7 gives 50% maximal proliferation with 200 pg/ml and a range of 10 pg/ml–100 ng/ml IL-4.

Murine IL-4 is normally measured using T-cell lines such as CTLL-2, HT-2, BCL-1 or AC-2. With HT-2 or CTLL lines their IL-2 responsiveness can be overcome by inclusion of anti-IL-2 or anti-IL-2 receptor antibodies in the assay medium (Mosmann and Fong, 1989). Recently, an interesting hIL-4-responsive recombinant cell line CTh4S has been created by transfecting the murine CTLL line with the human IL-4 receptor.

INTERLEUKIN-5

Interleukin-5 is produced by activated T cells. Human IL-5 is active on murine cells, but with a greatly reduced specific activity; murine IL-5 is active on human cells. The most common assay for IL-5 is the proliferation of murine BCL1 cells. BCL1 cells are passaged as a splenic tumour in BALB/c mice. The cells are purified from spleen cell suspensions by Ficoll gradient and T-cell depletion and anti-T cell MAbs and complement. Proliferation in response to IL-5 can be measured by MTT or ^{3}H-thymidine incorporation following a 2-day culture. A 50% maximal response is seen with 250 pg/ml mIL-5, with a range of 25 pg/ml–1 ng/ml. The assay is a thousand times less sensitive to hIL-5. Murine IL-4 and GM-CSF also stimulate BCL1 whereas TGF-β and IFN-γ inhibit IL-5 responses (O'Garra). IL-5 can also be measured by stimulating the formation of eosinophil colonies in an agar colony assay or by estimation of eosinophil peroxidase (O'Garra and Sanderson, 1987). Human IL-5 also stimulates the proliferation of TF-1 cells (Fig. 2).

INTERLEUKIN-6

Interleukin-6 is a single gene product that is produced by many cell types in response to a variety of immunological or pathological stimuli. The most potent sources include endotoxin-stimulated monocytes, or IL-1-stimulated fibroblasts. Human and murine IL-6 are equally active on murine cells; murine IL-6 is not active on human cells. IL-6 has biological effects on most cell types, and many of these effects have formed the basis of bioassays. However, because of their sensitivity and specificity most workers now only use a murine hybridoma assay. A number of hybridoma lines have been described, the most commonly used are B-9 and 7TD1 (Van Snick et al., 1986; Helle et al., 1988). These cells are maintained in IL-6, washed prior to assay, samples added and proliferation measured 3 days later by MTT or ^{3}H-thymidine incorporation. A 50% maximal response is seen at 2–3 pg/ml, with a range of 500 fg/ml–15 pg/ml. The only other cytokine which mildly stimulates these cells is mIL-4. The assay is robust enough to detect IL-6 in clinical samples such as rheumatoid synovial fluids. No inhibitors of IL-6 have been described; the receptor is shed by cells, but stimulates target cells by binding free IL-6 and then associating with the 130 kDa IL-6 signalling molecule.

INTERLEUKIN-7

Interleukin-7 is produced by bone marrow stromal cells. Assay of human and murine IL-7 can be achieved using murine B cell lines such as IxN/2b (Park et al., 1990).

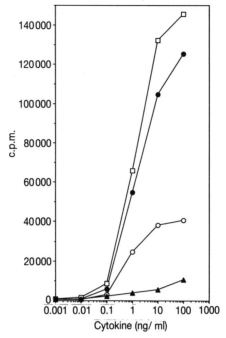

Fig. 2. The effect of IL-3 (●), IL-4 (▲), IL-5 (○) and GM-CSF (□) on the proliferation of the erythroleukaemic cell line TF1.

Proliferation can be measured using MTT or ^{3}H-thymidine. Maximal responses of 50%
are obtained with 25–50 pg/ml, with a range of response between 10–100 pg/ml. No
information is yet available on the specificity of this assay line. IL-7 can also be
measured by using nonadherent pre-B cells from long-term Whitlock-Witte bone
marrow cultures which proliferate in response to IL-7 (Namen *et al.*, 1988).

INTERLEUKIN-8

Interleukin-8 is a member of the chemokine supergene family comprising a number of
small (7–15 kDa) peptides with chemoattractant or mitogenic properties for a range of
target cells (see Table 2 and Matsushima and Oppenheim, 1989). IL-8 is produced by
monocytes, and fibroblasts, endothelial or epithelial cells stimulated with virus, IL-1 or
TNF. Human IL-8 is active on rodent and rabbit neutrophils. IL-8 assays are normally
performed on human peripheral blood leukocytes. Chemokinesis assays using buffy
coat leukocytes migrating out of agarose gel spots in 96-well plates are probably the
most straightforward systems (Camp *et al.*, 1983). Cell migration can be determined by
measuring the diameter of cell migration on a projected image of the well; a digitizing
tablet speeds data handling. Boyden chamber systems, which measure cell migration
through porous filters, are also used and are commercially available (reviewed by
Bignold, 1988). Using neutrophils 50% maximal responses are seen at 2 ng/ml with a
range of response from 200 pg/ml–20 ng/ml. T cells give responses at 100-fold lower
doses. Other factors such as C_{5a} des-arg and LTB4 and fMLP are also neutrophil
chemoattractants. No IL-8 inhibitors have yet been described.

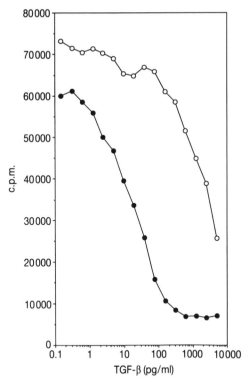

Fig. 3. The inhibition of IL-5-driven proliferation of TF1 cells by TGF-β (●), and its reversal by antibody to TGF-β (○).

Table 2. Assays for chemokines.

Chemokine	Chemotaxis assay	Other assay
IL-8	PMN, Baso, Lympho	Angiogenic
MIP-1α	B, Eosino, Tcyt	Stem cell inhibition
MIP-1β	T memory	Haemopoiesis
MIP-2	PMN	Myelopoiesis
GRO/MGSA	PMN	Fibroblast, melanoma growth
MCP-1,2,3	Mono	Mono, Baso activation
RANTES	Mono, T memory, Eosino	Baso, Eosino activation
PF-4	Mono, PMN	Anti-coagulant, Angiogenic inhibition
βTG	PMN	PMN Activation
NAP-2	PMN	PMN Activation
I-309	Mono	Unknown
γIP10	Mono, T	Lymphocyte adhesion

INTERLEUKIN-9

Interleukin-9 is produced by activated T cells. Murine IL-9 stimulates human cells but not vice versa. The mIL-9 can be measured by increased proliferation of certain T helper cell lines (Renauld *et al.*, 1990). The human IL-9 can be assayed using long-term cultured peripheral blood leukocytes which have been maintained by PHA, IL-4 and irradiated allogeneic feeder cells. IL-9 enhances erythroid burst-forming activity in the presence of erythropoietin (EPO) (Donahue *et al.*, 1990). Alternately, the MO-7e line proliferates in response to IL-9 with a 50% maximal response at 50 pg/ml, and a range of 0.01–10 ng/ml.

INTERLEUKIN-10

Interleukin-10 is produced by B and T helper lymphocytes, and suppresses the release of cytokines particularly IFN-γ and IL-12. It is also reported to be a cofactor for the proliferation of mast cells and thymocytes (Moore *et al.*, 1990). The human counterpart is strongly homologous to the murine IL-10 and acts on murine cells; mouse IL-10 is not active on human cells. IL-10 can be assayed using inhibition of IFN-γ production by mouse T cells (Fiorentino *et al.*, 1989) or by using the murine mast cell line MC/9 (Vieira *et al.*, 1991) which has a 50% maximal response at 400 pg/ml and a range of 0.1–100 ng/ml.

INTERLEUKIN-11

Interleukin-11 is produced by fibroblasts and stromal cells and stimulates B-cell proliferation and megakaryocyte production (Paul *et al.*, 1990). Human and murine IL-11 can be measured using the proliferation of IL-6-dependent murine plasmacytoma lines such as T1165 (Nordan and Potter, 1986). A subclone of this line T10, can be used in a 2-day proliferation assay with a 50% maximal response of 200 pg/ml and a range of 0.1–50 ng/ml. This line also responds to IL-6, but requires 2.5 ng/ml to give 50% maximal proliferation.

INTERLEUKIN-12

Interleukin-12 is a heterodimeric cytokine produced by macrophages and B cells which stimulates interferon-γ production by T and NK cells (Chan *et al.*, 1991) and the generation of TH1 lymphocytes (Scott, 1993). The murine protein is active on human cells but not vice versa (Schoenhaut *et al.*, 1992). IL-12 can be measured using proliferation of human 4-day PHA-activated lymphoblasts; 50% maximal proliferation is obtained with 3.5×10^{-9} M IL-12 (Stern *et al.*, 1990).

INTERLEUKIN-13

Interleukin-13 is produced by activated TH2 lymphocytes and stimulates monocytes to differentiate to a dendritic phenotype and B lymphocyte proliferation and IgG and IgE secretion (properties shared with IL-4). Mouse IL-13 is active on human cells. IL-13 can be measured by proliferation of the TF-1 cell line with 50% maximal proliferation at 2×10^{-11} M, or proliferation of activated human B lymphocytes, as for IL-4 (McKenzie *et al.*, 1993).

LEUKAEMIA INHIBITORY FACTOR

Leukaemia inhibitory factor (LIF) is produced by T cells and a range of tumour cell types. Human LIF is active on murine cells. LIF was originally defined by a bioassay which measures the differentiation of the mouse M1 leukaemia cell line in a colony assay format (Gearing, D.P. *et al.*, 1987). This assay is slow and nonspecific also responding to IL-6 and IFN-β. Sensitivity is 500 pg/ml giving 50% maximal response with a range of 100 pg/ml–2.5 ng/ml. The only specific assay for LIF would involve supporting the growth of murine embryonic stem cells without causing differentiation. LIF can also be measured using DA1.a cells, a line that was originally used to measure mIL-3 but which also proliferates in response to G-CSF, mIL-4 and mGM-CSF (Gascan *et al.*, 1989), and also the TF-1 line which proliferates in response to LIF with a 50% maximal response of 5 ng/ml and a range of 0.1–100 ng/ml.

ONCOSTATIN M

Oncostatin M (OncoM) is produced by T cells and monocytes and stimulates fibroblast proliferation whereas it inhibits the growth of several tumour cell lines (Rose and Bruce, 1991). There is no murine homologue of OncoM. OncoM can be measured by growth inhibition of the A375M melanoma cell line, or by stimulation of proliferation of the TF-1 line (assay range 5 pg–5 ng/ml, 50% maximal response at 250 pg/ml).

ERYTHROPOIETIN

Erythropoietin regulates the growth and differentiation of erythroid precursor cells. Human EPO is active on rodent cells. EPO is produced by adult kidney or fetal liver cells. There are several assay systems for EPO, the most sensitive is the induction of proliferation of the human erythroleukaemic cell line TF-1 (Kitamura *et al.*, 1989) which gives 50% maximal response at about 10 pg/ml of EPO with a range of 2 pg/ml–100 pg/ml. As with other leukaemic lines TF-1 is not specific, responding to GM-CSF, IL-3, IL-4, IL-5 and IL-13. EPO can also be measured using phenylhydrazin-treated mouse spleen cells as a source of erythroid precursors which give 50% maximum proliferation at 100 pg/ml. Bone marrow colony assays can also be used to detect EPO either by monitoring colonies or burst-forming units of erythrocytes in methylcellulose cultures. Variation in batches of methylcellulose can be a problem, although pre-tested batches are now available commercially. These assays are slow and relatively insensitive, 5–10 ng/ml giving 50% maximal responses (Krumwieh *et al.*, 1988).

GRANULOCYTE COLONY STIMULATING FACTOR

Granulocyte colony stimulating factor (G-CSF) is a single gene product (177 or 179 amino acid differential splicing variants in human) produced by endotoxin stimulated monocytes and IL-1 or TNF stimulated endothelial cells, or fibroblasts. There is full cross-species activity between mouse and human G-CSF. Classically, G-CSF was identified using a 7-day agar colony assay with mouse bone marrow cells. A more rapid assay can be performed which measures the proliferation of low-density (Ficoll gradient) bone marrow cells in response to G-CSF. This assay gives 50% maximal proliferation at 500 pg/ml with a range of 10 pg/ml–1 mg/ml. More reproducible assays have been developed using murine cell lines such as WEHI 3BD+, which forms differentiated granulocytic colonies in agar in the presence of G-CSF with slight response to GM-CSF (Nicola *et al.*, 1983), or sub-clones of the NFS-60 line such as G-NFS-60 which are dependent for growth and survival on G-CSF. Proliferation over a 24 h period in response to G-CSF can be measured with 50% proliferation at 200 pg/ml and a range of 10 pg/ml–2 ng/ml. Responses are also seen to a lesser extent with mIL-3, M-CSF and IL-6.

GRANULOCYTE MACROPHAGE COLONY STIMULATING FACTOR

Granulocyte macrophage colony stimulating factor (GM-CSF) is produced by a range of cell types in response to multiple stimuli. Murine and human GM-CSF have no cross-species action. GM-CSF was originally characterized using an agar bone marrow colony assay in which it induces colonies containing macrophages, neutrophils, eosinophils and megakaryocytes. Proliferation assays have been developed for human GM-CSF using myeloid leukaemia cell lines such as AML-193, MO-7 or TF-1 (Lange *et al.*, 1987; Avanzi *et al.*, 1988; Kitamura *et al.*, 1989). Sensitivities of 50% maximal response at 50 pg/ml and ranges of 1 pg/ml–100 ng/ml are routinely achieved. Specificity is not a strong point of these assays with responses to IL-3, G-CSF for AML193, IL-3, IL-4, IL-6 and TNF-α for MO-7, and IL-3, IL-4, IL-5, IL-13 and EPO for TF-1.

For murine GM-CSF several proliferation-dependent cell lines are available including DA-1, FDC-P1 and BCL-1, but are again not specific, responding to IL-3, IL-4 and IL-5 (BCL-1 only).

MACROPHAGE COLONY STIMULATING FACTOR

Macrophage colony stimulating factor (M-CSF) is a single gene product which forms two different transcripts of 256 or 554 amino acids by alternative splicing. The two forms dimerize, with the larger forms being proteolytically cleaved and secreted from cells, the smaller becomes membrane associated and subsequently cleaved by proteases. M-CSF is produced by a range of cell types including monocytes, endothelial cells and fibroblasts in response to LPS, IL-1 or TNF. Human M-CSF is fully active on murine cells. M-CSF produces colonies of macrophages in bone marrow colony assays. Recently, murine cell lines including Bac.1 and M-NFS-60, which proliferate in response to M-CSF have been described (Morgan *et al.*, 1987; Nakoinz *et al.*, 1989). M-NFS-60 gives 50% maximal responses to 2.5 ng/ml M-CSF with a range from 10 pg/ml–10 ng/ml. Similar responses are seen to IL-6. G-CSF and murine IL-3 also cause proliferation of the line.

STEM CELL FACTOR

Stem cell factor (SCF) is produced by stromal cells and stimulates mast cell growth and synergizes with other haemopoietic cytokines to generate haemopoietic cells (Martin *et al.*, 1990; Metcalf and Nicola, 1991). Rodent SCF can be measured using the proliferation of the murine mast cell line MC/9 with 50% maximal stimulation at 5 ng/ml, human SCF is 800-fold less active on this line. Human SCF can be measured using bone marrow colony assays, or in the MO-7e assay (50% maximal at 10 ng/ml range 1–100 ng/ml).

TUMOUR NECROSIS FACTOR

There are three different tumour necrosis factor (TNF) gene products, TNF-α, lymphotoxin (TNF-β) and lymphotoxin-β (Browning *et al.*, 1993); all appear to exist as trimers. TNF from human cells is active on murine cells with slight reduction in specific activity. TNF shares many of the biological effects of IL-1 and as such they commonly interfere in bioassays. The most commonly used bioassay for TNF, which is unaffected by IL-1, is a cytotoxicity assay based on murine fibroblasts such as L929 or L-M cells. These cells deteriorate and die over a 3-day period in the presence of TNF. The speed and sensitivity are potentiated by actinomycin-D to give a 1-day assay which can, in our hands, detect as little as 2.5 pg/ml. Sensitivity levels do vary with cell isolates, passage number and temperature and other groups report sensitivities of up to 125 pg/ml for human TNF-α. Human TNF-β and mTNF have been reported to be more potent. The murine WEHI 164 clone 13 has been reported to be sensitive to 2 pg/ml of hTNF without actinomycin D; however, some authors have reported lower sensitivity (Meager *et al.*, 1989).

Soluble TNF receptors act as specific TNF inhibitors. Interferon γ may increase titres in murine samples by enhancing TNF receptor expression on the target cells.

INTERFERON-α/β

There are 15 different α interferons (IFNs) and one β interferon, all of which interact with the same receptor type. These interferons are produced by lymphocytes, monocytes and fibroblasts in response to viral or bacterial stimulation. Fibroblasts produce β interferon in response to IL-1. Interferons are species restricted, IFN-γ does not cross species at all, and the α IFNs are much less active across species. The most common and specific assay for interferons is the cytopathic effect reduction assay (Meager, 1987). In this assay interferon reduces the killing of a target cell line such as L929 (murine), HEp2C or A549 (human) cells by, for example, encephalomyocarditis virus. Cells are cultured as monolayers in 96-well plates in the presence of IFN samples for 24 h. Virus is added to the wells and the plates left for 24–48 h for optimal cell death to occur in untreated wells. Vital staining with a dye such as amido blue-black, followed by fixation, and solubilization of dye with 50 mM sodium hydroxide, allows quantification of cell survival by reading at 610 nm in an ELISA reader. These assays can reliably detect 100–200 pg/ml IFN.

INTERFERON-γ

Interferon-γ (IFN-γ) is produced by activated T cells and acts on a distinct receptor from the other IFNs. The assays described above for α and β IFNs also respond to IFN-γ. An alternative assay system involves measurement of induction of HLA-DR antigens on tumour cells by IFN-γ (Gibson and Kramer, 1989). Cells such as COLO 205 are incubated for 2 days in the presence of IFN in 96-well plates. After fixation with alcohol, HLA is detected with specific monoclonal antibody and labelled second antibody using an ELISA reader. Only IL-1 and IFN-β give slight induction of HLA in this assay; however, may other cytokines can modulate the response to IFN-γ, e.g. TNF and IL-1 synergize and IFN-α and G-CSF antagonize. A 50% maximal response is found at 1 ng/ml with a range of 250 pg/ml–10 ng/ml.

TRANSFORMING GROWTH FACTOR β_1

Transforming growth factor (TGF-β_1) is one of four closely related gene products. TGF-β_1 is a disulphide-linked homodimer produced by monocytes, lymphocytes and platelets. The original assay for TGF-β was to induce colony growth of fibroblasts such as the normal rat kidney fibroblast NRK-49F in soft agar (Assoian *et al.*, 1983). Although sensitive (50% maximal response at 50 pg/ml), other factors such as EGF and TGF-α can interfere. For routine and rapid assay, the mink lung fibroblast MV-3D9 line can be used (Like and Massague, 1986). TGF-β inhibits the proliferation of this line, assessed by reduction of ^{3}H-thymidine incorporation after 72 h. This assay gives 50% maximal response at 200 pg/ml, with a range of 40 pg/ml–5 ng/ml for β_1 and β_2. TGF-β also reduces the IL-5-driven proliferation of TF-1 cells (Randall *et al.*, 1993). An enhanced sensitivity can be obtained in this assay.

MIGRATION INHIBITION FACTOR

Migration inhibition factor (MIF) is a single gene product of activated T cells which may form multimers. The standard assays measure the decrease in migration of peripheral blood monocytes from agarose drops or from capillary tubes (Harrington and Stastny, 1973). IFN-γ, TNF and IL-4 also inhibit monocyte migration. There is no information on the sensitivity of the assays.

CHEMOKINES

The chemokine family of cytokines has several members in addition to IL-8 including RANTES, macrophage chemotactic protein (MCP)-1, MCP-2, MCP-3, macrophage inflammatory protein (MIP)-1α, MIP-1β, MIP-2, I-309, platelet factor 4 (PF-4), GRO/MGSA, γIFN-inducible protein-10 (γIP10) and β-thromboglobulin (β-TG) (Oppenheim *et al.*, 1991). Each of these molecules is chemoattractant for particular cell types and can be measured using standard chemoattraction assays (Van Damme and Conings, 1992; Westwick, 1992). Each chemokine also has either activating, proliferative or antiproliferative properties for specific cell lineages. The chemokines and their individual chemoattractant and other assay targets are described in Table 2.

SUMMARY

The problems of nonspecificity and effects of inhibitors described above mean that bioassay results are rarely unambiguous. Properly validated two-site immunoassays with appropriate standards are at present the only specific assay systems in common use, even though they may also be inhibited by the same binding proteins or soluble receptors that interfere in bioassays. Current advice must be to take note of known cross reactions and inhibitors when choosing assays, to employ specific neutralizing antibody controls in bioassays, and when possible to measure cytokines by at least two different methods to be confident of the result.

GENERAL REFERENCES

Clements, M.J., Morris, A.G. and Gearing, A.J.H., eds (1987). *Lymphokines and Interferons: A practical approach.* IRL Press, Oxford.
Balkwill, F.R., ed. (1991). *Cytokines: A practical approach.* IRL Press, Oxford.

Oppenheim, J.J., Rossio, J.L. and Gearing, A.J.H. (1993). *Clinical Applications of Cytokines: Role in Pathogenesis, Diagnosis and Therapy*, Oxford University Press, NY.

Thorpe, R.C., Wadhwa, M., Bird, C.R. and Mire-Sluis, A.R. (1992). *Blood Reviews* **6**, 133–148.

REFERENCES

Avanzi, G.C., Lista, P., Giovinazzo, B., Miniero, R., Saglio, G., Benetton, G., Coda, R., Cattoretti, G. and Pegoraro, L. (1988). *B. J. Haematol.* **69**, 359–366.

Assoian, R.K., Komoriya, A., Meyers, C.A., Miller, D.M. and Sporn, M.B. (1983). *J. Biol. Chem.* **258**, 7155–7159.

Baldino, F. and Lewis, M.E. (1989). In: *Methods of Neuroscience, Gene probes* (ed. P.M. Conn), pp. 282–292. New York, Academic Press.

Bignold, L.P. (1988). *J. Imm. Methods* **108**, 1–19.

Bird, C.R., Wadhwa, M. and Thorpe, R.C. (1991). *Cytokine* **3**, 562–567.

Browning, J.L., Ngam-ek, A., Lawton, P. *et al.* (1993). *Cell* **72**, 847–856.

Callard, R.E., Shields, J.G. and Smith, S.H. (1987). In: *Lymphokines and Interferons: A Practical Approach* (eds M.J. Clements, A.G. Morris and A.J.H. Gearing), IRL Press, Oxford, pp. 345–364.

Camp, R.D.R., Mallet, A.I., Woolard, P.M., Brain, F.D., Kobza-Black and Greaves, M.W. (1983). *Prostaglandins* **26**, 431–447.

Cannon, J.G., Van Der Meer, J.W.M., Kwiatkowski, D., Endres, S., Lonneman, G., Burke, J.F. and Dinarello, C.A. (1988). *Lymphokine Res.* **7**, 457–467.

Chan, S.H., Perussia, B., Gupta, J.W., Kobayashi, M., Pospisil, M., Young, H.A., Wolf, S., Young, D., Clark, S.C. and Trinchieri, G. (1991). *J. Exp. Med.* **173**, 869–878.

Custer, M.C. and Lotze, M.T. (1990). *J. Imm. Methods* **128**, 109–119.

Cosman, D. (1993). *Cytokine* **5**, 95–106.

Damme, J. van and Conings, R. (1991). In: *Cytokines: A Practical Approach* (ed. F.R. Balkwill), IRL Press, Oxford, pp. 187–196.

Dinarello, C.A. (1989). In: *Interleukin 1, Inflammation and Disease* (eds R. Bomford and B. Henderson), Elsevier, Amsterdam, pp. 177–190.

Donahue, R.E., Yang, Y.C. and Clark, S.C. (1990). *Blood* **75**, 2271–2275.

Eastgate, J.A., Symons, J.A., Wood, N.C., Grinlington, F.M., Di Giovine, F.S. and Duff, G.W. (1988). *Lancet* **2**, 706–709.

Finney, D.J. (1978). *Statistical Methods, Biological Assay*. Academic Press.

Fiorentino, D.F., Bond, M.W. and Mosmann, T.R. (1989). *J. Exp. Med.* **170**, 2081.

Gascan, H., Moreau, J.F., Jaques, Y. and Soulilou, J.P. (1989). *Lymphokines Res.* **8**, 79–84.

Gatanaga *et al.* (1990). *Proc. Natl Acad. Sci. USA* **87**, 8781.

Gearing, A.J.H. and Thorpe, R. (1988). *J. Imm. Methods* **114**, 3–9.

Gearing, A.J.H. and Thorpe, R. (1989). In: *Interleukin 1, Inflammation and Disease* (eds R. Bomford and B. Henderson), Elsevier, Amsterdam, pp. 79–91.

Gearing, A.J.H., Bird, C.R., Bristow, A., Poole, S. and Thorpe, R. (1987). *J. Imm. Methods* **99**, 7–11.

Gearing, A.J.H., Bird, C.R., Priest, R., Cartwright, J.E., Wadhwa and Thorpe, R. (1989). *Lancet* **2**, 1011–1012.

Gearing, A.J.H., Fincham, N.J., Bird, C.R., Wadhwa, M., Meager, A., Cartwright, J.E. and Camp, R.D.R. (1990). *Cytokine* **2**, 68–75.

Gearing, D.P., Gough, N.J., King, J.A., Hilton, D., Nicola, N.A., Simpson, R.J., Nice, E.C., Kelso, A. and Metcalf, D. (1987). *EMBO J.* **6**, 3995–4002.

Gery, L., Gershon, R.K. and Waksmann, B.H. (1972). *J. Exp. Med.* **136**, 128–135.

Gibson, U.E.M. and Kramer, S.M. (1989). *J. Imm. Methods* **125**, 105–115.

Gillis, S., Ferm, M.M., Ou, W. and Smith, K.A. (1978). *J. Immunol.* **120**, 2027–2033.

Harrington, J.T. and Stastny, P. (1973). *J. Immunol.* **110**, 752–759.

Helle, M., Boeje, L. and Aarden, L.A. (1988). *Eur. J. Immunol.* **18**, 1535–1538.

Hopkins, S.J. and Humphreys, M. (1989). *J. Imm. Methods* **120**, 271–277.

Kitamura, T., Tange, T., Terasawa T., Chiba, S., Kuwaki, T., Miyagawa, K., Piao, Y., Miyazono, K., Urabe, A. and Takaku, F. (1989). *J. Cell Physiol.* **140**, 323–334.

Krumwieh, D., Arnold, I. and Seiler, F.R. (1988). *Develop. Biol. Standard.* **69**, 15–22.

Labalette-Houache, M., Torpier, G., Capron, A. and Dessaint, J.P. (1991). *J. Imm. Methods* **138**, 143–153.

Lange, B., Valtieri, M., Santoli, D., Caracciolo, D., Mavilio, F., Gemperlein, I., Griffin, C., Emmannuel, B., Finan, J., Nowell, P. and Rovera, G. (1987). *Blood* **70**, 192–199.

Lewis, C.E. (1991). In: *Cytokines: A Practical Approach* (ed. F.R. Balkwill), IRL Press, Oxford.

Lewis, C.E., McCarthy, S.P., Richards, P.S. *et al.* (1990). *J. Imm. Methods* **127**, 51–59.

Like, B. and Massague, J. (1986). *J. Biol. Chem.* **261**, 13426–13429.

McKenzie, A.N.J., Culpepper, J.A., de Waal-Malefyt, R., Brière, F., Punnonen, J., Aversa, G., Sato, A., Dang, W., Cocks, B.G., Menon, S., de Vries, J.E., Banchereau, J. and Zurawski, G. (1993). *Proc. Natl Acad. Sci. USA* **90**, 3735–3739.

Martin, F.H., Suggs, S.V., Langley, K.E. *et al.* (1990). *Cell* **63**, 203–211.

Matsushima, K. and Oppenheim, J.J. (1989). *Cytokine* **1**, 2–13.

Meager, A. (1987). In: *Lymphokines and Interferons: A Practical Approach* (eds M.J. Clements, A.G. Morris and A.J.H. Gearing), IRL Press, Oxford, pp. 129–147.

Meager, A. (1991). In: *Cytokines: A Practical Approach* (ed. F.R. Balkwill), ILR Press, Oxford, pp. 299–308.

Meager, A., Leung, H. and Wooley, J. (1989). *J. Imm. Methods* **116**, 1–17.

Metcalf, D. (1984). *The Haemopoietic Colony Stimulating Factors,* Elsevier, Amsterdam.

Metcalf, D. and Nicola, N.A. (1991). *Proc. Natl Acad. Sci. USA* **88**, 6239–6243.

Mire-Sluis, A.R. (1993). *Biologicals* **21**, 131–144.

Moore, K.W., Viera, P., Fiorentino, D.F., Trounstine, M.L., Khan, T.A. and Mosmann, T.R. (1990). *Science* **248**, 1230–1234.

Morgan, C., Pollard, J.W. and Stanley, E.R. (1987). *J. Cell Physiol.* **130**, 420.

Mosmann, T.R. (1983). *J. Imm. Methods* **65**, 55–59.

Mosmann, T.R. and Fong, T.A.T. (1989). *J. Imm. Methods* **116**, 151–159.

Nakoinz, I., Lee, M., Weaver, J.F. and Ralph, P. (1989). In: *7th International Congress of Immunology*, Gustav Fischer, Stuttgart, Abstr. 40–43.

Namen, A.E., Schmierer, A.E., Marh, C.J., Overell. R.W., Park, L.S., Urdal, D.L and Mochizuki, D.Y. (1988). *J. Exp. Med.* **167**, 988.

Naylor, M.S. and Balkwill, F.R. (1991) In: *Cytokines: A Practical Approach* (ed. F.R. Balkwill), IRL Press, Oxford, pp. 31–50.

Nicola, N.A., Metcalf, D., Matsumoto, M. and Johnson, G.R. (1983). *J. Biol. Chem.* **258**, 9017–9023.

Nordan, R.P. and Potter, M. (1986). *Science* 566–569.

O'Garra, A. and Sanderson, C.J. (1987). In: *Lymphokines and Interferons: A Practical Approach* (eds M.S. Clements, A.G. Morris and A.J.H. Gearing), IRL Press, Oxford, pp. 323–343.

Oppenheim, J.J., Zachariae C.O.C., Mukaida, N. and Matsushima, K. (1991). *Annu. Rev. Immunol.* **9**, 617–648.

Orrencole, S.F. and Dinarello, C.A. (1989). *Cytokine* **1**, 14–23.

Park, L.S., Friend, D., Sassenfeld, H.M. and Urdal, D.L. (1987). *J. Exp. Med.* **16**, 476–488.

Park, L.S., Friend, D.J., Schmierer, A.E., Dower, S.K. and Namen, A.E. (1990). *J. Exp. Med.* **171**, 1073–1089.

Paul, S.R., Bennett, F., Calvetti, J.A. *et al.* (1990). *Proc. Natl Acad. Sci. USA* **87**, 7512–7516.

Poole, S. (1991). In: *Cytokines: A Practical Approach* (ed. F.R. Balkwill), ILR Press, Oxford, pp. 269–278.

Randall, L.A., Wadhwa, M., Thorpe, C.R. and Mire-Sluis, A.R. (1993). *J. Imm. Methods* **164**, 61–67.

Renauld, J., Goethals, A., Houssiau, F., Van Roost, E. and Van Snick, J. (1990). *Cytokine* **2**, 9–13.

Rose, T.M. and Bruce, A.G. (1991). *Proc. Natl Acad. Sci. USA* **88**, 8641–8645.

Sander, B., Andersson, J. and Andersson, U (1991). *Imm. Rev.* **119**, 65–93.

Scott, P. (1993). *Science* **260**, 496–497.

Schoenhaut, D.S. *et al.* (1992). *J. Immunol.* **148**, 3433–3440.

Symons, J.A., Dickens, E.M., Di Giovine, F. and Duff, G.W. (1987). In: *Lymphokines and Interferons: A Practical Approach* (eds M.J. Clements, A.G. Morris, and A.J.H. Gearing), IRL Press, Oxford, pp. 269–289.

Stern, A.S. *et al.* (1990). *Proc. Natl. Acad. Sci. USA* **87**, 6808–6812.

Suda, T., Hodjkin, P., Lee F. and Zlotnik, A. (1989). *J. Imm. Methods* **120**, 173–179.

Testa, N.G. *et al.* (1991). In: *Cytokines: A Practical Approach* (ed. F.R. Balkwill), IRL Press, Oxford.

Van Snick, J., Cayphas, S., Vink, A., Uyttenhove, C., Coulie, P.G., Rubira, M.R. and Simpson, R.J. (1986). *Proc. Natl Acad. Sci. USA* **83**, 9679–9683.

Vieira, P., de Waal-Malefyt, R., Dang, M.N. *et al.* (1991). *Proc. Natl Acad. Sci. USA* **88**, 1172–1176.

Wadhwa, M., Bird, C.R., Tinker, A., Mire-sluis, A.R. and Thorpe, R. (1991) In: *Cytokines: A Practical Approach* (ed. F.R. Balkwill), IRL Press, Oxford.

Wadhwa, M., Thorpe, R.C., Bird, C.R. and Gearing A.J.H. (1990). *J. Imm. Methods* **128**, 211–217.

Yang, Y.C., Ricciardi, S., Ciarletta A. *et al.* (1989). *Blood* **74**, 1880–1884.

Zheng, R.Q.H., Abney, E., Chu, C.Q. *et al.* (1991). *Clin. Exp. Immunol.* **83**, 314–319.

Chapter 26

Cytokines and their Receptors as Potential Therapeutic Targets

R. Geoffrey P. Pugh-Humphreys[1] and Angus W. Thomson[2]

[1]Cell and Immunobiology Unit, Department of Zoology, University of Aberdeen, Scotland, UK, and [2]Departments of Surgery and Molecular Genetics & Biochemistry, University of Pittsburgh, PA, USA

GENERAL FEATURES OF CYTOKINES

Origins of Cytokine Research

The previous chapters in this book have been concerned with biochemical and biological considerations of individual cytokines and the nature of the interactions of cytokines with their respective receptors. This chapter not only addresses the pathophysiological roles of cytokines but also considers cytokines and their receptors as therapeutic targets in the treatment of various maladies.

Cytokines normally exert their diverse biological activities within the context of a cytokine network to maintain homeostatic mechanisms. Cytokine interactions play pivotal roles in many normal and pathological events, including the generation of immune responses, inflammatory reactions, remodelling of tissues, angiogenesis and neoplastic transformation of cells (Meager, 1990).

An imbalance in the production and/or action of cytokines within the network provides the basis for generating immune-deficiency states as well as pathological processes including inflammatory disorders, such as rheumatoid arthritis, fibrotic disorders, growth factor related diseases and neoplasia, all of which can be ameliorated by intervening in the production of cytokines using drugs and in the interaction of cytokines with their respective receptors through the use of antibodies, antagonists and other blocking factors (Gullick, 1991). We commence this review with a consideration of the cytokine network and its role in health and disease, and then review research work which has been concerned with cytokines and their receptors as potential therapeutic targets in the treatment of a variety of pathological states.

THE CYTOKINE NETWORK AND ITS ROLE IN HEALTH AND DISEASE

The cytokines are a family of pleiotropic cell-regulatory molecules that operate within a cytokine network. The term cytokine describes several small, 6–30 kDa glycosylated polypeptides including ILs, chemokines, growth factors, IFNs, TGFs, TNFs and CSFs (Arai *et al.*, 1990; Meager, 1990). Within multicellular systems, the component cells use cytokines as signalling molecules with which to communicate with other cells and alter their behaviour. The term cytokine was originally coined by Cohen (Cohen *et al.*, 1979) to describe soluble mediator substances produced by lymphoid and nonlymphoid cells that induce specific effects in target cells. During their biosynthesis within cells, post-translational modification of cytokine molecules occurs, involving glycosylation, addition of fatty acyl chains and, in the case of those cytokines that are synthesized as larger precursors, proteolytic cleavage of the polypeptide to the biologically active cytokine (Meager, 1990). Some cytokines may exist in more than one form; for instance the TGF-β family of multifunctional dimeric polypeptides, includes five structurally and functionally related isoforms called TGF-β_1, TGF-β_2, TGF-β_3, TGF-β_4 and TGF-β_5 which influence cell proliferation, differentiation and extracellular matrix production (Miyazono and Heldin, 1991; Johnson *et al.*, 1993). All the isoforms of TGF-β are secreted as inactive, latent complexes. TGF-β_1 is secreted as a large precursor protein containing 390 amino acids and consists of a latency-associated 40 kDa N-terminal peptide, an active 25 kDa homodimer and a 125–160 kDa binding protein linked by disulphide bonds to the latency associated peptide (Miyazono and Heldin, 1991). The active 25 kDa homodimer is released from the inactive precursor through proteolytic cleavage by plasmin (Lyons *et al.*, 1990), which may represent a means of regulating the effects of TGF-β molecules. Some cytokines may remain anchored within the plasma membrane of the producer cell and exert their effects on target cells by direct intercellular contact (Dainiak, 1990). These cytokines can be cleaved extracellularly by proteases and subsequently released in soluble form (Dainiak, 1990). Cytokines such as TGF-β and FGF-2 bind to proteoglycans and glycosaminoglycans located at cell surfaces (Andres *et al.*, 1992) and the cell-surface glycopolymers may be involved in the presentation of cytokines between neighbouring cells (Tanaka *et al.*, 1993).

Cytokines are a diverse group of polypeptides which are extremely potent, often being active at nanomolar or picomolar concentrations (Meager, 1990). Based on their molecular conformations the cytokines can be separated into three classes: the α-helical cytokines (IFN-α, IFN-β and IFN-γ, IL-2, IL-3, IL-4, IL-5, IL-6, IL-7, G-CSF, M-CSF, GM-CSF); the β structural cytokines (IL-1α, and IL-β, TNF-α, LT and the FGFs) and the α-plus-β cytokines (IL-8, PF-4, IFN-γ and gro).

Cytokines can also be grouped together into superfamilies and subfamilies on the basis of amino acid sequence homologies, structural and functional similarities, and/or common signal transduction mechanisms. For instance, on the basis of their structural and functional similarities, and a common signal transduction mechanism, the cytokines LIF, G-CSF, IL-6, oncostatin M and ciliary neurotropic factor (CNTF) have all been grouped into a common cytokine family (Rose and Bruce, 1991; Hilton, 1992). Based on their amino acid sequence homologies, a group of 10 or more proinflammatory cytokines (chemokines) have been designated the PF-4 cytokine superfamily (Schall, 1991) which is subdivided into the C–C and C–X–C subfamilies, according to the spacing of conserved cysteine residues within the primary amino acid sequences; the C–C subfamily is called the RANTES/sis cytokine family and includes HC14, I-309, MCP-1, MIP-α, MIP-β, MCAF and RANTES, whereas the C–X–C subfamily includes IL-8, MGSA/gro, PF-4 and β-TG (Schall, 1991).

CYTOKINE GENE EXPRESSION AND REGULATION

The genes encoding cytokines are under the control of multiple transcription factors and regulatory elements (Muegge and Durum, 1990). Cytokine genes are usually transcriptionally inactive and their expression is stringently regulated by extracellular signals; for example, IL-1 induces the expression of genes encoding IL-1, IL-2 and IL-6 (Muegge and Durum, 1990) and IFN-γ and IL-2 synergize in inducing the expression of genes encoding IL-1α, IL-1β, TNF-α and IP-10 (Hermann *et al.*, 1989; Narumi *et al.*, 1990). Cytokine gene expression is controlled by transcription factors like AP-1, OTF, NF-IL6, IRF-1 and NF-κB and stimuli which elicit cytokine production do so either by inducing the *de novo* expression of transcription factors (e.g. IRF-1), or by post-translation activation of factors, such as NF-κB, which regulates the expression of genes for cytokines such as IL-1, IL-2, IL-6, IFN-γ (Muegge and Durum, 1990; Bose, 1992; Akira *et al.*, 1993).

The eukaryotic transcription factor NF-κB is a heterodimeric complex of two proteins (p50, p65) belonging to the *rel* oncogene family of transcription factors (Bose, 1992). Within eukaryotic cells NF-κB is associated with an inhibitor protein complex called IκB to form an inactive NF-κB/IκB complex, and IκB can be phosphorylated by a number of protein kinases (including protein kinases A and C) that can transduce cytokine receptor signals (Blank *et al.*, 1992). Probably mediators of the NF-κB 'activation' signal are kinases (Blank *et al.*, 1992), and various agents (mitogens, LPS, cytokines, viruses) activate NF-κB by inducing its release from the NF-κB/IκB complex following phosphorylation of IκB (Blank *et al.*, 1992). The NF-κB then translocates to the nucleus where it binds as a heterodimer of p50, p65 to its decameric 10 bp κB motifs in the *cis* enhancer and promoter elements of genes for cytokines (Muegge and Durum, 1990; Narumi *et al.*, 1992). The identification of transcription factors as regulatory molecules in gene expression indicates that these proteins could be potential targets for therapeutic intervention (Peterson and Baichwal, 1993).

Within tissues, cytokines control the expression of genes involved in the biosynthesis of extracellular matrix molecules, integrins and those enzymes regulating matrix reorganization, and in these ways the local actions of cytokines, mediated by autocrine or paracrine mechanisms, are of major importance in maintaining and regulating cell and tissue homeostasis (Lee and Han, 1990; Wong and Wahl, 1990).

THE ACTION OF CYTOKINES IN THE CYTOKINE NETWORK

Cytokines normally operate within the context of a cytokine network (Balkwill and Burke, 1989; Meager, 1990) in which upregulation and downregulation of cytokine production and/or activities contributes to the operation of the cytokine network between different cell types (see Fig. 1, Table 1).

Cytokines can affect multiple cell types and produce antagonistic, synergistic and overlapping effects. For instance, cytokines can downregulate the production of other cytokines e.g. TFG-β depresses the synthesis of IL-1, IL-2, IL-6, IL-7, TNF-α and other proinflammatory cytokines. IL-10 downregulates the production of TNF-α, IL-1, IL-6, IL-8, GM-CSF and G-CSF, but upregulates the synthesis of IL-1 antagonists, thereby exerting an anti-inflammatory effect. IL-1 and TNF-α stimulate the production of each

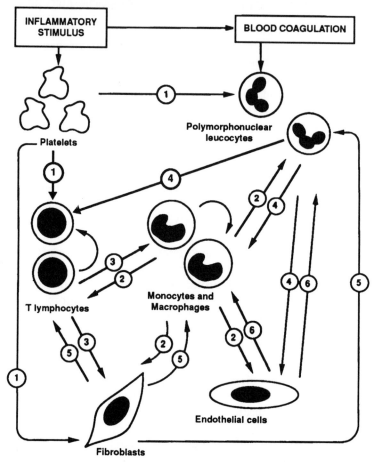

Fig. 1. Diagrammatic representation of the complex series of interactions between numerous cell types, depicted as a series of arrows, involved in such events as inflammation, the various phases of the wound-healing process and tissue repair. These interactions are made possible through the release and recognition of cytokines acting in autocrine and paracrine fashions. The arrows are numbered and the cytokines involved in the interactions are listed in Table 1 (modified after Wong and Wahl, 1990).

other, as well as the production of IL-2, IL-6, IL-8 and PDGF. An inhibition of the production of IL-1, TNF-α or IL-6, reduces the activities of the other two. Although IL-1 and TNF-α do not influence each other's specific biological activities, IL-1 and TNF-α are strongly synergistic for the induction of GM-CSF production. In other instances cytokines can antagonize the effects of other cytokines, for example in mice IFN-α antagonizes the effects of IL-4 on B cells (Coffman *et al.*, 1988; Vitetta *et al.*, 1989).

The cytokine network rapidly mobilizes and amplifies inflammatory, immunological and tissue repair processes, in an attempt to restore homeostasis within damaged or infected tissue (Meager, 1990). Dysfunction in the regulatory mechanisms governing the production and actions of cytokines within the network causes an imbalance in the network, which can have profound pathological consequences and can lead to the pathogenesis of a plethora of diseases (Meager, 1990; Mire-Sluis, 1993).

Table 1. Cytokines involved in the interactions between the principal cells depicted in Fig. 1.

1. Platelet-derived cytokines
   PDGF-A and -B   TFG-β FGF-2

2. Monocyte/macrophage-derived cytokines
   PDGF-A and -B   TGF-α and -β IL-1α and β IL-6
   IL-8   TNF-α IFN-α IFN-β
   GM-CSF   FGF-2   EGF   IGF-1

3. T-helper cell-derived cytokines
   IL-2   IL-3   IL-4   IL-5
   IL-6   IL-8   IL-10   GM-CSF
   IFN-γ TNF-α LT

4. PMN leukocyte-derived cytokines
   IL-1β IL-6   IL-8   G-SCF
   M-CSF   GM-CSF   TNF-α

5. Fibroblast-derived cytokines
   IL-1α and β IL-6   IL-7   IL-8
   PDGF-A and B   G-CSF   M-CSF   GM-CSF
   TGF-α TGF-β

6. Endothelial cell-derived cytokines
   IL-1α and β IL-6   IL-8   G-CSF
   M-CSF   GM-CSF   TNF-α PDGF-A and -B
   FGF-2

Table 2. Cytokines which act as competence or progression factors.

Competence factors	Progression factors
PDGF-A	EGF
PDGF-B	NGF
TGF-β	FGFs
IL-1α and β	TGF-2
IL-4	IFG-1 and 2
IL-6	IL-2
IL-8	IL-3
IFN-α	IL-5
IFN-β	G-CSF
IFN-γ	M-CSF
TNF-α	GM-CSF
LT	EPO

Cytokines act on other cells to promote activation or stimulate cell proliferation and/or differentiation. Cytokines that are responsible for inducing cell activation and/or differentiation can be regarded as competence factors which commit cells to proceed from G0 (the quiescent stage) to the S phase of the cell cycle, whereas cytokines that induce proliferation and/or differentiation can be regarded as progression factors which complement the action of competence factors and allow cells to proceed through the G1 phase to the S phase and then go through G2 to the M phase (see Table 2). The competence cytokines may act not only as co-stimulators of cellular responses but also to induce the formation of other cytokines: for example, IL-1 induces the formation of PDGFs in fibroblasts, of GM-CSF in endothelial cells and of IL-2 in T lymphocytes. A cytokine may not induce the synthesis of another cytokine itself, but may prime a cell to become responsive to a coinducer, e.g. IFN-γ can prime monocytes/macrophages to produce TNF-α or LT in response to stimulation with LPS, IFN-γ or IL-2 (Adams and Hamilton, 1992).

Within the cytokine network we now know that a single cytokine (e.g. IL-1 or IL-6) can interact with more than one type of cell (e.g. fibroblasts, endothelial cells, macrophages, hepatocytes), a single cytokine can have multiple biological activities (e.g. the CSFs are polyfunctional and not only control cell proliferation, but also regulate cell differentiation, commitment, maturation induction and functional activity of mature, postmitotic haemopoietic cells; Cowling and Dexter, 1992; Metcalf, 1992), a single cell, e.g. fibroblast, can interact with more than one cytokine (e.g. TNF-α, IL-1, TGF-β, FGFs), many cytokines have overlapping activities (e.g. IFN-γ and IL-4), and a single cytokine may induce or inhibit the expression of a gene encoding another cytokine.

Because cytokines have overlapping spectra of activities it is sometimes difficult to distinguish which cytokine within the network is responsible for eliciting a specific response. For example, IL-1 induces many pathophysiological effects (Dinarello, 1991) that are also induced by TNF-α (Beutler, 1990) and IL-6 (Akira et al., 1993). IL-6 is produced by activated monocytes and fibroblasts, and its expression in fibroblasts is induced by TNF-α and PDGFs. The induction of cytokine synthesis by other cytokines can promote amplification of biological responses such as those important in the development of inflammatory responses at sites of tissue injury (Wong and Wahl, 1990).

CYTOKINE RECEPTORS

Cytokine receptors which display structural similarities have been separated into families, namely the haemopoietic cytokine receptor (HCR) family (IL-2R (β and γ chains), IL-3R (α and β chains) and IL-6Rgp130, IL-7R, IL-9R, EPO-R, G-CSFR, GM-CSFR (α and β chains) and LIF-R); the family of IFN receptors (IFNα-R; IFNβ-R and IFNγ-R); the tumour necrosis factor/nerve growth factor receptor family (TNF-R1, TNF-R2 and NGF-R); the TGF-β receptor family; the family of receptors for cytokines of the PF-4/IL-8 supergene (chemokine) family, and the family of receptors for growth factors (EGF-R, PDGF-R, IGF-1R) (Yarden and Ullrich, 1988; Foxwell et al., 1992; Massague, 1992; Minami et al., 1992). Alternatively, cytokine receptors have also been grouped into the cytokine receptor family, the immunoglobulin superfamily and the tyrosine kinase receptor family (see Table 3).

The receptors for cytokines such as IL-1, IL-3, IL-4, IL-6, IFN-γ, EPO and GM-CSF are single polypeptides and all have an extracellular domain, a single transmembrane domain and a cytoplasmic domain (Arai et al., 1990). The IL-1R (types 1 and 2), IL-6R and IFN-γR belong to the Ig superfamily of receptors which are characterized by having three extracellular Ig-like domains, a short transmembrane domain and cytoplasmic domains of variable lengths (Foxwell et al., 1992). Within the cytokine receptor superfamily both the Class 1 receptors (e.g. EPO-R, G-CSFR, GM-CSFR, IL-3R, IL-4R, IL-6R, IL-7R and IL-2Rβ) and the Class 2 receptors (e.g. IFN-α-Rβ and IFN-γR)

Table 3. Receptor families.

Receptor family		Immunoglobulin superfamily	Tyrosine Kinase receptor family
IL-2Rβ	EPO-R	IL-1R1	SCF-R (c-kit)
IL-3R	LIF-R	IL-1R2	EGF-R
IL-4R	G-CSFR	SCF-R (c-kit)	PDGF-R (αα, αβ ββ)
IL-5R	GM-CSFR	G-CSFR	M-CSFR
IL-6R	TNF-R1	M-CSFR (c-fms)	
IL-7R	TNF-R2	PDGF-R (αβ)	
	IFN-γR		
	EGF-R		
	IFN-α-Rβ		

(Foxwell *et al.*, 1992) share ligand-binding domains which allows binding of variously shaped and sized helical cytokines that display a 'recognition α-helix' (Bazan, 1990).

Whereas most cytokine receptors are single-chain polypeptides, other cytokine receptors, such as the receptors for colony stimulating factors, consist of α and β subunits (Nicola and Metcalf, 1991). In humans, GM-CSFR and IL-3R share a common β subunit (Lopez *et al.*, 1989), whereas in mice GM-CSFR and IL-5R share a common β subunit (Minami *et al.*, 1992). The HCR family contains polypeptides that do not bind cytokines directly (e.g. IL-6Rgp 130 and the common β chains of IL-3R, IL-5R and GM-CSFR) (Foxwell *et al.*, 1992). Although the HCRs are responsible for the binding of a single cytokine, some of the receptors (e.g. IL-2R, IL-3R, IL-5R, IL-6R and GM-CSFR) require additional proteins to confer high-affinity binding. For instance, the high-affinity IL-2R is a heterotrimer of three polypeptides IL-2Rα (p55); (also called the Tac antigen), IL-2Rβ (p75) and IL-2Rγ (p64). IL-2Rα and IL-2Rβ bind IL-2 with low (K_d 10^{-8} M) and intermediate (K_d 10^{-9} M) affinity respectively, whereas the heterotrimer of IL-2Rα/β/γ binds IL-2 with high (K_d 10^{-11} M) affinity (Takeshita *et al.*, 1992). A number of cytokine receptors (e.g. IL-6R, oncostatin M receptor and LIF-R) interact with the nonligand binding protein gp130 to form a high-affinity complex involved in signal transmission via the cytoplasmic portion of gp130 (Akira *et al.*, 1993). The binding of cytokines to the ligand binding sites on cytokine receptors is the first step in a complex series of signal transduction events which ultimately affect gene expression within target cells (Arai *et al.*, 1990).

The cytoplasmic domains of some cytokine receptors (e.g. the receptors for EGF, PDGF and IGF-1 and M-CSFR), have functional tyrosine kinase activity, whereas those receptors lacking intrinsic enzyme activity are coupled via G proteins to enzymes such as adenylate cyclase (e.g. IL-1R types 1 and 2) and phospholipase C (PLC) (e.g. IL-4R and IL-8R) (Meager, 1990) (see Table 4). Those receptors which transduce their signals via PLC, stimulate PLC-mediated hydrolysis of phosphatidyl inositol (PIP2) to form inositol trisphosphate (IP3) and diacyl glycerol (DAG) which cause the release of calcium from intercellular stores (IP3) and activation of protein kinase C (PKC) (DAG) (Arai *et al.*, 1990; Meager, 1990). The generation of cyclic AMP (cAMP) by adenylate cyclase causes activation of serine–threonine kinases (A-kinases) (Arai *et al.*, 1990). IP3, DAG, calcium and cAMP are important second messengers involved in intracellular signal transduction (Arai *et al.*, 1990; Meager, 1990). The intracellular signal transduction mechanisms mediated by cytokine receptors may also involve cytoplasmic

Table 4. Signal transduction mechanisms associated with cytokine receptors.

Intrinsic tyrosine kinase	Linked to cytoplasmic tyrosine kinases	G protein linked	Linked to PLC activation	Linked to PIP2 hydrolysis	Linked to Ca++ influx
SCF-R (c-kit)	IL-2Rαβγ	IL-1R1	IL-1R2	IL-7R	IL-8R1
EGF-R	IL-3R	IL-1R2	IL-4R	IFNγ-R	IL-8R2
PDGF-R (αα, αβ, ββ)	IL-4R	IL-8R1	IL-8R	EGF-R	IFNγ-R
M-CSFR (c-fms)	IL-5R	IL-8Rw			SCF-R (c-kit)
	IL-7R	G-CSFR			EGF-R
	TNF-R1				
	TNF-R2				

tyrosine kinases (including several members of the src family of tyrosine kinases, such as p56lck, p59fyn and p56lyn), transcription of proto-oncogenes (e.g. c-*fos*, c-*myc*, c-*myb*), activation of the ubiquitous cytoplasmic kinase, Raf-1, activation of A-kinases, and activation of both the phosphatidyl inositol-3-kinase (PI3 kinase) and the ras protein (p21ras) (Minami *et al.*, 1992) (see Fig. 2). PKC mediated activation of NADP oxidase is involved in the generation of superoxide anions (O_2^-) which are subsequently converted to reactive oxygen intermediates (ROIs) by superoxide dismutase (SOD). ROIs cause deregulation of intracellular Ca^{++} levels ($[Ca^{++}]_i$), initiate a variety of intracellular events, including activation of protein kinases and phospholipases, as well as induce the expression of the proto-oncogenes c-*fos*, c-*jun* and c-*myc* (Maki *et al.*, 1992). Oxygen radicals may also be mediators of the NF-κB activation signal (Blank *et al.*, 1992). Those cytokine receptors that activate plasma-membrane-bound calcium channels via G proteins (see Fig. 2 and Table 4) cause an influx of Ca^{++} ions which function in intracellular signal transduction events (Arai *et al.*, 1990).

Some cytokine receptors can exist in more than one form. For instance, there are two forms of the IL-1R, the type 1 (60 kDa) and the type 2 (80 kDa) receptors. Both receptors are separate gene products, can bind IL-1α and IL-1β with high affinity, and both are capable of mediating IL-1α/β transmitted signals (Solari, 1990; Dinarello, 1991). IL-1R1 is expressed on T cells, synoviocytes, chondrocytes and hepatocytes, whereas IL-1R2 is expressed on B cells, neutrophils and bone-marrow cells (Dinarello, 1991). Although some cells can coexpress both of the IL-1 receptors (Solari, 1990), the type 2 receptor appears to predominate (Giri *et al.*, 1992). TNF-α exerts its pleiotropic effects via two high-affinity receptors, identified as TNF-R1 (55 kDa) and TNF-R2 (75 kDa), which are found on many different cell types, and the cytotoxic and proliferative responses of cells to TNF-α may be segregated between the two TNF receptors (Barrett *et al.*, 1991). Five TGF-β receptors have been identified and are designated type I (55–65 kDa), type II (70–85 kDa), type III/betaglycan (250–310 kDa), type IV (60 kDa) and type V (400 kDa) (Massagué, 1992). The type I and type II receptors bind all isoforms of TGF-β with equal affinity and the effects of TGF-βs are transduced by the type I and type II receptors in most normal cells (Massagué, 1992). Although the type I receptor does not possess kinase activity, the type II receptor possesses a cytoplasmic domain with serine–threonine kinase activity (Lin *et al.*, 1992). The type III receptor is a proteoglycan called betaglycan and is functionally distinct from the type I and type II

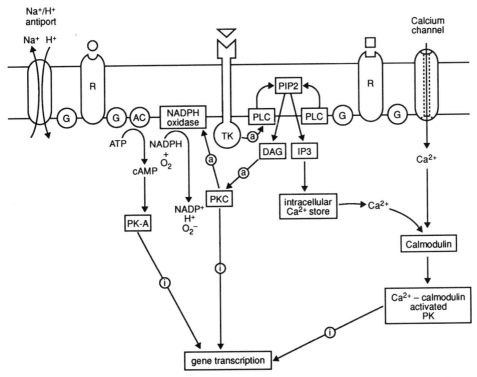

Fig. 2. Simplified representation of transmembrane signalling events following the interactions of ligands (O, ▽, ▢), including cytokines, with membrane receptors (R). Some of the receptors are coupled to intercellular effector systems through G proteins which can either activate membrane bound enzymes or enhance the operation of transmembrane ion transport systems (the Na^+H^+ antiport or calcium channels). Ligand engagement of those membrane receptors with intrinsic tyrosine kinase (TK) domains results in activation of TK activity. Activation of membrane-bound adenylate cyclase (AC) by G proteins results in the production of the second messenger cyclic AMP (cAMP), whereas stimulation of membrane-bound phospholipase C (PLC) by either G proteins or activated TK results in phosphoinositide (PIP2) turnover within the plasma membrane leading to the formation of the second messengers diacyl glycerol (DAG) and inositol trisphosphate (IP3). The IP3 induces the mobilization of Ca^{++} ions from intracellular Ca^{++} stores. The cAMP, DAG and intracellular free Ca^{++} ions activate (—(a)→) various protein kinases (PK-A, PKC and Ca^{++}-calmodulin activated PKs respectively) which in turn induce (—(i)→) gene expression within the nucleus. PKs can also activate membrane bound NADPH oxidase leading to the formation of superoxide anions (O_2^-) which can act as intracellular signalling moieties.

receptors; it is a membrane proteoglycan containing 853 amino acids which carries GAG chains. The type III receptor constitutes the predominant binding receptor of mesenchymal cells, and the cytoplasmic portion lacks a signalling motif (Segarini, 1991).

A number of cytokine receptors (e.g. IL-1R2, IL-2R (α and β chains), IL-4R, IL-6R, IL-7R, IL-9R, G-CSFR, gp130, IFN-γ-R and TNF-R1/R2) exist in both membrane anchored and soluble forms (Fernandez-Botran, 1991; Akira *et al.*, 1993). The soluble receptors have ligand-binding domains with binding affinities comparable to the membrane-bound receptors, but lack the transmembrane and intracytoplasmic domains, and arise either by proteolytic cleavage of the membrane-bound receptor or by translation from separate mRNA transcripts encoding soluble receptors (Fernandez-Botran, 1991). For instance, sIL-2R (p55) and sTNF-Rs arise by proteolytic cleavage of membrane-bound receptors (receptor shedding), whereas sIL-4R and sIL-7R arise by translation from alternatively spliced mRNA (Fernandez-Botran, 1991). Soluble receptors can serve as inhibitors for their respective cytokine ligands, and can be used to monitor the severity and clinical progression of infectious diseases, autoimmune diseases and malignancy (Fernandez-Botran, 1991; Mire-Sluis, 1993).

The selective responses of cells to cytokines are dictated, in part, by the repertoire of cytokine receptors expressed on cells, which in turn is dependent upon the type of target cell and its stage of differentiation (Arai et al., 1990). The level of surface expression of cytokine receptors is also determined by the balance between the rates of insertion into the plasma membrane (following de novo synthesis or receptor recycling) and the loss of receptors owing to receptor shedding or internalization (Arai et al., 1990). Whereas the expression of some receptors (e.g. IL-1R1, IL-1R2, IL-4R and IL-6R) appears to be constitutive, the expression of other cytokine receptors can be upregulated or downregulated following exposure of cells to cytokines (Arai et al., 1990; Fernandez-Botran, 1991; Foxwell et al., 1992). In some cases cytokines can modulate the expression of their own receptors; for instance, upregulation of the expression of their corresponding receptors is induced by IL-2 (Lee et al., 1990), IL-4 and GM-CSF (Fan et al., 1992), whereas G-CSF can downregulate the expression of its receptor. The CSF receptors are able to transmodulate each other's surface expression in a hierarchical and unidirectional fashion (Nicola and Metcalf, 1991). The expression of GM-CSFR on murine macrophages may be regulated by G proteins and PKC, whose activities are in turn linked to the regulatory pathways of other cytokine receptors (Fan et al., 1993).

Functional pleiotropy and redundancy are characteristic features of cytokines within the cytokine network (Balkwill and Burke, 1989; Arai et al., 1990). Some cytokine receptors can couple to multiple signal transduction systems, and the pleiotropic functions of cytokines on different target cells may be mediated by the coupling of the high-affinity receptors to different signal-transducing molecules within each type of target cell (Arai et al., 1990; Miyajima et al., 1992). Alternatively, cytokine receptors can couple to the same signal transduction system via common transducers, and the association of the signal transducer protein gp130 with several different cytokine receptors would explain why several different cytokines can elicit the same responses within a given target cell type (Arai et al., 1990; Foxwell et al., 1992). Although the majority of cytokine receptors occur as single polypeptide chains, others contain subunits, and the sharing of a common β subunit by some receptors (e.g. GM-CSFR, IL-3R and IL-5R) may provide the structural basis for the pleiotropic actions of cytokines within the cytokine network (Arai et al., 1990; Meager, 1990).

THE ACTION OF CYTOKINES WITHIN TISSUES AND BODY FLUIDS

In the complex milieu of tissues, the actions of cytokines will be affected by macromolecules present within the microenvironment, which consists of a solid phase (the extracellular matrix or ECM) and a plasma-derived tissue fluid phase. Certain cytokines engage in the process of 'crinopexy' and become bound to, and stabilized within, the ECM. For instance TGF-β and FGF-2 bind to proteoglycans and glycosaminoglycans (GAGs) within the ECM, and it is the GAGs that modulate the biological activities of FGF-2 (Givol and Yayon, 1992). The ECM is a complex and dynamic reservoir of cytokines, and cells can access these cytokines by mediating limited degradation of the ECM through the release of plasminogen activator (PA), which converts plasminogen to plasmin, and through the release of the endoglycosidase heparanase; the expression of urokinase type PA (u-PA) leading to the activation of plasmin can liberate both FGF-2 and TGF-β from the ECM (Falcone *et al.*, 1993). The liberation of cytokines sequestered within the ECM plays an important role in angiogenesis and repair of wounded tissues (Vlodavsky *et al.*, 1991). The plasma-derived tissue fluid contains a number of cytokine-binding proteins which can modulate the activities of cytokines *in vivo*, and these include soluble cytokine receptors such as sIL-2Rp55, sIL-4R, sIL-6R, sIL-7R, sIFN-γR and sTNF-αR (Fernandez-Botran, 1991), IgG (Edgington, 1993), autoantibodies (Bendtzen *et al.*, 1990) and other proteins such as α_2-macroglobulin (James, 1990) which can bind cytokines including IL-1, IL-6, IL-2 and PDGF (James, 1990). The soluble cytokine receptors may not only regulate the levels of biologically active cytokines within tissue and body fluids, but also exert a regulatory effect upon the intensity of inflammatory and immune responses, and this raises the possibility of using soluble cytokine receptors as immunomodulating agents in the treatment of auto-immune and inflammatory diseases (Fernandez-Botran, 1991; Mire-Sluis, 1993). The autoantibodies and α_2-macroglobulin may afford cytokines some protection from biochemical degradation by enzymes present within tissue and body fluids (James, 1990).

Other proteins within biological fluids which can influence the action of cytokines, but which do not bind cytokines *per se*, include receptor-binding antagonists which competitively inhibit the binding of a cytokine to its receptor by competing for the same binding site on the receptor, e.g. IL-1Ra (Arend, 1993). IL-1Ra is a naturally occurring inhibitor within serum, synovial fluids and urine which competes with IL-1α and IL-1β for their receptor and acts as an IL-1 receptor antagonist. IL-1Ra does not bind to IL-1α or β (Poutsiaka *et al.*, 1992). IL-1Ra is an 18–22 kDa glycoprotein produced by monocytes following their exposure to agents that stimulate IL-1 production, and forms part of an endogenous negative-feedback mechanism of IL-1 production (Ulich *et al.*, 1991). IL-1Ra is considered a member of the IL-1 gene family and has been purified and its cDNA cloned. IL-1Ra binds to both IL-1R1 and IL-1R2, yet lacks the agonist activity of IL-1α and β, and blocks the proinflammatory activities of IL-1α and β while not appearing to compromise host immune responsiveness (Dinarello and Thompson, 1991; Arend, 1993). The elevated production of IL-1Ra and its increased titre within the circulation appears to be a natural host response in certain clinical conditions, such as endotoxaemia, sepsis and rheumatoid arthritis, and reduces the severity of these diseases (Dinarello and Thompson, 1991; Arend, 1993).

CYTOKINES IN INFLAMMATION AND IMMUNITY

The multifunctionality of cytokines is amply illustrated in the molecular and cellular events associated with inflammation, angiogenesis and wound repair, and the host immune response (see Fig. 3). The inflammatory response is a host defence reaction which mobilizes leukocytes to tissues traumatized either by invasion of potentially pathogenic microorganisms (viruses, bacteria, fungi) and parasites, or as a consequence of hypersensitivity reactions or invasion by malignant neoplasms, or alternatively to

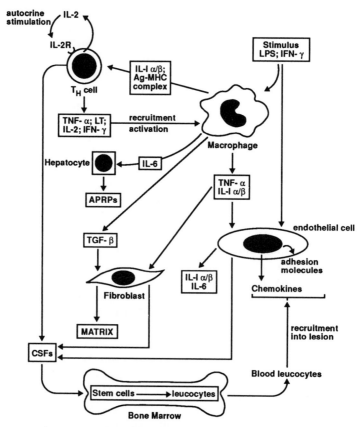

Fig. 3. A diagrammatic representation of the interactions between endothelial cells, fibroblasts, T-helper lymphocytes and cells of the monocyte-macrophage lineage in the generation of cytokines, especially colony stimulating factors (CSFs), and acute-phase reactant proteins (APRPs) during the host response to an inflammatory stimulus. The cytokines involved in these interactions, particularly the effects of cytokines (IL-1α/β and TNF-α) on vascular endothelial cells which promote transendothelial leukocyte migration into an inflammatory lesion, as well as the effects of CSFs in promoting leukopoiesis within the bone marrow during host inflammatory reactions, are indicated.

tissues damaged by chemicals or physical trauma (Wong and Wahl, 1990; Whaley and Burt, 1992). Within developing inflammatory lesions blood plasma, containing fibrinogen and fibronectin, extravasates and clots extravascularly to form a hydrated fibrin–fibronectin gel. This gel serves as a provisional matrix which is subsequently invaded by inflammatory leucocytes (PMN leukocytes, monocytes and lymphocytes), fibroblasts and capillary endothelial cells; these events are regulated by cytokines released by both platelets and inflammatory leucocytes (Nathan, 1990; Wong and Wahl, 1990).

Infection and injury are associated with increases in the numbers of circulating PMN leucocytes and monocytes in response to CSFs generated within inflammatory lesions (Wong and Wahl, 1990). Both the PMN leucocytes (Lloyd and Oppenheim, 1992) and the monocytes-macrophages (Nathan, 1990) release cytokines that coordinate and regulate inflammatory and immune responses within inflammatory lesions (Nathan, 1990; Wong and Wahl, 1990; Adams and Hamilton, 1992). PMN leukocytes and monocytes are recruited into lesions where they debride the lesion of infectious agents by their phagocytic activities, and where monocyte-derived macrophages participate in tissue repair and remodelling by releasing cytokines which induce fibroblast chemotaxis, activation and proliferation (e.g. IL-1α/β, TGF-β) (Nathan, 1990; Adams and Hamilton, 1992) and which are mediators of general inflammation. These subsequently stimulate the production of IL-1α/β, IL-6, IL-8, M-CSF, GM-CSF, IFN-α and IFN-β (Wong and Wahl, 1990). These cytokines are produced early in the response to injury and infection, and exert proinflammatory activities (Wong and Wahl, 1990; van Deuren et al., 1992). IL-1α/β, IL-6 and TNF-α induce the production of haemopoietic colony stimulating factors by fibroblasts, endothelial cells and bone-marrow stromal cells (Wong and Wahl, 1990). IL-1α/β and IL-6 are hepatocyte stimulating factors and induce the production by hepatocytes of many acute-phase reactant proteins (APRPs) (e.g. C-reactive protein, α_1-acid glycoprotein, α_1-antitrypsin, haptoglobin, serum amyloid A protein and fibrinogen) as well as fibronectin (Beutler, 1990; Hagiwara et al., 1990; Akira et al., 1993).

Both macrophages and endothelial cells produce many cytokines which orchestrate many facets of inflammatory reactions. Endothelial cells are both a source and a target for cytokines (Mantovani and Dejana, 1989; Pober and Cotran, 1990), and, following their exposure to IL-α/β and TNF-α, they participate in inflammatory reactions through the release of CSFs, as well as the generation of chemokines and the upregulated expression of endothelial-leukocyte adhesion molecules (selectins, integrins and immunoglobulin-related molecules) which regulate transendothelial traffic of leukocytes into inflammatory lesions (Mantovani and Dejana, 1989; Pober and Cotran, 1990).

The host immune response within an inflammatory lesion involves interactions between T and B lymphocytes, macrophages and other effector cells, and is determined, in part, by the pattern of cytokines produced by different subsets of T lymphocytes (Mosmann and Moore, 1991) (Fig. 4). Clonal proliferation of antigen-specific T cells occurs following their stimulation by an APC, involving presentation of antigen–MHC complexes to the T-cell receptor (TCR) and the simultaneous release of IL-1; these stimuli induce the expression by the T cells of IL-2 and IL-2R, and the autocrine interaction between IL-2 and IL-2R is subsequently translated into a signal-transduction event within the T cell (Altman et al., 1990; Isakov, 1993).

CD4$^+$T cells differentiate into either T_{H1} or T_{H2} cells (see Fig. 4). IL-12 is produced by monocytes, macrophages, B lymphocytes and other accessory cells in response to infection by bacteria and parasites, and is an obligatory factor in the generation of T_{H1} cells (Trinchieri, 1993). T_{H1} cells secrete IL-2 and IFN-γ and mediate cell-mediated immune reactions (Mosmann and Moore, 1991), whereas T_{H2} cells secrete IL-4, IL-5, IL-6 and IL-10 which induce humoral immune responses with selective production of IgG, IgE and IgA isotypes (Coffman et al., 1993). IFN-γ plays an obligatory role in the induction of cytolytic activity in NK cells, LAK cells and cytotoxic T lymphocytes (Tc or CTLs), and IL-2 participates in the activation and tumoricidal activation of NK cells and LAK cells (Rosenberg, 1988). IFN-γ and TNF-α alone, or in combination, can also enhance the cytotoxic actions of CTLs, NK cells and LAK cells (Balkwill, 1989a).

Both T_{H1} cells and T_{H2} cells appear able to regulate each other's functions (Mosmann and Moore, 1991). The fact that IL-4 and IL-10 produced by T_{H2} cells inhibit the activities of T_{H1} cells, whereas IFN-γ produced by T_{H1} cells suppresses the activities of

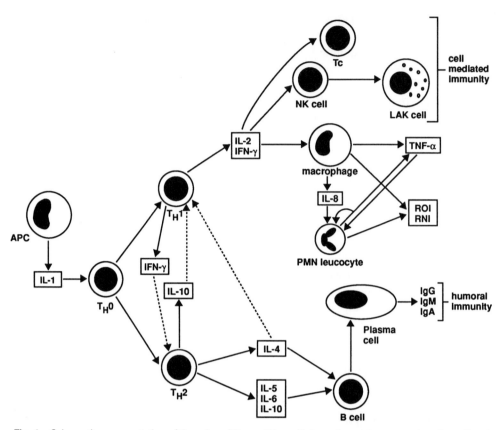

Fig. 4. Schematic representation of the roles of T_{H1} and T_{H2} cells in orchestrating events in cell-mediated and humoral immune responses, respectively through the release of cytokines. Through the release of IL-2 and IFN-γ, T_{H1} cells activate T_c cells, NK cells to become effector cells, whereas macrophages and PMN leukocytes are activated to release TNF-α, ROI and RNI which participate in the killing of neoplastic cells, micro-organisms and parasites. Through the release of cytokines (IL-4, IL-5, IL-6, IL-10), T_{H2} cells promote the differentiation of B cells into antibody-secreting plasma cells. Both T_{H1} and T_{H2} cells regulate each other's functions through the suppressive effects (- - - - - -) of IFN-γ and IL-4/IL-10, respectively.

T_{H2} cells, provides an explanation for the inverse relationship observed between cell-mediated and humoral immune responses (Bretscher *et al.*, 1992). However, T_{H1} and T_{H2} cells represent opposite ends of the T_H cell spectrum and it is an oversimplification to state that these cells have totally distinct patterns of cytokine secretion since both T_{H1} and T_{H2} cells produce IL-3, GM-CSF and TNF-α (Mosmann and Moore, 1991). Through the production of IL-3, IL-4, IL-5 and GM-CSF, T_{H2} cells are involved in the pathogenesis of allergic inflammatory reactions (Ricci *et al.*, 1993). The action of IL-10 as a powerful inhibitor of the secretion of the proinflammatory cytokines IL-1α/β, IL-6, IL-8 and TNF-α, as well as being a mediator of IL-1Ra expression, makes IL-10 an important regulator of inflammatory and immune responses (Howard and O'Garra, 1992). IL-12 agonists and antagonists which would modulate T_{H1} cell responses could provide useful therapeutic agents in patients with clinical cancers, allergic reactions, autoimmune diseases and immunodeficiencies (Trinchieri, 1993).

The progression of AIDS is accompanied by a profound depletion of immunoprotective T_{H1} cells, B-cell activation and hypergammaglobulinaemia; the T_{H1}/T_{H2} switch is a critical factor in the progression of AIDS symptoms within HIV-infected individuals and is characterized by loss of IL-2 and IFN-γ production by T_{H1} cells and an increased production of IL-4 and IL-10 by T_{H2} cells (Clerici and Shearer, 1993). The administration of anti-IL-4 and anti-IL-10 antibodies may restore T_{H1} responses within infected patients and thus provide an essential initial step in attempts to immunize patients with HIV vaccines (Graham et al., 1992; Clerici and Shearer, 1993).

Macrophages play an important role in the afferent and efferent arms of host immune responses through their actions as antigen processing, presenting and cytokine secreting cells (Steinman, 1991; Stein and Keshav, 1992), as well as their capacity to act as effector cells in host defence against infections with viruses (Gendelman and Moraham, 1992), bacteria (Speert, 1992), parasites (Sadick, 1992) and against malignancy (Nathan, 1990). The effector functions of macrophages are modulated by cytokines produced by T_H cells (Nathan, 1990; Adams and Hamilton, 1992), and macrophages activated by cytokines such as IFN-γ play a major role in host defence against infection and cancer through the production of ROI (e.g. superoxide anions, OH^- and H_2O_2), reactive nitrogen intermediates (RNI) (e.g. nitric oxide, nitrite and nitrate) and TNF-α (Nathan, 1990, 1992; Adams and Hamilton, 1992). ROI plays an important role in the bactericidal activities of macrophages (Speert, 1992).

Nitric oxide ($\cdot$NO) is a highly reactive product of activated macrophages, and is derived by the oxidative cleavage of guanidino nitrogens from L-arginine leaving L-citrulline as a coproduct of L-arginine metabolism (Nathan, 1992). There are two forms of $\cdot$NO, a constitutive form and an inducible form produced by inflammatory leukocytes after stimulation with LPS and cytokines; $\cdot$NO is an important modulator of inflammatory and immune responses (Nathan, 1992). IFN-γ enhances the synthesis of $\cdot$NO by macrophages through an inducible IFN-γ-mediated increase in the availability of tetrahydrobiopterin which is required as a cofactor for inducible biosynthesis of $\cdot$NO (Nathan, 1992). In the presence of oxygen, $\cdot$NO is rapidly converted to other reactive intermediates, nitrite and nitrate (Ignarro, 1989). Macrophage-derived $\cdot$NO not only kills intracellular parasites (Liew et al., 1990; Sadick, 1992) and neoplastic cells (Nathan, 1990, 1992), but also regulates the progression of specific lymphocyte responses (Nathan, 1992). Activated macrophages can enhance and depress immune responses through the release of cytokines and $\cdot$NO; although macrophages produce a number of cytokines that induce T-cell proliferation and activation during immune responses, the simultaneous release of $\cdot$NO by macrophages renders lymphocytes anergic or hyporesponsive to the actions of the macrophage-derived cytokines (Nathan, 1992).

The local, paracrine effects of macrophage-derived TNF-α are often beneficial to the host (Cerami, 1992) and include actions which directly influence the host's immune response, such as inducing effector-cell activation, induction of cell-surface MHC molecule expression, cytokine induction and receptor modulation, and degranulation of cytotoxic effector cells (Cerami, 1992). TNF-α also affords a protective effect against neoplastic cells, parasites and facultative intracellular microorganisms (Liew et al., 1990; Nathan, 1990; Pesanti, 1991; Sadick, 1992). A number of cytokines including IFN-β, IFN-γ, TNF-α and TGF-β exert an antiviral role (Ramsay et al., 1993). IL-2 can induce an antiviral activity through the chemotactic recruitment and activation of NK cells. NK cells not only kill virus-infected cells, but also secrete IFN-γ and TNF-α. Following Class I MHC-restricted recognition of virus infected cells, CD8$^+$ CTLs also release antiviral cytokines such as IFN-γ and TNF-α within virus-infected tissues, thereby mediating an antiviral effect (Ramsay *et al.*, 1993).

IL-4 produced by T$_{H2}$ cells is an important anti-inflammatory cytokine which suppresses proinflammatory activities of macrophages by downregulating the production of IL-1β and TNF-α (Essner *et al.*, 1989; Hart *et al.*, 1989), G-CSF and GM-CSF (Hamilton *et al.*, 1992), PGE$_2$ (Hart *et al.*, 1989), IL-6 (Cheung *et al.*, 1990), IL-8 (Standiford *et al.*, 1990), H$_2$O$_2$ (Lehn *et al.*, 1989), superoxide anions (Abramson and Gallin, 1990) and monocyte-derived procoagulant activity (Szabo and Miller-Graziano, 1990). IL-4 also decreases the adhesion of monocytes to endothelial cells (Elliott *et al.*, 1991) and hence depresses the traffic of monocytes into inflammatory lesions.

Following neutralization of the inflammatory agent by PMN leukocytes and macrophages within an inflammatory lesion, the lesion resolves. The fibrin–fibronectin gel is degraded and replaced first by loose, vascularized connective tissue (called granulation tissue) and later by dense, collagenous, hypocellular and hypovascular scar tissue (Whaley and Burt, 1992). The formation of granulation tissue, which involves fibroblast proliferation (fibroplasia), the biosynthesis of matrix molecules by fibroblasts and endothelial cells, as well as angiogenesis, is regulated by cytokines released by platelets and inflammatory leukocytes and that include PDGF, EGF, IGF-1, FGFs, TGF-α and TGF-β (Wong and Wahl, 1990; Kovacs, 1991).

TGF-α, TGF-β, FGFs and IGF-1 exert powerful effects upon tissue cells within inflammatory lesions (Wong and Wahl, 1990; Kovacs, 1991). TGF-α is a structural and functional homologue of EGF and, along with EGF, IGF-1, FGF-2 and PDGF, contributes to angiogenesis and fibroplasia; TGF-α is also immunosuppressive (Wong and Wahl, 1990). The TGF-β family of cytokines function as both inhibitory and stimulating factors in inflammatory and immune responses (Massague, 1992; Weinberg *et al.*, 1992). TGF-β_1 stimulates chemotactic recruitment of fibroblasts and inflammatory leukocytes, followed by a wave of cytokine secretion from monocytes and fibroblasts (Wong and Wahl, 1990). TGF-β_1 is predominantly a growth-inhibitory cytokine which strongly stimulates the production of matrix molecules (including interstitial collagens, elastin, glycoproteins, proteoglycans and GAGs) and the formation of granulation tissue (Wong and Wahl, 1990). Recent evidence (Reddy and Howe, 1993) suggests that the growth-inhibitory effects of TGF-β_1 are associated with a late G1 cell cycle arrest involving inhibition of the activity of the protein kinase p34^{cdc2}. The FGF family, which comprises seven structurally and functionally related polypeptides (FGF1–7) (Goldfarb, 1990), are potent inducers of proliferation of fibroblasts and endothelial cells, and, because of their strong chemotactic effects on endothelial cells, are also classified as angiogenic factors (Folkman and Shing, 1992) (Table 5). FGF-2 is a key cytokine in angiogenesis and stimulates the expression of plasminogen activator and neutral metalloproteinases by endothelial cells (Rifkin *et al.*, 1990). Under the influence of TGF-β fibroblasts synthesize protease inhibitors (Overall *et al.*, 1991) which moderate the actions of the proteases.

Coincident with fibroplasia there is proliferation of small blood vessels (angiogenesis) during granulation tissue formation. New blood vessels arise from existing blood vessels, and this is preceded by dissolution of the basal lamella of venules followed by invasion of cords of migratory endothelial cells into the surrounding connective tissue

Table 5. Angiogenic factors and diseases related to angiogenesis.

Purified angiogenic factors	Angiogenesis-related diseases
Angiogenin	Diabetic retinopathy
Angiotrophin	Neovascular glaucoma
Platelet-derived endothelial-cell growth factor (PD-ECGF)	Trachoma
	Retrolental fibroplasia
FGF-1	Psoriasis
FGF-2	Pyogenic granuloma
TNF-α	Burn granulations
TGF-α	Hypertrophic scars
TGF-β	Delayed wound healing
EGF	Atherosclerotic plaques
	Haemangioma
	Angiofibroma
	Tumour growth
	Arthritis

(Klagsbrun and Folkman, 1990). The endothelial cells produce a number of proteolytic enzymes which enable them to degrade both the basal lamella and the connective tissue matrix during angiogenesis (Matrisian, 1992). The cords of endothelial cells eventually organize into capillaries to form a vascular network within the granulation tissue (Klagsburn and Folkman, 1990; Wong and Wahl, 1990). Following successful elimination of the injurious agent by phagocytic cells, an inflammatory lesion undergoes resolution, which involves removal of granulation tissue and angiogenic blood vessel atrophy (devascularization) and their replacement with collagen-rich scar tissue (Whaley and Burt, 1992). If the inflammatory agent persists, the inflammatory lesion becomes chronic, does not heal, and the granulation tissue not only persists, but may hypertrophy.

TGF-β_1 plays a dual role during the course of inflammatory reactions, being proinflammatory at first and immunosuppressive later (Wahl, 1992). Dysregulated production of TGF-β_1 is usually associated with fibrotic and proliferative inflammatory diseases (Kilkarni and Karlsson, 1993). For instance, a central pathological feature of glomerulonephritis is the excessive accumulation of ECM within the glomeruli due to overexpression of TGF-β (Okuda et $al.$, 1990). Administration of antibodies to TGF-β to glomerulonephritic rats suppresses glomerular matrix production and accumulation (Border et $al.$, 1990). The proteoglycan decorin, an ECM component induced by TGF-β, binds TGF-β and neutralizes its biological activity, thereby acting as a natural regulator of TGF-β activity (Border et $al.$, 1990). Decorin has been shown to protect against scarring in experimental glomerulonephritis in rats (Border et $al.$, 1992) and may prove useful in the clinical treatment of diseases associated with overexpression of TGF-β in organs such as kidney, lung and liver.

CYTOKINES AND THE PATHOGENESIS OF DISEASES

Cytokines play a pivotal role in maintaining homeostatic mechanisms required for the well-being of the host, but any imbalance in the production and action of cytokines and/ or their receptors and cellular response elements, will disturb homeostatic processes

Table 6. Diseases related to excessive fibroblast growth factor activity.

Atherosclerosis
Rheumatoid arthritis
Cirrhosis
Psoriasis
Sarcoidosis
Idiopathic pulmonary fibrosis
Tumour development

Table 7. Fibrotic disorders (inappropriate deposition of fibrotic tissue or unresolved inflammatory response).

Pulmonary fibrosis
Scleroderma
Rheumatoid arthritis
Cirrhosis

and have pathological consequences (Duff, 1989; Meager, 1990). TNF-α is a cytokine with pleiotropic effects upon cell growth, inflammation and immune responsiveness (Cerami, 1992). Whereas the local effects of TNF-α are often beneficial to the host, when generated at higher concentrations within chronic inflammatory lesions the proinflammatory effects of TNF-α often become systemic. Infusion of bacterial endotoxin causes a sharp rise in TNF-α concentrations within the plasma and induces many of the symptoms of sepsis (Cannon et al., 1990; Martich et al., 1991). Infusion of TNF-α duplicates the symptoms, and elicits the same cascade of mediators as those encountered in sepsis (Marks et al., 1990; van den Poll et al., 1990), indicating the pathogenic role of TNF-α in sepsis. Antibodies to TNF-α can protect against the lethal effects of endotoxaemia (Beutler, 1990; Opal et al., 1991; Cerami, 1992). In bacterial meningitis, the severity of inflammation correlates with the concentration of TNF-α within the cerebrospinal fluid (Beutler, 1990; Cerami, 1992). TNF-α also plays a disease-promoting role in severe murine malaria, involving a lethal neurological syndrome with all the clinical and histopathological features of cerebral malaria (Curfs et al., 1990; Grau et al., 1990). TNF-α induces a shedding of TNF-α receptors which can complex with circulating TNF-α, and serve to limit the severity of TNF-α-induced pathophysiological effects (Engelmann et al., 1990; van der Poll et al., 1992).

Thus, cytokines can be viewed as double-edged swords, benefiting the host when their production and actions are regulated, but posing a threat to the host when their production and actions are unregulated. Such imbalances can have profound influences on acute and chronic inflammation and can contribute to the pathogenesis of diseases related to angiogenesis (Table 5), excessive fibroblast growth factor activity (Table 6) and fibrotic disorders (Table 7), as well as to the pathogenesis of autoimmune diseases such as rheumatoid arthritis, and the development of malignant tumours (Balkwill, 1989a; Meager, 1990; Mire-Sluis, 1993).

CYTOKINES AND RHEUMATOID ARTHRITIS

The synovium within normal joints covers all intra-articular structures, except articular cartilage, and consists of a layer of fibrous tissue containing synoviocytes which consists of type I macrophage-like synoviocytes, type II synoviocytes which are HLA-DR positive, and type III fibroblast-like synoviocytes (Ziff, 1990). Rheumatoid arthritis is a chronic inflammatory autoimmune disease of joints which is initiated by certain antigens and viruses, such as Epstein-Barr virus and human parvoviruses, and endogenous antigens, such as IgG and type II collagen. It is believed that the type II synoviocytes process and present antigens along with the HLA-DR molecules to $CD4^+$ T cells within the rheumatoid synovium, and that the T cells release IFN-γ and TNF-α (Brennan et al., 1989) (see Fig. 5). In response to stimulation with IFN-γ and TNF-α the type III synoviocytes release three electrophoretically distinct species of MCP-1 (Arend, 1993). MCP-1 is a potent chemotactic and activating cytokine for monocytes and plays an important role in recruiting inflammatory monocytes to the rheumatoid joint (Arend, 1993). TGF-β produced by the synovial macrophages is not only chemotactic for monocytes, but also induces the production of IL-1 and TNF-α within these cells (Arend, 1993). The IL-1, IL-6, IL-8, CSFs and TNF-α detected within rheumatoid joints are produced by type I synoviocytes and by monocytes within the synovial fluid (Harris, 1990b; Arend, 1993). The cytokines IL-1, TNF-α and IFN-γ induce ·NO synthesis by endothelial cells, macrophages and PMN leukocytes, and the elevated serum and synovial fluid nitrite levels in rheumatoid and osteoarthritic patients compared with matched control individuals reflects elevated production of ·NO within the inflamed synovium (Farrell et al., 1992).

IL-1 has an autocrine effect upon its own synthesis by articular chondrocytes (Seid et al., 1993), smooth muscle cells and endothelial cells (Warner et al., 1987a,b), synoviocytes and monocytes (Dinarello, 1991), and therefore contributes to the amplification of IL-1 production within arthritic joints. IL-1 also induces overproduction of IL-8 (Larsen et al., 1989) which is produced by fibroblasts (Larsen et al., 1989), endothelial cells (Strieter et al., 1989), chondrocytes (van Damme et al., 1990) and monocytes (Mukaida et al., 1989; Seitz et al., 1991). IL-1 also induces overproduction of CSFs (Seelentag et al., 1989), which have been detected within the rheumatoid synovium (Firestein et al., 1990). The CSFs amplify the disease process by stimulating the production of IL-1 (Lindemann et al., 1988), upregulating HLA-DR expression on type II synoviocytes and enhancing the production and activation of monocytes (Xu et al., 1989; Harris, 1990b).

Macrophages within the synovium orchestrate the disease process through the release of cytokines (Harris, 1990b), and PDGF and FGFs produced by the macrophages stimulate the proliferation of synovial fibroblasts (Beutler, 1990), whereas TGF-β stimulates the production of ECM by the fibroblasts (Wong and Wahl, 1990). These events, along with the TNF-α-mediated stimulation of an angiogenic response within the synovial vasculature, are responsible for the proliferation of the type III synoviocytes (Harris, 1990b). The synovium becomes hyperplastic, contains large numbers of perivascular lymphoid nodules, and is thrown into villous folds that project into the synovial cavity. A pannus of granulation tissue extends from the inflamed synovium and grows over, and erodes, the articular cartilage; the subchondral bone also undergoes resorption by osteoclasts (Harris, 1990b; Reid, 1992). The biological processes that

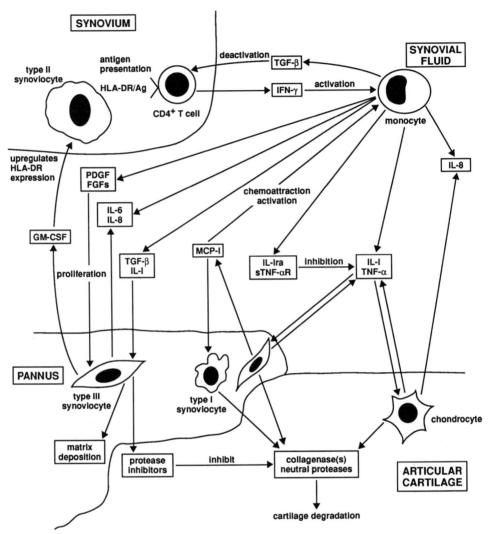

Fig. 5. Diagrammatic representation of key cellular interactions involving chondrocytes, CD4[+]T cells and synoviocytes (types I, II, III) involved in facets of the pathogenesis of rheumatoid arthritis within articulated joints, which are orchestrated by inflammatory monocytes and which are mediated by monocyte-derived cytokines (IL-1, IL-6, IL-8, TNF-α, PDGF, FGFs and TGF-β). The proinflammatory effects of cytokines such as IL-1 and TNF-α are partially inhibited by the endogenous inhibitors IL-1Ra and sTNF-αR. The continued influx of inflammatory monocytes into the inflamed joint in response to the chemotactic protein MCP-1 generated by type I synoviocytes amplifies the pathogenic events within the rheumatoid joint. Articular cartilage erosion results from the stimulation by IL-1 and TNF-α of the production of proteases (collagenase(s) and neutral proteases) by type I synoviocytes and chondrocytes. The actions of the proteases are regulated by the production of protease inhibitors. Pannus tissue formation results from stimulation of proliferation of type III synoviocytes by PDGF and FGFs and the TGF-β and IL-1-mediated deposition of extracellular matrix by the type III synoviocytes. The production of GM-CSF by type III synoviocytes induces the upregulation of HLA-DR molecule expression on type II synoviocytes, thereby enhancing their ability to present autoantigens to CD4[+]T cells within lymphoid follicles in the inflamed synovium of arthritic joints.

contribute to cartilage destruction in rheumatoid arthritis involve interactions between the cytokines IL-1 and TNF-α and the various cell types found within the rheumatoid joints. TNF-α stimulates the production of PGE$_2$ and collagenase by synovial fibroblasts and articular cartilage chondrocytes (Dayer et al., 1985; Husby and Williams, 1988; Yocum et al., 1989). Along with IL-1 and TNF-α, MCP-1 also induces the release of metalloproteinases by macrophages (Firestein et al., 1990). CSFs and IL-6 induce bone resorption by stimulating the differentiation of osteoclasts (Macdonald et al., 1986).

TGF-β reduces the expression of collagenases within fibroblasts while increasing the production of protease inhibitors such as PAI-1 and tissue inhibitor of metalloproteinases (Overall et al., 1989, 1991), and these inhibitors reduce the intensity of collagen degradation within the articular cartilage. Nevertheless, degradation of the collagen by the actions of metalloproteinases and neutral proteases within the articular cartilage generates arthritogenic collagen peptide autoantigens which amplify the inflammatory autoimmune reaction (Harris, 1990b). The accumulation of activated macrophages generating IL-1 and TNF-α is believed to aggravate the inflammatory cycle within the rheumatoid synovium (Firestein et al., 1990), and once initiated, the disease process appears to be self-perpetuating (Harris, 1990b). The presence of endogenous inhibitors such as soluble cytokine receptors and IL-1Ra serve to limit the actions of the proinflammatory cytokines, and hence limit the severity of the disease (Harris, 1990b; Dinarello, 1991; Fernandez-Botran, 1991; Arend, 1993).

CYTOKINES AND CANCER

Neoplastic cells frequently contain the cellular homologues of retroviral oncogenes, and the regulation of cell proliferation becomes deranged when these genes are activated (Balkwill, 1989a,b; Marshall, 1989). Some of the oncogenes stimulate cell proliferation by encoding growth factors, growth factor receptors or components of the signal transduction pathway (Marshall, 1989; Travali et al., 1990). For instance, the oncogenes hst and int-2 encode the FGFs, c-sis encodes the B chain of PDGF, c-erb-B encodes the EFG-R, and c-fms encodes M-CSFR; the oncogenes erb-B2 and met encode proteins which are truncated receptors with tyrosine kinase activity. Oncogenes which encode components of the signal transduction pathway include ras (which encodes G proteins), jun, fos and myc (which encode components of transcription factors) and src, lck and abl (which encode cytoplasmic tyrosine kinases).

Amplification of oncogene expression within neoplastic cells may be responsible for the expression of genes, including cytokine genes, within neoplastic cells (Nishizawa et al., 1990; Suzuki et al., 1991). For instance, the tax gene not only regulates HTLV gene expression within infected T cells, butt also transactivates the expression of genes for IL-2 and IL-2R (Siekevitz et al., 1987; Ballard et al., 1988), GM-CSF (Nimer et al., 1989), IL-3, IL-4 (Ratner, 1989) as well as overexpression of c-sis (Ratner, 1989) and c-fos (Fujii et al., 1988). The overexpression of c-fos, c-sis and GM-CSF gene within HTLV-infected T cells may be involved in the deregulation of cell growth in leukaemogenesis (Feuer and Chen, 1992). M-CSF is generated by human acute myelogenous leukaemia (AML) cells (Rambaldi et al., 1988) and ovarian and breast carcinoma cells (Ramakrishnan et al., 1989) and various sizes of M-CSF transcripts have been identified in human neoplastic cells (Wong et al., 1987; Rajavashisth et al., 1987).

Differential splicing of mRNA is thought to be responsible for the production of the multiple M-CSF transcripts (Ladner *et al.*, 1987), and studies within murine systems have indicated cell-type-specific preferential expression of the different M-CSF transcripts (Pollard *et al.*, 1987).

The oncogene *erb*-B2 encodes the EGF-R (Marshall, 1989) which is overexpressed in many human neoplastic cells and is of prognostic significance in certain types of malignancy (Harris, 1990a; Gullick, 1991). Cells with an elevated surface expression of EGF-R have a high tumorigenic potential (Velu, 1990), and there is evidence that the EGF-R is involved in an autocrine stimulatory loop which enhances the growth of malignant cells (di Marco *et al.*, 1989; Kurachi *et al.*, 1991; Modjtahedi *et al.*, 1993). Coexpression of growth factors and their corresponding receptors occurs rarely in normal tissue cells, but occurs more frequently in malignant cells, thereby establishing an autocrine circuit of growth stimulation (Perosio and Brooks, 1989; Roberts and Sporn, 1990). Haemopoietic growth factor receptors for IL-3, GM-CSF and G-CSF are expressed on the surfaces of AML and acute lymphocytic leukaemia (ALL) cells, and autocrine growth stimulation renders these leukaemia cells independent of exogenous growth factor stimulation, and is a critical step in the genesis of myeloid leukaemias (Lowenberg and Touw, 1993).

Certain oncogenes encode growth factor receptors with structural lesions, including truncated receptors that lack a ligand binding site but retain high intrinsic kinase activity in the cytoplasmic domain; such truncated receptors divert the malignant cells to a mode of continuous proliferation (Roberts and Sporn, 1990). Infection of cells with oncogenic viruses alters the growth properties of the infected cells; for instance, the genome of the myeloproliferative leukaemia virus (MPLV) encodes a fusion protein, consisting of an envelope protein coupled to a truncated haemopoietin receptor, and this mutated form of the receptor may be involved in the leukaemic transformation of haemopoietic cells (Souyri *et al.*, 1990).

A neoplasm consists of neoplastic cells and stromal cells (e.g. fibroblasts, endothelial cells and inflammatory leukocytes), and the complex process of development of a neoplasm involves autocrine and paracrine interactions between the numerous cell types which produce, and respond to, a variety of cytokines (van den Hooff, 1988; Balkwill, 1989a,b, 1990; Pugh-Humphreys, 1992). The stromal response is an important growth determinant for neoplastic lesions (van den Hooff, 1988; Pugh-Humphreys, 1992), and although initiated and propagated by different mechanisms, the processes of granulation tissue formation within inflammatory lesions and the development of the neoplastic stroma share many features, including fibroplasia and angiogenesis (Dvorak, 1986; Whalen, 1990; Pugh-Humphreys, 1992). CSFs produced by cells within neoplastic lesions stimulate the production of inflammatory leukocytes from stem cells within the bone marrow and spleen, resulting in peripheral blood leukocytosis and splenomegally due to myelomonocytic hyperplasia (Feuer and Chen, 1992; Pugh-Humphreys, 1992). Neoplastic lesions produce a plethora of cytokines which influence the recruitment into, and activation of leukocytes within, the stroma; these leukocytes, along with the endothelial cells and fibroblasts produce cytokines (van den Hooff, 1988; Balkwill, 1989a,b, 1990; Whalen, 1990; Pugh-Humphreys, 1992).

The development of solid neoplasms is angiogenesis dependent (Denekamp, 1990; Klagsburn and Folkman, 1990), and the development of the vasculature, as well as the production of abundant peritumoural connective tissue (called the desmoplastic response), result from the secretion by neoplastic cells and/or stromal cells of angiogenic cytokines such as TGF-α, TGF-β, PDGF, EGF, IGF-1 and FGFs (van den Hooff, 1988; Klagsburn and Folkman, 1990; Clarke *et al.*, 1992; Pugh-Humphreys, 1992). FGF-2 is a potent angiogenic cytokine, and the deranged expression of FGF-2 by retinoblastoma, melanoma, osteosarcoma and hepatoma cells may induce both autocrine growth stimulation of these cells and angiogenesis. It is believed that aberrant autocrine regulation of neoplastic cell growth may involve alterations in TGF-β secretion or activity, or loss of TGF-β receptor expression on neoplastic cells (Roberts and Sporn, 1990). The actions of the TGF-βs are regulated by oestrogen (Arrick *et al.*, 1990) and the anti-neoplastic effects of the anti-oestrogen Tamoxifen in patients with breast carcinomas have been ascribed to an increase in the secretion of locally active TGF-β_1 from breast carcinoma cells (Knabbe *et al.*, 1987) and stromal fibroblasts (Coletta *et al.*, 1990). Since the metastatic behaviour of malignant neoplasms, such as breast carcinomas, is strongly linked to the degradation of basal lamellae by collagenases (Liotta *et al.*, 1991) and since TGF-β_1 inhibits the synthesis of collagenases (Moses, 1990), then stimulation of TGF-β_1 synthesis and activity probably explains the anti-neoplastic effects of Tamoxifen.

Neoplasms can be regarded as cytokine generating units; although the cytokines generated exert autocrine and paracrine effects within the microenvironment of a neoplastic lesion, some cytokines, such as IL-6 and TNF-α, may spill over into the circulation and exert systemic physiological effects within the host which are characteristic of malignancy (Balkwill, 1989a,b, 1990). IL-6 is a multifunctional cytokine (Akira *et al.*, 1993) and appears to be important in the pathogenesis of myelomas and lymphocytic leukaemias where the IL-6 generated by the neoplastic cells acts as a growth stimulant. IL-6 is present in the serum of myeloma patients with progressive disease, and may be responsible for the osteolysis and hypercalcaemia found in 20–50% of patients with myelomas, since IL-6 induces the differentiation of osteoclasts which cause bone resorption. These patients could benefit from therapy with antibodies directed against IL-6 or IL-6R (Akira *et al.*, 1993; Sato *et al.*, 1993a) or with IL-6 antagonists (Mire-Sluis, 1993).

TNF-α has been detected within the circulation of cancer patients (Balkwill, 1989a, b, 1990, 1993) and is detectable in a variety of neoplastic cells (Cordingley *et al.*, 1988; Hoang *et al.*, 1989; Lindemann *et al.*, 1989; Kobari *et al.*, 1990; Naylor *et al.*, 1990; Sappino *et al.*, 1990). Although TNF-α can exert cytostatic and cytotoxic effects upon neoplastic cells *in vitro* and *in vivo* (Balkwill, 1989a; Nathan, 1990), there is evidence that TNF-α can enhance the proliferation of neoplastic cells in a dose-dependent fashion (El-Badry *et al.*, 1989; Goillot *et al.*, 1992) and may even induce tumour angiogenesis (Klagsburn and Folkman, 1990). TNF-α is also involved, along with IL-1, in inducing the cachectic state within cancer patients (Balkwill, 1989a, 1990). Although at one time TNF-α was advocated as a therapeutic agent in the treatment of cancer, the clinical trials on the therapeutic effects of TNF-α in cancer patients have been disappointing (Lienard *et al.*, 1992; Spriggs and Yates, 1992) and TNF-α may even exert adverse effects (Balkwill, 1993). An alternative therapeutic strategy would involve the administration of antibodies directed against TNF-α or its receptors, or the administration of inhibitors or antagonists such as mutant TNF-α molecules (Ostade *et al.*, 1993).

There are reports that generation of systemic immunity to neoplastic cells has been achieved following vaccination of hosts with neoplastic cells genetically engineered to produce different cytokines (Russell, 1990) such as IL-2 (Fearon *et al.*, 1990; Gansbacher *et al.*, 1990), IL-4 (Golumbeck *et al.*, 1991), IL-7 (Aoki *et al.*, 1992; McBride *et al.*, 1992), TNF-α and IFN-γ (Watanabe *et al.*, 1989; Gansbacher *et al.*, 1990). However, these studies did not establish whether the generation of the systemic immunity observed was due to the cytokines secreted by the neoplastic cells, or to the exposure by moribund neoplastic cells of antigens to the immune system during primary rejection of the neoplastic cells. Hock *et al.* (1993) report that J558L murine plasmacytoma cells engineered to produce IL-2, IL-4, IL-7, TNF-α and IFN-γ were no more effective as immunogens in the generation of systemic immunity within Balb/c mice, than the parental J558L cells admixed and administered with the adjuvant *Corynebacterium parvum*.

CYTOKINES AND THEIR RECEPTORS AS THERAPEUTIC TARGETS

Although there are numerous clinical applications for cytokines in the therapy of diseases (Balkwill, 1989a; Dallman and Clark, 1992), the involvement of cytokines in the pathogenesis of diseases has prompted the development of strategies for targeting cytokines and their receptors as therapeutic manoeuvres for inhibiting cytokine action in the treatment of cytokine-mediated disease processes. The actions of cytokines can be inhibited at several levels (see Fig. 6) through the use of (1) signal transduction inhibitors (i.e. inhibitors of second messenger production), (2) drugs which function as transcription and translation inhibitors, (3) agents which prevent cytokine action by binding soluble cytokines (e.g. monoclonal antibodies (mAbs), soluble cytokine receptors, cytokine binding proteins), and (4) agents which interfere with the binding of cytokines to their receptors (e.g. mAbs or antagonists).

INTERFERING WITH THE ACTIONS OF CYTOKINES BY THE USE OF SIGNAL TRANSDUCTION INHIBITORS

Signal transduction inhibitors are low-molecular-weight, nonprotein drugs which interfere with the generation of intracellular signals following cytokine-receptor binding. Both PKC and PTK are targets for inhibitor development since they are involved in the signal transduction mechanisms associated with cytokine receptors.

In the case of receptors belonging to the HCR family, binding of the cytokine (e.g, IL-2, IL-3, IL-4, IL-5, IL-6, IL-7, GM-CSF, EPO and CNTF) to the respective receptor, activates intracellular PTKs which catalyse the tyrosine-specific phosphorylation of cytoplasmic proteins, some of which may be downstream signalling molecules such as serine–threonine kinases (e.g. c-raf), or p21ras. Inhibitors of PTK activity, such as herbimycin A, block the formation of the GTP-bound form of p21 ras (activated ras) when cells are stimulated by IL-3, IL-5, GM-CSF and EPO (Satoh *et al.*, 1992). PTK inhibitors, such as the tyrphostins, block the actions of tyrosine kinases associated with growth factor receptors (e.g. PDGF-R and EGF-R) and are potential antiproliferative agents (Levitzki, 1990). PKC inhibitors such as chelerythrine and hypericin have been used clinically in the treatment of diseases including periodontal inflammatory disease (chelerythrine; Cerna, 1989), and as anti-viral agents (hypericin; Takahashi *et al.*, 1989;

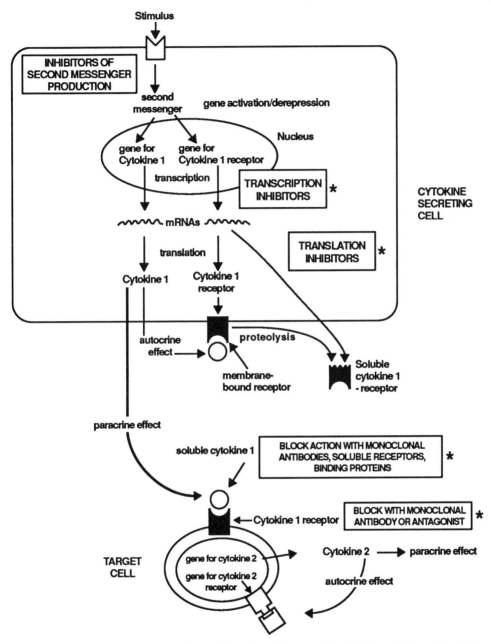

Fig. 6. Diagrammatic representation of the actions of cytokines on cells within the cytokine network. The activation of cytokine and cytokine receptor genes with cytokine-secreting cells, and the sites of interference with gene expression using inhibitors of second-messenger production as well as transcription and translation inhibitors, are indicated. Cytokine-secreting cells not only release cytokines which can exert autocrine or paracrine actions, but they can also synthesize cytokine receptors, some of which are membrane bound but can be cleaved extracellularly to be released as soluble cytokine receptors, whereas others are released directly as soluble receptors. The interactions of cytokines with cells can be blocked using antibodies directed either against the cytokines and/or against their receptors. Cytokines can induce the release of other cytokines within target cells through activation of the relevant cytokine genes.

Carpenter and Kraus, 1991). Both PKC and PTK inhibitors have proved useful in the treatment of osteosarcomas, SLE and cerebral malaria (Mire-Sluis, 1993).

IMMUNOSUPPRESSIVE DRUGS THAT INTERFERE WITH CYTOKINE PRODUCTION OR THE RESPONSES OF LYMPHOCYTES TO GROWTH FACTORS

The structurally distinct fungal metabolites cyclosporin A (CsA) and FK 506 are potent immunosuppressive agents that mediate their antilymphocytic activity by a strong inhibitory action on T cell cytokine production (reviewed by Ryffel, 1989; Thomson, 1990). The inhibitory effect of these drugs on T-cell driven responses is due to their capacity to suppress the activation of certain cytokine genes, including those encoding IL-2, IL-3, IL-4, IL-5, IFN-γ and GM-CSF. Inhibition of the production of IL-2 contributes much of the immunosuppressive activity both of CsA and FK 506, including inhibition of the clonal expansion of T cells (CD4$^+$ and CD8$^+$ subsets), upregulation of IL-2R expression, production of other proinflammatory cytokines such as IFN-γ, stimulation of B cells and monocytes, and support for the development of cytotoxic T lymphocytes.

Detailed studies on the modes of action of CsA and FK 506 at the molecular level have revealed that neither agent is, by itself, antilymphocytic. Rather, each of these drugs is now perceived as a molecular adaptor that mediates the interaction between its respective intracellular drug-binding protein (or immunophilin) and its ultimate individual target molecule. In the case of CsA, the appropriate family of drug-binding proteins is the cyclophilins and in the case of FK 506, the FK 506-binding proteins (FKBPs). Intensive research on the mode of action of FK 506 and CsA (Liu *et al.*, 1991; Liu, 1993) has revealed that the heterodimeric, Ca^{++}/calmodulin-regulated phosphatase calcineurin is a major common target of the CsA-cyclophilin A and FK 506-FKBP12 drug–immunophilin complexes *in vitro* (note, cyclophilin A and FKBP12 are the predominant immunophilin isoforms that bind CsA and FK 506, respectively). Although rapamycin, a powerful immunosuppressant related structurally to FK 506, also binds to FKBP, it fails to inhibit calcineurin activity and acts on T-cell proliferation by a quite distinct molecular mechanism (see below).

It is now recognized that calcineurin is a key enzyme in the T-cell signal transduction cascade following T-cell receptor (TCR) activation (Clipstone and Crabtree, 1992; Liu *et al.*, 1992; O'Keefe *et al.*, 1992). Furthermore, inhibition of calcineurin phosphatase activity, and not CsA affinity for cyclophilin A, correlates with the suppression of early T cell activation events (Nelson *et al.*, 1993). Among the most important conclusions from these observations is that interaction of drug–immunophilin complexes with calcineurin and inhibition of its phosphatase activity provides a molecular basis for the inhibitory effect of CsA or FK 506 on expression of genes encoding IL-2 and other cytokines.

Since both CsA and FK 506 inhibit, specifically, the TCR-mediated transcription of the IL-2 gene, its promoter region and in particular, the binding site for the nuclear factor of activated T-cells (NFAT), has been the focus of intensive investigation. NFAT is a T-cell-specific transcription factor, the activity of which correlates with the extent of IL-2 gene transcription following activation of the TCR. NF-AT has two components— a nuclear (n) subunit (NF-ATn) and a cytoplasmic (c) component (NF-ATc). An important finding is that the CsA/FK 506 drug–immunophilin complexes, which form

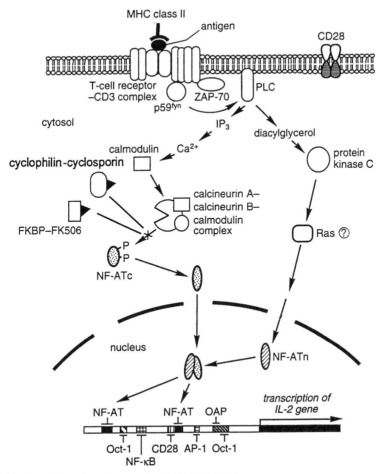

Fig. 7. Molecular actions of cyclosporin A and FK 506. The T-cell receptor-mediated signal transduction pathway leading to IL-2 transcription is shown with the recently identified signal transducing molecules highlighted. PLC, phospholipase Cγ1; IP$_3$, inositol-1,4,5-trisphosphate; NF-ATc, the cytoplasmic component of the nuclear factor of activated T cells; NF-ATn, the nuclear component of NF-AT; FKBP, FK 506 binding protein. Reproduced from Liu J., *Immunology Today* **14**, 293, 1993 with kind permission of the author and Elsevier Science Publishers Ltd.

pentameric complexes with calcineurin (A and B) and calmodulin (see Fig. 7) block the assembly of functional NF-AT (Flanagan *et al.*, 1991). It appears that this is achieved by inhibition of translocation of the pre-existing NF-ATc from the cytoplasm to the nucleus. NF-ATn is transcriptionally inactive in all cells other than activated T cells and is induced by signals from the TCR. Its appearance is not blocked by FK 506 or CsA. Current thinking is that FK 506 and CsA block the dephosphorylation by calcineurin of NF-ATc, a step that is required for its translocation to the nucleus.

This model has gained credence from the finding of McCaffrey *et al.* (1993) that NF-ATc is indeed a phosphoprotein in resting T-cells and can be dephosphorylated by calcineurin. Moreover, the same group has shown that dephosphorylation of NF-ATc by calcineurin in cell lysates can be inhibited by a specific peptide inhibitor of

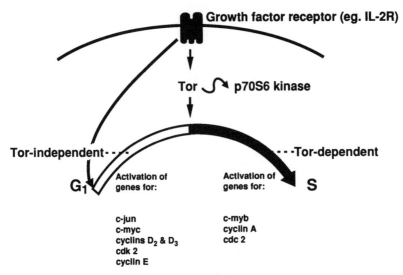

Fig. 8. A model for the mechanism of action of rapamycin. IL-2-mediated signalling activates two distinct pathways: a target of rapamycin (Tor)-independent pathway and a Tor-dependent pathway. The Tor-dependent pathway is simply defined as being inhibited by rapamycin. Rapamycin blocks cell cycle progression at a point where many early to mid-G1 cell-cycle-regulatory proteins have accumulated (cyclins D2, D3 and E) yet are unable to execute their function without an additional triggering event(s). The activation of the cyclin E/CDK2 kinase complex, which is blocked by rapamycin, could be the triggering event required for progression into the S phase of the cell-cycle. For details see Flanagan and Crabtree (1993).

calcineurin or by pretreatment of the cells with CsA or FK 506. These data suggest both that NF-ATc may be the direct substrate of calcineurin and that it may serve as the ultimate protein messenger of the signal transduction cascade from the cell surface TCR to the nucleus.

In T-cells, activation of the genes both for IL-2 and its receptor determines the progression of the cell from the G0 to the G1 phase of the cell cycle. G1 to S stage progression is then regulated by IL-2. The powerful immunosuppressive drug rapamycin (Morris, 1992) is a close structural analogue of FK 506 and binds to the same immunophilin (FKBP) as FK 506, forming a drug–immunophilin (rapamycin-FKBP) complex (Schreiber, 1991). However, this complex does not inhibit calcineurin activity (Liu *et al.*, 1991) or G0 to G1 progression, as defined by the expression of IL-2 or IL-2R. Recently, however, it has been shown that rapamycin potently inhibits the rapid activation of p70S6 kinase following IL-2 stimulation of T-cells and consequently, G1-to-S phase progression (Chung *et al.*, 1992; Kuo *et al.*, 1992). Although this finding implicates p70S6 kinase activation as important in Ca^{++}-independent signalling leading to cell proliferation, there is no evidence that p70S6 kinase is involved directly in S-phase entry. Conversely, recent results obtained using the murine helper T-cell clone D10, have demonstrated that the IL-2-stimulated expression of a serine–threonine kinase p34 cdc2, that is known to be required for cell cycle progression and may be essential for G1 to S transition, is a target of rapamycin (Flanagan and Crabtree, 1993).

A model for the action of rapamycin is shown in Fig. 8. In this model (for further details see Flanagan and Crabtree, 1993 and Flanagan *et al.*, 1993), IL-2 signalling via the IL-2R activates both target of rapamycin (Tor)-independent and Tor-dependent

Table 8. The use of mAbs directed against cytokines in the treatment of diseases.

Disease/Disorder	Pathogenic Cytokine	Therapeutic intervention
Myeloma	IL-6	anti-IL-6-mAb
Breast carcinoma	TGF-β	anti-TGF-β mAb
Fibrosis	TGF-β	anti-TGF-β mAb
Lymphoid leukaemia	TNF-α	anti-TNF-α mAb
Rheumatoid arthritis	TNF-α	anti-TNF-α mAb
Multiple sclerosis	TNF-α	anti-TNF-α mAb
Septic shock	TNF-α	anti-TNF-α mAb

pathways. It is thought that rapamycin blocks G1 to S progression at a point where many early to mid-G1 cell-cycle-regulatory proteins (cyclins D2, D3 and E) have accumulated, yet are unable to fulfil their function without additional triggering events. Activation of the cyclin E/cdk2 complex, which is blocked by rapamycin, may be the triggering event required for progression into S phase.

Rapamycin is clearly a valuable tool for analysis of autocrine growth-factor receptor-induced signalling events and their linkage to downstream targets that regulate cell cycle S-phase entry. The reliance of T lymphocytes on a single (IL-2–IL-2R) signalling pathway renders these cells uniquely susceptible to the growth-inhibitory properties of rapamycin.

The recent discovery that calcineurin and p70S6 kinases are important signalling mediators clearly emphasizes the utility of immunosuppressive drugs as probes of lymphocyte signal transduction in addition to their important roles as clinical immuno-suppressive agents.

AGENTS THAT PREVENT CYTOKINE ACTION BY BINDING SOLUBLE CYTOKINES

Monoclonal Antibodies (mAbs)

Monoclonal antibodies directed against specific cytokines have been used in the treatment of a number of diseases (see Table 8). However, since murine monoclonal antibodies are immunogenic in humans, their therapeutic value in the clinic has been disappointing, and consequently attempts have been made to engineer the antibodies to make them more human-like to improve their clinical performance. The most complete humanization of a murine antibody is achieved by grafting the CDRs from a murine antibody framework to create a functional antigen-binding site in a reshaped human antibody (Riechmann et al., 1988; Kettleborough et al., 1991).

A human IgG$_1$ mouse Fv chimaeric antibody directed against TNF-α, called cA2 and produced commercially by Celltech, is currently being used as an immunomodulating agent in the therapy of rheumatoid arthritis (cited in Mire-Sluis, 1993).

Soluble Cytokine Receptors

The circulating levels of certain soluble cytokine receptors, e.g. sIL-2R, are elevated in clinical patients with certain disease states (see Table 9), and there is reason to believe that soluble cytokine receptors may function as physiological modulators of cytokine

Table 9. Disease states associated with elevated plasma levels of soluble IL-2 receptors.

Lymphoblastic lymphomas
Non-Hodgkins' lymphoma
B-cell chronic lymphocytic leukaemia (B-CLL)
Hairy cell leukaemia
Rheumatoid arthritis
Systemic lupus erythematosus (SLE)
Atopic eczema
Type 1 diabetes
Psoriasis
Malaria
Tuberculosis
Acquired immunodeficiency syndrome (AIDS)

Table 10. The use of soluble cytokine receptors in the treatment of diseases.

Disease/Disorder	Pathogenic Cytokine	Therapeutic intervention
Myeloma	IL-6	sIL-6R
Myeloid leukaemia	IL-1	sIL-1R
Lymphoid leukaemia	IL-2	sIL-2R
Rheumatoid arthritis	IL-1	sIL-1R
Ankylosing spondylitis	IL-1	sIL-1R
Type 1 diabetes	IL-1	sIL-1R
	IL-4	sIL-4R
Systemic lupus erythematosus	IL-2	sIL-2R
Multiple sclerosis	IL-1	sIL-1R
Septic shock	IL-1	sIL-1R

action and could have clinical significance as cytokine inhibitors (Fernandez-Botran, 1991). Soluble receptors which bind a range of cytokines, including IL-1, IL-2, IL-4 and IL-6, may be used as immunomodulating agents (Fernandez-Botran, 1991) and are undergoing clinical trials in the treatment of a number of diseases (see Table 10) (Mire-Sluis, 1993).

Although soluble cytokine receptors can inhibit the binding of cytokines to their respective membrane-anchored receptors, there are instances where the soluble receptors can enhance the action of the respective cytokine. For instance, sIL-6R enhances the action of IL-6 when the Il-6/sIL-6R complex associates with the plasma membrane-anchored gp130 signal transducer; under these circumstances the IL-6/sIL-6R complex can mimic the actions of OM, LIF or CNTF (Akira *et al.*, 1993).

Cytokine binding Proteins

In addition to autoantibodies and α_2-macroglobulin which can bind cytokines, biological fluids also contain other cytokine binding proteins which may be derived from cytokine receptors. For instance the 30 kDa, highly glycosylated TNF-α binding protein (TNF-BP) found in human fluids is a polypeptide derived from the transmembrane TNF-receptor molecules and can block the inflammatory and harmful effects of TNF-α (Fernandez-Botran, 1991).

AGENTS THAT INTERFERE WITH THE BINDING OF CYTOKINES TO THEIR RECEPTORS

Antibodies to Cytokine Receptors as Immunomodulating Agents

An ideal immunosuppressive therapy should be effective in controlling the overall immune response as well as targeting selectively only those lymphoid cells that are committed to participate in the undesired immune reaction. Whereas conventional immunosuppressive drugs (e.g. prednisolone, hydrocortisone and dexamethasone) exact unwanted side effects on nonlymphoid tissues, the introduction of T-cell-specific mAbs as pharmacological tools has obviated many of these effects by providing a far more target-directed form of immunosuppressive therapy (Stroobant, 1990).

IL-2 and IL-2R: Model Targets for Therapeutic Intervention

The interaction of IL-2 with IL-2R plays an essential role in both the proliferation and differentiation of allostimulated T cells (Smith, 1989). High-affinity IL-2R are only transiently expressed upon T cells during the antigen-driven proliferative burst, and mAbs directed against the IL-2R should target recently activated T cells (as well as LAK cells and NK cells); these cells mediate hypersensitivity and autoimmune reactions, and thus IL-2R is a promising target for selective immunosuppressive therapy (Diamantstein et al., 1989). Immunosuppression has been achieved through the use of antibodies directed against IL-2R (Kelley et al., 1988; Kupiec-Weglinski et al., 1989), and in a number of instances the immunosuppressive effects of the anti-IL-2R antibodies have been enhanced by the simultaneous administration of cyclosporin A (Kupiec-Weglinski et al., 1989, 1991a,b; Hancock et al., 1990; Tanaka et al., 1990; Ueda et al., 1990; Higuchi et al., 1991; Steinbruchel et al., 1991, 1992).

Monoclonal antibodies to IL-2R prolong allograft survival across MHC barriers within various animal species (Strom et al., 1988; Thedrez et al., 1989; Okada et al,. 1992; Steinbruchel et al., 1992; van Gelder et al., 1992) and suppress both graft-versus-host (GVH) diseases (Herve et al., 1990, 1992; Blaise et al., 1991) and certain autoimmune reactions (Braley-Mullen et al., 1991). Treatment of mice with the anti-IL-2R mAb, AMT-13, not only prolonged the survival of cardiac allografts, but also caused an increase in the serum levels of sIL-2R (Burkhardt et al., 1989). The 20-fold increase in the titre of sIL-2R in the serum of AMT-13-treated mice is believed to play a role in the immunosuppressive action of AMT-13. Activated T cells and macrophages play an important role in the induction of streptozotocin-induced diabetes in C57BL/6J mice, and the anti-IL-2R mAb M7/20, which recognizes the α-subunit of IL-2R, inhibits autoimmune insulitis in nonobese diabetic (NOD) mice and lupus nephritis within NZB $\times$ NZW F_1 murine hybrids (Kelley et al., 1988).

Following the administration of the first or second dose of murine anti-IL-2R mAbs (e.g. OKT3 and 16H5) to patients, there are elevations in the serum levels of TNF-α, IFN-γ and IL-2 which induce unwanted systemic effects, such as chills, tremors, fever, nausea and vomiting, and neurotoxicity (Horneff et al., 1991). In addition, the formation of neutralizing anti-idiotypic antibodies is a further limiting factor in the use of murine mAbs for immunosuppressive therapy in humans; consequently chimaeric mouse/human anti-IL-2R mAbs have been constructed which are not only less immunogenic than the murine anti-IL-2R mAbs, but are more effective immunological reagents which inhibit human T-cell proliferation (Rose *et al.*, 1992) and elicit ADCC activity not observed with the original murine monoclonals (Waldmann *et al.*, 1990). The hyperchimaeric anti-IL-2Rα (anti-Tac) mAb is more than 95% human and has minimal immunogenicity in humans (Hale *et al.*, 1988; LoBuglio *et al.*, 1989), providing a versatile reagent with clinical applications in the treatment of lymphoid malignancies, allograft rejection, GVH disease and autoimmune diseases (Mire-Sluis, 1993). Humanized anti-Tac monoclonals armed with β-emitting strontium-90 or α-emitting bismuth-212 have been used clinically in radio-isotope therapy of T-cell leukaemias (Pastan *et al.*, 1992).

Antibodies to TNF Receptors and other Cytokine Receptors

Antibodies to TNF receptors can be agonistic as well as antagonistic (Engelmann *et al.*, 1990). Antagonistic antibodies to TNF-R1 completely block several TNF-α activities (Espevik *et al.*, 1990; Shalaby *et al.*, 1990; Naume *et al.*, 1991), whereas monoclonals directed against TNF-R2 only partially antagonize TNF-α activities (Hohmann *et al.*, 1990; Shalaby *et al.*, 1990; Naume *et al.*, 1991). These observations suggest that TNF-R1 is the biologically relevant receptor, and that the binding of TNF-α to TNF-R2 is not sufficient to initiate TNF-α responses within target cells (Thoma *et al.*, 1990). Polyclonal antibodies directed against TNF-R1 and TNF-R2 have been described which behave as specific receptor agonists, and each induces a subset of TNF-α activities (Tartaglia *et al.*, 1991). In mice, TNF-R1 signals cytotoxic effects, fibroblast proliferation and the induction of both NF-κB and manganese-activated superoxide dismutase (MnSOD), while TNF-R2 signals proliferation in thymocytes and T_c cells (Tartaglia *et al.*, 1991). Thus the two TNF receptors are responsible for distinct TNF-α activities.

Not only do antibodies to TNF receptors have agonist activities, but mAbs to the β chain of the IL-2R can also act as agonists in the induction of biological activity in macrophages (Belosevic and Nacy, 1990). The murine monoclonal PM-1 directed against IL-6R, inhibits IL-6 functions and displays anti-tumour activity against multiple myeloma cells (Hirata *et al.*, 1989). The PM-1 mAb has been reshaped and humanized (Sato *et al.*, 1993) and should prove efficacious in the clinical treatment of human multiple myeloma.

CYTOKINE ANTAGONISTS AS THERAPEUTIC REAGENTS

Alternative strategies for blocking cytokine action involve the use of proteins that bind specific cytokine receptors, but which lack the agonist activity of cytokines.

IL-1Ra as a Therapeutic Reagent

IL-1 induces a number of pathophysiological effects during the development of various diseases, and strategies for inhibiting the activities of IL-1 provide a focal point for the therapy of a number of clinical diseases (Dinarello, 1991; Dinarello and Thompson, 1991).

IL-1 plays a major role in the pathogenesis of chronic synovisitis, as well as in damage to articular cartilage and bone within rheumatoid joints (Harris, 1990b; Arend, 1993).

Table 11. The use of IL-1Ra in the treatment of diseases.

Disease/Disorder
Myeloid leukaemia
Rheumatoid arthritis
Ankylosing spondylitis
Type 1 diabetes
Multiple sclerosis
Asthma
Septic shock

The balance between the amounts and secretion of IL-1 and its antagonist, IL-1Ra, may be a critical determinant in the clinical course of rheumatoid arthritis; those patients with high concentrations of IL-1Ra but low concentrations of IL-1β in the synovial fluid have rapid resolution in attacks of rheumatoid arthritis, whereas in the reverse situation, the patients have long intervals to recovery from attacks of rheumatoid arthritis (Miller *et al.*, 1993). Administration of exogenous IL-1Ra, which acts as a natural IL-1 antagonist within rheumatoid joints (Arend, 1993), not only inhibits the influx of inflammatory leukocytes into the synovium and joint cavity, but also blocks the IL-1-mediated degradation of proteoglycans within the articular cartilage (Henderson *et al.*, 1991) and therefore beneficially influences the clinical course of the disease (Arend, 1993). In addition to the treatment of rheumatoid arthritis, IL-1Ra has found clinical application in the treatment of a number of other diseases (see Table 11).

Cytokine Peptides and Muteins as Cytokine Antagonists

IL-1 peptides have been generated which act as IL-1 antagonists. The *C*-terminal portion of mature IL-1β retains some biological activity and an IL-1β subpeptide consisting of residues 237–269 antagonizes the effects of IL-1β on T cells (Palaszynski, 1987) whereas a 21-amino-acid subpeptide (residues 165–186) of human IL-1β exhibits fibroblast stimulatory properties (Herzbeck *et al.*, 1989). A nonapeptide of IL-1β consisting of residues 163–171 activates T cells, stimulates GAG synthesis, recruits anti-tumour reactivity *in vivo*, but lacks the proinflammatory and pyrogenic activities of IL-1. A pentapeptide, consisting of amino acids 165–169 is more potent than the nonapeptide.

PDGF acts as an autocrine or paracrine modulator of neovascularization and can act synergistically with other cytokines (e.g. FGF-2, TGF-β and insulin-like growth factor 1 (IGF-1)) in the process of neovascularization (Satoh *et al.*, 1992). Coexpression of the PDGF-β chain and the PDGF-R has been demonstrated in hyperproliferating micro-vascular endothelial cells in malignant gliomas (Hermansson *et al.*, 1988). The basic *C*-terminal sequence 211 amino acids within PDGF-A is involved in the binding of PDGF-A to cell-surface heparin sulphate proteoglycans (LaRochelle *et al.*, 1990a,b; Ostman *et al.*, 1991) and a peptide identical to this *C*-terminal region is able to compete with, and displaces, attached forms of PDGF and other growth factors (Khachigian *et al.*, 1992; Raines and Ross, 1992) and could have clinical application in the control of angiogenesis-related diseases.

Various muteins of IL-1α/β have been generated by amino acid substitutions within the intact molecules. A single point-mutation of aspartic acid 151 to tyrosine in mature IL-1β generates a mutein that functions as a receptor antagonist for both IL-1α and β. N-terminal mutations have yielded IL-1β muteins with altered biological properties and receptor-binding characteristics (Huang et al., 1987). A single point-mutation of arginine 127 to glycine in human IL-1β results in a 100-fold loss of bioactivity in the IL-1β mutein on T cells without diminishing receptor–ligand binding, and this mutein could function as an IL-1 receptor antagonist. A potent TNF-α antagonist called a TNF-R immunoadhesin, constructed by gene fusion of the extracellular portion of type 1 TNF-R with the constant domains of human IgG heavy chains (TNFR-IgG), has been shown to be effective in protection against endotoxic shock in mice and may have application in the prevention and therapeutic treatment of sepsis in the clinic (Ashkenazi et al., 1991; Mire-Sluis, 1993).

Suramin as a Cytokine Antagonist

Suramin is a polysulphonated naphthyl urea that interferes with the cell proliferation-inducing activities of various growth factors (including IGFs, EGF, PDGF, IL-2, TGF-β and FGFs) by inhibiting the binding of these factors to their respective receptors (Mills et al., 1990; Pollak and Richard, 1990; Foekens et al., 1992; Vignon et al., 1992). Suramin exerts its effect either by directly complexing with the growth factors, or by modifying the respective cell-surface receptors (Coffey et al., 1987). However, direct intracellular effects of suramin cannot be excluded since suramin is internalized and can inhibit the activities of a number of intracellular enzymes (including DNA polymerase, terminal deoxynucleotide transferase, hexokinase and succinic dehydrogenase; Hawking, 1978; Jindal et al., 1990) as well as block the activity of PKC, which is involved in the intracellular signal transduction pathway of growth factors such as the FGFs (Hensey et al., 1989) and the expression of mRNA for FGF receptors (Kasayama et al., 1993).

Suramin inhibits the proliferation of a variety of malignant cells in vitro (Freuhauf et al., 1990; Olivier et al., 1990; Foekens et al., 1992, 1993; Vignon et al., 1992) and consequently has generated much interest in suramin as an anti-tumour agent. Other clinical applications of suramin centre on its ability to interfere with growth factor activity; for instance, FGFs are involved in angiogenesis through stimulation of endothelial-cell proliferation and motility (Klagsbrun and Folkman, 1990) and suramin may have application in the treatment of pathological conditions that are angiogenesis related, in particular inhibition of FGF-2-dependent tumour angiogenesis (Pesenti et al., 1992). Suramin inhibits the proliferation of fibroblasts in response to monocyte-derived growth factors (Kelley and Hildebran, 1987) and may have clinical application in the treatment of those fibrotic disorders which develop within several organ systems and which involve cytokine-driven proliferation of fibroblasts and excessive deposition of extracellular matrix (Kovacs, 1991).

Immunotoxins and Chimaeric Cytotoxic Cytokines as Novel Therapeutic Reagents

The presence of cytokine receptors on the surfaces of diseased cells can be exploited in novel forms of disease therapy using mutant or chimaeric cytokines coupled to toxins.

Pseudomonas exotoxin (PE) is a single-chain toxin secreted by *Pseudomonas aeruginosa* and must be endocytosed in order to kill a target cell; a 40 kDa protein (PE40) derived from PE has been used to generate an immunotoxin by coupling it to antibodies (Pastan *et al.*, 1992). Single-chain antigen-binding antibodies have been constructed by linking the Fv region of antibodies (consisting of two 110-amino-acid fragments from the *N*-termini of the H and L chains) via a linking peptide of approximately 15 amino acids. Several single-chain immunotoxins have been generated from these single-chain antibodies, which have a high affinity for antigens and have PE40 fused to their carboxyl ends (Pastan *et al.*, 1992). The single-chain immunotoxins have been used to direct toxins such as PE40 to target cells, and include an anti-Tac (Fv)–PE40 complex which binds to the IL-2R on human adult T-cell leukaemia cells and inhibits their proliferation (Pastan *et al.*, 1992).

Chimaeric cytotoxins have been made by fusing the PE40 gene to cDNAs coding for cytokines such as IL-2, IL-4, IL-6, FGF-1, IGF-1 and TGF-α (Pastan *et al.*, 1992). These cytotoxins can be used to kill target cells bearing the receptors for the respective cytokines. TGF-α–PE40 targets epidermoid carcinoma cells and adenocarcinoma cells and proliferating smooth muscle cells, whereas IL-6–PE40 targets myeloma and hepatoma cells. IL-2–PE40 targets adult T-cell leukaemia cells and lymphoma cells and has been used in the treatment of inflammatory diseases such as autoimmune arthritis, uveitis and encephalitis (Pastan *et al.*, 1992).

REFERENCES

Abramson, S.L. and Gallin, J.J. (1990). *J. Immunol.* **144**, 625–630.

Adams, D.O. and Hamilton, T.A. (1992). In *The Macrophage* (eds C.E. Lewis and J.O'D. McGee), IRL Press, Oxford, pp. 77–114.

Akira, S., Taga, T. and Kishimoto, T. (1993). *Adv. Immunol.* **54**, 1–78.

Altman, A., Coggeshall, K.M. and Mustelin, T. (1990). *Adv. Immunol.* **48**, 227–360.

Andres, J.L., De Falcis, D., Noda, M. and Massagué J. (1992). *J. Biol. Chem.* **267**, 5927–5930.

Aoki, T., Tashiro, K, Miyatake, S.-I., Kinashi, T., Nakano, T., Oda, Y., Kikuchi, H. and Honjo, T. (1992). *Proc. Natl Acad. Sci. USA* **89**, 3850–3854.

Arai, K., Lee, F., Miyajima, A., Miyatake, S., Arai, N. and Yokota, T. (1990). *Annu. Rev. Biochem.* **59**, 783–836.

Arend, W.P. (1993). *Adv. Immunol.* **54**, 167–227.

Arrick, A.B., Karc, M. and Derynck, R. (1990). *Cancer Res.* **50**, 299–303.

Ashkenazi, A., Marsters, S.A., Capon, D.J., Chamow, S.M., Figari, I.S., Pennica, D., Goeddel, D.V., Palladino, M.A. and Smith, D.H. (1991). *Proc. Natl Acad. Sci. USA* **88**, 10535–10539.

Balkwill, F.R. (1989a). *Cytokines in Cancer Therapy*, Oxford University Press, Oxford.

Balkwill, F.R. (1989b). *Br. Med. Bull.* **45**, 389–400.

Balkwill, F.R. (1990). In: *Peptide Regulatory Factors* (ed. A.R. Green), Edward Arnold, London, pp. 50–59.

Balkwill, F.R. (1993). *Immunol. Today* **14**, 149–150.

Balkwill, F.R. and Burke, F. (1989). *Immunol. Today* **10**, 299–304.

Ballard, D.W., Bohnlein,E., Lowenthal, J.W., Wano, Y., Franzen, B.R. and Green, W.C. (1988). *Science* **241**, 1652–1655.

Barrett, K., Taylor-Fishwick, D.A., Cope, A.P., Kissonerghis, A.M., Gray, P.W., Feldmann, M. and Foxwell, B.M. (1991). *Eur. J. Immunol.* **21**, 1649–1656.

Bazan, J.F. (1990). *Proc. Natl Acad. Sci. USA* **87**, 6934–6938.

Belosevic, M. and Nacy, C.A. (1990). *Cell Immunol.* **128**, 635–640.

Bendtzen, K., Svenson, M., Jønsson, V. and Hippe, E. (1990). *Immunol. Today* **11**, 167–170.

Beutler, B. (1990). In: *Peptide Growth Factors and Their Receptors* 2 (eds M.B. Sporn and A.B. Roberts), Springer, London, pp. 39–70.

Blaise, D., Olive, D., Hirn, M., Viens, P., Lafage, M. and Attal, M. (1991). *Bone Marrow Transpl.* **8**, 105–111.

Blank, V., Kourilsky, P. and Israel, A. (1992). *TIBS* **17**, 135–140.
Border, W.A., Okuda, S., Languino, L.R., Sporn, M.B. and Ruoslahti, E. (1990). *Nature* **346**, 371–374.
Border, W.A., Noble, N.A., Yamamoto, T., Harper, J.R., Yamaguchi, Y., Pierschbacher, M.D. and Ruoslahti, E. (1992). *Nature* **360**, 361–364.
Bose, H.R. (1992). *Biochim. Biophys. Acta* **1114**, 1–17.
Braley-Mullen, H., Sharp, G.C., Bickel, J.T. and Kyriakos, M. (1991). *J. Exp. Med.* **173**, 899–912.
Brennan, F.M., Chantry, D., Jackson, A., Maimi, R. and Feldmann, M. (1989). *Lancet* **ii**, 244–247.
Bretscher, P.A., Wei, G., Menon, J.N. and Bielefold-Ohmann, H. (1992). *Science* **257**, 539–542.
Burkhardt, K., Mandel, T.E., Diamantstein, T. and Loughnan, M.S. (1989). *Immunology* **66**, 183–189.
Cannon, J.G., Tompkins, R.G. and Gelfland, G.A. (1990). *J. Inf. Dis.* **161**, 79–84.
Carpenter, S. and Kraus, G.A. (1991). *Photochem. Photobiol.* **53**, 169–174.
Cerami, A. (1992). *Clin. Immunol. Immunopath.* **62**, S3–S10.
Cerna, H. (1989). *Acta Univ. Palacki Olomuc. Fac. Med.* (Czech.) **123**, 293–302.
Cheung, D.L., Hart, P.H., Vitti, G.F., Whitty, G.A. and Hamilton, J.A. (1990). *Immunology* **71**, 70–75.
Chung, J., Kuo, C.J., Crabtree, G.R. and Blenis, J. (1992). *Cell* **69**, 1227–1236.
Clarke, R., Dickson, R.B. and Lippman, M.E. (1992). *Crit. Rev. Oncol. Hematol.* **12**, 1–23.
Clerici, M. and Shearer, G.M. (1993). *Immunol. Today* **14**, 107–111.
Clipstone, N.E. and Crabtree, G.R. (1992). *Nature* **357**, 695–697.
Coffey, R., Leof, E., Shipley G. and Moses, H.L. (1987). *J. Cell Physiol.* **132**, 143–148.
Coffman, R.L., Seymour, B.W., Lebman, D.A., Hiraki, D.D., Christiansen, J.A. and Shrader, B. (1988). *Immunol. Rev.* **102**, 5–28.
Coffman, R.L., Lebman, D.A. and Rothman, P. (1993). *Adv. Immunol.* **54**, 229–270.
Cohen, S., Pick, E. and Oppenheim, J.J. (1979). In: *Biology of the Lymphokines* (eds S. Cohen, E. Pick and J.J. Oppenheim), Academic Press, New York, pp. 1–7.
Colletta, A.A., Wakefield, L.M., Howell, F.V., van Roozendaal, K.E.P., Danielpour, D., Ebbs, S.R., Sporn, M.B. and Baum, M. (1990). *Br. J. Cancer* **62**, 405–409.
Cowling, G.J. and Dexter, T.M. (1992). *TIB Tech.* **10**, 349–357.
Curfs, J.H.A., van der Meer, J.W.M, Sauerwein, R.W. and Eling, W.M.C. (1990). *J. Exp. Med.* **172**, 1287–1291.
Dainiak, N. (1990). *Prog. Clin. Biol. Res.* **352**, 49–64.
Dallman, M.J. and Clark, G.J. (1992). In: *The Molecular Biology of Immunosuppression* (ed. A.W. Thomson), Wiley, Chichester, pp. 55–78.
Dayer, J-M., Beutler, B. and Cerami, A. (1985). *J. Exp. Med.* **162**, 2163–2168.
Denekamp, J. (1990). In: *Genes and Cancer* (eds. D. Carney and K. Sikora), Wiley, Chichester, pp. 191–200.
Di Marco, E., Pierce, J.A. and Fleming, T.P. (1989). *Oncogene* **4**, 831–838.
Diamantstein, T., Kupiec-Weglinski, J.W., Strom, T.B. and Tilney, N.L. (1989). *Exp. Clin. Endocrinol.* **93**, 114–124.
Dinarello, C.A. (1991). *Blood* **8**, 1627–1652.
Dinarello, C.A. and Thompson, R.C. (1991). *Immunol. Today* **12**, 404–410.
Duff, G.W. (1989). In: *Peptide Regulatory Factors* (ed. A.R. Green), Edward Arnold, London, pp. 112–120.
Dvorak, H.F. (1986). *N. Engl. J. Med.* **315**, 1650–1659.
Edgington, S.M. (1993). *BioTechnol.* **11**, 676–681.
El-Badry, O.M., Romanus, J.A., Helman, L.J., Cooper, M.J., Rechler, M.M. and Israel, M.A. (1989). *J. Clin. Invest.* **84**, 829–839.
Elliott, M.J., Gamble, J.R., Parks, L.S., Vadas, M.A. and Lopez, A.F. (1991). *Blood* **77**, 2739–2745.
Engelmann, H., Novick, D. and Wallach, D. (1990). *J. Biol. Chem.* **265**, 1531–1536.
Espevik, T.M., Brockhaus, M., Loetscher, H., Nonstad, U. and Shalaby, R. (1990). *J. Exp. Med.* **171**, 415–426.
Essner, R., Rhoades, K., McBride, W.H., Morton, D.L. and Economou, J.S. (1989). *J. Immunol.* **142**, 3857–3861.
Falcone, D.J., McCaffrey, T.A., Haimovitz-Friedman, A. and Garcia, M. (1993). *J. Cell Physiol.* **155**, 595–605.
Fan, K., Ruan, Q.Y., Sensenbrenner, L. and Chen, B.D.M. (1992). *Blood* **79**, 1679–1685.
Fan, K., Barendsen, N., Sensenbrenner, L. and Chen, B.D.M. (1993). *J. Cell Physiol.* **154**, 535–542.
Farrell, A.J., Blake, D.R., Palmer, R.M.J. and Moncada, S. (1992). In: *The Biology of Nitric Oxide 2. Enzymology, Biochemistry and Immunology* (eds S. Moncada, M.A. Marletta, J.B. Hibbs Jr. and E.A. Higgs), Portland Press, London and Chapel Hill, pp. 276–277.

Fearon, E.R., Pardoll, D.M., Itaya, T., Golumbeck, P., Levitsky, H.I., Simons, J.W., Karasuyama, H., Vogelstein, B. and Frost, P. (1990). *Cell* **60**, 397–403.

Fernandez-Botran, R. (1991). *FASEB J.* **5**, 2567–2574.

Feuer, G. and Chen, I.S.Y. (1992). *Biochim. Biophys. Acta* **1114**, 223–233.

Firestein, G.S., Alvaro-Garcia, J.M. and Maki, R. (1990). *J. Immunol.* **144**, 3347–3353.

Flanagan, W.M. and Crabtree, G.R. (1993). *Ann. NY Acad. Sci.*

Flanagan, W.M., Corthesy, B., Bram, R.J. and Crabtree, G.R. (1991). *Nature* **352**, 803–807.

Foekens, J.A., Sieuwerts, A.M., Stuurman-Smeets, M.J., Dorssers, L.C.J., Berns, E.M.J.J. and Klijn, J.G.M. (1992). *Int. J. Cancer* **51**, 439–444.

Foekens, J.A., Sieuwerts, A.M., Stuurman-Smeets, E.M.J., Peters, H.A. and Klijn, J.G.M. (1993). *Br. J. Cancer* **67**, 232–236.

Folkman, J. and Shing, Y. (1992). *J. Biol. Chem.* **267**, 10931–10934.

Foxwell, B.M.J., Barrett, K. and Feldmann, M. (1992). *Clin. Exp. Immunol.* **90**, 161–169.

Freuhauf, J.P., Myers, C.E. and Sinha, B.K. (1990). *J. Natl Cancer Inst.* **82**, 1206–1209.

Fujii, M., Sassone-Corsi, P. and Verma, I.M. (1988). *Proc. Natl Acad. Sci. USA* **85**, 8526–8530.

Gansbacher, B., Zier, K., Daniels, B., Cronin, K., Bannerjy, R. and Gilboa, E. (1990). *J. Exp. Med.* **172**, 1217–1224.

Gendelman, H.E. and Morahan, P.S. (1992). In: *The Macrophage* (eds C.E. Lewis and J. O'D. McGee), IRL Press, Oxford, pp. 157–195.

Giri, J.G., Robb, R., Wong, W.L. and Horuk, R. (1992). *Cytokine* **4**, 18–23.

Givol, D. and Yayon, A. (1992). *FASEB. J.* **6**, 3363–3369.

Goillot, E.,Combaret, V., Ladenstein, R., Baubet, D., Blay, J.-Y., Philip, T. and Favrot, M.C. (1992). *Cancer Res.* **52**, 3194–3200.

Goldfarb, M. (1990). *Cell Growth Differ.* **1**, 439–445.

Golumbeck, P.T., Lazenby, A.J., Levitsky, H.I., Jaffee, L.M., Karasnyama, H., Baker, M. and Pardoll, D.M. (1991). *Science* **254**, 713–716.

Graham, B.S., Belshe, R.B. and Clements, M.L. (1992). *J. Inf. Dis.* **166**, 244–252.

Grau, G.E., Bieler, G. and Pontaire, P. (1990). *Immunol. Lett.* **25**, 189–194.

Gullick, W. (1991). *Br. Med. Bull.* **47**, 87–98.

Hagiwara, T., Suzuki, H., Kono, I., Kashiwagi, H., Akiyama, Y. and Onozaki, K. (1990). *Am. J. Path.* **136**, 39–47.

Hale, G., Dyer, M.J., Clark, M.R., Phillips, J.M., Riechmann, L. and Waldmann, H. (1988). *Lancet* **ii**, 1394–1399.

Hamilton, J.A., Whitty, G.A., Royston, A.K.M., Cebon, J. and Layton, J.E. (1992). *Immunology* **76**, 566–571.

Hancock, W.W., Di Stefano, R., Braun, P., Schweizer, R.T., Tilney, N.L. and Kupiec-Weglinski, J.W. (1990). *Transplantation* **49**, 416–421.

Harris, A.L. (1990a). *Cancer Cells* **2**, 321–323.

Harris, E.D. (1990b). *N. Engl. J. Med.* **322**, 1277–1289.

Hart, P.H., Vitti, G.F., Burgess, D.R., Whitty, G.A and Hamilton, J.A. (1989). *Proc. Natl Acad. Sci. USA* **86**, 3803–3807.

Hawking, F. (1987). *Adv. Pharmacol. Chemother.* **15**, 289–322.

Henderson, B., Thompson, R.C., Hardingham, T. and Lewthwaite, J. (1981). *Cytokine* **3**, 246–249.

Hensey, C.F., Boscoboinik, D. and Azzi, A. (1989). *FEBS Lett.* **258**, 156–158.

Hermann, F., Cannistra, S.A., Lindemann, D.B., Rambaldi, A., Mertelsmann, R.H. and Griffin, J.D. (1989). *J. Immunol.* **142**, 139–143.

Hermansson, M., Nister, M., Betsholtz, C., Heldin, C.-H., Westermark, B. and Funa, K. (1988). *Proc. Natl Acad. Sci. USA* **85**, 7748–7752.

Herve, P., Wijdenes, J., Bergerat, J.P., Bordigoni, P., Milpied, N., Cahn, J.Y., Clement, C., Beliard, R., Morel-Fourrier, B., Racadot, E., Troussard, X., Benz-Lemoine, E., Gand, C., Legros, M., Attal, M., Kluft, M. and Peters, A. (1990). *Blood* **75**, 1017–1023.

Herve, P., Flesch, M., Tiberghien, P., Wijdenes, J., Racadot, E., Bordigoni, P., Plouvier, E., Stephen, J.L., Bourdeau, H., Holler, E., Lioure, B., Roche, C., Vilmer, E., Bemeocq, F., Kuentz, M. and Cahn, J.Y. (1992). *Blood* **79**, 3362–3368.

Herzbeck, H., Blum, B., Rönspeck, W., Frenzel, B., Brandt, E., Ulmer, A.J. and Flad, H.-D. (1989). *Scand. J. Immunol.* **30**, 549–562.

Higuchi, M., Diamantstein, T., Osawa, H. and Caspi, R.R. (1991). *J. Autoimmun.* **4**, 113–124.

Hilton, D.J. (1992). *TIBS* **17**, 72–76.

Hirata, Y., Taga, T., Hibi, M., Nakano, N., Hirano, T. and Kishimoto, T. (1989). *J. Immunol.* **143**, 2900–2907.

Hoang, T., Levy, B., Onetto, N., Haman, A. and Rodriquez-Cimadevilla, J.C. (1989). *J. Exp. Med.* **170**, 15–26.

Hock, H., Dorsch, M., Kunzendorf, U., Uberla, K., Quin, Z., Diamantstein, T. and Blankenstein, T. (1993). *Cancer Res.* **53**, 714–716.

Hohmann, H.-P., Brockhaus, M., Baeuerle, P.A., Remy, R., Kolbeck, R. and van Loon, A.P.G.M. (1990). *J. Biol. Chem.* **265**, 22409–22417.

Horneff, G., Krause, A., Emmich, F., Kalden, J.R. and Burmester, G.R. (1991). *Cytokine* **3**, 266–267.

Howard, M. and O'Garra, A. (1992). *Immunol. Today* **13**, 198–200.

Huang, J.J., Newton, R.C., Horuk, R., Matthew, J.B., Corington, M., Pezzella, K. and Lin, Y. (1987). *FEBS Lett.* **223**, 294–298.

Husby, G. and Williams, R.C. (1988). *J. Autoimmun.* **1**, 363–371.

Ignarro, L.J. (1989). *FASEB J.* **3**, 31–36.

Isakov, N. (1993). *Mol. Immunol.* **30**, 197–210.

James, K. (1990). *Immunol. Today* **11**, 163–166.

Jindal, H.K., Anderson, C.W., Davis, R.G. and Vishwanatha, J.K. (1990). *Cancer Res.* **50**, 7754–7757.

Johnson, M.D., Jennings, M.T., Gold, L.I. and Moses, H.L. (1993). *Human Pathol.* **24**, 457–462.

Kasayama, S., Saito, H., Kouhara, H., Sumitani, S. and Sato, B. (1993). *J. Cell Physiol.* **154**, 254–261.

Kelley, J. and Hildebran, J.N. (1987). *Amer. Rev. Resp. Dis.* **135**, A65.

Kelley, V.E., Gaulton, G.N., Hattori, M., Ikegami, H., Eisenbarth, G. and Strom, T.B. (1988). *J. Immunol.* **140**, 59–61.

Kettleborough, C.A., Saldanha, J., Heath, V.J., Morrison, C.J. and Bendig, M.M. (1991). *Protein Eng.* **4**, 773–783.

Khachigian, L.M., Owensby, D.A. and Chesterman, C.N. (1992). *J. Biol. Chem.* **267**, 1660–1666.

Kilkarni, A.B. and Karlsson, S. (1993). *Am. J. Path.* **143**, 3–9.

Klagsbrun, M. and Folkman, J. (1990). In: *Peptide Growth Factors and Their Receptors 2* (eds M.B. Sporn and A.B. Roberts), Springer, London, pp. 549–586.

Knabbe, C., Lippman, M.E. and Wakefield, L.M. (1987). *Cell* **48**, 417–428.

Kobari, L., Weil, D., Lemoine, F.M., Dubois, C., Thiam, D. and Baillou, C. (1990). *Exp. Hematol.* **18**, 1187–1192.

Kovacs, E.J. (1991). *Immunol. Today* **12**, 17–23.

Kuo, C.J., Chung, J., Fiorentino, D.F., Flanagan, W.M., Blenis, J. and Crabtree, G.R. (1992). *Nature* **358**, 70–73.

Kupiec-Weglinski, J.W., van der Meide, P., Stunkel, K.G., Tanaka, K., Diamantstein, T. and Tilney, N.L. (1989). *Transplant Proc.* **21**, 992–993.

Kupiec-Weglinski, J.W., Sablinski, T., Hancock, W.W., DiStefano, R., Mariani, G., Mix, C.T. and Tilney, G.L. (1991a). *Transplantation* **51**, 300–305.

Kupiec-Weglinski, J.W., Sablinski, T., Hancock, W.W., Mix, C.T. and Tilney, G.L. (1991b). *Transplant Proc.* **23**, 285–286.

Kurachi, H., Morishige, K., Amemiya, K., Adachi, H., Hirota, K., Miyake, A. and Tanizawa, O. (1991). *Cancer Res.* **51**, 5956–5959.

Ladner, M.B., Martin, G.A., Noble, J.A., Nikoloff, D.M., Tal, R., Kawasaki, E.S. and White, T.J. (1987). *EMBO J.* **6**, 2693–2698.

LaRochelle, W.J., Giese, N., May-Siroff, M., Robbins, K.C. and Aaronson, S.A. (1990a). *Science* **248**, 1541–1544.

LaRochelle, W.J., Giese, N., May-Siroff, M., Robbins, K.C. and Aaronson, S.A. (1990b). *J. Cell Sci.* **13** (Suppl.) 31–42.

Larsen, C.G., Anderson, A.O., Oppenheim, J.J. and Matsuchima, K. (1989). *Immunology* **68**, 31–36.

Lee, D.C. and Han, V.K.M. (1990). In: *Peptide Growth Factors and Their Receptors 2* (eds. M.B. Sporn and A.B. Roberts), Springer, London, pp. 611–654.

Lehn, M., Weiser, W.Y., Engelhorn, S., Gillis, S. and Remold, H.G. (1989). *J. Immunol.* **143**, 3020–3024.

Levitzki, A. (1990). *Biochem. Pharmacol.* **40**, 913–918.

Lienard, D., Lejeune, F., Delmotte, J.J., Renard, N. and Ewalenko, P. (1992). *J. Clin. Oncol.* **10**, 52–60.

Liew, F.Y., Millot, S., Parkinson, C., Palmer, R.M.J. and Moncada, S. (1990). *J. Immunol.* **144**, 4794–4797.

Lin, Y.H., Wang, X.-F., Ng-Eaton, E., Weinberg, R.A. and Lodish, H.F. (1992). *Cell* **68**, 775–785.

Lindemann, A., Reidel, D., Oster, W., Mertelsmann, R. and Herrmann, F. (1988). *Eur. J. Immunol.* **18**, 369–374.

Lindemann, A., Ludwig, W.D., Oster, W., Mertelsmann, R. and Herrmann, F. (1989). *Blood* **73**, 880–884.

Liotta, L.A., Steeg, P.S. and Statler-Stevenson, W.G. (1991). *Cell* **64**, 327–336.

Liu, J. (1993). *Immunology Today* **14**, 290–294.

Liu, J., Albers, M.W., Wandless, T.J., Luan, S., Alberg, D.G., Belshaw, P.J., Cohen, P., MacKintosh, C., Klee, C.B. and Schreiber, S.L. (1992). *Biochemistry* **31**, 3896–3901.

Liu, J., Farmer, J.D. Jr., Lane, W.S., Friedman, J., Weissman, I. and Schreiber, S.L. (1991). *Cell* **66**, 807–815.

Lloyd, A.R. and Oppenheim, J.J. (1992). *Immunol. Today* **13**, 169–172.

LoBuglio, A.F., Wheeler, R.H., Trang, J., Haynes, A., Rogers, K., Harvey, E.B., Sun, L., Ghrayeb, J. and Khazaeli, M.B. (1989). *Proc. Natl Acad. Sci. USA* **86**, 4220–4224.

Lopez, A.F., Eglinton, J.M., Park, L.S., Clark, S. and Vadas, M.A. (1989). *Proc. Natl Acad. Sci. USA* **86**, 7022–7026.

Lowenberg, B. and Touw, I.P. (1993). *Blood* **81**, 281–292.

Lyons, R.M., Keski-Oja, J. and Moses, H.L. (1990). *J. Cell. Biol.* **110**, 1361–1367.

McBridge, W.H., Thacker, J.C., Comora, S., Economou, J.S., Kelley, D., Hogge, D., Dubinett, S.M. and Dougherty, G. J. (1992). *Cancer Res.* **52**, 3931–3937.

MacDonald, B.R., Mundy, G.R., Clark, S., Wang, E.A., Kuehl, T.J., Stanley, E.R. and Roodman, G.D. (1986). *J. Bone Mineral Res.* **1**, 227–233.

Maki, A., Berezesky, I.K., Fargnoli, J., Holbrook, N.J. and Trump, B.F. (1992). *FASEB J.* **6**, 919–924.

Mantovani, A. and Dejana, E. (1989). *Immunol. Today* **10**, 370–375.

Marks, J.D., Berman-Marks, C., Luce, J.M., Montgomery, A.B., Turner, J., Metz, C.A. and Murray, J.F. (1990). *Am. Rev. Respir. Dis.* **141**, 94–97.

Marshall, C.J. (1989). In: *Oncogenes* (eds D.M. Glover asnd B.D. Hames), IRL Press, Oxford, pp. 1–21.

Massagué, J. (1992). *Cell* **97**, 1067–1073.

Martich, G.D., Danner, R.L., Ceska, M. and Suffredini, A.F. (1991). *J. Exp. Med.* **173**, 1021–1024.

Matrisian, L.M. (1992). *BioEssays* **14**, 455–463.

McCaffrey, P.G., Perrino, B.A., Soderling, T.R. and Rao, A. (1993). *J. Biol. Chem.* **268**, 3747–3752.

Meager, A. (1990). In: *Cytokines,* Open University Press, Milton Keynes.

Metcalf, D. (1992). *TIBS* **17**, 286–289.

Miller, L.C., Lynch, E.A., Isa, S., Logan, J.W., Dinarello, C.A. and Steere, A.C. (1993). *Lancet* **341**, 146–148.

Mills, G.B., Zhang, N., May, C., Hill, M. and Chung, A. (1990). *Cancer Res.* **50**, 3036–3042.

Minami, Y., Kono, T., Yamada, K. and Taniguchi, T. (1992). *Biochim. Biophys. Acta* **1114**, 163–177.

Mire-Sluis, A. (1993). *TIBTech.* **11**, 74–77.

Miyajima, A., Hara, T. and Kitamura, T. (1992). *TIBS* **17**, 378–382.

Miyazono, K. and Heldin, C.-H. (1991). In: *Clinical Application of TGF-β*, Ciba Foundation Symposium 157, Wiley, Chichester, pp. 81–92.

Modjtahedi, H., Eccles, S., Box, G., Styles, J. and Dean, C. (1993). *Br. J. Cancer* **67**, 254–261.

Morris, R.E. (1992). *Transplant. Rev.* **6**, 39–87.

Moses, H.L. (1990). In: *Growth Factors. From Genes to Clinical Application* (ed. V.R. Sara), Raven, New York, pp. 141–155.

Mosmann, T.R. and Moore, K.W. (1991). In: *Immunoparasitology Today* (eds C. Ash and R.B. Gallagher), Elsevier, Cambridge, pp. A49–A53.

Muegge, K. and Durum, S.K. (1990). *Cytokine* **2**, 1–8.

Mukaida, N., Shiroo, M. and Matsushima, K.R. (1989). *J. Immunol.* **143**, 1366–1371.

Narumi, S., Finke, J.H. and Hamilton, T.A. (1990). *J. Biol. Chem.* **265**, 7036–7041.

Narumi, S., Tebo, J.M., Finke, J.H. and Hamilton, T.A. (1992). *J. Immunol.* **149**, 529–534.

Nathan, C.F. (1990). In: *Peptide Growth Factors and their Receptors* (eds M.B. Sporn and A.B. Roberts), Springer, London, pp. 427–462.

Nathan, C.F. (1992). *FASEB J.* **6**, 3051–3064.

Naume, B., Shalaby, R., Lesslauer, W. and Espevik, T. (1991). *J. Immunol.* **146**, 3045–3048.

Naylor, M.S., Stamp, G.W.H. and Balkwill, F.R. (1990). *Cancer Res.* **50**, 4436–4440.

Nelson, P.A., Akselband, Y., Kawamura, A., Su, M., Tung, R.D., Rich, D.H., Kishore, V., Rosborough, S.L., DeCenzo, M.T., Livingston, D.J. and Harding, M.W. (1993). *Immunol.* **150**, 2139–2147.

Nicola, T. and Metcalf, D. (1991). *Cell* **67**, 1–4.

Nimer, S.D., Gasson, J.C., Hu, K., Smalberg, I., Williams, J.L., Chen, I.S.Y. and Rosenblatt, J.D. (1989). *Oncogene* **4**, 671–676.

Nishizawa, M., Tsuchiya, M., Watanabe-Fukunaga, R. and Nagata, S. (1990). *J. Biol Chem.* **265**, 5897–5902.

O'Keefe, S.J., Tamura, J., Kincaid, R.L., Tocci, M.J. and O'Neill, E.A. (1992). *Nature* **357**, 692–694.

Okada, M., Senoo, Y. and Teramoto, S. (1992). *Acta Med. Okayama,* **46**, 37–44.

Okuda, S., Languino, L.R., Ruoslahti, E. and Border, A.W. (1990). *J. Clin. Invest.* **86**, 453–462.

Olivier, S., Formento, P., Fischel, J.L., Etienne, M.C. and Milano, G. (1990). *Eur. J. Cancer* **26**, 867–871.

Opal, S.M., Cross, A.S., Sadoff, J.C., Collins, H.H., Kelly, N.M., Victor, G.H., Palardy, J.E. and Bodmer, M.W. (1991). *J. Clin. Invest.* **88**, 885–890.

Ostman, A., Andersson, M., Betsholtz, C., Westermark, B. and Heldin, C.-H., (1991). *Cell Reg.* **2**, 503–512.

Overall, C.M., Wrana, J.L. and Sodek, J. (1989). *J. Biol. Chem.* **264**, 1860–1869.

Overall, C.M., Wrana, J.L. and Sodek, J. (1991). *J. Biol. Chem.* **266**, 14064–14071.

Palaszynski, E.W. (1987). *Biochem. Biophys. Res. Commun.* **147**, 204–209.

Pastan, I., Chaudhary, V. and Fitzgerald, D.J. (1992). *Annu. Rev. Biochem.* **61**, 331–354.

Perosio, P.M. and Brooks, J.J. (1989). *Lab. Invest.* **60**, 245–253.

Pesanti, E.L. (1991). *J. Inf. Dis.* **163**, 611–616.

Pesenti, E., Sola, F., Mongelli, N., Grandi, M. and Spreafico, F. (1992). *Br. J. Cancer* **66**, 367–372.

Peterson, M.G. and Baichwal, V.R. (1993). *TIB Tech.* **11**, 11–18.

Pober, J.S. and Cotran, R.S. (1990). *Physiol. Rev.* **70**, 427–451.

Pollak, M. and Richard, M. (1990). *J. Natl Cancer Inst.* **82**, 1349–1352.

Pollard, J.W., Bartocci, B., Arceci, R., Orlofsky, A., Ladner, M.B. and Stanley, E.R. (1987). *Nature* **330**, 484–486.

Poutsiaka, D.D., Clark, B.D., Vannier, E. and Dinarello, C.A. (1991). *Blood* **78**, 1275–1281.

Pugh-Humphreys, R.G.P. (1992). *FEMS Microbiol. Immunol.* **105**, 289–308.

Raines, E.W. and Ross, R. (1992). *J. Cell Biol.* **116**, 533–543.

Rajavashisth, T.B., Eng, R., Shadduck, R.K., Waheed, A., Ben-Avram, C.M., Shively, J.E. and Lusis, A.J. (1987). *Proc. Natl Acad. Sci. USA* **84**, 1157–1161.

Ramakrishnan, S., Xu, F.S., Brandt, S.J., Niedel, J.E., Bast, R.C. and Brown, E.L. (1989). *J. Clin. Invest.* **83**, 921–926.

Rambaldi, A., Wakamiya, N., Vellenga, E., Horiguchi, J., Warren, M.K., Kufe, D. and Griffin, J.D. (1988). *J. Clin. Invest.* **81**, 1030–1035.

Ramsay, A.J., Ruby, J. and Ramshaw, I.A. (1993). *Immunol. Today* **14**, 155–157.

Reddy, K.B. and Howe, P.H. (1993). *J. Cell. Physiol.* **156**, 48–55.

Reid, R.P. (1992). In: *Muir's Textbook of Pathology,* 13th edn (eds R.N.M. MacSween and K. Whaley), Edward Arnold, London, pp. 946–1011.

Ricci, M., Rossi, O., Bertoni, M. and Matucci, A. (1993). *Clin. Exp. Allergy* **23** 360–369.

Riechmann, L., Clark, M., Waldmann, H. and Winter, G. (1988). Nature **332**, 323–327.

Rifkin, D.B., Moscatelli, D, Bizik, J., Quarto, N., Blei, F. and Dennis, P. (1990). *Cell Differ.* Dev. **32**, 313–318.

Roberts, A.B. and Sporn, M.B. (1990). In: *Peptide Growth Factors and Their Receptors.* 1 (eds. M.B. Sporn and A.B. Roberts), Springer, London.

Rose, B., Gillespie, A., Wunderlich, D., Kelley, K., Dzuiba, J., Shedd, D., Cahill, K. and Zerler, B. (1992). *Immunology* **76**, 452–459.

Rose, T.M. and Bruce, A.G. (1991). *Proc. Natl Acad. Sci. USA* **88**, 8641–8645.

Rosenberg, S.A. (1988). *Immunol. Today* **9**, 58–62.

Russell, S.J. (1990). *Immunol. Today* **11**, 196–200.

Ruffel, B. (1989). *Pharmacol. Rev.* **41**, 407–422.

Sadick, M.D. (1992). In: *The Macrophage* (eds C.E. Lewis and J. O'D., McGee), IRL Press, Oxford, pp. 265–284.

Sappino, A.P., Schürch, W. and Gabbiani, G. (1990). *Lab. Invest.* **63**, 144–161.

Sato, K., Tsuchiya, M., Saldanha, J., Koishihara, Y., Ohsugi, Y., Kishimoto, T. and Bendig. M.M. (1993a). *Cancer Res.* **53**, 851–856.

Sato, N., Beitz, J.G., Kato, J., Yamamoto, M., Clark, J.W., Calabresi, P. and Frackleton, A.R. (1993b). *Amer. J. Path.* **142**, 1119–1130.

Satoh, T., Uehara, Y. and Kaziro, Y. (1992). *J. Cell. Biol.* **267**, 2537–2541.

Schall, T.J. (1991). *Cytokine* **3**, 165–183.

Schreiber, S.L. (1991). *Science* **251**, 283–287.

Seelentag, W., Mermod, J.J. and Vassalli, J.P. (1989). *Eur. J. Immunol.* **19**, 209–212.

Segarini, P.R. (1991). In: *Clinical Applications of TGF-β.* Ciba Foundation Symposium 157. Wiley, Chichester, pp. 29–51.

Seid, J.M., Rohman, S., Graveley, R., Bunning, R.A.A.D., Nordmann, R., Wishart, W. and Russell, R.G. (1993). *Arthritis Rheum.* **36**, 35–43.

Seitz, M., Dewald, B., Gerber, N. and Baggiolini, M. (1991). *J. Clin. Invest.* **87**, 463–469.

Shalaby, M.R., Sundan, A., Loetscher, H., Brockhaus, M., Lesslauer, W. and Espevik, T.M. (1990). *J. Exp. Med.* **172**, 1517–1520.

Siekevitz, M., Feinberg, M.B., Holbrook, N., Wong-Staal, F. and Greene, W.C. (1987). *Proc. Natl Acad. Sci. USA* **84**, 5389–5393.

Smith, K.A. (1989). *Annu. Rev. Cell Biol.* **5**, 397–425.

Solari, R. (1990). *Cytokine* **2**, 21–28.

Souyri, M., Vignon, I., Penicolelli, J.-F., Heard, J.M., Tambourin, T. and Wendling, F. (1990). *Cell* **63**, 1137–1147.

Speert, D.P. (1992). In: *The Macrophage* (eds C.E. Lewis and J. O'D. McGee), IRL Press, Oxford, pp. 215–263.

Spriggs, D.R. and Yates, S.W. (1992). In: *Tumor Necrosis Factors: The Molecules and Their Emerging Role in Medicine* (ed. B. Beutler), Raven Press, New York, pp. 383–406.

Standiford, T.J., Streiter, R.M., Chensue, S.W., Westwick, J., Kasahara, K. and Kunkel, S.L. (1990). *J. Immunol.* **145**, 1435–1439.

Stein, M. and Keshav, S. (1992). *Clin. Exp. Allergy* **22**, 19–27.

Steinbruchel, D.A., Koch, C., Kristensen, T. and Kemp, E. (1991). *Scand. J. Immunol.* **34**, 627–633.

Steinbruchel, D.A., Larsen, S., Kristensen, T., Starklint, H., Koch, C. and Kemp, E. (1992). *Acta Path. Microbiol. Immunol. Scand.* **100**, 682–694.

Steinman, R. (1991). *Annu. Rev. Immunol.* **9**, 271–296.

Strieter, R.M., Kunkel, S.L., Showell, H.J., Remick, D.G., Phan, S.H., Ward, P.A. and Marks, R.M. (1989). *Science* **243**, 1467–1469.

Strom, T.B., Kelley, V.E., Murphy, J.R., Osawa, H., Tilney, N.L. and Shapiro, M.E. (1988). In: *Interleukin 2* (ed. K.A. Smith), Academic Press, New York, pp. 223–236.

Stroobant, P. (1990). In: *Genes and Cancer* (eds D. Carney and K. Sikora), Wiley, Chichester, pp. 237–241.

Suzuki, A., Takahashi, T., Okuno, Y., Nakamura, K., Tashiro, H., Fukumoto, M., Konaka, Y. and Imura, H. (1991). *Int. J. Cancer* **48**, 428–433.

Szabo, G. and Miller-Graziano, C.L. (1990). *Transplantation* **50**, 301–309.

Takahashi, I., Nakanishi, S., Kobayashi, E., Nakano, H., Suzuki, K. and Tamaoki, T. (1989). *Biochem. Biophys. Res. Commun.* **165**, 1207–1212.

Takeshita, T., Asao, H., Ohtani, K., Ishii, N., Kumaki, S., Tanaka, N. *et al.* (1992). *Science* **257**, 379–382.

Tanaka, K., Tilney, N.L., Stunkel, K.G., Hancock, W.W., Diamantstein, T. and Kupiec-Weglinski, J.W. (1990). *Proc. Natl Acad. Sci. USA* **87**, 7375–7379.

Tanaka, Y., Adams, D.H. and Shaw, S. (1993). *Immunol. Today* **14**, 111–115.

Tartaglia, L.A., Weber, R.F., Figari, I.S., Reynolds, C., Palladino, M.A. and Goeddel, D.V. (1991). *Proc. Natl Acad. Sci. USA* **88**, 9292–9296.

Thedrez, P., Paineau, J., Jacques, Y., Chatal, J.F., Pelegrin, A., Bouchaud, G. and Soulillou, J.P. (1989). *Transplantation* **48**, 367–371.

Thoma, B., Grell, M., Pfizenmaier, K. and Sheurich, P. (1990). *J. Exp. Med.* **172**, 1019–1023.

Thomson, A.W. (1990). *Transplant. Rev.* **4**, 1–13.

Travali, S., Koniecki, J., Petralia, S. and Baserga, R. (1990). *FASEB J.* **4**, 3209–3214.

Trinchieri, G. (1993). *Immunol. Today* **14**, 335–338.

Ueda, H., Hancock, W.W., Cheung, Y.C., Diamantstein, T., Tilney, N.L. and Kupiec-Weglinski, J.W. (1990). *Transplantation* **50**, 545–560.

Ulich, T.R., Yin, S., Guo, K., del Castillo, J., Eisenberg, S.P. and Thompson, R.C. (1991). *Amer. J. Path.* **138**, 521–524.

van Damme, J., Bunning, R.A.D., Coning, R., Russell, R.G.G. and Opdenakker, G. (1990). *Cytokine* **2**, 106–111.

van den Hooff, A. (1988). *Adv. Cancer Res.* **50**, 159–196.

van der Poll, T., Büller, H.R., ten Cate H., Wortel, C.H., Bauer, K.A., van Deventer, S.J.H., Deventer, S.J.H. van, Hack, C.E., Sauerwein, H.P., Rosenberg, R.D. and ten Cate, J.W. (1990). *N. Engl. J. Med.* **322**, 1622–1627.

van der Poll, T., Jansen, J., van Leenen, D., Levi, M., Brockhaus, M. and van Deventer, S.J.H. (1992). *Eur. Cytokine Netw.* **3**, 214–219.

van Deuren, M., Dofferhoff, A.S.M. and van der Meer, J.W.M. (1992). *J. Pathol.* **168**, 349–356.

Velu, T. (1990). *Mol. Cell Endocrinol.* **70**, 205–216.

Vignon, F., Prebois, C. and Rochefort, H. (1992). *J. Natl Cancer Inst.* **84**, 38–42.

Vitetta, E.S., Fernandez-Botran, R., Myers, C.D. and Sanders, V.M. (1989). *Adv. Immunol.* **45**, 1–105.

Vlodavsky, I., Fuks, Z., Ishai-Michaeli, R., Bashkin, P., Levi, E. and Korner, G. (1991). *J. Cell Biochem.* **45**, 167–176.

Wahl, S.M. (1992). *J. Clin. Immunol.* **12**, 61–74.

Waldman, T.A., Grant, A., Tendler, C., Greenberg, S., Goldman, C. and Bamford, R. (1990). *J. Clin. Immunol.* **10** (Suppl. 6), 19S–28S.

Warner, S.J.C., Auger, R.R. and Libby, P. (1987a). *J. Exp. Med.* **165**, 1316–1331.

Warner, S.J.C., Auger, R.R. and Libby, P. (1987b). *J. Immunol.* **139**, 1911–1917.

Watanabe, Y., Kuribayashi, K., Miyatake, S., Nishihara, K., Nakayama, E.-I., Taniyama, T. and Sakata, T.-A. (1989). *Proc. Natl Acad. Sci. USA* **86**, 9456–9460.

Weinberg, A.D., Whitham, R., Swain, S.L., Morrison, W.J., Wyrick, G., Hoy, C., Vandenbark, A. and Offner, H. (1992). *J. Immunol.* **148**, 2109–2117.

Whalen, G.F. (1990). *Lancet* **336**, 1489–1492.

Whaley, K. and Burt, A.D. (1992). In: *Muir's Textbook of Pathology*, 13th edn (eds R.N.M. MacSween and K. Whaley), Edward Arnold, London, pp. 112–165.

Wong, G.G., Temple, P.A., Leary, A.C., Witek-Giannotti, J.S., Yang, Y.-C., Ciarletta, A.B., Chung, M., Murtha, P., Kriz, R., Kaufman, R.J., Ferenz, C.R., Sibley, B.S., Turner, K.J., Hewick, R.M., Clark, S.C., Yanai, N., Yokota, H., Yamada, M., Saito, M., Motoyoshi, K. and Takaku, F. (1987). *Science* **235**, 1504–1508.

Wong, H. and Wahl, S.M. (1990). In: *Peptide Growth Factors and Their Receptors 2* (eds M.B. Sporn and A.B. Roberts), Springer, London, pp. 509–548.

Xu, W.D., Firestein, G.S., Taetle, R., Kaushansky, K. and Zvaifler, N.J. (1989). *J. Clin. Invest.* **83**, 876–882.

Yarden, J. and Ullrich, A. (1988). *Annu. Rev. Biochem.* **57**, 443–479.

Yocum, D.E., Esparza, L., Durby, S., Benjamin, J.B., Volz, R. and Scuderi, P. (1989). *Cell Immunol.* **122**, 131–145.

Ziff, M. (1990). *J. Rheumatol.* **17**, 127–133.

Chapter 27

The Phylogeny of Cytokines

C.J. Secombes

Department of Zoology, University of Aberdeen, Aberdeen AB9 2TN, UK

INTRODUCTION

The largest dichotomy in animal defences occurs at the level of the vertebrates (Klein, 1989); only vertebrates possess anticipatory immune responses characterized by the presence of lymphocytes able to undergo proliferation in response to specific antigens, true lymphoid organs housing these cells and specific antibody/immunoglobulin. In addition, vertebrates, like invertebrates, possess nonanticipatory (nonspecific) immune responses based upon phagocytes, NK cells and a large variety of soluble non Ig factors. Invertebrates also demonstrate responses that mimic anticipatory responses, but recently it has been argued that these are fundamentally different from lymphocyte-mediated immune responses.

Lymphocyte heterogeneity appears to exist throughout the vertebrates, with a conclusively demonstrated thymus-dependent subpopulation equivalent to mammalian T cells being present in amphibians and higher vertebrates (Roitt et al., 1989). In fish it has been more difficult to confirm the presence of a thymus-dependent subpopulation, but surface Ig$^-$ and surface Ig$^+$ subpopulations functionally equivalent to T and B cells are present (Graham and Secombes, 1990a). Thus, the large number of cytokines that are considered to be T-lymphocyte products may be present throughout the vertebrates. Indeed, many may prove to be unique to the vertebrates, particularly those crucial for lymphocyte responses. Conversely, cytokines released from cells of the nonspecific defences or important in their regulation may well be present in invertebrates, or have a functionally equivalent analogue. In this chapter what is known about nonmammalian cytokines is reviewed under three categories: interferons, interleukins and phagocyte-modulating cytokines.

INTERFERONS

IFNs are substances able to inhibit virus replication and in mammals three classes exist, α (leukocyte), β (fibroblast) and γ (immune), based upon their biological and biochemical properties and gene sequences (see Chapter 14). IFN-α and IFN-β have many similarities and are grouped together as type 1 IFN. They are both induced in cells infected with virus, are acid stable and probably any cell type can produce them. In

Table 1. Physicochemical characterization and species specificity of purified type 1 interferon from rainbow trout fibroblasts.

Treatment	Type of cells protected	IFN activity (units/ml)	Reduction in IFN activity (%)
None	Trout	8831	0
None	Goldfish	449	95
pH2	Trout	9120	−3
25°C	Trout	8710	1
56°C	Trout	5623	36
65°C	Trout	398	96
Trypsin	Trout	1023	88

Adapted from DeSena and Rio (1975), *Infect. Immun.* **11**, 815–822, with permission.

contrast, IFN-γ is unrelated to type 1 IFNs, is induced following antigen or mitogen (Con A, PHA) stimulation of T lymphocytes and has a wide spectrum of biological activities, including macrophage activation and upregulation of class II MHC antigens. It is therefore referred to as type 2 IFN. IFNs appear to be unique to vertebrates, with all classes possessing type 1 gene sequences and (with the exception of amphibia, for which experimental data are lacking) secreting IFN molecules in response to virus infection or mitogen stimulation. The possible divergence of IFN-α from IFN-β at the level of the reptiles has also been indicated.

Type 1 IFN

Fish
It is well established that fish fibroblast or epithelial cell lines can secrete IFN molecules in response to virus infection *in vitro* (Gravel and Marlsberger, 1965; DeSena and Rio, 1975), particularly when confluent before infection. IFN activity can be detected in the supernatants 24–72 h postinfection, as assessed by their ability to reduce viral cytopathic effects (CPE) in cell lines pretreated with the supernatants for 24 h prior to addition of a challenge virus. This IFN activity is acid (pH 2) stable, relatively temperature resistant but destroyed by trypsin treatment (Table 1)—all properties typical of a type 1 IFN. In addition, this activity is species-specific with respect to the cell line being protected but nonspecific with regard to the challenge virus, i.e. it can provide protection against a virus unrelated to that which induced it.

Similarly, *in vivo* studies have shown that IFN activities with biological properties identical to those described above can be detected in the serum of fish following natural or experimental viral infection (Dorson *et al.*, 1975). In the latter case IFN activity is detectable within 1 day postinfection, begins to decrease by 4 days and is undetectable by day 14. The IFN is protective *in vivo*, as demonstrated by an increased survival of rainbow trout alevins bath-challenged with viral haemorrhagic septicaemia (VHS) virus following an injection of IFN-containing serum, compared with fish injected with control serum (Fig. 1) (DeKinkelin *et al.*, 1982). Separation of the serum into light and heavy (antibody) fractions reveals that protection is not associated with the latter fraction. The IFN activity is short-lived following passive transfer, being undetectable 6-8 h postinjection. Protection is also seen against infectious pancreatic necrosis (IPN)

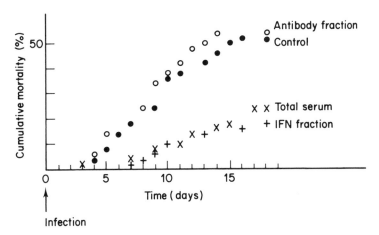

Fig. 1. Protection of young rainbow trout against VHS virus by transfer of IFN. Two groups of 50 fish were injected intraperitoneally with 20–30 IFN units contained in either serum or its low-molecular-weight fraction. Two control groups received either the high-molecular-weight serum fraction of the IFN-containing serum or whole normal trout serum. All groups were then infected immediately by immersion in VHS virus and the mortalities noted (from DeKinkelin *et al.* (1982), *Dev. Comp. Immunol. (Suppl.)* **2**, 167–174, with permission).

virus *in vivo*, demonstrating that the *in vivo* antiviral activity is also nonspecific in nature.

Physicochemical analysis of these *in vitro* and *in vivo* induced IFNs has shown large differences. Serum IFN possesses a molecular mass of 26 kDa, a pI of 5.3 and a sedimentation coefficient of 2.3 (Dorson *et al.*, 1975), whereas fibroblast IFN has a molecular mass of 94 kDa and a pI of 7.1 (DeSena and Rio, 1975).

Cross-hybridization studies with a human IFN-β cDNA probe show that IFN-ß sequences are present in bony fish (Wilson *et al.*, 1983; Tengelsen *et al.*, 1991). Thus, a distinct IFN-β gene probably arose before the divergence of fish and amphibia. However, studies with a human IFN-α cDNA probe have failed to reveal hybridization (Wilson *et al.*, 1983).

Amphibia

Crosshybridization studies with a human IFN-β cDNA probe reveal IFN-β sequences in frog (*Xenopus*) DNA (Wilson *et al.*, 1983). However, as in bony fish, no hybridization occurs with a human IFN-α cDNA probe.

Reptiles

Tortoise (*Testudo graeca*) kidney and peritoneal cell cultures and turtle (*Terrapene carolina*) heart-cell cultures can secrete IFN activity in response to virus infection (Galabov, 1981; Mathews and Vorndam, 1982). Using peritoneal cells, IFN production commences as early as 2 h postinfection at 37°C, increasing to a maximum at 8 h. At 26°C IFN release is delayed until 8 h, but at 20°C and 8°C no IFN release occurs. In the tortoise IFN activity can also be induced in response to polyI:polyC or *Serratia marcescens* endotoxin, even at temperatures as low as 8°C (although greatly reduced and delayed). The tortoise IFN, irrespective of the type of inducer, is acid stable (pH 2), relatively heat-resistant but sensitive to trypsin treatment, whereas turtle IFN is sensitive to both heat and trypsin. As in fish, protection of cell lines against viral CPE by reptilian IFN is species-specific but nonspecific with regard to the challenge virus. Fractionation of the tortoise IFN-containing supernatants by gel chromotography shows a single peak of IFN activity with a molecular mass of 58.5 kDa from virus-treated cells, and two peaks of activity with molecular masses of 43.5–62 kDa and 102–144 kDa from endotoxin or polyI:polyC-treated cells.

Crosshybridization of a human IFN-α cDNA probe with lizard (*Lacerta viridis*) DNA reveals faint but consistently labelled DNA fragments (Wilson *et al.*, 1983). Thus, different classes of type 1 IFN are likely to be present in amniotes. Human IFN, however, has no antiviral effects on tortoise kidney cells.

Birds

In birds IFN activity is readily demonstrated in allantoic fluid from eggs inoculated with virus for 48 h (Moehring and Stinebring, 1981). Indeed, hens' eggs were the first source of IFN. IFN is also produced in adult birds following intravenous inoculation with virus. In addition, virally induced IFN is produced by chicken embryo fibroblast and macrophage cultures between 1 and 4 days postinfection. In the latter case, yields of IFN can be increased if inactivated viruses are used for infection or if the cells are treated with low doses of IFN for 2–4 h prior to infection. The IFN activity is pH stable, relatively heat-resistant and trypsin sensitive (Lampson *et al.*, 1965) as in other vertebrate classes, indicating that it is a type 1 IFN. Considerable interspecies activity is found between avian IFNs and an 'order specificity' is apparent (Moehring and Stinebring 1970). Thus, cells and IFN preparations from a particular species within an avian order (e.g. Galliformes) can crossreact to various extents with other species in that order but not with species in other orders (Table 2). In agreement with this, no crossreactivity of avian IFN with mammalian cells occurs. Physicochemical analysis of chicken type 1 IFN shows that it has a molecular mass of 26–38 kDa and a pI of 7–8 (Lampson *et al.*, 1965).

In addition to its antiviral activity, avian type 1 IFN is also able to induce macrophage activation, as evidenced by induction of cytostatic activity against a T-lymphoblastoid cell line and enhanced cell spreading (Von Bulow *et al.*, 1984). Cytostasis-inducing activity of fibroblast-derived IFN is some 20–30 fold lower than its antiviral activity, whereas with macrophage-derived IFN the relative levels of the two activities are much closer. This suggests that heterogeneity exists within this avian IFN type. That different types of class 1 IFN are present in birds is also supported by crosshybridization studies using human IFN-α and IFN-β cDNA probes, which both react with chicken DNA (Wilson *et al.*, 1983).

Type 2 IFN

Fish

In rainbow trout IFN activity is present in 48 supernatants from Con-A-pulsed head kidney leukocytes (Graham and Secombes, 1990b). The highest degree of protection of trout epithelial (RTH) cells against the CPE of IPN virus is seen using relatively low virus titres, 5×10^3 TCID$_{50}$/well and lower. IFN activity in these crude preparations is significantly decreased following exposure to acid conditions (pH 2) or

Table 2. Order specificity of type 1 interferon in birds.

Source of IFN	Galliformes						Anseriformes			Columbiformes
	Chicken	Turkey	Pheasant	Partridge	Quail	Guinea fowl	Pekin duck	Mallard duck	Goose	Common pigeon
Chicken (O)	+	+	-	+	+	+	-	ND	-	-
Turkey (O)	+	+	+	+	+	+	-	ND	-	-
Pheasant (O)	+	+	+	+	+	+	-	ND	ND	-
Partridge (O)	-	+	-	+	+	+	-	ND	ND	-
Quail (T)	-	-	-	-	+	-	ND	ND	-	-
Guinea fowl (O)	-	ND	-	ND	+	+	ND	ND	ND	ND
Pekin duck (O)	-	-	ND	ND	-	-	+	+	+	-
Mallard duck (O)	ND	-	ND	ND	ND	-	+	+	+	-
Goose (O)	-	-	ND	ND	-	-	+	+	+	-
Common pigeon (T)	-	-	ND	ND	ND	-	-	ND	-	+

O, produced *in ovo*; T, produced in tissue culture; + positive antiviral effect; – no antiviral effect; ND, not done. Adapted from Moehring and Stinebring (1970) *Nature* **226**, 360–361, with permission.

relatively high temperatures (60°C). However, some antiviral activity does remain in these supernatants, possibly owing to the presence of a small amount of type 1 IFN. Fractionation of the supernatants by HPLC size-exclusion chromatography reveals IFN activity in two protein peaks with molecular masses of 19 kDa and 32 kDa, with most activity being in the former peak. Exposure of the 19 kDa peak to acid conditions (pH 2), 60°C for 1 h and trypsin completely removes the antiviral activity. The acid- and temperature-sensitivity, combined with the mode of induction, suggest that this is a type 2 IFN. In addition, the IFN activity coelutes with MAF activity in this species, which is also acid- and temperature-sensitive (see below). Whether these two activities are due to the same molecular species awaits further study. Mammalian IFN-γ does not have an effect on fish cells, in that it does not increase the respiratory-burst activity of cultured rainbow trout macrophages (Nagelkerke, L. personal communication).

Birds

In chickens 24–72-h supernatants from Con-A-stimulated splenocytes and thymocytes contain IFN activity (Weiler and Von Bulow, 1987a). This activity increases with the length of time in culture with Con A over the 72-h period, is decreased in supernatants from leukocytes receiving a pulse exposure to Con A, and is dependent upon adherent cells. Indeed, addition of 5% autologous spleen cells to adherent cell-depleted splenic leukocytes fully restores IFN production and can increase thymocyte production 10-fold. As in fish, the Con-A-induced IFN is clearly sensitive to acid, temperature and trypsin but some antiviral activity remains (40%) following these treatments, possibly due to some type 1 IFN in the supernatants (Von Bulow et al., 1984).

In addition to their antiviral activity these supernatants possess potent MAF activity and are able to increase phagocytosis and induce cytostatic activity in cultured macrophages (Von Bulow et al., 1984). They can also induce the expression of Class II MHC (B-L) antigens on epithelial cells and inhibit the development of the obligate intracellular protozoan parasite Eimeria tenella in cultured chick kidney cells (Kogut and Lange, 1989). The MAF and anti-Eimeria activities are sensitive to acid and temperature, which suggests that a close relationship may exist between them and the IFN activity. Indeed, both the MAF and IFN activities are secreted from thymocytes, containing approximately 80% T cells, but not from bursal cell cultures containing 5% T cells, and thus appear to be T-cell products. This is in agreement with the suggestion that chicken Con-A-induced IFN activity is a type 2 IFN.

INTERLEUKINS

The term interleukin was introduced over a decade ago to describe cytokines able to act on leukocytes in a specific manner. The number of interleukins discovered has been increasing steadily, with thirteen currently recognized (Chapters 3–14) and possibly more receiving interleukin status in the near future (Chapter 28). Outside of the mammals few cytokines with interleukin activity have been described, probably owing to the lack of long-term lymphocyte cell lines, especially B-cell lines which are commonly used to detect the activity of several of the interleukins. Those that have been described appear to correlate functionally with IL-1 and IL-2, and both of these activities have been detected in fish, amphibia and birds. IL-1 activity, in particular, may be quite conserved phylogenetically, with several reports of invertebrates producing an IL-1-like protein. The biological activity and sources of these molecules are now considered in more detail.

IL-1

Stimulation of phagocytes with LPS has been the main approach taken to generate supernatants with IL-1-like activity. A thymocyte costimulation assay which examines thymocyte proliferation in the presence of submitogenic concentrations of T-cell mitogens (Con A, PHA), has commonly been used to test for IL-1 activity.

Invertebrates

Both Deuterostome* and Protostome invertebrates have been shown to produce molecules with IL-1-like activity. Within Deuterostomes, tunicates of the class Ascidiacea (Beck et al., 1989) and the starfish Asterias forbesi (Beck and Habicht, 1986), have had this activity detected using a murine thymocyte costimulation assay (where a two-to-threefold increase in proliferation is seen) and a fibroblast proliferation assay. In addition, the tunicate factor can increase vascular permeability when injected intradermally into rabbits. The function of these factors in Deuterostomes is not known.

IL-1-like activity can be detected in starfish freeze–thaw extracts of coelomyocytes (the principal phagocytes in this species) and coelomic fluid, or from tunicate tissue homogenates and blood. However, in the starfish samples activity is detectable only following fractionation by gel chromatography. The presence of activity in the blood and coelomic fluid suggests that the IL-1-like factor is a secreted protein, probably from the invertebrate phagocytes. The molecular masses of the secreted form are approximately 30 kDa and 20 kDa for the starfish and tunicate, respectively, with pI values of 4.8, 5.9 and 7.5, or 5.5 and 7.0. The intracellular activity from the starfish coelomocytes is more heterogeneous and can be detected at molecular weights of approximately, 10, 30 and 70 kDa (Beck and Habicht, 1986). Finally, both starfish and tunicate IL-1-like activities can be significantly neutralized using polyclonal antiserum to human IL-1.

In Protostomes, stimulation of haemocytes of the mussel Mytilus edulis with LPS induces cell-spreading in vitro and this can be inhibited with anti-IL-1α (Hughes et al., 1991). Human rIL-1α induces similar effects and immunoreactive IL-1 can be detected in concentrated haemolymph (Hughes et al., 1990). Such data support the notion that IL-1 is a functionally conserved molecule that has been important in the evolution of host defence mechanisms, although its exact role in invertebrates has not been elucidated.

Fish

The requirement for macrophages or monocytes in fish (catfish and salmonid) immune responses has been known for several years. In vitro studies have shown that proliferation in response to T-cell mitogens or allogeneic leukocytes (MLR), MAF production and secretion of anti-hapten antibodies are all accessory-cell-dependent (Graham and

---

*The Deuterostomes diverged at an early stage in evolution from the Protostome invertebrates, and are thought to be on the evolutionary line that gave rise to the vertebrates.

Secombes, 1990a; Clem *et al.*, 1991). Indeed, supernatants from LPS-stimulated monocytes or spontaneous monocyte-like cell lines of channel catfish allow macrophage-depleted lymphocytes to undergo Con-A-induced mitogenesis and *in vitro* antibody responses to both TD and TI antigens, without the need for intact accessory cells (Clem *et al.*, 1991). That this soluble factor is detectable by manipulation of mitogenesis assays is analogous to the situation with IL-1, but that it can replace the need for antigen processing and presentation by macrophages in the antibody response implies that this function can be carried out by other cell types in the presence of this cytokine. B cells and monocytes have both been shown to be very efficient antigen-presenting cells in fish, with T cells having a much weaker capacity (Vallejo *et al.*, 1992).

Supernatants containing murine or human IL-1 (but not rIL-1) can also substitute for intact accessory cells in fish, and in the latter case this effect can be inhibited using antibodies against human IL-1 (Hamby *et al.*, 1986; Clem *et al.*, 1991). Thus, fish lymphocytes appear to possess a receptor that can recognize and respond to IL-1. Anti-human IL-1α and IL-1β also inhibit the fish response to fish supernatants. Similarly, fish supernatants, in concert with PHA, can induce proliferation of murine thymocytes and IL-2 production by a murine T lymphoma (LBRM33-1AS).

An IL-1-like factor has also been found in supernatants from a carp (*Cyprinus carpio*) epithelial-cell line (Sigel *et al.*, 1986). This cytokine has been shown to be costimulatory in a murine thymocyte proliferation assay, to induce IL-2 production from murine T cells and to cause an increase in thromboxane production from rabbit corneal epithelial cells and chicken chondrocytes.

Fractionation of the fish monocyte-derived IL-1-like activity by gel filtration has shown two forms of the molecule, with molecular masses of approximately 15 kDa and 70 kDa (Clem *et al.*, 1991). The high-molecular-mass form is active on catfish cells but not mouse T cells, whereas the low-molecular-mass form has the reverse activity. Similar studies with culture supernatants from a mouse monocyte-cell line (P388D1) have also found IL-1 activity for catfish and mouse T cells in either a high- or low-molecular-weight fraction, respectively; both fractions react with anti-mouse IL-1α. Western blot analysis of the catfish material with anti-human IL-1 has shown that both forms possess α and β determinants. Furthermore, cytoplasmic mRNA from catfish monocytes hybridizes with a murine IL-1α cDNA probe, and the hybridizing species has a mobility similar to that observed with P388D1 cell mRNA. These findings suggest that a polymeric IL-1-like molecule may be required for the fish cells, and since mammalian rIL-1 is exclusively of low molecular weight this would explain why it is not active in fish.

Amphibia

In the frog *Xenopus laevis*, 24-h supernatants from LPS-stimulated adherent peritoneal cells (containing 50–80% macrophages) are active in a thymocyte-costimulation assay (Watkins *et al.*, 1987). Both adult and larval thymocyte proliferation is only marginal in response to the supernatants or low concentrations of PHA alone, or to a combination of LPS and PHA, but a marked costimulatory effect is seen when the supernatants plus PHA are used (Table 3). Culture with LPS for 48 h before harvesting the supernatants results in lower activity. These supernatants do not stimulate the proliferation of thymic lymphoblasts or support their long-term growth, which suggests that they do not contain T-cell growth factors (cf. IL-2). Furthermore, since LPS is not a T-cell mitogen

Table 3. Thymocyte costimulatory activity of 24-h supernatants from LPS-stimulated macrophages (SN) in two *Xenopus* clones.

Medium supplemented with	C.p.m. (+SEM) when assayed on thymocytes from	
	Adults	Larvae
Experiment 1[a]		
Nothing	480(131)	1886(1012)
PHA	1149(141)	1564(853)
SN	4650(413)	4331(1222)
SN + PHA	24605(1932)	8214(1663)
Experiment 1[b]		
Nothing	400(12)	913(153)
PHA	860(217)	1699(358)
SN	3437(85)	2855(309)
SN + PHA	10820(293)	7424(810)

[a]Clone LG-6 stage 60-61 larvae; outbred 10-month-old.
[b]Clone LG-17 stage 56-57 larvae; 7-month-old adults. From Cohen *et al.* (1987) In *Developmental and Comparative Immunology* (eds E.L. Cooper, C. Landet and J. Bierne), Alan R. Liss Inc, New York, pp. 53–68, with permission.

in amphibia, as in mammals, it seems likely that this costimulatory cytokine is a macrophage product.

Human IL-1-containing supernatants do not costimulate *Xenopus* thymocytes and *Xenopus* supernatants do not stimulate the mouse D.10.G4.1 cell line, suggesting a lack of crossreactivity *in vitro*. However, human rIL-1 does appear to have effects *in vivo*. During metamorphosis from tadpole to adult, high levels of endogenous corticosteroids are thought to impair T-cell functions, including an antigen-dependent thymus-suppressor function. Injection of human rIL-1 can restore this suppressor function in a dose-dependent manner, possibly by overcoming a lesion in the antigen-presenting cells (Highet and Ruben, 1987). Human rIL-1 also has effects *in vivo* in the common American newt (*Notophthalmus viridescens*), where it can substitute for carrier priming in anti-hapten responses (Ruben *et al.*, 1988).

Reptiles

Nothing is known about the production of IL-1 by reptile cells. However, the lizard *Dipsosaurus dorsalis* does appear to be able to respond to rabbit IL-1, as evidenced by induction of fever following an intracardiac injection (Bernheim and Kluger, 1977). The lizard can also produce an endogenous pyrogen in response to stimulation with thioglycollate or killed bacteria, but the relationship of this pyrogen to IL-1 is unclear.

Birds

In chickens 72-h supernatants from LPS-pulsed (4-h) adherent spleen cells are costimulatory for chicken thymocytes stimulated with Con A or PHA, enhancing the mitogen response approximately twofold (Hayara *et al.*, 1982). These supernatants also show costimulatory effects on the Con A response of mouse thymocytes, and mouse IL-1 is costimulatory in the chicken response. Mammalian IL-1 is also able to induce PGE_2 and

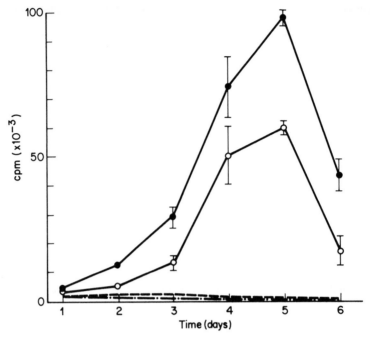

Fig. 2. Effect of growth-factor-containing supernatants on the kinetics of ^{3}H-thymidine uptake into carp lymphoblasts. Blast cells (2.5 × 10^4 per well) were incubated with growth-factor-containing supernatants from PHA-activated head kidney leukocytes (●), control supernatants from nonmitogen treated cells (– – –), control supernatants supplemented with PHA (○), or fresh medium (·–·–·). Both types of control cultures incorporated only low levels of ^{3}H-thymidine. PHA by itself was mitogenic for blasts, but significantly more incorporation was seen with the growth-factor containing supernatants (from Grondel and Harmsen (1984), *Immunology* **52**, 477–482, with permission).

cAMP formation from chicken ileal mucosa *in vitro* (Chang *et al.*, 1987), and to stimulate increases in short-circuit current (a measure of anion secretion). Since the latter is blocked using a specific inhibitor of cyclooxygenase it appears that IL-1 induces the formation of inflammatory mediators such as PGE$_2$ by activating arachidonic acid metabolism.

IL-2

Stimulation of leukocytes/lymphocytes with a T-cell mitogen has been the main approach adopted to generate supernatants containing IL-2-like activity in the lower vertebrates. Because of the essential role of IL-2 in T cell growth (see Chapter 4), a blast-cell assay is normally employed to test for IL-2 activity.

Fish

In carp, supernatants from leukocyte cultures stimulated by mitogen (PHA) or alloantigen (MLR) induce the proliferation of purified PHA-activated lymphoblasts (T-cell blasts?), analogous to the effect of IL-2 (Fig. 2) (Caspi and Avtalion, 1984; Grondel and Harmsen, 1984). Only cells that are already activated undergo proliferation in response to such supernatants; freshly harvested (virgin) leukocytes are not stimulated. Furthermore, adsorption of the supernatants with blast cells significantly reduces the activity of this growth factor, whereas adsorption with virgin leukocytes has little effect. Such data suggests that receptors for this factor are induced upon activation of the virgin cells. Supernatants from two-way MLR cultures show a lower and more variable growth-promoting effect than do those from mitogen-stimulated cultures (Caspi and Avtalion, 1984). As mitogens have a polyclonal stimulatory effect upon lymphocytes this may induce the secretion of more lymphokine, explaining the higher activity in such supernatants. The variability of the MLR supernatants may be due to variability of the histocompatibility antigens on the lymphocytes used for allogeneic stimulation, since outbred animals are used. Pooling supernatants from at least four donors in several combinations has been found to give more consistent results, and significant enhancement of the growth-promoting activity can be obtained by having PMA present in the MLR cultures.

Mouse IL-2 has no effect on carp lymphoblasts (Grondel and Harmsen, 1984), although supernatants containing human, rat and monkey IL-2 have been reported to stimulate their proliferation (Caspi and Avtalion, 1984). Human IL-2 has also been reported to increase specific cellular cytotoxicity by carp lymphocytes, but fails to increase binding to, or killing of, target cells by rainbow trout NK cells. Whether the positive effect of mammalian IL-2-containing supernatants is due solely to the activity of IL-2 is unclear, especially as more-purified preparations are often less active. The use of defined reagents is clearly warranted.

Amphibia

In the frog *X. laevis*, 24–28-h supernatants from splenic leukocytes stimulated with PHA, Con A and neuraminidase plus galactose (NAGO) are costimulatory in a thymocyte-proliferation assay (using adult or larval cell supernatants), induce the proliferation of PHA-induced lymphoblasts and splenocytes from coccobacilloid infected animals (Haynes *et al.*, 1992), and support the growth of alloreactive T-cell lines (Watkins and Cohen, 1987). Splenocytes from infected animals also show constitutive production of this factor. The supernatants do not induce proliferation of unstimulated splenocytes, and adsorption with splenocytes does not affect the IL-2-like activity. However, adsorption with blasts does reduce this activity, the decrease being proportional to the number of blasts used. Therefore, as in fish, it appears that only lymphoblasts can bind to, or react with, this growth factor, suggesting the presence of an inducible receptor on frog T cells. Similarly, in the Axolotl *Ambystoma americanum* splenic blasts can be costimulated with homologous or *Xenopus*-derived growth-factor-containing supernatants in combination with PHA (Koniski and Cohen, 1991).

Purification of the *Xenopus* growth factor by DEAE ion-exchange chromotography and SDS-PAGE have shown that it has a molecular weight of 16 kDa, and lectin affinity chromatography indicates it has a three-dimensional configuration of carbohydrates that is similar to human IL-2 (Watkins and Cohen, 1985; Haynes and Cohen, 1993a). SDS–PAGE analysis of labelled Axolotl growth factor containing supernatants reveals bands of 15, 45 and 60 kDa (Koniski and Cohen, 1991).

Evidence to suggest that T cells are involved in producing, as well as responding to, this amphibian growth factor comes from several sources. First, T-cell mitogens induce secretion of this factor. Second, supernatants (48–120-h) from MLR cultures of MHC-distinct *Xenopus* strains and from alloreactive T-cell lines stimulated with PHA or

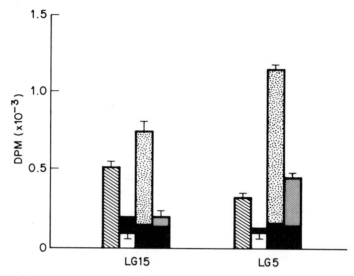

Fig. 3.   Effect of thymectomy on growth factor production by *Xenopus* splenocytes. Incorporation of ³H-thymidine into lymphoblasts from two different *Xenopus* clones (LG15 and LG5) following a 72-h incubation with medium (▨), PHA (☐) and 24-h supernatants from PHA-stimulated splenocytes obtained from normal (▦) or early thymectomized (▨) animals. The black shading represents the d.p.m. after adsorption of the PHA solution used with chicken erythrocytes (from Horton *et al.*, in preparation).

irradiated stimulator cells also have growth-promoting activity (Watkins and Cohen, 1987). Finally, thymectomy studies have shown that early thymectomy impairs production of this factor by PHA stimulation (Fig. 3). Thymocytes, however, apparently do not secrete this factor (Cohen *et al.*, 1987). Whether this is due to a complete inability of these cells to produce this factor or to an inefficient activation of the cells by low IL-1 secretion from thymic macrophages is unclear.

The *Xenopus* IL-2-like factor has no effect on human T-cell blasts or on a murine IL-2-dependent cell line, HT-2 (Watkins and Cohen, 1987). Crossreactivity of mammalian IL-2 and anti-IL-2 receptor (anti-Tac) antibody with the *Xenopus* cells, however, is subject to controversy. Some authors have elegantly shown, by flow cytometry and immunogold electron microscopy, that *Xenopus* splenocytes and PHA-stimulated thymocytes (when fixed with paraformaldehyde) bind both human rIL-2 and murine anti-Tac antibody (Fig. 4), and that rIL-2 will compete with the anti-Tac antibody for the binding sites (Ruben *et al.*, 1990, 1991). PHA activation of splenocytes increases the binding of anti-Tac and is inhibitable with cycloheximide, suggesting that this treatment induces the synthesis of new receptors. Immunoprecipitation of labelled PHA-stimulated thymocytes with the anti-Tac antibody reveals a molecule of approximately 55 kDa (Ruben *et al.*, 1991), similar to the human IL-2R Tac protein. Despite these findings, human rIL-2 and human or mouse IL-2-rich supernatants fail to stimulate proliferation of *Xenopus* blasts or T-cell mitogenesis *in vitro* (Watkins and Cohen, 1985). Nevertheless, factors such as PHA or phorbol dibutyrate (PDB), which do increase mitogenesis, increase the binding of anti-Tac (Ruben *et al.*, 1991), and factors such as dexamethasone or cyclosporin A, which inhibit PHA- or PDB-induced mitogenesis, decrease binding. *In vivo* it has been shown that injection of rIL-2 can: (1)

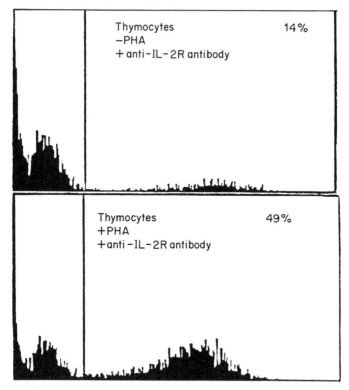

Fig. 4. The effect of PHA stimulation on the reactivity of *Xenopus* thymocytes with anti-human IL-2R antibody, analysed by flow cytometry. The histograms depict the relative cell number on the ordinate and log fluorescence intensity on the abscissa. The percentage of cells binding the antibody is shown in the upper right corner of each histogram (from Ruben *et al.* (1990), in *Defense Molecules* (eds J.J. Marchalonis and C. Reinisch), Alan R. Liss, New York, pp. 133–147. Reprinted by permission of John Wiley & Sons, Inc. All rights reserved).

substitute for carrier priming of helper function in anti-hapten responses; (2) increase (12-fold) the antibody response to TI-type 2 antigens; and (3) break hapten-specific tolerance (although not in thymectomized frogs) (Ruben, 1986; Ruben *et al.*, 1987). In addition, it can restore T-cell functions that are inhibited by high levels of endogenous corticosteroids during metamorphosis, as seen with human rIL-1.

In contrast, other authors have failed to immunoprecipitate molecules in the growth-factor-containing supernatants with anti-human IL-2 antibodies, to stain *Xenopus* splenic PHA blasts with human anti-Tac, and to immunoprecipitate cell-surface molecules with anti-Tac antibody (Haynes *et al.*, 1990). These authors suggest that binding only occurs following membrane damage and does not reflect ligand-binding on the cell surface. Until these controversies are resolved, whether IL-2 and its receptor are conserved phylogenetically must remain an enigma.

Reptiles

In the snake *Spalerosophis diadema*, supernatants from Con-A-stimulated splenocytes enhance the Con-A-induced proliferation of splenic lymphoblasts (El Ridi *et al.*, 1986).

Fractionation of these supernatants reveals activity in two peaks, with molecular masses of 15 kDa and 39–42 kDa. Only the low-molecular-mass protein is detectable by SDS–PAGE, which suggests that the high-molecular-mass molecule is possibly a polymer of the former. The pI values of these molecules lie in the ranges 5.5–5.8 and 6.4–6.6.

Birds

As in other vertebrate classes, supernatants from mitogen- or antigen-stimulated chicken splenocytes and peripheral-blood leukocytes (PBLs) contain IL-2-like activity (Schauenstein et al., 1982; Schnetzler et al., 1983). Such supernatants can induce the proliferation of Con-A-induced lymphoblasts, such costimulatory in a thymocyte proliferation assay and can maintain long-term cultured T cells. However, they do not induce proliferation of freshly isolated (unstimulated) splenocytes. Cyclosporin A (CsA) does not block this factor-mediated blast stimulation, suggesting that it acts specifically on activated T cells, which are unresponsive to the effects of CsA (Schnetzler et al., 1983); both cultured T cells and Con-A-induced blasts die within 1–2 days in the absence of this growth factor, demonstrating that their growth is totally factor-dependent. In addition, adsorption studies show that cultured T cells and Con-A-induced blasts can remove virtually all of this IL-2-like activity and thymocytes can remove about 45%, but virgin (unstimulated) PBL and bursal (B) cells remove insignificant amounts. Again, an inducible growth-factor receptor appears to be present on T cells. The use of T-cell mitogens to generate these growth-factor-containing supernatants, coupled with the fact that T-cell-enriched (84–88%) PBLs (Schnetzler et al., 1983) and PBLs from agammaglobulinaemic birds can also be used for this purpose (Vainio et al., 1986), suggests that this factor is a T-cell product.

IL-2-like activity is highest in 24-h supernatants, and Con A is slightly better at inducing its release than PHA. Treatment of lymphocytes with Con-A-coated chicken erythrocytes markedly enhances secretion of this IL-2-like molecule (Kromer et al., 1984). Activity of the supernatants is stable at $-20°C$ but is lost after 5 weeks at 4°C. The half-life at 40°C is approximately 10 ± 2 h, which is significantly shorter than for mammalian IL-2. Fractionation of the supernatants by gel chromatography reveals two major peaks of activity, with molecular masses of 9–13 kDa and 19.5–21.5 kDa, the former having a pI of 5.9. Using SDS–PAGE a single polypeptide of 13 kDa is found, indicating that the larger form may be a dimer of the 13 kDa molecule. The chicken IL-2-like factor is species-restricted, since it cannot induce proliferation of mouse or rat lymphoblasts. Mouse, rat and human IL-2 cannot induce proliferation of chicken lymphoblasts.

The IL-2-like factor appears to have a crucial role in T-cell activation in chickens, since there is a close correlation between proliferative responses of lymphocytes in culture and detectable growth-factor activity of the supernatants (Fig. 5) (Schauenstein and Kromer, 1987). Growth factor activity can be detected in cultures where the cells are not proliferating because of irradiation or cytostatic treatment, but proliferation cannot occur within the IL-2-like factor. This has also been shown for genetically determined high- and low-responsiveness to Con A of certain chicken strains, which parallels differences in the production and responsiveness to the growth factor. Similarly, during ontogeny of this species, the acquisition of proliferative responses to Con A is closely linked with the capacity to produce this IL-2-like factor. Thus, the

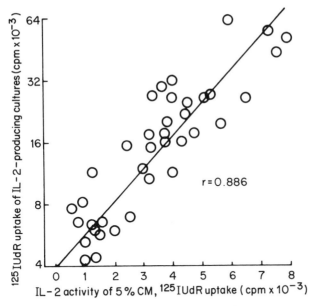

Fig. 5. Correlation of the proliferative response to Con-A (ordinate) and the production of IL-2 (abscissa) of individual chicken splenocyte cultures (from Kromer *et al.* (1984), *J. Immunol. Methods* **73**, 273–281, with permission).

production or secretion of this growth factor largely determines the magnitude of mitogen- or antigen-driven chicken T-cell responses.

Recently, a monoclonal antibody has been raised against Con-A-activated lymphoblasts that recognizes a chicken activated T-lymphocyte antigen (CATLA) (Schauenstein *et al.*, 1988). The CATLA molecule has been shown to have a molecular mass of 48–50 kDa by SDS–PAGE following immunoprecipitation of radiolabelled lymphocyte surface components. The number of splenocytes and PBLs expressing CATLA ranges from 1% of freshly isolated cells to 15–30% of 3-h Con-A-stimulated cells and more than 90% of 72-h Con-A-stimulated cells (Fig. 6). The presence of the anti-CATLA antibody markedly inhibits, in a competitive manner, the proliferative response of T lymphoblasts to the IL-2-like molecule. Similarly, pretreatment of lymphoblasts with this antibody reduces their ability to absorb the IL-2-like activity from conditioned media. Such data suggest strongly that CATLA is the chicken equivalent of an IL-2 receptor or an associated structure, and that the anti-CATLA antibody is equivalent to an anti-Tac antibody.

Pathological disturbances of T-cell regulations are known in chickens, particularly in the Obese strain (OS) of chickens which exhibit Hashimoto-like spontaneous autoimmune thyroiditis (SAT) (Schauenstein *et al.*, 1985; Kroemer and Wick, 1989). Animals suffering from SAT have elevated T-cell proliferation, IL-2 production and IL-2 receptor expression following mitogen stimulation. The hypersecretion of IL-2-like molecules is thought to be an accelerating factor modulating SAT, and not a secondary event of autoimmunity. Morphological studies have shown that lymphocytes infiltrating the thyroid which initiate the disease process, contain a high percentage of IL-2R-positive T cells and, if isolated, these thyroid-infiltrating lymphocytes can be

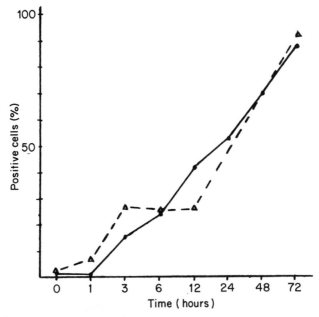

Fig. 6. The expression of chicken activated T-lymphocyte antigen (CATLA) on blood leukocytes (△) and splenocytes (●) at different times after stimulation *in vitro* with Con-A (2.5 μg/ml) (from Hala *et al.* (1986), *Eur. J. Immunol.* **16**, 1331–1336, with permission).

shown to secrete large amounts of IL-2 spontaneously. This T-cell defect appears to be encoded by a single recessive gene (Kroemer *et al.*, 1990). T-cell dysfunction has also been seen in avian scleroderma, where elevated IL-2 activity is seen in serum but blood leukocytes show impaired IL-2 production and IL-2R expression (Gruschwitz *et al.*, 1991).

IL-3

No reports of IL-3-like activity have been described other than in the mammals. A single report exists of the crossreactivity of mammalian IL-3 on chicken cells where, as with IL-1, IL-3 induces PGE_2 and cAMP formation and increases short-circuit current from isolated ileal mucosa (Chang *et al.*, 1987).

Other Interleukins

In fish, *in vitro* stimulation of immunoglobulin production by PHA has been shown and may be a result of interleukins secreted from T cells which subsequently influence B cells. Similarly, PMA/calcium-ionophore-induced T-like cell lines of channel catfish secrete factors that can enhance the mitogenic responses of B (and T) lymphocytes, but nonspecifically suppress *in vitro* antibody responses (Clem *et al.*, 1991). These putative interleukins do not function in mouse bioassays for B-cell growth factors (IL-4), and rIL-4 does not exhibit functional activity with fish cells.

In *Xenopus*, supernatants from PHA-stimulated splenocytes support the growth of homologous B cells (Cohen and Haynes, 1991). In addition, a striking costimulation of these supernatants with LPS and an anti-*Xenopus* IgM monoclonal antibody is seen.

Chicken supernatants from Con-A-stimulated splenocytes induce the formation of multinucleated giant cells in macrophage cultures (Weiler and Von Bulow, 1987b). This macrophage fusion factor (MFF) activity is optimal when added to 5–7-day-old cultures. MFF activity in mammals has been ascribed to IL-4 (McInnes and Rennick, 1988).

A variety of dialysable (<10 kDa) suppressive factors also exist in supernatants from mitogen- or specific-antigen-stimulated chicken leukocytes (Schauenstein and Kromer, 1987). Responses in both B cells (antibody secretion) and T cells (IL-2 production and responsiveness) are affected, in a nonspecific manner. Interestingly, in OS chickens with spontaneous autoimmune thyroiditis the suppressive activity is significantly reduced and accounts directly for the IL-2 hypersecretion and mitogen hyperactivity seen in this strain (Schauenstein *et al.*, 1985). This activity appears to be due to a macrophage product, since thymectomy, bursectomy and removal of nonadherent splenocytes do not influence suppressive activity.

To date, no other interleukin-like molecules are known in nonmammalian vertebrates.

PHAGOCYTE MODULATING CYTOKINES

It is well known that mammalian leukocytes can produce a diverse array of cytokines able to affect various phagocyte activities. These include factors able to enhance or inhibit their migration (chemokines and migration inhibition factors), to induce their proliferation (colony stimulating factors) or fusion (fusion factors), and to increase their killing activity (activating factors). As more purified cytokines have become available, some of these activities have been shown to be due to members of the interleukin and IFN cytokine groups, such as IL-4 and IFN-γ. Since few nonmammalian cytokines are well characterized, all of these activities are considered here.

Migration Inhibition Factors

Most studies of leukocyte migration inhibition factors (MIF) have employed the capillary tube technique. This involves centrifuging a capillary tube containing leukocytes in order to pellet the cells, cutting the tube at the cell–medium interface and then allowing the cells to migrate out into a culture dish containing medium for 18–24 h. The medium may contain preformed MIF (indirect assay) or, if *in-vivo*-sensitized leukocytes are used for migration, specific antigen to generate MIF *in situ* (direct assay). In either case the degree of migration inhibited is noted, usually by planimetry.

Invertebrates

Lysates from starfish *Asterias forbesi* coelomocytes (phagocytes) induce prompt aggregation of circulating coelomocytes when injected into the arm of intact starfish (Prendergast and Suzuki, 1970). The cells become fixed to the walls of the respiratory papulae for 20–40 min, after which they slowly disperse. When tested *in vitro* for MIF activity, significant inhibition of guinea-pig macrophage migration is seen. Exposure of

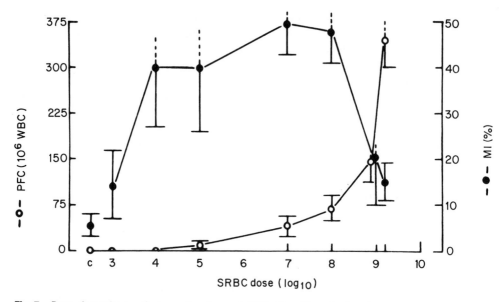

Fig. 7. Dose dependency of plaque-forming cell (PFC, O—O) and migration inhibition (MI, ●—●) responses to sheep red blood cells (SRBC) in *Tilapia mossambica*. Head kidney lymphocytes were assayed 5 days after immunization: C denotes control values (from Jayaraman *et al.* (1979). *Dev. Comp. Immunol.* **3**, 67–75. Reprinted by permission of John Wiley & Sons, Inc. All rights reserved).

the sea star factor (SSF) to a temperature of 56°C for 30 min completely destroys its MIF activity. Biochemical characterization of SSF has shown it to have a two-polypeptide chain structure with a molecular mass of 38 kDa and a pI of 8.2 (Prendergast and Liu, 1976).

Fish
MIF activity has been demonstrated in a large range of fish species using T-cell mitogens and a variety of antigens, including bacterial and parasite antigens, alloantigens and even autoantigens. Most studies have employed direct assays to detect MIF release from sensitized blood, head kidney or peritoneal leukocytes. Only few studies have used MIF-containing supernatants to confirm the presence of soluble mediators. For example, in carp, supernatants from blood leukocytes stimulated with 10 μg/ml Con-A for 24–48 h induce significant inhibition of head kidney leukocyte migration (Secombes, 1981). The migratory cells have been identified as macrophages by their morphology and characteristic adherence to the migration culture plates when these are inverted.

The ability to release MIF appears to vary inversely with the ability to secrete specific antibody. This occurs over a range of timings after immunization and antigen doses (Fig. 7), with MIF production predominating early in the immune response or in response to low antigen doses (Jayaraman *et al.*, 1979). Conversely, MIF production correlates very closely with allograft rejection in the garpike *Lepisosteus platyrhincus* (McKinney *et al.*, 1981) and with resistance against furunculosis in vaccinated brown trout, *Salmo trutta* (Smith *et al.*, 1980). Thus its detection is a good *in vitro* indicator of an ongoing cell-mediated immune response.

Supernatants from eel (*Anguilla japonica*) spleen, kidney or blood leukocytes incubated with specific antigen for 72 h can induce migration inhibition of guinea-pig peritoneal cells, suggesting a significant degree of conservation of MIF cytokines (Song *et al.*, 1989).

Amphibia

Both urodele (Axolotls) and anuran (frogs and toads) amphibians have been shown to produce MIF (Tahan and Jurd, 1979; Gearing and Rimmer, 1985a). MIF activity has been detected by direct and indirect assays, using antigen- and mitogen-stimulated splenocyte supernatants in the latter. In the axolotl *A. mexicanum*, splenocytes sensitized to *Mycobacterium tuberculosis* release MIF in direct assays following exposure to the purified protein derivative of tuberculin (PPD) (Tahan and Jurd, 1979). Sensitization can be transferred to unsensitized axolotls by injection of splenocytes (but not serum) from immunized donors, which suggests that this is a cell-mediated phenomenon. In the frog *Rana temporaria*, antigen-specific MIF release is seen 1–3 weeks postinjection in direct assays and is dependent upon the antigen concentration in the medium (Gearing and Rimmer, 1985a). In indirect assays MIF is detectable in 72-h supernatants from antigen-stimulated (primed) splenocytes and in 48-h supernatants from Con-A-stimulated control cells. In both assays its activity is blocked by α-L-fucose (but not by β-D-galactose) which is thought to compete with MIF for a cell-surface receptor.

Gel chromatography of the frog Con-A supernatants reveals MIF activity in the 27–50 kDa molecular mass range (Gearing and Rimmer, 1985a). Frog MIF activity does not appear to be species-specific, and a supernatant inducing 39% migration inhibition of *Rana* peritoneal cells will induce significant inhibition of rat (25%), *Xenopus* (15%) and carp (11%) leukocyte migration. Finally, injection of a MIF-rich mammalian preparation into *Rana esculenta* causes a marked reduction in the number of peritoneal macrophages, similar to that seen following injection of specific antigen into sensitized *Rana*. This macrophage disappearance reaction suggests that *Rana* cells can also react to mammalian MIF.

Reptiles

In the lizard *Calotes versicolor*, antigen-specific MIF release from sensitized splenocytes is detectable by direct assay 1–5 weeks after immunization or sensitization to skin allografts (Jayaraman and Muthukkaruppan, 1977, 1978). An inverse relationship exists between the migration inhibition response and humoral antibody response (Jayaraman and Muthukkaruppan, 1978): for example, low antigen doses result in a high degree of migration inhibition but low numbers of antibody-secreting cells, whereas high doses have the reverse effect. Addition of 5% sensitized splenocytes to unsensitized cells is sufficient to effect significant migration inhibition in the presence of antigen. Thymocytes from sensitized animals can also bring about this effect (although a higher cell ratio is required), suggesting active generation of MIF-producing cells in the thymus. Thymus-derived cells have also been implicated as the MIF-producing cells in cell-separation experiments. Only nylon–wool nonadherent splenocytes from immunized animals, that are sensitive to anti-thymocyte serum, are effective in inhibiting the migration of control splenocytes in the presence of specific antigen (Manickasundari *et al.*, 1984).

Birds

MIF production by sensitized avian leukocytes incubated with specific antigen can be demonstrated by both direct and indirect assays some 2–3 weeks after immunization (Vlaovic *et al.*, 1975; Trifonov *et al.*, 1977). Both splenocytes and blood leukocytes have been used in direct assays, and a positive correlation with wattle tests (a measure of chicken DTH) has been found (Vlaovic *et al.*, 1975). Using indirect assays, chicken splenocytes, thymocytes, bursal cells and ileocaecal tonsil lymphocytes have all been shown to secrete MIF, as evidenced by migration inhibition of target splenocytes, thymocytes, thrombocytes, bursacytes or peritoneal cells (Trifonov *et al.*, 1977; Stinson *et al.*, 1979; Martin and Glick, 1983). Turkey splenocytes and ileocaecal tonsil lymphocytes also secrete MIF, and in both species splenocyte migration is inhibited to a greater extent than that of peritoneal cells. The ability of B cells to secrete a MIF is rather intriguing. Bursal MIF does not appear to be identical to thymocyte-derived MIF, in that it has a wider target specificity (Martin and Glick, 1983). However, as with mammalian MIF, both cytokines have a molecular mass range of 10–50 kDa, are sensitive to chymotrypsin and neuraminidase treatment but are relatively stable to heat and pH. In contrast to other vertebrate groups, avian MIF is species-specific. Turkey MIF has no effect on the migration of chicken or goose peritoneal and spleen cells, and chicken MIF has no effect on turkey or goose cells (Trifonov *et al.*, 1977).

Chemokines

The migration of leukocytes has been studied in two main ways. In the agarose method, cells migrate from a well cut in an agarose gel towards wells containing the various stimuli. In the Boyden-chamber method, cells migrate from one compartment, through a micropore filter, towards a blind compartment containing the stimuli. Whether an increased migration is chemotactic (directed) or chemokinetic (random) can be determined by the Boyden-chamber method, which permits migration to occur with increasing concentration of the stimulus in the presence or absence of a gradient (checkerboard assay). Since this has not been carried out with nonmammalian cytokines, the term chemotactic factor (CTF) used throughout this section is not intended to imply that a distinction between these activities has been demonstrated.

Fish

That fish can produce cytokines able to influence leukocyte migration has been demonstrated in carp (Howell, 1987). CTF-containing supernatants can be generated by incubation of sensitized kidney cells from carp immunized for 1–2 weeks, with specific antigen for 24–48 h at 28°C. Alternatively, the mitogen PHA can be used to generate such supernatants in the same manner. In a Boyden-type assay both types of supernatants induce significant migration of kidney cells from unsensitized animals, but require rather long migration times (16–22 h). This factor is possibly equivalent to MCP-1/MCAF (Matsushima and Oppenheim, 1989).

Amphibia

In amphibia, supernatants (48–72 h) from mitogen- and specific-antigen-stimulated splenocytes of *R. temporaria* are able to increase the migration of peritoneal cells in

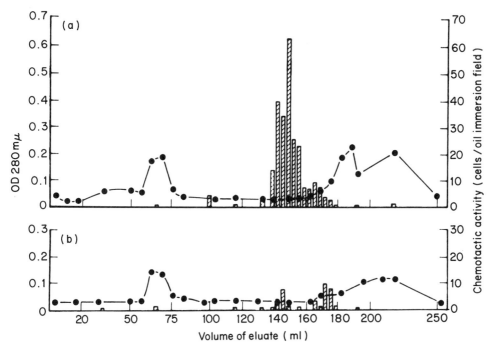

Fig. 8. Fractionation of chemotactic activity in 48-h supernatants from (a) Con-A stimulated chicken splenocytes or (b) nonmitogen-treated cells reconstituted with Con-A, by gel chromatography. Fractions were tested for absorbance (●——●) and monocyte chemotactic activity (▨). The highest column in graph (a) has a molecular mass of 12.5 kDa (from Altman and Kirchner (1974). *Immunology* **26**, 393–405, with permission).

both the agarose and Boyden-type assays (Gearing and Rimmer, 1985b). Predominantly polymorphonuclear leukocytes migrate in response to these supernatants, possibly owing to a faster migration rate. Fractionation of the supernatants reveals that the CTF activity has a molecular mass range of 16–27 kDa.

Birds

Chicken supernatants from splenocytes, thymocytes and blood leukocytes incubated with Con A (5–10 µg/ml) for 48 h significantly increase the migration of monocytes (Altman and Kirchner, 1974). Similarly, lymphocytes from chick embryos stimulated with mitogen *in vivo* are able to produce a factor that enhances eosinophil migration *in vitro*, using either embryonic or adult eosinophils (Moriya and Ichikawa, 1981).

The production of chicken monocyte CTF correlates with a delayed skin-reaction (wattle swelling), which suggests that it is a good *in vitro* correlate of delayed hypersensitivity in this species (Altman and Kirchner, 1974). Physicochemical analysis of this cytokine has shown that, like human CTF, it has a molecular mass of 12.5 kDa (Fig. 8), is relatively heat- and freeze–thaw stable, is resistant to neuraminidase digestion but not to trypsin or pepsin digestion. These latter findings show that chicken CTF is a protein which does not require a terminal sialic acid moiety for its activity, in agreement with mammalian studies. No crossreactivity is apparent for chicken CTF with human, guinea-pig and rabbit monocytes, or for human and guinea-pig CTF with chicken monocytes (Altman and Kirchner, 1974).

The Con-A-induced monocyte CTF is not produced by bursal cells but is produced by spleen cells from agammaglobulinaemic chickens (Altman and Kirchner, 1972), suggesting that it is a T-cell product. The eosinophil CTF, however, appears to be produced by thymocytes or splenocytes in response to Con-A and by bursal cells in response to LPS.

Macrophage Activating Factors

Macrophage activating factors (MAF) are cytokines able to upregulate macrophage bactericidal or tumoricidal activity. A variety of other functions and features may also be affected by such cytokines, but are not sufficient evidence on their own that macrophage activation has been achieved. Thus, only factors able to increase macrophage killing or killing mechanisms are considered in this section.

Fish

In rainbow trout, peritoneal washes from fish primed and boosted intraperitoneally with *Aeromonas salmonicida* are able to increase respiratory-burst activity in control macrophages (Chung and Secombes, 1987). Antibodies do not appear to be involved in this phenomenon, since the peritoneal washes and serum from the same fish do not contain detectable agglutinating antibodies against *A. salmonicida*.

More conclusive evidence that fish can produce a soluble macrophage activating cytokine comes from *in vitro* mitogen studies. Supernatants from Con-A-pulsed kidney leukocytes can significantly increase the spreading, phagocytosis, respiratory-burst activity and bactericidal activity of target macrophages from control fish, particularly when using a virulent strain of *A. salmonicida* in the last case (Graham and Secombes, 1988). Stimulation of MAF release is enhanced using PMA with Con A to stimulate kidney leukocytes, and these supernatants also significantly increase macrophage acid phosphatase levels. The target macrophage require at least 48 h of continuous exposure to MAF to become activated; pulse exposure or shorter incubation times have little effect.

The MAF activity is acid- (pH 2), temperature- (60°C) and trypsin sensitive but relatively freeze–thaw resistant (Graham and Secombes, 1990b). It is not significantly enriched following Con-A-affinity chromatography. However, it can be partly purified by HPLC size-exclusion chromatography, where it is found in the 19- and 32-kDa protein peaks. The predominant and most consistent MAF activity resides in the former peak, as with IFN activity (see above).

That fish MAF is a lymphokine has been suggested by panning experiments using a monoclonal antibody against trout Ig (Graham and Secombes, 1990a). Only purified lymphocytes lacking surface Ig can secrete MAF (Fig. 9), although they require the presence of accessory cells (which do not secrete MAF).

Birds

In chickens, MAF activity is detectable in 24–72-h supernatants from Con-A-stimulated splenocytes or thymocytes, antigen-stimulated immune T lymphocytes and a T-

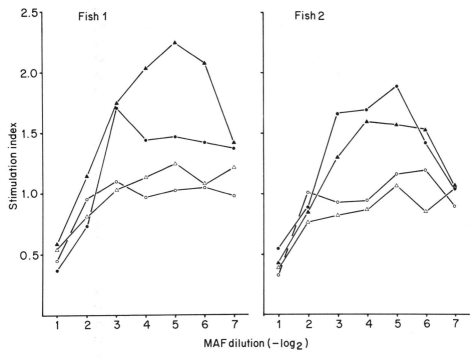

Fig. 9. MAF production by unfractionated rainbow trout blood leukocytes (●), macrophages (○), sIg⁻ lymphocytes plus macrophages (▲) and sIg⁺ lymphocytes plus macrophages (△). MAF activity was assessed by the respiratory-burst activity of target macrophages following a 48-h incubation with the MAF-containing supernatants. The results were expressed as a stimulation index by dividing the value from macrophages incubated with test supernatants with that from macrophages incubated with control supernatants obtained from leukocytes not stimulated with Con-A/PMA (from Graham and Secombes (1990), *Dev. Comp. Immunol.* **14**, 59–68, with permission).

lymphoblastoid cell line, JMV-1 (Weiler and Von Bulow, 1987a,b; Lillehoj *et al.*, 1989). Conversely, Con-A-treated bursal cells and adherent cell-depleted splenocytes do not produce MAF. Both cytostatic activity for a different lymphoblastoid cell line (MDCC-RP1) and anti-*Eimeria* activity are induced in macrophages over an 18–48-h incubation with the supernatants. Increased cell-spreading, giant-cell formation and phagocytic activity are also seen (Weiler and Von Bulow, 1987b). Injection (intraperitoneal, intramuscular or intravenous) of these crude MAF-containing supernatants into chickens 1–5 days before or 1 day after an experimental challenge confers significant protection against avian coccidiosis (*Eimeria* spp.), as evidenced by reduced oocyst production, lesion score and mortality (Lillehoj *et al.*, 1989). Cell-mediated immune responses are thus implicated as a major mechanism of host protective immunity against eimerian infections.

Chicken MAF is clearly a lymphokine secreted by T cells. As cytostatic activity, like IFN activity in these supernatants, is acid (pH 2), temperature (56°C) and trypsin sensitive there is possibly a close link between the molecules effecting these functions (cf. type 2 IFN) (Weiler and Von Bulow, 1987a). However, the induction of giant-cell

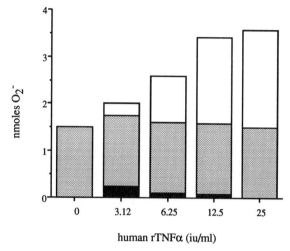

Fig. 10. Respiratory-burst activity (superoxide anion production) of rainbow trout head kidney macrophages treated with human rTNF and 1 : 2 diluted MAF individually and together to show their synergistic effect. Values represent the mean for four fish. ■, rTNF alone; ▦, MAF alone; □, synergy between MAF and rTNF (from Hardie *et al.* (in press). *Vet. Immunol. Immunopathol.*, with permission).

formation may indicate that a separate MAF is present, possibly equivalent to IL-4 or a colony stimulating factor which are known to have these activities in mammals.

Tumour Necrosis Factor

TNF is the principal mediator of the host response to gram-negative bacteria and is typically released from LPS-stimulated macrophages and monocytes (Abbas *et al.*, 1991). It can exert a paracrine and autocrine effect on leukocytes during inflammatory reactions, and can act as an endogenous pyrogen (see Chapter 16). Many of its effects are enhanced by IFN-γ, possibly through its ability to increase TNF-receptor expression.

Invertebrates
Human rTNF induces cell spreading in haemocytes of the mussel *M. edulis*, and this can be inhibited with anti-TNF (Hughes *et al.*, 1990). Immunoreactive TNF can also be detected in concentrated haemolymph by ELISA. That mussel haemocytes may themselves produce TNF has been suggested from two observations; first, that stimulation *in vitro* with LPS induces haemocyte spreading which can be inhibited with anti-TNF, and second, a reduction in haemocyte number in response to injection with LPS into the posterior adductor muscle of this species can also be inhibited with anti-TNF (Hughes *et al.*, 1991).

Fish
Human rTNF synergizes with rainbow trout MAF to elevate macrophage respiratory burst activity (Fig. 10). This effect is inhibited with anti-TNF but not by treatment with polymixin B (Hardie *et al.*, 1993). Human rTNF also synergizes with mitogenic stimuli to heighten proliferative responses of trout head kidney leukocytes.

Birds

A partial gene sequence of a chicken TNF/LT homologue is in the EMBL database but the sequence is unpublished and there are no details of how it was obtained.

Others

Isolated SSF from coelomocyte lysates of the starfish *A. forbesi* inhibits the lymphokine-induced expression of class II MHC antigens on murine macrophages *in vitro* (Donelly *et al.*, 1985). Intraperitoneal injection of SSF also reduces class II MHC antigen expression on peritoneal exudate macrophages in *Listeria*-infected mice. The presence of indomethacin reverses this effect, suggesting that SSF affects arachidonic acid metabolism in macrophages, which in turn inhibits class II MHC antigen expression. In this same species, 48-h supernatants from mixed (xenogeneic) cultures of nonadherent axial organ* (AO) cells are mitogenic for the entire AO population but not for adherent and nonadherent cells cultured separately (Luquet *et al.*, 1989). The released molecules are probably glycoproteins with a molecular mass in excess of 10 kDa. Whether this is due to an interleukin-like molecule or a colony-stimulating-like molecule is not known.

TGF-β has been cloned from birds (TGF-β_4) and amphibians (TGF-β_2, TGF-β_5), and these forms have some 60% to 80% amino acid sequence identity to mammalian TGF-βs (Haynes and Cohen, 1993b). In *Xenopus* rTGF-β_2 and rTGF-β_5 have a mesoderm-inducing activity on amphibian ectoderm (Roberts and Sporn, 1990) and rTGF-β_1 and rTGF-β_5 inhibit T-cell growth factor-induced proliferation of splenic blasts (Haynes and Cohen, 1993b). In addition, supernatants from mitogen-stimulated *Xenopus* splenocytes contain TGF-β_5 activity, as determined with specific antisera and a mink lung fibroblast assay. A novel fibroblast growth factor has also been cloned in *Xenopus* (XeFGF), and is closely related to FGF-4 and FGF-6 (Isaacs *et al.*, 1992). rXeFGF has a mesoderm-inducing activity and can influence the anteroposterior axis in gastrula stage *Xenopus* embryos.

CONCLUSIONS

To date, the majority of nonmammalian cytokines discovered appear to have functional similarities to mammalian cytokines (e.g. IFN, MIF, IL-1, MCP-1, TGF-β) but few studies have looked for molecular homology. With the increasing number of reagents available to characterize these cytokines, such as cDNA probes, it should be possible to confirm their relationships with their mammalian counterparts, shedding light on the evolutionary origin of particular cytokine families. Undoubtedly, some will prove to be a vertebrate innovation appearing coincidentally with the first appearance of lymphocytes. Others may be phylogenetically older. Of particular interest will be cytokines that are found to be unique to a particular animal group, whether they prove to be known mammalian cytokines present only in advanced vertebrates or novel cytokines in animals that have evolved independently of the line giving rise to mammals. With

---

*A tissue involved in the defence system of this organism and considered to be an ancestral lymphoid organ.

respect to lymphocyte products, it is already known that the number of Ig classes increases through the vertebrates (from one in fish to five in mammals), yet fish IgM appears to be capable of performing many of the functions ascribed to various mammalian antibody classes. If the same situation has occurred during the phylogeny of the lymphokines it may be possible for fish to possess only restricted numbers of lymphokines without being deficient functionally. The establishment recently of long-term lymphocyte-cell lines from fish (Clem *et al.*, 1991) is an important advance in this area, since these cells can act both as a source of cytokines and as target cells to detect cytokines. There is clearly still much to be learned about the origins of cytokines.

REFERENCES

Abbas, A.K., Lichtman, A.H. and Pober, J.S. (1991). *Cellular and Molecular Immunology*. W.B. Saunders Company, Boston, 417 pp.
Altman, L.C. and Kirchner, H. (1972). *J. Immunol.* **109**, 1149–1151.
Altman, L.C. and Kirchner, H. (1974). *Immunology* **26**, 393–405.
Beck, G. and Habicht, G.S. (1986). *Proc. Natl Acad. Sci. USA.* **83**, 7429–7433.
Beck, G., Vasta, G.R., Marchalonis, J.J. and Habicht, G.S. (1989). *Comp. Biochem. Physiol.* **92B**, 93–98.
Bernheim, H.A. and Kluger, M.J. (1977). *J. Physiol.* **267**, 659–666.
Caspi, R.R. and Avtalion, R.R. (1984). *Dev. Comp. Immunol.* **8**, 51–60.
Chang, E.B., Wang, N.S. and Mayer, L.F. (1987). *Gastroenterology* **92**, 1342.
Chung, S. and Secombes, C.J. (1987). *J. Fish Biol.* **31A**, 51–56.
Clem. L.W., Miller, M.W. and Bly, J.E. (1991). In: *Phylogenesis of Immune Functions* (eds G.W. Warr and N. Cohen), CRC Press, Boca Raton, FL, pp. 191–213.
Cohen, N. and Haynes, L. (1991). In: *Phylogenesis of Immune Functions* (eds G.W. Warr and N. Cohen), CRC Press, Boca Raton, FL, pp. 241–268.
Cohen, N., Watkins, D. and Parsons, S.V. (1987). In: *Developmental and Comparative Immunology* (eds E.L. Cooper, C. Langlet and J. Bierne), Alan R. Liss Inc., New York, pp. 53–68.
DeKinkelin, P., Dorson, M. and Hattenberger-Baudouy, A.M. (1982). *Dev. Comp. Immunol.* **2** Suppl., 167–174.
DeSena, J. and Rio, G.J. (1975). *Infect. Immun.* **11**, 815–822.
Donnelly, J.J., Vogel, S.N. and Prendergast, R.A. (1985). *Cell. Immunol.* **90**, 408–415.
Dorson, M., Barde, A. and DeKinkelin, P. (1975). *Ann. Microbiol. Inst. Pasteur* **126**B, 485–489.
El Ridi, R., Wahby, A.F. and Saad, A.-H. (1986). *Dev. Comp. Immunol.* **10**, 128.
Galabov, A.S. (1981). *Methods Enzymol.* **78A**, 196–208.
Gearing, A. and Rimmer, J.J. (1985a). *Dev. Comp. Immunol.* **9**, 291–300.
Gearing, A. and Rimmer, J.J. (1985b). *Dev. Comp. Immunol.* **9**, 281–290.
Graham, S. and Secombes, C.J. (1988). *Immunology* **65**, 293–297.
Graham, S. and Secombes, C.J. (1990a). *Dev. Comp. Immunol.* **14**, 59–68.
Graham, S. and Secombes, C.J. (1990b). *J. Fish. Biol.* **36**, 563–573.
Gravel, M. and Malsberger, R.G. (1965). *Ann. NY Acad. Sci.* **126**, 555–565.
Grondel, J.L. and Harmsen, E.G.M. (1984). *Immunology* **52**, 477–482.
Gruschwitz, M.S., Moormann, S., Kromer, G., Sgonc, R., Dietrich, H., Boeck, G., Gershwin, M.E., Boyd, R. and Wick, G. (1991). *J. Autoimmunity* **4**, 577–593.
Hala, K., Schauenstein, K., Neu, N., Kroemer, G., Wolf, H., Boeck, G. and Wick, G. (1986). *Eur. J. Immunol.* **16**, 1331–1336.
Hamby, B.A., Huggins, E.M., Jr, Lachman, L.B., Dinarello, C.A. and Sigel, M.M. (1986). *Lymphokine Res.* **5**, 157–162.
Hardie, L.J., Chappell, L.H. and Secombes, C.J. (1994). *Vet. Immunol. Immunopathol.* **40**, 73–84.
Hayara, Y., Schauenstein, K. and Globerson, A. (1982). *Dev. Comp. Immunol.* **6**, 785–789.
Haynes, L. and Cohen, N. (1993a). *Developmental Immunol.*
Haynes, L. and Cohen, N. (1993b). *Developmental Immunol.*
Haynes, L., Moynihan, J.A. and Cohen, N. (1990). *Immunol. Letters* **26**, 227–232.
Haynes, L., Harding, F.A., Koniski, A.D. and Cohen, N. (1992). *Dev. Comp. Immunol.* **16**, 453–462.

Highet, A.B. and Ruben, L.N. (1987). *Immunopharmacology* **13**, 149–155.

Howell, C.J. St. G. (1987). *Dev. Comp. Immunol.* **11**, 139–146.

Hughes, T.K. Jr, Smith, E.M., Chin, R., Cadet, P. Sinisterra, J., Leung, M.K., Shipp, M.A., Scharrer, B. and Stefano, G.B. (1990). *Proc. Natl Acad. Sci. USA* **87**, 4426–4429.

Hughes, T.K. Jr., Smith, E.M., Barnett, J.A., Charles, R. and Stefano, G.B. (1991). *Dev. Comp. Immunol.* **15**, 117–122.

Isaacs, H.V., Tannahill, D. and Slack, J.M.W. (1992). *Development* **114**, 711–720.

Jayaraman, S. and Muthukkaruppan, V.R. (1977). *Dev. Comp. Immunol.* **1**, 133–144.

Jayaraman, S. and Muthukkaruppan, V.R. (1978). *Immunology* **34**, 231–246.

Jayaraman, S., Mohan, R. and Muthukkaruppan, V.R. (1979). *Dev. Comp. Immunol.* **3**, 67–75.

Klein, J. (1989). *Scand. J. Immunol.* **29**, 499–505.

Kogut, M.H. and Lange, C. (1989). *J. Interferon Res.* **9**, 67–77.

Koniski, A.D. and Cohen, N. (1991). *Dev. Comp. Immunol.* **15**, S55 C9.

Kromer, G. and Wick, G. (1989). *Immunol. Today* **10**, 246–251.

Kromer, G., Gastinel, L.N., Neu, N., Auffray, C. and Wick, G. (1990). *Autoimmunity* **6**, 215–233.

Kromer, G., Schauenstein, K. and Wick, G. (1984). *J. Immunol. Methods* **73**, 273–281.

Lampson, G.P., Tytell, A.A., Nemes, M.M. and Hilleman, M.R. (1965). *Proc. Soc. Exp. Biol. Med.* **118**, 441–448.

Lillehoj, H.S., Kang, S.Y., Keller, L. and Sevoian, M. (1989). *Exp. Parasitol.* **69**, 54–64.

Luquet, G., Lemaitre, J. and LeClerc, M. (1989). *Lymphokine Res.* **8**, 451–458.

McInnes, A. and Rennick, D.M. (1988). *J. Exp. Med.* **167**, 598–611.

McKinney, E.C., McLeod, T.F. and Sigel, M.M. (1981). *Dev. Comp. Immunol.* **5**, 65–74.

Manickasundari, M., Selvaraj, P. and Pitchappen, R.N. (1984). *Dev. Comp. Immunol.* **8**, 367–374.

Martin, D.E. and Glick, B. (1983). *Cell. Immunol.* **79**, 383–388.

Mathews, J.H. and Vorndam, A.V. (1982). *J. Gen. Virol.* **61**, 177–186.

Matsushima, K. and Oppenheim, J.J. (1989). *Cytokine* **1**, 2–13.

Moehring, J.M. and Stinebring, W.R. (1970). *Nature* **226**, 360–361.

Moehring, J.M. and Stinebring, W.R. (1981). *Methods Enzymol.* **78A**, 189–192.

Moriya, O. and Ichikawa, Y. (1981). *Microbiol. Immunol.* **25**, 417–421.

Prendergast, R.A. and Liu, S.H. (1976). *Scand. J. Immunol.* **5**, 873–880.

Prendergast, R.A. and Suzuki, M. (1975). *Nature,* **227**, 277–279.

Roberts, A.B. and Sporn, M.B. (1990). In: *Peptide Growth Factors and Their Receptors*, (eds M.B. Sporn and A.B. Roberts), Springer-Verlag, New York, pp. 417–472.

Roitt, I.M., Brostoff, J. and Male, D.K. (1989). *Immunology*, 2nd edn., Churchill Livingstone, London.

Ruben, L.N. (1986). *Immunol. Lett.* **13**, 227–230.

Ruben, L.N., Clothier, R.H., Mirchandani, M., Wood, P. and Balls, M. (1987). *Immunology* **61**, 235–241.

Ruben, L.N., Beadling, C., Langeberg, L., Shiigi, S. and Selden, N. (1988). *Thymus* **11**, 77–87.

Ruben, L.N., Langeberg, L., Lee, R., Clothier, R.H., Malley, A., Holenstein, C. and Shiigi, S. (1990). In: *Defense Molecules* (eds J.J. Marchalonis and C. Reinisch), Alan R. Liss Inc., New York, pp. 133–147.

Ruben, L.N., Langeberg, L., Malley, A., Clothier, R.H., Beadling, C., Lee, R. and Shiigi, S. (1991). *Immunol. Lett.* **24**, 117–126.

Schauenstein, K. and Kromer, G. (1987). In: *Avian Immunology: Basis and Practice, Vol. 1* (eds A. Toivanen and P. Toivanen), CRC Press, Boca Raton, FL, pp. 213–227.

Schauenstein, K. Globerson, A. and Wick, G. (1982). *Dev. Comp. Immunol.* **6**, 533–540.

Schauenstein, K., Kromer, G., Sundick, R.S. and Wick, G. (1985) *J. Immunol.* **134**, 872–879.

Schauenstein, K., Kromer, G., Hala, K., Bock, G. and Wick, G. (1988). *Dev. Comp. Immunol.* **12**, 823–831.

Schnetzler, M., Oommen, A., Nowak, J.S. and Franklin, R.M. (1983). *Eur. J. Immunol.* **13**, 560–566.

Secombes, C.J. (1981). Ph.D Thesis, University of Hull, UK.

Sigel, M.M., Hamby, B.A. and Huggins, E.M., Jr. (1986). *Vet. Immunol. Immunopathol.* **12**, 47–58.

Smith, P.D., McCarthy, D.H. and Paterson, W.D. (1980). In: *Fish Diseases, 3rd COPRAQ Session* (ed. W. Ahne), Springer-Verlag, Berlin, pp. 113–119.

Song, Y.-L., Lin, T. and Kou, G.-H. (1989). *J. Fish Diseases* **12**, 117–123.

Stinson, R.S., Mashaly, M.M. and Glick, B. (1979). *Immunology* **36**, 769–774.

Tahan, A.M. and Jurd, R.D. (1979). *Dev. Comp. Immunol.* **3**, 299–306.

Tengelsen, L.A., Trobridge, G.D. and Leong, J.C. (1991). In: *Proc. 2nd Int. Symp. on Viruses of Lower Vertebrates*, pp. 219–226.

Trifonov, S., Sotirov, N. and Filchev, A. (1977). *Cell. Immunol.* **32**, 361–369.

Vainio, O., Ratcliffe, M.J.H. and Leanderson, T. (1986). *Scand. J. Immunol.* **23**, 135–142.

Vallejo, A.N., Miller, N.W. and Clem, L.W. (1992). *Annu. Rev. Fish Dis.* **2**, 73–89.

Vlaovic, M.S., Buening, G.M. and Loan, R.W. (1975). *Cell. Immunol.* **17**, 335–341.

Von Bulow, V., Weiler, H. and Klasen, A. (1984). *Avian Pathol.* **13**, 621–637.

Watkins, D. and Cohen, N. (1985). *Dev. Comp. Immunol.* **9**, 819–824.

Watkins, D. and Cohen, N. (1987). *Immunology* **62**, 119–125.

Watkins, D., Parsons, S.C. and Cohen, N. (1987). *Immunology* **62**, 669–673.

Weiler, H. and Von Bulow, V. (1987a). *Vet. Immunol. Immunopathol.* **14**, 257–267.

Weiler, H. and Von Bulow, V. (1987b). *Avian Pathol.* **16**, 439–452.

Wilson, V., Jeffreys, A.J., Barrie, P.A., Boseley, P.G., Slocombe, P.M., Easton, A. and Burke, D.C. (1983). *J. Mol. Biol.* **166**, 457–475.

Chapter 28

Future Cytokines: Interleukin 2001

Scott K. Durum

Laboratory of Molecular Immunoregulation, National Cancer Institute,
National Institutes of Health, Frederick, MD, USA

INTRODUCTION

A man goes to a fortune teller. She looks into her crystal ball and says 'I'm afraid I have really bad news. Tomorrow your wife will leave you, set fire to the house on the way out, and the IRS will send you an enormous bill for overdue taxes.' But the man doesn't show the least concern and says 'That's pretty bad all right, but I'm afraid it already happened yesterday.' The exasperated fortune teller picks up the crystal ball, slaps it in irritation and says 'Damn thing stopped again.'

Similarly, in cytokinology, the immediate past has been full of surprises, and who can imagine the future? To be sure, the future will be eventful, for from our immediate experience, we have to conclude that the creator must have had an inordinate fondness for cytokines, having made so many that do so many things. Metchnikoff poked a rose thorn into a starfish and observed a cellular reaction. A century later, this simple inflammatory reaction has been intensively dissected, and cytokines are major components of it. Today, cytokine research accounts for nearly 2% of the entire biomedical literature, has spawned a biotech industry, and by 2001 I am predicting a cytokine theme park where you can ride the α helix, slide the β sheet, and experience giant holographic tumour cells undergoing apoptosis.

But are there any more fundamentals to be learned about cytokines? There is a great deal to be learned. We do not even know all the elements (cytokines) that control cells, and until we know all the elements we cannot finally approach a grand cytokine unification theory. Most of cytokine research will continue to focus on the biological activities of these molecules, which often follows the formula: interleukin X induces/inhibits expression of interleukin Y (receptor) in Z cells. But there will be a lot of other directions in cytokine research and, over the next few pages, I will outline a few of these for the next decade or so, including new cytokines, crystallography, antagonists, cytokine design, viruses, postreceptor mechanisms, evolution, neuroendocrinology, transgenics, clinical and agricultural applications.

The Cytokine Handbook, 2nd ed.
ISBN 0–12–689661–5

NEW CYTOKINES

In the animal kingdom, every year, scientists discover three new bird species, 15 mammalian species and thousands of insect species. New cytokines, in the last decade, were cloned at an average rate of five to 10 a year. There will continue to be much interest in cloning new cytokines. We once asked a workshop of about a hundred people (at the Leukocyte Culture Conference at Banff, UK, in 1988) how many labs had a mystery cytokine they were working on. Most of the hands went up. Most new cytokines have been found in industry and, given the potential profit in a patentable cytokine, there are strong incentives in industry to discover new cytokines. There are also professional rewards for academics who discover and develop a new cytokine, for each one has the potential to open a new field of study.

How many more cytokines are there? Today more than 100 have been cloned, including the interleukins, IFN, CSFs, TNFs, LIF, TGFs, chemokines, and various growth factors. Hundreds more probably exist.

There have been several discovery techniques that will continue to be used. The classical method is to discover a biological activity, purify the protein, sequence it, search a cDNA library and get the full sequence; then one verifies that one has the right gene by expressing it and showing activity or by making antibodies to the cloned product and blocking the activity of the starting crude supernatant. The first inter-leukins (IL-1, IL-2, IL-3) and interferons (IFN-α, IFN-β, IFN-γ) were cloned this way. A shortcut has been to omit the initial protein purification, and instead to clone in an expression library, testing the supernatants for the designated biological activity. A number of the interleukins (e.g. IL-4 and IL-5) and receptors (e.g. IL-1 and GM-CSF) have been cloned using the expression library approach, and the orphan receptors have recently been used to clone their ligands this way (e.g. c-kit, CD30 and CD40). Another discovery technique has been to clone inducible RNAs with no initial regard to function. This has led to a number of new cytokines (e.g. γ-IP10, RANTES and IL-13), which in most cases have eventually been ascribed a function, such as chemotaxis in the case of γ-IP10 and RANTES. IL-12 was especially difficult to clone because its two chains are encoded by separate genes. A surprising feature of the cytokines is that each is so unique that new ones have not been cloned based on homology to old ones—there is much more homology among the cytokine receptors than among the cytokines themselves.

How will we know when the last cytokine is cloned? The human genome project will signal the end of searching for new human cytokines; this project will undoubtedly turn up numerous cytokines, and for each one it will need to be shown which cells produce it and what it does functionally.

Will every cytokine in man have a counterpart in all other species? I suppose not. Moreover, in some cases the interspecies counterparts have had so little in common, that it was not possible to clone them by homology. It is interesting that in some cases of human versus mouse genes (e.g. IL-3 and IFN-γ), there was much more in common in noncoding parts of the genes (5' and introns) than in the coding parts. This implies that regulation of a cytokine gene is more conserved than the actual protein structure, and invokes the concept that nature does not define a cytokine by its structure, but rather defines a cytokine by when it is made and what it does.

CYTOKINES WE NEED

In particle physics, someone predicts the existence of a particle because it is needed to explain something, then someone (else) sets out to find it experimentally. Using this approach, an objective of cytokine research is to find cytokines that control specific cell proliferation and differentiation at will. We want to make more of the good things in life, like nerve, muscle, skin, kidney, liver, teeth, and pancreas. And we want to make less of the bad things in life, like tumours, fat, pannus, plaque and senescence. Thus, our current state of knowledge of every physiological system is missing key regulatory elements.

The immune system presents immunologists with phenomena that do not seem to be controlled by our pharmacopoeia to date. To give just one example, there is a major gap in determining what controls the production of T lymphocytes. Whereas other blood cells have a corresponding CSF, where is the T-CSF? Such a cytokine could be very useful in treatment of AIDS and cancer, as an adjunct to radiation and chemotherapy, and could be used to improve bone-marrow transplantation. Why has the 'T-CSF' not been found yet? Probably because there is no simple *in vitro* assay system for producing T cells. The other haemopoietic cells can be produced from bone-marrow cultures *in vitro*, and it was feasible to purify their CSFs using this assay. But an *in vitro* technique for generating T cells from precursors has not been found, and thus a T-CSF, if it exists, would have to be assayed *in vivo*, and this would be a very difficult molecule to purify.

FUTURE RESEARCH

Unforeseeable advances in technology have had critical impacts on cytokine research. The most important technology was gene cloning and the second was the development of monoclonal antibodies. Transgenes, homologous recombination and drug design are the new technologies of our day that will have great impact on this field. We cannot even imagine what new technologies could emerge tomorrow to revolutionize cytokine research, and such unpredictable advances make the future in the field, well, unpredictable. However, even limited by today's technologies, the following trends are foreseeable.

Crystallography

Crystallography studies have shown important properties of the cytokines. For example, IL-1, TNF-α, and TNF-β are β-pleated sheets, whereas IL-2–6, M-CSF, G-CSF, GM-CSF and erythropoietin are α helical. A common structural motif, the TGF-β fold, was discovered to be shared also with EGF; this was not evident from primary sequence. Cocrystallizing growth hormone with its receptor revealed that one growth hormone molecule binds two receptor molecules, and this has led to a general model of receptor crosslinking being a mode of signalling for many cytokines. Further crystallography studies will show how cytokines engage their receptors and lead to rational drug design for antagonists and agonists.

Antagonists

Antagonists for the cytokines will be applied increasingly to treat autoimmune diseases such as rheumatoid arthritis, systemic lupus erythematosis, multiple sclerosis, and diabetes and to various inflammatory states such as sepsis, burn, shock and trauma disorders. Such antagonists can be designed from crystallography data. Other approaches to antagonist design are based on peptides related to the known primary sequence of the cytokine (for example some muteins of IL1-α, IL-2 and IL-4 have antagonist activity). Random screening of broths has been used, for example, to identify an antagonist for the peptide bombesin. Natural physiological antagonists are already known for several of the cytokines, these include the IL-1-like IL-1 inhibitor, and the soluble forms of the receptors for IL-1, TNF, IFN-γ, IL-4 and IL-7. Perhaps many cytokines will have natural physiological competitive inhibitors. Moreover, there have been a few observations of other proteins in physiological fluids that bind a cytokine but do not necessarily antagonize the activity of the cytokines. The case of IL-6 is particularly interesting, in that the artificially engineered IL-6 receptor has the remarkable property of binding IL-6 in solution, then the complex binds to the cell and, via a second chain, transduces its signal.

Cytokine Design

Cytokine design is being used to make molecules with altered function. For example it would be desirable to delete some functions. Multiple functions have already been achieved, such as the fusion products of IFN with TNF, GM-CSF with IL-3, and IL-2 or IL-6 with bacterial toxins. Thus, in the latter cases, cytokine receptors are exploited to deliver toxins to specific cell types (normal or tumour cells). One could also use the cytokine receptors to import other intracellular agents of interest, such as viruses, proteins or DNA. Similarly, one could introduce transgenes that couple a cytokine promoter to the gene for an intracellular toxin—this would delete any cell that would ordinarily express the cytokine gene.

Viruses

Viruses are known to exploit cytokine machinery. For example, the coding region of IL-10 has apparently fused with a viral product in EBV. The CSF-1 receptor is part of a viral oncogene. Vaccinia virus produces an EGF-like factor. Poxvirus produces a TNF receptor, a soluble IL-1 receptor, and an inhibitor of the IFN-β-converting enzyme. Several other viruses, such as HTLV and HIV, are known to exploit the same transcription factors that cytokine genes use. HIV can divert T cells from the T_{H1} to the T_{H2} pattern of cytokine production. Thus, viruses, long known to use intracellular components for their transcription and translation, are now being appreciated to also appropriate extracellular machinery, the cytokines.

Postreceptor Mechanisms

Post-receptor mechanisms are not understood for any cytokine. We are long overdue for a breakthrough on this front and it is likely that novel mechanisms are involved, including new kinases, G proteins, lipases and who knows? Second messenger pathways could be targets for clinically useful drugs, considering the success of glucocorticoids or cyclosporin which operate on second-messenger pathways in inflammation and immunity. It will be interesting to see whether there are some common pathways that are used by different receptors. The transcription factors that are activated by cytokines have been somewhat easier to study than the earlier postreceptor events, and much progress is being made in this area. However a fuller understanding of the most complicated cellular responses, replication and differentiation, still seem remote goals.

Evolution

Evolution of the cytokines has not received much attention to date, and it would be of great interest to determine their origin. For example, it is difficult to understand how the IL-1s, the TNFs and IL-6, which are so structurally different, came to be produced under such similar circumstances and have such similar activities. Will PCR or some such technique eventually give us the detailed understanding of how molecules evolve new structures? Is there an easy way to pinpoint an ancestral function in, say starfish, by something like gene targeting (discussed below)?

One theory of cytokine evolution that I have heard from several sources is that they could have evolved from adhesion molecules. The idea is that in multicellular organisms, (1) one cell needs to stick to another cell—we could call this the first-generation cytokine receptor; (2) the second-generation improvement would be for the cell to know that it is stuck to the right cell, (and not the wrong cell)—hence, the receptor becomes a real receptor with signal transduction ability; (3) the third-generation improvement would be for the cell to release the cytokine—a molecule packed with information, like a message in a bottle, to communicate with a distant cell. Perhaps this phylogeny is recapitulated in those cytokines that are produced both as membrane and released forms (such as CSF-1, SCF and TNF).

Neuroendocrine Functions

Neuroendocrine connections of cytokines have been pointed out. This seems to be the twilight zone of cytokine research, yet the pyrogenic actions of several cytokines has been known for some time, and action on the pituitary also seems clear. There have been some claims that cytokines (e.g. TNF and IL-1) and receptors are produced by neuronal tissue in the brain. Although there is cause for skepticism about this, if a neurotransmitter can take the form of a gas like NO, why not a cytokine?

Transgenic Experiments

Transgenic experiments have been performed increasingly, and manipulating the genome will certainly play a big role in future cytokine research; this role seems limited purely by imagination. Clinical applications will certainly be found for introducing cytokine transgenes into somatic cells, as discussed in a later section. Introducing genes into animal germlines has been possible for several years. Overexpression of many of the cytokines in mice has been done and all sorts of pathologies have been noted to result from this, for example, IFN-α led to testicular atrophy, GM-CSF to blindness, IL-2 to alopecia, IL-4 to immunosuppression, IL-6 to lymphoplasia, and IL-7 to lymphoma. Many of the cytokines are lethal if transgene expression is controlled by a strong promoter (e.g. IL-1, IL-4, TNF and TGF-β). However, the overexpression experiments have not taught us much about the normal physiological roles of the cytokines, and they have not been good disease models, since they do not mimic relevant pathologies. Another possible approach is to eliminate all cells producing a particular cytokine by connecting the cytokine promoter to a toxin gene (such as diphtheria toxin which acts intracellularly).

Gene targeting by homologous recombination should be far more informative as to the real physiological significance of cytokines. Mice have been produced which lack IL-2, IL-4, IL-10 and TGF-β_1 and many more will soon be available. The findings using these 'knockout' mice have been much debated, particularly by scientists whose expectations were not borne out, but admittedly there are shortcomings even to this elegant approach. Developmental roles of some cytokines may be discovered in future knockout experiments, for example, chemotactic cytokines might control the movement of cells during embryogenesis.

The next step with knockout mice would be to put the missing gene back, but under a different promoter to ask for example, what if only CD8 (but not CD4) cells made IL-2, or what if T_{H2} (not T_{H1}) cells made IL-2? A major issue addressed by the cytokine knockouts is the issue of redundancy—there is considerable overlap in cytokine production and activities (for example IL-1, IL-6 and TNF), and the question is, does each one have a sufficiently unique role that its absence will be noticed? Probably it will, considering the results with TGF-β: there are three TGF-β isoforms, but knocking out just one produced a lethal chronic inflammatory disease. A disappointment from the cytokine knockouts is the general lack of follow-up publications. It looks like the animals are not being distributed for widespread study, which is a real pity since these animals are an important scientific resource that can only be effectively exploited using multiple approaches.

Clinical Applications

Clinical applications are progressing and many trials will follow to assess the multitude of potential uses for these powerful molecules. New trials are launched every day, for example IFN trials have begun for multiple sclerosis. There is much room for optimism with so many activities of cytokines to explore, and a number of useful applications are already approved, for example the use of IFN for chronic hepatitis.

However, there have been very discouraging side-effects in man that were not anticipated, for example the vascular-leak syndrome seen with IL-2 and the hypotension with IL-1. An example of unanticipated *in vivo* side effects was seen in our laboratory: *in vitro*, IL-1 strongly promoted the growth of immature thymocytes, but when we gave IL-1 to whole animals the thymus shrunk dramatically, probably as an indirect effect of IL-1 induction of glucocorticoids or prostaglandins. One generalization that can be made with cytokine therapy is that cytokines work best when administered locally, rather than by flooding the body systemically (either in a therapeutic bolus or in overexpression from a transgene). Thus, far more applications will be found for local administrations than for systemic ones.

An example of the success of such a local administration is the recent finding that TNF given in isolated limb perfusion dramatically reduced tumour mass when given combined with chemotherapy; TNF is much too toxic if given systemically in man to achieve an effective dose.

Blocking the cytokines holds great promise for treating a number of diseases. Preliminary results with anti-TNF antibody for rheumatoid arthritis look good. Graft-versus-host disease responded remarkably to anti-TNF antibody, gastrointestinal symptoms were reduced dramatically, but returned when the antibody was discontinued. Septic shock, a likely candidate for anti-cytokine therapy, responds well in animal models; human trials have not shown efficacy in blocking just IL-1 or TNF alone, but combinations of blockers for IL-1, TNF, IL-6 and IFN-γ ought to work with some fine-tuning.

AIDS is a cytokine deficiency disease. The missing CD4$^+$ T cells are needed for cytokine production which then probably drives cytotoxic T-cells and inflammatory cells. The deficient cytokines in AIDS appear to be the T$_{H1}$ group, which decline even before symptoms appear, whereas the T$_{H2}$ cytokines actually increase (at least until the late stage when T$_{H2}$ cells also decline); so the problem is missing cytokines, probably IL-2 and IFN-γ. The challenge is to work out how to deliver the missing cytokines with a vehicle as precise as an antigen-specific CD4$^+$ T cell. One possibility would be to transfect the patient's own CD8$^+$ cells with IL-2 and IFN-γ genes controlled by the perforin promoter.

Several other chronic infectious diseases may use this strategy of stimulating a T$_{H2}$ imbalance over T$_{H1}$. There is evidence for this in leprosy and leishmaniasis. Thus, the relevant infectious agents may induce a kind of immunological tolerance by selectively expanding T$_{H2}$ cells. Although T$_{H2}$ cells promote antibody production, which is certainly an important defence mechanism against some infectious agents, it has no efficacy against these intracellular agents; in these situations, T$_{H2}$ cells have a suppressive effect, via IL-4 and IL-10, on T$_{H1}$ cells. It is the T$_{H1}$ cells that may be required to clear these infectious agents, and hence, these parasites (and HIV and other viruses noted above) may have evolved elegant strategies for suppressing them.

A congenital cytokine deficiency disease is the X-linked immunodeficiency that results in defective IL-2 receptor γ chain. It has been speculated that other ligands may also use this receptor chain, so the deficiency may be in more cytokines than just the IL-2 system. It is likely that other cytokine deficiency diseases remain to be identified—the knockout mice will give clues about what to look for.

Thus, infectious diseases, immunodeficiencies, autoimmunity and inflammatory diseases offer many therapeutic targets for cytokines or their inhibitors. Therapies can include giving the cytokines as proteins or genes, as well as inhibitors directed at the cytokine, the receptor or the signal-transduction pathway.

Cancer treatments exploiting cytokines as adjuncts to chemotherapy make sense: cytokines can be used to protect the host or sensitize the tumour to drugs. For example, IL-1 protects the host from haemopoietic damage and from alopecia induced by chemotherapy. IFN-γ augments the anti-tumour activity of 5-fluorouracil. TNF, as noted above, augments chemotherapy in an isolated limb. While chemotherapy looks reasonable, immunotherapy is another matter. Much effort has been directed towards using cytokines to stimulate host immunological rejection of tumours, this works in mice, but not yet in humans. I suspect this is because human tumours simply lack recognizable antigens, whereas many mouse tumours express endogenous retroviral antigens. Cancer is caused by genetic events that are unlikely to create new antigens, the exceptions being the idiotypes on B lymphomas and the viral antigens on EBV lymphomas.

Agricultural Applications

Agricultural applications of cytokines are receiving considerably more interest. Probably agricultural-grade cytokines and antagonists will be used—there are a lot of milk cows with arthritis and mastitis. Transgenes will be widely applied. However, the state of Wisconsin has banned the use of hormones to increase bovine milk production, and the use of steroids to increase cattle muscle mass is banned in some countries. From this we should anticipate resistance to our efforts to improve upon nature.

CONCLUSION

Will there be a cooling-off of cytokine research? I think that if more therapeutic applications are not found soon, that much of the economic incentive will be lost, along with public funding. It was disheartening to learn that IFN-α, formerly the drug of choice for hairy-cell leukaemia, has at some centres been supplanted by other drugs that have advantages over the cytokine. Clinical applications are the fuel that drives this field, and cytokines, with their myriad of potential uses, must be expediently taken to the clinic in order to sustain the momentum.

It appears however, that the future of cytokine research will be rewarding and relatively secure. It is not clear whether there will continue to be a field of study dedicated to cytokines. The question is whether there is some advantage to considering the study of cytokines as a speciality field, *per se*, or whether cytokines ought to (or will) be studied as parts of many fields. Studies of cytokines as such has been an advantage to date: we have studied their similarities (TNF has similar activities to IL-1), differences (TNF has a different receptor from that of IL-1) and interactions (TNF induces IL-1). In the future however, when there are hundreds of cytokines, will there be any common ground, any need for cytokine books (like this one) and journals, for cytokine meetings and courses? Will there be anyone who can know and integrate information on them all? Perhaps not, but like Endocrinology, which was launched in 1917, Cytokinology will occupy at least another generation of scientists and clinicians to produce, scientifically characterize and evaluate clinically the potential of these powerful molecules.

ACKNOWLEDGEMENTS

I thank Drs Kathrin Muegge, Howard Young, Jo Oppenheim, Lou Matis and Dan Longo for their comments on this manuscript.

Subject Index

Numbers in italics refer to illustrations or tables.

Acute-phase reactions, IL-6, 156–157
Adhesion molecules
  IL-4 effects on, 111
  IL-5 effects on, 138–139
Adipose, effects of TNF-α, 296
Adult T-cell leukaemia (ATL)
  TGF-β in, 331
Agricultural applications, 600
AIDS, 539, 601
  cytokine immunotherapy, 482–483
  GM-CSF use in, 361
Allergic inflammatory reactions, 538
Amphibia
  chemokines, 586–587
  IFNs, 569
  IL-1, 574–575
  IL-2, 577–579
  MIF production, 585
Angiogenesis, 540–*541*
  in solid neoplasms, 546–547
Animal models, 462–463, 482
  anti-IL-1RI antibodies, 49–50
  anti-IL-2R mAb, 555
  chemokines in tumour transduction, 439
  CSF-1 in fibroblasts, 401
    action in female reproductive tract, 408–411
    regulation of mononuclear phagocytes, 405, 407
  G-CSF, 376
  GM-CSF, 355–356
    in transgenic mice, 356
  IFNs as antiviral agents, 274
  IL-1 production, 38
  IL-1Ra blockade, 46–47
  IL-3, 86–87, 93–94
  IL-4, 106, 107
  IL-5
    B-cells of mice, 139–141
    in transgenic mice, 136
  IL-7, and transgenic mice, 177–178
  IL-9 and mouse T-cell oncogenesis, 216–217
  IL-10
    minus mice, anti-IL-10 treatment, 233
    in mouse immune response, 231
  IL-12, mouse, 253–255
  knockout mice, 9, 10, 600
  TGF-β systems, 331
    transgenic mice, 334
  TNF-β activity, transgenic mice, 314

Antagonistic interactions, cytokine, 7
  IL-4, 104
Antagonists, 556–559, 598
Anti-CD40 antibody, 104–105, 106
Anti-IgM antibody, 103, 104
Anti-IL-1RI antibodies, 49–50
Anti-IL-2 receptor antibody see Anti-Tac antibody
Anti-IL-2R mAbs, 555–556
Anti-IL-3 antibodies, 93–94
Anti-IL-4 antibody, 106, 107
Anti-IL-6 antibody, 154
Anti-IL-10 antibody and IL-10 minus mice, 233
Anti-inflammatory effect, IL-4, 110, 468
Anti-Tac antibody, 59–60, 61, 556, 578
Antibacterial activity, PF4, 443
Antibodies
  to cytokine receptors, 555
  to TNF receptors, 556
Antibody formation
  effects of IFNs on, 281–282
Antigen
  presentation
    IL-4 enhancement of B to T-cells, 103
  receptor triggering, 103–104, 105
  specific, cytotoxic activity
    IL-4 effects, 108
Antiproliferative effects
  of IFNs, 282
  of TGF-β, 327, 328, 329, 335, 475
Antitumour activity
  IL-4, 113–114, 118–119, 468
  IL-6, 470
  IL-12, 254
  PF4, 443
  rHuIL-4, 116
  TNF-α, 297
  see also Neoplasia
Antiviral role, IFNs in, 273–277, 478, 539–540
Apoptosis
  induction by TNF-α/β, 311
  protection by GM-CSF, 352
Arachidonic acid
  IL-1 signal transduction, 36, 37
Assays see Biological: assays; Immunological: assays
Atherosclerosis and haemopoietic growth factors, 491
Autoimmune diseases
  IL-2, role of, 467

Autoimmune diseases (*contd.*)
  IL-6, role of, 158–159
  TNF-α/β, role of, 313

B-cells
  activation of CD40 dependent, 104–105
  IFNs and differentiation of, 281
    IFN-γ, expression of class II MHC antigens, 278
  IL-2 and IL-2R action, 68
  IL-4 effects on, 102–106, 112
  IL-5 effects on, 139–141
  IL-6 effects on, 153–154
    abnormalities in chronic inflammation, 158–159
  IL-7 effects on, 173–175
  IL-9 effects on, 215–216
  IL-10 effects on, 226–227, 229–230
  production of TNF-β, 306
  regulation of growth and differentiation, 12–14
  response to IL-3, 83–84
Basophils
  chemokine effects on, 435–436
  IL-5 effects on, 139
Betaglycan (TGF-β type III receptor), 324
Binding
  affinities
    IL-2R subunits for IL-2, 64–65
    IL-3/IL-3 receptor, 91, 93
    IL-4/IL-4 receptor, 100
    IL-8 receptor, 192
    TNF-α receptors, 291
  direct, studies of chemokine, 444–445
  G-CSF to receptor, 377
  proteins, TGF-β, 323–329
  of soluble cytokines, 553–554
Biochemical
  characterization
    of IL-8, 188–191
    of TGF-β, 321
  pathways, IL-4 action, 112–113
  properties
    of G-CSF, 371–373
    of G-CSF receptor, 377
    of IL-10, 223–224
Biological
  actions
    of G-CSF, 375–377
    of GM-CSF, 351–359
  activities of IFN-α/β, 274
  assays, 507–522
    choice of, 509–510
    for IL-9, *213*
    readouts, 507–508
  effects
    of IL-1, 39–42

  of IL-4, *117*, 118
  of IL-6, *153*–157
  of IL-8, 193–195
  of IL-9, 214–218
  of TNF-α, 293–297
  function of TNF-α receptors, 292
  roles, TNF-β, 313–315, 326
  specificity of eosinophilia, 133–134
Biology
  CSF-1, 404–412
  IL-2, 67–69
    molecular, 57–59
  IL-2R, 67–69
Biosynthesis, CSF-1, 388–391
Birds
  chemokines, *587*–599
  IL-1, 575–576
  IL-2, 580–583
  MAF production, 588–590
  MIF production, 586
  Type 1 IFNs, 570, *571*
  Type 2 IFNs, 572
Blocking IL-1, 37
  strategies for, 44–52
Bone differentiation, TGF-β in, 333
Bone-marrow
  cultures
    IL-3 and IL-6, 155
    IL-5 eosinophil production, 134–135
  transplantation, 155
    GM-CSF in graft failure, 360
Boyden chamber, 432, 508
Breast cancer and TGF-β1, 336, 547

C10, mouse, 431
c-kit signalling pathways, 89
Cachexia, TNF-α induced, 299
Calcineurin, 550
cAMP
  induction by IL-4, 112
  role in IL-1 production, 44
Cancer, cytokines and, 545–548
  see also Neoplasia
Cardiovascular system, TNF-α effects on, 295
Cartilage differentiation, TGF-β in, 333
Catabolic effects
  of IL-1, 40–41
  of TNF-α, 299
CD40-dependent activation, IL-4 on B-cells, 104–105, 106
Cell
  expression, GM-CSF, 345–347
  interactions with cytokines, *529*
  populations, new cytotoxic, 480–481
  production, cytokine, 5
  proliferation, TGF-β effects on, 326–329

responses to cytokines, 534
sensitivity to IL-2, 68–69
sources
    of CSF-1, 404–405
    of IL-4, 101–102
    and targets for chemokines, *452*
    of TNF-α, 291
    of TNF-β, 306
surface phenotypic modulation, IL-12 on NKs,
    249
targets of IL-3, 81–84, 87
Cellular
    adhesion
        in leukocyte trafficking, 437–438
    production of cytokines, control of, 493
Central nervous system
    IL-1 effects on, 40
    TNF-α effects on, 294
Chemoattraction *in vitro*, monocytes and
    neutrophils, *433*
Chemokines, 419–453
    assays for, *517*, *522*
    C–C, 198, 426–431, 433
    C–X–C, 197–198, 421–426
        nonplatelet, 424–426
    in disease, 450–453
    effects on blood leukocytes, 432–437
        trafficking of, 437–438, *440*, 441
    gene organization, 431
    history of, 420–431
    phylogeny of, 586–588
    receptor-ligand interactions, 444–450
    superfamily, *421*
    in tumour biology, 439, 441
Chemoprotective effects, GM-CSF 355–356
Chemotactic activity
    TGF-β, 330
Chicken activated T-lymphocyte antigen
    (CATLA), 581, *582*
Chimaeric cytotoxins, 558–559
Chondrocytes in rheumatoid arthritis, *544*
Chronic inflammatory disease (CID), 21–23,
    601
    IL-4 usage in, 119
    IL-6 and B-cell abnormalities, 158–159
    proliferative, 159
Chronic lymphatic leukaemia (CLL)
    IL-7 and, 180
Circulating
    CSF-1, in regulation mononuclear phagocytes,
        406
    levels
        IL-1, human, 38
        IL-1Ra, 49, 51
        IL-1β, 49
Cisplatin, 495

Clinical
    applications
        CSF-1, 412
        cytokines, 600–602
        G-CSF, 376–377
        rhGM-CSF, 359–361
    implications, IL-2, 72–74
    significance IL-3, 93–94
    trials
        hyper-IgE patients, 107
        IFN-β in multiple sclerosis, 478
        IL-1Ra blockade, 47–48
        rHuIL-4, 114–118
Cloning
    of IL-7, 169–171
    of IL-8, 191
    of IL-9, 210
    of IL-10, recombinant, 224–225
    of IL-12, 240–241
    TGF-β, 320
Clonogenicity
    GM-CSF and progenitor cells, *in vitro*, 352
Colony stimulating factors *see* CSFs; CSF-1
Combination therapy, cytokine, 251, 479, 480, *481*
    IL-3/GM-CSF, 490
Congenital cytopenias, GM-CSF in, 358, 360
Conversion assays, IL-1 and, 512
Corticosteroids, and IL-5, 129
Crystal structure of hIL-5, *131*
Crystallography, 597
CSF-1, 387–412
    assays for, 520
    biology of, 404–412
    biosynthesis and structure, 388–391
    gene, 388, *390*, 391
    receptor *see* CSF-1R
    signal transduction, 394, 398–404
CSF-1R, 387–388, 500
    biology of, 405–412
    biosynthesis and structure, 391–394
    gene, *394*
CSF-2RA gene, 351
CSFs, 3
    cross-species comparisons of, *344*
    in macrophage activation, 14
    production in neoplasia, 546
    response to infection and injury, 536–537
    see also G-CSF; GM-CSF; IL-5
CTAP III, 423
Cyclosporin, 496
    A and FK 506: 550, *551*
Cytokine
    antagonists, 556–559
    binding
        proteins, 554
        to receptors, interference of, 555–556

Cytokine (*contd.*)
  cascade, 462, 480
  cell production, 5
  definition, *4*
  diversity, 149–150
  genes
    control of expression, 493–495
    regulation of, 527
  immunology, 1–15
  immunotherapy, prospects for human, 461–483
    drug delivery, 481–482
  networks, 6–10, 462, 525–526
    action of, 527–530, *549*
    TNF-α and, *298*
  nomenclature, 3–4
  receptor family, 5, 9, 147–149, 530–534
    interactions, 498–500
    as potential therapeutic targets, 525–559
  research, 1–3, 525–526
  standards and reference reagents, *511*
  sub/superfamilies, 526
Cytokines
  action of, in tissues and body fluids, 534–535
  as adjuvants, 482
  and cancer, 545–548
    see also Neoplasia
  cell interactions with, *529*
  detection of, in cells and tissues, 509
  endogenous production, 493–496
    modification of, 495–496
  future, 479–482, 595–602
  general features of, 525
  in inflammation and immunity, 535–541
  molecular genetics of, 21–28
  new, 496–498, 596
  and pathogenesis of diseases, 541–542
  pharmacology of, 491
  phylogeny of, 567–592
  as potential therapeutic targets, 525–559
  prediction of patient responses to, 479–480
  rheumatoid arthritis and, 474, 479, 543–545
Cytotoxic T-lymphocytes (CTLs)
  IL-6 induction of differentiation, 155
  IL-7 generation of, 178–179
  role of cytokines in generation, 12

D10 proliferation assay, 512
Deglycosylated molecules, 496
Deuterostome invertebrates, IL-1 in, 573
Differentiation
  B-cell
    IFN effects on, 281
    IL-4 effects on, 105–106
    role of cytokines, 12–14
  G-CSF effects on, 380, *381*
  GM-CSF effects on, 353–354

IFN effects on, 281, 283
IL-6 effect on cell, 156, 157
Dimerization of G-CSF receptor, 380–381
Direct binding studies, chemokine, 444–445
Downregulation
  of *c-kit*, IL-3, 89–90
  of IL-1 effects, 464
  of IL-2 effects, 467
  of IL-6 effects, 470
  of other cytokines, 527–528
DTH reactions, IL-10 effects on, 231, 233

ELISAs for cytokine receptors, 509
Embryonic development, TGF-β in, 332–333
Endocrinological effects
  IL-1, 41
  TNF-α, 296
Endothelial cells
  and coagulation, TNF-α effects, 293–294
  GM-CSF production, 346–347
  IL-4 effects on, 111–112
  in inflammatory reactions, 537
Eosinophilia, 133–139, 141
Eosinophils
  activation of, 137–138
  chemokine effects on, 436
  production of, IL-5, 134–137
Epithelia, TGF-β synthesis, 333–334
Epithelial cells
  IL-4 effects on, 112
Epithelial-derived neutrophil attractant-78
    (ENA-78), 425
Erythropoiesis, TGF-β gene effects on, 476
Erythropoietin, assays for, 519
Evolution, cytokine, 599
Ex vivo assays, 509
Exon structure, hIL-5Rα chain, *132*
Extracellular matrix (ECM), 534–535

Familial clustering, multifactorial diseases, *21*
Female reproductive tract, CSF-1 action, 408–411
Fetal T-cells, IL-7 effects on, 175
Fever induction
  by chemokines, 442
  by IL-1, 32, 36, 37, 40
Fibroblasts
  CSF-1 production, 401
  GM-CSF induction, 347
  IL-4 effects on, 111
  TGF-β effects on, 336
Fish
  chemokines, 586
  IL-1, 573–574
  IL-2, 576–577
  MAF production, 588, *589*
  MIF production, 584–585

TNF, 590
Type 1 IFN, 568–569
Type 2 IFN, 570, 572

G-CSF, 371–382
   assays for, 519–520
   biochemical properties, 371–373
   biological activities
      in vitro, 375–376
      in vivo, 376–377
   blocking of expression, 494–495
   current and projected usage, 490
   gene, properties of, 373, *375*
   receptor, 371, 377–381
Gene therapy, murine model IL-12, 254–255
Genes
   cytokine and CIDs, 22–23
      control of expression, 493–495, 527
   knockout studies, 9–*10*
   transcription
      in CIDs, 22–23
      regulation of, IL-2R, 71
Genetics
   molecular, of cytokines, 21–28
Glomerulonephritis, 541
   IL-6 and, 159
Glycosylation patterns, IL-3, 85–86
GM-CSF, 343–351
   amplification of eosinophil precursors, 135
   assays for, 520
   biological action
      in vitro, 351–354
      in vivo, 354–359
   cell expression, *345*–347
   clinical
      applications, 359–361
      results, 93
   current and predicted usage, 490
   functional regions of promoters, 494
   gene, 347, 348, 349–351
   receptor, 130, 347–349, 498, *499*, 500
      similarity with IL-5, 133
      see also CSF-2RA
   signal transduction, 349
   structure, 343–345
   structure–function analysis, 497
gp130 in signal transduction, 150–*152*
Graft failure, GM-CSF in, 360
Graft-versus-host disease, IL-3 and, 87
Granulation tissue, formation of, 540–541
Granulocyte chemotactic protein-2 (GCP-2), 425
Granulocyte Colony Stimulating Factor *see* G-CSF
Granulocyte-Macrophage Colony Stimulating
      Factor *see* GM-CSF
Granulocytes
   IL-4 effects on, 110–111

neutrophils, G-CSF effects, 375, 376
   terminal differentiation, 380
GRO, 192, *196*, 197
Growth
   of B-cells
      IL-4 effects, 13, 103–105
      regulation of, 12–14
   factors, 3, 4, 5
      haemopoietic, 489–501
      induction of IFN-*α/β*, 268
      in neoplasias, 546
   hormone, prolactin and G-CSF receptors,
      381
   see also PDGF; TGF-*β*, TGF-*β*1

Haematological malignancy
   GM-CSF in, 360
   and IL-7, 180
Haemopoiesis
   chemokine effects on, 441–442
   cytokine receptors in normal, 498
   IL-1 effects on, 464
   IL-4 effects on, 109
   IL-6 effects on, 155–156, 469–470
   steady-state
      links between stress and, 89–90
      role of IL-3, 88, 89
   see also Leukaemia
Haemopoietic
   effects
      IL-1, 41–42
      TNF-*α*, 296–297
   growth factors, 489–501
      current and projected use, 490–491
      endogenous production, 493–496
      modes of administration, 491–496
   progenitors
      and GM-CSF, 351–352
      and IL-4, 468
      and IL-9, 218
Haemopoietic cytokine receptor (HCR) family,
      530, 531
Headache, rHuIL-4 induced, 114, 116
Hepatitis B, IFNs and, 478
Hepatocytes
   IL-1 effects on, 40
   IL-4 effects on, 112
   TNF-*α* effects on, 294, 295
Herpes viruses, IL-10 related genes, 225–226
Histocompatibility antigens, cytokine regulation of
      class II, 14–15
HIV
   GM-CSF and, 361
   IL-4 and, 110
   IL-6 and, 146
   rIL-13 and, 259

HIV (*contd.*)
  TGF-β and, 331
  TNF-β and, 314
Hormones, 4–5
  steroid, 495–496
Host defence mechanisms, 535, *536*
  and GM-CSF, 352
  IL-1 effects on, 51
  IL-1Ra effect on, 51–52
Human T-cell leukaemia virus-1 (HTLV-1) and
    TNF-β, 306, 314
Hypoglycaemia, and rHuIL-4, 114
Hypotension
  IL-1 induced, 32, 39
  TNF-α induced, 295

I-309, 428–429
IFN-α/IFN-β
  assays for, 521
  effects on antibody formation and B-cell
    differentiation, 281
  gene
    human, 265–*266*
    mouse, *266*–267
    regulation of expression, 270–271
  immunotherapy with, 476
  induction of synthesis, 267–268
    molecular mechanism, 269–271
  modulation of MHC antigen expression, 278–
    279
  receptor, 271–272
IFN-γ, 2, 267, 268–269
  assays for, 521–522
  effects on antibody formation and B-cell
    differentiation, 281
  and IL-10, 227, 228
  immunotherapy with, *477*
  modulation of MHC antigen expression, 277–278
  receptor, 272
  stimulation of TNF receptors, 9
IFN-τ, 267
IFN-ω gene cluster, 265–*266*
IFN regulatory factor-1 (IRF-1), 350
IFNs, 265–283,
  as antiviral agents, 273–277
  effects on tumour cells, 282–283
  in human immunotherapy, 476–479
    combination therapy, 479
  induction of synthesis, 267–271
  macrophage activity, stimulation of, 279–280
  and major histocompatibility antigens, 277–279
  modulation of B, T, and NK cells, 280–282
  phylogeny of
    type 1, 568–570, *571*
    type 2, 570, *572*
  receptors, 271–272

signalling pathways, 272–273
  structure of, 265–267, 279–280
Ig isotype production
  cytokine regulation of, 13–14
IgA production, IL-5 enhancement, 140
IgE
  and anti-IL-6 antibody, 154
  induction by IL-13, 258
  modulation of production by IL-9, 215–216
  regulation by IL-4, 106–107
IL-1, 2, 31–52
  assays for, 510, 512
  balance with IL-1Ra, 48–49
  biological effects, 39–42
  comparison with TNF and IL-6, 42
  gene, 32–34
    cluster, 26–27
    expression, 39, 43–53
  in human immunotherapy, 463–465
  as mediator of disease, 37–39
  phylogeny of, 573–576
  receptor *see* IL-1R; IL-1Ra
  signal transduction, 36–37
  stimulatory effect of, 8
  structure of, 32–34
  toxicity, 32, 36, 39
    prevention of effects, 43–51
IL-1 converting enzyme (ICE), 33, 45
IL-1α, 32–34, 44
  toxicity, 39
IL-1β, 32–34, 44
  circulating levels, 49
  toxicity, 39
IL-1R, 34–*35*
  blockade, 50
  regulation of, 36
IL-1Ra, *23*, 26, 33, *35*
  balance with IL-1, 48–49
  production of, 48
  specific receptor blockade, 45–48
  as therapeutic reagent, 556–557
IL-2, 2, 11, 57–74
  assays for, 512–513
  binding affinities for, and IL-2R subunits, 64–
    65
  biology, 67–69
    molecular, 57–59
  combined with IL-12, 247, 248, 250–251
  dependence on IL-6, 154
  gene, 58, 68
  in human immunotherapy, 465–467
  pathology and clinical implications, 72–74
  phylogeny of, 576–582
  receptor *see* IL-2R; IL-2Rα; IL-2Rβ; IL-2Rγ
  structure of, 57–*59*
IL-2/IL-2R system, function of, 67–72

IL-2R, 11, 57–74
  biology, 67–69
  model targets for therapeutic intervention, 555–556
  multimolecular complex, 64–67
  signal transduction, 69, 71–72, *73*
IL-2Rα, 57
  binding affinities, 64, 65, 66
  composition, 59–61
IL-2Rβ, 57
  binding affinities, 64–66
  composition, 61–*62*
IL-2Rγ, 57
  binding affinities, 64, 65–66
  composition, 62–*63*
IL-3, 81–94
  amplification of eosinophil precursors, 135
  assays for, 513
  cell targets, 81–84, 87
  clinical significance, 93–94
  in normal and immunologically stimulated
    animals, 86–87
  phylogeny of, 582–583
  receptor, 85, 90, 91, 94, 130
  role of, in haemopoiesis, 88, 89
  in the serum, 87
  signal transduction, 90–93
  source of, 86
  structure of, 84–86
IL-4, 99–119
  anti-inflammatory actions, 540
  assays for, 513–515
  biochemical pathways, 112–113
  biological effects, *117*, 118
  cell sources of, 101–102
  clinical aspects, 113–118
  effects on
    B-cells, 11, 102–106, 112
    myelomonocytic cells, 109–111
    T-cells, 107–109
  in human immunotherapy, *467*–468
  IgE regulation *in vivo*, role of, 106–107
  molecular aspects of, 99–100
  receptor, 100–101
IL-5, 127–141
  assays for, 515
  eosinophilia, 133–139
  gene, 128–129
  receptor *see* IL-5Rα
  relationship to IL-3, 84
  source of, 141
  structure of, 129–130
IL-5Rα, 130–133
IL-6, 145–161
  assays for, 515
  biological activity, *153*–157

comparison with IL-1, 42
in disease, 157–160
gene, 146–147
in human immunotherapy, 469–470
and neoplasia, 159–160, 547
receptor *see* IL-6Rα
structure of, 145–147
IL-6Rα, 147–149
IL-7, 160–181
  assays for, 515–516
  cloning and purification, 169–171
  effects on
    B-cells, 173–175
    monocytes, 177
    NK cells, 177
    T-cells, 11, 175–177
  gene, 171
    transfection of tumour, 179–180
  and immunotherapy, 178–180, 470–471
  as a lymphopoietin, 172–173
  receptor, 171–172
  source of, 174
  transgenic animals, 177–178
IL-8, 185–199
  assays for, 516
  biochemical characterization, 188–191
  biological activities, 193–195
  cellular sources of, *186*–*187*, 188
  direct binding studies, 444–445
  gene, 191
  induction by IL-1, 32, 50
  in inflammation, 453
  in leukocyte trafficking, 438
  receptor, 192
  role of in pathology, 199
  signal transduction, 192–193
  similarity to inflammatory proteins, 195–196
  structure, 191
IL-9, 209–220
  bioassays for, 212–*213*, 517–518
  biological activities of, 214–218
  cloning of, 210
  gene, 209, 211–212
  and haemopoietic progenitors, 218
  receptor, 218–219
IL-10, 105, 223–234
  assays for, 518
  biochemical properties, 223–224
  effects *in vivo*, 232–233
  expression of, in immune responses, 231–232
  functions of, 227–230
  herpes viruses, related genes, 225–226
  in human immunotherapy, 471–472
  receptor, 226
  recombinant cloning, 224–225
IL-11, assays for, 518

IL-12, 149, 228, 239–255
    assays for, 518
    effects
        in vivo, 253–255
        on NK cells, 246–249
        on T-cells, 249–253
    gene, 240
    in human immunotherapy, 492
    molecular characterization and cloning of, 240–
        241
    production of, 241–245
    receptor (IL-12R), 246
IL-13, 257–259
    assays for, 518
    gene, 257, *258*
IL-14, 259–*260*
IL-15, 261–262
Immune responses
    IL-2, 466
    IL-6, 153–155
    IL-10, 231–232
    IL-12 and T$_{H1}$ stimulation, 251–253
    TGF-β, 329–332, 336
Immunity, cytokines in, 535–541
Immunoassays, 508
Immunological
    assays, 507–522
    effects, rHuIL-4, 116
Immunology
    introduction to cytokines, 1–15
Immunoregulatory actions of cytokines, 11–15
    TNF-α, 475
Immunosuppression
    with anti-IL-2R antibodies, 555
    PF4 alleviation, 443
Immunosuppressive drugs 550–553
Immunotherapy
    anti-tumour, IL-7, 178–180
    prospects for human cytokine, 461–483
        future developments, 479–483
Immunotoxins, 558–559
Infection and injury, cytokine response to, 536–537
Inflammation
    cytokine activation at site of, 462, 535–541
    TGF-β role in, 330, 331, 540, 541
    TNFα, 473
Inhibitory actions, in cytokine production, 8
    TGF-β, 330
Integrins, TGF-β effects on, 326
Interferons *see* IFNs
Interleukins *see* IL-1 etc
Intracellular signalling pathways, 6, 7
Invertebrates
    IL-1, 573
    MIFs, 583–584
    TNF, 590

IP-10, 197–198, 424
Isotype switching, 13–14
    and IL-4, 106
    and IL-13, 258

Kinetic studies, CSF-1, 399
Knockout mice, 600
    TGF-β1, 9, 10

LAK cells
    activity and IL-12, 246–248
    and IL-2, 68, 465
    and IL-4, 109
    and IL-7, 178
Latent TGF-β binding protein (LTBP), 321, 322
Leukaemia
    adult T-cell (ATL), 331
    chronic lymphatic (CLL), 180
    myeloid, 94, 357, 377, 470, 477
    role of GM-CSF in pathogenesis, 357–358
Leukaemia inhibitory factor (LIF), 150–*151*
    assays for, 519
Leukocyte adhesion inhibitor (LAI), 193
Leukocytes, chemokine effects on, 432–438, *440*,
    441
Liver, TNF-α effects on, 294–295
Local
    effects, IL-1, 32
    therapy, 492–493, 600, 601
Low-dose therapy, 492
Lymphocytes, chemokine effect on, 434–435
Lymphoma, induction by IL-9, 216–217
Lymphopoietin, IL-7, 172–173
Lymphotoxin-α (LT-α) *see* TNF-β
Lymphotoxin-β (LT-β), 305

Macrophage activating factors (MAFs)
    phylogeny of, 588–590
Macrophage colony stimulating factor (M-CSF) *see*
    CSF-1
Macrophage inflammatory proteins (MIP-1α/MIP-
    1β), 427–428, 434, 435
    direct binding studies, 444–445
    in haemopoiesis, 441–442
    signal transduction, 446
Macrophages
    activation by cytokines, 14–15
    CSF-1R
        cultured, 407
        female reproductive tract, 410
        pathological and physiological roles, 407
        proteins, 403
        in signalling, 402, 404
    G-CSF expression, 373
    GM-CSF production, 346
    in host immune responses, 539

IFN stimulation, 279–280
IFN-γ action on, 277
IL-3 effects on, 82
IL-4 effects on, 109–110
inhibition by IL-10, 227–228, 252
production of IL-12, 252
in rheumatoid arthritis, 543
as source of TNF-α, 291
TGF-β effects on, 331
treatment of, with IL-13, 258
tumoricidal activity, 14, 279–280
Major histocompatibility complex (MHC)
antigens and IFNs, 277–279
association with CID, 21–22
and TNF, 23–24
Markers, disease severity
IL-1 gene polymorphism, 27–28
Mast cells
IL-3
effects and, 82
growth of dependent, 88
interaction with fibroblasts, 89
as source of, 86
IL-9 effects on, 214
IL-10 stimulation of, 229
Mastocytosis and IL-9, 214–215
Megakaryocytes, IL-6 effect on, 156
Megakaryopoiesis, PF4 inhibition of, 443
Melanoma
IL-2 and LAK cells, 465–466
TIL clone, IL-12 augmentation IL-2, *252*
TNF-α, 473
Melanoma growth-stimulatory activity (MGSA),
197, 424–425
Mesenchymal differentiation
TGF-β effects on, 332, 333
Migration inhibition factor (MIF), 2
assays for, 522
phylogeny of, 583–586
Modulation of cytokine production, IL-4,
118
Molecular
aspects of IL-4, *99–100*
biology of IL-2, 57–59
characterization
of chemokine receptors, 447
of IL-12, 240–241
genetics of cytokines, 21–28
mechanism of IFN α/β induction, 269–271
philosophy, cytokine actions, 7
structure TNF-β, 308, 310
Monoclonal antibodies (mAbs), 553
anti-IL-2R, 555–556
Monocyte chemotactic protein (MCP-1), 429–430,
433
direct binding studies, 444–445

in disease, 450–451
signal transduction, 445–446
Monocytes
effects of chemokines on, 432–434
gene expression in, 43
IL-1 secretion, 44
IL-4 effects on, 109–110
IL-7 effects on, 177
TGF-β activation of, 329, 330, 331
Multimolecular IL-2R complex, 64–67
Multiple sclerosis, IFN-β and, 478
Muscle, TNF-α effects on, 295–296
Myelodysplastic syndromes (MDS)
GM-CSF and, 358
Myeloid
cells
GM-CSF and, 352, 353
IL-4 action, 113
leukaemia
G-CSF, role of in, 377
GM-CSF, role of in, 357
IFN-α and, 477
IL-3 and, 94
IL-6 adjuvant therapy, 470
Myeloma
cells and IL-6, 160
multiple, 477
Myelomonocytic cells, effects of IL-4, 109–111
Mx protein, 276–277

Neoplasia, 545, 546–548
chemokines in tumour biology, 439, 441
CSF-1/CSF-1R, role of, 411
G-CSF and, 372
GM-CSF in pathogenesis of leukaemias, 357–358
IFN-γ, MHC class II antigen expression, 278
and IL-2, 465–466
and IL-4, 113–114, 118–119, 468
IL-7 action in mouse, 178–179
plasma cell and IL-6, 159–160
TGF-β in tumour development, 335–337
TNF-α in, 473, 547
see also Antitumour activity; Haematological
malignancy; Leukaemia; Melanoma
Networks, cytokine, 6–10, 462, 525–526
action of, 527–530, *549*
TNF-α and, *298*
Neuroendocrine functions, 599
Neutrophil activating protein-2 (NAP-2), 192, *196*,
197, 423
Neutrophilic granulocytes, G-CSF effects, 375, 376
on terminal differentiation, 380
Neutrophils, effects of chemokines on, 432–434
Nitric oxide ($\cdot$NO), 539
NK cells
IFNs effects on, 281–282

NK cells (*contd.*)
  IL-4 effects on, 109
  IL-7 effects on, 177
  IL-12 effects on, 246–249
  inhibition of, by IL-10, 229
Nomenclature, cytokine, 3–4
Nuclear factor of activated T-cells (NF-AT), 550–552

Oligo-adenylate synthesis, 275–276
Oncogene expression, IFN effects on, 282–283
  amplification of, 545–546
Oncogenesis
  IL-9 and mouse T-cells, 216–217
Oncostatin M, assays for, 519
Ontogeny
  IL-4 effects
    on B-cells, 102
    on T-cells, 108
OSM, 150–*151*

p55 (TNF-β receptor), 307, 310
p56^lck, 70, 72
p75 (TNF-β receptor), 307, 310
p500, 428
Parasites, destruction by IFN-activated macrophages, 280
Patient responses to cytokines, prediction of, 479–480
Peptides and muteins as antagonists, 557–558
Phagocyte modulating cytokines, 583–591
Phagocytes, regulation of mononuclear by CSF-1, 405–408
Phagocytosis, Fc receptor-mediated, 279
Pharmacology of cytokines, 491
Phosphorylation
  IL-4 induction in B-cells, 112
  in signalling
    IL-2R, 69–70
    IL-3, 91–92
  see also Tyrosine phosphorylation
Phylogeny of cytokines, 567–592
Placenta
  development of, mouse, CSF-1/CSF-1R, *408*
  mature, CSF-1, 410
Plasma cell neoplasia and IL-6, 159–160
Platelet α granule proteins, 421–423
Platelet-derived growth factor (PDGF)
  TGF-β effects on, 327
Platelet factor 4 (PF4), 421–423
  activities of, 442–443
Polymorphism, disease-related, 22
  IL-1 gene cluster, 26–27
  TNF, 23–25
Post receptor mechanisms, 598–599
pRB and TGF-β, 328

Pre-B-cells, 171, 173, 174
Pregnancy
  CSF-1 synthesis
    human, 410–411
    mouse, 408, *409*
  IL-10 expression, 232
Pro-B-cells, 173, 174
Protein kinase, 276
Protostomes, IL-1 in, 573
Pseudomonas exotoxin (PE), 559
Purification
  IL-7, 169–171
  IL-8, 189

Radioprotection
  GM-CSF and, 355–356
  IL-1 and, 464
RANTES, 429
  chemoattraction of eosinophils to, 436
  direct binding studies, 444–445
  in signal transduction, 446
Rapamycin, 550, 552–553
Receptor-based assays, 509
Receptors
  cytokine, 5, 147–149
    interactions, 498–500
    as potential therapeutic targets, 525–559
    transmodulation of, 9
  families of, *531*
  growth factor, oncogene encoded, 546
  soluble, 50–51, 533–534, 535
    in prevention of cytokine action, 553–554
Red blood cells, and receptor chemokine interactions, 449–450
Regulation
  B-cell growth and differentiation, 12–14
  of cytokine genes, 527
  differential, of TGF-β isoforms, 321
  of human IFN α/β expression, 270–271
  of Ig isotype production, 13–14
  of IL-1 receptors, 36
  of IL-2R gene transcription, 71
  of IL-2Rβ gene expression, 61–62
  IL-9 expression, 212
  of *in vivo* role of IL-4 IgE, 106–107
  of mononuclear phagocytes by CSF-1, 405–408
  of T-cell growth and differentiation, 11–12
  of TNF-β gene, 311–313
Reptiles
  IL-1, 575
  IL-2, 579–580
  MIF production, 585
  Type 1 IFN, 569–570
Retroviral vectors and IL-12, 241, *244*
Rheumatoid arthritis, 479, 543–545
  anti-TNF monoclonal antibody therapy, 474

rhGM-CSF in clinical use, 359–361
rHuIL-4, clinical trials, 114–118

Saragramostim *see* rhGM-CSF
'Second-generation' cytokines, 496, 497–498
Secretion
  of IL-1, 44–45
Septic shock, TNFα in, 298–299
Sequence analysis
  chemokines
    C–C, *427*
    C–X–C, *426*
    receptors, *448*
  CSF-1, 388, *390*, 391, *392–393*
  CSF-1R, *395–397*
  G-CSF, 372
    gene, 375
    receptor, 378
  IFN α/β receptor, 271
  IL-2, *58*
  IL-2R α, *60*
  IL-2R β, 61, *62*
  IL-2R γ, *63*
  IL-5, *130*, 133
    gene, 128–129
  IL-7, *170*, 171
  IL-8, 189, *190*, 191
    and related chemokines, *196*
  IL-9, *210*
    receptor, 219
  IL-10, 225
  IL-12, *242–243*
    gene, 240–241
  IL-13 gene, 257, *258*
  IL-14, *260*
  IL-15, *261–262*
  TGF-β, 320, 321
  TNF-β, 308–*309*
    gene, 312
Serum, animal, IL-3 in, 86, 87
Shock
  induced by IL-1 infusion, 39–40
  TNF-α, induction of, 295
  septic, 298–299
Signal transduction, 5, 531–*532*, 534
  c-kit signalling pathways, 89
  chemokine, 445–447
  CSF-1, 394, 398–404
  G-CSF receptor, 380
  GM-CSF, 349
  gp130, 150–*152*
  IFN signalling pathway, 272–273
  IL-1, 36–37
  IL-2R, 69, 71–72, *73*
  IL-3, 90–93

IL-6, 148
  receptor complex, 151–153
IL-8, 192–193
IL-9 receptor, 219
inhibitors of, 548–550
TNF-α, 292
TNF-β signalling mechanisms, 310, 311, 325
transmembrane signalling, *533*
Single-agent therapy, G-CSF and GM-CSF, 490
Skin reactivity of IL-8, 194, *195*
Soluble cytokine receptors, 50–51, 533–534, 535
  in prevention of cytokine action, 553–554
Standardization of assays, 510
Stem cell factor (SCF), assays for, 520
Stem cells
  IL-3 action, 81, 84, 89–90
Stimulatory actions in cytokine production, 8
Stress
  link with steady-state haemopoiesis, 89–90
Stromal cells
  IL-5 dependence, 136
  as source of IL-7, 174, 175
Structure
  CSF-1, 388–391
  G-CSF, *374*
    receptor, 378–379
  GM-CSF, 343–345
  IFNs, 265–267
  IL-1, 32–34
  IL-2, 57–*59*
  IL-2R
    influence on signalling function, 71–72
    subunit cooperation and ligand binding, 65–67
  IL-3, 84–86
  IL-5 protein, 129–130
  IL-6, 145–147
  IL-8, 191
  TGF-β, 320–321
  TNF-α, 289–290
  TNF-β protein, 307–310
Structure–function analysis
  chemokine receptor-ligand, 447, 449
  cytokine, 496–497
Subcutaneous administration
  IL-3, 88
  rhGM-CSF, 359
  rHuIL-4, 114, 116
Suramin as antagonist, 558
Synergistic interactions, cytokine, 6–7, 42, 84, 111, 155, 214, 249, 250, 353, 354, 466
  see also combination therapy, cytokine
Synoviocytes and rheumatoid arthritis, 543, *544*
Systemic effects
  anti-IL-1R mAbs, 555
  GM-CSF, 491–492

Systemic effects (*contd.*)
  IL-1, 32, 36, 39
    prevention of, 43–51
    reduction of, 466
  IL-2, 68
  IL-8, 194
  rhGM-CSF, 359–360
  rHuIL-4, 114–116
  TGF-β, 475
  TNF-α, 294–297
    reduction of, 474
Systemic inflammatory response syndrome (SIRS),
    37–38
  IL-1Ra blockade, 47–48

T-cell activation gene 3 (TCA 3), 428, 429, 434
T-cell leukaemia/lymphoma syndrome, IL-2R α,
    72–73
T-cells
  chemokine effect on, 435
    C–C, 431
  differentiation of, role of cytokines, 12
  in eosinophilia, 133
  in host immune response, 537
  IFN modulation of activity, 280–281
  IFN-γ
    expression of class II MHC antigens, 278
    synthesis by cytotoxic/suppressor cells, 269
  IL-2 effects on, 67–68
  IL-3
    effects on, 83
    as source of, 86
  IL-4
    effects on, 107–109
    as source of, 101–102
  IL-5 production, 127, 129, 141
  IL-6
    activation by, 154
    production, 146
  IL-7
    effects on, 175–177
    enhancement of proliferation, 178–179
    expression of receptor, 171
  IL-9 production, 212, 216–218
  IL-10
    production, 226
    selective inhibition/enhancement of 228–229
  IL-12 effects on, 249–253
    cytolytic activity, 251
    proliferation, 249–251
  production, GM-CSF, 346
  regulation of growth and differentiation, 11–12
  TNF-β, release from, 306
  see also cytotoxic T-lymphocytes
T-helper 1 (T$_{H1}$) cells
  in CIDs, 601

IFN-γ and, 269
IL-4 and, 101–102, 103, 108
IL-9 and, 214
IL-10 and, 223, 227, 228, 230, 232
IL-12 stimulation of, 251–253
response to infection, 537, *538*, 539
T-helper 2 (T$_{H2}$) cells
  in CIDs, 601
  IFN-γ and, 269
  IL-4 and, 101–102, 103, 108
  IL-9 and, 214
  IL-10 and, 223, 230, 232
  response to infection, 537, *538*
T-suppressor cells, IFN effect on, 280–281
TGF-α, 3
TGF-β, 3, 319–337
  in cytokine production, 8
  in immune system, 329–332
  in mesenchymal differentiation, 322, 333
  in normal mammalian development, 332–335
  receptors and binding proteins, 323–329
    in development, 334
  role of associated proteins, 322–323
  structure, 320–321
  superfamily, 320, 475–476
  in T-cell regulation, 12
  in tumour development, 335–337
TGF-β1, 526
  assays for, 522
  in breast carcinomas, 336, 547
  effects on inflammatory lesions, 540, 541
  knockout mice, 9, 10
β-thromboglobulin (β-TG), 421, 423
Thymectomy studies, IL-2 in amphibia, *578*
Thymocytes
  IL-1 effects in amphibia, 574, *575*
  IL-4 effects on, 107–108
  IL-6 effects on, 155
  IL-7 effects on, 175–176
Tissue localization in eosinophilia, 138–139
TNF, 2
  assays for, 521
  comparison with IL-1 and IL-6, 42
  gene, *24*, 25
  and the MHC, 23–24
  phylogeny of, 590–591
  polymorphism, 23–25
  receptors, 9
    antibodies to, 556
  stimulatory effect of, 8
TNF-α, 289–300
  biological effects, 293–297
  biosynthesis, 290–291
  in diseases, *300*
  in human immunotherapy, 472–475
  interaction with other cytokines, 298

local paracrine effects, 539
and neoplasia, 547
polymorphism, *25*
proinflammatory effects, 542
receptors, 291–292
in septic shock, 298–299
structure, 289–290
tolerance to effects, 297
TNF-β, 305–315
activities and mechanism, 310–311
biological roles, 313–315, 326
cells of origin, 306
gene structure and regulation, 311–313
in human immunotherapy, 472–475
polymorphism, 24
protein structure, 307–310
receptors, 306–307
Toxicity
anti-IL-2R mAbs, 555
GM-CSF, 359–360, 491–492
IL-1, 32, 36, 39–40
prevention of effects, 43–51
reduction of, 466
IL-2, 68
IL-8, 194
rhGM-CSF, 359–360
rHuIL-4, 114–116
TGF-β family, 475
TNF-α, 294–297
reduction of, 474
Transcription
activation of IL-2R α gene, 60
factors, 495, 496, 527, 550
of GM-CSF, 347
and IFN synthesis, 269, 270
of IL-1, 43–44
regulation of gene
IL-2/IL-2R, 71
TNF-α/TNF-β, 312
Transfection
IL-7, of tumour, 179–180
Transformed cells, cytokine receptors in, 498, 500

Transforming growth factor-β *see* TGF-β
Transgenic experiments, 599–600
IL-7 and, 177–179
see also Animal models
Translation
of IL-1, 43, 44
product from IL-2R α gene, 60
Transmodulation of cytokine receptors, 9
Transplantation
bone-marrow
GM-CSF in graft failure, 360
studies
leukaemia, 357
over-expression GM-CSF, 356
Tumour
cells, expression of chemokines, 439, 441
transduction models, chemokines in, 439
Tumour necrosis factors *see* TNFs
Type I TGF-β receptor, 325
Type II TGF-β receptor, 324
Type III TGF-β receptor, 324
Tyrosine phosphorylation
CSF-1/CSF-1R induction, 399, 401, 402, 403
IL-3 stimulation, 91–92
IL-6 induction, 151
IL-7 induction, 172

Ulcerative colitis, disease markers, *28*

Vascular wall
effects of IL-1, 41
see also Endothelial cells
Viruses and cytokine actions, 598
induction of IFNα/β, 268
VNTR polymorphism, 26

Wound healing, PF4 and, 422–423

X-linked severe combined immunodeficiency (X-SCID)
IL-2R γ in, 73–74